Managing Acute Decompensated Heart Failure

Managing Acute Decompensated Heart Failure

Editors

Christopher M. O'Connor MD, FACP, FACC
Professor of Medicine
Duke University Medical Center
Durham, North Carolina, USA

Wendy Gattis Stough PharmD
Assistant Clinical Professor in Medicine
Duke University Medical Center
Durham, North Carolina, USA

Mihai Gheorghiade MD, FACC
Professor of Medicine
Northwestern University
Chicago, Illinois, USA

Kirkwood F. Adams Jr. MD
Associate Professor of Medicine and Radiology
The University of North Carolina School of Medicine
Chapel Hill, North Carolina, USA

informa
healthcare

New York London

First published in 2005 by the Taylor & Francis Group, LLC.

This edition published in 2011 by Informa Healthcare, Telephone House, 69-77 Paul Street, London EC2A 4LQ, UK.

Simultaneously published in the USA by Informa Healthcare, 52 Vanderbilt Avenue, 7th Floor, New York, NY 10017, USA.

Informa Healthcare is a trading division of Informa UK Ltd. Registered Office: 37–41 Mortimer Street, London W1T 3JH, UK. Registered in England and Wales number 1072954.

A CIP record for this book is available from the British Library.

Library of Congress Cataloging-in-Publication Data available on application

ISBN-13: 9781841843742

Orders may be sent to: Informa Healthcare, Sheepen Place, Colchester, Essex CO3 3LP, UK
Telephone: +44 (0)20 7017 5540
Email: CSDhealthcarebooks@informa.com
Website: http://informahealthcarebooks.com/

For corporate sales please contact: CorporateBooksIHC@informa.com
For foreign rights please contact: RightsIHC@informa.com
For reprint permissions please contact: PermissionsIHC@informa.com

Contents

Part V: Issues in the Management of Acute Heart Failure

Acknowledgement

The editors acknowledge Deana Betterton-Lewis for her dedicated editorial work on this textbook.

Contributors

Kirkwood F Adams, Jr MD
Associate Professor of Medicine and Radiology
Director, UNC Heart Failure Program
Division of Cardiology
The University of North Carolina School of Medicine
Chapel Hill, North Carolina
USA

Sana M Al-Khatib MD, MHS, FACC
Assistant Professor of Medicine
Department of Medicine/Division of Cardiology
Duke University Medical Center
Duke Clinical Research Institute
Durham, North Carolina
USA

Aysha Arshad MBBS, FACC
Attending Electrohysiologist, St Luke's-Roosevelt Hospital Center
Assistant Professor of Medicine, Columbia University College of Physicians and Surgeons
Division of Cardiology, St Luke's-Roosevelt Hospital Center
New York, New York
USA

Catalin F Baicu PhD
Assistant Professor of Medicine
Division of Cardiology
Department of Medicine
University of South Carolina
Charleston, South Carolina
USA

Guido Boerrigter MD
Instructor in Medicine
Division of Cardiovascular Diseases
Mayo Clinic and Mayo Clinic College of Medicine
Rochester, Minnesota
USA

Jamieson M Bourque MD, MHS
Research Associate
Department of Internal Medicine
Duke University Medical Center
Durham, North Carolina
USA

David Bragin-Sánchez MD
Cardiomyopathy and Cardiac Transplant Cardiologist
Cardiovascular Center of Puerto Rico and the Caribbean
San Juan, Puerto Rico
USA

Robert Brewer MD
Senior Cardiothoracic Surgeon
Division of Cardiothoracic Surgery
Henry Ford Health System
Detroit, Michigan
USA

John C Burnett, Jr MD
Professor of Medicine and Physiology
Division of Cardiovascular Diseases
Mayo Clinic and Mayo Clinic College of Medicine
Rochester, Minnesota
USA

Patricia P Chang MD, MHS, FACC
Assistant Professor
Director, Cardiomyopathy and Transplant Service
Division of Cardiology, Department of Medicine
The University of North Carolina at Chapel Hill
Chapel Hill, North Carolina
USA

Jun Ratunil Chiong MD
Assistant Professor of Medicine
University of Florida
Division of Cardiology
Jacksonville, Florida
USA

John G F Cleland MD, FRCP, FACC, FESC
Professor of Cardiology
Department of Cardiology
University of Hull
Kingston-Upon-Hull
UK

Robert J Cody MD
Professor of Internal Medicine
Division of Cardiovascular Medicine
University of Michigan Health System
Ann Arbor, Michigan
USA

Gadi Cotter MD
Assistant Clinical Professor of Medicine
Department of Medicine/Division of Clinical Pharmacology
Duke University Medical Center
Durham, North Carolina
USA

Vincent Dor MD
Professor of Cardiothoracic Surgery
Centre Cardio-Thoracique de Monaco
Monaco

Mark H Drazner MD, MSc
Medical Director, Parkland Memorial Hospital CHF Clinic
Associate Professor of Medicine
Donald W Reynolds Cardiovascular Clinical Research Center
Division of Cardiology, University of Texas Southwestern Medical Center
Dallas, Texas
USA

Mark E Dunlap MD
Director, Heart Failure Program and Associate Chief of Cardiology
Louis B Stokes Veterans' Affairs Medical Center
Associate Professor of Medicine, Physiology and Biophysics
Case Western Reserve University
Cleveland, Ohio
USA

Michael D Faulx MD
Chief Fellow, Cardiology
University Hospitals of Cleveland
Case Western Reserve University
Cleveland, Ohio
USA

G Michael Felker MD, MHS
Assistant Professor of Medicine
Division of Cardiology
Duke University Medical Center
Durham, North Carolina
USA

Gregg C Fonarow MD
Professor of Medicine, UCLA Division of Cardiology
The Eliot Corday Chair in Cardiovascular Medicine and Science
Director, Ahmanson–UCLA Cardiomyopathy Center
University of California Los Angeles
Los Angeles, California
USA

Gary S Francis MD
Professor of Medicine
Lerner College of Medicine of Case Western Reserve University
Cleveland Clinica Foundation
Cleveland, Ohio
USA

Joëlle Y Friedman MPA
Project Leader
Center for Clinical and Genetic Economics
Duke Clinical Research Institute
Duke University Medical Center
Durham, North Carolina
USA

Laura H Gaulden RN, MSN, ANP
Clinical Operations Director
Duke Heart Failure Program
Duke University Medical Center
Durham, North Carolina
USA

Jalal K Ghali MD
Professor of Medicine
Associate Director, Cardiology Section
Director, Heart Failure and Cardiovascular Research Program
Louisiana State University Health Sciences Center
Shreveport, Louisiana
USA

Mihai Gheorghiade MD, FACC
Professor of Medicine
Associate Chief of Cardiology
Northwestern University, Feinberg School of Medicine
Chicago, Illinois
USA

Jana Glotzer RN, MSN, CCRN, ACNP, CHF
Acute Care Nurse Practioner
UNC Heart Failure Program
The University of North Carolina at Chapel Hill
Chapel Hill, North Carolina
USA

William B Haynos MD
Heart Failure Treatment Program
Department of Internal Medicine, Roy J Carver College of Medicine
The University of Iowa
Iowa City, Iowa
USA

Adrian F Hernandez MD
Assistant Professor of Medicine
Division of Cardiology
Duke University Medical Center
Durham, North Carolina
USA

Shahriar Iravanian MD
Medicine Resident, St Luke's-Roosevelt Hospital Center
Division of Medicine, St Luke's-Roosevelt Hospital Center
New York, New York
USA

Wei Jiang MD
Assistant Professor of Medicine, Psychiatry and Behavioral Science
Department of Internal Medicine, Psychiatry and Behavioral Science
Duke University Medical Center
Durham, North Carolina
USA

Edo Kaluski MD, FACC
Director of the Coronary Care Unit
Asaf Harofeh Medical Center
Zrifin and The Sackler School of Medicine, University of Tel Aviv
Tel Aviv
Israel

Jason N Katz MD
Chief Medicine Resident
Department of Internal Medicine
University of Texas Southwestern Medical Center
Dallas, Texas
USA

Dalane W Kitzman MD
Professor of Internal Medicine
Sections of Cardiology and Geriatrics
Director of Echocardiography
Wake Forest University School of Medicine
Winston-Salem, North Carolina
USA

Robert C Kowal MD, PhD
Electrophysiologist, Clinical Associate Professor of Medicine
Baylor University Medical Center
University of Texas Southwestern Medical Center
Dallas, Texas
USA

Ranga R Krishnan MD
Professor and Chairman
Department of Psychiatry and Behavioral Sciences
Duke University Medical Center
Durham, North Carolina
USA

Marvin W Kronenberg MD
Professor of Medicine and Radiology
Division of Cardiovascular Medicine
Department of Medicine
Vanderbilt University School of Medicine
Nashville, Tennessee
USA

Krishna Lalukota MBBS, MRCP
Department of Cardiology
University of Hull
Kingston-Upon-Hull
UK

Alan S Maisel MD
Professor of Medicine
University of California, San Diego
Director, Coronary Care Unit and Heart Failure Research Program
San Diego VA Healthcare Center
San Diego, California
USA

Mandeep R Mehra MD
Vice Chairman, Department of Cardiovascular Medicine
Medical Director, Cardiomyopathy and Heart Transplantation Center
Ochsner Clinic Foundation
New Orleans, Louisiana
USA

Carmelo A Milano MD
Associate Professor of Surgery
Division of Thoracic Surgery
Duke University Medical Center
Durham, North Carolina
USA

Alan B Miller MD
Professor, Internal Medicine/Cardiology
University of Florida
Jacksonville, Florida
USA

Olga Milo-Cotter MD
Durham, North Carolina
USA

Debra K Moser DNSc, RN, FAAN
Professor and Gill Chair of Nursing
University of Kentucky, College of Nursing
Lexington, Kentucky
USA

Rimbida Obeleniene MD
Division of Cardiology
St Luke's-Roosevelt Hospital
New York, New York
USA

Christopher M O'Connor MD, FACP, FACC
Professor of Medicine
Chief, Division of Clinical Pharmacology
Director, Duke Heart Failure Program
Duke University Medical Center
Durham, North Carolina
USA

E Magnus Ohman MD, FACC
Ernest and Hazel Craige Professor of Cardiovascular Medicine
Chief of Division of Cardiology
Department of Medicine/Division of Cardiology
The University of North Carolina at Chapel Hill
Chapel Hill, North Carolina
USA

Ron Oren MD
Professor of Clinical Medicine
University of Iowa
Heart Failure Treatment Program
University of Iowa Hospitals and Clinics
Iowa City, Iowa
USA

Cesare Orlandi MD, FACC
Vice President, Clinical Development
Otsuka Maryland Research Institute
Rockville, Maryland
USA

J Herbert Patterson PharmD, FCCP, BCPS
Associate Professor of Pharmacy and Research Associate Professor of Cardiology
University of North Carolina at Chapel Hill
School of Pharmacy
Division of Pharmacotherapy and Experimental Therapeutics
Chapel Hill, North Carolina
USA

Ileana L Piña MD, FACC
Professor of Medicine
Section of Medicine, Cardiology, Heart Failure and Case Western Reserve University
Louis B Stokes Veterans Medical Center
Food and Drug Administration (FDA) Consultant
Chair, Heart Failure Section, American Heart Association
Cleveland, Ohio
USA

Maurizio Porcu MD
Director, Division of Cardiology, Heart Failure and Cardiac Transplant Program
Azienda Ospedaliera "G Brotzu" – San Michele
Cagliari
Italy

Joseph G Rogers MD
Medical Director, Cardiac Transplant Program
Department of Medicine/Division of Cardiology
Duke University Medical Center
Durham, North Carolina
USA

Lynn P Roser RN, MSN
Associate Professor of Nursing
Bluegrass Community and Technical College
Doctoral Student, University of Kentucky College of Nursing
Lexington, Kentucky
USA

Hani N Sabbah PhD, FACC, FCCP, FAHA
Professor of Medicine and Director of Cardiovascular Research
Division of Cardiovascular Medicine
Henry Ford Health System
Detroit, Michigan
USA

Jonathan D Sackner-Bernstein MD
Director, Clinical Research
Heart Failure and Cardiomyopathy Center
North Shore University Hospital
Manhasset, New York
USA

Kevin A Schulman MD
Professor of Medicine
Center for Clinical and Genetic Economics
Duke Clinical Research Institute
Duke University Medical Center
Durham, North Carolina
USA

Anne-Marie Seymour PhD
Department of Biological Sciences
University of Hull
Kingston-Upon-Hull
UK

Ashish S Shah MD
Division of Thoracic Surgery
Department of General and Thoracic Surgery
Duke University Medical Center
Durham, North Carolina
USA

Victor G Sharov MD, PhD
Senior Staff Investigator
Division of Cardiovascular Medicine
Henry Ford Health System
Detroit, Michigan
USA

Norman A Silverman MD
Division Head, Cardiothoracic Surgery
Division of Cardiothoracic Surgery
Henry Ford Health System
Detroit, Michigan
USA

Jonathan S Steinberg MD, FACC
Chief, Division of Cardiology
Director, Arrhythmia Service St Luke's-Roosevelt Hospital Center
Professor of Medicine, Columbia University College of Physicians and Surgeons
Division of Cardiology, St Luke's-Roosevelt Hospital Center
New York, New York
USA

William G Stevenson MD
Associate Professor of Medicine
Harvard Medical School
Director, Clinical Cardiac Electrophysiology Program
Brigham and Women's Hospital
Boston, Massachusetts
USA

Wendy Gattis Stough PharmD
Assistant Clinical Professor in Medicine
Department of Medicine
Division of Cardiology
Duke University Medical Center
Durham, North Carolina
USA

W H Wilson Tang MD
Associate Staff
Section of Heart Failure and Cardiac Transplant Medicine
Cleveland Clinic Foundation
Assistant Professor in Medicine
Cleveland Clinic Lerner College of Medicine
Cleveland, Ohio
USA

Elaine J Tanhehco PhD
Associate Staff Investigator
Division of Cardiovascular Medicine
Henry Ford Health System
Detroit, Michigan
USA

Victor F Tapson MD
Professor of Medicine, Pulmonary and Critical Care Medicine
Director, Pulmonary Vascular Disease Center
Duke University Medical Center
Durham, North Carolina
USA

John R Teerlink MD, FACC, FAHA, FESC
Associate Professor of Medicine
Director of Heart Failure
School of Medicine, University of California
Section of Cardiology, San Francisco Veterans Affairs Medical Center
San Francisco, California
USA

Eric J Velazquez MD
Assistant Professor of Medicine
Department of Medicine/Division of Cardiology
Duke University Medical Center
Director, Heart Failure Research
Duke Clinical Research Institute
Durham, North Carolina
USA

Hector O Ventura MD
Cardiomyopathy and Heart Transplantation Center
Ochsner Clinic Foundation
Clinical Professor of Medicine
Tulane University School of Medicine
New Orleans, Louisiana
USA

Carson S Webb MD
Cardiology Fellow
Division of Cardiology
Department of Medicine
University of South Carolina
Charleston, South Carolina
USA

David J Whellan MD, MHS
Asistant Professor of Medicine
Director of Clinical Trial Outcomes, Department of Medicine
Director of Clinical Research, Jefferson Heart Institute
Jefferson Medical College
Thomas Jefferson University
Philadelphia, Pennsylvania
USA

Jonathan E E Yager MD
Cardiology Fellow
Division of Cardiology
Duke University Medical Center
Durham, North Carolina
USA

Clyde Yancy MD, FACC, FAHA
Professor of Internal Medicine/Cardiology
Carl H Westcott Distinguished Chair in Medical Research
Associate Dean of Clinical Affairs, St Paul University Hospital
Medical Director, Heart Failure/Transplantation
University of Texas Southwestern Medical Center
Dallas, Texas
USA

Cheryl Hoyt Zambroski PhD, RN
Assistant Professor of Nursing
University of Louisville School of Nursing
Louisville, Kentucky
USA

Michael R Zile MD
Charles Ezra Daniel Professor of Medicine
Division of Cardiology
Department of Medicine
University of South Carolina
Charleston, South Carolina
USA

Foreword

In the past decade, a growing number of cardiologists have become concerned about the disparity in attention to clinical trials and guidelines among the different presentations of cardiovascular disease. During this time, the pattern of these discrepancies has become clear. For several decades, ST-segment-elevation acute myocardial infarction had been a focus of clinical trials, resulting in the entry of tens of thousands of patients into randomized trials and, consequently, the establishment of effective therapies that have become standards of care. Similar activity occurred in the field of chronic heart failure, with the subsequent definition of effective patterns of care based on evidence. In contrast, patients with non-ST-segment-elevation acute coronary syndromes and acute heart failure, though seen in large numbers in practice, were rarely entered into clinical trials.

Drs. O'Connor, Stough, Gheorghiade, and Adams were key leaders in calling attention to the deficit of evidence for practice in caring for patients with acute heart failure, and this text is definitive proof of the success of their efforts. Through a series of meetings with thought leaders, government agencies, and leaders in the medical products industry, they have directed attention to the topic of acute heart failure. A similar effort has been underway for non-ST-elevation acute coronary syndromes, with similar results. In both areas, we can now rest assured that the clinical community is convinced of the importance of the problem and the critical necessity of producing evidence through clinical trials and epidemiological studies.

Beginning with the Outcomes of a Prospective Trial of Intravenous Milrinone for Exacerbations of Chronic Heart Failure (OPTIME-CHF) trial, a series of studies has now identified a variety of therapies that seem to have little to offer patients with acute heart failure. Other therapies are promising—but as yet unproven—in the acute phase of heart failure. These trials have not only served the purpose of informing the practice community about therapies, but they have also refocused attention on the complexity of the pathophysiology and clinical epidemiology of acute heart failure.

This textbook begins, appropriately, with a definition of the problem, including its scope and epidemiology. The huge number of acute heart failure patients will seem startling to those who have not considered this issue before. However, practitioners who see patients in general medicine or cardiology practice are aware of the onslaught of patients with this problem.

The book then moves on to common complications and comorbid conditions. Given the older age of most patients with acute heart failure, it is not surprising that understanding issues such as renal insufficiency, respiratory insufficiency, diabetes, and stroke is so important in caring for these patients. For the most part, decision-making regarding mechanical complications and arrhythmias in the acute phase of the heart failure admission remains an art rather than a science, but the growing volume of clinical epidemiological studies is producing a clear picture of critical decision points that will be amenable to developing definitive evidence for practice.

The text then provides an in-depth review of the pharmacological therapy for acute heart failure. The lack of proven, effective medical therapies remains a major concern in this arena. Milrinone and dobutamine have fallen into disfavor due to negative or unfavorable studies, while many other medications, such as nesiritide and endothelin antagonists, have shown promising but unproven benefit. The good news is that major clinical outcome studies are under way evaluating both of these exciting new therapies.

A particularly interesting twist in this book is the focus on integrative care of the patient. The chapters on psychosocial aspects, nursing care, and disease management clarify many critical issues about the total care of the patient and family that are usually ignored or given short shrift in most medical textbooks. These chapters in particular represent the selfless manner in which O'Connor, Stough, Gheorghiade, and Adams have developed teams dedicated to every aspect of the needs of patients with heart failure.

We hope that future editions of this book will document significant progress in the pursuit of evidence upon which to base practice. It has been a pleasure to participate in the development of a new field of cardiology with O'Connor, Stough, Gheorghiade, and Adams. We hope that *Managing Acute Decompensated Heart Failure* will become an essential companion to practitioners caring for patients with this increasingly common, difficult, and fatal disease.

Robert M Califf, MD,
Duke Clinical Research Institute,
Durham, NC

Robert O Bonow, MD,
Northwestern Memorial Hospital,
Chicago, IL

July 2005

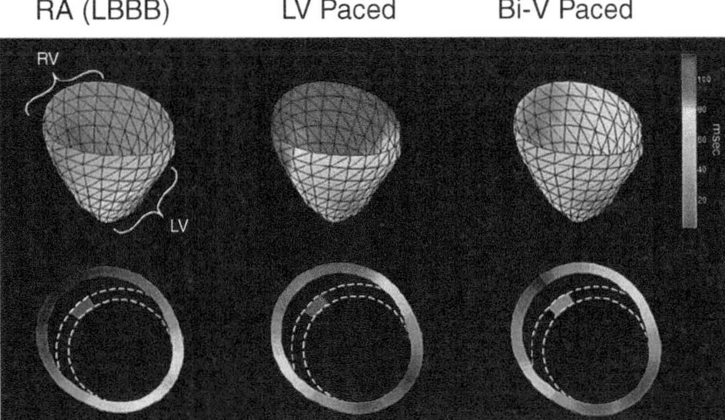

Figure 25.1. *Electrical response with different pacing modes. Top row: Electrical epicardial activation map of whole heart for three pacing modes. Activation time is color coded (blue early → red late). With right atrial (RA) pacing (left bundle branch block [LBBB]), electrical activation spreads from right to left, whereas LV pacing reversed the pattern but did not reduce conduction delay. Biventricular (BV) pacing, however, showed improved electrical synchrony. Bottom row: Short-axis slice demonstrating that activation time at the endocardial septum was similar to that at epicardial electrodes over the same region. (With permission from Leclercq* et al.[74])

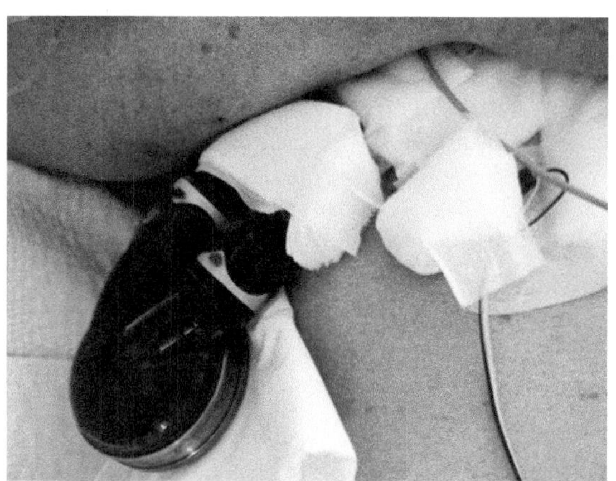

Figure 29.3. *A newer paracorporeal device, compatible with the ABIOMED BVS 5000®, the AB5000™ circulatory support system eliminates extensive blood tubing and may be less prone to thromboembolic complications*

Figure 29.4. *The Thoratec® extracorporeal ventricular assist device. (Reprinted with permission from Thoratec Corporation.)*

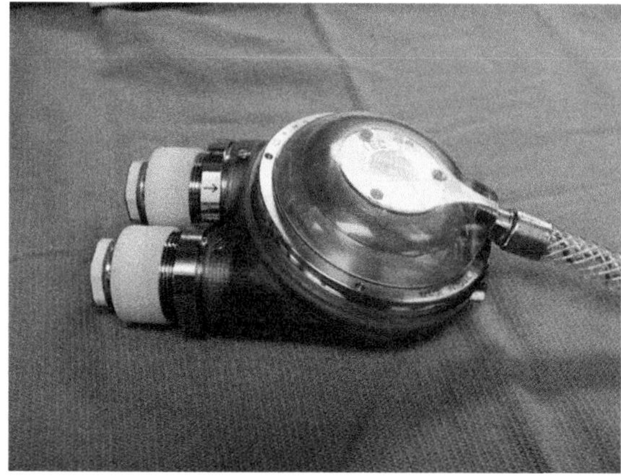

Figure 29.5. *A newer console allows patients greater mobility and the potential for home discharge. (Reprinted with permission from Thoratec Corporation.)*

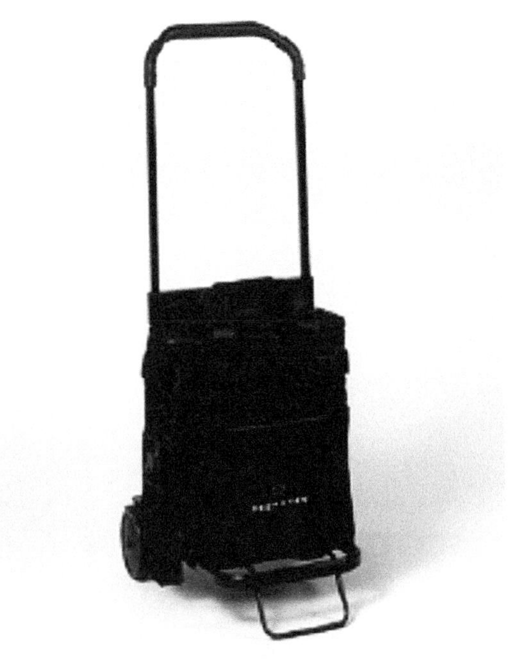

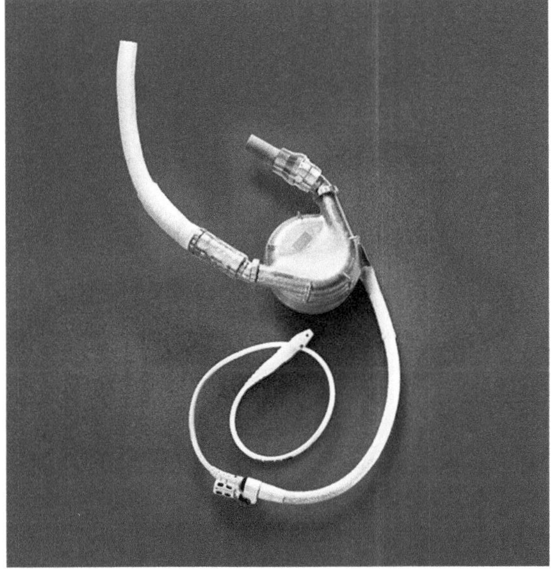

Figure 29.6. *The textured lining of the HeartMate® ventricular assist device generates a pseudointimal layer and contributes to decreased thromboembolic complications. (Reprinted with permission from Thoratec Corporation.)*

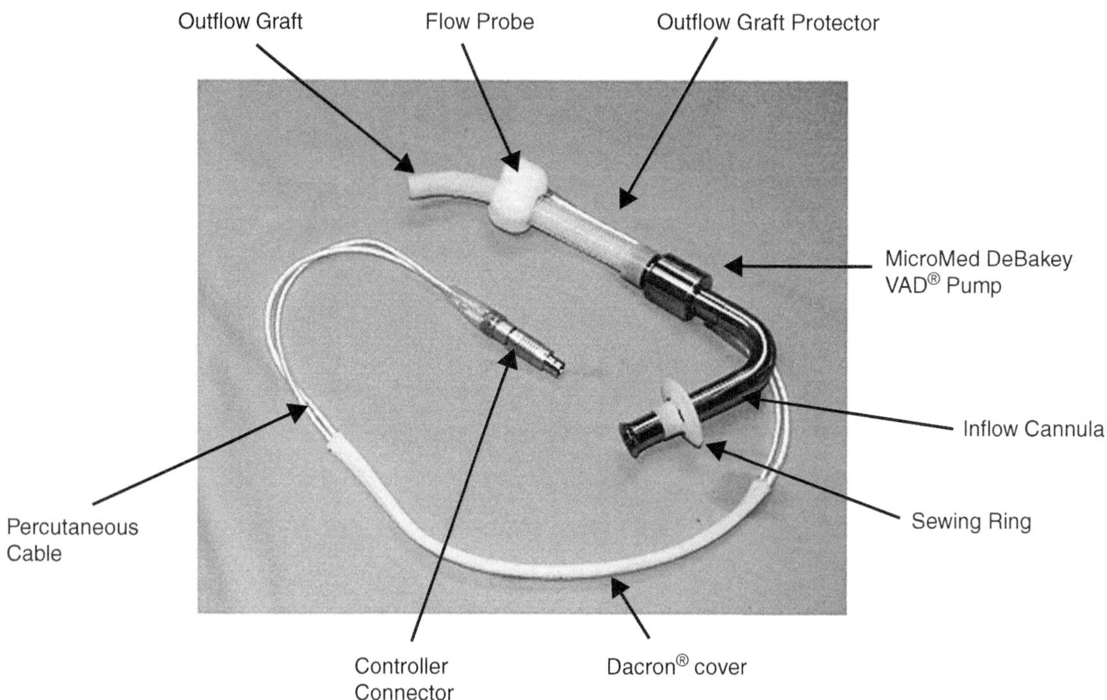

Figure 29.7. *The MicroMed DeBakey® ventricular assist device axial flow pump represents the next generation in devices. These blood pumps are smaller, quiet and more efficient then previous devices. (Reprinted with permission from MicroMed Technology, Inc.)*

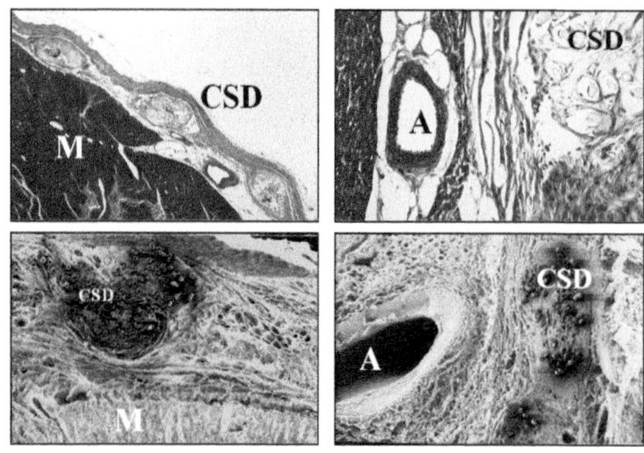

Figure 31.2. *Top left: Trichrome stained section of left ventricular myocardium from a dog treated for 3 months with the cardiac support device (CSD). The CSD is encapsulated by thin layers of mature connective tissue (blue-green). There is a clear demarcation between the CSD and the myocardium (M, dark red) with no evidence of invasion of the myocardium by connective tissue. Top right: An epicardial artery (A) coursing between the CSD and the epicardial myocardium is normal in appearance. Bottom panels: Scanning electron micrograph from a dog with heart failure treated for 3 months with the CSD. The micrograph depicts a single CSD fiber consisting of multiple filaments, the adjacent connective tissue, underlying epicardial myocardium and an epicardial artery (A) coursing between the CSD and the epicardial myocardium*

PART I

Epidemiology and Pathophysiology

CHAPTER 1

The history of acute heart failure management: how far have we come?

Hector O Ventura, Mandeep R Mehra

Introduction

Our understanding of the basic mechanisms associated with the development of heart failure and advances in modern pharmacology have reduced the morbidity and mortality for patients who have this disorder.

Prior to the twentieth century, heart failure was known as *dropsy*. This term was used to describe the presence of generalized swelling, which was a clinical result of the syndrome. Thus, the treatment modalities available for dropsy, whether surgical or medical, were aimed at an "emptying of the system" or relieving fluid retention. These remedies were crude in composition, unpredictable in action, and associated with untoward side effects. Bloodletting, by venesection, leeches, hydragogue cathartics, squill, or mercury, was a common method for alleviating the patient's symptoms.[1–3]

The first important innovation in the medical treatment of heart failure was the discovery of the pharmacologic properties of foxglove by William Withering in the eighteenth century. His classic monograph, *An Account of the Foxglove*, published in 1785,[4] describes how he had learned from an old countrywoman (the so-called "Shropshire maid") that tea made from the leaves of the purple foxglove plant was "good for the dropsy."

For many years, digitalis was the only valuable drug for the treatment of heart failure. It was not until 1919 that the diuretic properties of mercury were demonstrated in patients with syphilis, severe rheumatic heart disease, and anasarca. This led to the synthesis of the organic mercurial diuretics.[2,5,6]

This chapter provides an historical overview of the therapeutic strategies intended to alleviate salt and water retention in patients with heart failure. The fundamental basis by which these therapies were prescribed related to the concept that heart failure was an abnormality of cardiac function in which reduced ejection and impaired filling led to circulatory responses such as salt and water retention. This paradigm dominated the thinking throughout the first half of the twentieth century, until the utilization of vasodilatory agents in the 1970s.[7,8]

Bloodletting

Bloodletting is one of the oldest remedies known to man. In the past, some commonly used methods for bloodletting included general bloodletting by venesection or arteriotomy and local bloodletting by scarification with wet cupping, cauterization, and leeches.[1] According to Heath's *Dictionary of Practical Surgery*:

> Bloodletting is said to be general when the blood is taken from a vein or artery so that the amount in the vascular system is

> materially diminished as shown by diminution on the tension of the blood vessels: it is termed local when, by means of leeches, cupping, or scarification, blood is taken in smaller quantities, with a view of relieving limited congestion and vascular tension.[9]

One of the reasons that the practice of bloodletting continued for so long is that the procedure is actually beneficial in reducing the fluid overload associated with heart failure. Early physicians, however, did not have the physiological understanding to determine the conditions for which bloodletting was medically indicated. Therefore, this procedure was used for almost everything, including agitated psychoses when a drop in blood pressure resulted in sedation. It was John Pancoast, who reported the reason by which bloodletting was beneficial in patients with dropsy, "the diminution of the mass of the blood, by which overloaded capillary or larger vessels of some affected part may be relieved, the modification of the force and frequency of the heart's action."[10]

From the time of the Egyptians, through Avicenna and Hippocrates, to the beginning of the twentieth century, bloodletting was used in various forms for the treatment of fluid retention. The following sections review the therapeutic use of bloodletting in patients with heart failure throughout history, focusing on some important contributions.

Bloodletting in Roman times

From 100 BC to AD 476, the Roman Empire dominated the known world. The medicine practiced in Rome was largely of Greek origin with excellent clinical descriptions. However, the treatment strategies used were largely ineffective and consisted of simple measures such as changes in diet, rest, and bloodletting. However, the Romans did make great progress in the field of public health and sanitation and they founded the first hospitals.[11] Perhaps one of the most famous names from this period is Celsus (25 BC to AD 40).

Aurelius Cornelius Celsus

Aurelius Cornelius Celsus, the Roman encyclopedist, wrote a detailed account of medical practice in his treatise *De Medicina*. He describes two basic kinds of therapeutic methods:

> Now every corporeal aid either diminishes substance or adds to it, either draws it out or represses it, either cools or warms, either hardens or softens ... Substance is withdrawn by blood letting, cupping, purging, vomiting, rubbing, rocking, and by bodily exercises of all kinds, by abstinence, by sweating.[12]

In relation to heart failure and its treatment, the following passages are clear and excellent descriptions of dyspnea and its treatment strategy:

> When moderate and without any choking, it is called dyspnoea; when more severe, so that the patient cannot breathe without making a noise and gasping, asthma; but when in addition the patient can hardly draw his breath unless with the neck outstretched, orthopnea. Of these the first can last a long while, the two following are as a rule acute.
>
> Blood-letting is the remedy unless anything prohibits. Nor is that enough, but also the bowels are to be relaxed by milk, the stool being rendered ... as the body becomes depleted by the measures the patient begins to draw his breath more readily. Moreover, even in bed the head is to be kept raised.[13]

Celsus also describes the technique of bloodletting as follows:

> Blood letting by the incision of the vein, is no novelty ... now if the object be to relieve the whole body; it ought to be drawn from the arm, if to relieve a part, then from that part itself, or certainly from that nearest to it.[14]

Celsus's prescription of bloodletting and the fact that there is an improvement in breathing suggests that some of the patients suffered from dyspnea associated with heart disease. Interestingly, he also utilized a very current treatment for pulmonary edema and cardiac asthma, which is to keep the head raised.

In another chapter of his book, Celsus describes the technique of paracentesis for "dropsical patients." He stated that, "the tap should be done below the navel at the distance of about four digits to the left."[15]

Bloodletting in the Middle Ages

In the Middle Ages, cauterization was another technique used to relieve patients with fluid retention. It was used as a topical stimulant to attract fluid to the area involved.[1,16] Its use is represented in the following passage discussing the disease of Alexius I, ruler of the Byzantine Empire from AD 1081 to 1118. His daughter, who watched Alexius's attending physicians during their deliberations about her father's disease, describes the following:

> [They] felt his pulse and found all kind of irregularities … his heart, they said, was inflamed and was attracting all the superfluous matter from the rest of the body … every day it grew worse, attacking him no longer at intervals but relentlessly, with no interruption. He was unable to lie on either side, so weak that every breath involved great effort … his condition was serious for never for one moment could he breathe freely. He was forced to sit upright to breathe at all … but his stomach was visibly enlarged to a great size and his feet also swelled up and fever laid him low, some of the doctors with scant regard to fever had recourse to cauterization.[16]

Bloodletting in the Renaissance

Although significant advances in the knowledge of human anatomy occurred during the Renaissance, heart failure remained a poorly understood syndrome.[17] At the beginning of the seventeenth century, *Exercitatio Anatomica de Mortu Cordis et Sanguinis in Animalibus* (*On the Motion of the Heart and Blood in Animals*) by William Harvey was published and paved the way to understanding the syndrome of heart failure. Through experiments in animals, this text demonstrates that blood circulated constantly and that the heart was a pump. Harvey writes, "it must therefore be concluded that the blood in the animal body moves around in a circle continuously, and that the action or function of the heart is to accomplish this by pumping."[18] This description produced a paradigm shift in medicine, since the heart was previously thought to be a furnace to heat the blood. After the publication of Harvey's treatise, the heart became known as a pump to bring blood to the tissues.[7]

Using Harvey's paradigm, Giorgio Baglivi in his treatise *De Praxi Medica* (*On the Practice of Medicine*), which appeared first in 1669, illustrated the first acceptable clinical description of pulmonary edema and attempted to establish a mechanism by which it occurs.[19] He writes:

> Next to be considered is a dangerous disease of the lungs which is called suffocative catarrh. It is caused chiefly by stagnation of the blood in the lungs and about the pericardium … In this kind of catarrh the patient has a cold, and pain in the chest, and difficulty in breathing; also interrupted speech, anxiety, cough, stertor, a widely spaced low pulse, foam at the mouth, and the like … The foam at the mouth is caused by impaired circulation of blood about the lungs and consequent circulation of the lymph in the upper parts of the body near the face; hence this [kind of] catarrh comes from sudden stagnation of blood in the vicinity of the heart and lungs, and not from phlegm running down from head as the ancients believed to be the condition in this disease. An instant remedy for this disease during the paroxysm is repeated bloodletting … the disease is very precipitous; unless phlebotomy is done immediately the blood coagulates more and stagnates. Thus the opportunity for cure is lost. The blood should be reduced in amount, the clotting should be undone and a bland sweat should be produced.

In another passage of his treatise Baglivi writes about asthma:

> If anyone in the evening at bedtime, or specially after three or four hours of sleep, is

> suddenly aroused by severe asthma or is taken with suffocation and opens the window and wants fresh air, consider it certain that he is suffering from dropsy of the chest ... dysuria is beneficial to asthmatics; if the dysuria ceases suddenly, the patients is seized with asthma again. Furthermore, this gives additional confirmation to what I have repeatedly observed, namely in the diseases of the chest the treatment should lead toward the urinary passages.

Later in the *Appendix on Asthma*, Baglivi states:

> It may be granted that bloodletting cures asthmatic paroxysm immediately. However, frequent bloodlettings weaken the tone of the blood more, and enfeeble it; and for this reason the disease ends in generalized dropsy. Therefore the cause of the asthma should be corrected, instead of being caressed by frequent phlebotomy.[19]

Several inferences can be drawn from Baglivi's discussion. First, Baglivi gives an excellent and clear description of patients with pulmonary edema and the attack of nocturnal dyspnea. Second, he relates the production of dyspnea and pulmonary edema to an impaired circulation of blood to the lungs, an explanation based on Harvey's ideas. Finally, Baglivi recommends the use of urgent phlebotomy to reduce blood volume for the treatment of pulmonary edema. The latter comment provides an early example of a physiologic approach to therapy in heart failure. In addition, he also cautions against the use of repeated bloodlettings and perhaps erroneously relates this therapy to the production of chronic fluid retention. It is more likely that the patient, despite the repeated phlebotomies, progresses to chronic heart failure. Interestingly, he emphasizes that frequent phlebotomies cause only symptomatic relief, but the treatment should be directed to the underlying cause of asthma. More intriguing is the statement:

> Dysuria is beneficial to asthmatics; if the dysuria ceases suddenly, the patient is seized with asthma again. Furthermore, this gives additional confirmation to what I have repeatedly observed, namely in the diseases of the chest the treatment should lead toward the urinary passages.

Jarcho analyzed this particular remark and concluded that perhaps Baglivi intended to write "diuresis." If that is the case, Baglivi demonstrates the association between decrease in diuresis and dyspnea and in addition he points out that the treatment of the diseases of the chest should be focused on increasing urine output.[19]

Bloodletting in the nineteenth century

The nineteenth century was a period of great progress in cardiology. Several diagnostic tools were introduced, such as the stethoscope and sphygmomanometer, among others, to aid in the objective assessment of cardiac diseases.[20] The understanding of the pathophysiology of heart failure continued to evolve, including the recognition of hypertrophy, cardiac enlargement, valvular heart disease, and ischemic heart disease as underlying causes of heart failure. Despite the evolution of the concept of heart failure, therapeutic options remained limited to the removal of fluids using bloodletting, starvation, and purgation.[21]

James Hope

James Hope, one of the most famous English cardiologists, published his book, *A Treatise on the Diseases of the Heart and Great Vessels*, in 1831.[22] This book contained several classic descriptions of the signs and symptoms of heart failure. It also added to the understanding of hypertrophy and dilatation of the heart, described the mechanism by which edema develops, and created the concept of backward failure. According to Hope, "The overworked ventricle first hypertrophies and then dilates. As it dilates the blood gets dammed up behind it and an increased venous pressure is transmitted ultimately to the capillaries where the edema is formed." Hope's treatment of this disorder was based on removing fluids by bleeding, puncturing, diaphoretics, emetics, purgatives, and expectorants.[22]

Hope also used a combination of "three grains

of calomel (blue pill), one or half of one of digitalis and one of scillae (squill) given 3 or 4 times a day," for the treatment of dropsy.[22]

The Irish School of Medicine

In general, the Irish School of Medicine was opposed to the use of bloodletting in great quantities and one of the champions of this theory was Dominic Corrigan. He stated that, "Bleeding after bleeding, blister after blister were repeated, starvation enforced and digitalis exhibited, until the patient was reduced to such weakness that he had scarcely strength to rise himself in bed."[23]

The review of the treatment of heart failure, specifically the chapter on "treatment of the weak and probably dilated heart in connexion with enlargement of the liver and pulmonary disease," in William Stokes's masterpiece *The Diseases of the Heart and the Aorta* demonstrates Stokes's aversion to the use of bloodletting and the importance of the use of mercury instead.[2,24] He states that:

> We should avoid all reducing measures; we must endeavour to improve the condition of the blood, and, by stimulants and tonics, increase the power of the weakened and atrophied muscular fibres ... although the great principles of treatment are the same in the weakened and dilated heart such as occurred in the case of Mr. Colles, and in either form of fatty heart, yet in one important particular we find them to differ. I allude to the beneficial action of mercury in relieving many of the symptoms, and removing the consequences of the first of these diseases.[24]

However, in another passage, Stokes recommends the use of bloodletting especially in acute decompensation:

> Mr. Colles ... from about the year 1834 was the subject of a chronic bronchitis, with occasional exacerbation of the disease in the acute form. During these attacks the pertinent symptoms were dyspnea and palpitation, and the treatment adopted was to employ small general bleedings.[25]

Reginald S. Southey

In 1877, an interesting development in the treatment of fluid retention was the invention, by English physician Reginald Southey, of small rubber tubes that were placed in the lower extremities to relieve severe edema.[26] Although early on these tubes, known as Southey's tubes, were used for the treatment of anasarca related to kidney failure, their use evolved in the next century to the treatment of obstinate edema in heart failure when other medical therapies failed.

Bloodletting in the twentieth century

William Osler

William Osler was born and educated in Canada and became the first professor of Medicine at Johns Hopkins University. At the end of the nineteenth century, he published his book, *The Principles and Practice of Medicine*, in which he described the natural history of heart failure, focusing on cardiac hypertrophy. Cardiac hypertrophy is either adaptive or maladaptive during the evolution of a patient's history.[27] Osler stated that, "The course of any case of cardiac hypertrophy may be divided into three stages: 1) the period of development, 2) the period of full compensation and 3) the period of broken compensation."[27]

The treatment of the stage of broken compensation (acute decompensated heart failure [ADHF]) is depicted in the following passage. He recommends venesection or depletion of the bowels only in this period.[27]

> Among the first indications are shortness of breath on exertion or attacks of nocturnal dyspnea ... dilatation of the heart, the gallop rhythm, or various forms of arrhythmia, with or without the existence of dropsy. Under these circumstances the following measures are to be carried out
>
> 1 Rest
> 2 Relief of the embarrassed circulation
>   (a) *By venesection.* In cases of dilatation, from whatever cause ... when signs of venous engorgement are marked and when there is orthopnea with

cyanosis, the abstraction of from twenty to thirty ounces of blood is indicated. This is the occasion in which timely venesection may save the patient's life. It is a condition in which I have had most satisfactory results from venesection. I have on several occasions regretted the postponement, particularly in instances of acute dilatation and cyanosis in connection with emphysema.

(b) *By depletion through the bowels*. This is particularly valuable when dropsy is present. Of the various purges the salines had to be preferred, and may be given by Matthew Hay's method. Half an hour before breakfast from half an ounce to an ounce and a half of Epsom salts may be given in a concentrated form. This usually produces three to five liquid evacuations.

Paul Dudley White

Paul Dudley White published the first edition of his important treatise in cardiology, *Heart Disease*, in 1932.[28] Referring to the treatment of heart failure, he established very clearly the use of "various mechanical therapeutic measures." Among the types of treatments, he described venesection as:

> not often necessary in the treatment of congestive heart failure, but sometimes as an emergency measurement it gives relief and probably saves a few lives. It was much more often necessary in the days before there was a proper appreciation of how to give digitalis—that is before the time of more or less universal digitalization and maintenance of digitalis effect. Venesection is applicable to two types of patients: first, the cardiac patient with acute and fulminating congestive heart failure, as in cases of cardiac asthma and of marked venous congestion with tachycardia, and second, the chronic cardiac patient who has obstinate edema and persistently high venous pressure (over 20 cm of water in arm vein) in spite of rest, digitalis, diuretics, and other therapy. Blood should be removed from the arm vein by knife or needle in amounts between 250 and 500 mL (½ to 1 pint). The procedure may be repeated at intervals as needed, but it should not be done unless the venous pressure is elevated.

White also described the use of "bloodless bloodletting" utilizing upper and lower extremity bands in patients with decompensated heart failure:

> Another way by which temporarily the heart may be relieved of excess blood, reported to be helpful in acute heart failure like cardiac asthma, is constriction of the proximal parts of all four extremities by blood pressure cuffs or similar bands, cutting temporarily the venous circulation.

Paul Wood

In the 1950s, Paul Wood, the director of the Institute of Cardiology in London, published his textbook, *Diseases of the Heart and Circulation*.[29] Similar to White, besides medical therapy, he utilized venesection, venous tourniquets in patients with pulmonary edema, and acupuncture of the extremities, as well as Southey's tubes for treating massive edema. The following excerpts are from his textbook:

> Venous tourniquets may be applied around the thighs to trap blood in the legs or venesection may be preferred.

> Venesection deserves a better reputation. It has fallen out of favour because similar results may be obtained by means of certain drugs, but it offers a quick and sure way of lowering the venous pressure and should not be abandoned. About 600 to 750 mL of blood may be withdrawn.

> When edema is gross and fails to respond, it may necessary to resort to acupuncture. A triangular cutting needle is used and about a dozen punctures are made in each leg ... Southey's tubes constitute a cleaner way of removing fluid on the same principle.

Phlebostasis

Another treatment used in the twentieth century was so-called "bloodless bloodletting" or *phlebostasis*. This was accomplished by inflating cuffs on the extremities and then allowing the air from the cuffs to escape very slowly or by using tourniquets in patients with cardiac asthma.

A specific case of the use of phlebostasis is depicted by Dr. Heinrich Stern, a physician who wrote an interesting treatise, *The Theory and Practice of Bloodletting*, in 1915.[30] He described the following case:

> male patient, 58 years old; consulted me first in December 24, 1912. He complained chiefly of asthmatic attacks coming on after exertion … the amount of his twenty-four hours' urine hardly ever exceeded one liter … the physical examination showed … the area of cardiac dullness was markedly increased toward the left as well as toward the right … the systolic blood pressure was 240 mm Hg … On application of phlebostasis for three minutes relieved the attacks of cardiac dyspnea for a number of weeks.

In his treatise, Dr. Stern also reviews the literature on the use of bloodletting either by venesection, leeches, or phlebostasis for heart failure.[30] Several remarks, especially on the use of bloodletting by James McKenzie, and other recommendations are important to note:

> Bloodletting should be performed rapidly by either venesection or leeches when the right heart is distended …
>
> Bloodletting acts instantaneously … in pulmonary edema.
>
> In pronounced cases of decompensation the most stressing and alarming symptoms, particularly cardiac asthma, are almost instantly removed by a timely bloodletting … congestive cardiac states, on the other hand, require repeated withdrawals of blood.
>
> I wish to emphasize again that in patients with congestion … medicinal or other therapeutic agents generally exert a more prompt and lasting influence after than before bloodletting.
>
> As individuals with congenital heart disease do not bear well the abstraction of blood, amounts not exceeding 75 mL should be removed at one time …
>
> The primus of modern cardiologists, James McKenzie, holds bloodletting in high esteem in the treatment of the diseases of the heart, deploring, however, the temporary character of relief which it affords … in extreme cases, McKenzie says, it merely delays the end.
>
> McKenzie employs bloodletting when there is distress in breathing, on account of great distension of the right heart …
>
> McKenzie concludes that instantaneous alleviation [with bloodletting] of the distressing phenomena is frequently very striking, particularly in cases with auricular fibrillation, and cases with high blood pressure and extreme failure of the heart.
>
> Several authors bear witness that cardiopaths treated with "bloodless bloodletting" note a subjective improvement of their condition.
>
> There is no doubt that phlebostasis will serve a good purpose in most cases of heart disease in which bloodletting is indicated.

Digitalis

An Account of the Foxglove

The publication of *An Account of the Foxglove, and Some of its Medical Uses: With Practical Remarks on Dropsy, and Other Diseases* by William Withering marks one of the defining moments for the treatment of patients with heart failure.[4] In this book,

Withering describes in detail his experience with digitalis, including the evaluation of the dose response and the description of the beneficial and toxic effects of the drug.

This section describes some of the most important passages from Withering's book, which has become one of the classic monographs in the history of cardiology and pharmacology. The following passage illustrates both a record of the early use of digitalis in a patient with heart failure and an interesting example of the practice of medicine in the late eighteenth century.[31]

> On the 25th of July I was desired to meet Dr. Darwin at the lady's house. I found her nearly in a state of suffocation; her pulse extremely weak and irregular, her breath very short and laborious, her countenance sunk, her arms of a leaden colour, clammy and cold. She could not lye down in bed, and had neither strength nor appetite, but extremely thirsty. Her stomach, legs and thighs were greatly swollen, her urine very small in quantity, not more than a spoonful at a time, and that very seldom. It had been proposed to scarify her legs, but the proposition was not acceded to. She had experienced no relief from any means that had been used ... In this situation of things I knew of nothing likely to avail us, except the Digitalis: but I hesitated to propose, from an apprehension that little could be expected from anything; that an unfavourable termination would tend to discredit a medicine which promised to be a great benefit to mankind, and I might be censured for a prescription which could not be countenanced by the experience of any other regular practitioner. But these considerations soon gave way to the desire of preserving the life of this valuable woman, and accordingly I proposed the Digitalis to be tried; adding, that I sometimes found it to succeed when other, even the most judicious methods had failed ...
>
> The patient took five of (digitalis) draughts, which made her very sick, and acted powerfully upon the kidneys, for within the first twenty-four hours she made upwards of eight quarts of water. The sense of fullness and oppression across the stomach was greatly diminished, her breath was eased, her pulse became more regular, and the swelling of her legs subsided.

This case clearly represents a patient with heart failure (right and left) and atrial fibrillation (irregular pulse). Although we do not know the anatomical diagnosis of this patient, but it might represent the natural history of rheumatic heart disease (mitral stenosis) in which slowing the heart rate leads to clinical improvement.

In the next passage, Withering gives an explanation of the types of patients who seemed to respond, and at the end of his book he lists the side effects and signs of overdose, the method of securing the optimal dose by dose titration against the onset of the first adverse effect, and finally the inferences of his experience.[32]

> The Foxglove when given in a very large and quickly-repeated doses, occasions sickness, vomiting, purging, giddiness, confused vision, objects appearing green or yellow; increased secretion of urine, with frequent motions to part with it, and some times inability to retain it; slow pulse, even as slow as 35 in a minute, cold sweats, convulsions, syncope, death ... [The direction requires] ... attention to the state of the pulse, and it was moreover of consequence not to repeat the doses too quickly, but to allow sufficient time for the effects of each to take place, as it was found very possible to pour an injurious quantity of the medicine, before any of the signals for forbearance appeared.

According to Withering, the inferences are:

> I. That the Digitalis will not universally act as a diuretic.
> II. That it does do so more generally than any other medicine.
> III. That it will often produce this effect after every other probable method has been fruitlessly tried.

IV. That if it fails, there is but little chance of any other medicine succeeding.
V. That in proper doses, and under the management now pointed out, it is mild in its operation, and gives less disturbances to the system, than squill, or almost any other active medicine.
VI. That when dropsy is attended by palsy, unsound viscera, great debility, or other complication of disease, neither Digitalis, nor any other diuretic can do more than obtain a truce to the urgency of the symptoms; unless by gaining time, it may afford opportunity for other medicines to combat and subdue the original disease.
VII. That the Digitalis may be used in every species of dropsy, except the encysted.
VIII. That it may be made subservient to the cure of diseases, unconnected with dropsy.
IX. That it has a power over the motion of the heart, to a degree yet unobserved in any other medicine, and that this power may be converted to salutary ends.

Withering thought that digitalis was mainly a diuretic but he also thought that it had cardiac activity. His ninth inference states that digitalis "has a power over the motion of the heart, to a degree yet unobserved in any other medicine, and that this power may be converted to salutary ends."

More than 200 years have passed since the publication of Withering's masterpiece and digitalis is still used today in the treatment of heart failure. We have learned more about the effects of digitalis, but the principles of its use which are clearly delineated in his book have stood the test of time. *An Account of the Foxglove* represents one of the first clinical trials and the first piece of what today is called evidence-based medicine when the only treatment used before that time was bloodletting. The introduction of digitalis into the medical armamentarium represents a defining moment for the treatment of heart failure and is a real triumph in the practice of medicine.

Use of digitalis after the publication of Withering's Book

Unfortunately, despite the fact that Withering had delineated clear guidelines for the use of digitalis, those guidelines were not followed during the next century. Therefore, the important therapeutic actions of digitalis in heart failure were not appreciated until the end of the nineteenth century and the beginning of the twentieth century.[33]

In the same year that Withering died, 1799, John Ferriar was the first to describe the cardiac effects of digitalis. He wrote, "the extractions from the leaf furnish us a means of regulating the pulse to our wish and supporting it in a given state of velocity as long as we may judge it proper . . . ."[33]

The entire nineteenth century was associated with several clinical and animal studies on digitalis. Some of these studies are worth mentioning. Fothergill in England poisoned a heart with aconite and watched its contractility improve with digitalis. Frank's experiments in 1895 demonstrated that digitalis increased the cardiac output in the abnormal heart without any effects in the normal hearts of frogs. This study was confirmed by others, concluding that digitalis in the abnormal heart not only increased cardiac output, but also decreased right atrial pressure.[33]

The steps taken to discover the active ingredient of foxglove are beyond the scope of this chapter, but suffice it to say that *digitalis lanata*, a plant related to foxglove, produced an entirely new glycoside called digoxin, the one used today for the treatment of heart failure.[33]

In the earlier part of the twentieth century, James McKenzie and Thomas Lewis established the effects of digitalis in humans. They suggested that the primary action of digitalis was to slow ventricular rate. Therefore, it was beneficial in patients with heart failure and atrial fibrillation.[33]

Clinical uses of digitalis in heart failure

The use of digitalis in the treatment of patients with heart failure is clearly described in some of the most prestigious textbooks in cardiology published prior the 1960s. In 1932, Paul White stated that digitalis had been used mainly from the dried leaves of the second-year growth of the plant.[34] Several preparations such as pills, capsules, tincture, infusion, and suppositories were in existence and tests were established to achieve a practical standard strength for universal use. Regarding the action of digitalis on the heart, he notes three effects:

> (a) In the first place it depresses the pacemaking function of the sinoauricular node and also the auriculoventricular node, with the resulting tendency from the heart rate to be slowed … (b) a second effect of digitalis on the heart is on conduction. This occurs all through the heart muscle with increase in the refractory period of the auricular and ventricular muscle, so that auricular flutter is converted into auricular fibrillation … it is this depressant influence of digitalis on conduction that explains at least half of the virtue of the drug. It has long been known that there is one type of patient with congestive heart failure especially helped by digitalis therapy, sometimes with astounding success; this type is the patient who has also auricular fibrillation with more or less rapid ventricular rate … (c) a third effect of digitalis on the heart is on contraction.

The therapeutic indications for the use of digitalis, according to White, were as follows:

> congestive heart failure with or without auricular fibrillation, auricular flutter … as a therapeutic test when it is uncertain whether or not there is a slight degree of congestive heart failure, or perhaps as a means of warding off impending failure … the most common method of administration is by mouth … For the very few individuals with congestive heart failure for whom digitalis is urgently needed because of their grave or almost moribund condition, the drug can be given intravenously in the same dosage that is used by mouth, but more rapidly … there is only one drug besides digitalis which has digitalis-like action that it is ever worthwhile. That is strophanthin or ouabain. It is necessary only in emergency treatment.

White also gives the clinical parameters to be followed when a patient with congestive heart failure receives digitalis or strophanthin: "1) the apex heart rate and pulse deficit, especially if there is atrial fibrillation, 2) the loss of weight and urine output as compared to fluid intake and 3) subjective symptoms of improvement."[34]

In his textbook on cardiology, Paul Wood states that digitalis should be used in heart failure with or without atrial fibrillation.[35] He also describes the properties by which digitalis exerts its activity, "it lowers the venous pressure, raises the blood pressure, slows the heart rate, relieves hepatic distension, increases the vital capacity, shortens the pulmonary circulation time, increases the cardiac output and encourages diuresis."

Wood states that ouabain can be used in cardiogenic shock, but cautions against the use of intravenous digitalis in patients with acute pulmonary edema, he states: "Strophanthin and digitalis are probably best avoided in view of their pressor actions, indeed, paroxysmal cardiac dyspnea may occasionally be initiated by intravenous digoxin." Wood's view of avoiding digitalis in pulmonary edema, presumably in patents with hypertension and heart failure, is still in use today.

The role of digitalis in the treatment of acute heart failure is limited and it is more suitable for chronic therapy. Recently, digitalis has been shown to be beneficial in improving symptoms and hospitalizations of patients with heart failure, and toxicity is rarely seen.[36] Withering's prediction "That it [digitalis] has a power over the motion of the heart, to a degree yet unobserved in any other medicine, and that this power may be converted to salutary ends" has become a reality, in the treatment of heart failure today.

Diuretics

Mercury

William Cullen was the Professor of Chemistry at Edinburgh University and one of Withering's mentors. In 1789, he published a work entitled A

Treatise on Materia Medica, in which he described the properties of mercury. Cullen states:

> I shall treat of this medicine as fully as I can, as it is the most useful and universal medicine I known ... Universally mercury in its active state seems to be the stimulus to every sensible and moving fibre of the body to which is immediately applied: and in consequence, it is particularly a stimulus to every excretory of the system to which it is applied externally or internally.[37]

Cullen concluded that this particular ability of mercury to "increase the excretory ability of the system to which is applied" made mercury a very powerful therapeutic agent in the practice of medicine.[37]

Mercury (calomel) also called the "blue pill" was used for centuries in combination with digitalis and squill for the treatment of heart failure.[2] Several authors, including Hope, Corvisart, Stokes, and Blackall, among others, advocated its use as a therapeutic agent for patients with edema.

John Blackall

John Blackall made some interesting observations regarding the clinical characteristics and treatment of dropsy. In his book, *Observations on the Nature and Cure of Dropsies*, he made several important observations regarding the use of mercury for the treatment of fluid retention. First, he tried to establish some rules for which patients should be given mercury.[38] He states, "In dropsy the mineral [mercury] is given in a manner equally indiscriminate and in larger doses, and with such opposite success, as to make it highly desirable that its exhibition should, if possible, be not conjectural, but defined and guided by some plain rules." He adds:

> Some firmness of the general habit will, I believe, be the best encouragement to it ... yet I think the characters of the urine are most easily understood, and the least liable to nay misconception. If that discharge errs chiefly by want of dilution, the presence of bile, mercury is likely to render great service to the obstructions which are probably present, particularly those of the liver, and also to prove a true diuretic; and the swellings never pass off so readily and freely ... If on the contrary, the habit is so depraved that the coagulable part of the blood already passes off the kidneys, the operation of this mineral is obviously equivocal and hazardous.[38]

This interesting description demonstrates that the evaluation of the urine was a very important and more objective tool for prescribing mercury, since this agent only worked in cases of dropsy in which the urine did not coagulate or did not contain albumin. The latter were cases of renal disease. It was several years later that Richard Bright reported the association between albuminuria and fullness of the pulse, dropsy, and hardening of the kidneys—the so-called Bright disease. For patients in which the urine did not contain albumin, mercury was a true diuretic and it was beneficial in patients with dropsy. The allusion to the "obstruction of the liver" is probably related to liver enlargement secondary to fluid retention in heart failure.

Alexander Philip Wilson Philip

The main problem with the use of calomel was its toxicity, which ranged from lack of appetite, nausea, excess salivation, severe gastrointestinal irritation, lack of concentration, and mobility of the teeth to anxiety, insomnia, and depression. Therefore, some of the more practical physicians in the eighteenth and nineteenth centuries advocated the use of calomel in small doses.

In a book published in 1834 entitled, *On the Influence of Minute Doses of Mercury*, Dr. Alexander Philip Wilson Philip, a practicing physician in England, stated that, "I was led to them [minute doses of mercury] by observing that in lessening the dose and increasing its frequency, in proportion as we lessen the immediate, we increase the alterative, effects."[39] In relation to the mechanism by which mercury exerted beneficial effects on people with dropsy, Dr. Philip added that "the most remarkable of the effects peculiar to mercury, is its influence on the liver," and to prove this point he described a case as follows:

> Mr. Hobson had for thirty-four years labored under the symptoms of diseased heart, to which all the powers of his constitutions were yielding. He had become pale and edematous ... I [Dr. Philip] was led ... to regard the affection of the heart as chiefly sympathetic to the function of the liver, which was more or less, and occasionally much disordered. For many months he steadily pursued the plan of treatment ... taking half a grain of blue pill three times a day combined with such other means as tended to restore the digestive organs, and relieve the occasional more severe attacks ... I had the satisfaction to see him relieved from every symptom.[40]

Dr. Philip believed that the mechanism by which calomel relieved fluid retention was associated with an effect on the digestive system, mainly in the liver.

William Stokes

In his famous treatise, William Stokes describes the case of Abraham Colles and the use of mercury in his treatment. First, Dr. Stokes introduces the concept using mercury for symptomatic relief specifically when the patient has hepatomegaly and pulmonary disease as compared to cases with simple fatty degeneration. This is an important observation since mercury is prescribed when the patient is in an edematous state. Interestingly, he cautions against the use of "reducing measures" (bloodletting). He adds:

> It is remarkable, that although the beneficial action of mercury in this affection is known to many practical physicians, but little information can be found on the subject in any of our medical works ... I do not wish it to be believed that by mercury we can cure dilatation of the heart; but many years' experience has convinced me that by the use of this remedy we can delay its production, remove the irregular action which assists in causing the disease, and, above all, prolong the patient's life, and again and again relieve him from dropsy, and from pulmonary and hepatic congestions, even when they have arrived at a point which threatens speedy dissolution.[41]

In the following passage, Stokes describes the guidelines by which mercury should be used in patients with heart failure and congestion:

> The more common examples of weakened hearts in which so much benefit is derived from mercurial action. In such cases the following circumstances are to be met with:
>
> 1) The patient is generally advanced in life, most of the cases being in persons of from 50 to 70 years of age.
> 2) These individuals are originally of healthy constitution and strong habit of body.
> 3) They are liable to some degree of gout, which malady, after having long occurred in its more regular form, becomes masked or imperfect.
> 4) They are subject to bronchitis, which, during the aggravation of symptoms, increases as to resemble suffocative catarrh.
> 5) The liver is permanently enlarged, yet in many no appearance of jaundice exists. The hepatic tumour is generally indolent, and the epigastric veins are seldom varicose.
> 6) Two conditions of the heart may be observed. In both there is permanent irregularity, always augmented during the paroxysm of suffering; but in one class of patients the physical signs indicate hypertrophy with valvular disease, while in the other the signs are those which have been indicated in the chapter on Dilatation of the Heart, unattended by any direct indication of valvular disease.[41]

Stokes also attempts to establish the dose and the mechanism by which mercury relieves symptoms of congestion and is very close to understanding the diuretic effect of the drug. The fact that mercury increases the production of urine is a very important observation, since today it is known that the diuretic effect is the mechanism of the action of the mercurial agents. In addition, he establishes the use of mercury in combination with digitalis. He states:

> The quantity of the remedy which is required, as we might expect, varies in different cases. In some it is requisite to establish ptyalism, while in others the relief of the heart and the disappearance of the dropsy, are observed after the use of a very mild course ... if any of the characteristic action of mercury can be perceived unless we include diuresis. In other cases it will be necessary to use diuretics following on the mercurial action, and in this way we often observe a singularly abundant secretion of urine, attended by rapid subsidence of the dropsy and visceral oppression. We should use various combinations of the vegetable and saline diuretics; and even digitalis, in connexion with diuretics of the tonic and stimulating class, may be employed. The success of diuretics appears to turn upon their being preceded by mercury ... but the truth is, that in these cases we are not to be over-timid in the repetition of mercurial medicines; for there is nothing more remarkable than the power which the patients exhibit of bearing repeated courses of mercury not only without injury, but with extraordinary benefit to their general health ... there has been no unhealthy action on the mouth, no periostitis, cutaneous eruptions, or tremors.

He adds:

> It need hardly be observed, that the time at last arrives when, as in the case of Dr Colles, the system no longer responds to the action of medicine, and the patient sinks with dropsy and pulmonary congestion.[42]

Mercurial diuretics

It was not until 1920, that Saxl and Heilig, in a classic manuscript, reported the diuretic effect of merbaphen (Novasurol), which contained mercury in complex organic combination and was originally introduced as an antisyphilitic agent.[5] Alfred Vogl,[6] an American student in the Wenckebach clinic from 1919 to 1920, described the manner in which this finding was accomplished. He and the nurse noticed that when Novasurol was given to two patients with syphilis, it produced an increase in urinary output. After this observation, he proceeded to give Novasurol, the wonder drug, to a patient with heart failure. He states:

> Soon afterwards there was admitted to our wards a boy with a huge rheumatic heart and tricuspid insufficiency, in severe, waterlogged failure, almost anuric and obviously terminal. The case seemed hopeless and he suffered cruelly. In sympathy and desperation, we tried our wonder drug. He received this injection and unfortunately expired the following day. Before his death, however, he passed three liters of urine. Post mortem examination confirmed the clinical diagnosis and revealed no evidence of syphilis.

This case represents the first use of an organic mercurial agent in the treatment of heart failure.

Novasurol was painful and toxic, and was soon replaced by the more potent yet more benign Salyrgan. These agents became widely used in the 1940s as an adjunct therapy in heart failure. However, they were given only parenterally, which was a major drawback for patients who needed chronic therapy. Adverse reactions associated with the use of the organic mercurial diuretics were very similar to the old inorganic compounds. These included stomatitis, colitis, albuminuria, hematuria, and sudden death. A test dose of 0.5 mL was utilized 24 hours before the full therapeutic dose was given and the patients were observed for side effects. Combinations with theophylline resulted in a less painful and more effective agent.[43]

Mercurial diuretics exerted their action on patients with fluid retention and heart failure mainly by decreasing the reabsorption of sodium, potassium, and chloride in the tubular system of the kidneys, thereby reducing edema. The decline in blood volume and venous pressure was secondary to the renal action. The effects were gradual, beginning 1 to 2 hours after the injection.[43]

Oral diuretics

The development of orally active diuretics started in the mid-1940s. At that time, several reports demonstrated that sulfanilamides and sulfonamides were specific inhibitors of carbonic anhydrase. These studies led to the demonstration that sulfanilamide was a weak natriuretic-diuretic agent in patients with heart failure.[2] In 1958, after several years of research, Beyer *et al.* reported on the diuretic and saluretic properties of a sulfonamide called chlorothiazide. This compound became the first orally-active diuretic and in a very short time the thiazides became an important component of diuretic therapy for patients with hypertension or heart failure.[2]

Loop diuretics

The introduction of diuretics that act within the loop of Henle—loop diuretics—dramatically affected the ability of clinicians to improve the symptoms of heart failure with minimum toxicity.[2,44] They were eagerly accepted because they could be given orally as well as parenterally and also because they possessed potent diuretic capabilities. Furosemide, one of the first loop diuretics to be developed, was, and still is, utilized intravenously in patients with pulmonary edema or decompensated heart failure to decrease excessive lung water through natriuresis and diuresis. The most important effect of furosemide in the acute management of acute decompensated heart failure (ADHF) probably relates to its substantial hemodynamic effects. Furosemide has been shown to reduce cardiac filling pressures secondary to a vasodilatory effect.[45,46] The same effect was observed in patients with acute myocardial infarction (AMI) and heart failure.[47] Conversely, a vasoconstrictor effect with a reduction in cardiac output has been reported with the use of furosemide, due to diuretic-induced neurohormonal activation.[48] Other loop diuretics utilized in the treatment of heart failure are bumetanide and torsemide (in the 1980s).[44] Loop diuretics, although very effective, should be judiciously employed because they can cause hypotension and because of their kaliuretic effect they can cause hypokalemia, activation of neurohormones and cardiac arrhythmias.[2,45,48]

Other Therapeutic Measures

Oxygen and morphine, as well as other diuretics, such as carbonic anhydrase and theobromine inhibitors, have been used down the centuries for patients with ADHF and pulmonary edema. Oxygen and morphine are still in use today. Conversely, aminophylline, a therapeutic agent, that was very popular from the 1950s until the 1970s, is no longer used in patients who present with acute pulmonary edema. In his cardiology textbook, Paul Wood describes the effects of aminophylline in patients with paroxysmal cardiac dyspnea as follows:

> theophylline-ethylene-diamine (aminophylline) 0.24 to 0.48 gram intravenously, lowers the venous pressure immediately, relieves bronchial spasm, and may have a direct stimulating action on the heart ... will produce dramatic improvement ... aminophylline suppository of 0.14 gram. At night will prevent both Cheyne-Stokes breathing and paroxysmal nocturnal dyspnea, and in doing so may earn the patient's thanks for a good night sleep.[49]

Another agent used in the treatment of acute pulmonary edema was, and still is, sublingual nitroglycerin. In 1957, Johnson *et al.*[50] demonstrated that the symptomatic relief obtained by the use of nitroglycerin in patients with paroxysmal dyspnea and acute pulmonary edema was related to a rapid decrease in pulmonary artery and pulmonary capillary wedge pressures. Johnson *et al.* concluded that, "the clinical and physiologic data obtained after nitroglycerin administration suggest that this drug has an important place in the management of patients with pulmonary-artery hypertension and paroxysmal dyspnea associated with failure of the left ventricle."[50]

Conclusion

In summary, this historical overview describes some, but not all, of the therapies that have been used in the treatment of heart failure from ancient times until the 1970s. In 1997, the editor of the *Lancet*, Richard Horton, wrote, "Medicine pays almost exclusive homage to the shock of the new ... we place constant emphasis on novelty ... this is an era of the instantaneous and the immediate."[51] It seems that medicine's concern with the "new" leaves little space for history. We do not subscribe to this point of view. As T. S. Eliot wrote, "the historical sense involves the perception not only of the pastness of the past, but of its presence."[52] Thus, one cannot appreciate the present separate from the milieu of the past. The newly developed strategies for the treatment of acute heart failure will be detailed in this book. However, the successes of our present days are rooted in the past and that it is why a historical overview of past therapies for patients with acute heart failure is crucial to recognize not only how far we have come but also how much we can accomplish in the future.

References

1. Seigworth GR. Bloodletting over the centuries. N Y State J Med 1980; 80: 2022–2028.
2. Ventura HO, Mehra MR, Young JB. Treatment of heart failure according to William Stokes: the enchanted mercury. J Card Fail 2001; 7: 277–282.
3. Ventura HO, Mehra MR. Colles–Stokes contributions to the concept of heart failure. Am J Cardiol 1998; 81: 1470–1473.
4. Withering W. An Account of the Foxglove and Some of Its Medical Uses with Practical Remarks on Dropsy and Other Diseases (Robinson: Birmingham, 1785).
5. Saxl P, Heilig R. Über die diuretische Wirkung von Nuvasurol und anderen Quecksilberinjektionen (The diuretic effects of Novasurol and other mercury injections). Wien Klin Wochnschr 1920; 33: 943–944.
6. Vogl A. The discovery of the organic mercurial diuretics. Am Heart J 1950; 39: 881–883.
7. Katz AM. Evolving concepts of heart failure: cooling furnace, malfunctioning pump, enlarging muscle. Part I. J Card Fail 1997; 4: 319–334.
8. Cohn JN, Franciosa JA. Vasodilator therapy for heart failure: (first of two parts). N Engl J Med 1977; 297: 27–31.
9. Heath C. Dictionary of Practical Surgery (Smith, Elder, & Co.: London, 1886), 162.
10. Pancoast J. Treatise of Operative Surgery (Carey & Hart: Philadelphia, PA, 1844), 15.
11. Majors RH. Medicine in the Roman Empire. In: Majors RH (ed.) A History of Medicine (Charles C Thomas: Springfield, IL, 1954), 162–219.
12. Celsus A. De Medicina. Translated by Collier GF, (Longman & Co.: London, 1838), IV, 130.
13. Celsus A. De Medicina. Translated by Collier GF, (Longman & Co.: London, 1838), IV, 132–133.
14. Celsus A. De Medicina. Translated by Collier GF, (Longman & Co.: London, 1838), II, 52.
15. Celsus A. De Medicina. Translated by Collier GF, (Longman & Co.: London, 1838), VII, 292.
16. Lutz JE. An XII century description of congestive heart failure. Am J Cardiol 1988; 61: 494–495.
17. Jarcho S. A summary of this story. In: The Concept of Heart Failure: From Avicenna to Albertini (Harvard University Press: Cambridge, MA, 1980), XX, 362–363.
18. Harvey W. Exercitatio Anatomica de Mortus Cordis et Sanguinis in Animalibus (English translation with annotations by CD Leake) (Charles C. Thomas: Springfield, IL, 1928), 7.
19. Jarcho S. Georgio Baglivi and the practice of medicine. In: The Concept of Heart Failure: From Avicenna to Albertini (Harvard University Press: Cambridge, MA, 1980), 228–236.
20. Acierno LJ. Diagnostic techniques. In: Acierno LJ (ed.) The History of Cardiology (The Parthenon Publishing Group Ltd: New York, 1994), 447–501.
21. Katz AM. Evolving concepts of heart failure: cooling furnace, malfunctioning pump, enlarging muscle. Part II: Hypertrophy and dilatation of the failing heart. J Card Fail 1998; 4: 67–68.
22. Hope J. A Treatise on the Diseases of the Heart and Great Vessels (John Churchill: London, 1839), 407–412.
23. Baldry PE. Pump failure. In: The Battle Against Heart Disease (Cambridge University Press: London, 1971), 152–156.
24. Stokes W. Treatment of the weak and probably dilated heart in connexion with enlargement of the liver and pulmonary disease. In: Stokes W (ed.) The Diseases of the Heart and the Aorta, 1st edition (University Press: Dublin, 1853), 352–356.
25. Stokes W. Disease of the muscular structures of the heart. In: Stokes W (ed.) The Diseases of the Heart

and the Aorta, 1st edition (University Press: Dublin, 1853), 255–298.

26. Southey R. Chronic parenchymatous nephritis of right kidney. Left kidney small and atrophied. Old scrofulous pyelitis. Trans Clin Soc London 1877; X: 152–156.
27. Osler W. The Principles and Practice of Medicine (D. Appleton & Co.: New York, 1892), 624–626.
28. White PD. Congestive heart failure. In: Heart Disease (MacMillan: New York, 1932), 588–589.
29. Wood P. Heart failure. In: Wood P (ed.) Diseases of the Heart and Circulation (Eyre & Spottiswoode: London, 1957), 311.
30. Stern H. Circulatory disturbances (heart). In: The Theory and Practice of Bloodletting (Rebman Co.: New York, 1915), 133–147.
31. Withering W. An Account of the Foxglove, and Some of its Medical Uses: With Practical Remarks on Dropsy and Other Diseases (Robinson: Birmingham, 1785), 2–3.
32. Withering W. An Account of the Foxglove, and Some of its Medical Uses: With Practical Remarks on Dropsy and Other Diseases (Robinson: Birmingham, 1785), 184–192.
33. Acierno LJ. Pharmacologic modalities. In: Acierno LJ (ed.) The History of Cardiology (The Parthenon Publishing Group Ltd: New York, 1994), 716–718.
34. White PD. Congestive heart failure. In: Heart Disease (Macmillan: New York, 1932), 576–585.
35. Wood P. Heart failure. In: Wood P (ed.) Diseases of the Heart and Circulation (Eyre & Spottiswoode: London, 1957), 297–300.
36. The Digitalis Investigation Group. The effect of digoxin on mortality and morbidity in patients with heart failure. N Engl J Med 1997; 336: 525–533.
37. Cullen W. A Treatise on Materia Medica (C. Elliot: Edinburgh, 1789), 442–454.
38. Blackall J. Observations on the Nature and Cure of Dropsies (James Webster: Philadelphia, PA, 1820), 121–122.
39. Philip APW. On the Influence of Minute Doses of Mercury Combined with the Appropriate Treatment of Various Diseases in Restoring Functions of Health, and the Principles on Which it Depends (I) (Duffy Green: Washington, DC, 1834), 7–13.
40. Philip APW. On the Influence of Minute Doses of Mercury Combined with the Appropriate Treatment of Various Diseases in Restoring Functions of Health, and the Principles on Which it Depends (III) (Duffy Green: Washington, DC, 1834), 59.
41. Stokes W. Treatment of the weak and probably dilated heart in connexion with enlargement of the liver and pulmonary disease. In: Stokes W (ed.) The Diseases of the Heart and the Aorta, 1st edition (University Press: Dublin, 1853), 354.
42. Stokes W. Treatment of the weak and probably dilated heart in connexion with enlargement of the liver and pulmonary disease. In: Stokes W (ed.) The Diseases of the Heart and the Aorta, 1st edition (University Press: Dublin, 1853), 355–356.
43. Goodman LS, Gilman A. Diuretics. In: The Pharmacological Basis of Therapeutics: A Textbook of Pharmacology, Toxicology and Therapeutics for Physicians and Medical Students, 6th edition. (MacMillan: New York, 1941), 639–651.
44. Brater DC. Diuretic therapy. N Engl J Med 1998; 339: 387–395.
45. Lal S, Murtagw JG, Pollock A *et al.* Acute hemodynamic effects of furosemide in patients with normal and raised left atrial pressures. Br Heart J 1969; 31: 711–717.
46. Cody RJ. Clinical trials of diuretic therapy in heart failure: research directions and clinical considerations. J Am Coll Cardiol 1993; 22: 165A–171A.
47. Taylor SH. Diuretics in post infarction heart failure. Cardiovasc Drugs Ther 1993; 7: 5–9.
48. Francis GS, Siegel RM, Goldsmith SR *et al.* Acute vasoconstrictor response to intravenous furosemide in patients with chronic congestive heart failure. Ann Intern Med 1985; 103: 1–6.
49. Wood P. Heart failure. In: Wood P (ed.) Diseases of the Heart and Circulation (Eyre & Spottiswoode: London, 1957), 309–310.
50. Johnson JB, Gross JF, Hale E. Effects of sublingual administration of nitroglycerin on pulmonary artery pressure in patients with failure of the left ventricle. N Engl J Med 1957; 251: 1114–1117.
51. Horton R. A manifesto for reading medicine. Lancet 1997; 349: 872–874.
52. Eliot TS. Tradition and the individual talent. In: The Sacred Wood: Essays on Poetry and Criticism (Methuen: London, 1920).

CHAPTER 2

Acute heart failure: nomenclature, pathophysiology, and outcome measures

Gadi Cotter, Wendy Gattis Stough, G Michael Felker, Eric J Velazquez, Adrian F Hernandez, Joseph G Rogers, Mihai Gheorghiade, Kirkwood F Adams, Jr, Christopher M O'Connor

Acute Heart Failure: The Problem

Acute heart failure (AHF) is the most common reason for hospital admission in patients over the age of 65, accounting for 1 000 000 admissions, over 6 000 000 hospital days, and $12 billion in costs.[1,2] The prognosis of patients admitted with AHF is dismal, with a 20% readmission rate and a 20% mortality rate within 6 months after admission.[3] However, data are lacking on the pathogenesis, etiologic factors, risk stratification, and effective treatment of AHF. Most studies in AHF are small single-center studies, retrospective registries, or industry- or government-sponsored trials with selective eligibility criteria. A comprehensive evaluation of this syndrome in "real life" is still lacking. A major barrier to advancing our understanding of this syndrome has been defining AHF and differentiating it from decompensated chronic heart failure.

Recently, effective treatments have been developed for chronic heart failure including beta blockers, angiotensin-converting enzyme (ACE) inhibitors, biventricular pacing, and automatic implantable cardioverter-defibrillators (AICDs) for the prevention of lethal arrhythmias. The implementation of these novel treatments has affected the outcome of chronic heart failure, but not AHF. In the recently published Ontario registry,[3] these measures helped to decrease the one-year mortality of patients admitted with AHF (Figure 2.1). However, in the past two decades, the 30-day mortality of AHF has remained largely unchanged at > 10%. A better understanding of the pathophysiological core processes contributing to AHF and a better definition of its specific outcome measures may lead to the development of specific treatments to improve the significant adverse outcome related to this disease.

Nomenclature and Definitions

AHF is not a disease but rather it is a syndrome caused by different mechanisms. In many patients, AHF is the end result of slowly deteriorating chronic heart failure related mostly to non-adherence to diet, pharmacologic therapy, or fluid restriction, or due to disease progression. This type of AHF is referred to as acute decompensated heart failure (ADHF) and it can often be managed in the outpatient setting by administration of diuretics, resumption of proper diet and fluid restriction, and improved pharmacotherapy.

Conversely, the rapidly progressive syndrome of severe acute dyspnea leading to respiratory failure commonly encountered in emergency settings is most likely caused by a combination of systemic inflammatory and neurohormonal activation, increased vascular resistance, and diastolic left ventricular (LV) failure. This syndrome may be more accurately defined as acute cardiovascular failure.

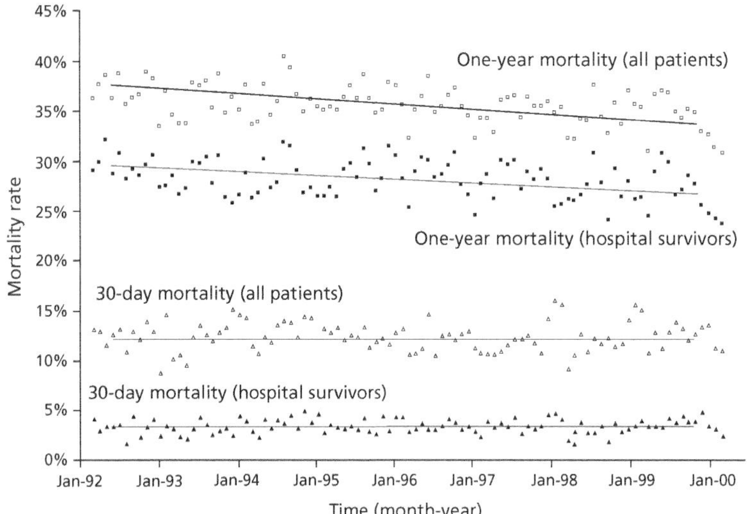

Figure 2.1. *One-month and one-year mortality in patients with acute heart failure (With permission from Lee* et al.[3]*)*

To avoid confusion, throughout this chapter, we will refer to this syndrome as AHF. This nomenclature is used primarily for historical reasons and does not accurately describe the true nature of the acute cardiovascular failure syndrome.

Classification schemes have been developed in an effort to categorize patients with AHF.[4] The wet–dry/warm–cold schema was developed using a cohort of patients with advanced cardiomyopathy (two-thirds men, mean left ventricular ejection fraction [LVEF] of 23%, and mean age of 55 years). While the patients in this cohort were severely ill and experiencing an acute decompensation of chronic heart failure, they differ from the majority of patients presenting with AHF. First, the "wet" definition in this classification includes pulmonary congestion (usually due to *fluid re-distribution* from the periphery to the lungs) as well as peripheral edema and ascites (related to *fluid overload* which is more common in acute decompensation of chronic heart failure) and therefore cannot be regarded as one entity. Second, according to the hemodynamic data generated by some recent studies of AHF, the overwhelming majority of patients with AHF are in the "wet" (pulmonary edema but not peripheral edema) and "cold" (vasoconstricted) category at admission. These patients transition to the "wet" and "warm" category after receiving vasodilators.[5] Finally, only a negligible minority of patients with real-world AHF will be "dry" at admission, and most of these will be in the ADHF group.

In patients with AHF, two terms are used to describe the most severe types of this syndrome: pulmonary edema and cardiogenic shock. Pulmonary edema is a subtype of AHF in which the backward failure symptoms are especially severe, usually leading to respiratory failure and oxygen desaturation to < 90%, necessitating invasive or non-invasive respiratory support. Cardiogenic shock is the most severe subtype of AHF in which extreme failure of LV contractility and inability to mount an appropriate vasoconstrictive response leads to progressive forward failure, multi-organ failure, and death.

Clinical Characteristics of Patients Admitted with Acute Heart Failure and Differences from Chronic Heart Failure

Historically, AHF has been regarded as a simple exacerbation of chronic heart failure, occurring in patients with the more severe forms of LV dysfunction. However, as recent studies have shown (Table 2.1), the characteristics of patients with

Table 2.1. *Baseline characteristics of patients admitted with acute heart failure*

Characteristic	Canada[3] AHF	EuroHeart[7] AHF	ADHERE[8] AHF (n > 100 000)	CHARM[10] CHF (7 599)	OPTIMIZE-HF* AHF (n = 34 059)	IMPACT-HF Registry[9] CHF (n = 567)	OPTIME-CHF[58] ADHF (n = 951)
Age (yrs)	76±11	71	75.2	71	73±15	71±12	66±14
Female %	50%	50%	52%	50%	52%	48%	33.9%
EF > 40%	50%	50%	40%	50%	50%	EF > 50% (25%)	0%
Renal Failure	—	17%	14%	17%	19%	23.5% (eGFR < 60 mL/min)	> 50%
DM	34%	27%	44%	27%	42%	45.1%	44%
Hypertension	—	—	72%	—	71%	64.7%	68%
IHD	37%	31%	37%	61%	50%	48.7%	52%
AF	30%	42%	30%	42%	30%	35.4%	34%

Notes: ADHF = acute decompensated heart failure; AF = atrial fibrillation; AHF = acute heart failure; CHF = chronic heart failure; DM = diabetes mellitus; EF = ejection fraction; eGFR = estimated glomerular filtration rate; IHD = ischemic heart disease.
*W.A. Gattis Stough, unpublished data, 2004.

AHF are different from those with chronic heart failure. In the last year, a few major studies were published examining the fundamental characteristics of patients admitted with AHF.[3,6–9] These studies demonstrated that the mean age of patients admitted with AHF is 71 to 76 years, half of the patients are women, and half have preserved LVEF (> 40%). These characteristics contrast with those of patients with chronic heart failure who are generally younger, more often men, and have a lower EF.[10] Typically, patients admitted with AHF have only mild background chronic heart failure, if any. In the European registry[7] and the Acute Decompensated Heart Failure National Registry (ADHERE™),[8] the index admission was the first time that heart failure was diagnosed in 25% to 27% of the patients. In the recent Initiation Management Predischarge: Process for Assessment of Carvedilol Therapy for Heart Failure (IMPACT-HF) study and registry, 70% of patients were in heart failure New York Heart Association (NYHA) class I or II at discharge and 30-day follow-up.[9]

Acute Heart Failure in Women and Minorities

In previous AHF registries, significant differences have been detected between women and men. In the OPTIMIZE-HF registry (Organized Program to Initiate Lifesaving Treatment in Hospitalized Patients with Heart Failure) (OPTIMIZE-HF Steering Committee, unpublished report, 2004) and other AHF registries, women presenting with AHF are older, more likely to be hypertensive, and less likely to have ischemic heart disease (IHD). Their LVEF also tends to be higher than that of men.[6–8] Despite these differences, the short-term and long-term outcomes for women and men are similar. In the ADHERE™ registry, Yancy and Chang[11] have compared the characteristics and outcome of African Americans (n = 6331) versus non-African Americans (n = 26 715) admitted with AHF. This analysis has demonstrated that as compared to non-African Americans, African Americans with AHF are younger, have more background hypertension, smoking, diabetes mellitus, renal failure, and a lower LVEF. Despite the higher degree of comorbidity, their adjusted risk of in-hospital mortality was lower. Conversely, in a smaller study, Mehta *et al.*[12] observed higher re-admission rates in African American patients. Jimenez *et al.*[13] analyzed the characteristics and outcome of Hispanic Americans (n = 1662) comparing them to African Americans (n = 12 914) and Caucasians (n = 47 202) in the ADHERE™ registry. Hispanic Americans were younger, more likely to be men, and had more background diabetes mellitus and hyperlipidemia. Their in-hospital mortality was intermediate (32%) between that of Caucasians (47%) and African Americans (21%).

Pathophysiology of Acute Heart Failure

AHF is induced by a combination of hemodynamic mechanisms including reduced cardiac contractility, increased diastolic dysfunction, peripheral vasoconstriction, and fluid and sodium retention leading to both forward (decreased perfusion) and backward (pulmonary congestion) failure. This chapter will discuss these major effectors and their contribution to the heart failure syndrome, briefly describe the different phases of the AHF syndrome, and finally address the causes for the decreased contractility, diastolic dysfunction, and vasoconstriction observed in patients with AHF.

Hemodynamic measures: severe vasoconstriction superimposed on low and decreasing contractility

Our knowledge of the hemodynamic events leading to AHF is limited by the selective use of right heart catheterization and Swan–Ganz catheters in patients with AHF, due to the invasive nature of the procedures, and the limited data supporting the clinical utility of these devices. These issues were emphasized by the results of the Evaluation Study of Congestive Heart Failure and Pulmonary Artery Catheterization Effectiveness (ESCAPE) study which demonstrated no short-term or long-term benefit of right heart catheterization in patients with severe decompensated heart failure.[14] Most patients undergoing right heart catheterization are critically ill, with acute decompensation of severe chronic heart failure. Thus, its application in AHF is not well defined. Pulmonary capillary wedge pressure (PCWP) has been considered the most important hemodynamic variable in patients with AHF. Although in the ESCAPE trial PCWP was a strong independent predictor of death and readmission (V. Hasselblad, unpublished data, 2004), some recent studies have found no correlation between admission PCWP and outcome.[15,16]

In recent years, accumulated evidence has suggested that measuring cardiac output (CO), and calculating cardiac power output (CPo, the product of simultaneously measured CO and mean arterial pressure [MAP]; CPo = MAP*CO) and systemic vascular resistance (SVR), might be important in the diagnosis, risk stratification, and monitoring of patients with AHF.[17] The introduction of the concept of cardiac power output (CPo) into clinical practice two decades ago provided a non-invasive method for directly measuring cardiac function. In patients with chronic heart failure, cardiac power reserve (i.e., CPo increase during stress) was found to be the best predictor of outcome.[18] Patients presenting with AHF have significant activation of neurohormonal and inflammatory mediators, leading to a significant inotropic and chronotropic response. Hence, most of their myocardial contractile reserve is recruited, and a measurement of CPo during the acute event is representative of their entire recruitable cardiac contractility during the event. In a recent study,[15] CPo and vascular resistance were measured in 100 patients with AHF monitored by Swan–Ganz catheters at baseline and for 30 hours. In analyzing the hemodynamic data from this study, we found that the only hemodynamic measurement at baseline that predicted recurrent AHF events was CPo. We found that decreased CPo at baseline was related to a 4-fold increase in the rate of recurrent AHF events (Figure 2.2). No other hemodynamic variable measured at baseline was correlated with outcome. Moreover, during the hours prior to the AHF event, CPo continued to decline in patients with recurrent heart failure events while increasing in patients without such events. The difference between these two groups increased throughout follow-up (Figure 2.3).

In another study,[16] Torre-Amione *et al.* found that the combination of CPo < 0.6 Watt at admission and further deterioration of CPo during the

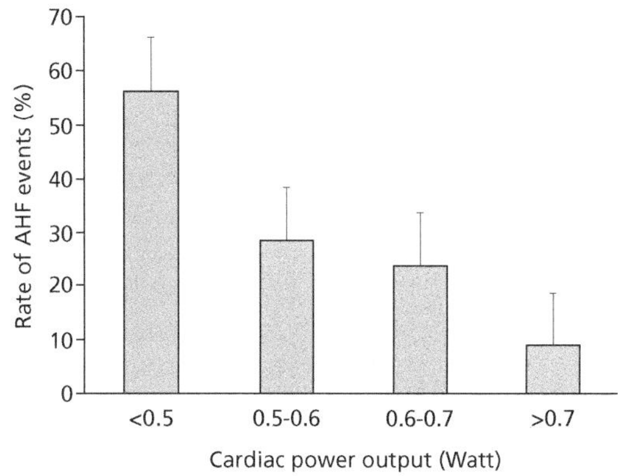

Figure 2.2. *Recurrent acute heart failure by baseline cardiac power quartiles (With permission from Cotter* et al.[14])

Abbreviations: AHF = acute heart failure.

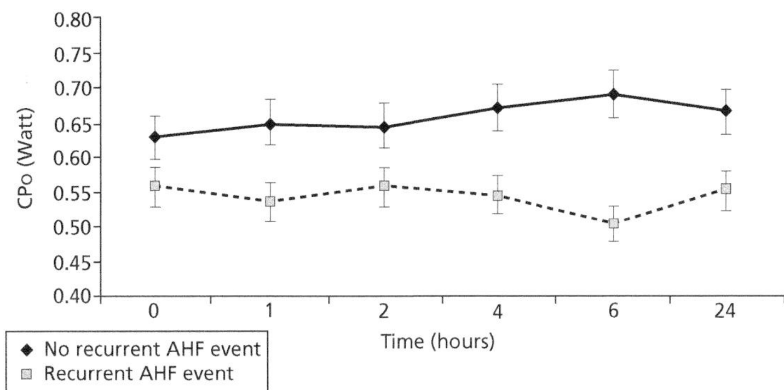

Figure 2.3. *Cardiac power changes during 24 hours of hemodynamic monitoring in patients with and without acute heart failure events during monitoring (With permission from Cotter* et al.[14]*).*

Abbreviations: AHF = acute heart failure; CPo = cardiac power output.

first 6 hours of monitoring was the strongest independent predictor of an AHF event during 7 and 30 days of follow-up and 6-month mortality. However, PCWP at admission and its change during the first hours of monitoring was not an independent predictor of AHF events.

Superimposed on this low and decreasing CPo, a steep increase in SVR to typically > 7000 dyn prior to the AHF event was also observed (Figure 2.4). This increase in SVR is the cause for the high blood pressure observed in many patients with AHF on admission. In a recent community-based registry of 340 consecutive admissions for AHF to a community hospital,[19] the mean blood pressure at admission was 164 (±33)/88 (±20) mm Hg. In the ADHERE™ registry,[8] the admission systolic blood pressure was > 140 mm Hg in 50% of the patients.

These core hemodynamic events lead to an acute afterload mismatch superimposed on a progressively failing left ventricle. This induces an acute increase in left ventricular end-diastolic pressure (LVEDP), and hence PCWP, as well as a decrease in cardiovascular flow (CO).

Echocardiographic measures: a disease of diastolic dysfunction?

Traditionally, echocardiographic LVEF has been regarded as an important measure of LV contractility. However, its exact correlation with hemodynamic measures of contractility (such as CPo) and outcome are not known. In many patients admitted with AHF, LVEF is the only echocardiographic measure reported, and other measures of contractility (such as tissue Doppler), and measures of diastolic dysfunction are not routinely assessed.

Surprisingly, echocardiographic assessment of patients with AHF has not been studied in detail. In the only significant study reported to date, Gandhi *et al.*[20] reported echocardiographic findings in a small cohort of 38 patients admitted with AHF accompanied by high blood pressure. They assessed ejection fraction (EF), valvular function, and simple echocardiographic measures of diastolic dysfunction at admission and recovery. The authors found that there was no change in EF or valvular function, while some measures of diastolic dysfunction were more severe at admission than at 3-day follow-up.

Uriel *et al.* recently evaluated the clinical, hemodynamic, and neurohormonal correlations of EF in patients with AHF.[21] Their data are limited by the retrospective nature of EF retrieval. However, the results of this study show that EF is only weakly correlated with hemodynamic measures of contractility (i.e., CPo), as well as outcome. In another study, Logeart *et al.*[22] demonstrated that EF has no value in predicting the short-term prognosis of patients with AHF. Therefore, the role of echocardiographic evaluation of LVEF in patients with AHF is not known.

The inability of preliminary studies to show changes in EF during the course of admission for AHF, as well as the low correlation between EF and hemodynamic measures of contractility and short-term outcome, may be related to the size of the studies, the retrospective data analysis, or a more fundamental problem of this evaluation. In previous studies, it was demonstrated that more

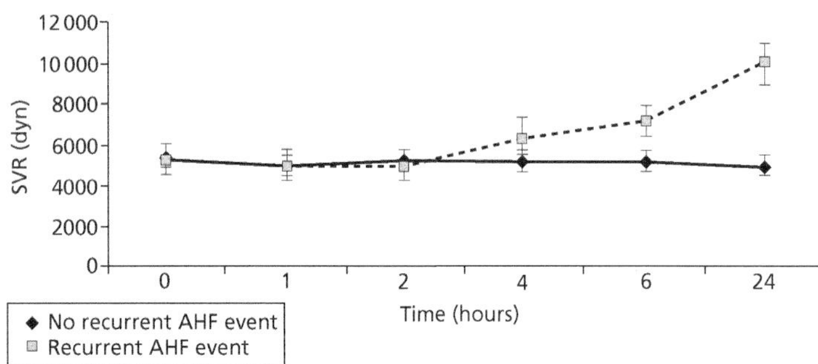

Figure 2.4. *Vascular resistance changes during 24 hours of hemodynamic monitoring in patients with and without acute heart failure events during monitoring (With permission from Cotter* et al.[14]*).*
Abbreviations: AHF = acute heart failure; SVR = systemic vascular resistance.

subtle measures of LV function, such as tissue Doppler,[23] were better correlated with LV contractility, which is impaired even in patients with apparently preserved EF.[24] Hence, these measures could show better correlation with disease severity and outcome in patients admitted with AHF.

As noted by Gandhi *et al.*[20] and Logeart *et al.*,[22] the most important echocardiographic measure that correlated with disease progression and outcome in AHF is diastolic dysfunction. In a recent review, Banerjee *et al.*[25] suggested that acute exacerbation of diastolic dysfunction may be one of the core echocardiographic findings in patients with AHF. However, it is difficult to conclude from these studies whether diastolic dysfunction is the primary effector or simply a marker of severity related to other more important pathophysiological processes, such as decreased cardiac contractility (CPo) and afterload mismatch imposed by an acute increase in SVR, atrial tachyarrhythmias, or fluid overload. Further detailed studies in which many echocardiographic variables are repeatedly measured throughout the course of the AHF event are needed to elucidate the role of echocardiographic evaluation in patients with AHF.

Fluid and sodium overload

Fluid and sodium overload due to non-adherence to sodium restriction, fluid restriction, or pharmacologic therapy, may cause a slow deterioration in the condition of many patients with significant systolic chronic heart failure. This type of ADHF is clinically distinct and develops gradually over days or weeks. It is commonly treated in the outpatient clinic, with higher diuretic doses, optimized evidence-based pharmacotherapy, fluid restriction, and diet modification.

The role of fluid and sodium overload in the pathogenesis of the more abrupt syndrome of AHF is less clear. It is our hypothesis that the genesis of this rapid onset pulmonary congestion is related mostly to *fluid re-distribution* rather than *fluid accumulation*. This redistribution is induced by the decreased LV contractility and increased SVR leading to afterload mismatch, acute diastolic dysfunction, and increased LV filling pressure. These hemodynamic alterations translate backwards to the lungs, causing fluid redistribution. However, since this issue has not been studied in detail, it is possible that some volume and sodium overload occurs during the initial stages of AHF, initiating a cascade of neurohormonal activation and triggering the AHF event.

Mechanisms of pulmonary congestion

The combination of hemodynamic events that lead to increased LV filling pressures and acute diastolic dysfunction subsequently cause significantly increased pulmonary venous pressure, which is the main reason for the acute pulmonary congestion observed in patients with AHF.

Under normal circumstances, the alveolar space is kept free of fluids by an active process of sodium ion (Na^+) and perhaps chloride ion (Cl^-) transport. Fluid is regularly transudated from the pulmonary capillaries through the thin gas exchange apparatus (composed of the capillary endothelial and type I alveolar cells) and into the alveoli. This process is slowed considerably due to the tight gap junctions existing between the cells, which reduce potential fluid transudation. Some fluid, however, escapes this mechanism and reaches the alveoli.

In the past, the common paradigm suggested that this fluid was removed from the alveoli by a simple osmotic pressure gradient. However, 20 years ago, Matthay *et al.*[26] demonstrated that alveolar fluid clearance is not affected by the Starling forces, but it is an active process of Na^+ transport leading to fluid clearance. Na^+ from the alveolar fluid enters the type II alveolar cells through amiloride-sensitive channels and co-transport with glucose, hydrogen ions (H^+), amino acids, phosphorous, and other as yet undefined mechanisms. It is then extruded at the basal side of the cells by an active process, mainly through the action of the sodium–potassium adenosine triphosphatase pump (Na, K-ATPase).[27] The fluid follows the Na^+ by a simple osmotic mechanism, which is at least partially mediated by aquaporins. Some fluid reabsorption also occurs in the airways, although in these regions, active Cl^- reabsorption probably plays a role in the overall fluid clearance.[28]

Therefore, fluid can accumulate in the alveolar space only when this protective mechanism fails.

This occurs when fluid is transudated into the alveolar space at an increased rate and overwhelms the active reabsorption mechanism, or when active fluid clearance mechanisms become less effective. In patients with AHF, the increase in LV pressure induced by the hemodynamic changes, translates into an increase in pulmonary venous pressure. This pressure is transduced backwards to the pulmonary capillaries, leading to increased fluid transudation into the pulmonary interstitium and alveoli. This process exceeds the capacity of the alveolar reabsorptive mechanism and leads to fluid accumulation which disrupts the alveolar gas exchange mechanism.

Phases of acute heart failure

Initiation phase

The combination of altered hemodynamic processes leads to the genesis of the initial phase of AHF (Figure 2.5), and it comprises both *"backward failure"* (increased LV filling pressure leading to pulmonary congestion and hypoxia) and *"forward failure"* (decreased perfusion of peripheral tissues). On echocardiography, the combination of these events may manifest as acute diastolic dysfunction.

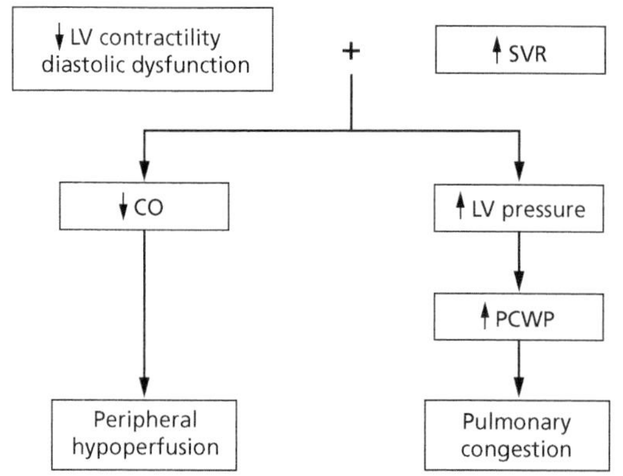

Figure 2.5. *The initiation phase of acute heart failure*

Abbreviations: CO = cardiac output; LV = left ventricular; PCWP = pulmonary capillary wedge pressure; SVR = systemic vascular resistance.

Amplification phase

Once initiated, the AHF process is amplified through several mechanisms (Figure 2.6):

1. *Myocardial necrosis and progressive LV failure*: Myocardial necrosis, as measured by troponin release, is a common event in patients with AHF. The Pilot Randomized Study of Nesiritide versus Dobutamine in Heart Failure (PRESERVD-HF), the first study to address this issue in a prospective manner, observed that nearly 50% of patients with AHF have detectable cardiac troponin at baseline, which in PRESERVD-HF was within 24 hours of hospital admission. In addition, of those patients who did not have detectable cardiac troponin levels at baseline, almost 20% developed detectable troponin during the hospitalization. The source of this troponin release is not clear. In many patients, AHF occurs along with significant coronary artery disease (CAD). In these patients, the hypoxia, acidosis, increased LV diastolic pressure, and reduced CO occurring during AHF can induce myocardial ischemia. However, the definition of such acute ischemic events in patients with AHF is challenging since troponin increase is observed in many patients with heart failure without ischemia and sometimes without CAD.[29] Therefore, an AHF event may be analogous to an acute coronary syndrome (ACS) event. In many patients, these events are associated with frank myocardial necrosis and ischemia, and further deteriorating myocardial contractility, and contractility reserve, contributing to the progressive process of heart failure.
2. *Right ventricular (RV) failure*: Increased fluid content in the lungs and decreased oxygen (O_2) saturation induce pulmonary vasoconstriction. This process leads to an increase in RV pressure that compromises LV function through the ventricular interaction mechanism.[30] Furthermore, it is possible that in some cases an acute event of RV failure (caused by pulmonary embolism) triggers an AHF event in patients with significantly reduced LV reserve.
3. *Respiratory failure*: Decreased oxygenation, presence of acidosis, and reduced CO may lead

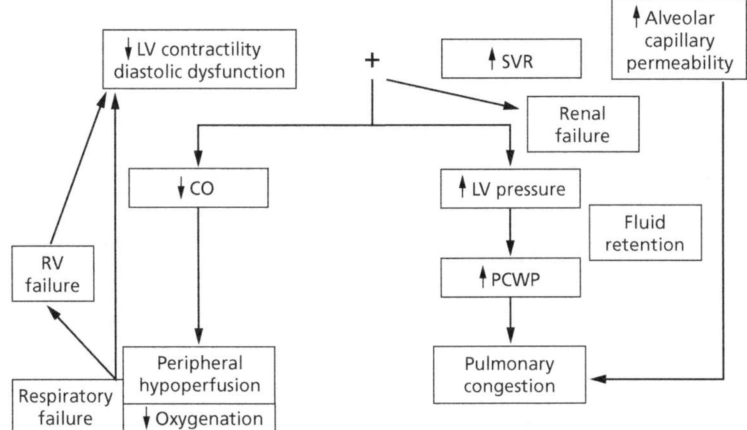

Figure 2.6. *The amplification phase of acute heart failure*

Abbreviations: CO = cardiac output; LV = left ventricular; PCWP = pulmonary capillary wedge pressure; RV = right ventricular; SVR = systemic vascular resistance.

to depressed central respiratory drive, failure of the respiratory muscles, and eventually respiratory failure superimposed on cardiovascular failure.

4. *Leakage of the alveolar-capillary membrane and decreased alveolar fluid clearance*: In the setting of AHF, an acute inflammatory reaction may lead to prolonged leakage of the alveolar-capillary membrane. The presence of this process has not been proven. However, if this acute inflammatory response occurs, it may contribute to the initial event as well as to the known tendency of patients admitted with AHF to develop recurrent events during the days following the initial event.[31] Furthermore, the significant hypoxia present during the initiation of the AHF event may depress the rate of alveolar fluid clearance, further enhancing pulmonary congestion.[28]
5. *Renal failure*: Patients with AHF who develop acute renal failure during the course of their admission (defined by an increase of at least 0.3 mg/dL in serum creatinine) have worse outcomes.[32] The exact cause for the renal failure is not known, although it occurs more frequently in patients who are older and have diabetes mellitus, hypertension, prior renal failure, or prior heart failure. Although acute renal failure during an AHF event may be related to many mechanisms, it has been suggested[33] that renal impairment in patients with heart failure is closely connected to the hemodynamic manifestations of decreased contractility. Hence, acute renal failure in the presence of AHF may be a simple measure of severity. Regardless of the mechanism, the occurrence of acute renal failure during an AHF event may lead to fluid retention, activate neurohormonal deleterious mechanisms, lead to resistance to treatment,[34]and further deteriorate the AHF event.
6. *Arrhythmias*: Arrhythmias, especially atrial tachyarrhythmias, are very common in patients with AHF. Recently, Benza *et al.*[35] have shown that the occurrence of new arrhythmias, mainly atrial arrhythmias, was a strong predictor of recurrent events and death. Hence, development of arrhythmia during the AHF event is an important reason for further deterioration in these patients.

Final vicious cycle

As the vicious cycle leading to AHF progresses, the patient deteriorates into a state of severe cardiovascular failure with low CO, reduced oxygenation, significantly activated neurohormonal and inflammatory modulators, increased SVR, decreased peripheral perfusion, myocardial ischemia, respiratory failure, and, if untreated, death (Figure 2.7).

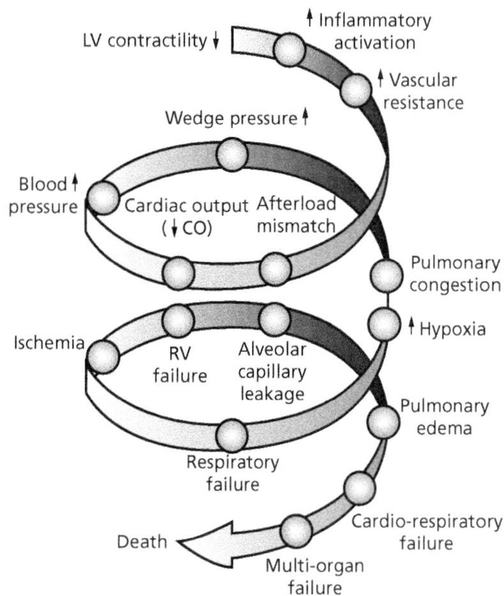

Figure 2.7. *The common final pathway of acute heart failure*

Mechanisms for the initial decrease in cardiac contractility and increase in vascular resistance

AHF is caused by a deteriorating chain of events culminating in a vicious cycle of progressive backward and forward failure. A few mechanisms have been described as initiating this chain of events including fluid overload, myocardial ischemia, arrhythmias, dyssynchronization, use of RV pacemakers, and neurohormonal and inflammatory activation.

Acute ischemia and acute heart failure

Most patients admitted for AHF have chronic IHD (Table 2.1). However, as previously suggested, the diagnosis of an ACS during an AHF event is challenging. An increase in troponin may occur in many patients with AHF, even if CAD does not exist. Hence, troponin increase alone cannot be regarded as absolute evidence of an ACS during AHF. Similarly, electrocardiographic changes during an AHF event are not universally indicative of acute ischemia.[36] Therefore, the diagnosis of ACS during an AHF event requires evidence of a combination of substantial clinical, electrocardiographic, and enzymatic changes. By using threshold enzymatic changes indicative of an ACS during an AHF event, in our experience,[9] ACS and significant troponin increase occur in only 20% of patients admitted with AHF. Similarly, in the large European registry,[7] 32% of patients admitted with heart failure had significant chest pain at admission, but frank acute myocardial infarction (AMI) was diagnosed in only 12%. Hence, ACS occurs in less than 30% of patients with AHF.

Surprisingly, the characteristics of patients admitted with AHF who also have ACS have not been studied in detail. Gattis *et al.* recently reported the outcome of a small cohort of patients (n < 200) admitted with AHF accompanied by ACS.[37] During the first 72 hours after enrollment, 3% of patients died, 12% sustained a recurrent event of heart failure, and 12% had recurrent ischemia, of which 3% were frank MIs. In these patients, troponin increase was a strong predictor of adverse outcome.[38]

More data exist describing the occurrence of AHF during admission for ACS. Khot *et al.*[39] reported on the incidence and outcome of clinical heart failure (by Kilip class) in a large cohort of patients (n > 20 000) with non-ST-elevation ACS enrolled in the Global Utilization of Streptokinase and t-PA for Occluded Coronary Arteries (GUSTO IIb), Paragon A and B, and Platelet IIb/IIIa Unstable Angina: Receptor Suppression of Using Integrilin Therapy (PURSUIT) studies. AHF (Kilip class ≥ 2) was observed in 11% of the patients leading to a 9% 1-month mortality and 16% 6-month mortality—more than triple the mortality observed in patients without heart failure. AHF was correlated with 30% of the overall mortality in the study, being the strongest independent negative prognostic factor in the cohort. Equally, James *et al.*[40] reported a significant association between increased levels of N-terminal pro-brain natriuretic peptide (NT-proBNP) at admission and adverse outcome in patients admitted for ACS enrolled in the GUSTO IV study, including a very significant correlation with 1-year mortality. Therefore, in a recent editorial, Velazquez and Pfeffer suggested that the interaction between ACS and AHF is a dangerous combination leading to high morbidity and mortality.[41]

Mechanical lesions and acute heart failure

In some patients, especially those who develop AHF during an ACS, the decreased myocardial effective contractility (CPo) is caused by a significant mechanical lesion that evolves or deteriorates rapidly. The different possible mechanical causes for AHF are listed in Table 2.2. The most common include acute mitral regurgitation (MR) due to ischemic or non-ischemic papillary muscle rupture, mechanical valve malfunction due to thrombosis or pannus, infective endocarditis leading to new onset of valvular regurgitation or, less commonly, significant exacerbation of stenosis, ventricular septal rupture due to an ACS, and aortic dissection causing severe ischemia or aortic regurgitation.

Arrhythmias in acute heart failure

The contribution of arrhythmias to the pathophysiology of AHF has not been studied in detail. Most registries (Table 2.1) have reported that atrial fibrillation occurs in 30% to 42% of patients admitted with AHF.[6–8] The rate of ventricular tachyarrhythmias, bradyarrhythmias, and conduction disturbances is not reported in most studies. Recently, Cleland *et al.*[7] reported on the incidence of arrhythmias in > 11 000 patients admitted with AHF. Their study demonstrated that 42% of patients had atrial fibrillation at admission, of which approximately half did not previously have chronic atrial fibrillation. A quarter of these patients had atrial fibrillation that was judged to be rapid and presumably the cause of the AHF event. In the same study, malignant ventricular tachyarrhythmias were reported in 8% of patients. Due to the retrospective nature of the study, the investigators were not able to show a cause and effect relationship between arrhythmias and the occurrence of heart failure or its outcome. Recently, Benza *et al.*[35] have shown that the occurrence of new arrhythmias, mainly atrial fibrillation, was a strong predictor of recurrent events and death in patients with AHF. Hence, arrhythmias, some of a transient nature, may sometimes cause steep decreases in cardiac contractility (and hence CPo) and diastolic dysfunction, leading to the AHF event.

Table 2.2. *Common valvular or mechanical lesions that may lead to acute heart failure*

- Significant aortic stenosis or regurgitation
- Significant mitral stenosis or regurgitation
- Mechanical valve malfunction (thrombosis or pannus formation or leakage)
- Acquired ventricular septal defect (associated with myocardial infarction)
- Infective endocarditis
- Aortic dissection

Ventricular dyssynchrony and pacemakers in acute heart failure

It has become apparent in recent years that the synchronization of cardiac contraction including atrioventricular, interventricular (right and left ventricle), and intraventricular (different segments of the left ventricle) is an important determinant of cardiac contractility.[42–46] Initially, dyssynchrony was shown to contribute significantly to cardiac dysfunction in patients with chronic heart failure and wide QRS complex by electrocardiography. However, in recent years, by using more advanced echocardiographic measures, especially tissue Doppler, dyssynchrony has also been demonstrated to exist in many patients with heart failure and narrow QRS complexes.[42–44] Dyssynchrony, especially of the intraventricular type, has been repeatedly shown to be associated with adverse outcomes in patients with chronic heart failure.[42,45] Its treatment with biventricular pacemakers improved this outcome somewhat.[42–46] The importance of this mechanism in patients with AHF has not been examined, although theoretically, acute changes in cardiac contractility and conduction may induce dyssynchrony. In support of this concept, Brophy *et al.* found that intraventricular conduction delay is associated with more adverse outcome in patients admitted with AHF.[47] Furthermore, RV pacing, which is known to induce dyssynchrony leading to hemodynamic deterioration[48,49] as well as adverse outcome[50,51] in patients with chronic heart failure, was found in a preliminary study by Cotter *et al.* to be related with increased 30-day mortality in patients admitted with AHF (odds ratio [OR], 6.1; confidence interval [CI], 1.3–24.5) (G. Cotter, unpublished data, 2004). No other study has evaluated the interaction of AHF and RV pacing or dyssynchrony in detail. Therefore, this important pathophysiological mechanism should be studied in patients with AHF, since it represents a potentially treatable cause of this syndrome.

Neurohormonal and inflammatory activation in acute heart failure

Recent studies have shown that pro-inflammatory cytokines, neurohormones, and selectins are involved in the heart failure syndrome. Highly significant correlations were demonstrated between the levels of specific neurohormones, cytokines, and adhesion molecules and the severity of chronic heart failure and its outcome. The interaction between inflammation and AHF is complex and has not been studied in detail. Fontana *et al.*[52] found increased levels of endogenous opioids and noradrenaline in patients with AHF. Pohar and Horvat[53] showed that these levels decreased during treatment with diuretics. Sato *et al.*[54] found significant elevations of interleukin-6 (IL-6), IL-4 and C-reactive protein (CRP) in patients with pulmonary edema. In a recent community-based registry of 340 consecutive patients admitted with AHF, Cotter *et al.* found that the leukocyte count at admission was relatively high (9600±3600), and correlated with admission systolic blood pressure ($R = 0.31$, $P < 0.001$) (G. Cotter, unpublished data, 2004). The correlation with systolic blood pressure suggests that the increased leukocyte count may be related to the vasoconstriction observed in patients with AHF.

Milo *et al.* recently concluded a small study examining a series of neurohormonal and inflammatory markers as well as adhesion molecules in patients with AHF,[55] comparing patients with and without acute ischemia during the AHF event. The results of this study showed that all three neurohormones measured (norepinephrine, B-type natriuretic peptide [BNP], and endothelin-1 [ET-1]) were significantly increased during the acute phase of pulmonary edema (P. Edem in figure), both at time 0 (before treatment) and at 48 hours (Figure 2.8). At two-month follow-up, the levels of these markers decreased significantly to levels similar to the control group (patients with reduced LVEF but no previous AHF event).

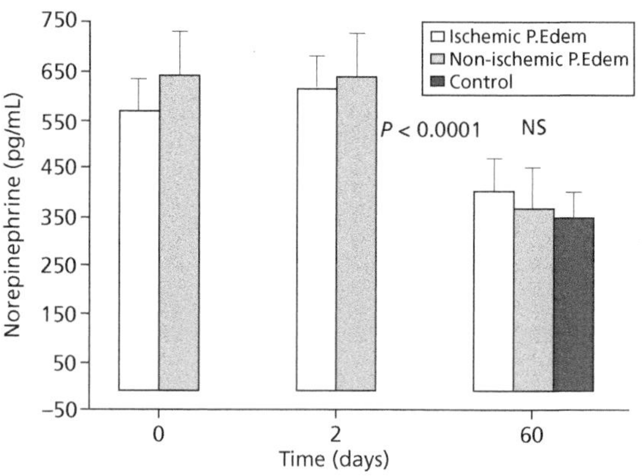

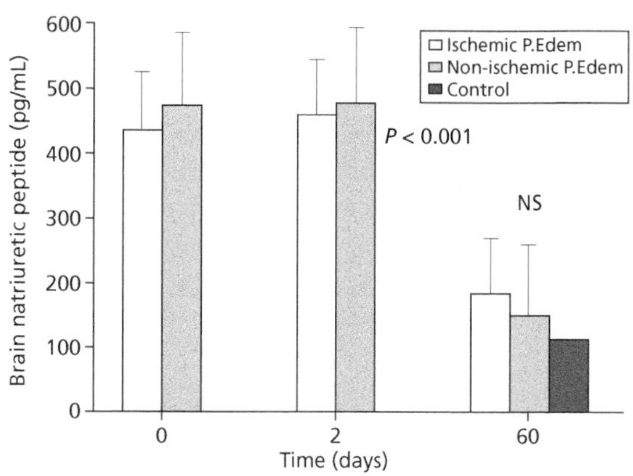

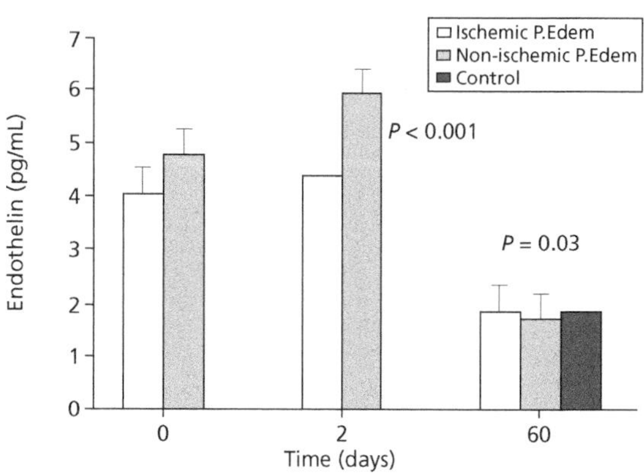

Figure 2.8. *Changes in neurohormonal markers in patients admitted with acute heart failure (With permission from Milo* et al.*[54]).*

Plasma levels of IL-6, CRP, and tumor necrosis factor-α (TNF-α) were significantly increased at both time 0 (before treatment) and at two days, in the two study groups, as compared to 60-day follow-up and control patients. At 60-day follow-up, however, IL-6 and CRP levels were significantly higher in patients with AHF without acute ischemia at presentation, as compared to patients with acute ischemic AHF and control patients (Figure 2.9).

Furthermore, findings of different patterns of inflammatory and neurohormonal activation in patients with AHF support the hypothesis that AHF involves different pathophysiological mechanisms. Milo *et al.* observed that patients with AHF without significant concomitant ischemia have higher increases in ET-1 during the acute event (Figure 2.8) and higher levels of IL-6 and CRP at 60 days (Figure 2.9).[55] Therefore, IL-6-related inflammatory activation leading to a steep increase in ET-1 may be an important mechanism of non-ischemic AHF.

In an analysis of the 50 patients enrolled in the PRESERVD-HF study (W. A. Gattis Stough, unpublished data, 2004), the same extent of neurohormonal-inflammatory activation was observed at admission. This neurohormonal-inflammatory activation persisted throughout the fifth day of hospitalization (Table 2.3). Therefore, this persistent neurohormonal inflammatory activation may have a role not only in the genesis of the AHF

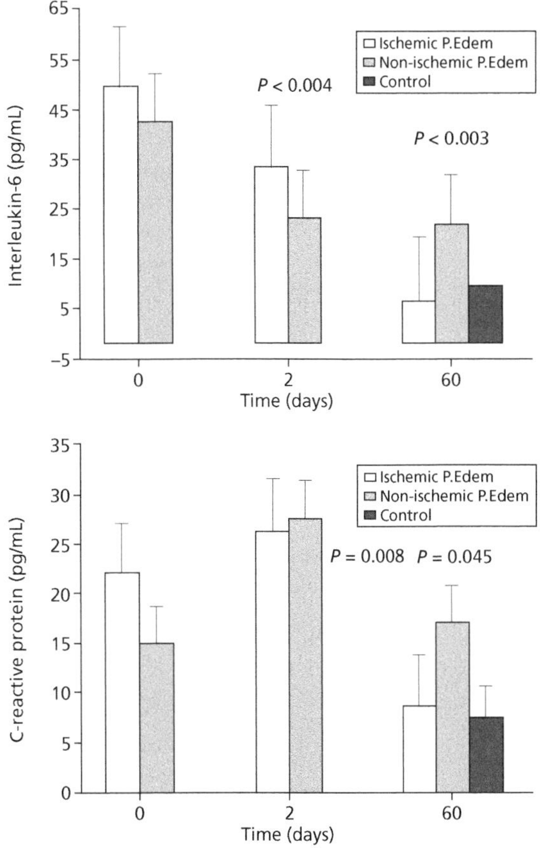

Figure 2.9. *Changes in inflammatory markers in patients admitted with acute heart failure (With permission from Milo* et al.*[54])*

Table 2.3. *Change in neurohormonal and inflammatory markers in patients with acute heart failure during admission*

Marker	Day 1	Days 4–6
B-type Natriuretic Peptide	178.5 pg/mL (49, 331)	168 pg/mL (53, 469)
Fatty Acid-Binding Protein	2192 pg/mL (1164, 3439)	1711 pg/mL (1227, 2855)
Aldosterone	20.1 pg/mL (16.71, 26.45)	20.455 pg/mL (14.06, 24.13)
Endothelin	4.08 pg/mL (2.48, 6.63)	4.425 pg/mL (1.9, 6.56)
Tumor Necrosis Factor	5.59 pg/mL (4.12, 9.46)	6.32 pg/mL (4.1, 8.14)
Interleukin-6	7.54 pg/mL (5.345, 12.46)	7.495 pg/mL (5.14, 12.67)
Interleukin-1	0.135 pg/mL (0.02, 0.28)	0.085 pg/mL (0.2, 0.27)
Interleukin-10	1.93 pg/mL (1.27, 2.98)	2.345 pg/mL (1.29, 3.74)

event, but also in the significant (approximately 30%) recurrent AHF rate observed during the first days of admission.

Platelet activation

In patients with chronic heart failure, many measures of platelet activation, especially P-selectin, have been shown to be increased and related with outcome.[56,57] Platelet activation, as measured by plasma and platelet-bound P-selectin, was examined in two studies. O'Connor *et al.* found a significant increase in both soluble and platelet-bound P-selectin in patients admitted with AHF as compared to controls (Figure 2.10).[56] In a second study, Milo *et al.* found the same increase when comparing values during an AHF event to values measured in the same patients at two-month follow-up.[55] This increase was related to poor outcome. This area needs to be further explored in order to determine the possible interactions between platelet activation and AHF, specifically the possible role of platelets in the vasoconstriction encountered in patients with AHF.

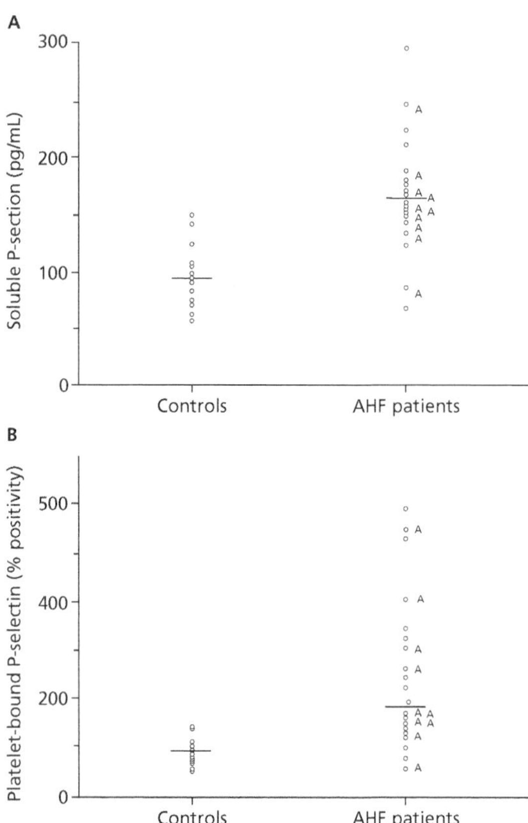

Figure 2.10. *Plasma P-selectin (A) and platelet-bound P-selectin (B) in patients with acute heart failure vs. controls (With permission from O'Connor* et al.[55])

Abbreviations: A = aspirin users; AHF = acute heart failure.

Outcome Measures and Their Predictors

Clinical measures

Mortality and readmission for heart failure

In previous studies, the main outcome measures assessed in patients admitted with AHF were recurrent hospitalizations and death. These two endpoints represent long-term outcome and may be more closely related to the severity of the patient's chronic heart failure than to the AHF event itself. Predictors of short-term and long-term mortality were assessed in a few studies[6,9] and some important variables were found to be correlated with long-term adverse outcomes. In the Canadian cohort, Lee *et al.*[6] reported that age, low blood pressure, low serum sodium, low hemoglobin, high serum urea nitrogen, and comorbid conditions (cerebrovascular disease, dementia, chronic obstructive pulmonary disease, hepatic cirrhosis, and cancer) were independent predictors of death at 30 days and one year. In an analysis of the IMPACT-HF study,[9] we found that renal failure, age, low blood pressure, history of depression, previous admissions due to heart failure, and use of nitrate treatment on admission were correlated with a higher rate of death or readmission at two months. In patients with ADHF enrolled in the Outcomes of a Prospective Trial of Intravenous Milrinone for Exacerbations of Chronic Heart Failure (OPTIME-CHF) study, age, NYHA class, anemia, blood pressure, sodium and blood urea nitrogen (BUN) were found to predict death and readmission for heart failure at two-month follow-up.[58] In these analyses, as well as other studies of AHF, the major clinical variables that emerge as strong predictors of long-term outcome in patients with AHF are age, renal failure, and anemia.

Age is an important predictor of outcome in all cardiovascular studies since it is related to more severe background characteristics. Therefore, it is not surprising that it is a major predictor of morbidity and mortality in patients with AHF, especially when taking into account their advanced age at admission.

Renal failure has been repeatedly shown to be associated with increased long-term morbidity and mortality in patients with chronic as well as AHF.[32,59] In the ADHERE™ registry, systolic blood pressure < 115 mm Hg, BUN > 43, and creatinine > 2.75 mg/dL were the strongest predictors of in-hospital mortality. In other recent studies, Shlipak *et al.*[32] and Cohen *et al.*[60] have shown that creatinine levels as low as 1.5 mg/dL confer an increased risk of morbidity and mortality in patients with AHF. The exact cause for the association between renal failure and poor outcome in patients with AHF is not known. However, renal failure may occur more frequently in patients with more severe AHF and, therefore, may be a marker of severity. In support of this concept, Ljungman *et al.*,[33] in a classic manuscript, demonstrated that creatinine clearance in patients with heart failure is closely related to impaired hemodynamics. On the other hand, renal failure in the setting of AHF may be associated with more fluid and sodium retention, neurohormonal activation, and resistance to treatment.[34] Hence, although the role of renal failure in the pathophysiology of AHF has to be studied in detail, the severity of renal failure is an important predictor of adverse outcome in patients with AHF.

Anemia has been repeatedly shown to be associated with adverse outcome in patients with AHF. In a recent manuscript, Felker *et al.*[61] demonstrated that anemia in patients with ADHF was associated with more adverse outcomes, even after controlling for many baseline characteristics. Again, the cause of this association is not known. It is possible that anemia is a marker of more severe activation of the inflammatory system or more advanced renal failure.

Conversely, many clinical characteristics assessed by physicians in the emergency room, such as NYHA class, were not found to predict outcome in patients with AHF. In the recently published Rapid Emergency Department Heart Failure Outpatient Trial (REDHOT),[62] it was reported that many such clinical variables were not well correlated with medium- and long-term outcome. Finally, ventricular dyssynchrony as evidenced by electrocardiogram (EKG)[47] or caused by RV pacing, may also confer increased risk of adverse outcome in AHF patients.

Early recurrent worsening heart failure

Recently, Torre-Amione *et al.* observed that in many cases the most common adverse outcome in patients with AHF is early recurrence of AHF. This includes all recurrent AHF events from admission through 7 to 30 days of follow-up. Recurrent AHF was defined as recurrent symptoms and signs of heart failure, pulmonary edema, or cardiogenic shock after initial stabilization, leading to administration or uptitration of an intravenous treatment, mechanical ventilation, circulatory support, readmission to the hospital after discharge, or death.[19]

Analyzing data from the placebo arms of three prospective studies of patients with AHF, Torre-Amione *et al.* found that the rate of early recurrent AHF was high (42% at 30 days after enrollment) and represented the main morbidity in the study.[63] Most of the events (Figure 2.11) occurred during the first seven days after enrollment, while the patient was still hospitalized for the initial episode. The recurrent AHF events presumably lead to more treatment and prolonged hospitalization.

Torre-Amione *et al.*[63] performed a multivariate analysis and found that the independent predictors for early recurrent AHF were related to a more severe admission AHF event, most notably oxygen saturation < 90% and the need for more intensive treatment for immediate stabilization, such as mechanical ventilation or intravenous treatment with dopamine. None of the measures known to predict worse outcome in patients with chronic heart failure (such as EF, age, renal failure, or diabetes) correlated with early recurrent AHF.

In both studies,[19,63] early recurrent AHF (within seven days of admission) was the strongest predictor of 1-month and 6-month mortality. In

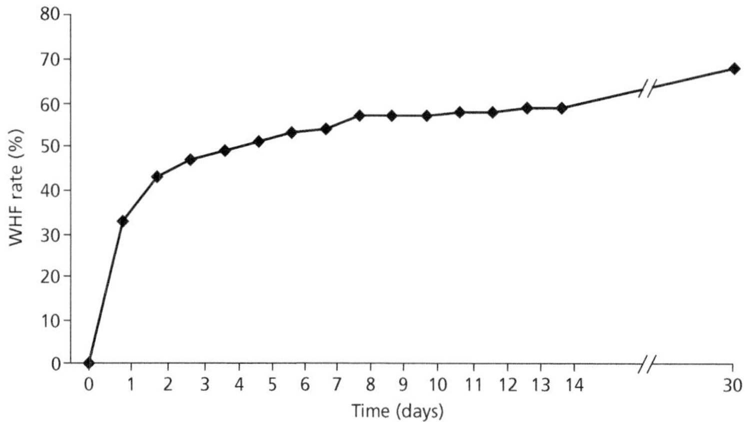

Figure 2.11. *Recurrent acute heart failure during the first month after admission due to acute heart failure*

Abbreviations: WHF = worsening heart failure.

the second prospective community-based study, by Torre-Amione *et al.*, of 340 patients admitted with clinical AHF,[19] early recurrent AHF was also found to be the most common morbidity. They followed the cohort for an average of 3 months and observed a mortality rate of 12.5%, of which 3.5% represented in-hospital mortality. This rate is very similar to the mortality rate of 3% observed in the ADHERE™ study.[8] The three variables emerging as the strongest independent predictors of death were dementia, 7-day recurrent AHF, and admission oxygen saturation. Furthermore, similar to the first study by Torre-Amione *et al.*,[63] early recurrent AHF emerged as a common, strong, independent, and potentially modifiable predictor of death in patients admitted with AHF (Figure 2.12, $P = 0.001$). Hence, in analogy to ACS, AHF emerges as a significant event in the course of heart failure. Each recurrent heart failure event is a marker of more severe disease and increased mortality. Furthermore, it is possible that by inducing myocardial necrosis, as manifested by the troponin spillage, each AHF event leads to progression in the heart failure process, explaining the significant association between recurrent AHF events and death.

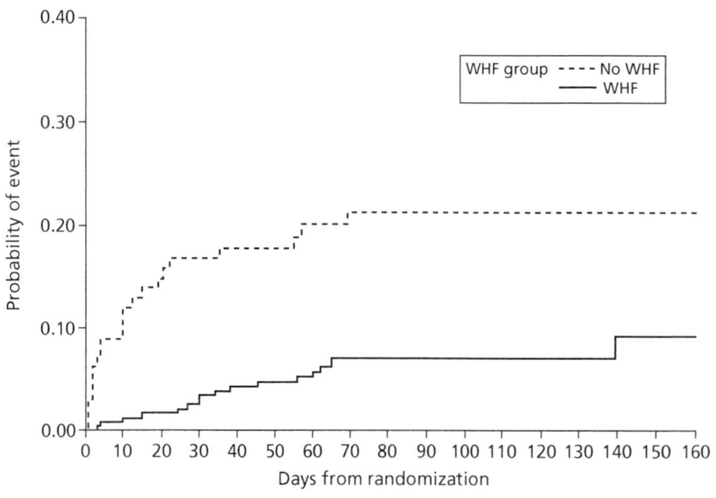

Figure 2.12. *Three-month mortality in patients admitted with recurrent acute heart failure within 7 days*

Abbreviations: WHF = worsening heart failure.

Symptom relief

Symptom relief, specifically improvement in dyspnea, is frequently used as an important measure in studies assessing new treatments for AHF. Although rapid improvement in symptoms is a desirable goal in managing patients with AHF, this measure should not become the only goal of treatment, nor should it be considered equal in significance to morbidity and mortality. This issue has gained much attention recently with the finding that many treatment modalities shown to improve symptoms in patients with AHF were shown to increase mortality. Continuing the analogy with ACS, it is obvious that chest pain relief is not assigned the same significance as reinfarction. Therefore, we believe that symptom relief should rank third in any study examining treatment of AHF after, and not combined with, mortality and morbidity.

Hemodynamic and neurohormonal measures

CPo measured at baseline and its changes during 6 hours of monitoring was found to be useful in the risk stratification of patients admitted with AHF (Figure 2.3).[16] However, calculation of CPo requires knowledge of CO, which until recently could be measured only invasively. In recent years, a few noninvasive devices have been developed, using bioimpedance, for the assessment of CO. Indeed, in the PREDICT trial,[64] stroke volume determination by thoracic bioimpedance was found to predict heart failure events within 2 weeks of measurement. Similarly, we have demonstrated that CPo determination using whole body bioimpedance is efficacious in predicting the outcome of patients with AHF.[65]

BNP was examined in the REDHOT study for its role in the risk stratification of patients with AHF in the emergency department.[62] Admission BNP > 200 pg/mL correlated with increased mortality at 90 days, but it did not correlate with recurrent heart failure events at 30 days and 90 days. Similarly, Logeart *et al.*[22] demonstrated that admission BNP levels have limited value in the risk stratification of patients with AHF, while predischarge measurements significantly correlated with outcome. Hence, BNP measured before discharge may have significant prognostic value in the long-term outcome of patients admitted with AHF.[22,62,66]

Recently, Cotter *et al.* examined the value of ET-1 in the risk stratification of patients with AHF.[67] In this study, ET-1 above the median at admission was associated with a more than doubled risk for AHF events within the first month after admission. Aronson and Burger[68] found that high admission ET-1 levels were the strongest neurohormonal predictors of mortality during one-year follow-up. However, at present, ET-1 levels cannot be measured in a clinical setting and hence are used only for investigational purposes.

Troponin increase has been shown in many studies to correlate with outcome in patients with AHF[38] (W.A. Gattis Stough, unpublished data, 2004). Although the exact cause for this relationship is not known, it has been suggested that acute ischemia, and sometimes diffuse myocardial necrosis, occur during an AHF event. Analogous to ACS, the more severe the damage is, the worse the long-term prognosis of the patient. Therefore, measurement of troponin release during the AHF event has significant prognostic value.

Conclusion

AHF is a distinctive, progressive cardiovascular syndrome leading to backward failure (pulmonary congestion) and forward failure (end-organ hypoperfusion), culminating in a vicious cycle of respiratory, cardiovascular, and multi-organ failure. Although in approximately 50% of cases, the main factors initiating this process are acute ischemia and arrhythmias, the cause of this syndrome in most patients is unknown. The role of novel potential mechanisms including neurohormonal and inflammatory activation (especially related to ET-1 and IL-6), diastolic dysfunction, and dyssynchrony needs to be explored in detail in large prospective studies.

Early recurrent AHF is an ominous sign in patients with AHF, leading to increased morbidity and mortality in both the short and long term. Early recurrent AHF may be the most important outcome measure in patients admitted with AHF.

However, its course, predictors, and contributing factors need to be explored in detail. Although some specific treatments (nesiritide and noninvasive ventilation [NIV]) were shown to be effective in the initial stabilization of these patients, more research is needed to identify effective treatments that improve the dismal outcomes associated with AHF.

References

1. American Heart Association. Heart Disease and Stroke Statistics—2003 Update. (American Heart Association: Dallas, TX, 2002).
2. Jessup M, Brozena S. Heart failure. N Engl J Med 2003; 348: 2007–2018.
3. Lee DS, Mamdani MM, Austin PC, *et al.* Trends in heart failure outcomes and pharmacotherapy: 1992 to 2000. Am J Med 2004; 116: 581–589.
4. Nohria A, Tsang SW, Fang JC, *et al.* Clinical assessment identifies hemodynamic profiles that predict outcomes in patients admitted with heart failure. J Am Coll Cardiol 2003; 41: 1797–1804.
5. Torre-Amione G, Young JB, Colucci WS, *et al.* Hemodynamic and clinical effects of tezosentan, an intravenous dual endothelin receptor antagonist, in patients hospitalized for acute decompensated heart failure. J Am Coll Cardiol 2003; 42: 140–147.
6. Lee DS, Austin PC, Rouleau JL, *et al.* Predicting mortality among patients hospitalized for heart failure: derivation and validation of a clinical model. JAMA 2003; 290: 2581–2587.
7. Cleland JG, Swedberg K, Follath F, *et al.* The EuroHeart Failure survey programme: a survey on the quality of care among patients with heart failure in Europe. Part 1: patient characteristics and diagnosis. Eur Heart J 2003; 24: 442–463.
8. Fonarow GC. The Acute Decompensated Heart Failure National Registry (ADHERE): opportunities to improve care of patients hospitalized with acute decompensated heart failure. Rev Cardiovasc Med 2003; 4: S21–S30.
9. Gattis WA, O'Connor CM, Gallup DS, *et al.* Predictors of 60-day death or rehospitalization in patients admitted with decompensated heart failure: insights from the IMPACT-HF trial. J Am Coll Cardiol 2003; 17: IV694 (Abstract).
10. McMurray JJ, Ostergren J, Swedberg K, *et al.* Effects of candesartan in patients with chronic heart failure and reduced left-ventricular systolic function taking angiotensin-converting-enzyme inhibitors: the CHARM-Added trial. Lancet 2003; 362: 767–771.
11. Yancy CW, Chang SF. Better outcomes in heart failure in African Americans despite negative risk factors: a report from the ADHERE™ registry. J Card Fail 2004. In press.
12. Mehta SK, Toto KH, Nelson LL, *et al.* Therapy of heart failure in African Americans: lessons from an urban public hospital. Congest Heart Fail 2004; 10: 40–43.
13. Jimenez J, Osorio JM, Andrade S, *et al.* Decompensated heart failure among Hispanic Americans: a report from the Acute Decompensated Heart Failure National Registry (ADHERE™). J Card Fail 2004; 4: S93 (Abstract).
14. Hill JA, Shah MR, Hasselblad V, *et al.* Pulmonary artery catheter use does not change the contribution of renal dysfunction to outcomes in patients with advanced heart failure: findings from ESCAPE. Circulation 2004; 110: III638 (Abstract).
15. Cotter G, Moshkovitz Y, Milovanov O, *et al.* Acute heart failure: a novel approach to its pathogenesis and treatment. Eur J Heart Fail 2002; 4: 227–234.
16. Torre-Amione G, Milo O, Kaluski E, *et al.* Hemodynamic variables (cardiac power) and their changes during 6 hours are the strongest predictors of short term outcome in acute heart failure. J Card Fail 2004; 10: S31 (Abstract).
17. Cotter G, Moshkovitz Y, Kaluski E, *et al.* The role of cardiac power and systemic vascular resistance in the pathophysiology and diagnosis of patients with acute congestive heart failure. Eur J Heart Fail 2003; 5: 443–451.
18. Cotter G, Williams SG, Vered Z, *et al.* Role of cardiac power in heart failure. Curr Opin Cardiol 2003; 18: 215–222.
19. Torre-Amione G, Kaluski E, Milo O, *et al.* Short term recurrent worsening heart failure is the most common morbidity in patients admitted with acute heart failure: time course and predictors of outcome. Eur J Heart Fail 2003; 1: 144 (Abstract).
20. Gandhi SK, Powers JC, Nomeir AM, *et al.* The pathogenesis of acute pulmonary edema associated with hypertension. N Engl J Med 2001; 344: 17–22.
21. Uriel N, Torre-Amione G, Milo O, *et al.* Echocardiographic ejection fraction in patients with acute heart failure: correlations with clinical, hemodynamic, and neurohormonal variables and short term outcome. Eur J Heart Fail 2004. In press.
22. Logeart D, Thabut G, Jourdain P, *et al.* Predischarge B-type natriuretic peptide assay for identifying patients at high risk of re-admission after decompensated heart failure. J Am Coll Cardiol 2004; 43: 635–641.

23. Greenberg NL, Firstenberg MS, Castro PL, *et al.* Doppler-derived myocardial systolic strain rate is a strong index of left ventricular contractility. Circulation 2002; 105: 99–105.
24. Bruch C, Gradaus R, Gunia S, *et al.* Doppler tissue analysis of mitral annular velocities: evidence for systolic abnormalities in patients with diastolic heart failure. J Am Soc Echocardiogr 2003; 16: 1031–1036.
25. Banerjee P, Clark AL, Nikitin N, *et al.* Diastolic heart failure: paroxysmal or chronic? Eur J Heart Fail 2004; 6: 427–431.
26. Matthay MA, Landolt CC, Staub NC. Differential liquid and protein clearance from the alveoli of anesthetized sheep. J Appl Physiol 1982; 53: 96–104.
27. Dada LA, Sznajder JI. Mechanisms of pulmonary edema clearance during acute hypoxemic respiratory failure: role of the Na,K-ATPase. Crit Care Med 2003; 31: S248–S252.
28. Matthay MA, Folkesson HG, Clerici C. Lung epithelial fluid transport and the resolution of pulmonary edema. Physiol Rev 2002; 82: 569–600.
29. Sato Y, Yamada T, Taniguchi R, *et al.* Persistently increased serum concentrations of cardiac troponin T in patients with idiopathic dilated cardiomyopathy are predictive of adverse outcomes. Circulation 2001; 103: 369–374.
30. Atherton JJ, Moore TD, Lele SS, *et al.* Diastolic ventricular interaction in chronic heart failure. Lancet 1997; 349: 1720–1724.
31. De Pasquale CG, Arnolda LF, Doyle IR, *et al.* Prolonged alveolocapillary barrier damage after acute cardiogenic pulmonary edema. Crit Care Med 2003; 31: 1060–1067.
32. Shlipak MG, Massie BM. The clinical challenge of cardiorenal syndrome. Circulation 2004; 110: 1514–1517.
33. Ljungman S, Laragh JH, Cody RJ. Role of the kidney in congestive heart failure. Relationship of cardiac index to kidney function. Drugs 1990; 39: 10–21.
34. Cioffi G, Stefenelli C, Tarantini L, *et al.* Hemodynamic response to intensive unloading therapy (furosemide and nitroprusside) in patients >70 years of age with left ventricular systolic dysfunction and decompensated chronic heart failure. Am J Cardiol 2003; 92: 1050–1056.
35. Benza RL, Tallaj JA, Felker GM, *et al.* The impact of arrhythmias in acute heart failure. J Card Fail 2004; 10: 279–284.
36. Littmann L. Large T wave inversion and QT prolongation associated with pulmonary edema: a report of nine cases. J Am Coll Cardiol 1999; 34: 1106–1110.
37. Gattis WA, O'Connor CM, Hasselblad V, *et al.* Usefulness of an elevated troponin-I in predicting clinical events in patients admitted with acute heart failure and acute coronary syndrome (from the RITZ-4 trial). Am J Cardiol 2004; 93: 1436–1437.
38. O'Connor CM, Gattis WA, Adams KF Jr., *et al.* Tezosentan in patients with acute heart failure and acute coronary syndromes: results of the Randomized Intravenous TeZosentan Study (RITZ-4). J Am Coll Cardiol 2003; 41: 1452–1457.
39. Khot UN, Jia G, Moliterno DJ, *et al.* Prognostic importance of physical examination for heart failure in non-ST-elevation acute coronary syndromes: the enduring value of Killip classification. JAMA 2003; 290: 2174–2181.
40. James SK, Lindahl B, Siegbahn A, *et al.* N-terminal pro-brain natriuretic peptide and other risk markers for the separate prediction of mortality and subsequent myocardial infarction in patients with unstable coronary artery disease: a Global Utilization of Strategies To Open occluded arteries (GUSTO)-IV substudy. Circulation 2003; 108: 275–281.
41. Velazquez EJ, Pfeffer MA. Acute heart failure complicating acute coronary syndromes: a deadly intersection. Circulation 2004; 109: 440–442.
42. Pitzalis MV, Iacoviello M, Romito R, *et al.* Cardiac resynchronization therapy tailored by echocardiographic evaluation of ventricular asynchrony. J Am Coll Cardiol 2002; 40: 1615–1622.
43. Sogaard P, Egeblad H, Kim WY, *et al.* Tissue Doppler imaging predicts improved systolic performance and reversed left ventricular remodeling during long-term cardiac resynchronization therapy. J Am Coll Cardiol 2002; 40: 723–730.
44. Cozma D, Kalifa J, Pescariu S, *et al.* Absence of correlation between QRS duration and echographic parameters of ventricular desynchronization: can we still trust the electrocardiographic criteria? Echocardiography 2004; 21: 205.
45. Bader H, Garrigue S, Lafitte S, *et al.* Intra-left ventricular electromechanical asynchrony: a new independent predictor of severe cardiac events in heart failure patients. J Am Coll Cardiol 2004; 43: 248–256.
46. Kass DA. Predicting cardiac resynchronization response by QRS duration: the long and short of it. J Am Coll Cardiol 2003; 42: 2125–2127.
47. Brophy JM, Deslauriers G, Rouleau JL. Long-term prognosis of patients presenting to the emergency room with decompensated congestive heart failure. Can J Cardiol 1994; 10: 543–547.
48. Hansen C, Sperzel J, Neumann T, *et al.* Acute hemodynamic effects of biventricular and left ventricular pacing in chronic pacemaker-dependent patients with advanced heart failure. Z Kardiol 2003; 92: 862–868.

49. Leon AR, Greenberg JM, Kanuru N, *et al.* Cardiac resynchronization in patients with congestive heart failure and chronic atrial fibrillation: effect of upgrading to biventricular pacing after chronic right ventricular pacing. J Am Coll Cardiol 2002; 39: 1258–1263.
50. Wilkoff BL, Cook JR, Epstein AE, *et al.* Dual-chamber pacing or ventricular backup pacing in patients with an implantable defibrillator: the Dual Chamber and VVI Implantable Defibrillator (DAVID) Trial. JAMA 2002; 288: 3115–3123.
51. Aukrust P, Ueland T, Lien E, *et al.* Cytokine network in congestive heart failure secondary to ischemic or idiopathic dilated cardiomyopathy. Am J Cardiol 1999; 83: 376–382.
52. Fontana F, Bernardi P, Pich EM, *et al.* Relationship between plasma atrial natriuretic factor and opioid peptide levels in healthy subjects and in patients with acute congestive heart failure. Eur Heart J 1993; 14: 219–225.
53. Pohar B, Horvat M. Influence of hemodynamic changes on neuroendocrine response in acute heart failure. Int J Cardiol 1997; 60: 263–271.
54. Sato Y, Takatsu Y, Kataoka K, *et al.* Serial circulating concentrations of C-reactive protein, interleukin (IL)-4, and IL-6 in patients with acute left heart decompensation. Clin Cardiol 1999; 22: 811–813.
55. Milo O, Cotter G, Kaluski E, *et al.* Comparison of inflammatory and neurohormonal activation in cardiogenic pulmonary edema secondary to ischemic versus nonischemic causes. Am J Cardiol 2003; 92: 222–226.
56. O'Connor CM, Gurbel PA, Serebruany VL. Usefulness of soluble and surface-bound P-selectin in detecting heightened platelet activity in patients with congestive heart failure. Am J Cardiol 1999; 83: 1345–1349.
57. Yin WH, Chen JW, Jen HL, *et al.* The prognostic value of circulating soluble cell adhesion molecules in patients with chronic congestive heart failure. Eur J Heart Fail 2003; 5: 507–516.
58. Felker GM, Leimberger JD, Califf RM, *et al.* Risk stratification after hospitalization for decompensated heart failure. J Card Fail 2004; 10: 460–466.
59. Yancy CW, Fonarow GC, Abraham WT, ADHERE™ Scientific Advisory Committee. Clinical differences between high and low mortality risk stratified patients hospitalized with acutely decompensated heart failure: ADHERE™ registry data. J Card Fail 2004. In press.
60. Cohen N, Gorelik O, Almoznino-Sarafian D, *et al.* Renal dysfunction in congestive heart failure, pathophysiological and prognostic significance. Clin Nephrol 2004; 61: 177–184.
61. Felker GM, Gattis WA, Leimberger JD, *et al.* Usefulness of anemia as a predictor of death and rehospitalization in patients with decompensated heart failure. Am J Cardiol 2003; 92: 625–628.
62. Maisel AS, Hollander JE, Guss D, *et al.* Primary results of the Rapid Emergency Department Heart Failure Outpatient Trial (REDHOT): a multicenter study of B-type natriuretic peptide levels, emergency department decision making, and outcomes in patients presenting with shortness of breath. J Am Coll Cardiol 2004; 44: 1328–1333.
63. Torre-Amione G, Kaluski E, Perchenet L, *et al.* Short-term recurrent worsening heart failure is the most common morbidity in patients admitted with acute heart failure, time course, predictors and outcome. J Card Fail 2004; 10: S38–S39 (Abstract).
64. Abraham WT, Trupp RJ, Mehra MR, *et al.* A multivariate impedance cardiography composite score can predict the occurrence of major heart failure events: the PREDICT study. Circulation 2004; 110: III597 (Abstract).
65. Torre-Amione G, Cotter G, Vered Z, Kaluski E, Stangl K. Whole-body electrical bio-impedance is accurate in non-invasive determination of cardiac output: a thermodilution controlled, prospective, double blind evaluation. J Am Coll Cardiol 2004; 43: 209 (Abstract).
66. Harrison A, Morrison LK, Krishnaswamy P, *et al.* B-type natriuretic peptide predicts future cardiac events in patients presenting to the emergency department with dyspnea. Ann Emerg Med 2002; 39: 131–138.
67. Cotter G, Kaluski E, Stangl K, *et al.* Endothelin-1 in acute heart failure: a significant predictor of outcome mediating the differential effect of high-dose versus low dose endothelin antagonism. Results from the tezosentan dose finding study. Circulation 2003; 17: IV694 (Abstract).
68. Aronson D, Burger AJ. Neurohormonal prediction of mortality following admission for decompensated heart failure. Am J Cardiol 2003; 91: 245–248.

CHAPTER 3

Clinical profile of the acute heart failure patient

Gregg C Fonarow, Kirkwood F Adams, Jr

Introduction

Heart failure is a chronic, progressive disease accounting for substantial morbidity and mortality.[1] There are currently 5 million Americans with chronic heart failure and these patients are at significant risk for decompensation and resulting hospitalization.[2] In the United States, hospitalizations for acute heart failure (AHF) have increased from 377 000 in 1979 to 999 000 in 2000.[2] AHF has emerged as a major public health problem and heart failure has become the leading cause of hospitalization in persons over 65 years of age.[1] It is estimated that there are 6.5 million hospital days attributed to AHF each year. For heart failure care, the major expenditure is on hospitalizations, with an estimated $12.7 billion spent on the inpatient management of AHF.[2] Patients hospitalized with AHF face a substantial risk of readmission, as high as 50% by 6 months after discharge.[3]

Until recently, the characteristics, management, and outcomes of patients hospitalized with AHF have been poorly defined, despite the high prevalence and public health importance of this syndrome. The clinical profile of these patients has been characterized by the description of patients enrolled in the relatively small number of clinical trials, retrospective analyses of hospital records, and administrative data sets.[1] A few single-center studies and multicenter registries have also evaluated patients hospitalized for AHF. Data from these studies have been potentially misleading because the included patients do not now appear representative of the patients routinely seen in clinical practice. Clinical trials typically enroll patients who are younger, have fewer comorbidities, and whose AHF is due to systolic dysfunction.[4,5] This profile is strikingly different from what has been observed in community cohorts and administrative datasets.[4] Data from national death indices or data captured from death certificates, neither of which are truly reliable data sources, are not truly helpful in that only very limited clinical and diagnostic data can be derived. Data collected from post-hoc review of patient charts at single referral centers are potentially biased towards inclusion of sicker patients referred for enrollment in clinical trials or evaluation for heart transplantation; thus they are not necessarily representative of the true cohort of patients hospitalized with AHF. As a result, data on characteristics and management of AHF patients have been incomplete. Recently, however, national registries have been created and detailed studies of Medicare datasets have been conducted, providing a much more comprehensive picture of the characteristics and outcomes of patients hospitalized with AHF.[6–9]

Characteristics of Patients Hospitalized with Acute Heart Failure

Clinical trials

In contrast to the large number of clinical trials on outpatients with chronic heart failure, there have been relatively few trials on patients hospitalized with AHF. Recent multicenter clinical trials have provided insights into the characteristics of patients hospitalized with AHF.[10,11] The Outcomes of a Prospective Trial of Intravenous Milrinone for Exacerbations of Chronic Heart Failure (OPTIME-CHF) evaluated 951 patients admitted with acute decompensated heart failure (ADHF) who were not in cardiogenic shock and randomized them to a 48-hour infusion of milrinone versus placebo added to usual care.[10] In this trial, the patients treated with milrinone fared worse than those receiving placebo and experienced a much higher incidence of atrial and ventricular arrhythmias, worsening heart failure, and a worrisome trend towards worse survival. The Vasodilation in the Management of Acute Congestive Heart Failure (VMAC) trial compared the hemodynamic and clinical response of intravenous nesiritide added to standard medical therapy with nitroglycerin and standard medical treatment in 498 patients from 55 centers in the United States.[11] There was a statistically significant benefit in the relief of dyspnea at 3 hours and a greater and more rapid sustained reduction in pulmonary capillary wedge pressures in instrumented patients.

The characteristics of patients enrolled in VMAC and OPTIME-CHF are shown in Table 3.1. In VMAC, the mean age was 62 years.[11] All patients had dyspnea at rest, or New York Heart Association (NYHA) class IV symptoms, at study entry; 84% had chronic decompensated heart failure that was classified as NYHA class III or class IV prior to decompensation; and most had clinical evidence of fluid overload (jugular venous distention [JVD] in 89%, rales in 73%, and pedal edema in 73%). Other important baseline clinical findings included an acute coronary syndrome in 12%, preserved systolic function (PSF) (ejection fraction [EF] > 40%) in 15%, renal insufficiency (serum creatinine ≥ 2.0 mg/dL) in 21%, and diabetes in 47%. Many patients had a history of significant arrhythmias including atrial fibrillation or atrial fibrillation/flutter (35%), nonsustained ventricular tachycardia (22%), sudden death (8%), ventricular fibrillation (6%), and sustained ventricular tachycardia (13%). The mean left ventricular ejection fraction (LVEF) was 27%. Mean systolic blood pressure at trial entry was 121 mm Hg.[11]

In OPTIME-CHF the mean age was 65 years.[10] At study entry, 47% of patients had dyspnea at rest (NYHA class IV symptoms). Most had clinical evidence of fluid overload with JVD in 73%, rales in 81%, and S3 in 58%. There was an ischemic etiology for heart failure in 51% of patients. Past medical history included hypertension in 67%, history of myocardial infarction (MI) in 48%, chronic lung disease in 23%, and diabetes in 44%. There was atrial fibrillation history in 32% of patients. The mean LVEF was 24%. Mean systolic blood pressure at trial entry was 120 mm Hg and mean serum creatinine was 1.5 mg/dL.[10]

The characteristics of patients in clinical trials appear to differ significantly from patients in community-based cohorts and national hospital registries.[4] The patients with AHF enrolled in these clinical trials have a mean age of 60 to 66 years, which is similar to outpatient trials. In contrast, national registries of hospitalized patients with AHF enrolled patients who were on average 10 years older. In the AHF trials, 69% to 71% of patients were men, similar to a review of 18 clinical outpatient chronic heart failure trials that included more than 1000 patients in which the percentage of male subjects was 60% to 89%. In contrast, in the registry population, 51% to 58% of the subjects were female. The prevalence of comorbid conditions such as hypertension, diabetes, atrial fibrillation, and ischemic heart disease also varied.[4]

National Heart Failure Study

The National Heart Failure Study described a contemporary national sample of elderly patients hospitalized with AHF.[8] The charts of 800 Medicare patients per state who were hospitalized with a principal diagnosis of heart failure between April 1998 and March 1999 were studied. There were

Table 3.1. *Characteristics of patients in acute heart failure clinical trials*

Characteristic	VMAC* (n = 489)	OPTIME-CHF† (n = 949)
Demographics		
Age (yr)	60(13) 62(15)*	66 (14)/65(15)†
White (%)	58	65
Black (%)	24	33
Female (%)	31	29
Heart Failure History		
NYHA Class II (%)	8	7
NYHA Class III (%)	42	46
NYHA IV (%)	42	47
Prior Hospitalizations	NA	1.9 (2.0)/2.1 (2.2)† (last year)
Left Ventricular Ejection Fraction		
EF (pre-hospital)	27 (14)	24 (8)
% EF ≥ 40% (pre-hospital)	13.3	NA
Medical History		
Coronary Artery Disease (%)	65	NA
Hypertension (%)	70	68
Myocardial Infarction (%)	46	48
Diabetes Mellitus (%)	47	44
Renal Insufficiency (%)	NA	NA
Ventricular Tachycardia (%)	13 (sustained)	NA
Ventricular Fibrillation (%)	6	NA
Atrial Fibrillation (%)	35	32
Baseline Medications		
ACE Inhibitors (%)	60	70
Diuretics (%)	86	90
Beta-Blockers (%)	33	22
Angiotensin Receptor Blockers (%)	10	13
Nitrates (%)	35	NA
Antiarrhythmics (%)	21	NA
Digoxin (%)	61	73
Physical and Laboratory Findings		
Systolic Blood Pressure, mm Hg	121 (22)	120 (18)/120(19)†
Serum Creatinine, mg/dL	NA	1.5 (0.5)/1.4(0.5)†
% Serum Creatinine > 2 mg/dL	21	NA

Data are expressed as mean (± SD), unless otherwise indicated.
*Based on data from the three treatment groups in the VMAC trial.[10]
†Data presented as placebo (n = 472)/milrinone (n = 477) for the OPTIME-CHF trial,[4] which excluded patients with serum creatinine > 3.0 mg/dL.
Abbreviations: ACE = angiotensin-converting enzyme; EF = ejection fraction; NA = not applicable, not assessed, or not reported; NYHA = New York Heart Association; OPTIME-CHF = Outcomes of a Prospective Trial of Intravenous Milrinone for Exacerbations of Chronic Heart Failure; SD = standard deviation; VMAC = Vasodilation in the Management of Acute Congestive Heart Failure trial.

34 587 patients in the sample, after the exclusion of patients who were < 65 years old, repeat discharges, discharged to another acute care facility or against medical advice, or receiving long-term hemodialysis.[8] The data set was analyzed for age-related trends in clinical characteristics.

The characteristics of these elderly hospitalized AHF patients are shown in Table 3.2. Mean age was 79 years with 49.2% of patients being age 80 or above.[8] In marked contrast to clinical trials, in this cohort 58.4% of hospitalized AHF patients were female. Comorbidities were very common in this

Table 3.2. *Characteristics of elderly patients hospitalized with acute heart failure in the National Heart Failure Study*

Variable	Value	No. of patients (%)
Age, yr (median, IQR)	79 (73, 85)	34 587 (100)
Sex (female) (%)	58.4	34 585 (100)
Ethnicity (%)		31 142 (90.0)
White	78.7	
African-American	9.2	
Other nonwhite	2.2	
Hispanic	3.2	
EF (mean %)	39	17 684 (51.1)
EF > 40% (%)	30.7	21 367 (61.8)
Laboratory		
Sodium (mmol/L)	138.5	33 784 (97.7)
Potassium (mmol/L)‡	4.2	30 689 (88.7)
BUN (mg/dL)	30.2	33 583 (97.1)
Creatinine (mg/dL)‡	1.5	29 403 (85.0)
Bilirubin (mg/dL)	0.8	19 597 (56.7)
Albumin (g/dL)	3.4	19 728 (57.0)
Cholesterol (mg/dL)	172.9	6 354 (18.4)
Left bundle branch block (%)	15.3	32 270 (93.3)
Most frequent comorbidities (%)		
Hypertension	60.6	34 587 (100)
CAD	55.7	34 587 (100)
Diabetes mellitus	38.1	34 587 (100)
COPD	32.9	34 587 (100)
Atrial fibrillation	29.5	32 270 (93.3)
Other comorbidities (%)		
History of stroke	18.0	34 587 (100)
Current smoker	8.8	32 629 (94.4)
Dementia	9.2	33 842 (87.6)
Admitted from LTC facility	10.0	36 412 (97.8)

Abbreviations: CAD = coronary artery disease; COPD = chronic obstructive pulmonary disease; EF = ejection fraction; IQR = interquartile range; LTC = long-term care.

*Number of patients ≥ 65 years old for whom data were available from the 34 587 charts abstracted.

‡The combination of measured and narrative information on EF provides sufficient data to determine whether EF is above or below 0.40 for 62% of the sample population.

patient cohort. About one-third of patients had chronic obstructive pulmonary disease (COPD), about 40% had diabetes, more than half had coronary heart disease (CHD), and more than half had a history of hypertension, but comorbidity rates declined with age. LVEF was < 40% in only 50.4% of patients in whom it was assessed. Patients > 80 years of age were less likely to have an underlying condition such as hypertension or coronary disease explaining the presence of heart failure (Table 3.3). Associated laboratory abnormalities were relatively constant across the age spectrum.[4] Very elderly patients with heart failure had similar serum creatinine levels to those aged 65 to 70 years. The likelihood that patients were in long-term care facilities before admission rose quite steeply with age.

These data demonstrate that elderly patients with AHF are a heterogeneous group and appear to differ substantially from patients enrolled in clinical trials. These AHF patients had more comorbid conditions, worse renal function, and more heart failure with preserved left ventricular (LV) systolic function than AHF patients enrolled in clinical trials. Little to no information was available in this data set regarding symptoms or physical examination at the time of presentation or during hospitalization.

Acute Decompensated Heart Failure Registry

The Acute Decompensated Heart Failure National Registry (ADHERE™) was developed as a large national multicenter observational study of characteristics, patterns of care, and outcomes of patients hospitalized with AHF to better define and improve the care of these patients.[9] The ADHERE™ Registry provides the most current and comprehensive analysis of the characteristics of patients hospitalized with AHF to date. The first patient was enrolled in the ADHERE™ Registry in October 2001. As of January 2004, over 100 000 patients have been enrolled through 263 participating academic and community hospitals. Representative hospitals from across the United States, including large and small, academic and community sites, were invited to participate. Patients were eligible for enrollment if they were admitted to the acute care hospital and had a discharge diagnosis of heart failure. This large database allows for subgroup analysis that typical clinical trials cannot accurately assess due to limited study size and population. Information on patient characteristics, treatments, and outcomes from initial presentation, throughout the hospitalization, and at discharge are entered into the ADHERE™ Registry database using a web-based electronic data capture (EDC) system via an electronic case report form. Timing of therapy is captured as well as clinical status at admission and discharge. Data reported in this chapter include enrollments from April 1, 2002, through March 31, 2003, as reported in the *ADHERE™ 3rd Quarter 2003 National Benchmark Report* (available at www.adhereregistry.com).

Demographic characteristics and medical history of ADHERE™ Registry patients (n = 52 047) are presented in Table 3.4. The mean age of patients was 75.2 years and more than half (52%) were female. Most patients were either white (73%) or black (19%), and most (78%) were covered by Medicare or Medicaid. The majority of hospitalized AHF patients (75%) had a history of heart failure. For 44% of patients, the number of prior hospitalizations for heart failure in the previous 6 months was not documented in the medical record. However, 23% of patients had documentation of hospitalization with this diagnosis within the prior 6 months. In that same period, 3% of patients had three or more heart failure-related hospitalizations (Table 3.4).

The combination of medical history, hospitalization history, and clinical presentation reveals that this population of heart failure patients is quite ill (Tables 3.4 and 3.5). At hospital admission, 72% of patients had a history of hypertension and 50% of AHF patients had a systolic blood pressure > 140 mm Hg. Several other conditions were common in the medical history of these patients. These include coronary artery disease (CAD) (58%), diabetes (44%), atrial fibrillation (31%), and COPD or asthma (31%), and chronic renal insufficiency (29%). Renal dysfunction is emerging as a critical feature of patients hospitalized with heart failure, as 29% of hospitalized AHF patients have a history of chronic renal insufficiency.

Table 3.3. *Characteristics in elderly patients hospitalized with acute heart failure in the National Heart Failure Study analyzed by age group*

	Age group						
	Total	**65-70**	**71-75**	**76-80**	**81-85**	**≥86†**	***P****
Total no.	20 388	3335	4102	4737	4213	3980	—
Men	8 834	1706	2040	2178	1684	1226	—
Women	11 553	1649	2062	2559	2529	2754	—
Female sex (%)	57	49	50	54	60	69	<0.0001
Race (%)							
White	85	78	83	87	88	89	
African-American	10	6	11	9	9	7	
Other	4	6	5	4	3	3	<0.0001
Cardiac history (%)							
Coronary disease	58	61	61	60	57	48	<0.0001
Myocardial infarction	31	34	34	34	29	27	<0.0001
Prior revascularization	29	37	36	33	26	12	<0.0001
Hypertension	64	65	65	65	63	60	<0.0001
Atrial fibrillation	31	24	29	32	34	37	<0.0001
Stroke	17	15	17	18	18	17	0.001
Other history (%)							
Chronic obstructive lung disease	32	36	38	33	30	22	<0.0001
Diabetes	38	51	46	41	32	22	<0.0001
Exclusionary comorbidity†	10	5	7	9	12	15	<0.001
Laboratory data							
Creatinine (mg/dL, mean)	1.7 ± 1.0	1.7 ± 1.0	1.7 ± 1.1	1.7 ± 1.0	1.7 ± 0.9	1.7 ± 0.8	NS
Potassium (mmol/L, median)	4.6	4.5	4.5	4.6	4.5	4.6	NS
Preserved left ventricular systolic function (%)							
Total	46	41	43	45	47	54	<0.0001
Men	35	31	34	34	36	43	0.0001
Women	55‡	51	52	54	54	60	0.0001

*P-value for trend across age groups.
†Dementia, metastatic malignancy, or hepatic failure.
‡$P < 0.0001$ compared to men.
With permission from Masoudi *et al.*[4]

Upon admission, most patients presented with dyspnea (89%, with dyspnea at rest in 36%), rales (67%), or peripheral edema (66%). Symptoms of fatigue were documented in 33% of patients. NYHA functional status was assessed and documented in the medical record in only 10% of patients. In those patients where NYHA was documented, 50% were reported to be class IV and 40%

Table 3.4. *Demographic characteristics and medical history of ADHERE™ enrollees*

Characteristics	No. of Patients (%) (n = 52047)
Median Age (yr)	75.2
Gender	
Male (%)	48
Female (%)	52
Race/Ethnicity	
Asian (%)	< 1
Black (%)	19
Hispanic (%)	2
White (%)	73
Other (%)	1
Primary Insurance	
Medicare (%)	72
Medicaid (%)	6
Commercial FFS/PPO (%)	8
HMO (%)	8
None/Self-Pay (%)	3
VA/Champus (%)	1
Other (%)	2
In Experimental Trial (%)	1
Heart Failure History	
Prior Heart Failure (%	75
Pre-hospital LVEF Assessed (%)	44 (n = 22857)
< 40% or Moderate-Severe Impairment (%)	59
Prior Cardiac Transplant	< 1
Listed for Cardiac Transplant (%)	1
Hospitalized for HF in Last 6 Months	
None (%)	9
1 Hospitalization (%)	15
2 Hospitalizations (%)	5
3 or More Hospitalizations (%)	3
No Mention of Hospitalizations (%)	44
Not Applicable, No History of HF (%)	25

Table 3.4. *continued*

Characteristics	No. of Patients (%) (n = 52047)
NYHA Class Assessed (%)	7 (n = 3849)
Baseline NYHA CLASS II (%)	21
Baseline NYHA CLASS III (%)	42
Baseline NYHA CLASS IV (%)	34
Medical History	
Coronary Artery Disease (%)	58
Myocardial Infarction (%)	32
Hypertension (%)	72
Hyperlipidemia/Dyslipidemia (%)	34
Cardiac Valvular Disease (%)	23
Stroke or TIA (%)	17
Atrial Fibrillation (%)	31
Ventricular Tachycardia (%)	8
Ventricular Fibrillation (%)	1
Pacemaker or ICD (%)	20
LVAD (%)	< 1
IABP (%)	< 1
Peripheral Vascular Disease (%)	18
Chronic Renal Insufficiency (%)	29
Chronic Dialysis (%)	5
Diabetes (%)	44
Insulin-Dependent Diabetes (%)	18
Liver Disease (%)	3
Thyroid Disease (%)	17
COPD or Asthma (%)	31
Active Malignancy (%)	5
Ever Smoked (%)	48
Current Smoker (%)	13

Abbreviations:
COPD = chronic obstructive pulmonary disease;
FFS = fee-for-service;
HF = heart failure;
HMO = health maintenance organization;
IABP = intraaortic balloon pump;
ICD = implantable cardioverter defibrillator;
LVAD = left ventricular assist device;
LVEF = left ventricular ejection fraction;
NYHA = New York Heart Association;
PPO = preferred provider organization;
TIA = transient ischemic attack;
VA = Veterans Affairs.

Table 3.5. *Clinical presentation and admitting diagnosis of ADHERE™ enrollees*

Symptom or Sign	No. of Patients (%) (n = 52 047)
Any Dyspnea	89
Dyspnea at Rest	36
Fatigue	33
Rales	67
Peripheral Edema	66
NYHA Class Assessed	10 (n = 5003)
Class II	9
Class III	40
Class IV	50
Systolic Blood Pressure Assessed	100 (n = 51 812)
SBP < 90 mm Hg	3
SBP 90-140 mm Hg	47
SBP > 140 mm Hg	50
Initial ECG Assessed	94 (n = 49 091)
Atrial Fibrillation	20
Other Abnormal Rhythm	26
Initial CXR Assessed	90 (n = 47 072)
Pulmonary Congestion	76
Initial Serum Sodium Assessed	98 (n = 51 109)
Sodium < 130 mmol/L	5
Mean Serum Sodium (mmol/L)	138
Initial Serum Creatinine Assessed	98 (n = 51 134)
Creatinine > 2.0 mg/dL	20
Initial BNP Assessed	30 (n = 15 850)
Median BNP (pg/mL)	839
LVEF Assessed	56 (n = 29 371)
< 40% or Moderate/Severe Impairment	47
Admitting Diagnoses	
Heart Failure	93
MI or Unstable Angina	4
Arrhythmia	3
Respiratory Infection	5
COPD/Asthma	12
Renal Insufficiency or Failure	14

Abbreviations: BNP = B-type natriuretic peptide; COPD = chronic obstructive pulmonary disease; CXR = chest x-ray; ECG = electrocardiogram; LVEF = left ventricular ejection fraction; MI = myocardial infarction; NYHA = New York Heart Association; SBP = systolic blood pressure.

were class III. The admitting diagnoses included heart failure in 93% of patients (Table 3.5).

An initial electrocardiogram (ECG) was assessed in 94% of patients and 20% of patients were in atrial fibrillation. An initial chest x-ray (CXR) was assessed in 90% of AHF patients and was interpreted as showing pulmonary congestion in 76%. The mean serum sodium on admission was 138 mmol/L with 5% of patients having sodium levels < 130 mmol/L. Upon hospitalization, 20% of AHF patients in the ADHERE™ trial had serum creatinine > 2.0 mg/dL and 14% had an admitting diagnosis of renal insufficiency or failure. Initial B-type natriuretic peptide (BNP) levels were assessed in 30% of patients and the mean level was 839 pg/mL.

There are significant differences in the clinical characteristics of AHF patients by gender, race and ethnicity. Data from these ADHERE™ AHF patients were analyzed according to gender.[12] Women accounted for 52% of admissions for AHF. There was no difference in race between the genders (Table 3.6). Women hospitalized with AHF were, however, older than men (mean age 74.6 years vs. 70.2 years; $P < 0.0001$). Based on their medical history, women were more likely to have a history of hypertension as compared with men (75% vs. 69%, $P < 0.0001$). CAD was more common in men than in women (64% vs. 51%, $P < 0.0001$).[12] Other risk factors for atherosclerosis, including smoking (17% vs. 10%, $P < 0.0001$), and hyperlipidemia (37% vs. 32%, $P < 0.0001$) were also more common in men than in women. The same percentage (44%) of men and women had diabetes. The incidence of atrial fibrillation was similar between the genders (31% of men, 30% of women). However, a history of prior ventricular arrhythmias was more common in men than in women (13% vs. 5%, $P < 0.0001$).

There were significant gender differences in clinical characteristics at presentation (Table 3.6). There were also differences in vital signs and laboratory values. Women had higher initial mean systolic blood pressures than men (148.4 mm Hg vs. 139.5 mm Hg, $P < 0.0001$). A significantly greater percentage of women had hemoglobin values < 12 g/dL than did men (51% and 39%, $P < 0.0001$). Mean hemoglobin values were

Table 3.6. *Clinical characteristics for acute heart failure analyzed by gender in ADHERE™*

Clinical characteristic	Men (n = 41 276)	Women (n = 44 340)	*P* value
Age (yr), mean	70.2 ± 13.9	74.6 ± 13.7	< 0.0001
LVEF (%), mean	32.9 ± 15.7	42.1 ±17.3	< 0.0001
EF > 40% (%)	28	51	< 0.0001
Atrial Fibrillation (%)	31	30	0.0040
CAD (%)	64	51	< 0.0001
Current Smoker (%)	17	10	< 0.0001
Diabetes Mellitus (%)	44	44	0.0434
Hyperlipidemia (%)	37	32	< 0.0001
Hypertension (%)	69	75	< 0.0001
ICD (%)	9	3	< 0.0001
Pacemaker (%)	19	14	< 0.0001
Renal Insufficiency (%)	33	27	< 0.0001
Thyroid Disease (%)	11	23	< 0.0001
Ventricular Tachycardia/ Fibrillation (%)	13	5	< 0.0001
Physical examination			
Mean SBP (mm Hg)	139.5 ± 322	148.4 ± 32.5	< 0.0001
Mean Pulse (bpm)	87.9 ± 21.6	89.1 ± 22	< 0.0001
Dyspnea (%)	89	90	< 0.0001
Edema (%)	67	65	< 0.0001
Fatigue (%)	33	32	0.0927
Rales (%)	66	70	< 0.0001
Mean QRS (ms/min)	119.9 ± 44.6	107.6 ± 42	< 0.0001
QRS > 120 (%)	39	28	< 0.0001
Chest X-ray Congestion (%)	66	70	< 0.0001
Pulmonary Edema (%)	84	86	< 0.0001
Laboratory results			
Mean BUN (mg/dL)	33.3 ± 21.9	3.3 ± 2.1	< 0.0001
Mean Creatinine (mg/dL)	1.9 ± 1.7	1.6 ± 1.5	< 0.0001
Mean Creatinine Clearance (calculated) (mL/min)	169.9 ± 188.5	118.5 ± 145.3	0.0005
Sodium < 130 mmol/L (%)	4	5	< 0.0001
Mean Hemoglobin (g/dL)	12.8 ± 2.7	12.1 ± 2.5	< 0.0001
Mean Hemoglobin < 12 g/dL (%)	39	51	< 0.0001

Abbreviations: bpm = beats per minute; BUN = blood urea nitrogen; CAD = coronary artery disease; EF = ejection fraction; ICD = implantable cardioverter defibrillator; LVEF = left ventricular ejection fraction; SBP = systolic blood pressure.

12.1 g/dL for women and 12.8 g/dL for men (*P* < 0.0001). Mean creatinine was 1.9 mg/dL in men and 1.6 mg/dL in women, and 24% of men had a creatinine level of > 2.0 mg/dL as compared with only 17% of women (*P* < 0.0001). Nevertheless, calculated creatinine clearance was worse in women (118.5 mL/min vs. 169.6 mL/min, *P* < 0.0001). Information on LV function was available in 79% of patients. In the ADHERE™ population, the mean LVEF was 37.4%. but men had a significantly lower mean LVEF (32.9%) than women (42.1%; only 28% of men had preserved

LV function (EF > 40%) as compared with 51% of women ($P < 0.0001$).[12] Men had a higher incidence of ventricular dyssynchrony (defined as a QRS duration > 120 ms) than women (39% vs. 28%, $P < 0.0001$).

There were also significant differences in the clinical characteristics of AHF by race and ethnicity. African-American patients with AHF were more likely to have a non-ischemic etiology and to be younger compared to Caucasian patients.[13]

Treatment of Patients Hospitalized with Heart Failure

The Emergency Department (ED) is clearly the treatment location to which most AHF patients initially present. In ADHERE™, 77% of all patients who were admitted for an acute episode of congestive heart failure initially presented to the ED, while 21% went directly to an inpatient unit.[14] An additional 2% were admitted to an inpatient unit on observation and less than 1% of patients were seen in an observation unit as their first point of care. Once hospitalized, only 14% of patients were admitted directly to an intensive care unit (ICU) setting. The vast majority of hospital care for heart failure was provided in telemetry (66%) and step down units (7%).

There are striking differences in the timing of the initiation of treatment between EDs and inpatient units. When diuretics are started in the ED, the mean door-to-needle time is 2.0 hours. If the diuretic is not started until the patient is admitted to an inpatient setting, the mean time to initiation of treatment is 7.7 hours. In ADHERE™, 64% of patients received intravenous diuretic therapy alone. Intravenous vasoactive therapy was used in 27% of all admissions. If intravenous vasoactive therapy is not started until after admission to an inpatient unit, the door-to-needle time is over 23 hours; whereas, if it is started in the ED, the time to treatment is 2 hours. When intravenous vasoactive therapy is initiated, the duration of therapy is approximately 3 days.[14]

Procedures occurring during hospitalization for AHF are shown in Table 3.7. Invasive hemodynamic monitoring was utilized in only 5% of the

Table 3.7. *Events and procedures during hospital stay for acute heart failure in ADHERE™*

Event or Procedure	All Patients % (n = 46 599)	ICCU/CCU Patients %* (n = 9110)
Death	4.1	10.8
Defibrillation or CPR	2	6
Mechanical Ventilation	5	24
Intraaortic Balloon Pump	1	2
PA Catheter	5	17
Dialysis	5	8
New Onset Dialysis	1	3
EP Study	4	6
Cardiac Catheterization	11	20
With PCI†	81	78
Without PCI†	19	22

Abbreviations: CCU = critical care unit; CPR = cardiopulmonary resuscitation; EP = electrophysiological study; ICU = intensive care unit; PA = pulmonary artery; PCI = percutaneous coronary intervention.
*Reflects events and procedures that occurred in patients who spent time in the ICU/CCU. The events and procedures recorded did not necessarily occur in the ICU/CCU.
†Of those who had cardiac catheterization.

hospitalizations. Diagnostic catheterization occurred in 11% of patients, with the majority of those who underwent catheterization also undergoing percutaneous coronary intervention (PCI). Electrophysiologic study was preformed in 4% of patients. Mechanical ventilation was required in 5% of patients. While 5% of patients had dialysis performed during hospitalization, in only 1% was this newly performed. The frequency of procedures is higher in patients hospitalized in the ICU, but interestingly the majority of patients hospitalized in the ICU were not mechanically ventilated nor invasively monitored (Table 3.7).

During the course of hospitalization, there was some improvement in chronic heart failure treatment regimens prior to discharge. Pre-hospitalization use of angiotensin-converting enzyme (ACE) inhibitor use (41%) or beta-blocker use (47%) increased to 55% and 58%, respectively, upon discharge from the hospital. Confining the analysis to the 12 754 patients with documented LVEF < 40%, beta-blockers were newly started in 27% of patients during the hospitalization, ACE inhibitors in 28%, and angiotensin receptor blockers (ARBs) in 4%.

In AHF patients with documented measurement of LV function, fully 49% of patients had PSF (LVEF ≥ 40%). These patients were older (76.3 years), more likely to be female (62%), and more likely to have a history of hypertension (77%) or diabetes (45%) than patients with reduced systolic function. More details on the characteristics of these patients is provided the "Acute Heart Failure and Preserved Systolic Function" section of this chapter.

Clinical Outcomes of Patients Hospitalized with Heart Failure

Hospital course and symptomatic status

In ADHERE™, 23% of patients received care in the ICU or critical care unit (CCU) and the median length of stay in the ICU or CCU was 2.5 days. The median length of stay in the hospital for all hospitalized patients was 4.1 days. Upon discharge, 44% of patients were asymptomatic. However, 30% were improved but still symptomatic. Less than 1% of patients were worse or had no change and 11% had no mention of status at discharge.

Hospital discharge and mortality outcomes

Patient outcomes varied tremendously. Some 63% of patients were discharged home and an additional 12% went home with additional care. Other patients were transferred to other hospitals (2%) or outpatient care (1%) or had unknown status (2%), and 16% went to hospice care. The in-hospital mortality rate was 4.1%. This mortality rate is well above that reported in heart failure clinical trials. In OPTIME-CHF, the inpatient mortality rate was 2.3% in the placebo plus standard care group.[10]

Mortality was significantly higher in men than in women (4.5% vs. 3.9%; $P = 0.0042$). This observation may be explained by the greater incidence in men of systolic dysfunction (25% of men had LVEF > 40% vs. 45% of women; $P < 0.0001$) and CAD (66% vs. 53%; $P < 0.0001$), which harbors a worse prognosis. One unexpected finding showed that, although African-American patients had greater renal insufficiency, advanced LV dysfunction, and evidence of pulmonary congestion, they had significantly better outcomes than non-African Americans.[13] Compared with non-African-American patients, mortality was more than 2-fold lower, and hospital stays were shorter ($P < 0.0001$ for both).

Outcome data on patients enrolled into the ADHERE™ database demonstrate that admission for heart failure is a high-risk event for patients, with death or significant adverse consequences for many. Treatment strategies that improve the outcome of ADHF should be identified and implemented in a very aggressive manner to address the striking risk of death observed in ADHERE™.

Performance Measures in Hospitalized Heart Failure Patients

ADHERE™ registry data on the Joint Commission on Accreditation of Healthcare Organizations

(JCAHO) Quality of Care Indicators show that only 30% of patients were receiving patient instructions on diet, weight monitoring, activity level, worsening symptoms, follow-up appointments, and medication management at discharge (JCAHO indicator HF-1).[9] Assessment of LV systolic function (HF-2) was either documented or scheduled in 83% of patients. Only 73% of eligible patients with LV systolic dysfunction received an ACE inhibitor at discharge (HF-3). Counseling on smoking cessation for current smokers (HF-4) was only given to 40% of eligible patients. These data suggest that there are substantial opportunities to improve the quality of care for patients hospitalized with AHF.

The combined findings of ADHERE™ and other studies of hospitalized patients with AHF regarding compliance with JCAHO heart failure care indicators, in-hospital mortality rate, significant morbidity, less than optimal treatment patterns, and the impact of early appropriate treatment on outcomes demonstrate the need for quality care improvements and interventions.

Outcome After Hospital Discharge

Clinical trials and registry data demonstrate that after AHF hospitalization patients are at particularly high risk for rehospitalization and mortality. For AHF patients, rehospitalization rates approach 50% at 6 months post-discharge.[3] In OPTIME-CHF, the 60-day death or rehospitalization rate was 35%.[10] In a large analysis of patients newly hospitalized with AHF in Canada, mortality rates were 11.6% and 30.1% at 30 days and 1 year post-hospitalization, respectively.[6] These rates are substantially higher than the annual mortality rates of 6% to 10% in stable ambulatory patients with chronic heart failure on beta-blockers and ACE inhibitors.[15]

Acute Heart Failure and Preserved Systolic Function (PSF)

An increasing number of patients hospitalized for AHF are found to have a normal or mildly reduced LVEF. The cause of AHF in these patients is thought to be related to LV diastolic dysfunction, though a number of mechanisms have been considered. The clinical profile of these patients has been characterized by retrospective analyses of hospital records and state data banks. A few single-center studies and multicenter registries have also evaluated patients hospitalized for heart failure with normal EF.[16] The characteristics of these patients from hospitalized cohorts were described in a recent review by Hogg *et al.*[17]

The proportion of patients hospitalized with AHF having PSF ranged from 24% to 55% (mean 41%).[17] These patients were older than those with reduced systolic function and were more likely to be female. MI (or any evidence of CHD) was much less common in patients with PSF than in those with reduced systolic function. Other evidence of atherosclerotic disease was also less common. Conversely, hypertension was more common in patients with PSF. In a multivariate analysis, Masoudi *et al.* reported that a history of hypertension was an independent predictor of PSF in patients hospitalized with AHF.[18] The incidence of atrial fibrillation was also more frequent in subjects with PSF, occurring in a quarter to a third of patients. In the Italian Network on Congestive Heart Failure (IN-CHF) registry, 16% of low LVEF patients had atrial fibrillation, compared to 25% of patients with an LVEF > 45%.[19] This raises the possibility that atrial fibrillation may be more likely to be a primary cause of AHF in patients with PSF, rather than a secondary problem. Diabetes mellitus was also common in both types of AHF.[17] However, this comorbidity was not more frequent in patients with PSF in many studies. Chronic lung disease was more common in patients with PSF, raising the concern of misdiagnosis. There was no clear difference in the frequency of renal impairment, creatinine concentration, or creatinine clearance between patients with AHF and PSF, and those with reduced systolic function.[17,18]

Patients with PSF have a better survival than patients with reduced systolic function at all time points from admission. Nevertheless, patients with PSF still have a high mortality following hospital admission, with rates of 40% to 50% after 4 to 5 years.[17] It is important to note that readmission rates in patients with PSF are very high, with 15%

to 25% of patients being readmitted within 6 months. The rehospitalization rates for any reason are 45% to 60% at 1 year.[17] It is clear that AHF, with or without reduced systolic function, has a poor prognosis. Philbin *et al.* showed that the 6-month rate of death or readmission was 50% in patients with PSF and 52% in those with reduced systolic function.[20]

In ADHERE™, among the 82% of patients with documented measurement of LV function, 49% of patients had PSF (LVEF > 40%). These patients were older (76.3 years), more likely to be female (62%) and more likely to have a history of hypertension (77%) or diabetes (45%) than patients with reduced systolic function.

A recent prospective registry provided additional information on this patient cohort. The New York Heart Failure Registry conducted a prospective multicenter registry in a large metropolitan area to define the clinical characteristics, hospital course, treatment, and factors precipitating decompensation in patients hospitalized for heart failure with a normal EF.[16] Patients hospitalized for heart failure at 24 medical centers in the New York metropolitan area and found to have a LVEF of > 50% within 7 days of admission were included in this registry. Of 619 patients, 73% were women, who were on average 4 years older than men (72.8 ± 14.1 years vs. 68.6 ± 13.8 years, $P < 0.001$). Black, non-Hispanic patients comprised 30% of the study population. They were 8 years younger than other patients (66.0 ± 14.2 years vs. 74 ± 13.5 years, $P < 0.001$). Comorbid conditions and their prevalence were: hypertension 78%, increased LV mass 82%, diabetes 46%, and obesity 46%. Before the clinical decompensation that precipitated hospitalization, 86% of patients had chronic symptoms compatible with NYHA functional class II to IV. Factors precipitating clinical decompensation were identified in 53% of patients. In-hospital mortality was 4.2%.

Conclusion

The national administrative databases and national registries are providing valuable information on current patient characteristics, management, and outcomes in an extensive and broad sample of patients who are hospitalized with AHF. There are substantial differences between these patient cohorts and those enrolled in clinical trials. A better understanding regarding the characteristics, treatments, and outcomes of patients hospitalized with AHF may help to delineate the best treatment practices. Important data on longitudinal trends in the characteristics, clinical care, and outcomes of patients admitted with heart failure are now being assessed. Because of the increasing burden of heart failure, further study and better understanding of the demographic variables, clinical characteristics, management, and outcomes of AHF are of critical importance.

References

1. Hunt SA, Baker DW, Chin MH, *et al.*, American College of Cardiology/American Heart Association. ACC/AHA guidelines for the evaluation and management of chronic heart failure in the adult: executive summary. A report of the American College of Cardiology/American Heart Association Task Force on Practice Guidelines (Committee to revise the 1995 Guidelines for the Evaluation and Management of Heart Failure). J Am Coll Cardiol 2001; 38: 2101–2113.
2. American Heart Association. Heart Disease and Stroke Statistics—2004 Update (American Heart Association: Dallas, TX, 2003).
3. Krumholz HM, Parent EM, Tu N, *et al.* Readmission after hospitalization for congestive heart failure among Medicare beneficiaries. Arch Intern Med 1997; 157: 99–104.
4. Masoudi FA, Havranek EP, Wolfe P, *et al.* Most hospitalized older persons do not meet the enrollment criteria for clinical trials in heart failure. Am Heart J 2003; 146: 250–257.
5. Krum H, Gilbert RE. Demographics and concomitant disorders in heart failure. Lancet 2003; 362: 147–158.
6. Jong P, Vowinckel E, Liu PP, Gong Y, Tu JV. Prognosis and determinants of survival in patients newly hospitalized for heart failure: a population-based study. Arch Intern Med 2002; 162: 1689–1694.
7. Baker DW, Einstadter D, Thomas C, Cebul RD. Mortality trends for 23505 Medicare patients hospitalized with heart failure in Northeast Ohio, 1991 to 1997. Am Heart J 2003; 146: 258–264.

8. Havranek EP, Masoudi FA, Westfall KA, *et al.* Spectrum of heart failure in older patients: results from the National Heart Failure project. Am Heart J 2002; 143: 412–417.
9. Fonarow GC, Adams K, Strausser PB. ADHERE™ (acutely decompensated heart failure national registry): rationale, design, and subject population. J Card Fail 2002; 8: S49 (Abstract).
10. Cuffe MS, Califf RM, Adams KF Jr., *et al.* Short-term intravenous milrinone for acute exacerbation of chronic heart failure: a randomized controlled trial. JAMA 2002; 287: 1541–1547.
11. Publication Committee for the VMAC Investigators (Vasodilation in the Management of Acute CHF): Intravenous nesiritide vs. nitroglycerin for treatment of decompensated congestive heart failure: a randomized controlled trial. JAMA 2002; 287: 1531–1540.
12. Moskowitz R, Galvao M, Galvin C, *et al.* Sex-based differences in patients hospitalized with acute decompensated heart failure. J Card Fail 2003; 9: S84 (Abstract).
13. Yancy CW, Chang SF. Better outcomes in heart failure in African Americans despite negative risk factors; a report from the ADHERE™ database. J Card Fail 2003; 9: S82 (Abstract).
14. Emerman CL, Peacock F, Fonarow GC. Effect of emergency department initiation of vasoactive infusion therapy on heart failure length of stay. Ann Emerg Med 2002; 40: S46 (Abstract).
15. Cohn JN, Tognoni G; Valsartan Heart Failure Trial Investigators. A randomized trial of the angiotensin-receptor blocker valsartan in chronic heart failure. N Engl J Med 2001; 345: 1667–1675.
16. Klapholz M, Maurer M, Lowe AM, *et al.*, New York Heart Failure Consortium. Hospitalization for heart failure in the presence of a normal left ventricular ejection fraction: results of the New York Heart Failure Registry. J Am Coll Cardiol 2004; 43: 1432–1438.
17. Hogg K, Swedberg K, McMurray J. Heart failure with preserved left ventricular systolic function; epidemiology, clinical characteristics, and prognosis. J Am Coll Cardiol 2004; 43: 317–327.
18. Masoudi FA, Havranek EP, Smith G, *et al.* Gender, age, and heart failure with preserved left ventricular systolic function. J Am Coll Cardiol 2003; 41: 217–223.
19. Tarantini L, Faggiano P, Senni M, *et al.* Clinical features and prognosis associated with a preserved left ventricular systolic function in a large cohort of congestive heart failure outpatients managed by cardiologists: data from the Italian Network on Congestive Heart Failure. Ital Heart J 2002; 3: 656–664.
20. Philbin EF, Rocco TA Jr., Lindenmuth NW, Ulrich K, Jenkins PL. Systolic versus diastolic heart failure in community practice: clinical features, outcomes, and the use of angiotensin-converting enzyme inhibitors. Am J Med 2000; 109: 605–613.

CHAPTER 4

Sex-related differences in heart failure

Jalal K Ghali

Introduction

A recent report entitled "Exploring the Biological Contributions to Human Health: Does Sex Matter?",[1] formulated by the Committee on Understanding the Biology of Sex and Gender Differences, proposed that cells from male and female organisms behave differently because of chromosomal and not necessarily hormonal influence, implying that every organ in the body, including the heart, had the potential to respond differently on the basis of sex.

Sex is defined as "The classification of living things, generally as male or female according to their reproductive organs and functions assigned by chromosomal complement"[1] and gender is defined as "A person's self-representation as male or female, or how that person is responded to by social institutions based on the individual's gender presentation."[1]

In the past two decades, women's health issues related to heart disease have received considerable interest. However, until recently, sex-related differences in patients with heart failure have received surprisingly little attention.[2–5] Under-representation of women in clinical trials has been a consistent finding in all heart failure trials and has resulted in a major limitation in our understanding of heart failure in women[2,3,6] (Table 4.1).[7–30] Furthermore, this limitation has been compounded by the tendency to extrapolate findings from heart failure clinical trials which were derived predominately from men and apply them to women.

This chapter reviews sex-related differences in epidemiology, pathophysiology, etiology, clinical characteristics, variables related to prognosis, outcome, and response to medications.

Epidemiology

The annual *Heart Disease and Stroke Statistics Update* prepared by the American Heart Association places the prevalence of heart failure at 4 900 000, including 2 400 000 males and 2 500 000 females.[31] A prevalence rate of 2.3% and 1.5% for white males and females, respectively, and 3.5% versus 3.1% for black males and females. This estimate is derived from the National Health and Nutrition Examination Survey (NHANES III), in which heart failure was self-reported among a sample of 39 695 individuals.[32,33] As documented in NHANES I,[34] conducted between 1971 and 1975, self-reported heart failure underestimated the presence of heart failure as validated by Framingham criteria by about 50%, a finding that led to the routine correction for under-reporting in self-reported studies. Recent data from the 1999 National Health Interview Survey[35] in which 30 801 adults were interviewed, estimated the prevalence of heart failure at 4 800 000. A higher prevalence in males was found only among persons

Table 4.1. *Age and sex in survival heart failure trials*

Trial	No. of patients	Age	No. of women (%)
Vasodilator Heart Failure Trial (V-HeFT) I[7]	642	58	—
Cooperative North Scandinavian Enalapril Survival Study (CONSENSUS)[8]	253	70	75 (30)
Vasodilator Heart Failure Trial (V-HeFT) II[9]	804	60	—
Studies of Left Ventricular Dysfunction Treatment (SOLVD-T)[10]	2569	61	504 (20)
Studies of Left Ventricular Dysfunction Prevention (SOLVD-P)[11]	4228	59	485 (11)
Prospective Randomized Milrinone Survival Evaluation Trial (PROMISE)[12]	1088	64	235 (22)
Congestive Heart Failure-Survival Trial of Antiarrhythmic Therapy (CHF-STAT)[13]	674	65	—
Prospective Randomized Amlodipine Survival Evaluation (PRAISE)[14]	1153	65	278 (24)
Flolan International Randomized Survival Trial (FIRST)[15]	471	65	112 (24)
Prospective Randomized Study of Ibopamine on Mortality and Efficacy (PRIME) II[16]	1906	65	374 (20)
Digitalis Investigation Group (DIG)[17]	6800	63	1519 (22)
Evaluation of Losartan in the Elderly (ELITE) I[18]	722	74	240 (33)
Vesnarinone Trial Investigators (VEST)[19]	3833	63	909 (23)
Cardiac Insufficiency Bisoprolol Study (CIBIS) II[20]	2647	61	515 (20)
Metoprolol Extended Release Randomized Intervention Trial in Heart Failure (MERIT-HF)[21]	3991	64	898 (23)
Assessment of Treatment with Lisinopril and Survival Study (ATLAS)[22]	3164	63	648 (20)
Randomized Aldactone Evaluation Study (RALES)[23]	1663	65	446 (27)
Evaluation of Losartan in the Elderly (ELITE) II[24]	3152	71	956 (30)
Beta-Blocker Evaluation of Survival Trial (BEST)[25]	2708	60	593 (22)
Valsartan Heart Failure Trial (Val-HEFT)[26]	5010	63	1002 (20)
Carvedilol Prospective Randomized Cumulative Survival Study (COPERNICUS)[27]	2289	66	465 (20)
Carvedilol or Metoprolol European Trial (COMET)[28]	3029	62	612 (20)
Candesartan in Heart Failure-Assessment of Reduction in Mortality and morbidity (CHARM)[29]	7599	66	2400 (32)
Comparison of Medical Therapy, Pacing, and Defibrillation in Chronic Heart Failure (COMPANION)[30]	1520	67	493 (32)
Total	64 967	64	14 649 (32)

aged 65 to 74 years (4.5% vs. 2.9%). The age-adjusted prevalence was 2.4% and 1.9% for white males and females, respectively, and 2.0% and 2.3% for black males and females.

In the Framingham Heart Study, 1075 heart failure cases developed among 10 333 participants over a 50-year period.[36] Although the incidence of heart failure changed little among men from the 1950s through the 1990s, it declined by one-third among women in the period from 1970 to 1999 as compared with 1950 to 1969. This finding is in contrast to the Rochester Epidemiology Project in which age- and sex-adjusted incidence of heart failure was not significantly different in the 1991 cohort (141 patients) compared with that in 1981 (107 patients).[37]

The Framingham data documented sex-related differences in the contribution of hypertension to heart failure, a 3-fold increase in the risk of developing heart failure in women compared to 2-fold increase in men.[38] Thus, the most plausible explanation for the disparity in heart failure incidence between the Framingham Study and the Rochester Project is the much longer duration of follow-up in the former, which permitted a much better control of blood pressure in the past three decades compared to the period from 1950 to 1969. The striking increase in the incidence of heart failure with aging has been well documented in all epidemiological studies, with the Framingham Study showing the incidence doubling each decade of life after age 45, and approaching 10 per 1000 population after age 65[39] (Figure 4.1). It is estimated that at

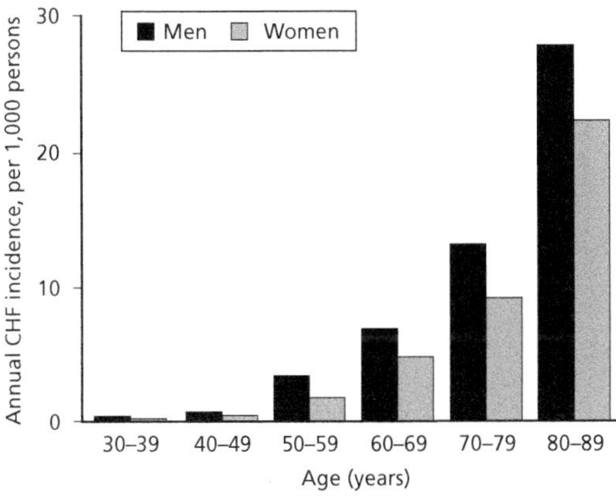

Figure 4.1. *Prevalence of heart failure by age and sex (The Framingham Study[39])*

age 40 years, the lifetime risk for developing heart failure is 21% for men and 20% for women.[40] A recent analysis of the National Hospital Discharge Survey (NHDS) showed that the increase in the rate of heart failure hospitalization over the period of 1990 to 1999 was confined to women but not to men, for whom the hospitalization rate was stable[41] (Figure 4.2).

Pathophysiology

The exclusive inclusion of patients with heart failure and impaired left ventricular ejection fraction (LVEF) into clinical trials led to the false impression that heart failure with preserved LVEF was rare. Currently, it has been well established that more than half the cases of heart failure in the community are associated with preserved LVEF.[42] Another consistent feature of all studies evaluating heart failure with preserved LVEF is the preponderance of women.[43] In the Framingham Heart Study, 65% of patients with heart failure and preserved LVEF were women,[44] a very similar figure to the 69% in the Rochester Epidemiology Project,[45] and the 67% in the Cardiovascular Health Study.[46] In the Strong Heart Study, the prevalence of patients with heart failure and preserved LVEF (defined as LVEF > 54%) who were women was 84%.[47]

In a recent study from a national sample of 37 500 Medicare beneficiaries hospitalized with heart failure,[48] left ventricular (LV) systolic function was assessed in 19 710 patients. Of those, preserved LVEF (as defined by LVEF > 50%) was present in 6700 (35%). The prevalence of women with heart

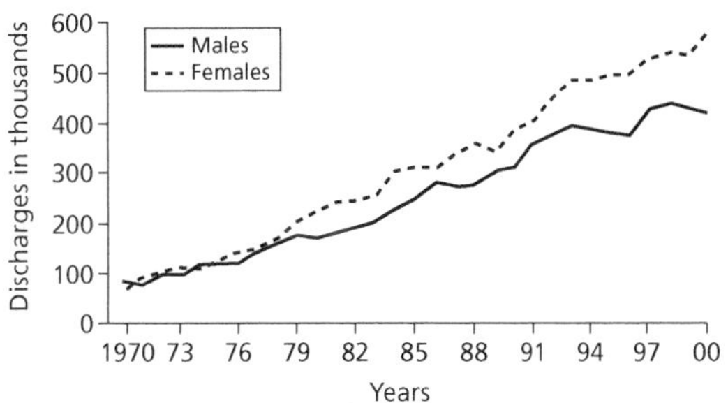

Figure 4.2. *NHANES III. Hospital discharges for heart failure by sex (1970–2000)*

failure and preserved LVEF was 79% compared to 49% in those with impaired LVEF. Not only was heart failure with preserved LVEF present almost twice as frequently in women as in men, but the strong association of female sex with preserved LVEF was persistent after adjustment for age.

The reasons for the preponderence of heart failure with preserved LVEF in women are not entirely clear. It is useful, however, to delineate some of the sex-related differences that could shed light on this issue. In a retrospective study of 586 women and 1081 men undergoing cardiac catheterization,[49] left ventricular end-diastolic volume (LVEDV) index was found to be lower in women, in spite of having similar left ventricular end-diastolic pressure (LVEDP), suggesting baseline differences in myocardial compliance or relaxation. Similarly, in elderly patients with aortic stenosis, women were found to have lower LV passive compliance than men, more concentric left ventricular hypertrophy (LVH), and better preserved LVEF as compared to men.[50] Higher LV systolic function has been reported in hypertensive women as compared to men.[51]

A better preservation of LV systolic function has been demonstrated in female rat hearts,[52] and in various models of heart failure including ischemic,[53] pressure overload,[54] or volume overload,[55] hearts in female rats showed a more favorable response to insult with development of appropriate hypertrophy, compared to significant dilatation in the hearts of male rats. Even when increased myocyte volume was noted in male and female decompensated hearts, myocyte volume was significantly larger in males at earlier stages, and reduced adaptive hypertrophy was noted only in males.[56]

An interaction of etiology was suggested by a study showing no sex-related differences in cellular remodeling among 50 patients with idiopathic cardiomyopathy, contrasted with significantly greater myocyte volume and length in males among 50 patients with ischemic cardiomyopathy.[57]

Clinical Characteristics

Sex-related differences in clinical characteristics of patients with heart failure and impaired LVEF were detailed in several reports (Figure 4.3, Table 4.2).[58–64]

In a study of a young population of 65 women and 238 men with idiopathic dilated cardiomyopathy (IDC), women were found to have higher a New York Heart Association (NYHA) class, larger cardiothoracic ratios, a higher prevalence of left bundle branch block (LBBB), and a shorter exercise duration.[58]

The University of North Carolina Heart Failure database included patients enrolled over a 10-year period with a documented assessment of LVEF.[59] Women (n = 177) were younger than men (n = 380), had a higher percentage of African Americans, were less likely to have ischemia or alcohol as an etiology, were more likely to have hypertension or valvular disease as an etiology, had a higher LVEF, and had a lower prevalence of atrial fibrillation.

The Flolan International Randomized Survival Trial (FIRST) enrolled 112 women and 359 men with advanced heart failure and a mean LVEF of 18%.[60] Women had a higher percentage of African Americans, lower prevalence of ischemia as an etiology, and higher heart rate. In the Cardiac Insufficiency Bisoprolol Study (CIBIS II), 2132 men and 515 women with heart failure and a mean LVEF of 28% were followed for 1.3 years.[61] Ischemic etiology was less prevalent in women who manifested a higher systolic blood pressure and higher prevalence of LBBB.

In the Metoprolol CR/XL Randomized Intervention Trial in Chronic Heart Failure (MERIT-HF), which has the largest database for women on beta-blockers, women (n = 898) were older than men (n = 3093), had a higher percentage of African Americans, less prevalence of ischemic etiology, had higher LVEF, higher systolic blood pressure and heart rate, were less likely to be current or former smokers, to have previous myocardial infarction (MI), and had higher prevalence of hypertension and diabetes, and lower prevalence of atrial fibrillation.[62]

In the Beta-Blocker Evaluation of Survival Trial (BEST) which enrolled patients with advanced heart failure, comparing women (n = 593) to men (n = 2115) showed that women were younger, had a higher percentage of African

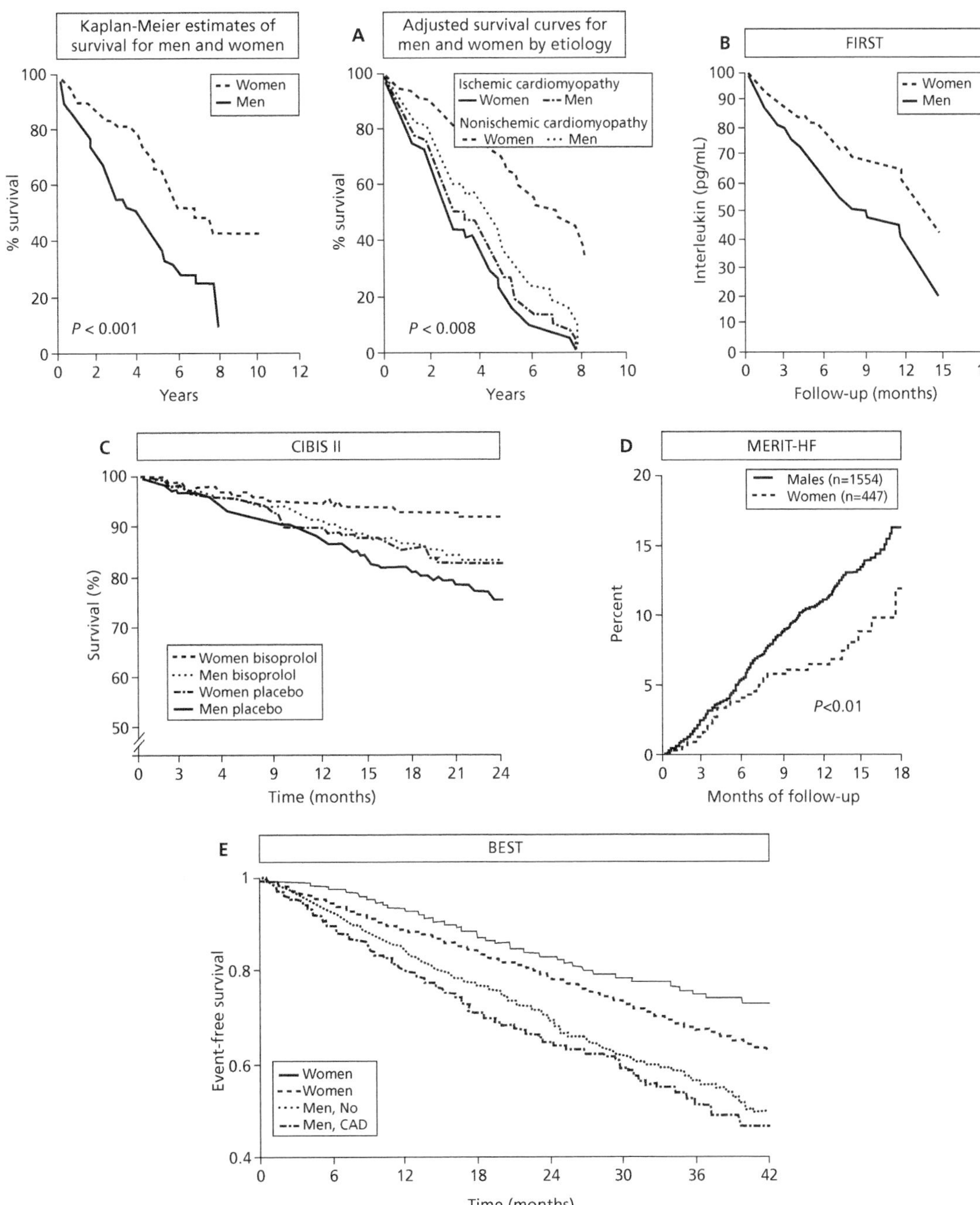

Figure 4.3. *Survival curves by sex.*

A *North Carolina Heart Failure Clinic*

B *Flolan International Randomized Survival Trial (FIRST)*

C *Cardiac Insufficiency Bisoprolol Study (CIBIS II)*

D *Metoprolol Extended-Release Randomized Intervention Trial in Chronic Heart Failure (MERIT-HF)*

E *Beta-blocker Evaluation of Survival Trial (BEST)*

Table 4.2. *Sex differences in patients with heart failure and impaired left ventricular ejection fraction*

	SPIC		UNC		FIRST		CIBIS II		MERIT-HF		BEST	
	Women (n = 65)	Men (n = 238)	Women (n = 177)	Men (n = 380)	Women (n = 112)	Men (n = 359)	Women (n = 515)	Men (n = 2132)	Women (n = 898)	Men (n = 3093)	Women (n = 593)	Men (n = 2115)
Age (yr)	45	42	49*	52	64	64	65†	60	65†	63	58*	61
NYHA III/IV (%)	48	38*	67	68	100	100	100	100	65†	57	100	100
Ischemic (%)			11†	37	44†	67	40†	52	58†	67	38†	64
HTN (%)			52*	76					51†	42	57	59
DM (%)			21	24	34	36	14	11	30†	23	36	35
Caucasian (%)			44†	58	74†	86	99	99	90†	95	62†	79
HR (bpm)					90*	86	81	80	84*	82	84†	81
LVEF (%)	28	29	24†	29	18	18	28	27	28.2†	27.6	25†	23
AF (%)	3	10	5*	12	15	24	17	20	10†	18	5†	13
LBBB (%)	41	29*					31†	25			34†	23
CTR (%)	0.56	0.53*									59†	55
Survival	Similar		Better (NI)		Better (NI)		Better		Better		Better (NI)	

Abbreviations: AF = atrial fibrillation; BEST = Beta-Blocker Evaluation of Survival Trial; bpm = beats per minute; CIBIS II = Cardiac Insufficiency Bisoprolol Study II; CTR = cardiothoracic ratio; DM = diabetes mellitus; FIRST = Flolan International Randomized Survival Trial; HR = heart rate; HTN = hypertension; LBBB = left bundle branch block; LVEF = left ventricular ejection fraction; MERIT-HF = Metoprolol CR/XL Randomized Intervention Trial in Heart Failure; NI = non-ischemic; NYHA = New York Heart Association; SPIC = Italian Multicenter Cardiomyopathy Study Group; UNC = University of North Carolina.

*$P \leq 0.05$

†$P < 0.005$

Americans, lower prevalence of ischemia and cardio-thoracic ratio, lower prevalence of atrial fibrillation, higher prevalence of LBBB and lower serum norepinephrine.[63]

In the Studies of Left Ventricular Dysfunction (SOLVD), women were more likely to have hypertension, less likely to have coronary artery disease (CAD) and coronary artery bypass grafting (CABG), and were more likely to have dyspnea and edema, third heart sound, and elevation of jugular venous pressure.[64]

Etiology and Risk Factors

There are significant differences in the prevalence of risk factors that lead to the development of heart failure between men and women.

Hypertension

Hypertension is more prevalent in women with heart failure with either preserved or impaired LVEF. In the Framingham study, the risk of developing heart failure conferred by hypertension (compared to normotensive) was about 3-fold in women compared to 2-fold in men.[38] Furthermore, hypertension exerted a higher population-attributable risk for heart failure in women (accounting for 59% of cases) compared to men (39%).[38] Cardiac adaptation to isolated systolic hypertension has been shown to differ by sex.[65]

Coronary artery disease

In patients with heart failure and impaired LVEF, the evidence is overwhelming that CAD is more prevalent among men than women.[60–64] It is interesting, however, that regardless of LVEF, women are more likely than men to develop heart failure post-MI.[66] Similarly, after CABG, women were more likely to develop heart failure despite equivalent or better LVEFs than men.[67,68]

Diabetes mellitus

The Framingham study found a doubling of the risk for developing heart failure in diabetic women compared to diabetic men.[39] The SOLVD data supported this finding with a higher prevalence of diabetes in women compared to men in the treatment and prevention arms as well as in the registry.[69] However, as shown in Table 4.2, other trials of patients with heart failure and impaired LVEF showed no difference in the prevalence of diabetes between men and women.[60–63]

Idiopathic dilated cardiomyopathy

The data are consistent and convincing of the lower prevalence of idiopathic dilated cardiomyopathy (IDC) in women, with a 2-fold to 4-fold higher prevalence of IDC in men as compared to women.[70–72]

Cigarette smoking

An under-appreciated risk factor for heart failure is cigarette smoking. Analysis of NHANES I revealed that cigarette smoking was associated with a 45% higher risk of heart failure in men, and an 88% higher risk of heart failure in women after adjusting for known risk factors including coronary disease.[73]

Alcohol

Consumption of large quantities of alcohol has been associated with a high prevalence of impaired LVEF.[74] It appears that women are more susceptible to the toxic effect of alcohol on LV systolic function as evident by developing impairment of LVEF at a lower level of alcohol consumption,[75] or lower lifetime dose of alcohol as compared to men.[76]

It is interesting to note that the Framingham study found moderate alcohol consumption to protect from the development of heart failure in men but not in women.[77]

Obesity

Recent data from Framingham showed that compared to women with a normal body-mass index (BMI), overweight women had a 50% greater risk of heart failure, and obese women had a doubling of the risk of heart failure. On the other hand, although no significant increase in risk of heart failure was observed in overweight men, a 90% increase in risk was noted in obese men.[78]

Medications

Angiotensin-converting enzyme inhibitors

Under-representation of women in trials that established the role of angiotensin-converting enzyme (ACE) inhibitors in heart failure with impaired EF has limited the ability to determine their benefit in women. In the Cooperative North Scandinavian Enalapril Survival Study (CONSENSUS), a 51% reduction in mortality was noted in the treated men versus a 6% reduction in women.[8] Similarly in the Survival and Ventricular Enlargement (SAVE) trial, the risk reduction of all-cause mortality in women was 2% as compared to 22% in men.[79] However, the small sample size of CONSENSUS and the lack of significant interaction between sex and captopril, as well as limited power in SAVE, did not permit a conclusion to be drawn.[80]

Combining the prevention and treatment arms of SOLVD provides the largest single experience with ACE inhibitor in patients with chronic heart failure. Interestingly, analysis of SOLVD by sex showed no benefit of the treatment in women (n = 980), compared to the substantial benefit in men (n = 5817).[81] Moreover, in pooling 30 studies of ACE-inhibitor use in heart failure, there was a 37% decrease in the risk of death and or hospitalization in men compared with a 22% decrease in women, and the 95% confidence interval (CI) for the effect in women was (0.59–1.04).[82] Admittedly, the direction of the benefit was similar to men and one should be very cautious in interpreting subgroup analysis. In addition, any conclusion should be based on the totality of evidence and the overall results of the study. There is a legitimate concern, however, that the magnitude of benefit with ACE inhibitors may be smaller in women. Unfortunately, this issue can never be resolved because of ethical considerations. Thus, as recommended by the guidelines, ACE inhibitors are mandatory for women with heart failure and low LVEF, although their beneficial effects may be attenuated compared to men.

Digitalis

A recent retrospective analysis assessing whether the effect of digoxin therapy varied based on sex was performed in the Digitalis Investigation Group (DIG) trial.[83] Among patients with heart failure and impaired LVEF, digoxin therapy was associated with an increased risk of death from any cause in women but not in men. Although adjustment was made for renal function, serum digoxin level was not measured, and the possibility that a higher serum digoxin level in women accounted for the increased mortality cannot be ruled out.

Beta-blockers

The beneficial effect of beta-blockers in women with heart failure and impaired LVEF has been documented. An analysis of the effect of the beta-blocker, metoprolol extended release, in women (n = 898) in the MERIT-HF database was published.[62] There was a significant 21% decrease in the primary endpoint of combined hospitalization and mortality with significant reductions in all-cause (19%), cardiovascular (29%), and heart failure (42%) hospitalization (Figure 4.4). Furthermore, in the subset of women with severe heart failure defined by NYHA class III or IV with LVEF < 25% (n = 183), there was a significant decrease in all-cause (44%), cardiovascular (57%), and heart failure hospitalization (72%) (Figure 4.4). Finally, pooling data from Carvedilol Prospective Randomized Cumulative Survival (COPERNICUS), CIBIS II, and MERIT-HF showed a decrease in total mortality in women, with a survival benefit similar to that achieved in men (Figure 4.5).[62] It is interesting to note that sex-related differences in pharmacokinetics and pharmacodynamics have been identified for metoprolol.[84]

Hormone replacement therapy

Two retrospective analyses have found a protective effect of hormone replacement therapy (HRT) in women older than 50 years with advanced heart failure and impaired LVEF.[85,86] Data combining three trials comparing vesnarinone and placebo showed a 38% reduction in mortality in HRT users (n = 237) compared to non-HRT users (n = 897).[85] Another analysis from BEST showed a 40% reduction in mortality in HRT users (n = 102) compared to non-HRT users (n = 333).[86] HRT has been shown to improve endothelial-dependent vasodilation in post-menopausal women,[87] and estrogen therapy

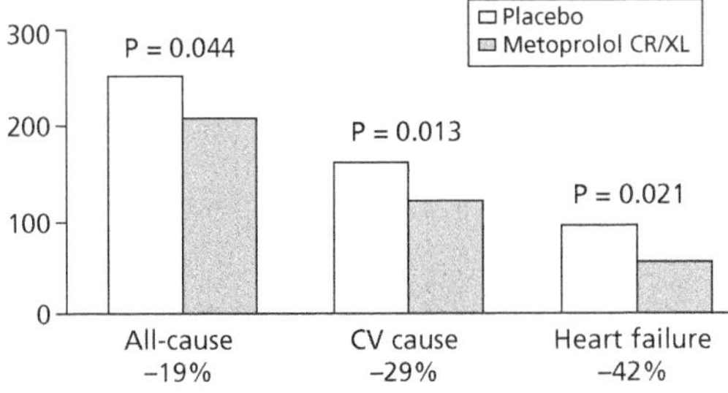

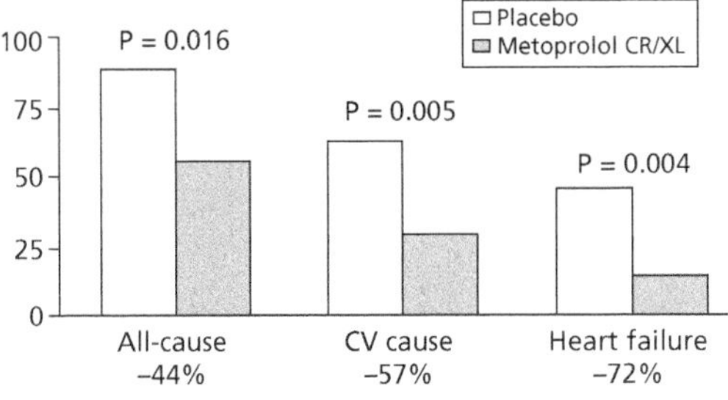

Figure 4.4. *MERIT-HF: Total number of hospitalizations for all-cause, cardiovascular (CV) cause, and worsening heart failure in all women (top), and in the subgroup of women with severe heart failure (New York Heart Association class III or IV and ejection fraction < 25%, bottom). Percent reductions calculated from rates defined as numbers per patient-year of follow-up (With permission from Ghali* et al.[62])

was associated with a reduced level of p38 mitogen-activated protein kinase that is thought to play an important role in the progression to heart failure.[88] A randomized trial in women with non-ischemic etiology is required to determine the potential role of HRT in women with heart failure and impaired LVEF.

Pattern of medications usage

In the Study of Patients Intolerant of Converting Enzyme Inhibitors (SPICE) registry[89] that enrolled 9580 patients with LVEF < 35%, 26% of which were women, ACE inhibitors, nitrates, acetylsalicylic acid, warfarin and antiarrhythmic agents were used less often in women. On the other hand, diuretics were taken more often by women. Under-use of ACE inhibitors by women has been reported in some[90,91] but not all studies.[92,93] In a study by Hood *et al.*, after adjusting for age, the under-utilization of ACE inhibitors by women was no longer noted.[94] It is possible that the initial prescription of ACE inhibitors in women is similar to that of men, and the reported underuse is related to higher incidence of side effects, especially cough, resulting in discontinuation.

Adverse events

In SOLVD, women were more likely to report side effects than men in the initial run-in phase

	No. randomized placebo/β-blockade	No. of deaths placebo/β-blocked
CIBIS II		
Females	258/257	35/18
Males	1062/1070	193/138
All	1320/1327	228/156
MERIT-HF		
Females	447/451	33/31
Males	1554/1539	184/114
All	2001/1990	217/145
COPERNICUS		
Females	228/237	35/23
Males	905/919	155/107
All	1133/1156	190/130
All 3 Studies		
Females	933/945	103/72
Males	3521/3528	532/359
All	4454/4473	675/431

Favors β-blockade | Favors placebo

0.0 1.0 1.8

Relative risk and 95% confidence interval

Figure 4.5. *Point estimates for hazard ratios and 95% confidence intervals for total mortality by gender and overall in CIBIS II, MERIT-HF and COPERNICUS (With permission from Ghali* et al.[62])

(8% vs. 5.8%)[95] as well as in the follow-up phase (26.4% vs. 21.3%).[96] Women reported cough twice as often as men (3% vs. 1.8% in the placebo group and 10% vs. 4.2% in the enalapril group).[96] In the combined Evaluation of Losartan in the Elderly Study (ELITE) I and II databases, women had a higher incidence of cough as well as higher withdrawal of therapy due to cough.[97]

Compliance

In a retrospective follow-up of 7247 outpatients, aged 65 to 99 years, with newly prescribed digoxin, better compliance was found in women as compared to men.[98]

Quality of Life

Limited data are available regarding sex-related differences in the quality of life of patients with heart failure. In a study of hospitalized patients[99] (90 women and 89 men), women had lower scores at baseline for vitality, physical function, and physical component summary scales, and at one year they showed less improvement in physical health status and perceived their quality of care to be lower than men. Another report compiling data from nine studies including 320 men and 320 women, with 3-month follow-up data[100] available on 163 men and 188 women, found emotional quality of life to be lower in women at baseline with significant and comparable improvement in quality of life at 3 months, confirming an earlier report, with a small sample (n = 103), of lower scoring in women in emotional well-being at baseline.[101] In a detailed report from SOLVD involving a large sample of 1382 patients (691 men and 691 women), age and EF matched, women had worse quality of life ratings than men for daily living and social activities.[102] Further studies are needed to explore the differences in quality of life and coping pattern in a sample that is well defined in terms of severity of heart failure, measures of LV function, and available support.

Exercise Training

Improvement in peak oxygen consumption (peak VO_2)[103] and 6-minute-walk[104] performance has been demonstrated in women with heart failure. Potential sex-related differences in exercise training have been suggested by reports showing that, in response to exercise, an increase in myosin heavy chain isoform 1 was found in men but not women,[105] and the suggestion that pathophysiological adaptations of skeletal muscles in women with heart failure are less pronounced as compared to those of men.[106,107]

Arrhythmias

An analysis of Holter monitor recordings in 159 men and 77 women hospitalized for heart failure revealed no differences in atrial ectopy, but a lower prevalence of complex ventricular ectopy and episodes of ventricular tachycardia in women.[108] In the same study, heart rate variability was assessed in 131 men and 68 women, and an attenuated sympathetic activation and parasympathetic withdrawal was found in women with non-ischemic etiology.[109] An earlier report from the Cardiovascular Health Study (CVHS) on 1372 patients showed a higher prevalence of ventricular arrhythmias and their association with impaired LV function in men.[110]

Morbidity

Hospitalization

Hospitalization for heart failure has been steadily increasing in the past two decades.[31,111–113] Although the prevalence of hospitalization is higher among men than women, especially at younger ages, this difference becomes much less pronounced in the elderly. However, because of the larger number of women with heart failure than men, greater numbers of women than men are hospitalized.[111–113] Several reports from a clinical trial,[63] a single center,[114] and the Connecticut Peer Review Organization data[115] indicate a similar hospital readmission rate between men and women. In a report from Medicare data on all survivors of hospitalization for heart failure from Connecticut[116] over a 4-year period (n = 17 448), men were more likely to be re-hospitalized than women (odds ratio

[OR], 1.16; 95 CI, 1.05–1.20). Men were reported to have a history of prior hospitalization more often than women,[117] and women were more likely[117] to have longer hospital stays than men.[118,119] NHDS data suggest that women are less likely than men to undergo invasive cardiac procedures provided to patients with heart failure.[113] Medicare data, however, show a similar pattern.[115] Both Medicare data[115] and NHDS data[113] suggest that women are more likely than men to be discharged to long-term care, a finding that may be related to the absence of a spouse, since more elderly women than men live alone.[120]

Thromboembolism

A retrospective analysis of SOLVD found a higher incidence of pulmonary embolism in women with heart failure and low EF in sinus rhythm compared to men.[121] This analysis also suggested that a decline in LVEF was independently associated with thromboembolism risk in women but not in men.

Transplantation

Heart transplantation is performed much more commonly on men than on women.[122] During the period from 1988 to 2003, women accounted for only 24% out of 34 288 transplants performed.[122] This finding may be explained by several factors including a higher prevalence of IDC in men as well as an earlier onset of ischemic heart failure with low LVEF in men. However, another possible contributing factor for under-representation of women is decreased willingness of women to undergo transplantation.[123]

Mortality

The better survival rate of women with heart failure compared to men is confirmed by epidemiological studies as well as heart failure survival trials.

The Framingham study provided the first evidence that women with heart failure, with either impaired or preserved LVEF, lived longer than men. The 5-year survival rate was 38% for women compared to 25% for men.[39] Similarly, the NHANES data showed consistently better survival for women, at 10 years as well as 15 years, whether heart failure was self-reported or based on clinical score.[34]

The Italian Network on Congestive Heart Failure provided data on 6428 consecutively seen outpatients with heart failure.[124] No difference in mortality was noted at 1-year follow-up. This study selected patients followed by cardiologists, of whom only 25% were women.

In patients with heart failure and impaired LVEF, the evidence is also strong in favor of a better survival in women. Although a study in a young population of 65 women and 238 men with IDC, who were enrolled consecutively, found no difference in 1-year survival rates between men and women,[58] several studies consistently reported better survival in women.[59–63] At the University of North Carolina Heart Failure Outpatient Clinic, 177 women and 380 men with heart failure and impaired LV systolic function were consecutively enrolled and followed for a mean of 2.4 years.[59] Compared to men, a significantly better survival rate was found in women. This survival advantage was confined to patients with non-ischemic etiology. Similar findings were reported from the Flolan International Randomized Survival Trial, in 112 women and 359 men with advanced heart failure and mean LVEF of 18%.[60] The survival rates in 515 women and 2132 men in CIBIS II confirmed better survival for women compared to men. However, this difference was predominantly noted in the undefined etiology group and no difference in survival was seen between women and men in the non-ischemic group.[61] Likewise, in MERIT-HF, women had a 37% lower risk of dying than men after adjusting for baseline differences including ischemic etiology.[62] Data from BEST on 593 women and 2115 men with advanced heart failure followed for a mean of two years showed a better rate of survival in women, confined to the non-ischemic patients.[63]

Findings from CIBIS II that no difference in survival was noted in the non-ischemic patients, and from MERIT-HF that the better survival of women was evident even after adjusting for ischemic etiology, should lead to the conclusion that the survival advantage of women cannot be explained entirely on the basis of higher prevalence of non-ischemic etiology. It is likely that other confounders not identified by measured baseline clinical and laboratory characteristics play a role.

In patients hospitalized for heart failure, the vast majority of studies have reported better survival in women. Data from the Canadian Institute for Health Information on 38 702 consecutive patients with a first-time admission for heart failure indicate better survival in women (n = 19 766) as compared to men (n = 18 936), with a decrease in the sex gap with advancing age.[125] In patients 75 years old or older, the sex gap in the risk of death at 1 year was 40% of the gap observed in patients younger than 75 years. Another interesting finding from this study was the decreasing sex gap in mortality with increasing comorbidities.

In the Scottish National Health Service Linked Patient Database of patients hospitalized for heart failure over a 10-year period, women (n = 35 507) accounted for 53% of all patients (n = 66 547).[117] Young women (< 64 years) had a higher 30-day mortality than men. However, women aged > 65 years, who form the majority of patients, had better 30-day mortality than men. One-year mortality also showed a lower case fatality rate for women (hazard ratio [HR] 0.87; 95% CI, 0.85–0.89) as compared to men.

The largest study on survival of hospitalized patients with heart failure reported on 170 239 Medicare patients, 67 years old or older, who had their first hospitalization for heart failure.[126] Six-year survival data showed that men had a 38% greater risk of mortality than did women.

In the EPICAL (EPidémiologie de l'Insuffisance Cardiaque Avancée en Lorraine) study,[127] 499 hospitalized patients with advanced heart failure, evidence of fluid retention, and LVEF < 30% were enrolled. In this study, the women were older than the men and had a higher 1-year mortality rate. However, when adjusted for age, the difference in mortality was no longer noted.

In the SOLVD Registry,[128] women (n = 1595) constituted 26% of the patients and were older than the men. This was the only study showing a higher 1-year mortality for women with heart failure as compared to men. It is possible that women were over-represented among the 14% of patients who entered the SOLVD Registry on the basis of hospital discharge diagnosis of heart failure confirmed by radiological evidence of venous congestion. Hospitalized patients were not required to have low LVEF, and would be expected to have worse prognosis than ambulatory patients.

Predictors of Mortality

Many clinical and laboratory characteristics have been found to be predictors of survival in patients with heart failure and impaired LVEF.[129] Some characteristics are expected to confer a better prognosis, namely, having a higher prevalence of non-ischemic etiology, higher LVEF,[130] lower occurrence of atrial fibrillation,[131] and lower plasma norepinephrine.[130] Some other characteristics, however, have been related to worse outcomes including higher heart rate,[132] cardiothoracic ratio,[130] and higher prevalence of LBBB.[133] However, the assessment of these characteristics were derived from clinical trials dominated by men. The existence of significant gender differences in clinical and laboratory characteristics would suggest that the predictive values of these characteristics may differ by sex. Therefore, a reassessment of the predictive value of these characteristics should be performed in women.

A multivariate analysis performed in BEST, which enrolled 593 women and 2115 men with advanced heart failure,[63] demonstrated that predictors of mortality were similar overall in men and women, including LVEF, the presence of coronary disease, age, systolic blood pressure, renal function, and diabetes. Atrial fibrillation, however, was found to be a predictor in women but not in men, confirming an earlier report on hospitalized patients with heart failure that showed a significant relationship between atrial fibrillation and mortality in women but not in men, and QRS duration and BMI were predictors only in men. A more interesting finding was that the predictive value of two variables differed in magnitude between men and women. For every 1% increase in LVEF there was an associated 4% decrease in mortality in women, compared with only a 1% decrease in mortality in men. Similarly, CAD conferred a 2.5-fold increase in the risk of death in women compared with a 1.5-fold increase in men. Thus, LVEF and CAD appear to be more powerful predictors of prognosis in women.

Conclusion

Women with heart failure differ significantly from men in their clinical and laboratory characteristics, risk factors and pathophysiology, predictors of prognosis and prognosis. The potential sex-related differences in response to various management strategies necessitate powering heart failure clinical trials to provide adequate understanding for the efficacy of the interventions in women. The notion that evidence based on interventions in men with heart failure could be translated to women, with the expectation of replicating the response in both direction and magnitude, should no longer be accepted.

References

1. Institute of Medicine. Exploring the Biological Contributions to Human Health: Does Sex Matter? (National Academy Press: Washington DC, 2001).
2. Ghali JK. A clinician's perspective on clinical trials. J Card Fail 2001; 7: 1–3.
3. Lindenfeld J, Krause-Steinrauf H, Salerno J. Where are all the women with heart failure? J Am Coll Cardiol 1997; 30: 1417–1419.
4. Petrie MC, Dawson NF, Murdoch DR, Davie AP, McMurray JJ. Failure of women's hearts. Circulation 1999; 99: 2334–2341.
5. Hoppe BL, Hermann DD. Sex differences in the causes and natural history of heart failure. Curr Cardiol Rep 2003; 5: 193–199.
6. Heiat A, Gross CP, Krumholz HM. Representation of the elderly, women, and minorities in heart failure clinical trials. Arch Intern Med 2002; 162: 1682–1688.
7. Cohn JN, Archibald DG, Ziesche S, *et al.* Effect of vasodilator therapy on mortality in chronic congestive heart failure: results of a Veterans Administration Cooperative Study. N Engl J Med 1986; 314: 1547–1552.
8. The CONSENSUS Trial Study Group. Effects of enalapril on mortality in severe congestive heart failure: Results of the Cooperative North Scandinavian Enalapril Survival Study (CONSENSUS). N Engl J Med 1987; 316: 1429–1435.
9. Cohn JN, Johnson G, Ziesche S, *et al.* A comparison of enalapril with hydralazine-isosorbide dinitrate in the treatment of chronic congestive heart failure. N Engl J Med 1991; 325: 303–310.
10. The SOLVD Investigators. Effect of enalapril on survival in patients with reduced left ventricular ejection fractions and congestive heart failure. N Engl J Med 1991; 325: 293–302.
11. The SOLVD Investigators. Effect of enalapril on mortality and the development of heart failure in asymptomatic patients with reduced left ventricular ejection fractions. N Engl J Med 1992; 327: 685–691.
12. The PROMISE Study Research Group. Packer M, Carver JR, Rodeheffer RJ, *et al.* Effect of oral milrinone on mortality in severe chronic heart failure. N Engl J Med 1991; 325: 1468–1475.
13. Singh SN, Fletcher RD, Fisher SG, *et al.* Amiodarone in patients with congestive heart failure and asymptomatic ventricular arrhythmia. Survival Trial of Antiarrhythmic Therapy in Congestive Heart Failure. N Engl J Med 1995; 333: 77–82.
14. Packer M, O'Connor CM, Ghali JK, *et al.* Effect of amlodipine on morbidity and mortality in severe chronic heart failure. Prospective Randomized Amlodipine Survival Evaluation Study Group. N Engl J Med 1996; 335: 1107–1114.
15. Califf RM, Adams KF, McKenna WJ, *et al.* A randomized controlled trial of epoprostenol therapy for severe congestive heart failure: The Flolan International Randomized Survival Trial (FIRST). Am Heart J 1997; 134: 44–54.
16. Hampton JR, van Veldhuisen DJ, Kleber FX, *et al.* Randomised study of effect of ibopamine on survival in patients with advanced severe heart failure. Second Prospective Randomized Study of Ibopamine on Mortality and Efficacy (PRIME II) Investigators. Lancet 1997; 349: 971–977.
17. The Digitalis Investigation Group. The effect of digoxin on mortality and morbidity in patients with heart failure. N Engl J Med 1997; 336: 525–533.
18. Pitt B, Segal R, Martinez FA, *et al.* Randomised trial of losartan versus captopril in patients over 65 with heart failure (Evaluation of Losartan in the Elderly Study, ELITE). Lancet 1997; 349: 747–752.
19. Cohn JN, Goldstein SO, Greenberg BH, *et al.* A dose-dependent increase in mortality with vesnarinone among patients with severe heart failure. Vesnarinone Trial Investigators. N Engl J Med 1998; 339: 1810–1816.

20. The Cardiac Insufficiency Bisoprolol Study II (CIBIS II): a randomised trial. Lancet 1999; 353: 9–13.
21. Effect of metoprolol CR/XL in chronic heart failure: Metoprolol CR/XL Randomised Intervention Trial in Congestive Heart Failure (MERIT-HF). Lancet 1999; 353: 2001–2007.
22. Packer M, Poole-Wilson PA, Armstrong PW, *et al.* Comparative effects of low and high doses of the angiotensin-converting enzyme inhibitor, lisinopril, on morbidity and mortality in chronic heart failure. ATLAS Study Group. Circulation 1999; 100: 2312–2318.
23. Pitt B, Zannad F, Remme WJ, *et al.* The effect of spironolactone on morbidity and mortality in patients with severe heart failure. Randomized Aldactone Evaluation Study Investigators. N Engl J Med 1999; 341: 709–717.
24. Pitt B, Poole-Wilson PA, Segal R, *et al.* Effect of losartan compared with captopril on mortality in patients with symptomatic heart failure: randomized trial: the Losartan Heart Failure Survival Study ELITE II. Lancet 2000; 355: 1582–1587.
25. Beta-Blocker Evaluation of Survival Trial Investigators. A trial of the beta-blocker bucindolol in patients with advanced chronic heart failure. N Engl J Med 2001; 344: 1659–1667.
26. Cohn JN, Tognoni G. Valsartan Heart Failure Trial Investigators. A randomized trial of the angiotensin-receptor blocker valsartan in chronic heart failure. N Engl J Med 2001; 345: 1667–1675.
27. Packer M, Fowler MB, Roecker EB, *et al.* Effect of carvedilol on the morbidity of patients with severe chronic heart failure: results of the carvedilol prospective randomized cumulative survival (COPERNICUS) study. Circulation 2002; 106: 2194–2199.
28. Poole-Wilson PA, Swedberg K, Cleland JGF, *et al.*, Carvedilol Or Metoprolol European Trial Investigators. Comparison of carvedilol and metoprolol on clinical outcomes in patients with chronic heart failure in the Carvedilol Or Metoprolol European Trial (COMET): randomised controlled trial. Lancet 2003; 362: 7–13.
29. McMurray J, Ostergren J, Pfeffer M, *et al.*, CHARM committees and investigators. Clinical features and contemporary management of patients with low and preserved ejection fraction heart failure: baseline characteristics of patients in the Candesartan in Heart failure-Assessment of Reduction in Mortality and morbidity (CHARM) programme. Eur J Heart Fail 2003; 5: 261–270.
30. Bristow MR, Saxon LA, Boehmer J, *et al.*, Comparison of Medical Therapy, Pacing, and Defibrillation in Heart Failure (COMPANION) Investigators. Cardiac-resynchronization therapy with or without an implantable defibrillator in advanced chronic heart failure. N Engl J Med 2004; 350: 2140–2150.
31. American Heart Association. Heart Disease and Stroke Statistics—2003 Update (American Heart Association: Dallas, TX, 2003).
32. Ansari M, Massie BM. Heart failure: How big is the problem? Who are the patients? What does the future hold? Am Heart J 2003; 146: 1–4.
33. DHSS. Vital and Health Statistics: Plan and Operation of the Third National Health and Nutrition Examination Survey, 1988–94 (Hyattsville, MD: National Center for Health Statistics, Centers for Disease Control and Prevention, US Dept of Health and Human Services; 1994), 407.
34. Schocken DD, Arrieta ML, Leaverton PE, Ross, EA. Prevalence and mortality rate of congestive heart failure in the United States. J Am Coll Cardiol 1992; 20: 301–306.
35. Ni, H. Prevalence of self-reported heart failure among US adults: results from the 1999 National Health Interview Survey. Am Heart J 2003; 146: 121–128.
36. Levy D, Kenchaiah S, Larson MG, *et al.* Long-term trends in the incidence of and survival with heart failure. N Engl J Med 2002; 347: 1397–1402.
37. Senni M, Tribouilloy CM, Rodeheffer RJ, *et al.* Congestive heart failure in the community: trends in incidence and survival in a 10-year period. Arch Intern Med 1999; 159: 29–34.
38. Levy D, Larson MG, Vasan RS, Kannel WB, Ho KK. The progression from hypertension to congestive heart failure. JAMA 1996; 275: 1557–1562.
39. Ho KKL, Pinsky JL, Kannel WB, Levy D. The epidemiology of heart failure: The Framingham Study. J Am Coll Cardiol 1993; 22: 6A–13A.
40. Lloyd-Jones DM, Larson MG, Leip EP, *et al.*, Framingham Heart Study. Lifetime risk for developing congestive heart failure: the Framingham Heart Study. Circulation 2002; 106: 3068–3072.
41. Koelling TM, Chen RS, Lubwama RN, L'Italien GJ, Eagle KA. The expanding national burden of heart failure in the United States: the influence of heart failure in women. Am Heart J 2004; 147: 74–78.
42. Redfield MM, Jacobsen SJ, Burnett JC, *et al.* Burden of systolic and diastolic ventricular dysfunction in the community: appreciating the scope of the heart failure epidemic. JAMA 2003; 289: 194–202.

43. Vasan RS, Benjamin EJ, Levy D. Prevalence, clinical features and prognosis of diastolic heart failure: an epidemiologic perspective. J Am Coll Cardiol 1995; 26: 1565–1574.
44. Vasan RS, Larson MG, Benjamin EJ, *et al.* Congestive heart failure in subjects with normal versus reduced left ventricular ejection fraction: prevalence and mortality in a population-based cohort. J Am Coll Cardiol 1999; 33: 1948–1955.
45. Senni M, Tribouilloy CM, Rodeheffer, *et al.* Congestive heart failure in the community: a study of all incident cases in Olmsted County, Minnesota, in 1991. Circulation 1998; 98: 2282–2289.
46. Kitzman DW, Gardin JM, Gottdiener JS, *et al.* Importance of heart failure with preserved systolic function in patients > or = 65 years of age. CHS Research Group, Cardiovascular Health Study. Am J Cardiol 2001; 87: 413–419.
47. Devereux RB, Roman MJ, Liu JE, *et al.* Congestive heart failure despite normal left ventricular systolic function in a population-based sample: the Strong Heart Study. Am J Cardiol 2000; 86: 1090–1096.
48. Masoudi FA, Havranek EP, Smith G, *et al.* Gender, age, and heart failure with preserved left ventricular systolic function. J Am Coll Cardiol 2003; 41: 217–223.
49. Mendes LA, Davidoff R, Cupples LA, Ryan TJ, Jacobs AK. Congestive heart failure in patients with coronary artery disease: the gender paradox. Am Heart J 1997; 134: 207–212.
50. Carroll JD, Carroll EP, Feldman T, *et al.* Sex-associated differences in left ventricular function in aortic stenosis of the elderly. Circulation 1992; 86: 1099–1107.
51. Gerdts E, Zabalgoitia M, Björnstad H, Svendsen TL, Devereux RB. Gender differences in systolic left ventricular function in hypertensive patients with electrocardiographic left ventricular hypertrophy (the LIFE Study). Am J Cardiol 2001; 87: 980–983.
52. Pfeffer JM, Pfeffer MA, Fletcher P, Braunwald E. Alterations of cardiac performance in rats with established spontaneous hypertension. Am J Cardiol 1979; 44: 994–998.
53. Litwin SE, Katz SE, Litwin CM, Morgan JP, Douglas PS. Gender differences in postinfarction left ventricular remodeling. Cardiology 1999; 91: 173–183.
54. Douglas PS, Katz SE, Weinberg EO, *et al.* Hypertrophic remodeling: gender differences in the early response to left ventricular pressure overload. J Am Coll Cardiol 1998; 32: 1118–1125.
55. Gardner JD, Brower GL, Janicki JS. Gender differences in cardiac remodeling secondary to chronic volume overload. J Card Fail 2002; 8: 101–107.
56. Tamura T, Said S, Gerdes AM. Gender-related differences in myocyte remodeling in progression to heart failure. Hypertension 1999; 33: 676–680.
57. Crabbe DL, Dipla K, Ambati S, *et al.* Gender differences in post-infarction hypertrophy in end-stage failing hearts. J Am Coll Cardiol 2003; 41: 300–306.
58. De Maria R, Gavazzi A, Recalcati F. *et al.* Comparison of clinical findings in idiopathic dilated cardiomyopathy in women versus men. The Italian Multicenter Cardiomyopathy Study Group (SPIC). Am J Cardiol 1993; 72: 580–585.
59. Adams KF Jr, Dunlap SH, Sueta CA, *et al.* Relation between gender, etiology and survival in patients with symptomatic heart failure. J Am Coll Cardiol 1996; 28: 1781–1788.
60. Adams KF Jr., Sueta CA, Gheorghiade M, *et al.* Gender differences in survival in advanced heart failure. Insights from the FIRST study. Circulation 1999; 99: 1816–1821.
61. Simon T, Mary-Krause M, Funck-Brentano C, Jaillon P. Sex differences in the prognosis of congestive heart failure: results from the Cardiac Insufficiency Bisoprolol Study (CIBIS II). Circulation 2001; 103: 375–380.
62. Ghali JK, Pina IL, Gottlieb SS, Deedwania PC, Wikstrand JC, MERIT-HF Study Group, Metoprolol CR/XL in female patients with heart failure: analysis of the experience in Metoprolol Extended-Release Randomized Intervention Trial in Heart Failure (MERIT-HF). Circulation 2002; 105: 1585–1591.
63. Ghali JK, Krause-Steinrauf HJ, Adams KF, *et al.* Gender differences in advanced heart failure: insights from the BEST study. J Am Coll Cardiol 2003; 42: 2128–2134.
64. Johnstone D, Limacher M, Rousseau M, *et al.* Clinical characteristics of patients in studies of left ventricular dysfunction (SOLVD). Am J Cardiol 1992; 70: 894–900.
65. Krumholz HM, Larson M, Levy D. Sex differences in cardiac adaptation to isolated systolic hypertension. Am J Cardiol 1993; 72: 310–313.
66. Tofler GH, Stone PH, Muller JE, *et al.* Effects of gender and race on prognosis after myocardial infarction: adverse prognosis for women, particularly black women. J Am Coll Cardiol 1987; 9: 473–482.
67. Hoffman RM, Psaty BM, Kronmal RA. Modifiable risk factors for incident heart failure in the coronary artery surgery study. Arch Intern Med 1994; 154: 417–423.
68. Jacobs AK, Kelsey SF, Brooks MM, *et al.* Better outcome for women compared with men undergoing coronary revascularization: a report from the Bypass

Angioplasty Revascularization Investigation (BARI). Circulation 1998; 98: 1279–1285.

69. Shindler DM, Kostis JB, Yusuf S, *et al.* Diabetes mellitus: a predictor of morbidity and mortality in the Studies of Left Ventricular Dysfunction (SOLVD) Trials and Registry. Am J Cardiol 1996; 77: 1017–1020.
70. Codd MB, Sugrue DD, Gersh BJ, Melton J 3rd. Epidemiology of idiopathic dilated and hypertropic cardiomyopathy: a population-based study in Olmstead County, Minnesota, 1975–1984. Circulation 1989; 80: 564–572.
71. Bagger JP, Baandrup U, Rasmussen K, Moller M, Vesterlund T. Cardiomyopathy in western Denmark. Br Heart J 1984; 52: 327–331.
72. Williams DG, Olsen EG. Prevalence of overt dilated cardiomyopathy in two regions of England. Br Heart J 1985; 54: 153–155.
73. He J, Ogden LG, Bazzano LA, *et al.* Risk factors for congestive heart failure in US men and women: NHANES I epidemiologic follow-up study. Arch Intern Med 2001; 161: 996–1002.
74. Urbano-Marquez A, Estruch R, Navarro-Lopez F, *et al.* The effects of alcoholism on skeletal and cardiac muscle. N Engl J Med 1989; 320: 409–415.
75. Urbano-Marquez A, Estruch R, Fernandez-Sola J, *et al.* The greater risk of alcoholic cardiomyopathy and myopathy in women compared with men. JAMA 1995; 274: 149–154.
76. Fernandez-Sola J, Estruch R, Nicolas JM, *et al.* Comparison of alcoholic cardiomyopathy in women versus men. Am J Cardiol 1997; 80: 481–485.
77. Walsh CR, Larson MG, Evans JC, *et al.* Alcohol consumption and risk for congestive heart failure in the Framingham Heart Study. Ann Intern Med 2002; 136: 181–191.
78. Kenchaiah S, Evans JC, Levy D, *et al.* Obesity and the risk of heart failure. N Engl J Med 2002; 347: 305–313.
79. Lorell BH. ACE inhibitors after myocardial infarction. N Engl J Med 1993; 328: 966–969. (Letter)
80. Pfeffer MA, Braunwald, E, Moye, LA. ACE inhibitors after myocardial infarction. N Engl J Med 1993; 328: 966–969 (Letter).
81. Limacher MC, Yusuf S, SOLVD Investigators. Gender differences in presentation, morbidity and mortality in the Studies Of Left Ventricular Dysfunction (SOLVD): a preliminary report. In: Wenger NK, Speroff L, Packard B (eds) Cardiovascular Health and Disease in Women (LeJacq Communications: Greenwich, CT, 1993), 345–348.
82. Garg R, Yusuf S, Overview of randomized trials of angiotensin-converting enzyme inhibitors on mortality and morbidity in patients with heart failure. Collaborative Group on ACE Inhibitor Trials. JAMA 1995; 273: 1450–1456.
83. Rathore SS, Wang Y, Krumholz HM. Sex-based differences in the effect of digoxin for the treatment of heart failure. N Engl J Med 2002; 347: 1403–1411.
84. Luzier AB, Killian A, Wilton JH, *et al.* Gender-related effects on metoprolol pharmacokinetics and pharmacodynamics in healthy volunteers. Clin Pharmacol Ther 1999; 66: 594–601.
85. Reis SE, Holubkov R, Young JB, *et al.* Estrogen is associated with improved survival in aging women with congestive heart failure: analysis of the vesnarinone studies. J Am Coll Cardiol 2000; 36: 529–533.
86. Lindenfeld J, Ghali JK, Krause-Steinrauf HJ. BEST investigators. Hormone replacement therapy is associated with improved survival in women with advanced heart failure. J Am Coll Cardiol 2003; 42: 1238–1245.
87. Lieberman EH, Gerhard MD, Uehata A, *et al.* Estrogen improves endothelium-dependent, flow-mediated vasodilation in post-menopausal women. Ann Intern Med 1994; 121: 936–941.
88. Haq S, Choukroun G, Lim H, *et al.* Differential activation of signal transduction pathways in human hearts with hypertrophy versus advanced heart failure. Circulation 2001; 103: 670–677.
89. Shah MR, Granger CB, Bart BA, *et al.* Sex-related differences in the use and adverse effects of angiotensin-converting enzyme inhibitors in heart failure: the Study of Patients Intolerant of Converting Enzyme Inhibitors registry. Am J Med 2000; 109: 489–492.
90. Clinical Quality Improvement Network Investigators. Mortality risk and patterns of practice in 4606 acute care patients with congestive heart failure. The relative importance of age, sex, and medical therapy. Arch Intern Med 1996; 156: 1669–1673.
91. Stafford RS, Saglam D, Blumenthal D. National patterns of angiotensin-converting enzyme inhibitor use in congestive heart failure. Arch Intern Med 1997; 157: 2460–2464.
92. Blackman IC, Bond, M, Bowling A, *et al.* Age and sex do not bias the use of angiotensin-converting enzyme inhibitors in acute myocardial infarction and congestive heart failure. J Am Geriatr Soc 2003; 51: 572–573 (Letter).
93. Echemann M, Zannad F, Briancon S, *et al.* Determinants of angiotensin-converting enzyme inhibitor prescription in severe heart failure with left

ventricular systolic dysfunction: the EPICAL study. Am Heart J 2000; 139: 624–631.
94. Hood S, Taylor S, Roeves A, *et al.* Are there any age and sex differences in the investigation and treatment of heart failure? A population based study. Br J Gen Pract 2000; 50: 559–563.
95. Kostis JB, Shelton BJ, Yusuf S, *et al.* Tolerability of enalapril initiation by patients with left ventricular dysfunction: results of the medication challenge phase of Studies of Left Ventricular Dysfunction (SOLVD). Am Heart J 1994; 128: 358–364.
96. Kostis JB, Shelton B, Gosselin G, *et al.* Adverse effects of enalapril in the Studies of Left Ventricular Dysfunction (SOLVD). SOLVD investigators. Am Heart J 1996; 131: 350–355.
97. Schleman K, Realson R, Robertson AD, Lindenfeld J. Cough is more common in women than men with heart failure regardless of medical therapy. J Am Coll Cardiol 2001; 37: 212A (Abstract).
98. Monane M, Bohn RL, Gurwitz JH, Glynn RJ, Avorn J. Noncompliance with congestive heart failure therapy in the elderly. Arch Intern Med 1994; 154: 433–437.
99. Chin MH, Goldman L. Gender differences in 1-year survival and quality of life among patients with congestive heart failure. Med Care 1998; 36: 1033–1046.
100. Riegel B, Moser DK, Carlson B, *et al.* Gender differences in quality of life are minimal in patients with heart failure. J Card Fail 2003: 9: 42–48.
101. Evangelista LS, Dracup K, Doering L, *et al.* Emotional well-being of heart failure patients and their caregivers. J Card Fail 2002: 8: 300–305.
102. Riedinger MS, Dracup KA, Brecht ML, Padilla G, Sarna L, Ganz PA. Quality of life in patients with heart failure: do gender differences exist? Heart Lung 2001; 30: 105–116.
103. Tyni-Lenné R, Gordon A, Europe E, Jansson E, Sylvén C. Exercise-based rehabilitation improves skeletal muscle capacity, exercise tolerance, and quality of life in both women and men with chronic heart failure. J Card Fail 1998; 4: 9–17.
104. Rostagno C, Galanti G, Romano M, Chiostri G, Gensini GF. Prognostic value of 6-minute walk corridor testing in women with mild to moderate heart failure. Ital Heart J 2002; 3: 109–113.
105. Keteyian SJ, Duscha BD, Brawner CA, *et al.* Differential effects of exercise training in men and women with chronic heart failure. Am Heart J 2003; 145: 912–918.
106. Duscha BD, Annex BH, Keteyian SJ, *et al.* Differences in skeletal muscle between men and women with chronic heart failure. J Appl Physiol 2001; 90: 280–286.
107. Duscha BD, Annex BH, Green HJ, Pippen AM, Kraus WE. Deconditioning fails to explain peripheral skeletal muscle alterations in men with chronic heart failure. J Am Coll Cardiol 2002; 39: 1170–1174.
108. Aronson D, Burger AJ. The effect of sex on ventricular arrhythmic events in patients with congestive heart failure. Pacing Clin Electrophysiol 2002; 25: 1206–1211.
109. Aronson D, Burger AJ. Gender-related differences in modulation of heart rate in patients with congestive heart failure. J Cardiovasc Electrophysiol 2000; 11: 1071–1077.
110. Manolio TA, Furberg CD, Rautaharju PM, *et al.* Cardiac arrhythmias on 24-h ambulatory electrocardiography in older women and men: the Cardiovascular Health Study. J Am Coll Cardiol 1994; 23: 916–925.
111. Ghali J, Cooper R, Ford E. Trends in hospitalization for heart failure in the United States, 1973–1986: evidence for increasing population prevalence. Arch Intern Med 1990; 150: 769–773.
112. Croft JB, Giles WH, Pollard RA, *et al.* National trends in the initial hospitalization for heart failure. J Am Geriatr Soc 1997; 45: 270–275.
113. Haldeman GA, Croft JB, Giles WH, Rashidee A. Hospitalization of patients with heart failure: National Hospital Discharge Survey, 1985–1995. Am Heart J 1999; 137: 352–360.
114. Burns RB, McCarthy EP, Moskowitz MA, *et al.* Outcomes for older men and women with congestive heart failure. J Am Geriatr Soc 1997; 45: 276–280.
115. Vaccarino V, Chen Y, Wang Y, Radford MJ, Krumholz HM. Sex differences in the clinical care and outcomes of congestive heart failure in the elderly. Am Heart J 1999; 138: 835–842.
116. Krumholz HM, Parent EM, Tu N, *et al.* Readmission after hospitalization for congestive heart failure among medicare beneficiaries. Arch Intern Med 1997; 157: 99–104.
117. MacIntyre K, Capewell S, Stewart S, *et al.* Evidence of improving prognosis in heart failure: trends in Case Fatality in 66 547 patients hospitalized between 1986 and 1995. Circulation 2000; 102: 1126–1131.
118. McMurray J, Morrison C. Increase in hospital admission rates for heart failure in The Netherlands, 1980–1993. Heart 1997; 78: 421–422.
119. Philbin EF, DiSalvo TG. Influence of race and gender on care process, resource use, and hospital-based outcomes in congestive heart failure. Am J Cardiol 1998; 82: 76–81.

120. Davis K. The Unfinished Agenda: Improving the Well-Being of Elderly People Living Alone. Final report of The Commonwealth Fund Commission on Elderly People Living Alone (The Commonwealth Fund: New York, 1993).
121. Dries DL, Rosenberg YD, Waclawiw MA, Domanski MJ. Ejection fraction and risk of thromboembolic events in patients with systolic dysfunction and sinus rhythm: evidence for gender differences in the studies of left ventricular dysfunction trials. J Am Coll Cardiol 1997; 29: 1074–1080.
122. Organ Procurement and Transplantation Network. Transplants in the U.S. by Recipient Gender. Available at: http://www.optn.org/latestData/rptData.asp. Accessed January 15, 2004.
123. Aaronson KD, Schwartz JS, Goin JE, Mancini DM. Sex differences in patients acceptance of cardiac transplant candidacy. Circulation 1995; 91: 2753–2761.
124. Opasich C, Tavazzi L, Lucci D, *et al.* on behalf of the Italian Network on Congestive Heart Failure (IN-CHF) Investigators. Comparison of one-year outcome in women versus men with chronic congestive heart failure. Am J Cardiol 2000; 86: 353–357.
125. Jong P, Vowinckel E, Liu PP, Gong Y, Tu JV. Prognosis and determinants of survival in patients newly hospitalized for heart failure: a population-based study. Arch Intern Med 2002; 162: 1689–1694.
126. Croft JB, Giles WH, Pollard RA, *et al.* Heart failure survival among older adults in the United States: a poor prognosis for an emerging epidemic in the Medicare population. Arch Intern Med 1999; 159: 505–510.
127. Zannad F, Briancon S, Juilliere Y, *et al.* Incidence, clinical and etiologic features, and outcomes of advanced chronic heart failure: The EPICAL Study. J Am Coll Cardiol 1999; 33: 734–742.
128. Bourassa MG, Gurné O, Bangdiwala SI, *et al.* Natural history and patterns of current practice in heart failure. The Studies of Left Ventricular Dysfunction (SOLVD) Investigators. J Am Coll Cardiol 1993; 22: 14A–19A.
129. Eichhorn EJ. Prognosis determination in heart failure. Am J Med 2001; 110: 14–35.
130. Cohn JN, Johnson GR, Shabetai R, *et al.* Ejection fraction, peak exercise oxygen consumption, cardiothoracic ratio, ventricular arrhythmias, and plasma norepinephrine as determinants of prognosis in heart failure. Circulation 1993; 87: V15–16.
131. Dries DL, Exner DV, Gersh BJ, *et al.* Atrial fibrillation is associated with an increased risk for mortality and heart failure progression in patients with asymptomatic and symptomatic left ventricular systolic dysfunction: a retrospective analysis of the Studies of Left Ventricular Dysfunction (SOLVD) trials. J Am Coll Cardiol 1998; 32: 695–703.
132. Lechat P, Hulot JS, Escolano S, *et al.* Heart rate and cardiac rhythm relationships with bisoprolol benefit in chronic heart failure in CIBIS II trial. Circulation 2001; 13: 1428–1433.
133. Baldasseroni S, Opasich C, Gorini M, *et al.*, Italian Network on Congestive Heart Failure Investigators. Left bundle-branch block is associated with increased 1-year sudden and total mortality rate in 5517 outpatients with symptomatic heart failure: a report from the Italian network on congestive heart failure. Am Heart J 2002; 143: 398–405.

CHAPTER 5

Heart failure in the elderly

Jalal K Ghali, Dalane W Kitzman

Introduction

It is often said that the definition of "elderly" changes with one's own age. It is certainly reasonable to think of differences in the cardiovascular systems of a 30-year-old and an 80-year-old patient. However, it is much more challenging to point to a specific age when the elderly could be defined. For the purposes of this chapter, the elderly are defined as 65 years or older and the very elderly as 80 years or older.

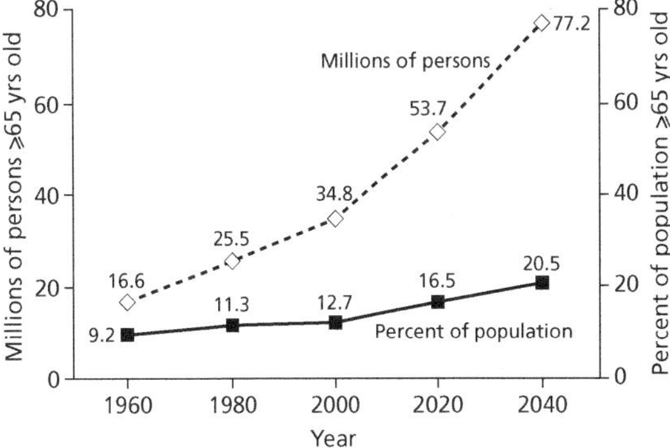

Figure 5.1. *Projected increases in the United States population 65 years of age or older (Data are from the U.S. Census Bureau)*

Epidemiology

The segment of American population that is 65 years old or older is the fastest growing population, with a projected increase from 12.7% (34.8 million) in the year 2000 to 16.5% (53.7 million) in the year 2020 (Figure 5.1).[1] Over 90% of all new cases of heart failure occur in patients 65 years old or older.[2] Therefore, heart failure has become primarily a disorder of the elderly population.

This is reflected in the marked increase in the incidence and prevalence of heart failure with aging. In the Framingham Heart Study, the incidence of heart failure increased from 2 cases per 1000 person-years in individuals younger than 60 years old to 10 per 1000 person-years for ages 70 to 79 years, and 25 per 1000 person-years for those 80 years old and older.[3] In the Cardiovascular Health Study, a population-based observational study of individuals > 65 years old, conducted in four communities, the incidence of heart failure was 10.6 per 1000 person-years at age 65, and 42.5 per 1000 person-years at age > 80 years.[4] In a population study in East London, the incidence increased from 0.02 cases per 1000 person-years in those aged 25 to 34 years to 11.6 in persons aged ≥ 85 years.[5] Similarly, the prevalence of heart failure increases sharply with age. In the Framingham study, the prevalence rises from < 1% in patients aged 45 to 54 to 5% in those aged 65 to 74, and 9% in patients 75 to 84 years old.[3] It essentially doubles every decade after the age of 45 (Figure 5.2). In the

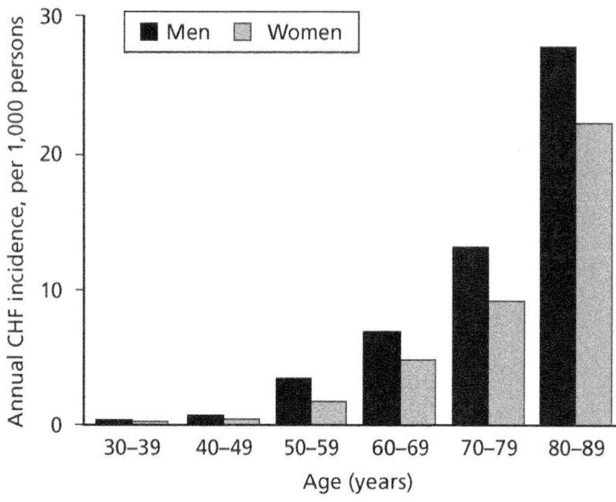

Figure 5.2. *Prevalence of heart failure by age and sex: the Framingham Study (With permission from Ho* et al.[3])

Olmsted County study, the prevalence of heart failure increased from 1.3% in patients 55 to 64 years old to 8.4% for those ≥ 75 years old.[6] In the Cardiovascular Health Study, the prevalence of heart failure tripled between the ages of 70 and 85 years (from 4.1% to 14.3% in women, and 7.8% to 17.4% in men).[7]

It is interesting to note that in the Olmsted County study, the mean age of patients was 76 years—similar to Framingham—and that not only did 88% of all new cases of heart failure occur in patients ≥ 65 years old, but the very elderly (≥ 80 years old) accounted for one-half of all new cases of heart failure.[2]

Changes in the Cardiovascular Systems with Aging

Efforts to identify the effect of aging on the cardiovascular system have encountered the inherent difficulties in separating changes induced by aging alone from those resulting from diseases and lifestyle changes, including deconditioning.

Changes in cardiovascular structure

The vasculature

With age, the endothelial cells in the intima of the arterial system become more heterogeneous in size, shape, and axial orientation, which may render the intraluminal blood flow less laminar.[8] Interestingly, impairment in endothelial function has also been described in the healthy, elderly population.[9]

In the media, thickening of the smooth-muscle layer, with greater fragmentation of elastin and increased calcification, contributes to decreased elasticity and compliance, especially of the aorta and great arteries.[8] Large-vessel wall thickening, however, results mainly from an increase in intimal thickness.[10] The carotid wall intimal media thickness increases 2-fold to 3-fold between the ages of 20 and 90, and a substantial increase in aortic root diameter occurs.[11] The age-associated increase in intimal media thickening is associated with increased vessel stiffness, as manifested by increased pulse wave velocity.[11] As the walls of large arteries become stiffer, systolic pressure increases and diastolic pressure decreases, resulting in a wide pulse pressure. It should be noted that the latter has been found to be a powerful predictor of the development of heart failure.[12]

Furthermore, the persistent rise of systolic blood pressure with aging, coupled with a leveling off of diastolic blood pressure to 60 mm Hg at age 50, and declining thereafter, leads to the emergence of isolated systolic hypertension as the most common form of hypertension in the elderly.[13]

The heart

Changes to the heart that occur with aging, which have been described, include enlargement of cardiac myocytes[14] and an increase in the amount and change in the properties of interstitial collagen, as well as fibrosis and amyloid deposition.[15,16]

Although the overall size of the heart does not increase with aging, a slight increase in left ventricular (LV) wall thickness does occur due to an increase in myocyte size, the left atrial dimension increases with age, and the pericardium becomes thicker and stiffer.[17]

Cardiovascular function

Resting left ventricular ejection fraction (LVEF) is preserved with aging.[18–20] However, there is a decrease in the maximum LVEF during upright exercise.[19] The inability to increase LVEF during exercise is due to a compromise in the ability to reduce end-diastolic volume (EDV) index. Thus, the stroke volume is preserved mainly because of an increase in EDV to a greater extent during exercise in older versus younger people.[20] Ejection of blood from the left ventricle into a stiffer aorta leads to a higher systolic blood pressure, which is more pronounced in the central aorta than in the periphery because of the superimposition of the direct pressure wave resulting from ejection of blood to the aorta and the reflected wave from the periphery.[11] The increased load on the left ventricle leads to increased LV wall thickness which appears to normalize LV wall stress, thus, maintaining a normal resting EF.

Relaxation of the myocardial muscle is prolonged and the maximal rate of early diastolic filling is reduced on average by 50% between the ages of 20 and 80 years.[21,22] This is compensated for by a greater contribution of atrial contraction to diastolic filling, leading to atrial enlargement and an exaggerated A wave. It should be noted that there is a widely held misconception that LV filling is impaired in the healthy elderly. In fact, during exercise, and despite a reduction in the maximal early diastolic filling rate, the LV end diastole is not reduced in healthy older patients but rather is greater in older than in younger men. In women, EDV is increased significantly by exercise with age.[19]

Sympathetic modulation

Several changes in the sympathetic nervous systems occur with aging. The activity of the sympathetic nervous system increases with aging, as evident by increasing circulating norepinephrine levels due to increased norepinephrine spillover as well as reduced clearance,[23,24] and as demonstrated by direct measurement of muscle sympathetic nerve activity.[25,26] Aging is also associated with the decreased density of myocardial beta-adrenergic receptors[27] and a decrease in plasma renin activity and angiotensin II.[28]

A diminished chronotropic and inotropic response to catecholamines has also been described. Infusion of beta-adrenergic agonists results in decreased heart rate and less increase in EF in older compared to younger patients, and less vasodilating effect.[29] However, as stated earlier, resting LVEF does not decline with age.

Heart rhythm

Heart rate variability declines with aging, predominantly because of a decline in parasympathetic function.[30,31] Isolated premature atrial beats were detected in 6% of healthy participants in the Baltimore Longitudinal Study on a resting electrocardiogram,[32] and in 88% during 24-hour ambulatory monitoring, and were not predictive over a 10-year period of cardiac events.[33] Similarly, in the Cardiovascular Health Study, supraventricular arrhythmias were detected in more than half the patients and were strongly associated with increasing age.[34] Similarly, an increase in the prevalence and complexity of ventricular arrhythmia was noted with aging, without having any adverse cardiac risk over a 10-year follow-up period.

Exercise

Aging is associated with a decline in maximal aerobic capacity averaging 10% per decade.[35,36] Several factors, all related to an age-related decrease in beta-adrenergic responsiveness, could potentially contribute to this effect. These factors include a decreased maximal heart rate, smaller increase in EF and diminished vasodilatory response to exercise.[37] However, these adverse effects on cardiac performance in exercise are compensated for by an increase in EDV maximizing the use of the Frank–Starling mechanism. The maximum heart rate decreases with exercise by about 30% between 20 and 85 years of age and it is the main reason for a 30% decline in maximum acute cardiac output reserve between 20 and 85 years.[19]

Non-cardiac factors, such as a decline in maximal skeletal muscle performance, a greater sense of muscle fatigue and discomfort, or an increase in the sensation of dyspnea, may also play a role in the decline of maximal aerobic capacity.[37]

Relevant changes in other organ systems

Several significant changes accompany aging in various organ systems that exert an influence on the development of manifestations of heart failure in the elderly and its management.

One of the most underestimated changes in the elderly is the decline in renal function. Due to the decrease in muscle mass, this decline is not reflected by measurement of serum creatinine, and calculation of creatinine clearance should be the routine in the elderly.[38] It has been estimated that glomerular filtration rates (GFRs) decline by an average of 8 cc/min per decade.[39] The decline in renal function leads not only to a decrease in the capacity of the elderly to handle volume overload, but contributes significantly to changes in the pharmacokinetics and pharmacodynamics of various medications.[40]

Renal function in the elderly patients with heart failure is markedly compromised.[41] There are age-associated changes, including a reduction in the GFR, decrease in tubular secretion and concentration ability due to a decrease in the number of renal glomeruli and tubules, and reduction in renal blood flow.[42]

Another change that is relevant to the use of diuretics in the elderly is impairment in the mechanism of thirst that may lead to intravascular volume depletion.[43]

In addition, there are a host of changes in the elderly that have practical impact on the management of heart failure, including hearing impairment and early stages of dementia that may render communication more challenging, visual impairment that may create difficulties in obtaining daily weight and complying with medications, and urinary incontinence that may impact on compliance with diuretics.

Risk factors

The specific risk factors for the development of heart failure in the elderly were evaluated in a study of 1749 individuals, aged 65 years or older, who were free of heart failure, myocardial infarction (MI) or angina.[44] During 10 years of follow-up, heart failure developed in 173 patients. Age, male gender, diabetes, wide pulse pressure, and body mass index (BMI) were all predictors of heart failure. Patients who had an MI during follow-up were at 20-fold greater risk of developing heart failure. Interestingly in that study, psychosocial factors, activities of daily living, and cognitive functions were not found to be predictors. In the Framingham Heart Study, hypertension preceded the development of heart failure in 91% of patients, with a high population attributable risk for heart failure, accounting for 39% of cases in men and 59% in women.[45] Thus, the traditional risk factors for heart failure are at play in the elderly.

In the Cardiovascular Health Study,[4] predictors of the development of heart failure in the elderly included age, coronary artery disease (CAD), systolic blood pressure, and interestingly, increased C-reactive protein (CRP). Among 732 elderly Framingham participants (mean age 78 years), elevated inflammatory markers including serum interleukin-6 (IL-6), CRP, and tumor necrosis factor-α (TNF-α) were associated with an increased risk for the development of heart failure.[46]

It is of no surprise that heart failure is a disease of the elderly. The major risk factors for heart failure, namely ischemia and hypertension, increase in prevalence with aging. Similarly, the prevalence of other risk factors for heart failure, including left ventricular hypertrophy (LVH), diabetes, and obesity, increases with aging. What is unique in the elderly population is a series of changes that render them susceptible to the development of heart failure. As described earlier, increasing vascular stiffness leads to increasing systolic blood pressure and LVH, among other things. The progressive slowing of early LV diastolic filling leads to more filling in later diastole, exaggerated atrial contraction, and left atrial enlargement and hypertrophy. The age-associated impairment in the ability to reduce end-systolic volume (ESV) with vigorous exercise leads to failure in increasing EF with exercise, so despite a greater increase in EDV during vigorous exercise, stroke volume and EF fail to do so. Furthermore, maximum heart rate decreases with vigorous exercise. Thus, the elderly population is more likely to manifest heart failure symptoms and signs in response to stressful events that could be well tolerated in a younger population. All these changes contribute to a lower threshold for the development of heart failure symptoms in the elderly because of a reduction in cardiac reserve.

It is of interest to note in this context that depression has been found to be a predictor of heart failure. In a follow-up study on 4538 elderly patients with systolic hypertension, depression was associated with a 3-fold increase in the development of heart failure.[47]

In another study on 2501 participants ≥ 65

years of age in the New Haven cohort of the Established Population for Epidemiological Studies in the Elderly,[48] 313 developed heart failure, and depression was found to be an independent risk factor for heart failure among elderly women but not elderly men.

Presentation of Elderly Patients with Heart Failure

Patients with heart failure present with signs and symptoms due to a congested state, low cardiac output state, or combined features of both. In the elderly, the previously mentioned changes and the limited reserve capacity may lead to different presentations. The most common symptom of heart failure—dyspnea—may be under-recognized in sedentary elderly patients because of limited physical activity or further restriction of physical activity that is ascribed to aging. Similarly, fatigue and weakness could be obscured by limiting activity. Symptoms such as minimal confusion, forgetfulness, or minimal mental disturbances could easily be interpreted as being due to aging rather than to low cardiac output. In addition, obtaining a detailed history may be difficult due to cognitive impairment. Nocturia is common in the elderly and might not trigger the suspicion of heart failure. Auscultatory findings in the lungs may be obscured by the presence of chronic obstructive pulmonary disease (COPD) or atelectasis. The presence of peripheral edema may be explained by chronic venous insufficiency rather than a sign of fluid overload. In addition, comorbidity is common. In a retrospective chart review of 34 587 patients who were 65 years old or older, hospitalized with heart failure, comorbidity was common.[49] Hypertension was present in 60% of patients, CAD in 55%, diabetes in 40%, COPD in one-third, and atrial fibrillation in one-third. More than twice as many patients were > 85 years old as compared with those 65 to 69 years old. Among patients > 85 years old, 18.4% were in long-term care facilities prior to admission.

Highlighting the difficulty in diagnosing heart failure in the elderly, a small retrospective study of 116 patients (median age 86; range 65 to 98 years) with an established diagnosis of heart failure during hospitalization,[50] found that only 28% were admitted primarily for heart failure. The majority (47%) were admitted for problems associated with mobility and self-care. None of the patients had heart failure as their only medical problem; lung disease was present in 30%, incontinence in 29%, cerebrovascular disease in 26%, and musculoskeletal problems in 41%. Cognitive impairment was present in 38% of the patients, and 35% had a Barthel activities of daily living score of 16 or less, implying possible difficulties with independent living. In addition, 39% were on psychotropic drugs. In a community-based epidemiological study of people ≥ 71 years, those with self-reported heart failure (n = 199) were at twice the risk for depression as compared to the rest of the community (n = 5926), highlighting the need to look for this association.[51]

Clinical features of outpatients

The clinical characteristics of elderly patients with heart failure and impaired LVEF are significantly different from younger patients. In the MERIT-HF study,[52] patients > 65 years (n = 1988) were compared to those < 65 years (n = 2009). Elderly patients had a higher prevalence of women, ischemic etiology, higher New York Heart Association (NYHA) functional class, higher systolic and lower diastolic blood pressure, lower heart rate, lower BMI, higher prevalence of history of MI and atrial fibrillation, and were less likely to receive angiotensin-converting enzyme (ACE) inhibitors. Similarly, in a cohort of 3327 outpatients with heart failure enrolled in the Registry of the Italian Network on Congestive Heart Failures,[53] patients ≥ 70 years (n = 1033) were more likely to be women, had a higher NYHA functional class, higher prevalence of ischemic etiology and atrial fibrillation and they received ACE inhibitors, beta-blockers and anticoagulants less frequently.

Hospitalization

The dominance of the elderly population in the steady increase in hospitalization for heart failure was recognized with the first publication describing the trends in hospitalization rate for heart failure for the period 1973–1986.[54] A similar finding was confirmed for subsequent years.[55–57] The *National Hospital Discharge Survey*[57] documented a significant increase in hospitalization for heart failure by age for the years 1990 and 2000 which was particularly pronounced between the ages of 65 to 74 and ≥ 75 years (Figure 5.3). A significant increase in hospitalization discharges were noted for men and women of all age groups. An interesting and consistent finding has been the high prevalence of women in patients with preserved left ventricular ejection fraction (PLVEF). In a cross-sectional study of a national sample of 19 710 Medicare patients hospitalized for heart failure, PLVEF was present in 35%, the majority of whom (79%) were women.[58]

In a web-based registry of patients hospitalized for heart failure, the Acute Decompensated Heart Failure National Registry (ADHERE™),[59] a total of 85 617 patient records were enrolled between October 2001 and October 2003. The mean age was 70 years for men and 75 years for women. Data on LVEF were available in 71% of the patients, and LVEF > 40% was present in 51% of women compared to 28% of men. Thus, in elderly patients hospitalized with acute heart failure, PLVEF appears primarily to involve women. (M. Galvao, personal communication, 2004).

Heart failure with preserved left ventricular ejection fraction

The high prevalence of heart failure with PLVEF in the elderly is well established.[4,6,7,59,60] In the Olmsted County study,[6] 43% of newly diagnosed patients with heart failure had PLVEF with a mean age of 78 years. In the Framingham study,[59] 51% had heart failure with PLVEF at a mean age of 73 years, and in the Cardiovascular Health study,[4] the percentage of heart failure patients with PLVEF was 63% at a mean age of 75 years.

A high preponderance of women was noted in these studies, ranging from 65% in Framingham[59] to 69% in the Olmsted County study, confirming findings from hospitalization discharges.[6] The underlying pathophysiology of this condition is diastolic dysfunction, as defined by increased resistance to LV filling resulting in elevated filling pressures.[61]

A distinction between heart failure with preserved versus impaired LVEF is important for several reasons. First is the recognition that heart failure with PLVEF is common in the elderly. It is easier to establish the diagnosis of heart failure when LVEF is impaired. However, in the presence of normal LVEF, and especially in view of the atypical presentation in the elderly, a high index of suspicion is required so the diagnosis of heart failure is not missed. It is worth mentioning here that with the widespread misuse of serum brain (b-type) natriuretic peptide (BNP) to aid in the diagnosis of heart failure, the level of BNP has been noted to be elevated in the elderly in the absence of heart failure.[62,63] Second, in the acute management of heart failure, the recognition of the presence of PLVEF is critical for using diuretics judiciously and avoiding overdiuresis that would lead to underfilling of the left ventricle and reduction of cardiac output and hypotension. Third, it is important for health care providers and the patient to know that LVEF is normal, considering the strong evidence that heart

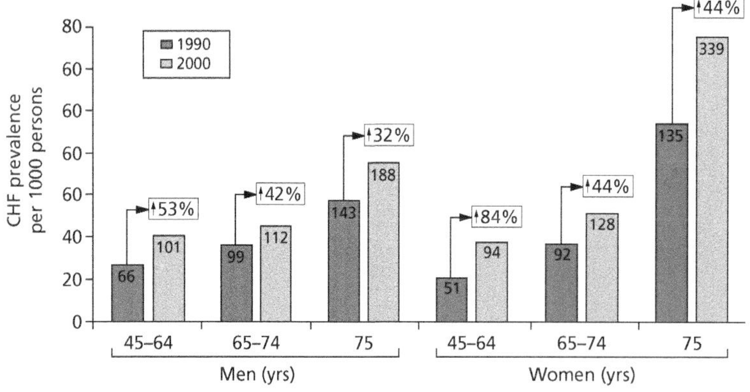

Figure 5.3. *Hospital discharges for heart failure by age: 1990 versus 2000*[57]

failure with PLVEF carries a less malignant prognosis as compared to impaired LVEF.[60,64] Finally, the results of the first large trial in patients with heart failure and PLVEF, the Candesartan in Heart Failure—Assessment of Reduction in Mortality and Morbidity (CHARM trial), in which 1514 patients were randomized to candesartan and 1509 to placebo, mean age 67 years and mean LVEF 54%, indicated that the angiotensin receptor blocker (ARB), candesartan, decreased cumulative hospitalization rate for heart failure as assessed by investigators. The total number of admissions for heart failure was lower with candesartan (n = 402) than placebo (n = 566) (P = 0.014) and so was the number of patients hospitalized for heart failure (n = 230) compared to placebo (n = 279) (P = 0.017).[66] Based on that study, and despite a lack of effect on mortality, this intervention should be considered in elderly patients with heart failure and PLVEF, to reduce hospitalization.

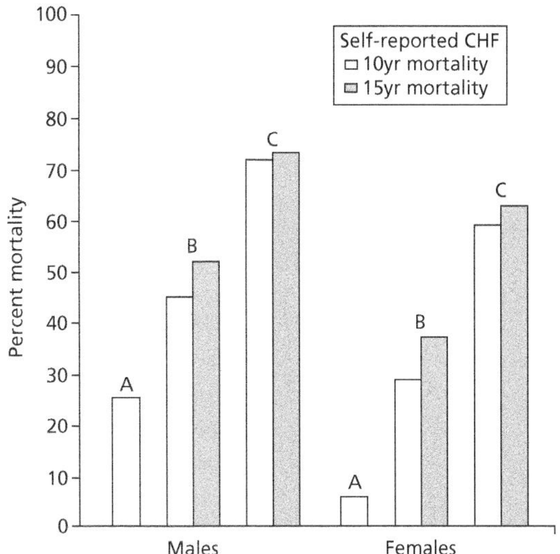

Figure 5.4. *Ten-year mortality rate of self-reported congestive heart failure (CHF). (A) 25 to 54 years, (B) 55 to 64 years, and (C) 65 to 74 years*

Prognosis

The grim prognosis for patients with heart failure was originally described by the Framingham investigators, showing an overall 1-year and 5-year mortality of 43% and 75% in men, and 36% and 62% in women, respectively.[3,65] Mortality increased with advancing age in both sexes (hazard ratio [HR] for men, 1.27 per decade of age; 95% confidence interval [CI], 1.09–1.47; HR for women 1.61 per decade of age; 95% CI, 1.37–1.90). Among participants 65 to 74 years who self-reported a history of heart failure in the First National Health and Nutrition Examination Survey, the 10-year mortality rate was 72% in men and 60% in women.[66] These mortality rates were remarkable higher than for younger patients (6% and 30% for women aged 25 to 54 and 55 to 64 years, respectively, and 25% and 45% for men aged 25 to 54 and 55 to 64 years, respectively (Figure 5.4).

In a national cohort of 170 239 Medicare patients ≥ 67 years who had no evidence of heart failure in 1984 or 1985 and who were discharged after first hospitalization for heart failure in 1986, the 6-year survival rate was 19% for black men, 16% for white men, 25% for black women and 23% for white women.[67]

The high mortality rate associated with heart failure in the elderly appears to have declined over the past decades. In the Framingham study, temporal trends in survival were examined during a 50-year interval from the 1950s through the 1990s.[68] Mean age at the diagnosis of heart failure was 63 years in the period from 1950 to 1969 and 80 years in the period from 1990 to 1999. During this period 1-year and 5-year mortality rates age-adjusted among men declined from 30% and 70%, respectively, to 28% and 59%, respectively. Among women, mortality rates declined from 28% and 57% to 24% and 45% respectively, for an overall improvement of 12% per decade for men and women.

A retrospective study in Scotland[69] showed that in a total of 66 547 patients, median age of 72 years in men and 78 years in women, admitted with heart failure between 1986 and 1995, 1-year case fatality (CF) was 27.2% in those aged < 55 years and 58.1% in those aged > 84 years. Thirty-day CF rate fell between 1986 and 1995 by 26% in men (P < 0.0001) and 17% in women (P < 0.0001). Median survival increased from

1.23 to 1.64 years. Similarly 1-year mortality for 23 505 Medicare patients hospitalized with heart failure declined by 14.6% ($P < 0.001$) between 1991 and 1997.[70]

Worsening renal function among hospitalized patients with heart failure is associated with worse outcome.[71] In a study of 1681 patients ≥ 65 years hospitalized with heart failure, worsening renal function occurred in 28% of patients and was associated with a significant increase in length of stay, hospital cost, and hospital mortality.[72]

Anemia has been associated with poor prognosis in heart failure.[73] In a consecutive sample of 2281 patients > 65 years (mean age 79 years), hospitalized with heart failure, each 1% lower hematocrit was associated with 2% greater 1-year mortality,[74] confirming this association in the elderly.

Another element that has not been given adequate attention is emotional support. A review of the records of 292 patients ≥ 65 years hospitalized with heart failure, who were participants of the New Haven, Connecticutt, Established Populations for the Epidemiologic Studies of the Elderly (EPESE), showed that the absence of emotional support, measured before admission was a strong independent predictor of fatal and non-fatal cardiac events in the year following discharge in elderly women but not elderly men.[75]

Precipitating Factors

Hospitalization is the single largest expenditure in the care of heart failure[76] and hospitalized patients face a 50% risk of subsequent hospitalization.[77] In addition, it is possible that the hemodynamic overload and neurohormonal activation associated with decompensation lead to further injury, and incremental damage to the left ventricle with each hospitalization (Figure 5.5).[78] Therefore, a meticulous search to identify potential precipitating factors and the implementation of preventive measures are mandatory for the proper management of heart failure.

Non-compliance, identified as the leading factor resulting in decompensation in a younger population[79] was found to be the most common factor leading to hospitalization (42% of cases), in a cohort of 179 patients, mean age 75 years, hospitalized over a 1-year period.[80]

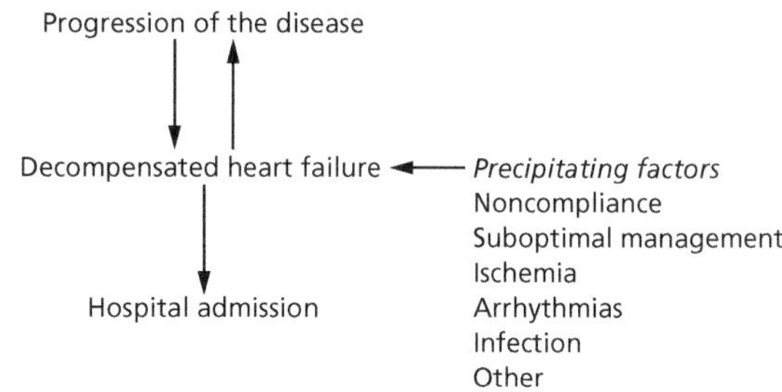

Figure 5.5. *Interplay between precipitating factors, decompensation and progression of the disease*

Non-compliance with diet is more pronounced in the elderly because of the difficulty and higher expense of preparing fresh food, and the higher utilization of processed food. Visual and hearing impairment, confusion, polypharmacy, side effects, and the cost of medications contribute to low adherence with the prescribed regimen of medications.

The occurrence of atrial fibrillation could precipitate heart failure because of loss of atrial contribution to late filling, very rapid ventricular response, or markedly slow rate. In a study of 154 patients hospitalized with heart failure, mean age 75 years, atrial fibrillation was thought to be the precipitating factor in 16% of patients.[81] The Framingham Study evaluated 1470 participants who developed new atrial fibrillation, heart failure or both.[82] Among 322 patients with both conditions, mean age 75 years, those with heart failure had a significant increase in mortality (men: HR 1.6, 95% CI 1.2–2.1; women: HR 2.7, 95%, CI 2.0–3.6) with the subsequent development of atrial fibrillation. Similarly, in those patients with atrial fibrillation, the development of heart failure was associated with increased mortality (men: HR 2.7%, 95% CI 1.9–3.7; women: HR 3.1, 95% CI 2.2–4.2). However, there is no evidence that maintaining sinus rhythm after the development of atrial fibrillation improves survival.

Management

The overall goals when treating heart failure are reducing symptoms, improving quality of life, slowing or reversing the progression of LV dysfunction, and improving survival. Achieving the first two goals is equally important in the young and old alike. However, with advancing age, the goal of prolonging survival may play a less prominent role.

The paucity of data on the pharmacological treatment effect in this group is striking. Underrepresentation of the elderly in heart failure clinical trials has been the rule.[83] The mean age of patients in survival heart failure trials is 63 years; this is in contrast to the mean age of patients with heart failure in the community which is 76 years.[2,3,5]

One cannot assume that a drug proven effective in a younger patient population will provide similar effectiveness in an older patient population. Changes in the vasculature, blood pressure, diastolic function, autonomic nervous system, and renal function, as well as the higher prevalence of comorbidities, noncompliance, changes in pharmacokinetics and pharmacodynamics of drugs, and higher risk of drug–drug interactions—all these factors underline the fallacy of the assumption that the results of trials conducted in a younger population should apply equally to the elderly.

Drug therapy in the elderly with heart failure

Drug therapy in the elderly is heavily influenced by factors unique to this population, including the higher prevalence of comorbidities, polypharmacy, environmental influences, and foremost, the effects of aging. The presence and interaction of these factors, to a different degree, contribute to the view that the elderly should be regarded as a more heterogeneous group, in which drug therapy should be individualized and the response of the patient closely monitored.

Distribution of a drug in the body depends on body composition, plasma protein binding, and blood flow to the organs.[40] The age-associated decrease in lean body mass and volume of total body water necessitates a reduction in the loading dose of water-soluble drugs like digoxin. On the other hand, because of increased body fat, lipid-soluble drugs have a larger volume of distribution.[42]

The two major routes for elimination of drugs are the kidneys and the liver. Reduction in drug elimination by the kidneys is well documented due to reduced GFR and decreased tubular secretion and concentration ability. These changes are due to an age-associated decrease in the number of renal glomeruli and tubules as well as a decrease in renal blood flow.[39] Thus, renal excretion of digoxin is decreased.

The use of ACE inhibitors may be associated with minimal but stable deterioration of renal function resulting from a reduction in GFR secondary to a decrease in the constriction of glomerular efferent arterioles. Although patients hospitalized with decompensated heart failure and impaired renal function may respond favorably to diuresis, vasodilators, or inotropes with subsequent improvement in renal function, not infrequently a deterioration of renal function may necessitate at least a temporary withholding of ACE inhibitors. The use of ACE inhibitors, ARBs, and aldosterone antagonists is more likely to be associated with hyperkalemia in the elderly.

The use of nonsteroidal antiinflammatory agents (NSAIDs) in the elderly is more likely to be associated with deterioration of renal function, fluid retention, and increased systemic vascular resistance resulting in decompensated heart failure.[84] The impact of selective cyclooxygenase-2 (COX-2) inhibitors on heart failure is not known. In a recent population-based retrospective study, NSAID-naïve patients 66 years or older who were started on rofecoxib (n = 14 583), celecoxib (n = 18 908), and non-selective NSAIDs (n = 5391) were compared to non-NSAID users as controls (n = 100 000). Relative to non-NSAID users, a higher risk for heart failure admission was found in users of rofecoxib and non-selective NSAIDs, (relative risk [RR]: 1.8, 95% CI, 1.5–2.2 and 1.4, 1.0–1.9), respectively, but not celecoxib (1.0, 0.8–1.3).[85] Thus, in this elderly population, significant differences were found between non-selective NSAIDs and individual COX-2-inhibitors. However, a prospective study to confirm this finding is lacking.

Diuretics

Several factors should be considered when administering diuretics to the elderly. Diuretic usage in the elderly may precipitate or exacerbate incontinence, and its potential occurrence should be specifically discussed with the patients. If feasible, adopting a gentle diuresis may help to minimize or prevent incontinence exacerbation. With aggressive diuresis, close monitoring of renal function is required due to the decline in renal function and the potential for deterioration of renal function. In elderly patients with heart failure and preserved LV systolic function, judicious use of diuretics is required to avoid hypotension. Furosemide withdrawal has been shown to improve postprandial hypotension, possibly by improving LV filling.[86] A small study of 17 patients ≥ 65 years with class IV heart failure demonstrated that continuous intravenous administration of furosemide was safe and effective.[87]

Digitalis

A subgroup analysis of the Digitalis Investigation Group (DIG) study examining the effect of age on response to digitalis showed that the beneficial effect of digitalis in reducing hospitalization was preserved in the elderly.[88] This analysis included 2092 patients between the ages of 70 and 79 years and 425 patients ≥ 80 years. It should be noted that the frequency of drug withdrawal due to side effects as well as hospitalization for suspected digitalis toxicity increased with age. With a decline in renal function, the dose of digitalis should be adjusted downward and the digitalis level should be kept below 1 ng/mL.[89]

Angiotensin-converting enzyme inhibitors

The elderly patients were under-represented in all clinical trials that assessed the benefit of ACE inhibitors in patients with systolic heart failure. A systematic review[90] of data from trials on patients with heart failure or LV dysfunction, including post-MI showed a significant reduction in mortality, MI, and hospital admission for heart failure in patients 65 to 75 years of age. A similar trend was noted for patients > 75 years of age.

Thus, ACE inhibitors should be prescribed to all patients with systolic heart failure. Special considerations in the elderly include paying more attention to the potential for orthostatic hypotension by measuring blood pressure in the standing position and closely following renal function and potassium levels.

Limited information is available on the effects of ACE inhibitors on the very old. In a retrospective cohort study[91] using the Systematic Assessment of Geriatric drug use via Epidemiology (SAGE) database, linking patient information with drug utilization data, 19452 patients with heart failure admitted to nursing homes were identified using either an ACE inhibitor (n = 4911) or digoxin (n = 14890). The mortality rate was 10% lower in ACE inhibitor users as compared to digoxin users (RR = 0.89, 95% CI, 0.83–0.95), and so was the rate of functional decline (RR = 0.74, 95% CI, 0.69–0.80), suggesting a beneficial effect of ACE inhibitors on survival and functional benefit in patients > 85 years with heart failure.

Beta-blockers

Despite the strong clinical evidence supporting the use of beta-blockers in systolic heart failure, these agents are underutilized in the elderly, probably because of concern about their safety and tolerability as well as the lack of definitive data regarding their benefit in this population.

In the three beta-blocker survival studies, the Cardiac Insufficiency Bisoprolol Study II (CIBIS II), Metoprolol CR/XL Randomized Intervention Trial in Congestive Heart Failure (MERIT-HF), and the Carvedilol Prospective Randomized Cumulative Survival (COPERNICUS) trial, the mean ages of patients were 61, 64, and 66 years, respectively. MERIT-HF, however, had a predefined data analysis plan in which subgroup analyses were pre-specified, including an analysis of the elderly for safety reasons.[52] Patients enrolled in MERIT-HF were 40 to 80 years old with LVEF ≤ 40%, and in NYHA class II-IV for at least three months prior to enrollment. In patients ≥ 65 years (n = 1582), total mortality was reduced in the metoprolol CR/XL group by 37% (95% CI 15–52, P = 0.0008), sudden death by 43% (CI 17–61, P = 0.003), and death from worsening heart failure by 61% (95% CI 32–77, P = 0.0005) (Figure 5.6). The number of hospitalizations for worsening heart failure was reduced by 38% (P = 0.0006). In total, there were 425 patients > 65 years with severe heart failure (NYHA class III or IV and EF < 25%) with a mean age of 72 (+ 4.1) years, and mean EF of 18% (± 4%). In this group, total mortality was

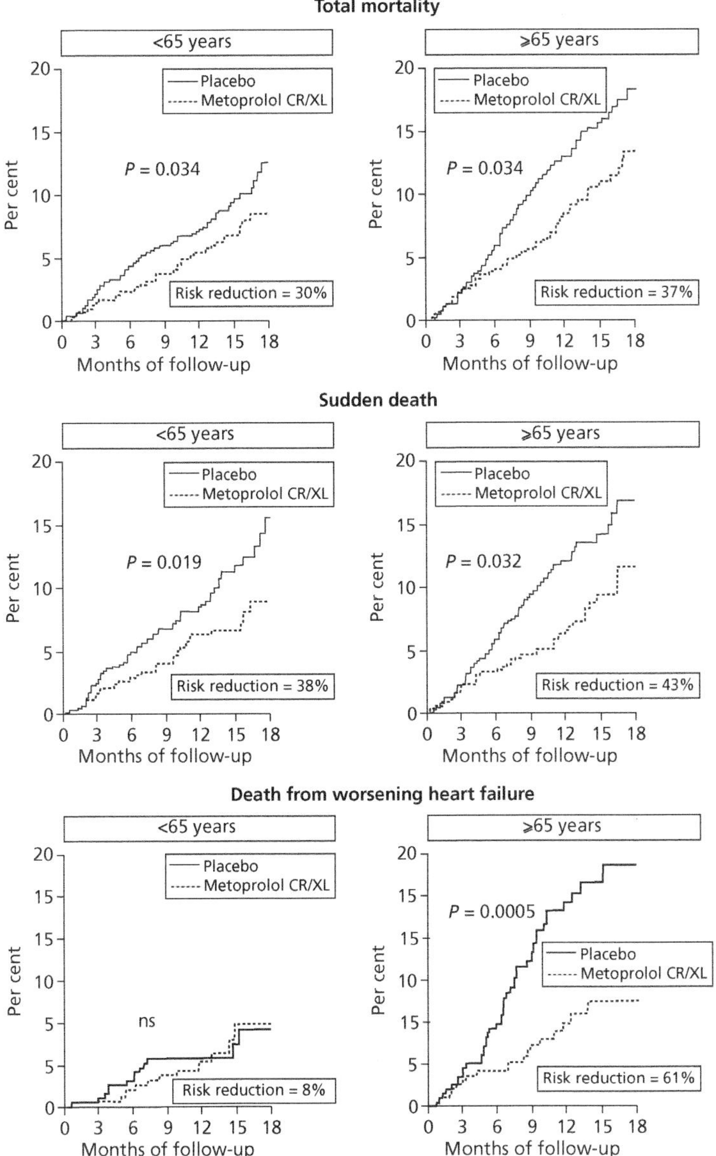

Figure 5.6. *Cumulative percentages of all-cause mortality (top), sudden death (middle), and death from worsening heart failure (bottom) in two age groups*

reduced by 36% ($P = 0.051$), and the combined endpoint of all-cause mortality and hospitalization due to worsening heart failure was reduced by 40% ($P = 0.031$).

It should be noted that beta-blockers were well tolerated as judged by fewer drug withdrawals as compared to placebo, regardless of severity of heart failure (Figure 5.7). An interesting observation from this analysis was the increase in systolic blood pressure by a few mm Hg in patients treated with beta-blockers.

Further support for the benefit of beta-blockers in the elderly comes from a population-based cohort of 11 942 patients ≥ 65 years (mean age of 79 years) with incident heart failure over a 5-year period.[92] The use of beta-blockers was associated with a substantial reduction in all-cause mortality (HR = 0.65, 95% CI 0.47–0.90).

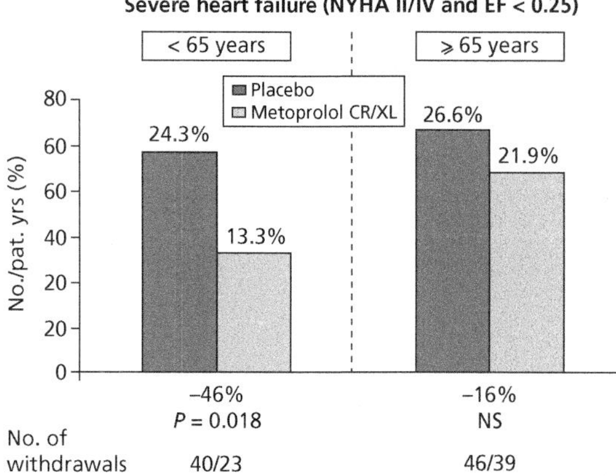

Figure 5.7. *Bar diagram illustrating yearly discontinuation rate of study medicine (all-cause) by age group in all patients randomized and in those with severe heart failure, defined as NYHA class III or IV and EF < 25% (lower panel)*

Abbreviations: EF = ejection fraction; ns = not significant; NYHA = New York Heart Association

A recent chart review study evaluated 11 854 hospitalizations for newly diagnosed heart failure over a 5-year period.[93] The mean age of patients was 79 years and the majority were ≥ 75 years. Comparing the prescription of both beta-blockers and ACE inhibitors/ARBs to no prescription demonstrated a 13.3% reduction in mortality (29.9% to 16.6%) for a relative adjusted risk reduction of 44%.

Devices

In patients with heart failure and impaired LVEF, resynchronization therapy has been proven to decrease hospitalization[94] and improve quality of life and exercise capacity.[95] The implantable defibrillator has been shown to decrease mortality.[94,96] The Comparison of Medical Therapy, Pacing, and Defibrillation in Chronic Heart Failure (COMPANION) study demonstrated this benefit in an elderly population (mean age of 67 years) with advanced heart failure.[94] It is critical that health care providers discuss the issues related to implanting a defibrillator in great detail with the patient and family members to ensure that the proper decision has been made. Unfortunately, when such a discussion has not taken place, the need may raise to turn off the defibrillator shortly after implantation.

Exercise training

Several studies have repeatedly confirmed that exercise in patients with heart failure improves exercise capacity and quality of life indicators.[97,98] The finding that exercise may improve diastolic filling[99] would suggest that elderly patients with heart failure may particularly benefit from exercise training. A small study involving 22 patients ≥ 75 years (mean of 81 years), with a mean LVEF of 27%, demonstrated a 20% increase in 6-minute walk distance with exercise, and the majority reported subjective improvement in well-being.[100]

The largest study of exercise training in heart failure included 180 patients, with a mean age of 65 years in the exercise arm (n = 90) and 66 years in the control (n = 91).[101] Patients were randomized into three months of supervised training and nine months of home-based training with usual care. The study showed improvement in peak oxygen uptake and strength during the supervised training, but little further improvement during the home-based training, suggesting the need for supervision and encouragement. More importantly, however, it showed the safety and feasibility of long-term exercise training. Special efforts are required to encourage elderly patients with heart failure to participate in exercise training.

Multidisciplinary disease management

A multidisciplinary disease management approach is very useful in addressing the multiple problems involved with compliance in the elderly, and has been demonstrated to improve quality of life, decrease hospitalization,[102] and potentially improve survival in elderly patients.[103]

Conclusion

Heart failure is a disease of the elderly. To provide optimal management of elderly patients with heart failure, an understanding of the age-related changes that occur in the structure and function of the cardiovascular system, as well as in other organs, and an appreciation of the cognitive and emotional state are needed. In addition, verification of the benefit of various management strategies requires adequate representation of the elderly in clinical trials.

References

1. National population projections. Washington, D.C.: Census Bureau, 2002. Available at: http://www.census.gov/population/www/projections/natproj.htm l. Accessed June 20, 2004.
2. Senni M, Tribouilloy CM, Rodeheffer RJ, *et al.* Congestive heart failure in the community: a study of all incident cases in Olmsted County, Minnesota, in 1991. Circulation 1998; 98: 2282–2289.
3. Ho KK, Pinsky JL, Kannel WB, Levy D. The epidemiology of heart failure: the Framingham Study. J Am Coll Cardiol 1993; 22: 6A–13A.
4. Gottdiener JS, Arnold AM, Aurigemma GP, *et al.* Predictors of congestive heart failure in the elderly: the Cardiovascular Health Study. J Am Coll Cardiol 2000; 35: 1628–1637.
5. Cowie MR, Wood DA, Coats AJ, *et al.* Incidence and etiology of heart failure; a population-based study. Eur Heart J 1999; 20: 421–428.
6. Redfield MM, Jacobsen SJ, Burnett JC Jr., *et al.* Burden of systolic and diastolic ventricular dysfunction in the community: appreciating the scope of the heart failure epidemic. JAMA 2003; 289: 194–202.
7. Kitzman DW, Gardin JM, Gottdiener JS, *et al.* Importance of heart failure with preserved systolic function in patients ≥ 65 years of age. CHS Research Group. Cardiovascular Heart Study. Am J Cardiol 2001; 87: 413–419.
8. Wei JY. Age and the cardiovascular system. N Engl J Med 1992; 327: 1735–1739.
9. Celermajer DS, Sorensen KE, Spiegelhalter DJ, *et al.* Aging is associated with endothelial dysfunction in healthy men years before the age-related decline in women. J Am Coll Cardiol 1994; 24: 471–476.
10. Virmani R, Avolio AP, Mergner WJ, *et al.* Effect of aging on aortic morphology in populations with high and low prevalence of hypertension and atherosclerosis: comparison between occidental and Chinese communities. Am J Pathol 1991; 139: 1119–1129.
11. Lakatta EG, Levy D. Arterial and cardiac aging: major shareholders in cardiovascular disease enterprises: Part II: the aging heart in health: links to heart disease. Circulation 2003; 107: 346–354.
12. Haider AW, Larson MG, Franklin SS, Levy D. Systolic blood pressure, diastolic blood pressure, and pulse pressure as predictors of risk for congestive heart failure in the Framingham Heart Study. Ann Intern Med 2003; 138: 10–16.
13. Franklin SS, Gustin W IVth, Wong ND, *et al.* Hemodynamic patterns of age-related changes in blood pressure. The Framingham Heart Study. Circulation 1997; 96: 308–315.
14. Olivetti G, Melissari M, Capasso JM, Anversa P. Cardiomyopathy of the aging human heart: myocyte loss and reactive cellular hypertrophy. Circ Res 1991; 68: 1560–1568.
15. Glenner GG. Amyloid deposits and amyloidosis: the beta-fibrilloses (second of two parts). N Engl J Med 1980; 302: 1333–1343.
16. Lie JT, Hammond PI. Pathology of the senescent heart: anatomic observations on 237 autopsy studies of patients 90 to 105 years old. Mayo Clin Proc 1988; 63: 552–564.
17. Fowler NO. The Pericardium in Health and Disease (Mount Kisco, NY: Futura Publishing Company, 1985).
18. Gerstenblith G, Frederiksen J, Yin FC, *et al.* Echocardiographic assessment of a normal adult aging population. Circulation 1977; 56: 273–278.
19. Fleg JL, O'Connor FC, Gerstenblith G, *et al.* Impact of age on the cardiovascular response to dynamic upright exercise in healthy men and women. J Appl Physiol 1995; 78: 890–900.
20. Rodeheffer RJ, Gerstenblith G, Becker LC, *et al.* Exercise cardiac output is maintained with advancing age in healthy human subjects: cardiac dilatation and increased stroke volume compensate for a diminished heart rate. Circulation 1984; 69: 203–213.
21. Schulman SP, Fleg JL, Goldberg AP, *et al.* Continuum of cardiovascular performance across a broad range of fitness levels in healthy older men. Circulation 1996; 94: 359–367.
22. Schulman SP, Lakatta EG, Fleg JL, *et al.* Age-related decline in left ventricular filling at rest and exercise. Am J Physiol 1992; 263: H1932–H1938.
23. Swinne CJ, Shapiro EP, Lima SD, Fleg JL. Age-associated changes in left ventricular diastolic performance during isometric exercise in normal subjects. Am J Cardiol 1992; 69: 823–826.
24. Ziegler MG, Lake CR, Kopin IJ. Plasma noradrenaline increases with age. Nature 1976; 261: 333–335.
25. Esler MD, Turner AG, Kaye DM, *et al.* Aging effects on human sympathetic neuronal function. Am J Physiol 1995; 268: R278–R285.
26. Ng AV, Callister R, Johnson DG, Seals DR. Age and

gender influence muscle sympathetic nerve activity at rest in healthy humans. Hypertension 1993; 21: 498–503.

27. White M, Roden R, Minobe W, *et al.* Age-related changes in beta-adrenergic neuroeffector systems in the human heart. Circulation 1994; 90: 1225–1238.
28. Tsunoda K, Abe K, Goto T, *et al.* Effect of age on the renin-angiotensin-aldosterone system in normal subjects: simultaneous measurement of active and inactive rennin, rennin substrate, and aldosterone in plasma. J Clin Endocrinol Metab 1986; 62: 384–389.
29. Stratton JR, Cerquerira MD, Schwartz RS, *et al.* Differences in cardiovascular responses to isoproterenol in relation to age and exercise training in healthy men. Circulation 1992; 86: 504–512.
30. O'Brien IAD, O'Hare P, Corrall RJM. Heart rate variability in healthy subjects: effect of age and the derivation of normal ranges for tests of autonomic function. Br Heart J 1985; 55: 348–354.
31. Pfeffer MA, Weinberg CR, Cook D, *et al.* Differential changes of autonomic nervous system function with age in man. Am J Med 1983; 75: 249–258.
32. Fleg JL, Kennedy HL. Cardiac arrhythmias in a healthy elderly population: detection by 24-hour ambulatory electrocardiography. Chest 1982; 81: 302–307.
33. Fleg JL, Kennedy HL. Long-term prognosis significance of ambulatory electrocardiographic findings in apparently healthy subjects ≥ 60 years of age. Am J Cardiol 1992; 70: 748–751.
34. Manolio TA, Furberg CD, Rautaharju PM, *et al.* Cardiac arrhythmias on 24-h ambulatory electrocardiography in older women and men: the Cardiovascular Health Study. J Am Coll Cardiol 1994; 23: 916–925.
35. Gerstenblith G, Lakatta EG, Weisfeldt ML. Age changes in myocardial function and exercise response. Prog Cardiovasc Dis 1976; 19: 1–21.
36. Dehn MM, Bruce RA. Longitudinal variations in maximal oxygen uptake with age and activity. J Appl Physiol 1972; 33: 805–807.
37. Lakatta EG. Cardiovascular regulatory mechanisms in advanced age. Physiol Rev 1993; 73: 413–467.
38. Shlipak MG. Pharmacotherapy for heart failure in patients with renal insufficiency. Ann Intern Med 2003; 138: 917–924.
39. Meyer BR, Bellucci A. Renal function in the elderly. Cardiol Clin 1986; 4: 227–234.
40. Montamat SC, Cusack BJ, Vestal RE. Management of drug therapy in the elderly. N Engl J Med 1989; 321: 303–309.
41. Cody RJ, Torre S, Clark M, Pondolfino K. Age-related hemodynamic, renal, and hormonal differences among patients with congestive heart failure. Arch Intern Med 1989; 149: 1023–1028.
42. Lindeman RD. Changes in renal function with aging: implications for treatment. Drugs Aging 1992; 2: 423–431.
43. Phillips PA, Rolls BJ, Ledingham JG, *et al.* Reduced thirst after water deprivation in healthy elderly men. N Engl J Med 1984; 311: 753–759.
44. Chen Y, Vaccarino V, Williams CS, Butler J, Berkman LF, Krumholz HM. Risk factors for heart failure in the elderly: a prospective community-based study. Am J Med 1999; 106: 605–612.
45. Levy D, Larson MG, Vasan RS, Kannel WB, Ho KKL. The progression from hypertension to congestive heart failure. JAMA 1996; 275: 1557–1562.
46. Vasan RS, Sullivan LM, Roubenoff R, *et al.* Inflammatory markers and risk of heart failure in elderly subjects without prior myocardial infarction: the Framingham Heart Study. Circulation 2003; 107: 1486–1491.
47. Abramson J, Berger A, Krumholz HM, Vaccarino V. Depression and risk of heart failure among older persons with isolated systolic hypertension. Arch Intern Med 2001; 161: 1725–1730.
48. Williams SA, Kasl SV, Heiat A, *et al.* Depression and risk of heart failure among the elderly: a prospective community-based study. Psychosom Med 2002; 64: 6–12.
49. Havranek EP, Masoudi FA, Westfall KA, Wolfe P. Spectrum of heart failure in older patients: results from the National Heart Failure Project. Am Heart J 2002; 143: 412–417.
50. Lien CT, Gillespie ND, Struthers AD, McMurdo ME. Heart failure in frail elderly patients: diagnostic difficulties, co-morbidities, polypharmacy and treatment dilemmas. Eur J Heart Fail 2002; 4: 91–98.
51. Turvey CL, Schultz K, Arndt S, Wallace RB, Herzog R. Prevalence and correlates of depressive symptoms in a community sample of people suffering from heart failure. J Am Geriatr Soc 2002; 50: 2003–2008.
52. Deedwania PC, Gottlieb S, Ghali JK, *et al.* Efficacy, safety and tolerability of beta-adrenergic blockade with Metoprolol CR/XL in elderly patients with heart failure. Eur Heart J 2004; 25: 1300–1309.
53. Opasich C, Tavazzi L, Lucci D, *et al.* Comparison of one-year outcome in women versus men with chronic congestive heart failure. Am J Cardiol 2000; 86: 353–357.
54. Ghali JK, Cooper R, Ford E. Trends in hospitalization for heart failure in the United States, 1973–1986: evidence for increasing population prevalence. Arch Intern Med 1990; 150: 769–773.

55. Croft JB, Giles WH, Pollard RA, *et al.* National trends in the initial hospitalization for heart failure. J Am Geriatr Soc 1997; 45: 270–275.
56. Haldeman GA, Croft JB, Giles WH, Rashidee A. Hospitalization of patients with heart failure: National Hospital Discharge Survey, 1985–1995. Am Heart J 1999; 137: 352–360.
57. CDC National Center for Health Statistics. National Hospital Discharge Survey (NHDS) 2002. Available at: http://www.cdc.gov/nchs/about/major/hdasd/nhds.htm. Accessed June 29, 2004.
58. Masoudi FA, Havranek EP, Smith G, *et al.* Gender, age, and heart failure with preserved left ventricular systolic function. J Am Coll Cardiol 2003; 41: 217–223.
59. Vasan RS, Larson MG, Benjamin EJ, *et al.* Congestive heart failure in subjects with normal versus reduced left ventricular ejection fraction. J Am Coll Cardiol 1999; 33: 1948–1955.
60. Hogg K, Swedberg K, McMurray J. Heart failure with preserved left ventricular systolic function; epidemiology, clinical characteristics, and prognosis. J Am Coll Cardiol 2004; 43: 317–327.
61. Zile MR, Brutsaert DL. New concepts in diastolic dysfunction and diastolic heart failure: Part I. Diagnosis, prognosis, and measurements of diastolic function. Circulation 2002; 105: 1387–1393.
62. Wang TJ, Larson MG, Levy D, *et al.* Impact of age and sex on plasma natriuretic peptide levels in healthy adults. Am J Cardiol 2002; 90: 254–258.
63. Redfield MM, Rodeheffer RJ, Jacobsen SJ, *et al.* Plasma brain natriuretic peptide concentration: impact of age and gender. J Am Coll Cardiol 2002; 40: 976–982.
64. Yusuf S, Pfeffer MA, Swedberg K, *et al.*, the CHARM Investigators and Committees. Effects of candesartan in patients with chronic heart failure and preserved left-ventricular ejection fraction: The CHARM-Preserved trial. Lancet 2003; 362: 777–781.
65. McKee PA, Castelli WP, McNamara PM, Kannel WB. The natural history of congestive heart failure: the Framingham Study. N Engl J Med 1971; 285: 1441–1446.
66. Schocken DD, Arrieta MI, Leaverton PE, Ross EA. Prevalence and mortality rate of congestive heart failure in the United States. J Am Coll Cardiol 1992; 20: 301–306.
67. Croft JB, Giles WH, Pollard RA, *et al.* Heart failure survival among older adults in the United States: a poor prognosis for an emerging epidemic in the Medicare population. Arch Intern Med 1999; 159: 505–510.
68. Levy D, Kenchaiah S, Larson MG, *et al.* Long-term trends in the incidence of and survival with heart failure. N Engl J Med 2002; 347: 1397–1402.
69. MacIntyre K, Capewell S, Stewart S, *et al.* Evidence of improving prognosis in heart failure: trends in case fatality in 66 547 patients hospitalized between 1986 and 1995. Circulation 2000; 102: 1126–1131.
70. Baker DW, Einstadter D, Thomas C, Cebul RD. Mortality trends for 23 505 Medicare patients hospitalized with heart failure in Northeast Ohio, 1991 to 1997. Am Heart J 2003; 146: 258–264.
71. Forman DE, Butler J, Wang Y, *et al.* Incidence, predictors at admission, and impact of worsening renal function among patients hospitalized with heart failure. J Am Coll Cardiol 2004; 43: 61–67.
72. Krumholz HM, Chen Y, Vaccarino V, *et al.* Correlates and impact on outcomes of worsening renal function in patients ≥ 65 years of age with heart failure. Am J Cardiol 2000; 85: 1110–1113.
73. Al-Ahmad A, Rand SM, Manjunath G, *et al.* Reduced kidney function and anemia as risk factors for mortality in patients with left ventricular dysfunction. J Am Coll Cardiol 2001; 38: 955–962.
74. Kosiborod M, Smith GL, Radford MJ, Foody JM, Krunholz HM. The prognostic importance of anemia in patients with heart failure. Am J Med 2003; 114: 112–119.
75. Krumholz HM, Butler J, Miller J, *et al.* Prognostic importance of emotional support for elderly patients hospitalized with heart failure. Circulation 1998; 97: 958–964.
76. American Heart Association. Heart Disease and Stroke Statistics—2004 Update (American Heart Association: Dallas, TX, 2003).
77. Krumholz HM, Parent EM, Tu N, *et al.* Readmission after hospitalization for congestive heart failure among Medicare beneficiaries. Arch Intern Med 1997; 157: 99–104.
78. Ghali JK. Decompensated heart failure revisited. Am J Med 2003; 114: 695–696.
79. Ghali JK, Kadakia S, Cooper R, Ferlinz J. Precipitating factors leading to decompensation of heart failure: traits among urban blacks. Arch Intern Med 1988; 148: 2013–2016.
80. Pitt B, Zannad F, Remme WJ, *et al.* The effect of spironolactone on morbidity and mortality in patients with severe heart failure. Randomized Aldactone Evaluation Study Investigators. N Engl J Med 1999; 341: 709–717.
81. Cocchi A, Zuccala G, Menichelli P, *et al.* Congestive heart failure in the elderly: an intriguing clinical reality. Cardiology in the Elderly 1994; 2: 227–232.

82. Wang TJ, Larson MG, Levy D, *et al*. Temporal relations of atrial fibrillation and congestive heart failure and their joint influence on mortality: The Framingham Heart Study. Circulation 2003; 107: 2920–2925.
83. Heiat A, Gross CP, Krumholz HM. Representation of the elderly, women, and minorities in heart failure clinical trials. Arch Intern Med 2002; 162: 1682–1688.
84. Lamy PP. Renal effects of nonsteroidal anti-inflammatory drugs: heightened risk to the elderly? J Am Geriatr Soc 1986; 34: 361–367.
85. Mamdani M, Juurlink DN, Lee DS, *et al*. Cyclo-oxygenase-2 inhibitors versus non-selective non-steroidal anti-inflammatory drugs and congestive heart failure outcomes in elderly patients: a population-based cohort study. Lancet 2004; 363: 1751–1756.
86. van Kraaij DJW, Jansen WMM, Bouwels LHR, Hoefnagels WHL. Furosemide withdrawal improves postprandial hypotension in elderly patients with heart failure and preserved left ventricular systolic function. Arch Intern Med 1999; 159: 1599–1605.
87. Howard PA, Dunn MI. Aggressive diuresis for severe heart failure in the elderly. Chest 2001; 119: 807–810.
88. Rich MW, McSherry F, Williford WO, Yusuf S. Digitalis Investigation Group. Effect of age on mortality, hospitalization and response to digoxin in patients with heart failure: the DIG Study. J Am Coll Cardiol 2001; 38: 806–813.
89. Rathore SS, Curtis JP, Wang Y, Bristow MR, Krumholz HM. Association of serum digoxin concentration and outcomes in patients with heart failure. JAMA 2003; 289: 871–878.
90. Flather MD, Yusuf S, Kober L, *et al*. Long-term ACE-inhibitor therapy in patients with heart failure or left-ventricular dysfunction: a systematic overview of data from individual patients. ACE-Inhibitor Myocardial Infarction Collaborative Group. Lancet 2000; 355: 1575–1581.
91. Gambassi G, Lapane KL, Sgadari A, *et al*. Effects of angiotensin-converting enzyme inhibitors and digoxin on health outcomes of very old patients with heart failure. SAGE Study Group. Systematic Assessment of Geriatric drug use via Epidemiology. Arch Intern Med 2000; 160: 2550.
92. Johnson D, Jin Y, Quan H, Cujec B. Beta-blockers and angiotensin-converting enzyme inhibitors/receptor blockers prescriptions after hospital discharge for heart failure are associated with decreased mortality in Alberta, Canada. J Am Coll Cardiol 2003; 42: 1438–1445.
93. Sin DD, McAlister FA. The effects of beta-blockers on morbidity and mortality in a population-based cohort of 11942 elderly patients with heart failure. Am J Med 2002; 113: 650–656.
94. Bristow MR, Saxon LA, Boehmer J, *et al*., Comparison of Medical Therapy, Pacing, and Defibrillation in Heart Failure (COMPANION) Investigators. Cardiac-resynchronization therapy with or without an implantable defibrillator in advanced chronic heart failure. N Engl J Med 2004; 350: 2140–2150.
95. Abraham WT, Fisher WG, Smith AL, *et al*., MIRACLE Study Group. Multicenter InSync Randomized Clinical Evaluation. Cardiac resynchronization in chronic heart failure. N Engl J Med 2002; 346: 1845–1853.
96. Moss AJ, Zareba W, Hall WJ, *et al*. Prophylactic implantation of a defibrillator in patients with myocardial infarction and reduced ejection fraction. N Engl J Med 2002; 346: 877–883.
97. Piepoli MF, Flather M, Coats AJ. Overview of studies of exercise training in chronic heart failure: the need for a prospective randomized multicenter European trial. Eur Heart J 1998; 19: 830–841.
98. Smart N, Marwick TH. Exercise training for patients with heart failure: a systematic review of factors that improve mortality and morbidity. Am J Med 2004; 116: 693–706.
99. Levy WC, Cerqueira MD, Abrass IB, *et al*. Endurance exercise training augments diastolic filling at rest and during exercise in healthy young and older men. Circulation 1993; 88: 116–126.
100. Owen A, Croucher L. Effect of an exercise programme for elderly patients with heart failure. Eur J Heart Fail 2000; 2: 65–70.
101. McKelvie RS, Teo KK, Roberts R, *et al*. Effects of exercise training in patients with heart failure: the Exercise Rehabilitation Trial (EXERT). Am Heart J 2002; 144: 23–30.
102. Rich MW, Beckham V, Wittenberg C, *et al*. A multidisciplinary intervention to prevent the readmission of elderly patients with congestive heart failure. N Engl J Med 1995; 333: 1190–1195.
103. Stewart S, Horowitz JD. Home-based intervention in congestive heart failure: long-term implications on readmission and survival. Circulation 2002; 105: 2861–2866.

CHAPTER 6

Pathophysiology of the spectrum of acute heart failure: de novo heart failure, decompensated heart failure, and advanced refractory heart failure

Gary S Francis, W H Wilson Tang, Kirkwood F Adams, Jr

Introduction

Acute heart failure (AHF) is defined as new-onset signs or symptoms of heart failure (from hours to days), or worsening signs and symptoms of previously stable heart failure whereby immediate evaluation and institution of therapy are appropriate. In many cases, AHF necessitates hospitalization for optimal management.[1] Up to and including the current era, problems with nomenclature have plagued the evolution of a clear definition of both chronic and AHF. Since there is no "gold standard" test that defines all types of heart failure, a consensus definition has been elusive.

AHF represents a heterogeneous cohort of patients, but the majority of patients (up to 75% of admissions for AHF) have a history of prior heart failure.[2] These patients, often referred to as having *acute decompensated heart failure* (ADHF), have underlying chronic stable heart failure, which for any number of reasons has become more symptomatic and requires evaluation and possible hospitalization. An important subgroup of these patients suffer from *advanced refractory heart failure* which is generally characterized by progressive left ventricular (LV) dysfunction and worsening symptoms despite aggressive medical management.

In contrast, new-onset or *de novo heart failure* occurs without known antecedent heart failure and likewise requires evaluation and possible hospitalization. In fact, certain etiologies of heart failure are more prone to de novo heart failure, such as acute myocardial infarction (MI), acute inflammatory myocarditis, certain toxic myocarditidies, peripartum cardiomyopathies, and acute valvular endocarditis. Furthermore, any process that results in a sudden loss of large amounts of contractile tissue can cause AHF, as can acute volume overloaded states, such as acute severe valvular insufficiency, acute renal failure, or excessive transfusion. However, the latter two examples could also be referred to as circulatory congestion states, as there may be no structural or functional abnormality of the heart.

Spectrum of Acute Heart Failure

In order to understand the pathophysiology of AHF, a review of the natural history of patients with this condition is warranted. In the past three years, we have learned a great deal from the Acute Decompensated Heart Failure National Registry (ADHERE™) regarding the demographics of patients admitted to the hospital with AHF.[3] This industry-sponsored registry is based on data from a comprehensive review of patients hospitalized for heart failure without regard for specific pharmacological treatments or particular clinical characteristics. Patient data have been collected in this ongoing study from over 275 academic and community-based hospitals across the United

States, with a total of over 170 000 patients with AHF currently enrolled. The latest figures indicate that patients hospitalized with heart failure are an elderly population (average age of 75 years), with a wide range of comorbid conditions (57% with coronary artery disease, 31% with a prior MI, 72% with hypertension, 44% with diabetes, 31% with chronic obstructive pulmonary disease, 30% with renal insufficiency, and 31% with atrial fibrillation). About half of the patients have preserved LV function. Interestingly, almost all patients had preserved blood pressures, with up to 50% of patients experiencing hypertension (systolic blood pressure > 140 mm Hg), suggesting the important role of diastolic dysfunction in the exacerbation of AHF.[2]

Pathophysiologic Considerations in Acute Heart Failure

Data from the ADHERE™ registry and other sources allows for a pathophysiologic classification of patients admitted with heart failure divided by the presence of preserved versus reduced left ventricular ejection fraction (LVEF). These two groups of patients, classically described as having heart failure due to predominately systolic or diastolic dysfunction, account for almost all cases of patients hospitalized for worsening heart failure. Other pathophysiological subsets are generally predominantly within the preserved LVEF group, such as acute pulmonary edema, or found most often in patients with reduced systolic function; for example, patients with low cardiac output syndrome. In the ADHERE™ registry, only about 5% of patients with AHF are managed in the hospital with a Swan–Ganz catheter, and only 20% are admitted to an intensive care unit.[2] Most go to a step-down or telemetry unit, where the average stay is about 4.1 days.

This chapter provides an overview of these two broad pathophysiological groups which are discussed in greater detail in subsequent chapters.

Patients with normal left ventricular ejection fraction

There is now a growing recognition that patients who present with acute severe pulmonary edema or decompensated heart failure often have a normal LVEF and are considered to have a predominant abnormality of diastolic function. They have what has come to be known as *diastolic heart failure*, which is both common (30–60% of cases of acute or chronic heart failure) and has a mortality only slightly less than patients with classic systolic dysfunction during long-term follow-up.[4]

In a recent review of 61 studies of patients with heart failure and preserved systolic function, there was great diversity in the criteria used to determine the presence of heart failure.[4] Even the very concept of diastolic heart failure has been challenged,[5,6] and the mechanism of diastolic heart failure remains under intense study.[7] Some have suggested that increased LV volume, and not LVEF, is what really characterizes the remodeled ventricle with systolic dysfunction.[8] Therefore, diastolic heart failure might best be defined as heart failure with a normal or small LV volume. However, disagreements about terminology persist.

Despite obvious uncertainties about the nomenclature, mechanisms, and treatment of patients with diastolic heart failure, there is no doubt that there are many such patients in the community.[9,10] These patients tend to be women and, as a group, are older than patients with systolic heart failure.[11] Morbidity and mortality rates are high, but not quite as high as patients with reduced systolic function.[12] The bedside clinical signs and symptoms of systolic and diastolic heart failure are indistinguishable,[13,14] and echocardiography and cardiac catheterization are most commonly used to help distinguish diastolic heart failure from systolic heart failure.

The presence of definite heart failure with an abnormal left ventricular end-diastolic pressure (LVEDP) and increased early and mid-diastolic pressure in the setting of a normal chamber size indicates increased LV diastolic stiffness,[15] and is typical of diastolic heart failure. Echocardiography is the most important laboratory test for the diagnosis of diastolic dysfunction.[16] Despite the enormous interest and controversy regarding the syndrome of diastolic heart failure, the natural history and treatment are rather similar to systolic heart failure.[17] Chronic diastolic heart failure commonly leads to ADHF.[18,19] Many, perhaps most, patients with flash pulmonary edema have preserved LV systolic function.[20] This has been known for many years.[21] Flash pulmonary edema tends to reoccur, and carries a high mortality. Such patients are often markedly hypertensive on presentation, both initially and on subsequent occurrences as seen in ADHERE™.[2] The acutely elevated blood pressure may be due to marked sympathetic activity, anxiety due to breathlessness, hypoxemia, and other factors. The severe hypertension aggravates diastolic dysfunction, leading to acute pulmonary edema.[18] Following restoration of normal blood pressure, the LVEF is usually found to be normal. In fact, LVEF is usually normal during the acute episode of hypertensive pulmonary edema, as well as after the congestion and blood pressures have been controlled (Figure 6.1).[19] These data suggest that transient systolic dysfunction and severe acute mitral regurgitation during the acute episode of acute pulmonary edema are infrequent. Patients with chronic, stable diastolic heart failure tend to have intermediate levels of plasma B-type natriuretic peptide (BNP), between those of normal patients and patients with stable systolic heart failure, but BNP levels can rise dramatically with acute decompensation.[22]

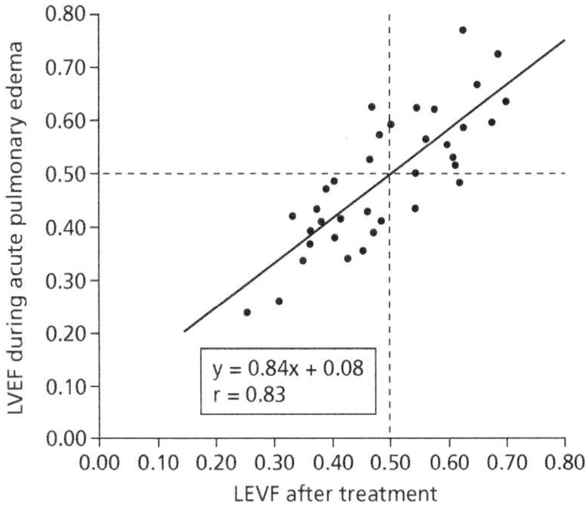

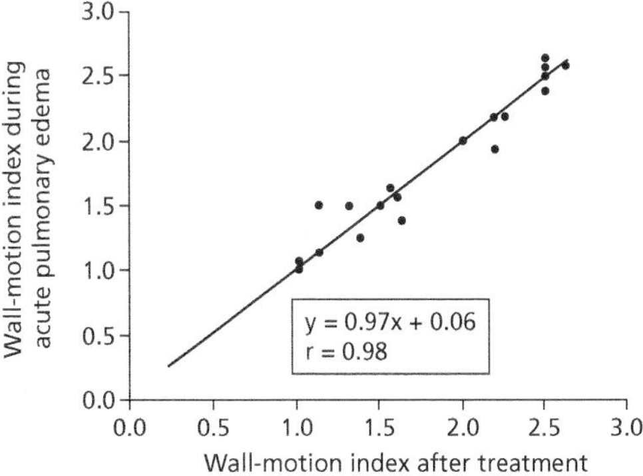

Figure 6.1. *Lack of alterations in global and regional myocardial systolic function in acute heart failure (With permission from Ghandi* et al.[18]*)*

The Working Group for the European Society of Cardiology have proposed three criteria for the diagnosis of diastolic heart failure: (1) signs and symptoms of heart failure; (2) the presence of normal LV systolic function; and (3) evidence of abnormal LV relaxation, filling, or diastolic stiffness.[23] In the strictest sense, there are problems with all proposed criteria for diastolic heart failure because contraction and relaxation are physiologically coupled in patients with and without heart failure.[24] The signs and symptoms of heart failure are nonspecific, and diastolic heart failure in isolation is rare. Because systolic impairment is mild, the assumption has been made that although patients have a combination of mild systolic and diastolic dysfunction, important elements relate to the poor relaxation and impaired filling due to diastolic dysfunction.[25,26]

Mechanisms that cause AHF in patients with predominantly diastolic heart failure are both intrinsic to the myocardium and extra-myocardial.[27] Extra-myocardial factors include altered loading conditions and abnormalities of the pericardium. Intrinsic myocardial factors are numerous and include alterations in calcium homeostasis, myofilaments, and energetics. The cardiac myocyte cytoskeleton may play an important role, and the interstitium and increased fibrosis likely play a critical role. More recently, alterations in myocyte microtubules, intermediate filaments, actin, titan, and nebulin have been observed in experimental heart failure. Undoubtedly, neurohormonal activation, nitric oxide, and oxidative stress also play some role. As with systolic heart failure, there is no single, fundamental abnormality that drives the process of acute diastolic heart failure. Multiple changes leading to stiffness of the peripheral vasculature and the heart itself are likely at fault.

Treatment will always consist of diverse strategies, including control of blood pressure, correction of myocardial ischemia,[28] control of circulating volume, relief of impaired relaxation, and reduction of rapid heart rate. Over time, regression of left ventricular hypertrophy (LVH) may be helpful. Patients with acute diastolic heart failure have similar, though not identical, pathophysiological characteristics as patients with acute systolic heart failure.[13,29,30] It is not very surprising that the signs and symptoms, natural history, and treatment of these two entities are very similar.

Patients with reduced left ventricular ejection fraction

The other pathophysiological subset of most importance in patients with AHF are those patients with reduced LVEF. Approximately half of these patients with AHF have a reduced LVEF, a dilated heart, and many have some degree of mitral insufficiency. Tissue and lung congestion are overwhelmingly present in this subset. Although common in academic medical centers, especially those specializing in cardiac transplantation, patients within this group presenting with hypotension and low-output syndrome are distinctly unusual. Data from the ADHERE™ registry suggests that this group of patients comprises less than 5% of patients admitted for worsening heart failure nationally.[3] In rare cases, some patients with ADHF due to LV systolic dysfunction will not have a dilated ventricle. Etiologies associated with impaired contractile function and normal left ventricular end-diastolic volume (LVEDV), including fulminant myocarditis, acute bacterial endocarditis with wide-open aortic regurgitation, acute MI, and chemotherapy-induced myocardial injury, may not have had time to dilate the left ventricle. There is no common phenotype that fits all cases. This categorization allows systolic heart failure that results in hospitalization to be divided into the following three categories:

1. New-onset systolic heart failure secondary to a major precipitating factor such as acute MI or acute inflammatory myocarditis. Severe acute contractile dysfunction is the major problem in these cases.
2. Acute decompensation of chronic heart failure that occurs weeks to days prior to hospital admission and is characterized predominantly by congestion, often due to dietary or medication noncompliance or previously undiagnosed heart failure which has not been medically treated.
3. End-stage heart failure with symptoms of both low output and congestion typically associated with marked reduction in systolic function (LVEF < 25%) that usually gradually worsens over days or weeks despite medical intervention and eventually responds poorly or not at all to conventional therapy.

The majority of patients with acute systolic heart failure demonstrate increased pulmonary capillary wedge pressure with a more variable change in cardiac index, though this is not always the case. In the Outcomes of a Prospective Trial of Intravenous Milrinone for Exacerbations of Chronic Heart Failure (OPTIME-CHF) trial, which enrolled patients with a history of advanced heart failure with impaired LVEF, 81% of the patients had rales and 72% had jugular venous distension.[31] Patients with rales and edema are sometimes referred to as "wet," while patients with preserved adequate forward flow are referred to as "warm."[32] Patients with low-output states who are vasoconstricted, "cold," and have a narrow pulse pressure and a blood pressure less than 100 mm Hg are perhaps more likely to be admitted to heart failure or heart transplant centers, as they are unusual in the ADHERE™ registry. In ADHERE™, only 3% of patients admitted with AHF have systolic blood pressures < 90 mm Hg.[2]

Precipitating factors in patients admitted with worsening heart failure

There are many factors responsible for precipitating acute systolic or diastolic heart failure, changing it from a chronic but stable condition to an acute problem that necessitates urgent care. The following factors may provoke AHF and, when possible, should be identified and treated:

- myocardial ischemia or MI
- excessive salt intake or dietary indiscretion

- noncompliance with medications
- iatrogenic volume overload, such as blood transfusion
- lack of patient knowledge about their heart failure condition
- arrhythmias, particularly atrial fibrillation
- comorbidities such as pneumonia, influenza, and uncontrolled diabetes mellitus
- adverse drug effects, particularly nonsteroidal antiinflammatory drugs (NSAIDs), alcohol, and abrupt withdrawal of some medications (such as digoxin).

Prognostic factors in acute heart failure

The role of worsening renal function in patients admitted with decompensated heart failure is receiving more attention. AHF is frequently associated with a rising serum creatinine, oliguria and reduced responsiveness to diuretic therapy.[2] This must be monitored carefully. Worsening renal function is an important marker for a poor prognosis and often heralds the onset of a low-output syndrome and sometimes a downward spiral toward death.[33,34]

Patients who develop a low-output syndrome are at much higher risk and may require temporary support as a bridge to cardiac transplantation. Once multi-organ failure develops, the prognosis is very poor, and the mortality rises steeply.[35] Data from the ADHERE™ registry have identified systolic blood pressure and reduced renal function as important predictors of outcome.[3] Previous hospitalization, symptoms for more than 18 months, ischemic cardiomyopathy, atrial fibrillation, heart rate > 100 beats per minute, and New York Heart Association (NYHA) classification are independently associated with an exacerbation of heart failure in outpatients being followed with stable symptoms.[36] Once hospitalized, failure to improve the hemodynamic profile has been associated with a worse prognosis.[37] The persistence of orthopnea following discharge from the hospital is an ominous sign.[37] Echocardiography also helps to determine prognosis: global LV impairment is worse than regional dysfunction; the larger the chamber size, the worse the prognosis; and the more the mitral or tricuspid regurgitation, the worse the prognosis.[38] Patients with right ventricular dysfunction as well as LV dysfunction have a worse prognosis.[39] Such prognostic information is very important for physicians in helping to guide patients toward more specific therapeutic strategies, such as bridging ventricular assist devices, LV restoration surgery or heart transplantation, comfort care measures, or hospice.

Conclusion

The pathophysiology of AHF is complex with multiple distinct clinical subsets present with overlapping mechanisms of disease. The emergence of heart failure with preserved LVEF as a very common syndrome has caused a reconsideration of the major elements of the pathophysiology of patients admitted for worsening heart failure. National database studies such as ADHERE™ have demonstrated that patients with low-output syndrome due to further impairment of LV systolic function are less common than expected, while patients who have their admission associated with worsening renal function, congestion, and frank hypertension, often despite multiple drug therapy, are much more common. Additional research into the pathophysiology of diastolic heart failure and advancing renal insufficiency in the setting of patients hospitalized for heart failure is warranted.

References

1. American Heart Association. Heart Disease and Stroke Statistics—2004 Update. (American Heart Association: Dallas, TX, 2003).
2. The ADHERE™ 1st Quarter 2004 National Benchmark Report. Available at: http://www.adheregistry.com. Accessed November 19, 2004.
3. Adams KF Jr., Fonarow GC, Emerman CL, *et al.* Characteristics and outcomes of patients hospitalized for heart failure in the United States: rationale, design, and preliminary observations from the first 100 000 Cases in the Acute Decompensated Heart Failure National Registry (ADHERE™). Am Heart J 2005; 149: 209–216.
4. Thomas MD, Fox KF, Coats AJ, Sutton GC. The epidemiological enigma of heart failure with preserved systolic function. Eur J Heart Fail 2004; 6: 125–136.

5. Sanderson JE. Diastolic heart failure: fact or fiction? Heart 2003; 89: 1281–1282.
6. Burkhoff D, Maurer MS, Packer M. Heart failure with a normal ejection fraction: is it really a disorder of diastolic function? Circulation 2003; 107: 656–658.
7. Kawaguchi M, Hay I, Fetics B, Kass DA. Combined ventricular systolic and arterial stiffening in patients with heart failure and preserved ejection fraction: implications for systolic and diastolic reserve limitations. Circulation 2003; 107: 714–720.
8. Konstam MA. "Systolic and diastolic dysfunction" in heart failure? Time for a new paradigm. J Card Fail 2003; 9: 1–3.
9. Redfield MM, Jacobsen SJ, Burnett JC Jr., *et al.* Burden of systolic and diastolic ventricular dysfunction in the community: appreciating the scope of the heart failure epidemic. JAMA 2003; 289: 194–202.
10. Vasan RS, Larson MG, Benjamin EJ, *et al.* Congestive heart failure in subjects with normal versus reduced left ventricular ejection fraction: prevalence and mortality in a population-based cohort. J Am Coll Cardiol 1999; 33: 1948–1955.
11. Masoudi FA, Havranek EP, Smith G, *et al.* Gender, age, and heart failure with preserved left ventricular systolic function. J Am Coll Cardiol 2003; 41: 217–223.
12. Hogg K, Swedberg K, McMurray J. Heart failure with preserved left ventricular systolic function; epidemiology, clinical characteristics, and prognosis. J Am Coll Cardiol 2004; 43: 317–327.
13. Kitzman DW, Little WC, Brubaker PH, *et al.* Pathophysiological characterization of isolated diastolic heart failure in comparison to systolic heart failure. JAMA 2002; 288: 2144–2150.
14. Goldsmith SR, Dick C. Differentiating systolic from diastolic heart failure: pathophysiologic and therapeutic considerations. Am J Med 1993; 95: 645–655.
15. Zile MR, Gaasch WH, Carroll JD, *et al.* Heart failure with a normal ejection fraction: is measurement of diastolic function necessary to make the diagnosis of diastolic heart failure? Circulation 2001; 104: 779–782.
16. Garcia MJ. Diastolic dysfunction and heart failure: causes and treatment options. Cleve Clin J Med 2000; 67: 727–729, 733–738.
17. Senni M, Redfield MM. Heart failure with preserved systolic function: a different natural history? J Am Coll Cardiol 2001; 38: 1277–1282.
18. Gandhi SK, Powers JC, Nomeir AM, *et al.* The pathogenesis of acute pulmonary edema associated with hypertension. N Engl J Med 2001; 344: 17–22.
19. Little WC. Hypertensive pulmonary oedema is due to diastolic dysfunction. Eur Heart J 2001; 22: 1961–1964.
20. Kramer K, Kirkman P, Kitzman D, Little WC. Flash pulmonary edema: association with hypertension and reoccurrence despite coronary revascularization. Am Heart J 2000; 140: 451–455.
21. Dodek A, Kassebaum DG, Bristow JD. Pulmonary edema in coronary-artery disease without cardiomegaly: paradox of the stiff heart. N Engl J Med 1972; 286: 1347–1350.
22. Yamaguchi H, Yoshida J, Yamamoto K, *et al.* Elevation of plasma brain natriuretic peptide is a hallmark of diastolic heart failure independent of ventricular hypertrophy. J Am Coll Cardiol 2004; 43: 55–60.
23. European Study Group on Diastolic Heart Failure. How to diagnose diastolic heart failure. Eur Heart J 1998; 19: 990–1003.
24. Vasan RS, Levy D. Defining diastolic heart failure: a call for standardized diagnostic criteria. Circulation 2000; 101: 2118–2121.
25. Eichhorn EJ, Willard JE, Alvarez L, *et al.* Are contraction and relaxation coupled in patients with and without congestive heart failure? Circulation 1992; 85: 2132–2139.
26. Grossman W, McLaurin LP, Rolett EL. Alterations in left ventricular relaxation and diastolic compliance in congestive cardiomyopathy. Cardiovasc Res 1979; 13: 514–522.
27. Zile MR, Brutsaert DL. New concepts in diastolic dysfunction and diastolic heart failure: Part I: diagnosis, prognosis, and measurements of diastolic function. Circulation 2002; 105: 1387–1393.
28. Kunis R, Greenberg H, Yeoh CB. Coronary revascularization for recurrent pulmonary edema in elderly patients with ischemic heart disease and preserved ventricular function. N Engl J Med 1985; 313: 1207–1210.
29. Grossman W. Diastolic dysfunction in congestive heart failure. N Engl J Med 1991; 325: 1557–1564.
30. Grossman W. Diastolic dysfunction and congestive heart failure. Circulation 1990; 81: III1–III7.
31. Cuffe MS, Califf RM, Adams KF Jr., *et al.* Short-term intravenous milrinone for acute exacerbation of chronic heart failure: a randomized controlled trial. JAMA 2002; 287: 1541–1547.
32. Nohria A, Lewis E, Stevenson LW. Medical management of advanced heart failure. JAMA 2002; 287: 628–640.
33. Gottlieb SS, Abraham W, Butler J, *et al.* The prognostic importance of different definitions of worsening renal function in congestive heart failure. J Card Fail 2002; 8: 136–141.
34. Forman DE, Butler J, Wang Y, *et al.* Incidence, predictors at admission, and impact of worsening renal

function among patients hospitalized with heart failure. J Am Coll Cardiol 2004; 43: 61–67.

35. Renlund DG. Building a bridge to heart transplantation. N Engl J Med 2004; 351: 849–851.
36. Opasich C, Rapezzi C, Lucci D, *et al.* Precipitating factors and decision-making processes of short-term worsening heart failure despite "optimal" treatment (from the IN-CHF Registry). Am J Cardiol 2001; 88: 382–387.
37. Lucas C, Johnson W, Hamilton MA, *et al.* Freedom from congestion predicts good survival despite previous class IV symptoms of heart failure. Am Heart J 2000; 140: 840–847.
38. Dhir M, Arora U, Nagueh SF. The role of echocardiography in the diagnosis and prognosis of patients with heart failure. Expert Rev Cardiovasc Ther 2004; 2: 141–144.
39. Gavazzi A, Berzuini C, Campana C, *et al.* Value of right ventricular ejection fraction in predicting short-term prognosis of patients with severe chronic heart failure. J Heart Lung Transplant 1997; 16: 774–785.

Chapter 7

Diastolic heart failure: diagnosis, prognosis, and treatment

Michael R Zile, Carson S Webb, Catalin F Baicu

Introduction

It is now abundantly clear that chronic heart failure caused by a predominant abnormality in diastolic function—*diastolic heart failure*—is common and causes a significant increase in morbidity and mortality. However, there is continued controversy surrounding the terminology used to describe patients with chronic heart failure and the criteria used for diagnosis of diastolic heart failure. As a result, clinical therapeutic trials have been slow to develop and difficult to design. Fortunately, these controversies are yielding to an emerging consensus. Recent clinical studies have provided sufficient data to develop standardized diagnostic criteria for diastolic heart failure. Experimental studies have provided increased insight into the mechanisms which cause diastolic heart failure. Together, these studies are being used to design targeted clinical trials to test effective treatments for diastolic heart failure. This chapter describes the criteria used to diagnose diastolic heart failure, the effects of diastolic heart failure on prognosis, and the approaches to treatment.

In the past three decades, clinicians and physiologists have re-examined their ideas about the pathophysiology of heart failure. A major focus of this deliberation has been clarifying the important distinctions between left ventricular (LV) systolic dysfunction and diastolic dysfunction (Figure 7.1). Systolic dysfunction is a defect in the ability of the myofibrils to shorten against a load; the ventricle loses its ability to eject blood into a high-pressure aorta and the ejection fraction (EF) falls. The term diastolic dysfunction implies that the myofibrils do not rapidly or completely return to their resting length; the ventricle cannot accept blood at low pressures, and ventricular filling is slow or incomplete unless atrial pressure rises. Cardiac structure and function differ substantially in systolic and diastolic dysfunction, but the clinical consequences—signs and symptoms of heart failure—are similar. A balanced view of the differences and similarities between these two conditions is essential to diagnosing and treating patients with heart failure.

Defining Diastolic Heart Failure

Differentiating diastolic dysfunction from diastolic heart failure

Heart failure is a clinical syndrome characterized by symptoms and signs of increased water retention in tissues and organs and decreased tissue and organ perfusion. Standardized criteria for diagnosing heart failure have been developed, perhaps the best validated of which come from the Framingham Study.[1] Defining the mechanisms that cause this clinical syndrome requires measurement of both systolic and diastolic function. When heart failure is accompanied by a predominant

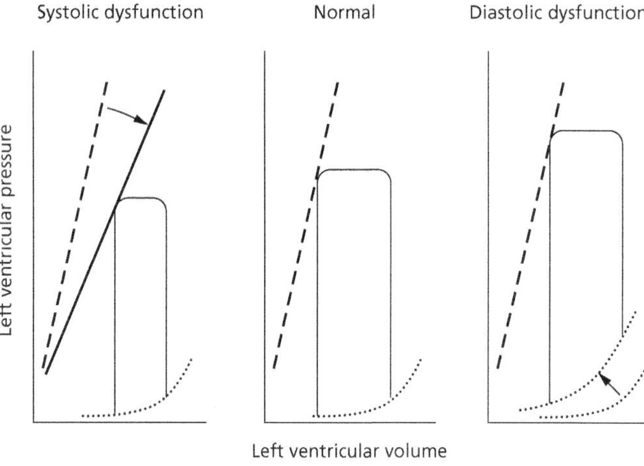

Figure 7.1. *Diagram of left ventricular (LV) pressure–volume loops in systolic dysfunction and diastolic dysfunction. In systolic dysfunction, contractility is depressed and the end-systolic pressure–volume line is displaced downward and to the right. In addition, there is diminished capacity to eject blood into a high-pressure aorta. In diastolic dysfunction, chamber stiffness is increased and the diastolic pressure–volume relation is displaced up and to the left. In addition, there is diminished capacity to fill at low diastolic pressures. The LV ejection fraction is low in systolic dysfunction and normal in diastolic dysfunction (Adapted, with permission, from Gaasch.[66])*

abnormality in diastolic function, this clinical syndrome is called *diastolic heart failure*.

Diastolic dysfunction is a condition in which abnormalities in mechanical function are present during diastole. Abnormalities in diastolic function can occur in the presence or absence of a clinical syndrome of heart failure and with normal or abnormal systolic function; whereas diastolic dysfunction describes an abnormal mechanical property, diastolic heart failure describes a clinical syndrome.

Diastolic heart failure is a clinical syndrome characterized by the symptoms and signs of heart failure, a preserved EF, and abnormal diastolic function. From a conceptual perspective, diastolic heart failure occurs when the ventricular chamber is unable to accept an adequate volume of blood during diastole at normal diastolic pressures and volumes sufficient to maintain an appropriate stroke volume. These abnormalities are caused by a decrease in ventricular relaxation, an increase in ventricular stiffness, or both. Diastolic heart failure can produce symptoms which occur at rest (New York Heart Association [NYHA] class IV), with less than ordinary physical activity (NYHA class III), or with ordinary physical activity (NYHA class II).

Thus, patients can have abnormal diastolic function without symptoms or signs of heart failure (asymptomatic diastolic dysfunction) or they can have abnormal diastolic function with both symptoms and signs of heart failure (diastolic heart failure).

Changes in left ventricular systolic and diastolic function in diastolic heart failure

A normal EF does not necessarily indicate the presence of normal myocardial or ventricular contractility.[2,3] Therefore, patients with diastolic heart failure (heart failure and preserved EF) may have relatively small but detectable abnormalities in selected measurements reflecting systolic function. However, there are no convincing data to support the idea that abnormalities in systolic function are responsible for the symptoms and signs of heart failure, or the pathophysiological remodeling that is seen in patients with diastolic heart failure. Patients with diastolic heart failure commonly have concentric remodeling characterized by normal LV volume, increased LV mass, increased wall thickness, decreased volume-to-mass ratio, and increased chamber and myocardial stiffness (Table 7.1). There is no conceptual framework to support the notion that abnormal systolic function contributes causally to this concentric remodeling. Therefore, the presence of abnormal indices of systolic function in patients with diastolic heart failure does not negate the fact that the predominant abnormality is diastolic dysfunction, nor does

Table 7.1. *Features differentiating systolic from diastolic heart failure*

Characteristic	Systolic heart failure	Diastolic heart failure
Demographics		
Age (mean)	61	72
Gender (% female)	35	66
Hypertension (%)	62	85
Coronary artery disease (%)	86	45
Symptoms and signs		
Exercise duration	↓	↓
Systolic blood pressure	↑	↑↑
Pulse pressure	↑	↑↑
Oxygen consumption (VO_2)	↓↓	↓↓
B-type natriuretic peptide	↑↑	↑
Systolic function		
Ejection fraction	↓↓	N – ↑
Stroke volume	N – ↓	N – ↓
Contractility	↓↓	N
Preload reserve	Exhausted	Limited
Diastolic function		
Left ventricular end-diastolic pressure	↑↑	↑↑
Relaxation time constant	↑	↑↑
Filling rate dynamics	Abnormal	Abnormal
Chamber stiffness	N – ↓	↑↑
Myocardial stiffness	N – ↑	↑
Remodeling		
Left ventricular end-diastolic volume	↑↑	N
Left ventricular end-systolic volume	↑↑	N
Left ventricular mass	↑ Eccentric LVH	↑ Concentric LVH
Relative wall thickness	↓	↑↑
Cardiomyocyte	↑ Length	↑ Diameter
Extracellular matrix collagen	↓	↑↑
Morbidity	↑↑	↑↑
Mortality	↑↑	↑

it support the idea that this abnormal systolic function is the mechanism responsible for the development of diastolic heart failure. Thus, heart failure in patients with diastolic heart failure is caused by a predominate abnormality in diastolic function.

Diagnosis of Diastolic Heart Failure

The Working Group for the European Society of Cardiology proposed that:

> a diagnosis of primary diastolic heart failure requires three obligatory conditions to be simultaneously satisfied: (1) presence of signs or symptoms of congestive heart failure (CHF); (2) presence of normal or only mildly abnormal left ventricular (LV) systolic function; (3) evidence of abnormal LV relaxation, filling, diastolic distensibility, or diastolic stiffness.[4]

These diagnostic criteria have been criticized for three reasons. The first obligatory condition requires the presence of either signs or symptoms of CHF. However, it is well recognized that the mere presence of breathlessness and fatigue are not specific for the presence of CHF. It would be more prudent to require signs and symptoms of CHF or to use specific diagnostic criteria such as the Framingham criteria. The second criticism involves the term *systolic function*. The working group defined systolic function as being normal when the LVEF is ≥ 45%. Because EF is not a measure of contractility or a load-independent measurement of systolic function, the second requirement would be more precise if it specified a normal EF.

Vasan and Levy suggested that these diagnostic criteria be divided into *definite*, *probable*, and *possible* diastolic heart failure.[5] *Definite* diastolic heart failure requires: (1) definitive evidence of CHF; (2) objective evidence of normal systolic function with an EF > 50% within 72 hours of the CHF event; and (3) objective evidence of diastolic dysfunction on cardiac catheterization. If objective evidence of diastolic dysfunction is lacking but the first two criteria are present, this fulfills the criteria for *probable* diastolic heart failure. If the first criterion is present and EF is > 50% but not assessed within 72 hours of the CHF event, this fulfills the criteria for *possible* diastolic heart failure. Possible diastolic heart failure can be upgraded to probable diastolic heart failure if one of a number of additional criteria is present.

The clinical application of these guidelines is limited because they are complex and empiric. However, subsequent studies suggested methods to simplify the diagnostic criteria and provided objective data for validation.[6,7] Studies by Ghandi *et al.* addressed the requirement for an EF ≥ 50% within 72 hours of the CHF event.[6] This study demonstrated that in patients presenting to the emergency room (ER) with acute pulmonary edema (APE) there were no significant differences between EF measured echocardiographically at the time of presentation to the ER when patients had active CHF and 72 hours after the event when patients were clinically stable and no longer in symptomatic heart failure. Therefore, under most circumstances, EF does not need to be measured coincident with the heart failure event.

Zile *et al.* examined the necessity of obtaining objective evidence of diastolic dysfunction.[7] In this study, patients with a history of CHF fulfilling the Framingham criteria and an EF ≥ 50% underwent diagnostic left heart catheterization and simultaneous Doppler echocardiography. None of these patients had evidence of coronary artery disease (CAD), valvular disease, hypertrophic obstructive cardiomyopathy, atrial fibrillation, pulmonary disease, or renal disease. Less than half of the patients had left ventricular hypertrophy (LVH), defined as LV mass ≥ 25 g/m^2. In this group of patients, 92% had at least one pressure-derived abnormality in diastolic function (including a left ventricular end-diastolic pressure [LVEDP] > 16 mm Hg), 94% had at least one Doppler echocardiographically-derived abnormality in diastolic function (including a deceleration time > 250 ms), and 100% had at least one pressure or Doppler abnormality in diastolic function. Therefore, objective measurements of LV diastolic function served to confirm rather than establish the diagnosis of diastolic heart failure. These investigators concluded that the diagnosis of diastolic heart failure can be made without measurement of diastolic function, if two criteria are present: (1) symptoms and signs of heart failure that meet the Framingham criteria; and (2) LVEF > 50%.

In spite of this data, clinicians and potential sponsors of clinical trials continue to express apprehension about a set of diagnostic criteria which uses a diagnosis by exclusion technique. Therefore, the search for a specific diagnostic test continues. Ideally, this would consist of a simple and widely available blood test, which could be performed at the point of care, was easy to interpret, and had a high sensitivity, specificity, and predictive accuracy. Some investigators suggest that the brain natruretic peptide (BNP) is just such a blood test.[8,9–18] Current studies suggest that BNP generally correlates with LV diastolic filling pressure, LV diastolic volume, LVEF, Doppler echocardiography indices of diastolic dysfunction, and severity of CHF. However, it is also clear that the relative levels of BNP are much greater in systolic heart failure (~500 pg/mL) than diastolic heart failure (~250 pg/mL, Triage BNP test, Biosite Diagnostics Inc.). The sensitivity, specificity, and predictive accuracy of BNP in diastolic heart failure are limited in part because BNP is altered by age, gender, pulmonary disease, renal disease, presence of LVH, and other factors.[9,10] These limitations make the determination of a discrimination limit or partition value, which distinguishes between normal and diastolic heart failure, difficult to chose. Therefore, the extent to which BNP will contribute to the diagnostic criteria for diastolic heart failure remains to be determined.

Prognosis for Diastolic Heart Failure

Prevalence

Early studies suggested that as many as one-third of patients presenting with overt CHF have a normal EF and, therefore, diastolic heart failure.[19–21] However, more recent studies have made it clear that both the incidence, prevalence, and prognosis of diastolic heart failure are dependent on age, gender, methods used to diagnose diastolic heart failure, study design, value of EF used as a cut-off value, and underlying clinical disease process causing diastolic heart failure.[22–35] While these determinants are largely interdependent, the most important determinant is likely to be patient age. Studies examining prevalence of diastolic heart failure in hospitalized patients, patients undergoing outpatient diagnostic screening, and prospective community-based studies have shown that the prevalence of diastolic heart failure approaches 50%.[22–35] Furthermore, a prevalence of 40% to 50% has been found in studies performed in the United States, Canada, South America, Europe, Asia, Australia, and Africa, which examined patients with diastolic heart failure.

These data apply to symptomatic patients with diastolic heart failure. What is the prevalence of asymptomatic patients with diastolic dysfunction? A recent study by Redfield *et al.* suggested that the prevalence of asymptomatic diastolic dysfunction may approach 20% in patients over the age of 45.[30]

Mortality

The prognosis of patients with diastolic heart failure, although less ominous than patients with systolic heart failure, does exceed age-matched control patients.[36–38] The annual mortality rate for patients with diastolic heart failure approximates 5% to 8%. In comparison, the annual mortality rate for patients with systolic heart failure approximates 10% to 15%, while age-matched control approaches 1%. In patients with diastolic heart failure, the prognosis is also affected by the pathologic etiology causing the disease. Thus, when patients with CAD are excluded, the annual mortality for isolated diastolic heart failure approximates 2% to 3%.[37,38] The other determinants of mortality include age, EF cut-off, and study design. Like prevalence, these are interactive with the most important determinant being age. In fact, one study suggested that in patients > 70 years old, the mortality rate for systolic and diastolic heart failure is nearly equivalent.[22–35] In the Candesartan in Heart failure–Assessment of Reduction in Mortality and morbidity–Preserved (CHARM-Preserved) study where the average age was 67 years, the annual mortality rate approached 5%.[39] Most published data indicate that patients with diastolic heart failure have a 20% to 30% 5-year mortality rate.

Morbidity

Morbidity from diastolic heart failure is quite high, requiring frequent outpatient visits, hospital admissions, and expenditure of significant health care resources. The 1-year readmission rate may approach 50% in patients with diastolic heart failure. This morbidity rate is nearly identical to patients with systolic heart failure.[24–37] The readmission rate for heart failure in the CHARM-Preserved study was 5% to 10% annually.[39]

Measurement of Diastolic Function

Measurements of diastolic function can be divided into two types: those which reflect the process of active relaxation, and those which reflect passive stiffness. This division is in some ways arbitrary because structures and processes which alter relaxation, can also result in measurable abnormalities in stiffness. However, this pragmatic division provides a necessary scaffold on which to develop methods of measurement.

Relaxation

Diastole encompasses the period during which the myocardium loses its ability to generate force and shorten and then returns to its resting force and length. Relaxation occurs in a series of energy-consuming steps beginning with the release of calcium from troponin C, detachment of the actin-myosin cross-bridge, phosphorylation of phospholamban, sarcoplasmic reticulum (SR) calcium adenosine triphosphatase (ATPase)-induced calcium sequestration into the SR, sodium/calcium exchanger-induced extrusion of calcium from the cytoplasm, slowing of cross-bridge cycling rate, and extension of the sarcomere to resting length.[40–44] Adequate energy supplies and the mechanisms to regenerate them must be present for this process to occur at a sufficient rate and extent.[41,43,44] The rate and extent to which these cellular processes occur determine the rate and extent of active ventricular relaxation. At the chamber level, this process results in LV pressure decline at constant volume (isovolumic relaxation), then LV chamber filling which occurs with variable LV pressures (auxotonic relaxation). Measurements made during auxotonic relaxation are affected both by active relaxation and passive stiffness.

Isovolumic relaxation can be quantified by measuring LV pressure using a high-fidelity micromanometer catheter and calculating the peak instantaneous rate of LV pressure decline, peak (-) dP/dt, and the time constant of isovolumic LV pressure decline, tau.[45–47] When the natural log of LV diastolic pressure is plotted versus time, tau equals the inverse slope of this linear relation. Stated in more conceptual terms, tau is the time that it takes for LV pressure to fall by approximately one-third of its initial value. When isovolumic pressure decline is slowed, tau is prolonged and the numeric value of tau increases. Noninvasive estimates of total isovolumic relaxation time (IVRT) can be made using echocardiographic techniques. No index of relaxation (isovolumic or auxotonic) can be considered an index of intrinsic relaxation rate unless loading conditions, and other modulators, are held constant or are at least specified. One practical way to overcome this limitation is to examine indices of relaxation over a range of loads. Afterload can be altered acutely using mechanical or pharmacological methods. Abnormal relaxation is indicated by the shift in the position of the relaxation rate versus afterload relationship where relaxation is slowed at any equivalent systolic stress.[48]

The auxotonic LV filling phases of diastole can be characterized using Doppler echocardiography, radionuclide, conductance, or magnetic resonance imaging (MRI) techniques. While each technique has advantages and disadvantages, all assess diastolic function by measuring indices of volume transients during ventricular filling. However, like all relaxation indices, auxotonic indices must be interpreted in light of simultaneous changes in load, both afterload and filling load (load present during filling).[48–50] For example, the precise pattern of early and late diastolic transmitral flow velocities depends on factors governing instantaneous atrial and LV pressures before and after mitral valve opening and the resultant atrial-ventricular pressure gradient (filling load). Thus, it is not surprising that interventions or pathologic conditions that increase left atrial pressure increase early transmitral flow velocities, while interventions that reduce left atrial pressure reduce early filling velocities. To correctly interpret changes in transmitral flow velocities, concomitant changes in filling load must be considered. Additional indices, which may be less sensitive to, and may indicate changes in, load include pulmonary venous flow rates, transmitral propagation velocity, and tissue Doppler velocity.[51–56]

Chamber stiffness

In addition to active relaxation, LV passive viscoelastic properties contribute to the process which returns the myocardium to its resting force and length. These passive viscoelastic properties are dependent on both intracellular and extracellular structures. Changes in the stiffness of the ventricular chamber can be assessed by examining the pressure and volume relationship during diastole. Chamber stiffness is determined by the stiffness of the constituent myocardium as well as the LV mass and LV mass/volume ratio.

Chamber stiffness can be quantified by examining the relationship between diastolic pressure and volume. The operating stiffness at any point along a given pressure–volume curve is equal to the slope of the tangent drawn to the curve at that point (dP/dV). Operating stiffness changes throughout filling; stiffness is lower at smaller volumes and higher at larger volumes (volume-dependent change in diastolic pressure and stiffness). Because the diastolic pressure–volume relationship is curvilinear and generally exponential, the relationship between dP/dV and pressure is linear. The slope (K_c) is called the modulus of chamber stiffness (or chamber stiffness constant) and it can be used as a single numeric value to quantify chamber stiffness. When overall chamber stiffness is increased, the pressure–volume curve shifts to the left, the slope of the dP/dV versus pressure relationship becomes steeper, and K_c increases (volume-independent change in diastolic pressure and stiffness). Thus, diastolic pressure can be changed either by a volume-dependent change in operating stiffness, or by a volume-independent change in the chamber stiffness.

Pathophysiology

The diastolic properties of the left ventricle are determined largely by the size or volume of the LV chamber, the thickness and physical properties of the ventricular wall, and the process of myocardial relaxation. Thus, a combination of increased myocardial mass and alterations in the extracellular collagen network may cause or contribute to an increase in passive elastic stiffness of the ventricle and a steep diastolic pressure–volume relation (Figure 7.1). Disorders of the active process of myocardial relaxation, acting alone or in concert with abnormal passive properties of the ventricle, can also stiffen the ventricle. As a result, LV compliance or distensibility is reduced, dynamics of filling are altered, and end-diastolic pressure is increased.[51,57–60] Under these circumstances, a relatively small increase in central blood volume can produce a substantial increase in LV diastolic pressures and consequently pulmonary venous hypertension and pulmonary edema. Chronic changes in venous and arterial compliance may also contribute to changes in the diastolic properties of the left ventricle.

Several factors can promote fluid retention and precipitate overt heart failure in patients with heart disease. Common precipitants include uncontrolled hypertension, atrial fibrillation, noncompliance with or inappropriate discontinuation of heart failure medications, myocardial ischemia, anemia, renal insufficiency, administration of nonsteroidal antiinflammatory drugs, or overindulgence in high-salt food.[61] The glitazones may have a similar effect.[62] Patients with LV diastolic dysfunction are especially sensitive to these precipitants because of the steep LV diastolic pressure–volume relation, which results in large changes in LV diastolic pressure with only small changes in volume. Thus, elevated LV diastolic and pulmonary venous pressures in patients with a normal EF, in the absence of valvular disease, are directly related to abnormalities in the diastolic properties of the ventricle (diastolic dysfunction).

Patients with diastolic heart failure, as well as those with diastolic dysfunction and little or no congestion, exhibit exercise intolerance for three principal reasons. First, elevated LV diastolic and pulmonary venous pressures cause a reduction in lung compliance, which increases the work of breathing and evokes the symptom of dyspnea. Second, a substantial number of patients who have LVH, a high relative wall thickness, and a small end-diastolic volume exhibit a low stroke volume and a depressed cardiac output.[63] A ventricle with a normal EF cannot produce a normal stroke volume if the chamber size is small. Third, these hearts exhibit a limited ability to utilize the Frank–Starling mechanism during exercise.[64,65] Such limited preload reserve, especially if coupled with the chronotropic incompetence that is seen with advancing age, limits cardiac output during exercise. This leads to lactic acid accumulation and structural, as well as functional, abnormalities of skeletal muscles. The result can be skeletal muscle fatigue in the legs and the accessory muscles of respiration. This latter mechanism helps to explain the poor relationship between exercise tolerance and changes in LV diastolic pressure. Other mechanisms, including physical deconditioning, contribute to exercise intolerance.

Management of Diastolic Heart Failure

Until recently, there have been no large randomized placebo-controlled trials that provide evidence-based therapeutic strategies in patients with diastolic dysfunction or diastolic heart failure. The CHARM-Preserved trial data indicate that treatment with candesartan reduces hospitalization rates in patients with diastolic heart failure.[39] The recommendations presented in this review are based on the results of small clinical studies, anecdotal experience, and an understanding of the pathophysiology of diastole.

In general, the management of diastolic heart failure has two objectives. The first is to reverse the consequences of diastolic dysfunction, including venous congestion and exercise intolerance. The second is to eliminate or reduce the factors that are responsible for diastolic dysfunction, including hypertrophy, fibrosis, and ischemia (Table 7.2).

Asymptomatic Diastolic Dysfunction

The prevalence of asymptomatic diastolic dysfunction is not known, but there is reason to believe that the condition is common, especially in people with hypertension or advanced age. The finding of diastolic dysfunction in an asymptomatic patient is a risk factor for the future development of CHF, and early identification of such patients provides a window of opportunity to prevent the progression of preclinical heart disease.[27,30,66] There are no data supporting treatment directed primarily at diastolic dysfunction. Rather, the goal should be aggressive management of hypertension and other potential causes of diastolic dysfunction.

Acute Diastolic Heart Failure

The initial management of acute heart failure and pulmonary edema consists of measures that relieve pulmonary congestion while maintaining oxygenation, arterial pressure, and perfusion of vital organs. With few exceptions, the initial treatment of patients with diastolic heart failure is similar to that used for systolic heart failure. Treatment is frequently initiated prior to hospitalization, often in an ambulance or hospital emergency department (ED).

Pre-hospital management

Airway management and the administration of oxygen should be the first consideration. A face

Table 7.2. *Management of diastolic heart failure*

Initial management	Long-term management
Treat the presenting syndrome	Consider mechanisms
■ pulmonary edema/congestive state	■ promote regression of left ventricular hypertrophy
■ systemic atrial hypertension	■ prevent/promote regression of fibrosis
■ myocardial ischemia	■ modify cellular/extracellular mechanisms
■ atrial fibrillation/tachycardia	
Clarify the diagnosis	Correct the pathophysiology
■ history and physical examination	■ salt restriction and diuretics
■ echocardiography	■ block the renin-angiotensin-aldosterone system
■ cardiac catheterization/angiography	■ maintain atrial contraction
■ biopsy	■ prevent excessive tachycardia
	■ treat hypertension
	■ prevent myocardial ischemia

mask is generally used, but there is evidence that continuous positive airway pressure (CPAP) can improve lung mechanics, lessen the work of breathing, and reduce the need for intubation.[67] Morphine reduces anxiety and has vasodilator properties, but its use can increase the need for mechanical ventilation. Administered intravenously in a dose of 3 mg to 5 mg over several minutes, morphine diminishes the patient's distress and reduces the work of breathing. Morphine achieves its beneficial hemodynamic effects by acting as a vasodilator and thereby pooling blood in the splanchnic circulation. Caution is necessary if pulmonary edema is associated with hypotension, stroke, or independent pulmonary disease, especially in patients with hypercapnia.

A second goal should be to reduce pulmonary venous pressure. This can be achieved safely and effectively with sublingual or intravenous nitroglycerin (10 µg/min to 50 µg/min depending on clinical response). The use of nitroglycerin avoids electrolyte disturbances seen when intravenous diuretics are administered as the initial treatment. When treatment with nitrates, furosemide, and morphine are compared, optimal clinical outcomes are seen with nitrates.[68] Moreover, the effects of nitrates are rapidly reversible in the event of hypotension. Rotating tourniquets can also effect a rapidly reversible reduction in central venous pressures. If the pre-hospitalization period is expected to be prolonged, the intravenous administration of nitroprusside (0.1 to 10 µg/kg/min) may be necessary in patients with severe hypertension, but there are no clear indications for angiotensin-converting enzyme (ACE) inhibitors or beta-adrenergic agonists during the pre-hospitalization period.

Initial hospital treatment

On admission to the ED, the diagnosis of heart failure should be confirmed, and associated or complicating problems should be investigated, including pneumonia, myocardial infarction, pulmonary embolism, and dissection of the aorta. At the same time, treatment should be initiated.

Preload reduction

A decrease in left atrial and pulmonary venous pressures is obviously desirable in patients with APE. In patients with LV systolic dysfunction and acute exacerbation of chronic heart failure (most of whom have an expanded central blood volume), a substantial reduction in pulmonary venous pressure can be achieved without a significant drop in arterial pressure. However, patients with diastolic heart failure often develop a dramatic decrease in arterial pressure when attempts are made to reduce preload. This occurs as a consequence of a steep LV diastolic pressure–volume relation; even a small reduction in diastolic volume can result in a relatively large reduction in LV diastolic pressure and systemic arterial pressure. Therefore, if there is reason to believe that diastolic heart failure is present, initial attempts at preload reduction should be conservative.

Diuretics are effective and commonly used in the initial treatment. Furosemide is administered intravenously at an initial dose of 40 mg to 80 mg; subsequent doses depend on the response to the initial dose. Intravenous nitroglycerin (10 µg/min to 50 µg/min), which is also used to reduce preload, has the advantage of being anti-ischemic and it does not result in electrolyte abnormalities. Nesiritide (0.015 µg/kg/min to 0.06 µg/kg/min) produces a dose-dependent decrease in pulmonary capillary wedge pressure (PCWP) and systemic vascular resistance (SVR), and an increase in cardiac output in patients with systolic heart failure.[69] There is little published data on patients with diastolic heart failure.

Afterload reduction

Many, if not most, patients with APE and diastolic heart failure are hypertensive.[6] Although nitroglycerin or nesiritide are both effective in reducing blood pressure and relieving pulmonary edema, nitroprusside is the vasodilator of choice when a substantial reduction in pressure is required. It is administered by intravenous infusion at a dose of 0.1 µg/kg/min to 10 µg/kg/min. The dose is adjusted to obtain the desired hemodynamic effects. Nitroprusside is used only in situations requiring short-term reductions in blood pressure; early arrangements should be made to substitute other antihypertensive agents. Beta-adrenergic receptor blockers may be used alone or in combination with nitroprusside.

Chronic Diastolic Heart Failure

Any attempt to develop a long-term therapeutic plan must be based on a careful consideration of the cause of the diastolic dysfunction and its potential response to treatment. In general, emphasis is placed on the control of arterial hypertension, management of the congestive state, maintenance of normal sinus rhythm, and prevention of myocardial ischemia. It is particularly important to avoid the known precipitants of heart failure.

Venous congestion

The renin-angiotensin-aldosterone system (RAAS) is activated in patients who have chronic heart failure, but the mechanisms that evoke its activation remain unclear in patients who have LV diastolic dysfunction. In some patients, myocardial ischemia, uncontrolled hypertension, and excessive dietary sodium may promote the development of congestion; whereas, in other patients, low SVR or low arterial pressure may contribute to salt and water retention.[70] Elevated venous pressure can directly cause renal sodium retention.[71] Despite a limited understanding of the pathogenesis of salt and water retention in patients with diastolic dysfunction, diuretics remain the mainstay of therapy for venous congestion. After the initial treatment, salt restriction is necessary, and long-term administration of a diuretic is usually required. Diuretics have the potential to reduce cardiac output, especially in patients with small LV chambers. With the exception of their antihypertensive effects, diuretics do not alter the primary disease processes that lead to diastolic dysfunction.

Thiazide diuretics (hydrochlorothiazide 25 mg to 50 mg p.o. q.d.) can suffice for management of mild heart failure, but the side effects of carbohydrate intolerance and hyperuricemia can be undesirable. Loop diuretics such as furosemide (40 mg to 240 mg p.o. q.d.) are more potent than the thiazide diuretics, especially when the glomerular filtration rate (GFR) is reduced. The combination of furosemide and a thiazide diuretic can be especially useful when edema is refractory to either agent alone. For patients who develop hypokalemia, the potassium-sparing diuretic spironolactone may be added. Aldosterone antagonists, such as spironolactone and eplerenone, also have the potential to retard the fibrosis that contributes to abnormal chamber stiffness. The reduction in blood volume produced by diuretics may trigger an increase in sympathetic tone and renin-angiotensin activation, which can lead to vasoconstriction and worsening of the pathophysiology. Some vasodilators, particularly nitrates and pure arteriolar vasodilators, evoke a similar response. ACE inhibitors and beta-blockers blunt the neurohormonal activation and decrease the salt and water retention that complicates the treatment of heart failure.

Atrial arrhythmias

Rapid atrial fibrillation in patients with LV diastolic dysfunction is usually accompanied by a substantial increase in ventricular diastolic and atrial pressures, leading to pulmonary edema and hypotension. Overt decompensation occurs because of inadequate time for complete ventricular relaxation, and also because of the loss of atrial mechanical function and its contribution to ventricular filling. An attempt to restore and maintain sinus rhythm is mandatory. Direct current cardioversion may be necessary on an emergency basis. In less urgent situations, electrical or chemical cardioversion can be performed after rate control with beta-blockers, calcium channel blockers, or digitalis.

Rate control

Tachycardia is poorly tolerated in most cardiac disorders. Atrial tachyarrhythmias, and even sinus tachycardia, have a negative impact on diastolic function for several reasons. A rapid heart rate causes an increase in myocardial oxygen demand and a decrease in coronary perfusion time, which can promote ischemic diastolic dysfunction even in the absence of CAD. In addition, tachycardia does not allow sufficient time for relaxation, and as a result there is incomplete relaxation between beats, which causes an increase in diastolic pressure relative to volume. Tachycardia also reduces the LV diastolic filling time and the coronary perfusion time. Accordingly, most clinicians use beta-blockers or calcium channel blockers to prevent excessive tachycardia and produce a relative bradycardia in patients who have diastolic dysfunction. However, bradycardia can result in a fall in cardiac output despite some potential for improved filling pressures. Such considerations underscore the need for individualizing therapeutic interventions that affect heart rate. An initial goal might be a resting rate of approximately 65 bpm to 70 bpm with a blunted exercise-induced increase in heart rate (and a blunted increase in blood pressure during exercise). Although the optimal heart rate for hypertrophic or failing hearts is not known, it is likely that such hearts would function most efficiently at relatively slow rates. This has several potentially beneficial effects that are largely related to the salutary effects on myocardial energetics and the prolonged diastolic interval that allows complete relaxation between beats. Furthermore, hypertrophied and failing hearts exhibit a flat or even negative force-frequency relationship, and in contrast to normal hearts, function may improve as the rate is slowed.[72,73]

Myocardial ischemia

Extensive clinical and experimental literature documents the deleterious effect of ischemia on diastolic function of the left ventricle. A transient increase in LV stiffness and diastolic pressure develops during myocardial ischemia caused by coronary spasm, exercise, rapid atrial pacing, angioplasty balloon inflation, and spontaneous angina.[74] Ischemia can be treated with nitrates, beta blockers, and calcium channel blockers, percutaneous coronary intervention (PCI), or coronary artery bypass grafting (CABG). When the signs of ischemic diastolic dysfunction are prominent, PCI or CABG is appropriate.[75] Yet, even after successful PCI or surgery, there may be recurrent episodes of heart failure.[76]

Hypertension and hypertrophy

Several factors contribute to the diastolic dysfunction seen in hypertensive heart disease.[77] First, the abnormal loading conditions imposed by arterial hypertension reduce LV relaxation and filling rates. Second, concentrically hypertrophied hearts exhibit increased passive stiffness (caused by a low LV volume–mass ratio and fibrosis of the myocardium) and impaired relaxation that is independent of hemodynamic loads. Third, limited coronary vascular reserve can be responsible for myocardial ischemia, even in the absence of epicardial coronary disease. Each of these factors should be considered in the treatment of patients with hypertensive heart disease and diastolic dysfunction. Abnormalities of diastolic function can be detected in asymptomatic hypertensive patients with or without measurable hypertrophy.[78] Adequate control of the arterial pressure in these patients with pre-clinical heart disease should favorably alter loading conditions in the short term, while promoting regression of hypertrophy in the long term.

Some studies of patients with hypertensive heart disease indicate that diastolic dysfunction improves as LVH regresses.[79,80] Other studies have confirmed improved diastolic function, prolonged exercise duration, and better heart failure scores in patients who have hypertensive heart disease and clinically significant LV diastolic dysfunction and are treated with verapamil. However, these clinical benefits were not closely related to changes in blood pressure or heart rate.[81] Differences in the effects of treatment on diastolic function probably depend on the amount of hypertrophy regression, alterations in LV loading conditions, direct myocardial effect of the antihypertensive agent, and possibly changes in coronary reserve.

Progressive interstitial fibrosis accompanies the hypertrophic response to systemic arterial hypertension. This abnormal accumulation of fibrillar collagen is a result of enhanced collagen synthesis or decreased degradation by cardiac fibroblasts which is related in part to the activity of the RAAS. The important functional consequences of progressive interstitial and perivascular fibrosis include increased myocardial stiffness and impaired coronary flow reserve. In experimental studies, ACE inhibitors, angiotensin receptor blockers (ARBs), or spironolactone appear to protect against this exaggerated fibrous tissue response.[82] Thus, the imperative to treat arterial hypertension may include prevention of the deleterious effects of angiotensin II and aldosterone. ACE inhibitors are widely used and effective antihypertensive agents that can produce regression of LVH, and a salutary effect on cardiac fibrosis may constitute an unexpected bonus. As a preventive or treatment strategy this has not yet been tested in humans with diastolic dysfunction.

Exercise intolerance

Patients who have a history of diastolic heart failure, even those who have diastolic dysfunction and little or no congestion, often exhibit substantial exercise intolerance. Given the limited understanding of the precise factors responsible for dyspnea and fatigue,[83,84] it has been difficult to develop a standard treatment plan for patients with LV diastolic dysfunction. Certainly, hypertension, myocardial ischemia, and clinically apparent congestion must be treated, but caution must be exercised to avoid even mild volume depletion that can contribute to reduced cardiac output. A most important, and largely ignored, treatment is directed against the deconditioning that is prominent in many patients with diastolic heart failure. Cardiac rehabilitation programs can be very helpful in this regard.[85] Although calcium channel blockers and beta-blockers improve symptoms in some patients with LV diastolic dysfunction, the benefit on exercise capacity is not always paralleled by improved measures of LV diastolic function. For example, in symptomatic patients with hypertrophic cardiomyopathy, a placebo-controlled double-blind comparison of the effects of verapamil and propranolol on exercise tolerance indicated that both agents produced an increase in exercise duration. However, relaxation rate increased with verapamil and decreased with propranolol.[86] The observation that such verapamil effects persist in the long term[87] and that it is effective in patients who have other causes of diastolic dysfunction[81] makes this agent a good choice for treatment of exercise intolerance. Beta-blockers are an acceptable alternative, despite a direct depressant effect on myocardial relaxation. ACE inhibitors or ARBs also have the potential to improve exercise tolerance in patients who have diastolic dysfunction. For example, treatment with losartan is associated with an increase in exercise capacity and improved quality of life in patients who have hypertensive cardiovascular disease and documented diastolic dysfunction.[88] These responses are similar to those observed in patients treated with verapamil.[81] The salutary effects of losartan and verapamil are related at least in part to their antihypertensive effect.

Positive inotropic drugs

Most patients with heart failure caused by LV systolic dysfunction benefit from treatment with positive inotropic agents. Such therapy is generally not used in the long-term treatment of patients with diastolic heart failure because the LVEF is preserved and there appears to be little potential for a beneficial effect. Moreover, positive inotropic agents have the potential to worsen the pathophysiologic processes that cause diastolic dysfunction. Digitalis, by inhibiting the sodium-potassium ATPase pump, augments intracellular calcium through a sodium-calcium exchange mechanism and enhances the contractile state. By doing so, digitalis produces an increase in systolic energy demands while adding to a diastolic calcium overload. These effects may not be clinically apparent in many circumstances, but during hemodynamic stress or ischemia, digitalis may promote diastolic dysfunction.[89] Data from the Digitalis Investigators Group (DIG) study, however, suggest that digitalis might have a beneficial effect on some clinical outcome measures, such as heart failure hospitalizations, despite a normal LVEF.[90] However, there appears to be a corresponding increase in endpoints related to myocardial ischemia and arrhythmias. Recognizing conflicting opinions on this issue, most clinicians do not use digitalis in patients with diastolic heart failure.

By increasing intracellular cyclic adenosine monophosphate (cAMP), beta-adrenergic agonists enhance calcium sequestration by the SR and thereby promote a more rapid and complete myocardial relaxation between beats.[91] Beta agonists can also increase venous capacitance, which leads to a reduction in ventricular filling pressures. Phosphodiesterase (PDE) inhibitors can produce similar salutary effects on myocardial relaxation and venous capacitance.[92] Unfortunately, all cAMP-dependent agents promote calcium influx into the cell and augment myocardial energy demands. Thus, dopamine, amrinone, and similar agents are only used in the short-term management of acute diastolic heart failure.

Differences between pharmacologic treatment of systolic and diastolic heart failure

With a number of notable exceptions, many of the drugs proposed to treat diastolic heart failure are the same as those used to treat systolic heart failure. However, the rationale for their use, the pathophysiologic process being altered by the drug, and the dosing regimen may be entirely different. For example, beta-blockers are now recommended for the treatment of both systolic and diastolic heart failure. In diastolic heart failure beta-blockers are used to decrease heart rate, increase the duration of diastole, and modify the hemodynamic response to exercise. However, in systolic heart failure, beta-blockers are used chronically to increase inotropic state and modify LV remodeling. In systolic heart failure, beta-blockers must be titrated slowly and carefully over an extended time period. This is generally not necessary in diastolic heart failure. Diuretics are used in the treatment of both systolic and diastolic heart failure. However, the doses used to treat diastolic heart failure are, in general, smaller than the doses used in systolic heart failure. Conversely, some drugs are used only to treat either systolic or diastolic heart failure, but not both. Calcium channel blockers, such as diltiazem, nifedipine, and verapamil, have no place in the treatment of systolic heart failure. By contrast, these drugs have been proposed as being useful in the treatment of diastolic heart failure.

Conclusion

Conceptually, an ideal therapeutic agent would target the underlying mechanisms causing diastolic heart failure. It might improve calcium homeostasis and energetics, blunt neurohumoral activation, or prevent and regress fibrosis. Fortunately, some pharmaceutical agents fitting these design characteristics are already in existence and many more are under development.

Unfortunately, randomized, double-blind, placebo-controlled multicenter trials examining the efficacy of these agents, used either alone or in combination, have been slow to develop. Difficulties preventing these studies have included lack of recognition of the importance of diastolic heart failure, inability to define a homogeneous study population, lack of agreement on the definition and diagnostic criteria for diastolic heart failure, and perception that there would be a marginal return on investment for funding these types of studies. However, there is now reason for a great deal of optimism. Diastolic heart failure is now recognized as an important problem. Guidelines for diagnosis have been developed, and the pharmaceutical industry has supported randomized, double-blind, placebo-controlled multicenter trials, and hopefully in the near future government agencies will as well.

A number of such trials are now underway.[93–96] Some trials target neurohumoral activation in the RAAS by inhibiting the ARB (Perindopril for Elderly People with Chronic Heart Failure [PEP-CHF], Irbesartan in Heart Failure with Preserved Systolic Function [I-Preserve], Hong Kong Diastolic Heart Failure study). Some trials target underlying structural mechanisms such as intracellular calcium homeostasis, using an agent which is proposed to improve SR calcium reuptake (MCC-135 GO1 study), or extracellular matrix collagen metabolism, using an agent which breaks advanced glycosylation end-product collagen cross-links (ALT-711 Diamond study). One study targets the beta-adrenergic nervous system (Study of Effects of Nebivolol Intervention on Outcomes and Rehospitalization in Seniors with Heart Failure [SENIORS]). With these studies, and others which are currently under development, an effective treatment for diastolic heart failure will be more completely defined.

References

1. McKee PA, Castelli WP, McNamara PM, Kannel WB. The natural history of congestive heart failure: the Framingham Study. N Engl J Med 1971; 285: 1441–1446.
2. Shimizu G, Zile MR, Blaustein AS, Gaasch WH. Left ventricular chamber filling and midwall fiber lengthening in left ventricular hypertrophy: conventional midwall measurements overestimates fiber velocities. Circulation 1985; 71: 266–272.

3. Aurigemma GP, Silver KH, Priest MA, Gaasch WH. Geometric changes allow normal ejection fraction despite depressed myocardial shortening in hypertensive left ventricular hypertrophy. J Am Coll Cardiol 1995; 26: 195–202.
4. European Study Group on Diastolic Heart Failure. How to diagnose diastolic heart failure. Eur Heart J 1998; 19: 990–1003.
5. Vasan RS, Levy D. Defining diastolic heart failure: a call for standardized diagnostic criteria. Circulation 2000; 101: 2118–2121.
6. Gandi SK, Powers JC, Nomeir A, *et al.* The pathogenesis of acute pulmonary edema associated with hypertension. N Eng J Med 2001; 344: 17–60.
7. Zile MR, Gaasch WH, Carroll JD, *et al.* Heart failure with a normal ejection fraction: is measurement of diastolic function necessary to make the diagnosis of diastolic heart failure? Circulation 2001; 104: 779–782.
8. Lubien E, DeMaria A, Krishnaswamy P, *et al.* Utility of B-natruretic peptide in detecting diastolic dysfunction: comparison with Doppler velocity recordings. Circulation 2002; 105: 595–601.
9. Wang TJ, Larson MG, Levy D, *et al.* Impact of age and sex on plasma natriuretic peptide levels in healthy adults. Am J Cardiol 2002; 90: 254–258.
10. Redfield MM, Rodeheffer RJ, Jacobsen SJ, *et al.* Plasma brain natriuretic peptide concentration: Impact of age and gender. J Am Coll Cardiol 2002; 40: 976–982.
11. Vasan RS, Benjamin EJ, Larson MG, *et al.* Plasma natriuretic peptides for community screening for left ventricular hypertrophy and systolic dysfunction. The Framingham Heart Study. JAMA 2002; 288: 1257–1259.
12. Maisel A. B-type natriuretic peptide levels: a potential novel "white count" for congestive heart failure. J Card Fail 2001; 7: 183–193.
13. Kazanegra R, Cheng V, Garcia A, *et al.* A rapid test for B-type natriuretic peptide correlates with failing wedge pressures in patients treated for decompensated heart failure: A pilot study. J Card Fail 2001; 7: 21–29.
14. Dao Q, Krishnaswamy P, Kazanegra R, *et al.* Utility of B-type natriuretic peptide in the diagnosis of congestive heart failure in an urgent-care setting. J Am Coll Cardiol 2001; 37: 379–385.
15. Maisel AS, Koon J, Krishnaswamy P, *et al.* Utility of B-natriuretic peptide as a rapid, point-of-care test for screening patients undergoing echocardiography to determine left ventricular dysfunction. Am Heart J 2001; 141: 367–374.
16. Andersson B, Hall C. N-terminal proatrial natriuretic peptide and prognosis in patients with heart failure and preserved systolic function. J Card Fail 2000; 6: 208–213.
17. Yamamoto K, Burnett JC, Bermudez EA, *et al.* Clinical criteria and biochemical markers for the detection of systolic dysfunction. J Card Fail 2000; 6: 194–200.
18. Yamanoto K, Burnett JC, Jougasaki M, *et al.* Superiority of brain natriuretic peptide as a hormonal marker of ventricular systolic and diastolic dysfunction and ventricular hypertrophy. Hypertension 1996; 28: 988–994.
19. Gaasch WH, Schick EC, Zile MR. Management of left ventricular diastolic dysfunction. In: Smith TW (ed.) Cardiovascular Therapeutics: a Companion to Braunwald's Heart Disease (W. B. Saunders Company: Philadelphia, PA, 1996), 237–242.
20. Zile MR. Diastolic heart failure: diagnosis, mechanisms, and treatment. Cardiology Rounds as Presented in the Rounds of the Cardiovascular Division of Brigham and Women's Hospital, Boston, Massachusetts. November, 1999; 3: 1–7.
21. Zile MR, Simsic JM. Diastolic heart failure: diagnosis and treatment. Clin Cornerstone 2000; 3: 13–24.
22. Philbin EF, Rocco TA. Use of angiotensin-converting enzyme inhibitors in heart failure with preserved left ventricular systolic function. Am Heart J 1997; 134: 188–195.
23. Senni M, Tribouilloy CM, Rodeheffer RJ, *et al.* Congestive heart failure in the community: a study of all incident cases in Olmsted County, Minnesota, in 1991. Circulation 1998; 98: 2282–2289.
24. Vasan R, Larson MG, Benjamin EJ, *et al.* Congestive heart failure in subjects with normal versus reduced left ventricular ejection fraction: prevalence and mortality in a population-based cohort. J Am Coll Cardiol 1999; 33: 1948–1955.
25. Kitzman DW, Gardin JM, Gottdiener JS, *et al.*, for the CHS Research Group. Importance of heart failure with preserved systolic function in patients >65 years of age. Am J Cardiol 2001; 87: 413–419.
26. Gottdiener JS, Arnold AM, Aurigemma GP, *et al.* Predictors of congestive heart failure in the elderly: the cardiovascular health study. J Am Coll Cardiol 2000; 35: 1628–1637.
27. Aurigemma GP, Gottdiener JS, Shemanski L, Gardin J, Kitzman D. Predictive value of systolic and diastolic function for incident congestive heart failure in the elderly: the cardiovascular health study. J Am Coll Cardiol 2001; 37: 1042–1048.
28. Dauterman KW, Massie BM, Gheorghiade M. Heart failure associated with preserved systolic function: a common and costly clinical entity. Am Heart J 1998; 135: S310–S319.

29. O'Conner CM, Gattis WA, Shaw L, Cuffe MS, Califf RM. Clinical characteristics and long-term outcomes of patients with heart failure and preserved systolic function. Am J Cardiol 2000; 86: 863–867.
30. Redfield MM, Jacobsen SJ, Burnett JC, *et al.* Burden of systolic and diastolic ventricular dysfunction in the community: appreciating the scope of the heart failure epidemic. JAMA 2003; 289: 194–202.
31. Petrie M, McMurray J. Commentary: changes in notions about heart failure. Lancet 2001; 358: 432.
32. Yip GWK, Ho PPY, Woo KS, Sanderson JE. Comparison of frequencies of left ventricular systolic and diastolic heart failure in Chinese living in Hong Kong. Am J Cardiol 1999; 84: 563–567.
33. Tsutsui H, Tsuchihashi M, Takeshita A. Mortality and readmission of hospitalized patients with congestive heart failure and preserved versus depressed systolic function. Am J Cardiol 2001; 88: 530–533.
34. Dauterman KW, Go AS, Rowell R, *et al.* Congestive heart failure with preserved systolic function in a statewide sample of community hospitals. J Card Fail 2001; 7: 221–231.
35. Gottdiener JS, McClelland RL, Marshall R, *et al.* Outcome of congestive heart failure in elderly persons: influence of left ventricular systolic function. The cardiovascular health study. Ann Intern Med 2002; 137: 631–639.
36. Setaro JF, Soufer R, Remetz MS, *et al.* Long-term outcome in patients with congestive heart failure and intact systolic left ventricular performance. Am J Cardiol 1992; 69: 1212–1216.
37. Judge KW, Pawitan Y, Caldwell J, *et al.* Congestive heart failure in patients with preserved left ventricular systolic function: analysis of the CASS registry. J Am Coll Cardiol 1991; 18: 377–382.
38. Brogen WC, Hillis LD, Flores ED, *et al.* The natural history of isolated left ventricular diastolic dysfunction. Am J Med 1992; 92: 627–630.
39. Yusuf S, Pfeffer MA, Swedberg K, *et al.* Effects of candesartan in patients with chronic heart failure and preserved left-ventricular ejection fraction: the CHARM-Preserved Trial. Lancet 2003; 362: 777–781.
40. Apstein CS, Morgan JP. Cellular mechanisms underlying left ventricular diastolic dysfunction. In: Gaasch WH, LeWinter MM (eds) Left Ventricular Diastolic Dysfunction and Heart Failure (Lea & Febiger: Philadelphia, PA, 1994), 3–24.
41. Ingwall JS. Energetics of the normal and failing human heart: focus on the creatine kinase reaction. Adv Org Biol 1998; 4: 117–141.
42. Solaro RJ, Wolska BM, Westfall M. Regulatory proteins and diastolic relaxation. In: Lorell BH and Grossman W (eds) Diastolic Relaxation of the Heart Kluwer Academic Publishers: Boston, 1994, 43–54.
43. Alpert NR, LeWinter M, Mulieri LA, Hasenfuss G. Chemomechanical energy transduction in the failing heart. Heart Fail Rev 1999; 4: 281–295.
44. Tian R, Nascimben L, Ingwall JS, Lorell BH. Failure to maintain a low ADP concentration impairs diastolic function in hypertrophied rat hearts. Circulation 1997; 96: 1313–1319.
45. Weiss JL, Fredericksen JW, Weisfeldt ML. Hemodynamic determinants of the time course of fall in canine left ventricular pressure. J Clin Invest 1976; 58: 83–95.
46. Smith VE, Zile MR. Relaxation and diastolic properties of the heart. In: Fozzard HA *et al.* (eds) The Heart and Cardiovascular System (Raven Press: New York, 1992), 1353–1367.
47. Mirsky I, Pasipoularides A. Clinical assessment of diastolic function. Prog Cardiovasc Dis 1990; 32: 291–318.
48. Zile MR, Nishimura RA, Gaasch WH. Hemodynamic loads and left ventricular diastolic function: factors affecting the indices of isovolumetric and auxotonic relaxation In: Gaasch WH, LeWinter MM (eds) Left Ventricular Diastolic Dysfunction and Heart Failure. (Lea and Febiger: Philadelphia, PA, 1994), 219–242.
49. Brutsaert DL, Sys SU. Diastolic dysfunction in heart failure. J Card Fail 1997; 3: 225–242.
50. Zile MR. Hemodynamic determinants of echocardiography derived indices of left ventricular filling. Echocardiography 1992; 9: 289–300.
51. Nishimura RA, Tajik J. Evaluation of diastolic filling of left ventricle in health and disease: Doppler echocardiography is the clinician's Rosetta Stone. J Am Coll Cardiol 1997; 30: 8–18.
52. Garcia MJ, Thomas JD, Klein AL. New Doppler echocardiographic applications for the study of diastolic dysfunction. J Am Coll Cardiol 1998; 32: 865–875.
53. Appleton CP, Firsterbreg MS, Garcia MJ, Thomas JD. The echo-Doppler evaluation of left ventricular diastolic function: a current perspective. Card Clinics 2000; 18: 513–546.
54. Ommen SR, Nishimura RA, Appleton CP, *et al.* Clinical utility of Doppler echocardiography and tissue Doppler imaging in the estimation of left ventricular filling pressures: a comparative simultaneous Doppler-catheterization study. Circulation 2000; 102: 1788–1794.
55. Garcia MJ, Smedira NG, Greenberg NL, *et al.* Color m-mode Doppler flow propagation velocity is a preload insensitive index of left ventricular relaxation:

animal and human validation. J Am Coll Cardiol 2000; 35: 201–208.
56. Nagueh SF, Zoghbi WA. Clinical assessment of LV diastolic filling by Dopper echocardiography. ACC Curr J Rev 2001; Jul/Aug: 45–49.
57. Glantz SA, Parmley WW. Factors which affect the diastolic pressure-volume curve. Circ Res 1978; 42: 171–180.
58. Gaasch WH, Levine HJ, Quinones MA, *et al.* Left ventricular compliance: mechanisms and clinical implications. Am J Cardiol 1976; 38: 645–653.
59. Grossman W, McLaurin LP. Diastolic properties of the left ventricle. Ann Intern Med 1976; 84: 316–326.
60. Zile MR, Brutsaert DL. New concepts in diastolic dysfunction and diastolic heart failure. Part 1: diagnosis, prognosis and measurements of diastolic function. Circulation 2002; 105: 1387–1393.
61. Tsuyuki RT, McKelvic RS, Arnold JM, *et al.* Acute precipitants of congestive heart failure exacerbations. Arch Intern Med 2001; 161: 2337–2342.
62. Wang CH, Weisel RD, Liu PP, *et al.* Glitazones and heart failure: critical appraisal for the clinician. Circulation 2003; 107: 1350–1354.
63. Aurigemma GP, Gaasch WH, McLaughlin M, *et al.* Reduced left ventricular systolic pump performance and depressed myocardial contractile function in patients >65 years of age with normal ejection fraction and high relative wall thickness. Am J Cardiol 1995; 76: 702–705.
64. Cuocolo A, Sax FL, Brush JE, *et al.* Left ventricular hypertrophy and impaired diastolic filling in essential hypertension: diastolic mechanisms for systolic dysfunction during exercise. Circulation 1990; 81: 978–986.
65. Kitzman DW, Higginbotham BM, Cobb FR, *et al.* Exercise intolerance in patients with heart failure and preserved left ventricular systolic function: failure of the Frank-Starling mechanism. J Am Coll Cardiol 1991; 17: 1065–1072.
66. Gaasch WH. Diagnosis and treatment of heart failure based on left ventricular systolic or diastolic dysfunction. J Am Med Assoc 1994; 271: 1276–1280.
67. Pang D, Keenan SP, Cook DJ, *et al.* The effect of positive pressure airway support on mortality and the need for intubation in cardiogenic pulmonary edema: a systematic review. Chest 1998; 114: 1185–1192.
68. Hoffmann JR, Reynolds S. Comparison of nitroglycerine, morphine, and furosemide in treatment of presumed prehospital pulmonary edema. Chest 1987; 92: 586–593.
69. Colucci WS. Nesiritide for the treatment of decompensated heart failure. J Card Fail 2001; 7: 92–100.
70. Anand IS, Chandrashekhar Y, Ferrari R, *et al.* Pathogenesis of congestive state in chronic obstructive pulmonary disease: studies of body water and sodium, renal function, hemodynamics and plasma hormones during edema and after recovery. Circulation 1992; 86: 12–21.
71. Firth JD, Raine AEG, Ledingham JGG. Raised venous pressure: a direct cause of renal sodium retention in edema. Lancet 1998; 1: 1033–1035.
72. Liu CP, Ting CT, Lawrence W, *et al.* Diminished contractile response to increased heart rate in intact human left ventricular hypertrophy: systolic versus diastolic determinants. Circulation 1993; 88: 1893–1906.
73. Mulieri LA, Hasenfuss G, Leavitt B, *et al.* Altered myocardial force-frequency relation in human heart failure. Circulation 1992; 85: 1743–1750.
74. Paulus WJ, Bronzwaer JGF, de Bruyne B, *et al.* Different effects of "supply" and "demand" ischemia on left ventricular diastolic function in humans. In: Gaasch WH, LeWinter MM (eds) Left Ventricular Diastolic Dysfunction and Heart Failure (Lea & Febiger: Philadelphia, PA, 1994), 286–305.
75. Kunis R, Greenberg H, Yeoh CG, *et al.* Coronary revascularization for recurrent pulmonary edema in elderly patients with ischemic heart disease and preserved ventricular function. N Engl J Med 1985; 313: 1207–1210.
76. Kramer K, Kirkman P, Kitzman D. Flash pulmonary edema: association with hypertension and reoccurrence despite coronary revascularization. Am Heart J 2000; 140: 451–455.
77. Hoit BD, Walsh RA. Diastolic function in hypertensive heart disease. In: Gaasch WH, LeWinter MM (eds) Left Ventricular Diastolic Dysfunction and Heart Failure (Lea & Febiger: Philadelphia, PA, 1994), 354–372.
78. Inouye I, Massie B, Loge D, *et al.* Abnormal left ventricular filling: an early finding in mild to moderate systemic hypertension. Am J Cardiol 1984; 53: 120–126.
79. Smith VE, White WB, Meeran MK, *et al.* Improved left ventricular filling accompanies reduced left ventricular mass during therapy of essential hypertension. J Am Coll Cardiol 1986; 8: 1449–1454.
80. Schulman SP, Weiss JL, Becker LC, *et al.* The effects of antihypertensive therapy on left ventricular mass in elderly patients. N Engl J Med 1990; 322: 1350–1356.
81. Setaro JF, Zaret BL, Schulman DS, *et al.* Usefulness of verapamil for congestive heart failure associated with abnormal left ventricular diastolic filling and normal left ventricular systolic performance. Am J Cardiol 1990; 66: 981–986.

82. Weber KT, Brilla CG. Pathological hypertrophy and cardiac interstitium: fibrosis and renin-angiotensin-aldosterone system. Circulation 1991; 83: 1849–1865.
83. Packer M. Abnormalities of diastolic function as a potential cause of exercise intolerance in chronic heart failure. Circulation 1990; 81: 78–86.
84. Chikamori T, Counihan PJ, Doi YL, *et al*. Mechanisms of exercise limitation in hypertrophic cardiomyopathy. J Am Coll Cardiol 1992; 19: 507–512.
85. Kitzman DW, Brubaker PH, Anderson RA, *et al*. Exercise training improves aerobic capacity in elderly patients with diastolic heart failure: a randomized, controlled trial. Circulation 1999; 100: 296 (Abstract).
86. Rosing DR, Kent KM, Maron BJ, *et al*. Verapamil therapy: a new approach to the pharmacologic treatment of hypertrophic cardiomyopathy. II. Effects on exercise capacity and symptomatic status. Circulation 1979; 60: 1208–1213.
87. Bonow RO, Dilsizian V, Rosing DR, *et al*. Verapamil-induced improvement in left ventricular filling and increased exercise tolerance in patients with hypertrophic cardiomyopathy: short and long term results. Circulation 1985; 72: 853–864.
88. Warner JG, Metzger DC, Kitzman DW, *et al*. Losartan improves exercise tolerance in patients with diastolic dysfunction and a hypertensive response to exercise. J Am Coll Cardiol 1999; 33: 1567–1572.
89. Lorell BH, Isoyama S, Grice WN, *et al*. Effects of ouabain and isoproterenol on left ventricular diastolic function during low-flow ischemia in isolated, blood-perfused rabbit hearts. Circ Res 1988; 63: 457–467.
90. Massie BM, Abdalla I. Heart failure in patients with preserved left ventricular systolic function: do digitalis glycosides have a role? Prog Cardiovasc Dis 1998; 40: 357–369.
91. Lang RM, Carroll JD, Nakamura S, *et al*. Role of adrenoceptors and dopamine receptors in modulating left ventricular diastolic function. Circ Res 1988; 63: 126–134.
92. Monrad ES, McKay R, Baim DS, *et al*. 1984. Improvement in indexes of diastolic performance in patients with congestive heart failure treated with milrinone. Circulation 1984; 70: 1030–1037.
93. Shibata MC, Flather MD, Bohm M, *et al*. Study of the effects of nebivolol intervention on outcomes and rehospitalization in seniors with heart failure (SENIORS): Rationale and design. Internat J Cardiol 2002; 86: 77–85.
94. Cleland JFG, Tendera M, Adamus J, *et al*., the PEP investigators. Perindopril for elderly people with chronic heart failure: the PEP-CHF study. Eur J Heart Fail 1999; 1: 211–217.
95. Sanderson JE. Letter to the editor. Eur J Heart Fail 2000; 2: 117.
96. Swedberg K, Pfeffer M, Granger C, *et al*., for the CHARM-programme investigators. Candesartan in heart failure: assessment of reduction in mortality and morbidity (CHARM): Rationale and design. J Card Fail 1999; 5: 276–282.

CHAPTER 8

Pathophysiology of the cardiorenal syndrome in acute heart failure

Guido Boerrigter, John C Burnett, Jr

Introduction

Heart failure is a common disease which, despite progress in medical and device-based therapies, continues to be associated with substantial morbidity and mortality. Heart failure is primarily characterized by impairment in cardiac function, which compromises the function of other organ systems and becomes a multisystem disorder. The kidney is the major organ in the control of body fluid and electrolyte homeostasis, and it is of particular importance in the pathogenesis of heart failure. While renal sodium and water retention are an attempt to maintain blood pressure and cardiac output, this can result in a vicious cycle by further increasing the load on an already failing heart.

Recent studies have shown that the kidney is an important factor in the compensation of heart failure. Indeed, in two retrospective analyses, impaired renal function was identified as a major predictor of mortality in patients with heart failure, more powerful even than New York Heart Association (NYHA) class and left ventricular ejection fraction (LVEF).[1,2] These studies underscore the importance of considering renal function in the management of heart failure.

This chapter briefly reviews the major physiological and pathophysiological characteristics of renal function in heart failure, defines the cardiorenal syndrome (CRS), which may represent an ominous stage of heart failure, and reviews strategies for the management of heart failure by improving renal function.

Cardiorenal Homeostasis

Besides cardiac function, intravascular volume is crucial for optimal cardiovascular homeostasis. The kidney is the primary organ involved in the regulation of fluid and electrolyte homeostasis and intravascular volume. To this end, the kidney integrates the input of various physiological factors, which include hemodynamic, hormonal, and neuronal factors (Figure 8.1). Under normal physiological conditions, about 20% of the cardiac output is directed to the kidneys to perform their important homeostatic function. Figure 8.2 shows a schematic of a nephron, the basic functional and structural unit of the kidney. Blood enters the glomerulus via the afferent arteriole, and a variable amount of plasma is filtered via endothelial cells, a basement membrane, and podocytes into the tubular space. Blood that is not filtered leaves the glomerulus via the efferent arteriole and subsequently flows through the peritubular vessels to the veins and back to the heart. The amount of plasma that is filtered in the glomerulus over time is the glomerular filtration rate (GFR); the ratio of GFR to renal plasma flow is the filtration fraction. Determinants of GFR are filtration pressure, which depends upon the hydrostatic and oncotic pressure gradients

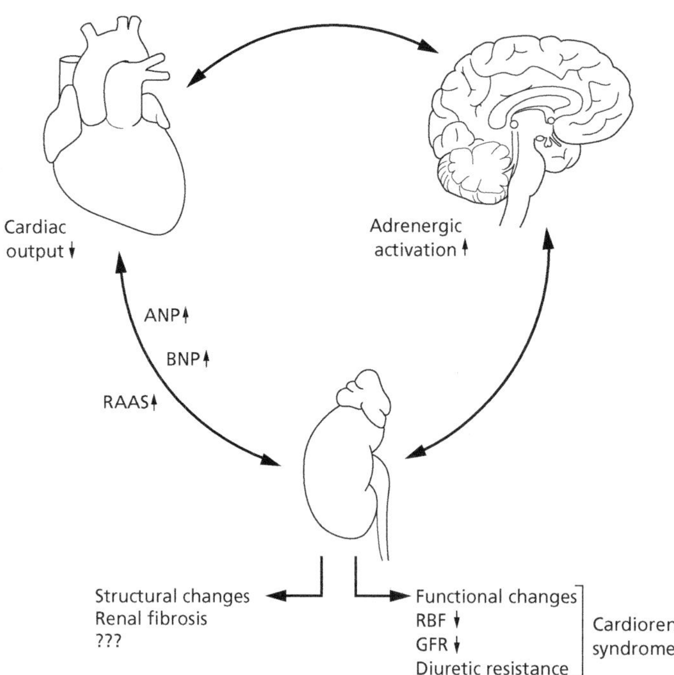

Figure 8.1. *Schematic of heart failure as a multisystem disorder with its specific consequences on renal function and structure. Heart failure and decreased cardiac output result not only in cardiac secretion of atrial natriuretic peptide (ANP) and B-type natriuretic peptide (BNP), but also in activation of the sympathetic nervous system and the renin-angiotensin-aldosterone system (RAAS), which can overwhelm the compensatory capacity of the natriuretic peptide system. Hemodynamic and neurohumoral changes ultimately contribute to the development of the cardiorenal syndrome with decreased renal blood flow and glomerular filtration rate, and diuretic resistance. Structural changes in the kidney that may be associated with the cardiorenal syndrome are not well defined.*

across the membrane, and the coefficient of filtration of the membrane. From the glomerulus, the filtrate flows through the proximal tubule, the loop of Henle, the distal tubule, and the collecting duct. The different sections of the tubule vary in permeabilities for water and solutes. Furthermore, the interstitial environment is different, with the highest osmotic pressures occurring in the renal medulla. An important intrarenal modulator of GFR is the juxtaglomerular apparatus, a structure that connects the distal tubule with the afferent arteriole. An increase in sodium delivery to the dis-

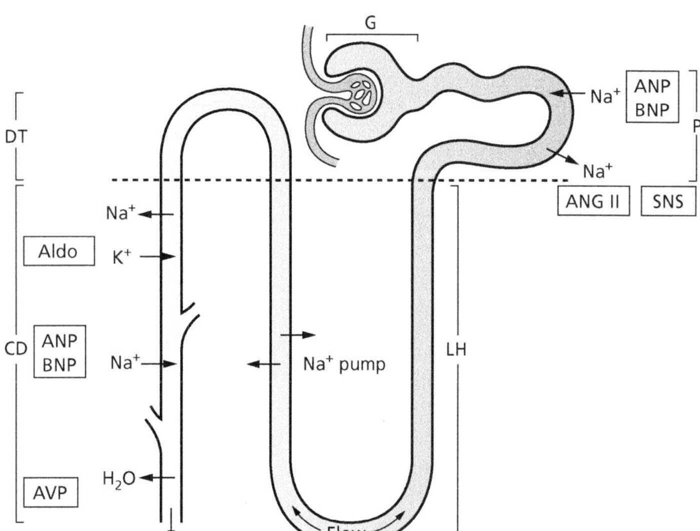

Figure 8.2. *Schematic of a single nephron, the basic functional unit of the kidney, with major sites of physiological regulation (With permission from Costello-Boerrigter et al.*[44]*)*

Abbreviations: Aldo = aldosterone; ANGII = angiotensin II; ANP = atrial natriuretic peptide; AVP = arginine vasopressin; BNP = B-type natriuretic peptide; CD = collecting duct; DT = distal tubule; G = glomerulus; LH = loop of Henle; PT = proximal tubule; SNS = sympathetic nervous system

tal tubule is sensed in the juxtaglomerular apparatus and leads to vasoconstriction of the afferent arteriole, decreasing blood flow into the glomerulus and effective filtration pressure, thus reducing GFR. This feedback mechanism is called tubuloglomerular feedback (TGF). A potential mediator of this feedback is adenosine.[3] It is well recognized that increased sodium delivery to the distal tubule leads to increased activation of adenosine triphosphate (ATP)-dependent ion pumps with a subsequent increase in adenosine. Tubuloglomerular feedback has important implications for the use of diuretic agents. As most conventional diuretics inhibit the tubular reabsorption of sodium and thus increase the tubular sodium concentration, TGF will reduce glomerular filtration and thus limit the efficacy of the diuretic. This may be further complicated by diuretic activation of aldosterone, which enhances sodium reabsorption in the inner medullary collecting duct. Of interest, the cardiac natriuretic peptide, atrial natriuretic peptide (ANP), inhibits TGF in experimental congestive heart failure (CHF), which may, in part, explain some of its renoprotective actions.

Different sections of the nephron display different permeabilities for water and solutes. The tubular cells contain a variety of channels that actively or passively reabsorb or secrete molecules. These channels are controlled by a variety of central nervous and hormonal factors and are a major target for pharmacological intervention. Water reabsorption occurs passively and is primarily a function of tubular permeability as well as osmotic and hydrostatic pressure differences.

The kidney is both a receiver and sender of neural and hormonal signals. Of special interest in heart failure, is the cardiorenal axis (Figure 8.3). If renal perfusion is low, renin is secreted by the kidney. Renin cleaves angiotensinogen to angiotensin I, which in turn is cleaved by the angiotensin-converting enzyme (ACE) to angiotensin II. Angiotensin II promotes vasoconstriction, sodium and water retention, and secretion of the mineralocorticoid aldosterone. In contrast, if the cardiac chambers are stretched, such as in volume overload with increased cardiac filling pressures, the heart secretes ANP and B-type natriuretic peptide (BNP) which promote vasodilation

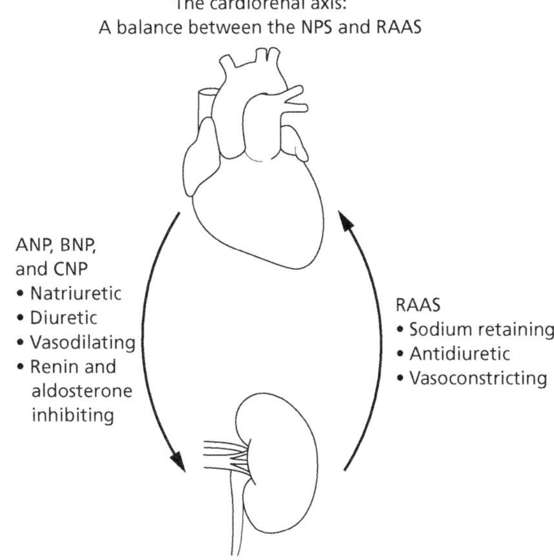

Figure 8.3. *Schematic of the cardiorenal axis*

Abbreviations: *NPS* = *natriuretic peptide system; RAAS* = *renin-angiotensin-aldosteron system*

as well as sodium and water excretion, together with suppression of aldosterone. Cardiac impairment with reduction in blood pressure, decrease in cardiac output, and increase in cardiac filling pressures have important consequences on the entire circulatory system and especially the kidneys. Therefore, we will review the most important compensatory mechanisms as they relate to the kidneys.

Symptomatic Heart Failure: Failure of the Kidneys to Compensate

By mechanisms which are multifactorial and not yet fully understood, the kidneys begin to retain sodium and water in progressive heart failure, thus fundamentally contributing to the evolution from asymptomatic to symptomatic ventricular dysfunction. First, the kidney has a substantial capability for autoregulation, such as keeping renal perfusion pressure constant even as systemic arterial pressure changes. However, in heart failure, these compensatory mechanisms are not enough and the drop in renal perfusion pressure results in a decrease in GFR and renal water and sodium excretion.

A hallmark of overt symptomatic heart failure is a more global activation of various neurohumoral systems, which can be categorized based upon their impact on renal sodium and water handling. Major neurohumoral systems that promote sodium and water reabsorption include the renin-angiotensin-aldosterone system (RAAS), the sympathetic nervous system (SNS), the arginine vasopressin (AVP) system, and the endothelin system. An important promoter of renal sodium and water excretion is the natriuretic peptide system (NPS), with its important components ANP and BNP. Given the importance of electrolyte and volume homeostasis, it is no wonder that there is extensive cross-talk between the heart and the kidney, which can be considered the 'cardiorenal axis.' If arterial baroreceptors signal an arterial underfilling, such as after hemorrhage, sodium- and water-retaining systems are activated to maintain or restore circulating volume and blood pressure.[4] In contrast, under conditions of cardiac overload, the cardiac peptides ANP and BNP are secreted and lead to sodium and water secretion. Under normal physiological conditions, renin and the natriuretic peptides should not be activated simultaneously. However, as heart failure is characterized by low renal perfusion and high cardiac filling pressures, there is simultaneous activation of sodium-retaining and natriuretic systems, resulting in conflicting input to the kidneys. There is evidence that the NPS plays an important role in the compensation of cardiac impairment in the early stages of heart failure.[5] However, with progression of heart failure, the sodium- and water-retaining systems overpower the capacity of the NPS to compensate, and symptoms ensue. Indeed, even diuretic therapy used in severe CHF may, via activation of the RAAS, attenuate the renal response to the natriuretic peptides.

Prognostic Relevance of Renal Dysfunction

Renal dysfunction has emerged as a major prognostic factor for mortality in heart failure in several studies.[1,2,6–8] Hillege *et al.* reported that GFR, estimated by the Cockcroft–Gault equation, was a more powerful independent predictor of mortality than LVEF and functional class (Figure 8.4).[1] Furthermore, Smilde *et al.* reported that estimated GFR was predictive of survival in patients with ischemic and nonischemic chronic heart failure as well as in patients with early heart failure (NYHA class II).[9,10] Gottlieb *et al.* reported that any increase in serum creatinine after hospital admission is predictive of higher mortality and extended hospital stay.[7] As the authors point out, this association suggests, but does not prove, that treatments aimed at maintaining or improving renal function may also improve prognosis. Most recently, Forman *et al.* have underscored the prognostic implications of worsening renal function in patients hospitalized for heart failure with respect

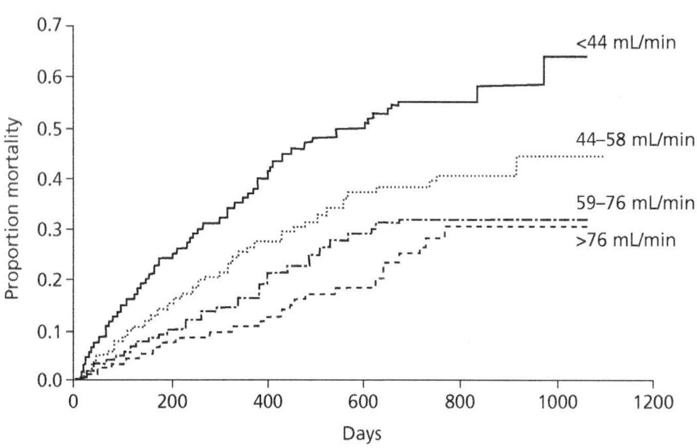

Figure 8.4. *Kaplan–Meier mortality curves for quartiles of glomerular filtration rate as estimated by the Cockcroft–Gault equation. Patients had heart failure (New York Heart Association class III or IV, left ventricular ejection fraction < 35%) and were enrolled in the Second Perspective Randomized study of Ibopamine on Mortality and Efficacy (PRIME-II) trial, which investigated the oral dopamine agonist ibopamine (With permission from Hillege* et al.[1]*)*

to in-hospital mortality, complications (shock, myocardial infarction [MI], stroke, major infections, clinically significant hypotension, and new onset atrial fibrillation with ventricular rates > 100 bpm), and length of stay.[8] This has heightened interest in what has been termed the cardiorenal syndrome (CRS).

Definition of Cardiorenal Syndrome

There are different definitions for the term cardiorenal syndrome. In a broader sense, it can be defined as a syndrome in which either the heart or the kidney fails to compensate for the functional impairment of the other organ, resulting in a vicious cycle that will ultimately lead to decompensation of the entire circulatory system. In a narrower sense, CRS can be defined as worsening renal function in patients hospitalized for heart failure who may be resistant to diuretics. Indeed, this population, which is at risk for worsening renal function while hospitalized, can be predicted by: (1) a history of heart failure or diabetes mellitus; (2) admission serum creatinine ≥ 1.5 mg/dL; and (3) systolic blood pressure >160 mm Hg.[8] Butler *et al.* performed a nested case-control study with 382 subjects who were hospitalized with heart failure, half of whom demonstrated worsening renal function, defined as a rise in serum creatinine of > 26.5 μmol/L (0.3 mg/dL). They found that, in addition to the factors mentioned above, the use of calcium channel blockers (25% vs. 10%) and the loop diuretic dose (199 ± 195 mg vs. 143 ± 119 mg) were higher in patients with worsening renal function.[11] As the authors conclude, further investigations are necessary to determine whether the use of calcium channel blockers or higher doses of loop diuretics are responsible for the decline in renal function or whether they are markers of higher risk.

Strategies for Targeting Cardiorenal Syndrome in Heart Failure Patients

There are not yet many studies on which to base treatment recommendations for CRS. Indeed, many heart failure trials exclude patients with reduced renal function. We will review potential strategies that could target the CRS in decompensated heart failure. Our focus will be on the most common forms of heart failure—ischemic and idiopathic. Other forms of heart failure, such as hypertrophic obstructive cardiomyopathy and valvular disease, may require quite different therapeutic approaches. Indeed, a high priority should be given to therapies that are able to improve cardiac function by directly targeting underlying cardiac disease. These interventions should also lead indirectly, via hemodynamic improvements, to an augmentation of renal function. As these strategies do not specifically target the kidney they are not discussed any further.

Conventional strategies for targeting cardiorenal syndrome in heart failure patients

Diuretics

Diuretics are used in heart failure to restore sodium and fluid homeostasis. Volume overload increases cardiac preload and afterload and can lead to further cardiac decompensation. Conversely, volume depletion should be avoided as it can lead to hypotension and impair cardiac function.

For many years, diuretics have been a mainstay in the treatment of heart failure and volume overload. In fact, when ACE inhibitors, beta-blockers, and aldosterone antagonists were evaluated in heart failure clinical trials, they were typically added on top of diuretic therapy. While symptomatic benefit of diuretic therapy is undeniable, there are no studies evaluating long-term morbidity and mortality with this pharmacological class.

Most of the conventional diuretics are saluretics; they actively inhibit the reabsorption of solutes while water excretion follows passively. In addition to the TGF mechanism, there are several characteristics of diuretics that are important in understanding how diuretic resistance (which some call the cardiorenal syndrome) develops and how to counter it.[12,13]

First, most diuretics have to be secreted into the tubular fluid to reach their site of action, which is the luminal side of the tubular cells. Thus, in renal insufficiency, the dose frequently has to be higher to achieve effective concentrations in the tubular fluid. Second, loop diuretics have a relatively short duration of action. When the tubular concentration declines, a period of sodium retention typically ensues, often termed post-diuretic sodium retention. This phenomenon can be countered by more frequent administrations or by continuous drug infusion. Third, different classes of diuretics inhibit different transport channels, which predominate at different sites along the nephron. Hence, some segments of the nephron will be sensitive to a specific diuretic while other nephron segments will be insensitive. The use of a loop diuretic increases sodium delivery to more distal nephron segments, which avidly reabsorb the sodium as they are insensitive to the loop diuretic. This not only counteracts the desired diuretic effect, it can lead to structural alterations such as hypertrophy and hyperplasia in distal nephron segments.[12] A combination of different classes of diuretics, specifically loop diuretics and thiazides, can increase the diuretic effect and overcome diuretic resistance in many cases; this is known as sequential nephron blockade. Fourth, diuretic-induced neurohumoral activation can counter the diuretic effect by decreasing GFR and promoting sodium and water reabsorption.

Loop diuretics

Loop diuretics are the most powerful saluretic agents, and their major site of action is the ascending limb of the loop of Henle. An appropriate dose must be determined for each patient, which will be higher in the presence of renal insufficiency. Loop diuretics have a relatively short half-life (a few hours) leading to post-diuretic sodium retention, and their action can be offset by increased sodium reabsorption in more distal nephron segments. More frequent administrations or continuous intravenous infusions can remedy the first problem, while the addition of a thiazide diuretic can remedy the second.

While loop diuretics can be very effective in patients with decompensated heart failure, the chronic administration of furosemide in a pig model of pacing-induced heart failure significantly accelerated the development of contractile and metabolic features of heart failure.[14] Furthermore, we have documented in human heart failure the decrease in GFR in response to acute furosemide, which can be attenuated with an angiotensin receptor antagonist.[15] Further studies have demonstrated other deleterious actions of furosemide on the kidney.[16] One could speculate that excessive loop diuretic therapy in patients with the CRS may actually contribute to the decline in renal function.

Thiazide and thiazide-like diuretics

Thiazides are less powerful saluretics than the loop diuretics and are generally associated with more potassium depletion for the same amount of diuresis. They act primarily on the distal convoluted tubule, but can also decrease reabsorption in the proximal tubule by inhibiting carbonic anhydrase. As monotherapy, they are generally ineffective if the GFR is below 30 mL/min. However, loop diuretics can lead to increased sodium reabsorption and tubular hypertrophy in more distal nephron segments. In this situation, the addition of a thiazide to a loop diuretic can induce a powerful diuresis. Dosing should be carefully monitored and electrolyte depletion must be avoided.

New therapeutic strategies

B-type natriuretic peptide

In 2001, nesiritide, a recombinant form of BNP, was the first new drug in 14 years to be approved in the United States for the treatment of patients hospitalized with heart failure. It is a balanced vasodilator but as it suppresses the SNS, this does not lead to tachycardia. In heart failure, there appears to be a resistance to endogenous BNP levels, which can be overridden by the administration of exogenous BNP. BNP is unique in that it has a variety of beneficial actions. It reduces cardiac preload by venodilation and natriuretic actions and decreases cardiac afterload by vasodilation. It is lusitropic, and it suppresses the SNS as well as renin and aldosterone secretion.[17–19] BNP is more effective than nitroglycerin in reducing pulmonary capillary wedge pressure (PCWP).[20,21] While BNP is a less powerful diuretic in heart failure than loop diuretics, it inhibits TGF and can enhance renal function, especially in combination with conventional diuretics.[22,23] Furthermore, in a subgroup analysis of patients with renal insufficiency (serum creatinine ≥ 2 mg/dL), nesiritide appeared to be safe and have similar beneficial actions as in patients without renal insufficiency.[24] In a different trial, patients who received BNP needed less diuretic than patients treated with standard therapy.[17] Similarly, BNP in experimental heart failure potentiated the diuretic effect of furosemide while at the same time preventing a furosemide-induced increase in plasma aldosterone (Figure 8.5).[23] However, in a small cross-over study (n = 15) specifically targeting patients with deteriorating renal function, nesiritide did not improve renal function (urinary sodium excretion, urine flow, GFR, or effective renal plasma flow) as compared to placebo.[25] A possible explanation is that the dose of the nesiritide infusion (0.01 μg/kg/min) was too low to overcome the renal resistance to nesiritide. Furthermore, the lack of a renal response contrasts with the beneficial hemodynamic effects in patients with renal dysfunction.[24] As the natriuretic peptide degrading enzyme, neutral endopeptidase (NEP) is especially abundant in the proximal tubule in the kidney, additional NEP inhibition might enhance the renal actions of exogenous BNP. While BNP is one of the most interesting recent additions to the pharmacological armamentarium of heart failure therapy, further studies are clearly needed to determine which patients are most likely to benefit from it and under what conditions.

While BNP was approved in the United States in 2001, ANP (carperitide) was approved for the treatment of acute decompensated heart failure (ADHF) in Japan in 1995.[26,27] Sward *et al.* reported that ANP enhanced renal excretory function, decreased the probability of dialysis, and improved dialysis-free survival in early, ischemic acute renal dysfunction after complicated cardiac surgery.[28] It remains to be established which natriuretic peptide has the best pharmacodynamic and pharmacokinetic profile for heart failure. Indeed, other naturally occurring natriuretic peptides or designer peptides may turn out to be best. Furthermore, chronic administration of BNP, in the form of chronic subcutaneous injection[29] or intermittent intravenous infusion on an outpatient basis,[30] are potential new strategies.

Vasopressin antagonists

Arginine vasopressin (AVP) is one of the various neurohormones activated in heart failure. AVP is vasoconstrictive via V_1a receptors and promotes free water reabsorption in the renal collecting duct

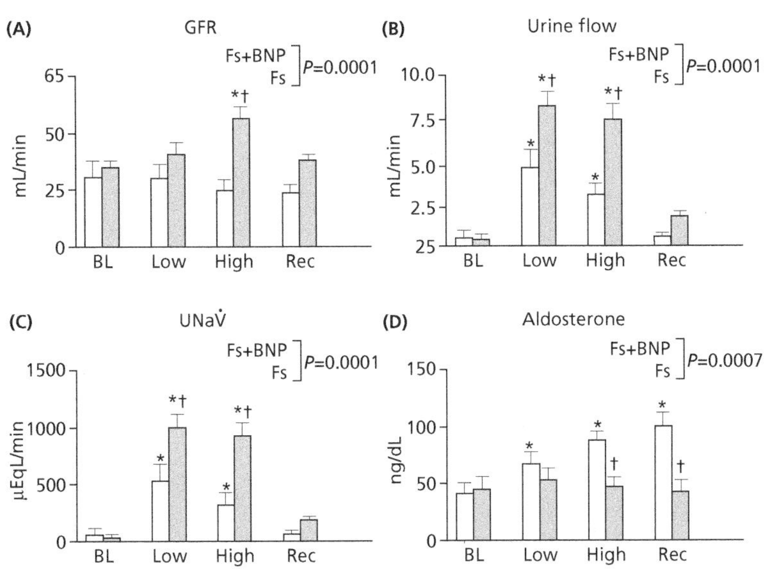

Figure 8.5. *Effect of furosemide with or without B-type natriuretic peptide (BNP) on renal function and plasma aldosterone levels. (A) glomerular filtration rate, (B) urine flow, (C) urinary sodium excretion, and (D) plasma aldosterone. Open bars: Furosemide group; closed bars: Furosemide + BNP group (with permission from Cataliotti* et al.[23]*)*

Abbreviations: BL = Baseline; Low = low-dose (2 pmol/kg/min) BNP + furosemide (1 mg/kg/h); High = high-dose (10 pmol/kg/min) BNP plus furosemide (1 mg/kg/h); Rec = recovery.

*$P < 0.005$ vs. BL

†$P < 0.001$ vs. furosemide

via V2 receptors, the activation of which induces the translocation of the water channel aquaporin-2 into the apical membrane. Both selective V2 antagonists, as well as dual V_1a/V_2 antagonists, are currently in clinical development.[31,32] While most of the conventional diuretics are saluretics, V2 receptor blockers act essentially as aquaretics; they promote free water excretion without (or with less) electrolyte loss.[33] This could be especially useful in patients with hyponatremia, a condition that limits the efficacy of conventional diuretics. In the Acute and Chronic Therapeutic Impact of a Vasopressin Antagonist in Congestive Heart Failure (ACTIV in CHF) trial (n = 319), the V_2 receptor antagonist tolvaptan resulted in a larger weight reduction at discharge in patients admitted to the hospital with ADHF.[34] During a 60-day follow-up period, tolvaptan treatment tended to improve mortality, which was significant in the subgroup with hyponatremia, renal dysfunction, or peripheral edema.

Adenosine antagonists

Adenosine is crucially involved in renal regulation, including the mechanism of TGF.[3] Lucas *et al.* reported that the selective A1 adenosine antagonist, BG9719, increased GFR, urine flow, and urinary sodium excretion in a pig model of pacing induced heart failure.[35] In addition, BG9719 increased diuresis when added to furosemide, and prevented the furosemide-induced decline in GFR in patients with heart failure (Figure 8.6).[36]

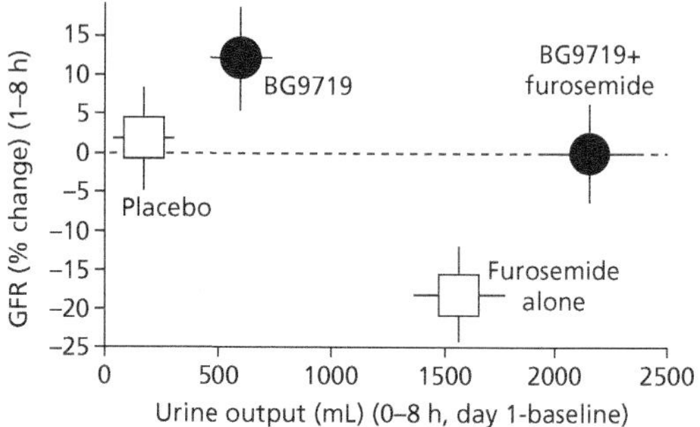

Figure 8.6. *Relationship between change in urine output and change in GFR for patients receiving the A1 adenosine receptor antagonist BG9719, which increased urine output when given with or without furosemide. The decrease in glomerular filtration rate with furosemide alone was not seen when BG9719 was given (With permission from Gottlieb* et al.[45])

Neutral endopeptidase inhibitors and vasopeptidase inhibitors

The natriuretic peptides are cleared from the circulation by either receptor binding, including a natriuretic peptide clearance receptor, or enzymatic degradation by neutral endopeptidase 24.11 (NEP). NEP inhibitors have been developed and they should increase the bioactivity of endogenous natriuretic peptides. It remains to be determined whether they are beneficial in the CRS or if they can reduce the dosing of exogenous BNP. The same is true for vasopeptidase inhibitors, which are molecules that simultaneously inhibit ACE and NEP. In the Inhibition of Metallo Protease by BMS-186716 in a Randomized Exercise and Symptoms Study in Subjects With Heart Failure (IMPRESS) trial (n = 573), the vasopeptidase inhibitor omapatrilat was superior to ACE inhibition with lisinopril in reducing the composite endpoint of death, admission, or discontinuation of study treatment for worsening heart failure.[37] The Omapatrilat versus Enalapril Randomized Trial of Utility in Reducing Events (OVERTURE) trial (n = 5770) compared omapatrilat with the ACE inhibitor enalapril in patients with heart failure.[38] Equal efficacy, related to the reduction of death or hospitalization for heart failure, was reported. Employing the endpoint criteria of the Studies of Left Ventricular Dysfunction (SOLVD) trial,[39] omapatrilat was associated with a statistically significant improvement compared to enalapril. It will be especially interesting to see whether these compounds can delay the progression of heart failure in earlier stages of the disease by enhancing the NPS and renal function. A potential problem with NEP inhibition is that NEP also degrades other hormones, such as the potent vasoconstrictor endothelin, which could offset some of the beneficial actions of natriuretic peptide enhancement.

Endothelin antagonists and endothelin-converting enzyme/neutral endopeptidase inhibitors

Endothelin-1 (ET-1) is a peptide hormone primarily secreted from endothelial cells, and it is the most potent endogenous vasoconstrictor known in humans so far. Given the beneficial effects of antagonizing other vasoconstricting systems in heart failure, antagonizing the endothelin system appeared to be a promising strategy. However, the results of chronic studies with endothelin antagonists in heart failure have been disappointing so far, with some studies suggesting increased sodium and water retention.[40] It remains to be determined whether short-term ET-blockade in ADHF is beneficial.[41]

Given that a potential problem of NEP inhibition is the simultaneous inhibition of endothelin degradation, while ET-antagonism has been associated with sodium and water retention, combined endothelin-converting enzyme (ECE)-NEP inhibitors could offer the benefits of both strategies while simultaneously counteracting the negative effects. Indeed, Mulder *et al.* reported that combined ECE-NEP inhibition improved LV dimensions, end-diastolic pressure, fractional shortening, and cardiac output compared to placebo and NEP inhibition alone.[42] Furthermore, Dickstein *et al.* reported that in heart failure patients, ECE-NEP inhibition increased ANP and BNP, and decreased cardiac filling pressures.[43]

Conclusion

In conclusion, the CRS has become an important focus of research in heart failure and it remains a very high priority and challenge for the practicing clinician. Several potential new therapeutic strategies for treating this serious disorder have emerged, which have to be evaluated in prospective clinical trials. If successful, we can expect some important changes in the management of heart failure in the future. As presumably the best way to deal with the CRS is to prevent it, additional studies should specifically investigate the impact of chronic therapeutic strategies on renal function.

References

1. Hillege HL, Girbes AR, de Kam PJ, *et al.* Renal function, neurohormonal activation, and survival in patients with chronic heart failure. Circulation 2000; 102: 203–210.
2. Dries DL, Exner DV, Domanski MJ, Greenberg B, Stevenson LW. The prognostic implications of renal insufficiency in asymptomatic and symptomatic patients with left ventricular systolic dysfunction. J Am Coll Cardiol 2000; 35: 681–689.
3. Thomson S, Bao D, Deng A, Vallon V. Adenosine formed by 5′-nucleotidase mediates tubuloglomerular feedback. J Clin Invest 2000; 106: 289–298.
4. Schrier RW, Abraham WT. Hormones and hemodynamics in heart failure. N Engl J Med 1999; 341: 577–585.
5. Stevens TL, Burnett JC Jr., Kinoshita M, Matsuda Y, Redfield MM. A functional role for endogenous atrial natriuretic peptide in a canine model of early left ventricular dysfunction. J Clin Invest 1995; 95: 1101–1108.
6. Krumholz HM, Chen YT, Vaccarino V, *et al.* Correlates and impact on outcomes of worsening renal function in patients > or = 65 years of age with heart failure. Am J Cardiol 2000; 85: 1110–1113.
7. Gottlieb SS, Abraham W, Butler J, *et al.* The prognostic importance of different definitions of worsening renal function in congestive heart failure. J Card Fail 2002; 8: 136–141.
8. Forman DE, Butler J, Wang Y, *et al.* Incidence, predictors at admission, and impact of worsening renal function among patients hospitalized with heart failure. J Am Coll Cardiol 2004; 43: 61–67.
9. Smilde TD, Hillege HL, Navis G, *et al.* Impaired renal function in patients with ischemic and nonischemic chronic heart failure: association with neurohormonal activation and survival. Am Heart J 2004; 148: 165–172.
10. Smilde TD, Hillege HL, Voors AA, Dunselman PH, van Veldhuisen DJ. Prognostic importance of renal function in patients with early heart failure and mild left ventricular dysfunction. Am J Cardiol 2004; 94: 240–243.
11. Butler J, Forman DE, Abraham WT, *et al.* Relationship between heart failure treatment and development of worsening renal function among hospitalized patients. Am Heart J 2004; 147: 331–338.
12. Reilly RF, Ellison DH. Mammalian distal tubule: physiology, pathophysiology, and molecular anatomy. Physiol Rev 2000; 80: 277–313.
13. Ellison DH. Diuretic therapy and resistance in congestive heart failure. Cardiology 2001; 96: 132–143.
14. McCurley JM, Hanlon SU, Wei SK, *et al.* Furosemide and the progression of left ventricular dysfunction in experimental heart failure. J Am Coll Cardiol 2004; 44: 1301–1307.

15. Chen HH, Redfield MM, Nordstrom LJ, Cataliotti A, Burnett JC Jr. Angiotensin II AT1 receptor antagonism prevents detrimental renal actions of acute diuretic therapy in human heart failure. Am J Physiol Renal Physiol 2003; 284: F1115–F1119.
16. Burnett JCJ, Costello-Boerrigter LC, Boerrigter G. Alterations in the kidney in heart failure: the cardiorenal axis in the regulation of sodium homeostasis. In: Mann DL (ed.) Heart Failure: A Companion to Braunwald's Heart Disease (W. B. Saunders: Philadelphia, PA, 2004), 279–289.
17. Colucci WS, Elkayam U, Horton DP, *et al.* Intravenous nesiritide, a natriuretic peptide, in the treatment of decompensated congestive heart failure. Nesiritide Study Group. N Engl J Med 2000; 343: 246–253.
18. Yamamoto K, Burnett JC Jr., Redfield MM. Effect of endogenous natriuretic peptide system on ventricular and coronary function in failing heart. Am J Physiol 1997; 273: H2406–H2414.
19. Brunner-La Rocca HP, Kaye DM, Woods RL, Hastings J, Esler MD. Effects of intravenous brain natriuretic peptide on regional sympathetic activity in patients with chronic heart failure as compared with healthy control subjects. J Am Coll Cardiol 2001; 37: 1221–1227.
20. Publication Committee for the VMAC Investigators (Vasodilation in the Management of Acute Heart CHF). Intravenous nesiritide vs nitroglycerin for treatment of decompensated congestive heart failure: a randomized controlled trial. JAMA 2002; 287: 1531–1540.
21. Elkayam U, Akhter MW, Singh H, Khan S, Usman A. Comparison of effects on left ventricular filling pressure of intravenous nesiritide and high-dose nitroglycerin in patients with decompensated heart failure. Am J Cardiol 2004; 93: 237–240.
22. Akabane S, Matsushima Y, Matsuo H, *et al.* Effects of brain natriuretic peptide on renin secretion in normal and hypertonic saline-infused kidney. Eur J Pharmacol 1991; 198: 143–148.
23. Cataliotti A, Boerrigter G, Costello-Boerrigter LC, *et al.* Brain natriuretic peptide enhances renal actions of furosemide and suppresses furosemide-induced aldosterone activation in experimental heart failure. Circulation 2004; 109: 1680–1685.
24. Butler J, Emerman C, Peacock WF, Mathur VS, Young JB, VMAC study investigators. The efficacy and safety of B-type natriuretic peptide (nesiritide) in patients with renal insufficiency and acutely decompensated congestive heart failure. Nephrol Dial Transplant 2004; 19: 391–399.
25. Wang DJ, Dowling TC, Meadows D, *et al.* Nesiritide does not improve renal function in patients with chronic heart failure and worsening serum creatinine. Circulation 2004; 110: 1620–1625.
26. Mizuno O, Onishi K, Dohi K, *et al.* Effects of therapeutic doses of human atrial natriuretic peptide on load and myocardial performance in patients with congestive heart failure. Am J Cardiol 2001; 88: 863–866.
27. Kikuchi M, Nakamura M, Suzuki T, *et al.* Usefulness of carperitide for the treatment of refractory heart failure due to severe acute myocardial infarction. Jpn Heart J 2001; 42: 271–280.
28. Sward K, Valsson F, Odencrants P, Samuelsson O, Ricksten SE. Recombinant human atrial natriuretic peptide in ischemic acute renal failure: a randomized placebo-controlled trial. Crit Care Med 2004; 32: 1310–1315.
29. Chen HH, Redfield MM, Nordstrom LJ, Horton DP, Burnett JC Jr. Subcutaneous administration of the cardiac hormone BNP in symptomatic human heart failure. J Card Fail 2004; 10: 115–119.
30. Yancy CW, Saltzberg MT, Berkowitz RL, *et al.* Safety and feasibility of using serial infusions of nesiritide for heart failure in an outpatient setting (from the FUSION I trial). Am J Cardiol 2004; 94: 595–601.
31. Gheorghiade M, Niazi I, Ouyang J, *et al.*, Tolvaptan Investigators. Vasopressin V2-receptor blockade with tolvaptan in patients with chronic heart failure: results from a double-blind, randomized trial. Circulation 2003; 107: 2690–2696.
32. Udelson JE, Smith WB, Hendrix GH, *et al.* Acute hemodynamic effects of conivaptan, a dual V(1A) and V(2) vasopressin receptor antagonist, in patients with advanced heart failure. Circulation 2001; 104: 2417–2423.
33. Burnett JC, Costello-Boerrigter LC, Smith WB, *et al.* Tolvaptan (OPC-41061), a V2 vasopressin receptor antagonist, protects against the decline in renal function observed with loop diuretic therapy. Circulation 2003; 108: 1841A (Abstract).
34. Gheorghiade M, Gattis WA, O'Connor CM, *et al.* Effects of tolvaptan, a vasopressin antagonist, in patients hospitalized with worsening heart failure: a randomized controlled trial. JAMA 2004; 291: 1963–1971.
35. Lucas DG Jr., Hendrick JW, Sample JA, *et al.* Cardiorenal effects of adenosine subtype 1 (A1) receptor inhibition in an experimental model of heart failure. J Am Coll Surg 2002; 194: 603–609.
36. Gottlieb SS, Brater DC, Thomas I, *et al.* BG9719 (CVT-124), an A1 adenosine receptor antagonist,

protects against the decline in renal function observed with diuretic therapy. Circulation 2002; 105: 1348–1353.

37. Rouleau JL, Pfeffer MA, Stewart DJ, *et al.* Comparison of vasopeptidase inhibitor, omapatrilat, and lisinopril on exercise tolerance and morbidity in patients with heart failure: IMPRESS randomised trial. Lancet 2000; 356: 615–620.
38. Packer M, Califf RM, Konstam MA, *et al.* Comparison of omapatrilat and enalapril in patients with chronic heart failure: the Omapatrilat Versus Enalapril Randomized Trial of Utility in Reducing Events (OVERTURE). Circulation 2002; 106: 920–926.
39. The SOLVD Investigators. Effect of enalapril on survival in patients with reduced left ventricular ejection fractions and congestive heart failure. N Engl J Med 1991; 325: 293–302.
40. Boerrigter G, Burnett JC. Endothelin in neurohormonal activation in heart failure. Coron Artery Dis 2003; 14: 495–500.
41. Torre-Amione G, Young JB, Colucci WS, *et al.* Hemodynamic and clinical effects of tezosentan, an intravenous dual endothelin receptor antagonist, in patients hospitalized for acute decompensated heart failure. J Am Coll Cardiol 2003; 42: 140–147.
42. Mulder P, Barbier S, Monteil C, *et al.* Sustained improvement of cardiac function and prevention of cardiac remodeling after long-term dual ECE-NEP inhibition in rats with congestive heart failure. J Cardiovasc Pharmacol 2004; 43: 489–494.
43. Dickstein K, De Voogd HJ, Miric MP, *et al.* Effect of single doses of SLV306, an inhibitor of both neutral endopeptidase and endothelin-converting enzyme, on pulmonary pressures in congestive heart failure. Am J Cardiol 2004; 94: 237–239.
44. Costello-Boerrigter LC, Boerrigter G, Burnett JC Jr. Revisiting salt and water retention: new diuretics, aquaretics, and natriuretics. Med Clin North Am 2003; 87: 475–491.
45. Gottlieb SS, Brater DC, Thomas I, *et al.* BG9719 (CVT-124), an A1 adenosine receptor antagonist, protects against the decline in renal function observed with diuretic therapy. Circulation 2002; 105: 1348–1353.

Part II

Diagnosis and Evaluations of the Acute Heart Failure Patient

CHAPTER 9

Evaluation of the acute heart failure patient: assessment of dyspnea and other physical examination parameters

John R Teerlink, Mark H Drazner

Introduction

One million patients are hospitalized each year in the United States with heart failure as the primary diagnosis and an additional 2 million patients are treated for heart failure as a secondary diagnosis during their hospitalization. The rapid and accurate assessment of these patients is critical to providing appropriate therapy. The history and physical examination, which may elicit the symptoms and signs crucial to diagnosis, are the first steps in this assessment. However, there has been limited research into the evaluation of the symptoms and signs of these patients. The aim of this chapter is to review the role of the history and physical examination in the care of the patient with acute decompensated heart failure (ADHF) and to briefly discuss the role that symptom assessments can play in clinical trials of new therapies for this indication.

Symptoms in Patients Presenting with Acute Decompensated Heart Failure

Until recently, most research in heart failure has focused on chronic heart failure and outpatient therapies, and while many studies of heart failure admissions have been performed, few contemporary reports have included extensive descriptions of the presenting symptoms. However, a consistent picture emerges from two large observational heart failure studies, ADHERE™ and EuroHeart Failure Survey, and a number of smaller investigations. A list of the more common presenting symptoms is provided in Table 9.1.

The Acute Decompensated Heart Failure National Registry (ADHERE™)[1] is an industry-sponsored, large, national, observational, multicenter study of the characteristics, patterns of care, and outcomes of patients hospitalized with ADHF. As of July 2003, 263 representative hospitals from across the United States—including large and small, as well as academic and community, sites—have enrolled patients who were admitted to an acute care hospital and had a discharge diagnosis of heart failure. In the most recent 12-month report,[2] the results from 58 919 discharges are presented, demonstrating that 89% of patients presented with dyspnea, 36% with dyspnea at rest, and 32% presented with fatigue. Information regarding other symptoms is not available in the report, and hopefully more complete details will be described in upcoming publications, but the report clearly establishes the primacy of dyspnea as a presenting symptom in these patients.

The EuroHeart Failure survey[3] screened all patients admitted to 115 participating centers in 24 European Society of Cardiology member countries over a 6-week period in 2000 to 2001, and included

Table 9.1. *Common presenting symptoms of decompensated heart failure*

Dyspnea (exertional, paroxysmal nocturnal dyspnea, orthopnea, dyspnea at rest, or florid pulmonary edema)
Cough
Wheezing
Foot and leg discomfort
Abdominal discomfort
Increased abdominal girth
Bloating
Early satiety or anorexia
Right upper quadrant pain or discomfort
Increased body weight
Fatigue
Depression
Altered mental status, confusion, or difficulty concentrating
Daytime drowsiness
Sleep disturbances
Palpitations
Dizziness, pre-syncope, or syncope

all patients with a diagnosis of heart failure during the index admission, previous diagnosis of heart failure, or treatment for heart failure or major ventricular dysfunction within 24 hours of death or discharge. There were 46 788 deaths or discharges screened, from which 11 327 patients were enrolled with heart failure. The mean age of these patients was > 70 years, about half of whom were women, and heart failure was the primary reason for admission in 40%. The most common presenting symptom was acute breathlessness, reported in almost 40% of the patients, while other manifestations of heart failure, such as increasing edema or exertional breathlessness, were present in 35%. Thus, in this large survey of patients, dyspnea and symptoms related to fluid overload predominated. However, almost one-fifth of the patients presented with acute coronary syndrome and almost 10% presented with rapid atrial fibrillation, reinforcing the need to elicit pertinent historical factors relating to these diagnoses.

Several other smaller studies have confirmed the predominance of dyspnea in patients with ADHF. In a single-center study of 282 consecutively admitted heart failure patients,[4] 98% of the patients presented with dyspnea on exertion, 86% with orthopnea, 72% with paroxysmal nocturnal dyspnea (PND), 41% with dyspnea at rest, and 8% with angina. In another single-center study of 181 patients admitted for heart failure,[5] 91% had dyspnea, while 35% reported having peripheral edema, and 33% reported a cough. Another small single-center study,[6] noted that of the 87 patients admitted with a diagnosis of heart failure, 98% presented with dyspnea, 25% with dyspnea at rest, 77% reported edema, 69% cough, and 41% weight gain. Although dyspnea is clearly the predominant symptom in these patients, the extent that ascertainment and methodologic biases influenced these results is unclear.

In addition to defining the prevalence of symptoms in ADHF patients, other studies have also addressed the question of whether there are differences in presenting symptoms between patients with preserved and reduced left ventricular (LV) systolic function. The ADHERE™ registry reports no difference in the proportion of patients with either preserved (LVEF ≥ 40%) or reduced (LVEF < 40%) LV function who present with dyspnea at rest (~ 40%). Two studies of 187[7] and 30[8] patients consecutively admitted for heart failure found no difference in the presenting symptoms between patients with reduced LV function (LVEF < 50%) and those with preserved LV function. A study of 225 patients[4] also demonstrated no significant difference in most symptoms related to dyspnea between patients with normal systolic function as compared to decreased systolic function, although patients with decreased systolic function reported angina more frequently. While the symptoms may be similar, there is evidence from a number of trials that severity is greater in patients with reduced LV function. In a study of 229 patients with heart failure,[9] 75% of the patients with reduced LV function were NYHA class IV, compared to 64% of the patients with preserved LV function; while another study reported that dyspnea was more severe in patients with reduced LV function.[10] A recent investigation[11] has reported greater reductions in quality of life in patients with reduced LV function, as measured by the SF-36® Health Survey and the Minnesota Living with Heart Failure Questionnaire (MLWHFQ). Thus, presenting symptoms do not appear to differ significantly between patients with preserved and reduced LV function, with the possible exception of angina, but symptoms do appear to be more severe in patients with reduced LV function.

Symptoms related to pulmonary congestion

As noted above, dyspnea is the most common presenting symptom in patients with ADHF, occurring in approximately 90% of the patients admitted for heart failure. Most of the literature on dyspnea is from pulmonary and critical care specialists. The American Thoracic Society has produced a consensus statement on the mechanisms, assessment, and management of dyspnea.[12] This group has defined dyspnea as "a term used to characterize a subjective experience of breathing discomfort that consists of qualitatively distinct sensations that vary in intensity." Unfortunately, this definition is very broad and of limited use in the clinical setting. Although it is an extremely prevalent acute and chronic symptom, the pathophysiology of dyspnea[13] is complex and poorly understood. This derives from the poor understanding of the neural pathways that mediate the sensation and the variety of disease states that appear to precipitate the symptom. The current prevailing theory posits that the symptom of dyspnea is the result of a perceived mismatch or dissociation between central respiratory motor activity and incoming afferent signals from receptors in the airways, lungs, and chest wall structures. In chronic heart failure, increased pulmonary capillary wedge pressure (PCWP) and decreased cardiac output contribute to this symptom, but it is clear that these are not the sole mechanisms.[14–17] Engorgement of pulmonary venous vasculature, interstitium, and lymphatics, as well as increased airway resistance and frank alveolar edema, interact with alterations in chest and skeletal musculature[18,19] and peripheral circulation to contribute to the sensation of dyspnea. As a subjective symptom, dyspnea presents in many ways, ranging from dyspnea on exertion to severe pulmonary edema.

Dyspnea on exertion[20] is a symptom that can be experienced by normal subjects,[21] but becomes clinically important when it occurs at an unexpectedly, or unacceptably, low workload. It is often the first type of dyspnea to be noted and can be an important early warning in gradually developing decompensation. While ADHF is a frequent cause, other etiologies must be considered, including reactive airway disease or other pulmonary disease, obesity or physical deconditioning, peripheral vascular disease, or anemia. Most importantly, dyspnea on exertion may represent an anginal equivalent, with ischemia inducing diastolic dysfunction and/or systolic LV dysfunction, or mitral regurgitation (MR) due to papillary muscle dysfunction or transient ventricular dilation. In addition to determining the underlying etiology, the workload under which the dyspnea occurs and the time course of the deterioration are important characteristics to elicit, particularly if reliable serial information is available.

Along with others,[22] we have noted that immediate dyspnea on light exertion (such as with dressing or brushing teeth) seems to be associated more frequently with markedly elevated LV filling pressures, while dyspnea at higher workloads may be the result of multiple abnormalities.

Other forms of dyspnea may precipitate presentation to the emergency room or acute care center. PND may occur in patients with severe heart failure, usually manifest by abrupt awakening about 1 to 2 hours after going to bed due to acute dyspnea which is relieved by sitting or getting up. A similar form of severe dyspnea is orthopnea, where the patient experiences dyspnea while in the recumbent position and finds relief only by elevating the thorax with extra pillows. Quantification of orthopnea is often measured in the number of pillows or the angle at which the patient sleeps. Both forms of dyspnea are felt to be related to increased venous return from the periphery in recumbency with consequent elevation of LV filing pressures. Finally, dyspnea at rest can be a prominent expression of severe pulmonary disease, but it may also represent severe heart failure.

Other symptoms related to pulmonary vascular congestion include cough, wheezing, and sleep disturbances. As noted previously, cough was noted to be present in 69% of patients with acute heart failure (AHF) in one study,[6] and although it is a frequent symptom in pulmonary disease, cough can occur in heart failure patients after exertion or with recumbency. Of note, cough due to pulmonary disease is often productive and leads to dyspnea, while in heart failure patients, dyspnea often precedes a nonproductive cough. Wheezing, or cardiac asthma, is another dyspnea equivalent and is often indistinguishable from reactive airway disease based on pulmonary physical examination findings. Other findings, such as a history of asthma or heart failure, or physical examination findings, such as elevated neck veins, peripheral edema or an S_3, will assist in the differentiation of the causes for the wheezing. Many different forms of sleep disturbances are present in patients with heart failure. AHF can result in frequent awakening from orthopnea or PND, as well as exacerbations of other forms of chronic sleep disorders.

Symptoms related to systemic venous congestion

Patients may also present with symptoms related to systemic venous congestion, including edema, weight gain, increasing abdominal girth, and discomfort. Although most practicing clinicians have been surprised by the degree of peripheral edema patients can ignore, eventually an inability to put on shoes, the development of skin breakdown or pain from taught edema will induce the most reticent patients to seek medical care. Chronic heart failure patients are usually instructed to carefully monitor their daily weights and adjust their diuretic regimen accordingly, but weight gain can still be a frequent presenting complaint in new onset, noncompliant, or deteriorating patients. Significant edema can occur centrally, so reports of abdominal discomfort and increasing abdominal girth may represent decompensation. The abdominal discomfort may be described as early satiety, a sense of bloating or fullness, diffuse nondescript aching, or even right upper quadrant pain (due to liver congestion). Inquiring about changes in belt size, or observation of the belt, can provide clues to the extent and rapidity of onset of the increased bowel edema and ascites.

Other symptoms of acute decompensated heart failure

Patients with ADHF may also present with other symptoms distinct from those caused by volume overload, including fatigue, depression, altered mental status, and sleep disorders. It is unclear how frequent these symptoms may be, given that they are often not recognized as being related to heart failure and are often not specifically elicited.

Fatigue is a common complaint in patients with chronic heart failure, but it can also be a frequent symptom in ADHF. Despite likely underreporting, almost one-third of patients reported fatigue on presentation in the ADHERE™ registry.[2] Initially, it was believed that fatigue was the result of decreased cardiac output, but the presence of fatigue in patients with preserved LV systolic function, and recent research revealing significant metabolic abnormalities, especially of skeletal muscle, have suggested that other mechanisms play an important role in the pathogenesis of fatigue. Abnormal skeletal muscle high energy phosphates have been demonstrated in many studies,[23–25] as well as changes in fiber distribution, innervation, and metabolism. These peripheral alterations are now felt to play a central role in the development of fatigue, and decompensation of heart failure can result in worsening of these abnormalities.

Depression is estimated to be present in about one-third of heart failure patients[26,27] and major depression is present in 40% of hospitalized patients with NYHA class IV heart failure.[28] Depression is a major concern for patients and is one of the most important factors affecting quality of life,[29] contributing to the patient's perception of other symptoms, such as dyspnea, and independently increasing mortality.[27] In addition, depression is strongly related to the extent and severity of physical symptoms,[30] suggesting an increased susceptibility to depression during acute exacerbations. While depression may be an unusual primary cause of admission in ADHF patients, recognition and treatment of the condition may hasten and improve recovery from the acute episode.

Patients with severely decompensated heart failure can also present with altered mental status or confusion. Heart failure patients can have a particularly high incidence of altered mental status due to the advanced age and multiple comorbidities evident in this population. Chronic heart failure, itself, appears to be independently associated with cognitive impairment[31,32] with multiple potential mechanisms, including hypotension, impaired cerebral circulation, vascular remodeling with abnormal endothelial function, silent cerebral infarction, atrial fibrillation, and hypercoagulable state.[33] ADHF can exacerbate pre-existing changes in cognitive function, such as in patients with Alzheimer's disease or ischemic dementia, as well as cause new evidence of cognitive impairment through significant uremia from renal failure (especially in patients with underlying renal dysfunction), cerebral hypotension due to low cardiac output or concomitant therapies, or other metabolic derangements. Thus, worsening heart failure can be a precipitant for altered mental status, especially in patients with severe chronic heart failure.

Sleep disturbances are a common problem in patients with chronic heart failure and can result in symptoms of marked drowsiness and fatigue. Acute exacerbations of heart failure can worsen these symptoms and severe drowsiness can be an unusual presentation of ADHF. Multiple factors can explain disrupted sleep patterns in these patients. As noted previously, progressive orthopnea and PND can result in decreased sleep, and nocturia, either induced by vascular redistribution while supine or persistent effects of diuretics, can also result in poor sleep. While these mechanisms are probably the most frequent cause of decreased sleep in the ADHF patient, there has been increasing recognition of sleep-disordered breathing in patients with chronic heart failure, especially obstructive and central sleep apnea. Obstructive sleep apnea[34] has been found in 11% to 37%[35,36] of heart failure patients undergoing polysomnography, but it appears to be predominantly a frequent comorbidity, rather than a pathophysiologic consequence of heart failure. In addition to weight reduction and avoidance of alcohol and sedatives, obstructive sleep apnea in heart failure patients also responds to continuous positive airway pressure (CPAP).[37] Central sleep apnea[38] has been found in 33% to 40%[35,36] of heart failure patients undergoing polysomnography and appears to be a result of the hemodynamic and neurohormonal perturbations caused by heart failure. Patients with severe central sleep apnea may report PND,[37] as well as daytime drowsiness, although snoring is less frequently reported. The degree of central sleep apnea is related to the severity of heart failure and is independently linked to increased mortality in these patients.[39,40] Presently, multiple studies are being performed to assess the efficacy of CPAP in these patients, including a large morbidity and mortality trial.[41] Thus, worsening of heart failure can result in disruption of sleep through multiple mechanisms, all of which can worsen during acute decompensation, and patients with ADHF can present with increasing daytime sleepiness and fatigue as manifestations of worsening heart failure.

Palpitations are a frequent symptom in patients with heart failure, although it is unclear how often they are the presenting symptoms in patients with ADHF. As noted in the EuroHeart Failure survey, 10% of patients with heart failure presented with rapid atrial fibrillation.[3] The character of the palpitations may give some clue to the underlying arrhythmia, with sensations of pauses and skipped or forceful beats suggesting premature atrial or ventricular complexes. Rapid palpitations can be irregular (as with atrial arrhythmias, such as atrial fibrillation, flutter or tachycardia) or regular (suggesting sinus, supraventricular, or ventricular tachycardias). Associated symptoms, including dizziness, pre-syncope and syncope, should be specifically elicited, and may be indicative of a more malignant arrhythmia, but none of these symptoms are specific enough to establish a diagnosis. Atrial fibrillation is a well-known precipitant of acute decompensation and, given its high prevalence in the heart failure population, should be actively sought as a contributing factor.

The Role of the History in the Assessment of the Patient with Acute Decompensated Heart Failure

Eliciting a history in the patient with ADHF is a staged process that evolves during the patient's admission and serves multiple purposes, including developing an accurate diagnosis, identification of precipitants, and providing an opportunity for patient education. Many patients are extremely symptomatic at presentation, when obtaining an in-depth history is frequently inappropriate, whereas further discussion can be performed after the acute symptoms are treated.

The initial history should focus on eliciting the symptoms of most prominent concern to the patient and providing information to make an accurate diagnosis. Specific inquiries regarding the presence of anginal chest pain or its equivalents are imperative, since myocardial ischemia and infarction can cause pulmonary edema and dyspnea that may overshadow the anginal symptoms. The rapidity of onset of the symptoms may give some insight into the likelihood of ischemia as a precipitant, although many patients with chronic heart failure seem to be much less sensitive to gradual decrements in their exercise tolerance until it reaches an individual threshold. Due to the important implications for therapies and prognosis, it is imperative that myocardial ischemia and infarction are fully considered as potential etiologies of the heart failure decompensation.

Differentiating heart failure from pulmonary disease, such as chronic obstructive pulmonary disease (COPD) exacerbation, is difficult based on history alone, although eliciting symptoms and signs of inflammation, such as fever, chills, myalgias, or cough with purulent sputum, can assist. A Bayesian approach can also be helpful, if prior histories of coronary artery disease (CAD), COPD exacerbation, systolic and/or diastolic dysfunction, accelerated hypertension, pulmonary emboli, or other conditions are present, but these morbidities coexist in many patients, limiting the usefulness of this approach. Multiple systems have been developed to assist with the diagnosis of heart failure (such as the Framingham criteria, NHANES clinical score, Boston criteria, study of men born in 1913, Walma score) and, in all of these systems, the presence of dyspnea is a major component. However, dyspnea alone can result in a high false positive rate and requires confirmation from other modalities.[42] Fortunately, the diagnosis need not be made solely on the basis of the history, but can be reinforced by the physical examination and other diagnostic tests.

In conjunction with questions attempting to establish the proper diagnosis, a careful history regarding precipitants for the heart failure decompensation should be obtained. Table 9.2 includes a listing of some of the common precipitants of AHF. In RESOLVD,[43] 143 of 768 heart failure patients with ejection fraction (EF) < 40% required hospitalization during the 43 weeks of the study. The precipitants of these hospitalizations were non-

Table 9.2. *Precipitants of decompensated heart failure*

Excess sodium or fluid intake

Medication noncompliance

Iatrogenic precipitants
- inappropriate reduction in heart failure medications
- volume overload

Uncontrolled hypertension

Myocardial ischemia or infarction

Valvular heart disease

Arrhythmia
- atrial fibrillation or flutter
- ventricular tachyarrhythmias
- bradyarrhythmias

Comorbidities
- fever, infection, or sepsis
- thyroid dysfunction
- anemia
- renal insufficiency
- nutritional deficiencies (i.e. thiamine)
- pulmonary disease (chronic obstructive pulmonary disease, pulmonary embolism, hypoxemia)

Adverse drug effects
- nonsteroidal antiinflammatory drugs
- alcohol
- negative inotropic agents (especially non-amiodarone antiarrhythmic agents, calcium channel blockers, etc.)
- corticosteroids

compliance with salt restriction (27%), other noncardiac causes (especially pulmonary infectious process, 24%), cardiac arrhythmias (22%), myocardial ischemia (12%), use of calcium channel blockers (15%) or antiarrhythmics (13%) in the past 48 hours, and inappropriate reductions in congestive heart failure (CHF) therapy (10%). Other studies have suggested that the use of nonsteroidal anti-inflammatory drugs can increase the risk of admission for heart failure as much as 10-fold.[44,45] Interestingly, many of these precipitants are modifiable, through increased education of both patients and physicians. An assiduous investigation into the precipitants may provide the best means to prevent future readmissions.

Many precipitants of ADHF are preventable. During the hospitalization, while the patient is more receptive, take the opportunity to educate them about how to modify their lifestyle and to avoid these episodes in the future.

As with all areas of medicine, an accurate and comprehensive history with a focus on acute symptoms is essential to appropriate care and treatment of the patient. In addition, the physical examination is especially important in the patient with possible ADHF.

Physical Examination of the Acute Heart Failure Patient

The value of the physical examination in the management of patients with cardiovascular disease has been questioned and some consider it to be an antiquated technique left over from olden times. Critics point out that the physical examination has poor operating characteristics as a diagnostic tool when directly compared to echocardiography[46] and B-type natriuretic peptide (BNP);[47] the latter diagnostic tools are viewed as modern or more sophisticated. Studies do demonstrate concerning deficiencies among young physicians in the ability to accurately perform a physical examination.[48–50] The basis of the decline in physical examination skills is likely multifactorial,[51–54] including a paucity of more senior physicians who have the skills needed to serve as teachers of physical examination techniques.[53] This observation is concerning as it portends exponential decay in physical examination skills with subsequent generations of physicians. Nevertheless, several recent studies have demonstrated that the physical examination continues to provide important prognostic value in the modern era in acute coronary syndromes,[55] asymptomatic LV dysfunction,[56] and symptomatic heart failure[57,58] and such data may reinvigorate interest in mastering physical examination skills.[59]

Within the broad arena of cardiovascular disease, chronic heart failure has emerged as a disease state in which there has been considerable interest in the physical examination. For example, in a recent series of letters by experts in the management of heart failure, many cited the integral role of the physical examination in their daily practice.[60] In this section, we will review aspects of a focused physical examination for a patient suspected of having ADHF.

General inspection

General inspection of the patient while obtaining the history is an efficient way to begin the physical examination. The presence of bitemporal wasting may alert the physician to cachexia and concomitant loss of true body weight which accompanies ADHF. Marked truncal obesity may suggest the possibility of obstructive sleep apnea. Total body anasarca and scleral icterus are other easily visible clues to the presence of ADHF. When considering cardiac transplantation as a therapeutic option, observing the patient's environment, such as whether family members are present or not, is helpful when evaluating the patient's social support.

Focused cardiac exam

Blood pressure

Measuring the blood pressure is a critical part in the evaluation of patients with heart failure. There are several aspects to measuring the blood pressure in this setting, including determining the systolic and diastolic blood pressure at rest and evaluating the changes in systolic blood pressure in response to normal respiration, standing up (orthostatic change), or the Valsalva maneuver.

The systolic blood pressure remains an important predictor of outcome in patients with advanced heart failure in the modern era.[61] In our experience, in patients with advanced heart failure, the systolic blood pressure can be < 80 mm Hg in the absence of lightheadedness in an ambulatory patient. Perhaps because this is not well appreciated by those who do not care for such patients on a routine basis, it is not unusual for us to detect a systolic blood pressure in this range (70 mm Hg to 79 mm Hg) when asked to evaluate a patient with advanced heart failure and progressive renal insufficiency of otherwise unknown basis. As with low blood pressure, the finding of a high systolic blood pressure is also important and provides the opportunity to improve a patient's clinical status by optimizing their antihypertensive regimen.

In addition to recording the systolic blood pressure, it is important to accurately measure the diastolic blood pressure so that one can know the width of the pulse pressure (systolic minus diastolic blood pressure). A low pulse pressure is a marker of a low cardiac output[62] and confers a relative risk of death of 2.5 in patients admitted with ADHF.[63] In our experience, it is extremely unusual to find the blood pressure recorded with a truly narrow pulse pressure (e.g., 90/78 mm Hg) on a vital signs flow sheet in the hospital, emphasizing the need to measure the blood pressure oneself. Not only is a low pulse pressure informative, but a high pulse pressure may alert the physician to a high output state, including the possibility of unrecognized thyrotoxicosis or anemia. Due to its importance, we recommend that every physician measure the resting blood pressure during their initial evaluation of a patient with ADHF.

Physicians can also gain important information by measuring the change in blood pressure in response to maneuvers such as breathing, standing (orthostatic changes), or the Valsalva maneuver. A decrease in systolic blood pressure of > 10 mm Hg during normal inspiration (pulsus paradoxus) raises the concern of cardiac tamponade which may mimic AHF. An orthostatic decline in blood pressure of > 10 mm Hg most often signals volume depletion, but the possibility of an autonomic neuropathy in a patient with diabetes or suspected amyloidosis should be considered. Measuring the blood pressure while the patient performs a Valsalva maneuver has proven useful to discriminate whether dyspnea is related to a pulmonary process or elevated left-sided filling pressures.[64–68] During the strain phase of the Valsalva maneuver (Figure 9.1), the systolic blood pressure first increases very briefly (2 to 3 beats) but then decreases below the baseline. However, in the presence of elevated left-sided filling pressures, the drop in blood pressure does not occur. The persistence of the blood pressure during the strain phase which occurs with elevated left-sided filling pressures has been termed the square-wave response (Figure 9.1). Not surprisingly, because the square-wave response represents elevated left-sided filling pressures, it has been correlated with elevations in natriuretic peptides.[69] In

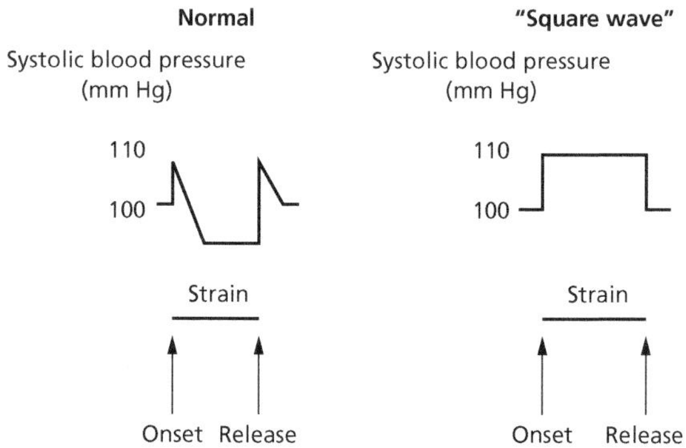

Figure 9.1. *Response of systolic blood pressure to the strain phase of the Valsalva maneuver. On the left, the normal biphasic response of systolic blood pressure is shown. On the right, the "square-wave" response is depicted. To perform this test, set the blood pressure cuff 10 mm Hg higher than the resting systolic blood pressure. Have the patient strain (or bear down) for 10 seconds. In this example, the patient is resting comfortably with a blood pressure of 100 mm Hg. The physician has the blood pressure cuff set at 110 mm Hg and thus hears nothing. In a healthy individual without heart failure, during the strain phase the blood pressure transiently (2 to 3 beats) increases. During this brief time, the physician would hear Korotkoff sounds which then disappear during the remainder of the strain phase as the blood pressure falls. In contrast, in the patient with heart failure and elevated left-sided filling pressures, the systolic blood pressure remains at 110 mm Hg, so the physician hears Korotkoff sounds throughout the 10 seconds of the strain phase.*

our clinical practice, we have found the Valsalva maneuver easy to perform, if the patient can cooperate with straining and does not have atrial fibrillation. The variable cycle length of atrial fibrillation can alter the systolic blood pressure and complicate the interpretation of the blood pressure response to the Valsalva maneuver.

Pulse and heart rate

Measuring the heart rate is critical in the initial assessment of patients with ADHF. Decompensation may be the result of bradycardia induced by digoxin toxicity (often in the presence of worsening renal function), hypothyroidism (especially in patients on amiodarone), beta-blockade, progressive conduction system disease, or an infiltrative process. Tachycardia is an equally important finding to note. It may signal occult infection, hyperthyroidism (especially in patients on amiodarone), anemia, pulmonary emboli, primary supraventricular or ventricular tachyarrhythmias, or simply be a marker of severely decompensated heart failure associated with a guarded prognosis.

Because many patients with ADHF are on telemetry, it may be tempting to look at the heart monitor to measure the heart rate rather than to palpate the radial artery. This, we believe, is a mistake because palpation of the pulse provides important information.

First, the overall strength of the pulse can be categorized as weak or strong, which provides insight into adequacy of cardiac output. Second, an alteration in the intensity of the pulse from strong to weak (mechanical alternans) has been shown to be common in heart failure and associated with abnormal cardiac structure and function.[70] Third, inequalities in pulse between extremities may be the first clue to the presence of peripheral vascular disease (which may suggest concomitant underlying CAD) or other aortic processes such as dissection or coarctation. The clinical relevance of such findings is highlighted by a recent patient we encountered with heart failure following coronary artery bypass surgery. In this patient, the absence of a left radial pulse alerted us to the presence of a proximal subclavian stenosis which compromised flow in the left internal mammary artery used to bypass the left anterior descending artery.

Jugular venous pressure

The jugular venous pressure (JVP) is perhaps the most useful physical examination finding for detecting ADHF. In addition, many physicians base their daily treatment decisions for patients hospitalized with ADHF on the JVP (i.e., continue diuresis until the JVP is no longer elevated).

Although JVP reflects the right atrial pressure, an elevated JVP is associated with elevated left-sided filling pressures as measured by the PCWP in patients with chronic heart failure.[62,71] In a series of 1000 patients with advanced heart failure referred for cardiac transplantation, the right atrial pressure and PCWP were similarly high or low 80% of the time, when the arbitrary cutoffs of 10 mm Hg and 22 mm Hg were used for a high right atrial pressure or PCWP respectively.[72] Additionally, changes in the right atrial pressure correlated with changes in the PCWP during intensive medical therapy. Although it may be anticipated that the presence of severe tricuspid regurgitation (TR) may impact the relationship of JVP and PCWP (leading the physician to overestimate the right atrial pressure and therefore the left-sided filling pressure), this is not a major clinical concern in patients with advanced heart failure, because severe TR is itself associated with an elevated PCWP.[72]

The JVP is measured in centimeters as 5+ (the vertical distance from the top of the pulsation in the jugular veins to the sternal angle of Louis). Multiplying this number by 0.75 converts it from centimeters to mm Hg.[22]

We have found the following principles helpful when assessing the JVP (Table 9.3). First, there is large variability between patients, presumably in part due to body habitus and venous anatomy, as to where the neck veins are visible. In some patients, they are obscured on the right side but easily visible on the left, whereas in others they are most evident in the midline. Thus, we routinely examine both sides of the neck when estimating JVP. Second, in some patients the external jugular veins are visible and the internal jugular veins cannot be seen. One must be careful that there is not a fixed obstruction of the external jugular vein leading to the false impression of increased right atrial pressure; seeing respirophasic changes in the filling of the external jugular vein reassures one

Table 9.3. *Practical tips when assessing the jugular venous pressure*

1. Look at both sides of the patient's neck.
2. Do not ignore the external jugular veins, especially when the internal jugular veins are not visible.
3. Assess the jugular venous pressure (JVP) with the patient at various angles off the horizontal (supine, 30 or 45 degrees off the horizontal, sitting, or standing) until the jugular venous pulsation is visible half-way up the neck.
4. Always assess the patient sitting upright or standing to exclude a very high JVP (which may be more difficult to detect when the patient is at a lower angle).
5. If the JVP does not appear elevated, press on the patient's abdomen or right upper quadrant to see if the abdominojugular response is present.
6. To distinguish the carotid from the jugular venous impulse, apply pressure with your hand 1 to 2 inches below the impulse. If the pulsation disappears, it was the jugular vein; if the pulsation persists, it was the carotid artery.

that this is not the case. Others emphasize the importance of seeing whether the external jugular veins fill from above or below after the veins are compressed, with the latter being associated with heart failure.[73] Third, the optimal angle between the patient's head and trunk and the horizontal plane (e.g., supine, 30 or 45 degrees off the horizontal, upright in bed, or standing) for viewing the jugular veins depends upon the pressure in the jugular veins. Because the JVP is not known before it is measured, it is therefore impossible to know what angle off the horizontal would be best to see the jugular veins in the individual patient being examined. Thus, we routinely examine the JVP with the patient's torso at different angles from the horizontal until we find the angle where the JVP is clearly seen halfway up the neck (midway between the clavicle and the jaw). Because of this need to move the patient through various angles off the midline, an electric hospital bed that allows the head of the bed to be moved is the ideal setting when first learning how to measure the JVP. Importantly, we have found that very high JVP may be hard to see when the patient is supine or at a low angle off the horizontal (especially in those where the external jugulars are not seen), and may only be visible when the patient is upright. In some of these patients, the most prominent sign of a markedly elevated JVP is a subtle wiggle of the ear lobe or base of the ear. Because these are the very patients in whom accurate estimation of the JVP is critical (since they are markedly decompensated), we recommend that one of the assessments of the neck veins in patients with suspected ADHF occur with the patient sitting upright to be certain that a very high JVP is not present. A convenient time to accomplish this is immediately following the history (since most patients are sitting up during the history). If the neck veins are not visible in the upright position, then they should be assessed subsequently with the patient at lower angles off the horizontal.

In our experience in training junior physicians in reading the neck veins, a common question is whether the visible pulsations in the neck are from the jugular vein or the carotid artery. Several maneuvers are helpful in making this distinction. The jugular veins have an easily visible respirophasic component and the carotids usually do not. A pulsation attributed to the jugular vein will change with different patient angles while a carotid arterial pulsation does not. If the impulse is no longer visible when the patient stands, it is likely to be the jugular vein and not the carotid. Similarly, by pressing on the liver or abdomen, there is usually a transient increase in the JVP, but not in the carotid pulse. The jugular vein has a more undulating character with two peaks while the carotid has a more brisk upstroke with a single peak. We have found the most helpful maneuver to distinguish between the jugular veins and the carotids to be manual compression of the neck 1 to 2 inches below the impulse. If the impulse is secondary to the jugular veins, it will no longer be visible, whereas if it is the carotid artery, the pulsation persists.

There are several caveats to using the JVP as a

noninvasive measure of the PCWP (Table 9.4). First, one must be careful in using the JVP to estimate the PCWP in patients with comorbidities such as obesity or lung disease. These processes can affect right ventricular (RV) function and therefore distort the relationship between right-sided and left-sided filling pressures. Second, 20% of patients referred for transplant have discordance between the JVP and PCWP.[72] When the clinical response to therapy guided by the JVP is unanticipated (e.g., development of hypotension and renal failure with diuresis in a patient with persistently elevated JVP), these data remind us that the JVP may not be reflective of the PCWP. Third, although the JVP and PCWP usually track together in chronic heart failure, in the setting of acute myocardial infarction (AMI), they often do not.[74] Thus, it is important to use the JVP as a noninvasive measure of the PCWP only in patients with decompensated chronic heart failure in the absence of myocardial infarction (MI). Finally, whether the JVP reflects the PCWP in heart failure in the setting of intact left ventricular ejection fraction (LVEF) (i.e., diastolic heart failure) is not known.

Table 9.4. *Limitations of the jugular venous pressure in assessing volume status in congestive heart failure*

1. The jugular venous pressure (JVP) may not reflect left-sided filling pressures in patients with dilated cardiomyopathy who also have pulmonary disease or obesity.
2. Although often useful in the clinical setting, the JVP is not a direct measure of left-sided cardiac filling pressures. Consider this possibility when the clinical response to therapies based on estimates of the JVP is unexpected (e.g., rising creatinine or hypotension with diuresis despite the persistence of elevated JVP).
3. Do not use the JVP to estimate left-sided filling pressures in acute myocardial infarction.
4. The relationship of the JVP to left-sided filling pressures has been assessed in systolic but not diastolic heart failure.

The response of the JVP to abdominal pressure (abdominojugular or hepatojugular response) is also informative as it also correlates with elevated left-sided filling pressures.[75] Here, a sustained increase of the JVP in response to abdominal pressure (e.g., pressing on the right upper quadrant or mid-abdomen for 10 to 15 seconds) should be sought rather than a transient flickering increase in the JVP. Of note, many patients with ADHF have hepatic congestion, and applying pressure in the right upper quadrant can cause splinting. When eliciting this sign, applying pressure in the mid-abdomen may avoid this concern.

In addition to being useful for detecting ADHF and in guiding diuretic therapy, elevated JVP also provides prognostic value in both chronic heart failure[57] and asymptomatic LV dysfunction.[56] Its presence is associated with an increased risk of adverse outcomes even after accounting for other measures of disease severity such as New York Heart Association (NYHA) functional class, LVEF, and serum sodium and creatinine.

Rales

Although inspiratory crackles or rales are often considered a classical finding of CHF, in the presence of decompensated, chronic heart failure, rales are often not heard,[62] likely due to exaggerated hypertrophy of lymphatics which keep the airspaces clear.

Enlarged lymphatics can, in fact, be seen on radiographic imaging studies.[76,77] In contrast, in the setting of flash pulmonary edema, as occurs with hypertensive crisis or acute coronary syndrome, patients will flood their lungs and crackles will be heard, sometimes to the apices. In patients with chronic heart failure with more gradual decompensation, crackles are usually not heard despite markedly elevated left-sided filling pressures. In this setting, the clue to volume overload is often elevated JVP and symptoms of decompensated CHF such as orthopnea. This observation has clinical utility. For example, in patients on amiodarone who develop increasing dyspnea, the presence of crackles throughout the lungs juxtaposed with flat neck veins on examination has alerted us to the probability of amiodarone pulmonary toxicity on more than one occasion.

Cardiac auscultation

Cardiac auscultation may lead the examiner to suspect an underlying valvular cardiomyopathy. In patients with ischemic or idiopathic dilated cardiomyopathy, severe mitral regurgitation (MR) may occur in concert with volume overload, but if it persists following optimization of filling pressures,[78] it may represent a target for surgical intervention.[79]

The presence of a third heart sound is a classical finding in patients with ADHF related to low ventricular compliance, increased ventricular filling pressures, or increased early diastolic filling rates.[80–83] To optimize detection of the third heart sound, the point of maximal impulse should be located and the bell of the stethoscope placed lightly over it with the patient in the left lateral decubitus position. We recognize, however, that the third heart sound can be difficult to hear because it is low pitched, and interobserver agreement on its presence is not good.[84–88] Nevertheless, it is an important sign to listen for in patients with heart failure as it provides important information when detected. Its presence has recently been shown to correlate with BNP levels,[89] an emerging adverse prognostic factor in heart failure. A third heart sound in patients with advanced LV dysfunction is associated with progression to symptomatic heart failure.[56] In those with symptomatic heart failure, it is independently associated with adverse outcomes including heart failure hospitalization and death from pump failure.[57]

Extremities

In assessing heart failure, the extremities are examined for two findings: temperature and edema. Determining whether the extremities are warm or cool is useful in assessing adequacy of cardiac perfusion. A cool lower leg with a palpable dorsalis pedis or posterior tibialis pulse (to rule out peripheral vascular disease) suggests a marginal cardiac index. Of note, the temperature should be assessed at the lower leg as opposed to the foot. It is also important to remember that the assessment of the temperature of the patient's extremity is relative to the temperature of the examiner's hands. Edema is another classical sign of decompensated CHF. However, edema has a reasonable positive predictive value for ADHF but a low sensitivity,[62,90,91] so its absence does not exclude that diagnosis. When edema is present, the jugular veins will usually be elevated as well.[62] If the JVP is not elevated, one should consider alternative causes such as venous insufficiency or thrombosis, nephrosis, cirrhosis, and edema associated with obesity.

Symptoms as an Endpoint in Acute Decompensated Heart Failure Trials

The history and physical examination assist in establishing an accurate diagnosis, with the ultimate goal of initiation of effective and safe therapies. Current therapies for ADHF have significant limitations and recently there has been considerable effort expended in developing new therapeutic approaches. Although clinical trial design for chronic heart failure is well established, ADHF presents some unique challenges in designing a clinical development program, especially in phase III efficacy trials.[92] This section will discuss the use of symptom assessments, with particular reference to dyspnea,[93] in clinical trials of ADHF therapies.

After establishing the proof of concept for a new therapy, drug development programs must address the regulatory requirements for drug approval as defined by the Food and Drug Administration (FDA) in the United States and the European Agency for the Evaluation of Medicinal Products (EMEA) in the European Union, either directly or via the recommendations of its Advisory Boards. Fortunately, these requirements are based upon the most appropriate scientific evaluation of the specific agent being studied. These requirements can evolve significantly over time, and in the field of ADHF they have evolved very rapidly. In 1988, intravenous milrinone was approved for the treatment of AHF patients, based largely on its hemodynamic effects, and, at that time, the ability to have a predictable hemodynamic response was sufficient for approval. The environment has changed significantly since then, and while it is still necessary for an agent to demonstrate predictable, beneficial hemodynamic effects (especially reduction in PCWP), it is no longer sufficient.

The regulatory agencies have attempted to provide some guidance for clinical trials in this area. In 1998, in response to issues regarding intravenous positive inotropes and other new agents for heart failure, the Cardiovascular and Renal Advisory Committee of the FDA produced a draft set of guidelines[94] which were greatly influenced by the mandate that therapies should make a patient feel better or live longer. These guidelines suggested that an intravenous agent for AHF should be able to demonstrate both favorable hemodynamic effects for 24 to 48 hours and a clinical benefit, in the context of no major short-term or long-term safety concerns. Many types of clinical benefit were discussed, but there were no definite recommendations of which symptom or clinical measure was preferable. The EMEA also released a set of guidelines that outlined specific recommendations for efficacy criteria in ADHF trials.[95] All-cause mortality is the preferred efficacy measure, but improvement in symptoms in the context of demonstrated hemodynamic benefit would also be acceptable evidence of efficacy. According to the EMEA, improvement in dyspnea is preferred for demonstration of symptomatic benefit. Both agencies (the FDA and the EMEA) stressed the importance of establishing the safety of any new therapy, and in trials that used symptom endpoints (i.e. dyspnea), reasonable assurance of a neutral effect on mortality would be required, in addition to a favorable adverse effect profile. This requirement can have dramatic impact on the sample size of a trial. Neither of the agencies have been enthusiastic about the use of surrogates as efficacy endpoints,[96] although there has been increasing pressure from investigators in support of PCWP and other physical parameters. While most researchers were quite adept at doing hemodynamic studies, even in unstable and critically ill patients, the requirement of demonstrating a clinical benefit in these patients has posed some challenges.

What are the types of clinical benefit that might be seen in patients with ADHF? In chronic heart failure trials, the reduction of mortality has become the main standard by which many therapies are ultimately judged. Many investigators felt that it was unreasonable to think that a therapy given for 24 to 48 hours would demonstrate a significant improvement in mortality in reasonably-sized studies, especially compared to placebo on top of standard therapy. While levosimendan raised the possibility of such a benefit, as a secondary endpoint compared to an active control of dobutamine,[97,98] efficacy in such active control trials has not previously been acceptable for approval in the United States, in the absence of placebo-controlled studies establishing a mortality effect for the active control. Thus, there remained the question of whether the positive effects on mortality with levosimendan were more a reflection of the adverse effects of dobutamine. A larger mortality trial of dobutamine versus levosimendan, the SURVIVE trial, is currently under way.

As in the chronic heart failure trials, a combined endpoint of morbidity and mortality could be considered to establish efficacy. Morbidity and mortality could be assessed by decreased intensive care unit (ICU) utilization, other specialized interventions, or hospitalization (either length of stay, readmissions, or a combination). This approach was pursued in the Outcomes of a Prospective Trial of Intravenous Milrinone on Exacerbations of Chronic Heart Failure (OPTIME-CHF) trial, where the efficacy of milrinone in reducing the number of days of cardiovascular hospitalization in a 60-day period was assessed.[99] OPTIME-CHF did not meet its primary endpoint, perhaps related to the increased adverse events of hypotension and new atrial fibrillation in the milrinone group.[100] Variations of a morbidity and mortality endpoint are currently being used in two major clinical trials. In the Randomized Evaluation of Intravenous Levosimendan Efficacy versus Placebo in the Short-term Treatment of Decompensated Chronic Heart Failure (REVIVE),[101] a "clinical course" endpoint[102] was developed which classified a patient as improved, unchanged, or worsened based upon global assessments at specific time points and their clinical status (worsening of heart failure or death) within a 5-day period. The Value of Endothelin Receptor Inhibition with Tezosentan in Acute heart failure Study (VERITAS) considers the time to worsening of heart failure or death within 7 days in tezosentan compared to placebo-treated patients as a co-primary endpoint.

Another clinical benefit that could be assessed is an improvement in end-organ function. For example, in patients with AHF and progressive renal dysfunction, the ability of an agent to treat the patient's heart failure and improve renal function could be a reasonable endpoint, although a change in renal function alone may not be acceptable from a regulatory standpoint. However, a therapy that is useful in this setting might also have broader impact on other outcomes, such as hospitalization. Progression to end-stage renal disease would also seem to be a reasonable component of a composite clinical endpoint.

Clinical benefit of an agent could be measured by assessing a change in the patient's symptoms or clinical status. As discussed previously, patients with ADHF will frequently present with a variety of symptoms, many of which would be reasonable targets for new therapies. However, the most prominent of these symptoms in ADHF patients is usually dyspnea. Dyspnea is the symptom that impels the patient to medical care and the symptom to which most of the acute interventions are directed. Thus, in all three of the most recent clinical development programs for new ADHF therapies, dyspnea has served as a prominent efficacy endpoint.[93]

Instruments to assess dyspnea

A number of instruments for the subjective assessment of dyspnea have been developed.[103] The early instruments attempted to standardize symptom reporting by relating the dyspnea to known activities. The first report of such a scale was in 1952, when patients were asked to rate the impact of dyspnea on activities, compared to age-matched healthy controls.[104] This scale was subsequently modified to emphasize the relation of dyspnea to walking distances or climbing stairs and was known as the Medical Research Council Scale.[105] Using these scales, one could compare the score from one visit to later visits to measure potential improvement. However, it has been suggested that this scale is not sensitive enough to assess the effects of a therapeutic intervention. Another instrument used a visual analog scale (VAS) in the form of an Oxygen Cost Diagram (OCD) consisting of 13 activities placed along a vertical 100-mm line in proportional ranking to the number of calories expended in performing the activity.[106] Sleeping was placed at the bottom and walking briskly uphill was at the top, and patients were asked to mark the level of activity that would cause dyspnea. The distance from the bottom to the patient's mark was the score (ranging from 0 to 100). More complicated assessments have been developed to attempt to account for the effort exerted by the patients. The Baseline Dyspnea Index (BDI) rates the patient's dyspnea on a 5-level scale (ranging from 0, or no impairment, to 4, or extraordinary or severe impairment),[107] during a brief interview which incorporates the measurement of functional impairment, the magnitude of effort, and the magnitude of the task. The BDI measures dyspnea at a single time point and another measure, known as the Transition Dyspnea Index (TDI),[108] was designed to measure changes from the baseline as measured by the BDI. This index is also derived from an extensive interview. Both the BDI and TDI have been validated in settings where their sensitivity to clinical interventions has been demonstrated in patients with interstitial lung disease[109] and with obstructive airway disease.[110] Finally, the University of California at San Diego Shortness of Breath Questionnaire (UCSDQ) is a 24-item questionnaire which measures dyspnea over a 1-week period, which has also been validated in patients with COPD.[111,112] All these measures of dyspnea share common features; they all assess dyspnea in the chronic setting, using activities of daily living as a gauge of exertion. However, the use of these daily activities does not account for the differences in effort extended during these activities.

Multiple instruments have been developed to attempt to standardize these dyspnea scores by using incremental exercise. Borg developed a scale ranging from 6 to 20 with which patients would rate their perceived dyspnea during physical exercise.[113] This scale was subsequently modified to a 10-point scale with specific descriptors associated with the numbers.[114] Another measure uses the Visual Analog Scale (VAS), a 100-mm horizontal or vertical line with specific anchor phrases at the ends of the lines. Although not standardized, examples of these phrases include "no shortness of breath" to "shortness of breath as bad as it can be," or "not breathless at all" to "extremely breathless." The patient marks this scale at pre-specified points during the incremental exercise, and changes in the scale or rates of change can be used to compare patients and interventions. These methods have been validated in multiple exercise studies, and are considered one of the best measures of dyspnea.

There have been a number of studies comparing these different instruments, although few have assessed them in the acutely dyspneic patient. In a study of patients with chronic disease,[115] 28 patients underwent symptom scores on both a VAS scale and 7-level Likert scale before and after an inpatient respiratory rehabilitation program. The VAS scale showed a greater standardized improvement in dyspnea, but was also accompanied by greater variation in response. They concluded that the ease of interpretation and administration of the Likert scales recommend its use in clinical trials. One study in normal subjects compared VAS scales, Borg scales, and Likert scales during submaximal exercise.[116] The VAS scale was the most reproducible and sensitive measure of changes in breathlessness, although the Borg scale was more sensitive to changes in fatigue.

The instruments discussed previously represent the main examples of those measures of dyspnea described in the literature. Unfortunately, most of them are directed to chronic dyspnea studies and the use of these instruments in the acute setting has not been validated. Furthermore, those instruments that required exercise are clearly not appropriate for the study of new agents in the ADHF patient. These measures all suffer from another significant limitation in that they fail to account for differences in the language that patients may use to describe their dyspnea. Patients with dyspnea due to heart failure tend to describe a sensation of rapid breathing with feelings of suffocation and air hunger, while those with asthma describe chest tightness, heavy and shallow breathing with incomplete exhalation and increased effort.[117,118] Additionally, there is evidence of ethnic differences in the description of dyspnea, which may further confound these instruments.[119] Confronted with these challenges, investigators in all three recent development programs chose very similar approaches, opting for relatively simple, direct questions using different, and not yet validated, versions of Likert scales.

Dyspnea as an endpoint: experience from three recent development programs

Three major clinical development programs for new ADHF agents have been undertaken in recent years. Each of these new agents, nesiritide,[120] levosimendan[121] and tezosentan,[122,123] has been demonstrated to produce significant beneficial effects on hemodynamics in patients with chronic and acute heart failure. Each agent has also been shown to significantly reduce dyspnea compared to its control group using a Likert scale.[120,121,124] However, dyspnea was not a primary endpoint in any of these studies, and there were many methodological flaws that limited the impact of these findings. All the studies limited the therapies that could be given to patients before and during the study, challenging the applicability and meaning of the results in a clinical setting. In addition, these studies were all hemodynamic investigations, with assessment of PCWP at multiple time points prior to the dyspnea assessment.

Each of these studies is confounded to various degrees by two separate, but related, issues: blinding and confounding bias. When a hemodynamically active therapy has such profound effects, it remains a question as to whether investigators and patients can remain blinded to therapy with regards to subjective assessments, especially when the hemodynamics are the main focus of the trial. In addition to possible problems with blinding, the biasing of the symptom assessments by these hemodynamic measures is an important consideration. Staff who care for patients with no improvement in hemodynamics could be reasonably expected to behave differently around the patient than those patients in whom the hemodynamics are improving. This nonverbal feedback to the patient has a high likelihood of biasing symptom assessments, even in the absence of direct feedback, which was not censored in these trials. This confounding bias would be expected to be particularly evident in physician assessments of patient symptoms, as was found in some of the studies. Additionally, these biases are compounded in some trials by the active role of the investigator in jointly determining with the patient the assessment of change in dyspnea.[121] These issues were given voice during the first Cardiovascular and Renal Advisory Committee meeting in January of 1999,[125] where nesiritide was not recommended for approval. Thus, while the symptom assessments in these trials were encouraging, the validity of these findings is reduced by the significant potential for unblinding and confounding biases.

Two major, contemporary trials attempted to address these issues. In response to suggestions from the regulatory agency and input from investigators, the Vasodilation in the Management of Acute CHF (VMAC) nesiritide trial was designed and conducted.[126] This elegant, though complicated, trial enrolled 489 patients with dyspnea at rest due to ADHF requiring hospitalization and treatment with intravenous therapy. Patients were stratified according to the treating physician's decision to use invasive pulmonary artery catheterization for management of the patient. The catheterized patients were eligible if PCWP $\geq$ 20 mm Hg, while non-catheterized patients had to have at least two distinct signs or symptoms of volume overload. Patients were randomized to placebo, nesiritide (either fixed or adjustable dose in the catheterized strata) or nitroglycerin infusions for the first 3 hours. After this initial placebo-controlled period, the placebo patients were randomly reassigned to either nesiritide or nitroglycerin (active control period). The primary endpoints were both the change in PCWP compared to placebo at 3 hours (catheterized patients) and the patient's self-evaluation of the change in dyspnea compared to placebo at 3 hours (all patients). The dyspnea assessment used a 7-point scale, asking the patient to rate the change in dyspnea as compared to start of therapy as markedly improved/moderately improved/minimally improved/no change/minimally worse/moderately worse/markedly worse. To reduce the effect of bias from hemodynamic results, study personnel and staff were explicitly instructed to not discuss the hemodynamic results with the patients and to perform the dyspnea assessment prior to obtaining the 3-hour hemodynamic measurements.

The results of VMAC demonstrated a significant improvement in both endpoints. Nesiritide significantly decreased PCWP as compared to both placebo and nitroglycerin at 3 hours (nesiritide: –5.8 mm Hg; nitroglycerin: –3.8 mm Hg; and placebo: –2.0 mm Hg) in the catheterized strata. Furthermore, nesiritide significantly improved dyspnea as compared to placebo at 3 hours in all the patients ($P = 0.03$), though not compared to nitroglycerin ($P = 0.56$); over 70% of nesiritide-treated patients rated their dyspnea as improved as compared to approximately 62% of the placebo group. Interestingly, less than 5% of all the groups rated their dyspnea as worse.

The VMAC study was the first positive trial in patients with ADHF using a clinical endpoint—the dyspnea assessment. The investigators limited confounders significantly in this trial, although some concerns about the bias introduced by combining the dyspnea assessments of the catheterized with the non-catheterized patients persisted. Due to the inclusion of an adjustable-dose group in the catheterized strata, more patients on nesiritide were catheterized compared to the other groups at 3 hours (124 nesiritide, 60 nitroglycerin, and 62 placebo patients), so that if invasive hemodynamics did bias the dyspnea assessment, the bias was in favor of nesiritide. In fact, nesiritide had no significant effect as compared to placebo on dyspnea in the non-catheterized patients at 3 hours. Although nesiritide had no significant effect on dyspnea at 24 hours versus nitroglycerin in all patients, nesiritide significantly improved dyspnea as compared to nitroglycerin in the subgroup of non-catheterized patients at 24 hours, suggesting a beneficial effect in the absence of invasive hemodynamics.[127] VMAC is a landmark study in regard to trial design for ADHF, and on the basis of this trial, nesiritide was approved by the FDA for treatment in this population.

The Randomized Intravenous TeZosentan (RITZ-1)[128] trial was designed to specifically address many of the issues discussed previously and this trial attempted to eliminate any confounding effects on the symptom assessments. RITZ-1 is the first clinical trial in ADHF to have a symptom assessment as its primary endpoint. This trial enrolled 669 patients who were admitted to the hospital for ADHF with dyspnea on minimal exertion or at rest, requiring intravenous therapy; patients requiring hemodynamic monitoring were excluded from the trial. Patients were randomized to either placebo or tezosentan infusions (50 mg/h) for at least 24 hours and up to 72 hours. The primary endpoint was the dyspnea assessment at 24 hours, using the 7-level scale as described previously (markedly improved/ moderately improved/ minimally improved/no change/minimally worse/ moderately worse/markedly worse), with an additional eighth category of "worst" for those patients who had deterioration of heart failure (as indicated by the investigator initiating intravenous rescue therapy), need for mechanical ventilation or circulatory support, or death. There was no significant difference in the dyspnea assessment in tezosentan-treated patients as compared to the placebo group at 24 hours of therapy. In view of the positive hemodynamic and dyspnea assessment results of the RITZ-2[124] trial, the results of RITZ-1 were quite surprising to many investigators and are being analyzed for possible explanations.

As discussed during the presentation of the RITZ-1 results at the Hotline session of the 23rd European Society of Cardiology Congress in 2001, there are at least four possible reasons for these disparate results. First, perhaps dyspnea is not a reasonable endpoint in these trials. It should be noted that no trial, with the possible exception of VMAC, has demonstrated a significant improvement in dyspnea with any agent in the absence of hemodynamic monitoring. Many have also suggested that this symptom is too subjective to be reliably measured in this patient population with the currently available research instruments. Second, perhaps tezosentan is not an effective agent for improving dyspnea in ADHF. However, if improvement in PCWP is related to improvements in dyspnea, the positive hemodynamic effects of tezosentan, as clearly demonstrated in RITZ-2, would suggest that it should be effective in improving dyspnea as well. Third, there are many reasons to believe that the patients in RITZ-1 were less symptomatic than in RITZ-2, with a much lower rate of deterioration, limiting the beneficial effect of any therapeutic intervention. Fourth, the dose of tezosentan was probably too high, so that the adverse effects outweighed the potential beneficial effects. Thus, in the trial that specifically investigated the effect on dyspnea of a therapy for ADHF, there was no observable beneficial effect.

Future Directions

The combined experience from these studies in ADHF has provided tremendous guidance for future development programs. Some common trends are evident in these studies, which suggest possible solutions. First, the potential for bias from hemodynamics and staff feedback is a significant problem in subjective symptom assessments. Ideally, trials would be performed in the absence of hemodynamic measurements. Second, patients must have prominent symptoms to enable improvement. It is clear that specific hemodynamic entry criteria can select patients with significant congestion, but these measures can confound later assessments. One option would be to use hemodynamic entry criteria, but then remove the pulmonary artery catheter, or not use it during a specified period. Another solution is to use well-defined symptoms or objective signs of congestion, perhaps combined with a heart failure score to select patients. Third, most patients improve with standard therapy. In the trials where standard therapy was allowed, such as the nesiritide comparator trial,[120] most patients receiving standard therapies improved and very few worsened. These results suggest that perhaps current therapies are fairly effective in treating ADHF, although this does not mean that there is no need for other therapies. Current therapies have significant limitations, including potentially increasing morbidity and mortality, which need to be addressed by novel approaches. Finally, the impetus to treat dyspnea is extremely high; as clinicians, none of us can stand idly by while our patients gasp for breath. Consequently, one could expect that there is a greater use of standard therapies, such as diuretics, in the control group in these studies, which might obscure beneficial effects of the study drug. One possible approach to this problem is to enroll patients very early in their hospital course and to incorporate a worsening of heart failure component to the endpoint. The clinical event of worsening of heart failure is the endpoint, but its trigger can be the determination by the investigator that the patient's condition has deteriorated to such an extent that they require additional intravenous therapies. Many of these design features are being incorporated in current and planned clinical trials that use dyspnea as a prominent component of an efficacy endpoint. For example, a co-primary endpoint in the VERITAS trial is the improvement in dyspnea in tezosentan-treated patients as compared to placebo-treated patients, as assessed by a 24-hour area under the curve analysis using VAS scales at multiple time points. It is clear that clinical trial design needs to continue evolving to effectively evaluate new therapeutic interventions for ADHF.

References

1. Fonarow GC. The Acute Decompensated Heart Failure National Registry (ADHERE™): opportunities to improve care of patients hospitalized with acute decompensated heart failure. Rev Cardiovasc Med 2003; 4: S21–S30.
2. Scios Inc. ADHERE™ Acute Decompensated Heart Failure National Registry. Second Quarter 2003 National Benchmark Report. Available at: http://www.adhereregistry.com/national_BMR/Q2_03_National_ADHERE_BMR.pdf. Accessed November 30, 2004.
3. Cleland JG, Swedberg K, Follath F, *et al.*, Study Group on Diagnosis of the Working Group on Heart Failure of the European Society of Cardiology. The EuroHeart Failure survey programme—a survey on the quality of care among patients with heart failure in Europe. Part 1: patient characteristics and diagnosis. Eur Heart J 2003; 24: 442–463.
4. Thomas JT, Kelly RF, Thomas SJ, *et al.* Utility of history, physical examination, electrocardiogram, and chest radiograph for differentiating normal from decreased systolic function in patients with heart failure. Am J Med 2002; 112: 437–445.
5. Friedman MM. Older adults' symptoms and their duration before hospitalization for heart failure. Heart Lung 1997; 26: 169–176.
6. Schiff GD, Fung S, Speroff T, McNutt RA. Decompensated heart failure: symptoms, patterns of onset, and contributing factors. Am J Med 2003; 114: 625–630.
7. Malki Q, Sharma ND, Afzal A, *et al.* Clinical presentation, hospital length of stay, and readmission rate in patients with heart failure with preserved and decreased left ventricular systolic function. Clin Cardiol 2002; 25: 149–152.
8. Vinch CS, Aurigemma GP, Hill JC, *et al.* Usefulness of clinical variables, echocardiography, and levels of brain natriuretic peptide and norepinephrine to distinguish systolic and diastolic causes of acute heart failure. Am J Cardiol 2003; 91: 1140–1143.
9. Varela-Roman A, Gonzalez-Juanatey JR, Basante P, *et al.* Clinical characteristics and prognosis of hospitalised inpatients with heart failure and preserved or reduced left ventricular ejection fraction. Heart 2002; 88: 249–254.
10. Smith GL, Masoudi FA, Vaccarino V, Radford MJ, Krumholz HM. Outcomes in heart failure patients with preserved ejection fraction: mortality, readmission, and functional decline. J Am Coll Cardiol 2003; 41: 1510–1518.
11. Kitzman DW, Little WC, Brubaker PH, *et al.* Pathophysiological characterization of isolated diastolic heart failure in comparison to systolic heart failure. JAMA 2002; 288: 2144–2150.
12. American Thoracic Society. Dyspnea. Mechanisms, assessment, and management: a consensus statement. Am J Respir Crit Care Med 1999; 159: 321–340.
13. Manning HL, Schwartzstein RM. Pathophysiology of dyspnea. N Engl J Med 1995; 333: 1547–1553.
14. Franciosa JA, Ziesche S, Wilen M. Functional capacity of patients with chronic left ventricular failure: relationship of bicycle exercise performance to clinical and hemodynamic characterization. Am J Med 1979; 67: 460–466.
15. Benge W, Litchfield RL, Marcus ML. Exercise capacity in patients with severe left ventricular dysfunction. Circulation 1980; 61: 955–959.
16. Francis GS, Goldsmith SR, Cohn JN. Relationship of exercise capacity to resting left ventricular performance and basal plasma norepinephrine levels in patients with congestive heart failure. Am Heart J 1982; 104: 725–731.
17. Franciosa JA, Park M, Levine TB. Lack of correlation between exercise capacity and indexes of resting left ventricular performance in heart failure. Am J Cardiol 1981; 47: 33–39.
18. Chua TP, Clark AL, Amadi AA, Coats AJ. Relation between chemosensitivity and the ventilatory response to exercise in chronic heart failure. J Am Coll Cardiol 1996; 27: 650–657.
19. Ponikowski P, Francis DP, Piepoli MF, *et al.* Enhanced ventilatory response to exercise in patients with

chronic heart failure and preserved exercise tolerance: marker of abnormal cardiorespiratory reflex control and predictor of poor prognosis. Circulation 2001; 103: 967–972.
20. Wasserman K, Casaburi R. Dyspnea: physiological and pathophysiological mechanisms. Annu Rev Med 1988; 39: 503–515.
21. Adams L, Chronos N, Lane R, Guz A. The measurement of breathlessness induced in normal subjects: individual differences. Clin Sci (Lond) 1986; 70: 131–140.
22. Nohria A, Lewis E, Stevenson LW. Medical management of advanced heart failure. JAMA 2002; 287: 628–640.
23. Wilson JR, Fink L, Maris J, *et al*. Evaluation of energy metabolism in skeletal muscle of patients with heart failure with gated phosphorus-31 nuclear magnetic resonance. Circulation 1985; 71: 57–62.
24. Massie B, Conway M, Yonge R, *et al*. Skeletal muscle metabolism in patients with congestive heart failure: relation to clinical severity and blood flow. Circulation 1987; 76: 1009–1019.
25. Massie BM, Conway M, Yonge R, *et al*. 31P nuclear magnetic resonance evidence of abnormal skeletal muscle metabolism in patients with congestive heart failure. Am J Cardiol 1987; 60: 309–315.
26. Koenig HG. Depression in hospitalized older patients with congestive heart failure. Gen Hosp Psychiatry 1998; 20: 29–43.
27. Murberg TA, Bru E, Svebak S, Tveteras R, Aarsland T. Depressed mood and subjective health symptoms as predictors of mortality in patients with congestive heart failure: a two-year follow-up study. Int J Psychiatry Med 1999; 29: 311–326.
28. Freedland KE, Rich MW, Skala JA, *et al*. Prevalence of depression in hospitalized patients with congestive heart failure. Psychosom Med 2003; 65: 119–128.
29. Dracup K, Walden JA, Stevenson LW, Brecht ML. Quality of life in patients with advanced heart failure. J Heart Lung Transplant 1992; 11: 273–279.
30. Friedman MM, Griffin JA. Relationship of physical symptoms and physical functioning to depression in patients with heart failure. Heart Lung 2001; 30: 98–104.
31. Zuccala G, Cattel C, Manes-Gravina E, *et al*. Left ventricular dysfunction: a clue to cognitive impairment in older patients with heart failure. J Neurol Neurosurg Psychiatry 1997; 63: 509–512.
32. Cacciatore F, Abete P, Ferrara N, *et al*. Congestive heart failure and cognitive impairment in an older population. Osservatorio Geriatrico Campano Study Group. J Am Geriatr Soc 1998; 46: 1343–1348.
33. Taylor J, Stott DJ. Chronic heart failure and cognitive impairment: co-existence of conditions or true association? Eur J Heart Fail 2002; 4: 7–9.
34. Bradley TD, Floras JS. Sleep apnea and heart failure: Part I: obstructive sleep apnea. Circulation 2003; 107: 1671–1678.
35. Javaheri S, Parker TJ, Liming JD, *et al*. Sleep apnea in 81 ambulatory male patients with stable heart failure: types and their prevalences, consequences, and presentations. Circulation 1998; 97: 2154–2159.
36. Sin DD, Fitzgerald F, Parker JD, *et al*. Risk factors for central and obstructive sleep apnea in 450 men and women with congestive heart failure. Am J Respir Crit Care Med 1999; 160: 1101–1106.
37. Harrison TR, King CE, Calhoun JA, Harrison WG. Congestive heart failure: Cheyne-Stokes respiration as the cause of dyspnea at onset of sleep. Arch Intern Med 1934; 53: 891–910.
38. Bradley TD, Floras JS. Sleep apnea and heart failure: Part II: central sleep apnea. Circulation 2003; 107: 1822–1826.
39. Lanfranchi PA, Braghiroli A, Bosimini E, *et al*. Prognostic value of nocturnal Cheyne-Stokes respiration in chronic heart failure. Circulation 1999; 99: 1435–1440.
40. Sin DD, Logan AG, Fitzgerald FS, Liu PP, Bradley TD. Effects of continuous positive airway pressure on cardiovascular outcomes in heart failure patients with and without Cheyne-Stokes respiration. Circulation 2000; 102: 61–66.
41. Bradley TD, Logan AG, Floras JS. Rationale and design of the Canadian Continuous Positive Airway Pressure Trial for Congestive Heart Failure patients with Central Sleep Apnea—CANPAP. Can J Cardiol 2001; 17: 677–684.
42. Mosterd A, Deckers JW, Hoes AW, *et al*. Classification of heart failure in population based research: an assessment of six heart failure scores. Eur J Epidemiol 1997; 13: 491–502.
43. Tsuyuki RT, McKelvie RS, Arnold JM, *et al*. Acute precipitants of congestive heart failure exacerbations. Arch Intern Med 2001; 161: 2337–2342.
44. Feenstra J, Heerdink ER, Grobbee DE, Stricker BH. Association of nonsteroidal anti-inflammatory drugs with first occurrence of heart failure and with relapsing heart failure: the Rotterdam Study. Arch Intern Med 2002; 162: 265–270.
45. Garcia Rodriguez LA, Hernandez-Diaz S. Nonsteroidal antiinflammatory drugs as a trigger of clinical heart failure. Epidemiology 2003; 14: 240–246.
46. Spencer KT, Anderson AS, Bhargava A, *et al*. Physician-performed point-of-care echocardiography using a laptop platform compared with physical

examination in the cardiovascular patient. J Am Coll Cardiol 2001; 37: 2013–2018.
47. Maisel AS, Krishnaswamy P, Nowak RM, *et al*. Rapid measurement of B-type natriuretic peptide in the emergency diagnosis of heart failure. N Engl J Med 2002; 347: 161–167.
48. St. Clair EW, Oddone EZ, Waugh RA, Corey GR, Feussner JR. Assessing housestaff diagnostic skills using a cardiology patient simulator. Ann Intern Med 1992; 117: 751–756.
49. Mangione S, Nieman LZ. Cardiac auscultatory skills of internal medicine and family practice trainees: a comparison of diagnostic proficiency. JAMA 1997; 278: 717–722.
50. Mangione S. Cardiac auscultatory skills of physicians-in-training: a comparison of three English-speaking countries. Am J Med 2001; 110: 210–216.
51. Craige E. Should auscultation be rehabilitated? N Engl J Med 1988; 318: 1611–1613.
52. Fletcher RH, Fletcher SW. Has medicine outgrown physical diagnosis? Ann Intern Med 1992; 117: 786–787.
53. Adolph RJ. In defense of the stethoscope. Chest 1998; 114: 1235–1237.
54. Weitz HH, Mangione S. In defense of the stethoscope and the bedside. Am J Med 2000; 108: 669–671.
55. Khot UN, Jia G, Moliterno DJ, *et al*. Prognostic importance of physical examination for heart failure in non-ST-elevation acute coronary syndromes: the enduring value of Killip classification. JAMA 2003; 290: 2174–2181.
56. Drazner MH, Rame JE, Dries DL. Third heart sound and elevated jugular venous pressure as markers of the subsequent development of heart failure in patients with asymptomatic left ventricular dysfunction. Am J Med 2003; 114: 431–437.
57. Drazner MH, Rame JE, Stevenson LW, Dries DL. Prognostic importance of elevated jugular venous pressure and a third heart sound in patients with heart failure. N Engl J Med 2001; 345: 574–581.
58. Brophy JM, Dagenais GR, McSherry F, Williford W, Yusuf S. A multivariate model for predicting mortality in patients with heart failure and systolic dysfunction. Am J Med 2004; 116: 300–304.
59. Rame JE, Dries DL, Drazner MH. The prognostic value of the physical examination in patients with chronic heart failure. Congest Heart Fail 2003; 9: 170–175, 178.
60. Leier CV, Young JB, Levine TB, *et al*. Nuggets, pearls, and vignettes of master heart failure clinicians. Part 2—the physical examination. Congest Heart Fail 2001; 7: 297–308.
61. Rouleau JL, Roecker EB, Tendera M, *et al*. Influence of pretreatment systolic blood pressure on the effect of carvedilol in patients with severe chronic heart failure: the Carvedilol Prospective Randomized Cumulative Survival (COPERNICUS) study. J Am Coll Cardiol 2004; 43: 1423–1429.
62. Stevenson LW, Perloff JK. The limited reliability of physical signs for estimating hemodynamics in chronic heart failure. JAMA 1989; 261: 884–888.
63. Aronson D, Burger AJ. Relation between pulse pressure and survival in patients with decompensated heart failure. Am J Cardiol 2004; 93: 785–788.
64. Gorlin R, Knowles JH, Storey CF. The Valsalva maneuver as a test of cardiac function. Am J Med 1957; 22: 197–212.
65. Zema MJ. Heart failure and the bedside Valsalva maneuver. Chest 1990; 97: 772–773.
66. Bernardi L, Saviolo R, Spodick DH. Do hemodynamic responses to the Valsalva maneuver reflect myocardial dysfunction? Chest 1989; 95: 986–991.
67. Schmidt DE, Shah PK. Accurate detection of elevated left ventricular filling pressure by a simplified bedside application of the Valsalva maneuver. Am J Cardiol 1993; 71: 462–465.
68. Givertz MM, Slawsky MT, Moraes DL, McIntyre KM, Colucci WS. Noninvasive determination of pulmonary artery wedge pressure in patients with chronic heart failure. Am J Cardiol 2001; 87: 1213–1215, A1217.
69. Rocca HP, Weilenmann D, Rickli H, Follath F, Kiowski W. Is blood pressure response to the Valsalva maneuver related to neurohormones, exercise capacity, and clinical findings in heart failure? Chest 1999; 116: 861–867.
70. Kodama M, Kato K, Hirono S, *et al*. Mechanical alternans in patients with chronic heart failure. J Card Fail 2001; 7: 138–145.
71. Butman SM, Ewy GA, Standen JR, Kern KB, Hahn E. Bedside cardiovascular examination in patients with severe chronic heart failure: importance of rest or inducible jugular venous distension. J Am Coll Cardiol 1993; 22: 968–974.
72. Drazner MH, Hamilton MA, Fonarow G, *et al*. Relationship between right and left-sided filling pressures in 1000 patients with advanced heart failure. J Heart Lung Transplant 1999; 18: 1126–1132.
73. Perloff JK. Physical Examination of the Heart and Circulation (W.B. Saunders: Philadelphia, PA, 2000).
74. Forrester JS, Diamond G, McHugh TJ, Swan HJ. Filling pressures in the right and left sides of the heart in acute myocardial infarction: a reappraisal of

central-venous-pressure monitoring. N Engl J Med 1971; 285: 190–193.
75. Ewy GA. The abdominojugular test: technique and hemodynamic correlates. Ann Intern Med 1988; 109: 456–460.
76. Slanetz PJ, Truong M, Shepard JA, *et al.* Mediastinal lymphadenopathy and hazy mediastinal fat: new CT findings of congestive heart failure. AJR Am J Roentgenol 1998; 171: 1307–1309.
77. Ngom A, Dumont P, Diot P, Lemarie E. Benign mediastinal lymphadenopathy in congestive heart failure. Chest 2001; 119: 653–656.
78. Rosario LB, Stevenson LW, Solomon SD, Lee RT, Reimold SC. The mechanism of decrease in dynamic mitral regurgitation during heart failure treatment: importance of reduction in the regurgitant orifice size. J Am Coll Cardiol 1998; 32: 1819–1824.
79. Bolling SF, Pagani FD, Deeb GM, Bach DS. Intermediate-term outcome of mitral reconstruction in cardiomyopathy. J Thorac Cardiovasc Surg 1998; 115: 381–386; discussion 387–388.
80. Shah PM, Yu, PN. Gallop rhythm: hemodynamic and clinical correlation. Am Heart J 1969; 78: 823–828.
81. Van de Werf F, Boel A, Geboers J, *et al.* Diastolic properties of the left ventricle in normal adults and in patients with third heart sounds. Circulation 1984; 69: 1070–1078.
82. Ishimitsu T, Smith D, Berko B, Craige E. Origin of the third heart sound: comparison of ventricular wall dynamics in hyperdynamic and hypodynamic types. J Am Coll Cardiol 1985; 5: 268–272.
83. Folland ED, Kriegel BJ, Henderson WG, Hammermeister KE, Sethi GK. Implications of third heart sounds in patients with valvular heart disease. The Veterans Affairs Cooperative Study on Valvular Heart Disease. N Engl J Med 1992; 327: 458–462.
84. Sloan AW, Campbell FW, Henderson AS. Incidence of the physiological third heart sound. Br Med J 1952; 2: 853–855.
85. Ishmail AA, Wing S, Ferguson J, *et al.* Interobserver agreement by auscultation in the presence of a third heart sound in patients with congestive heart failure. Chest 1987; 91: 870–873.
86. Gadsboll N, Hoilund-Carlsen PF, Nielsen GG, *et al.* Symptoms and signs of heart failure in patients with myocardial infarction: reproducibility and relationship to chest X-ray, radionuclide ventriculography and right heart catheterization. Eur Heart J 1989; 10: 1017–1028.
87. Westman EC, Matchar DB, Samsa GP, *et al.* Accuracy and reliability of apical S3 gallop detection. J Gen Intern Med 1995; 10: 455–457.
88. Lok CE, Morgan CD, Ranganathan N. The accuracy and interobserver agreement in detecting the 'gallop sounds' by cardiac auscultation. Chest 1998; 114: 1283–1288.
89. Marcus GM, Michaels AD, De Marco T, McCulloch CE, Chatterjee K. Usefulness of the third heart sound in predicting an elevated level of B-type natriuretic peptide. Am J Cardiol 2004; 93: 1312–1313.
90. Chakko S, Woska D, Martinez H, *et al.* Clinical, radiographic, and hemodynamic correlations in chronic congestive heart failure: conflicting results may lead to inappropriate care. Am J Med 1991; 90: 353–359.
91. Badgett RG, Lucey CR, Mulrow CD. Can the clinical examination diagnose left-sided heart failure in adults? JAMA 1997; 277: 1712–1719.
92. Teerlink JR. Clinical trial design in heart failure. In: Mann DL (ed.) Heart Failure: A Companion to Braunwald's Heart Disease (W.B. Saunders Company: Philadelphia, PA, 2004), 534–566.
93. Teerlink JR. Dyspnea as an endpoint in clinical trials of therapies for acute decompensated heart failure. Am Heart J 2003; 145: S26–S33.
94. United States Department of Health and Human Services. Food and Drug Administration. Center for Drug Evaluation and Research. Transcript of the 86th Meeting of the Cardiovascular and Renal Drugs Advisory Committee. Thursday, October 22, 1998. Available at: http://www.fda.gov/ohrms/dockets/ac/98/transcpt/3462t1.pdf. Accessed November 30, 2004.
95. Committee for Proprietary Medicinal Products (CPMP). Note for Guidance on Clinical Investigation of Medicinal Products for the Treatment of Cardiac Failure. Addendum on Acute Cardiac Failure (Draft; Report CPMP/EWP/2986/03/draft) (EMEA, The European Agency for the Evaluation of Medicinal Products: London, 2003).
96. Gheorghiade M, Adams KF, Gattis WA, *et al.* Surrogate endpoints in heart failure trials. Am Heart J 2003; 145: S67–S70.
97. Gomes UC, Cleland JG. Heart failure update. Eur J Heart Fail 1999; 1: 301–302.
98. Jones CG, Cleland JG. Meeting report—the LIDO, HOPE, MOXCON and WASH studies. Heart Outcomes Prevention Evaluation. The Warfarin/Aspirin Study of Heart Failure. Eur J Heart Fail 1999; 1: 425–431.
99. Cuffe MS, Califf RM, Adams KF Jr., *et al.* Rationale and design of the OPTIME–CHF trial: outcomes of a prospective trial of intravenous milrinone for

exacerbations of chronic heart failure. Am Heart J 2000; 139: 15–22.

100. Cuffe MS, Califf RM, Adams KF Jr., *et al*. Short-term intravenous milrinone for acute exacerbation of chronic heart failure: a randomized controlled trial. JAMA 2002; 287: 1541–1547.

101. Packer M, Colucci WS, Fisher L, *et al*. Development of a comprehensive new endpoint for the evaluation of new treatments for acute decompensated heart failure: results with levosimendan in the REVIVE-1 study. J Card Fail 2003; 9: S61 (Abstract).

102. Packer M. Proposal for a new clinical endpoint to evaluate the efficacy of drugs and devices in the treatment of chronic heart failure. J Card Fail 2001; 7: 176–182.

103. Ambrosino N, Scano G. Measurement and treatment of dyspnoea. Respir Med 2001; 95: 539–547.

104. Fletcher C. The clinical diagnosis of pulmonary emphysema: an experimental study. Proc Res Soc Med 1952; 45: 577–584.

105. Fletcher C, Elmes PC, Wood CH. The significance of respiratory symptoms and the diagnosis of chronic bronchitis in a working population. Br Med J 1959; 1: 257–266.

106. McGavin CR, Artvinli M, Naoe H, McHardy GJ. Dyspnoea, disability, and distance walked: comparison of estimates of exercise performance in respiratory disease. Br Med J 1978; 2: 241–243.

107. Mahler DA, Weinberg DH, Wells CK, Feinstein AR. The measurement of dyspnea: contents, interobserver agreement, and physiologic correlates of two new clinical indexes. Chest 1984; 85: 751–758.

108. Mahler DA, Rosiello RA, Harver A, *et al*. Comparison of clinical dyspnea ratings and psychophysical measurements of respiratory sensation in obstructive airway disease. Am Rev Respir Dis 1987; 135: 1229–1233.

109. Mahler DA, Harver A, Rosiello R, Daubenspeck JA. Measurement of respiratory sensation in interstitial lung disease: evaluation of clinical dyspnea ratings and magnitude scaling. Chest 1989; 96: 767–771.

110. Mahler DA, Matthay RA, Snyder PE, Wells CK, Loke J. Sustained-release theophylline reduces dyspnea in nonreversible obstructive airway disease. Am Rev Respir Dis 1985; 131: 22–25.

111. Eakin EG, Kaplan RM, Ries AL. Measurement of dyspnoea in chronic obstructive pulmonary disease. Qual Life Res 1993; 2: 181–191.

112. Eakin EG, Prewitt LM, Ries AL, Kaplan RM. Validation of the UCSD shortness of breath questionnaire. J Cardiopulm Rehab 1994; 14: 322–329.

113. Borg G. Perceived exertion as an indicator of somatic stress. Scand J Rehabil Med 1970; 2: 92–98.

114. Borg G. Simple rating methods for estimation of perceived exertion. Wenner-Gren Center International Symposium Series 1976; 28: 39–47.

115. Guyatt GH, Townsend M, Berman LB, Keller JL. A comparison of Likert and visual analogue scales for measuring change in function. J Chronic Dis 1987; 40: 1129–1133.

116. Grant S, Aitchison T, Henderson E, *et al*. A comparison of the reproducibility and the sensitivity to change of visual analogue scales, Borg scales, and Likert scales in normal subjects during submaximal exercise. Chest 1999; 116: 1208–1217.

117. Simon PM, Schwartzstein RM, Weiss JW, *et al*. Distinguishable types of dyspnea in patients with shortness of breath. Am Rev Respir Dis 1990; 142: 1009–1014.

118. Elliott MW, Adams L, Cockcroft A, *et al*. The language of breathlessness: use of verbal descriptors by patients with cardiopulmonary disease. Am Rev Respir Dis 1991; 144: 826–832.

119. Hardie GE, Janson S, Gold WM, Carrieri-Kohlman V, Boushey HA. Ethnic differences: word descriptors used by African-American and white asthma patients during induced bronchoconstriction. Chest 2000; 117: 935–943.

120. Colucci WS, Elkayam U, Horton DP, *et al*. Intravenous nesiritide, a natriuretic peptide, in the treatment of decompensated congestive heart failure. Nesiritide Study Group. N Engl J Med 2000; 343: 246–253.

121. Slawsky MT, Colucci WS, Gottlieb SS, *et al*. Acute hemodynamic and clinical effects of levosimendan in patients with severe heart failure. Study Investigators. Circulation 2000; 102: 2222–2227.

122. Torre-Amione G, Durand JB, Nagueh S, *et al*. A pilot safety trial of prolonged (48 h) infusion of the dual endothelin-receptor antagonist tezosentan in patients with advanced heart failure. Chest 2001; 120: 460–466.

123. Torre-Amione G, Young JB, Durand J, *et al*. Hemodynamic effects of tezosentan, an intravenous dual endothelin receptor antagonist, in patients with class III to IV congestive heart failure. Circulation 2001; 103: 973–980.

124. Torre-Amione G, Young JB, Colucci WS, *et al*. Hemodynamic and clinical effects of tezosentan, an intravenous dual endothelin receptor antagonist, in patients hospitalized for acute decompensated heart failure. J Am Coll Cardiol 2003; 42: 140–147.

125. United States Department of Health and Human Services. Food and Drug Administration. Center for Drug Evaluation and Research. Division of Cardio-

renal Drug Products. Transcript of the 87th Meeting of the Cardiovascular and Renal Drugs Advisory Committee. Friday, January 29, 1999. Available at: http://www.fda.gov/ohrms/dockets/ac/99/transcpt/3490t2.rtf. Accessed November 30, 2004.

126. Publication Committee for the VMAC Investigators. Intravenous nesiritide vs nitroglycerin for treatment of decompensated congestive heart failure: a randomized controlled trial. JAMA 2002; 287: 1531–1540.

127. Young JB, on behalf of VMAC Study Group. Sustained symptom improvement with nesiritide (B-type natriuretic peptide) compared to iv nitroglycerin in patients with acute decompensated heart failure. Circulation 2001; 104: II525 (Abstract).

128. Coletta AP, Cleland JG. Clinical trials update: highlights of the scientific sessions of the XXIII Congress of the European Society of Cardiology—WARIS II, ESCAMI, PAFAC, RITZ-1 and TIME. Eur J Heart Fail 2001; 3: 747–750.

CHAPTER 10

Biologic markers in acute heart failure

G Michael Felker, Adrian F Hernandez, Alan Maisel

What is a Biomarker?

In the most general terms, *biomarker* refers to a measurable biologic variable that is useful in the care of patients. In this sense, many traditional clinical variables, such as blood pressure, heart rate, or hemoglobin concentration could be considered biomarkers, although they are not frequently referred to as such. In common usage, *biomarker* has come to refer to measurable circulating factors that reflect ongoing physiologic or pathophysiologic processes and thus provide insight into diagnosis and management.

Some biomarkers, such as prostate specific antigen (PSA) in oncology and troponin in cardiology, have been well validated and have become widely accepted as important clinical tools. This success has led to great enthusiasm for investigation of the potential role of other biomarkers in other areas of medicine. Several features of heart failure make the identification of a useful biomarker for this disorder particularly appealing. The diagnosis of heart failure is based on the presence of an array of signs and symptoms, ranging from the readily apparent to the extremely subtle. Although multiple sets of diagnostic criteria have been proposed, there is still no "gold standard" for making the diagnosis. Despite a large body of research into risk stratification and prognostication in heart failure, triage of patients among available therapies remains highly subjective and imperfect.

In general, biomarkers have been evaluated used for five distinct purposes:

1. Detection of pre-clinical disease in asymptomatic persons—*screening*.
2. Diagnosis of clinical disease in patients with symptoms of uncertain cause—*diagnosis*.
3. Evaluation of prognosis in patients with clinical disease—*risk stratification*.
4. Guiding selection or titration of therapies in patients with known disease—*disease management*.
5. Serving as a surrogate endpoint in research studies.

All these potential applications have obvious relevance to the field of heart failure. In this context, this chapter will focus on current data on the uses of a variety of biomarkers in the diagnosis and management of patients with acute decompensated heart failure (ADHF), as well as new developments in genomics and proteomics that may speed identification of new biomarkers for this syndrome.

Natriuretic Peptides

Pathophysiology of heart failure and the natriuretic peptide family

The activation of physiologic compensatory mechanisms subsequent to myocardial injury, including the renin-angiotensin-aldosterone system (RAAS), the natriuretic peptide system, the sympathetic nervous system (SNS), endothelins, and other neurohormonal factors, has been well documented. The subsequent development of heart failure is complicated by a complex balance between vasodilatory and vasoconstrictive influences. Natriuresis, diuresis, and vasodilatory mechanisms work to relieve stress on the heart, but are essentially overwhelmed by the RAAS, SNS, and endothelins, leading to peripheral vasoconstriction and hemodynamic alterations. The end result is progressive deterioration of heart function with worsened symptoms of heart failure (i.e., dyspnea, peripheral edema, tachycardia, and volume overload). All three major natriuretic peptides share a common 17-amino-acid ring structure; atrial (A-type) natriuretic peptide (ANP) and brain (B-type) natriuretic peptide (BNP) are of myocardial cell origin, and C-type natriuretic peptide (CNP) is of endothelial origin.[1–3] All three peptides are secreted in an attempt to correct the vasoconstrictive, sodium-retaining, antidiuretic, and antifibrotic effects caused by the neurohormonal imbalance.

The major source of plasma BNP is the cardiac ventricles. This is unlike ANP, whose major storage sites include both the atria and ventricles.[3] Unlike ANP, which is mainly released from its storage granules in response to atrial wall tension, BNP (as the nucleic acid sequence of the *preproBNP* gene with high turnover of messenger RNA [mRNA] suggests) is synthesized in bursts by increased gene expression owing to stretch stimulus to the ventricular wall as preproBNP (132 amino acids) and then released in direct proportion to ventricular volume expansion and pressure overload from ventricular myocytes as a 76 amino acid N-terminal fragment (NT-BNP) and a 32 amino acid active hormone (BNP)[1,4,5]

Since ANP is stored in granules and released episodically, a minor stimulus, like exercise, can trigger the release of significant amounts of ANP into the bloodstream.[6] In contrast, BNP levels show only minor changes with vigorous exercise, making it unlikely that a normal patient would be classified as having congestive heart failure (CHF) based on a BNP level obtained after activity.[7] This suggests that BNP may be a more sensitive and specific indicator of ventricular disorders than other natriuretic peptides.[8] BNP levels accurately reflect the decompensated state of circulatory congestion.[9] BNP has been found to be an independent predictor of high left ventricular end-diastolic pressure (LVEDP) and is more useful than ANP or other neurohormones for assessing mortality in patients with chronic CHF.[9] The half-life of BNP is 22 minutes, and prior studies have established that BNP can accurately reflect pulmonary capillary wedge pressure (PCWP) changes every 2 hours.[10,11]

B-type natriuretic peptide in the diagnosis of heart failure

Shortness of breath is one of the most common presenting complaints to acute care settings. The presence of other comorbidities, such as chronic obstructive pulmonary disease (COPD), and the variability in physical findings of heart failure can led to substantial difficulties in making a definitive diagnosis in such patients. This clinical dilemma has led to substantial enthusiasm for BNP as an aid in the evaluation of patients presenting with unexplained dyspnea. In an initial study evaluating the role of BNP measurement in patients with unexplained dyspnea, Dao *et al.* found that BNP was a powerful predictor of a final diagnosis of heart failure (as determined by two cardiologists blinded to BNP results), with a plasma concentration of < 80 pg/mL having a negative predictive value of 98%.[12] A larger, multicenter prospective study using similar methodology, the Breathing Not Properly (BNP) Multinational study, confirmed the substantial value of BNP as an adjunct to the diagnosis of heart failure, and identified 100 pg/mL as the cut-off that maximized sensitivity and specificity based on receiver operator characteristic (ROC) curves.[13] Similar diagnostic utility of natriuretic peptide measurements have been demonstrated for levels of the inactive NT-BNP fragment, although optimal cut-off values differ for different assays.[14] Data from the Breathing Not Properly study suggest that BNP is more useful than other elements of the clinical evaluation in establishing a diagnosis of heart failure, but is most effective when combined with other components of the evaluation.[15] Recent data have also suggested that incorporation of BNP measurements into a diagnostic strategy may result in a significant reduction in health care costs.[16]

Enthusiasm for the measurement of natriuretic peptides in the diagnosis of heart failure must be tempered with an understanding of the potential limitations of the test. There is substantial overlap between ranges of BNP for patients with and without a final diagnosis of heart failure, potentially limiting the use of these measurements in an individual patient with intermediate levels of BNP. Available data suggest that BNP is particularly useful when values are low, making a diagnosis of decompensated heart failure as an explanation of dyspnea very unlikely (i.e., high negative predictive value). Traditional Bayesian analysis demonstrates that diagnostic testing is most useful in patients with an intermediate pre-test probability of the disease in question, suggesting that BNP levels are unlikely to alter the diagnosis in patients with a very high or low likelihood of heart failure based on routine clinical evaluation. Although BNP appears to be a useful adjunct to the diagnosis of heart failure, results of such testing must be interpreted in the context of the overall clinical evaluation, and such testing must augment rather than supersede careful clinical reasoning.[17]

BNP levels in hospitalized patients

It appears that BNP levels may be useful in targeting treatment of hospitalized CHF patients. Targeting treatment of disease using biomarkers has precedents—treatment of hypertension is targeted to blood pressure, diabetes to blood sugar, and hypercholesterolemia to cholesterol levels. The fact that BNP has a short half-life; has easy-to-measure levels; and is a surrogate for wedge pressure, volume, New York Heart Association (NYHA) functional class, and prognosis suggests its usefulness as a guide to therapy in heart failure.

Cheng *et al.* followed the course of 72 patients admitted with decompensated CHF using daily BNP levels and their relationship to 30-day readmission rates or death.[18] Patients who were most likely to have a cardiac event had higher BNP levels both at the time of admission and at discharge (Figure 10.1). Only 16% of patients with falling BNP levels during hospitalization had a subsequent cardiac event; whereas 52% of those with rising BNP levels during treatment had either readmission or cardiac death. Patients whose discharge BNP levels fell below 430 pg/mL had a reasonable likelihood of not being readmitted within the following 30 days. These data were supported by a recent study by Bettencourt *et al.* who found that failure of BNP levels to fall over the hospitalization

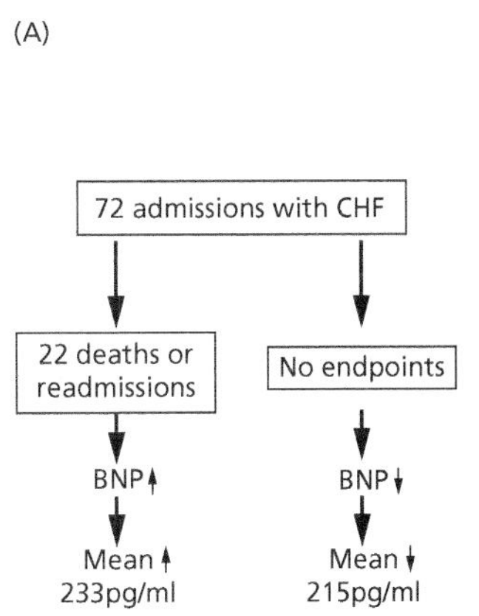

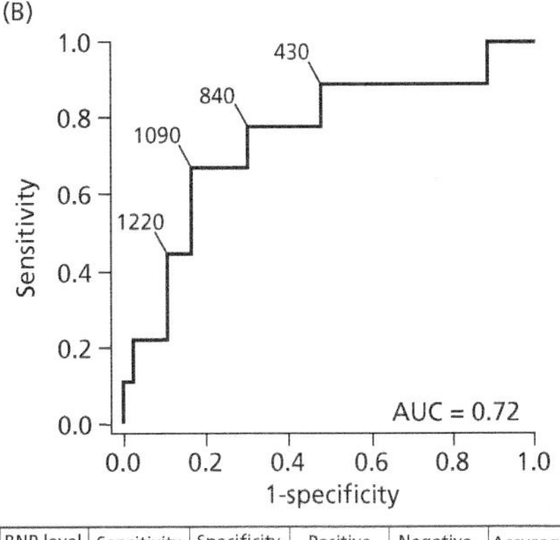

BNP level (pg/ml)	Sensitivity	Specificity	Positive predictive value	Negative predictive value	Accuracy (%)
430	89 (48–107)	52 (37–66)	25 (11–44)	96 (80–100)	58
800	78 (35–104)	68 (53–80)	30 (13–54)	94 (81–99)	69
950	67 (24–99)	74 (59–85)	31 (11–58)	92 (79–98)	92
1220	44 (7–55)	90 (78–85)	44 (7–85)	90 (78–90)	83

Figure 10.1. *Change in B-type natriuretic peptide (A) and outcome in decompensated heart failure (B) (With permission from Cheng* et al.[18])

period predicted death or rehospitalization and that discharge levels < 250 pg/mL predicted event-free survival.[19]

Does high BNP always mean high filling pressure?

Since a major stimulus for the release of BNP is increased wall tension, one might expect that BNP levels would correlate with elevated LV filling pressures. Indeed, there is a body of data to support that supposition. However, in the clinical setting, there are many occasions where a high BNP level is not associated with high filling pressures. Some of these situations include BNP elevations from right-sided failure secondary to cor pulmonale, pulmonary embolism, or primary or secondary pulmonary hypertension; acute or chronic renal failure; and rapid lowering of the wedge pressure with diuretics or vasodilators before a Swan–Ganz catheter is placed. Additionally, under some circumstances, BNP levels might be normal when the wedge pressure is high. This would most likely occur in acute mitral regurgitation (MR), where the increase in capillary pressure is upstream from the left ventricle, and in *flash* pulmonary edema, where the BNP might not have had time to be synthesized.

In a given patient, the BNP level does not always correlate to wedge pressure. However, in a patient admitted with CHF and high filling pressures secondary to volume overload, along with a high BNP level ("wet BNP"), a treatment-induced decrease in wedge pressure will almost always be associated with a rapid drop in BNP levels, as long as the patient is maintaining adequate urine output. Kazanegra *et al.* measured wedge pressure, hemodynamic measurements (PCWP, cardiac output, right atrial pressure, systemic vascular resistance [SVR]) and BNP levels every 2 to 4 hours for the first 24 hours and every 4 hours for the next 24 to 48 hours in patients admitted for decompensated CHF.[20] PCWP dropped from 33±2 mm Hg to 25±2 mm Hg over the first 24 hours, while BNP dropped from 1472±156 pg/mL to 670±109 pg/mL (Figure 10.2). The correlation between BNP levels and other indices of cardiac function-cardiac output (thermodilution), mixed venous oxygen saturation, and SVR was non-significant. It should be emphasized that patients with end-stage CHF admitted for transplant workup who are not acutely volume overloaded may not show a drop in BNP levels as the wedge pressure is lowered ("dry BNP").

Wet and dry BNP levels

The BNP level of a patient who is admitted with decompensated heart failure comprises two components: that of a baseline, euvolemic "dry BNP" level and that occurring from acute pressure or volume overload ("wet BNP" level). Figure 10.3 shows a hypothetical plot of dry BNP levels, NYHA class, and what happens when a patient decompensates. At the point of decompensation, a patient's BNP level will be a sum of their baseline BNP level plus what volume overload adds.

The lower the discharge "dry weight" BNP level is, the less likely the patient will be an early victim

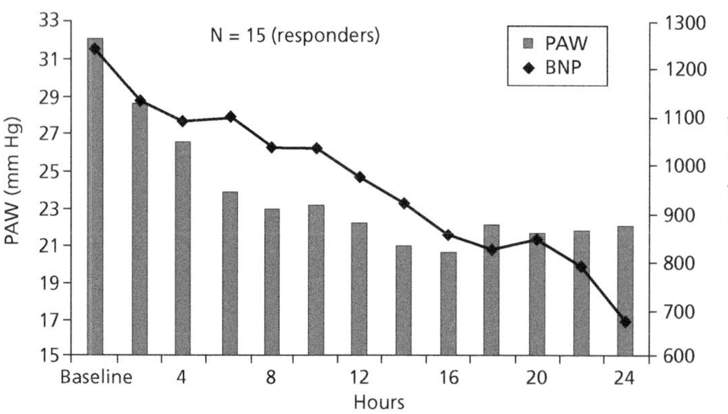

Figure 10.2. *Changes in B-type natriuretic peptide and pulmonary artery wedge levels during 24 hours of treatment (With permission from Kazanegra* et al.[20])

Abbreviations: BNP = B-type natriuretic peptide; PAW = pulmonary artery wedge.

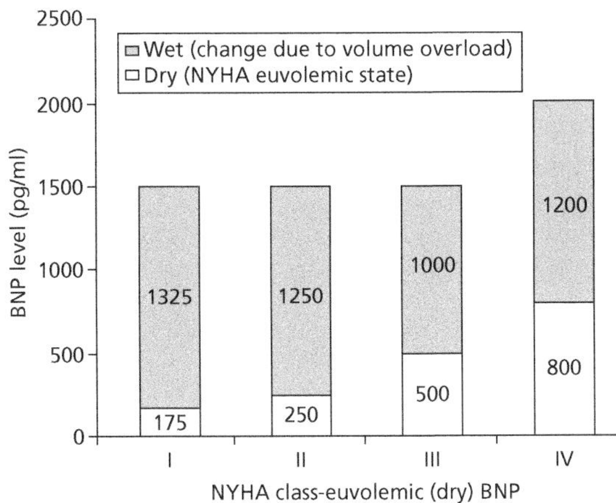

Figure 10.3. *In volume overloaded patients: B-type natriuretic peptide (BNP) level = baseline BNP (dry) plus change due to increase volume (wet)*

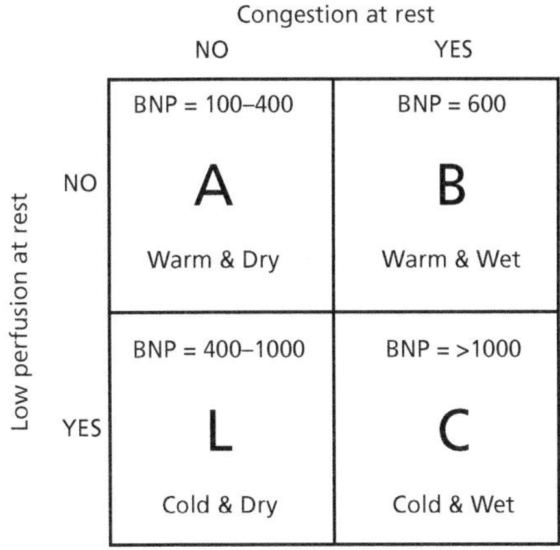

Figure 10.4. *B-type natriuretic peptide levels and rapid assessment of hemodynamic status. (With permission from Stevenson* et al.[21])

to rehospitalization. This is because a low BNP level (<200–300 pg/mL) represents a NYHA II patient and one that is more likely to be in a true euvolemic state. Knowing a patients' baseline "dry weight" BNP level is likely to be important in monitoring the patient in the first 30 days after discharge. Early elevations of BNP over baseline soon after discharge may trigger the need for more vigorous diuresis, additional vasodilators, or possibly outpatient Natrecor infusions.

Lynn Warner Stevenson has published a rapid assessment of hemodynamic status in order to stratify patients to treatment to diuretics, vasodilators, or inotropic agents.[21] We have updated this assessment by adding BNP ranges to this risk stratification scheme (Figure 10.4). Patients who are admitted to the hospital with either new onset or decompensated CHF are usually volume overloaded. Treatment in this setting includes diuretics and vasodilators when patients are "wet and warm." In our experience, almost all these patients have BNP levels > 600 pg/mL. In fact, if BNP levels were less than this, one would wonder how "wet" the patient truly was. Diuretics, inotropes, and vasopressors are often indicated when patients are classified as "wet and cold." These patients frequently have BNP levels > 1000 pg/mL. Patients that are "cold and dry" have BNP elevations secondary to systolic dysfunction, but perhaps BNP levels are not as high as the "cold and wet" patients. Finally, patients who are "warm and dry" are likely to have lesser elevations of BNP levels.

What if a BNP level does not fall with hospitalization?

There may be several explanations why elevated BNP levels do not fall with treatment in some patients with CHF. First and foremost, the high BNP level may actually be the patient's "dry" BNP level and will not be acutely lowered with diuretics or vasodilators. These patients tend to be NYHA class IV and have a poor prognosis.

Perhaps patients who have high BNP levels that do not respond to treatment should be considered for other more invasive types of therapies such as cardiac transplantation or use of ventricular assist devices. Patients with a wide QRS might be considered for biventricular pacing. In a recent trial of patients who received ventricular assist devices for end-stage heart failure, BNP levels appeared to fall as remodeling of the heart occurred, and an early decrease in BNP plasma concentration was indicative of recovery of cardiac function during mechanical circulatory support.[22] In any event, patients with high BNP levels at discharge are at increased risk, and if nothing else, are candidates for early follow-up and perhaps home nursing visits.

There are other reasons why a BNP level might not fall with treatment. It is possible that with parenteral diuretic treatment of the decompensated, pre-renal patient, further azotemia might occur. This will likely down-regulate BNP clearance receptors, and BNP levels will rise. In this setting, nesiritide infusions might be indicated. Another possible scenario is that a patient with left along with right heart failure and significant ascites and/or edema, may often diurese many liters before BNP levels actually drop. This is possibly because rather than lowering wedge pressure, the urine output is occurring secondary to mobilization of third-space fluid. Continuing diuresis or vasodilatation should eventually lower BNP levels. Finally, acute, severe pressure or volume overload might turn on the transcription of the mRNA for BNP to such a degree, that even upon initial lowering of the wedge pressure, BNP levels might sill be increasing.

Troponins

The troponin complex consists of three protein subunits: troponin I, troponin T, and troponin C. These proteins play a key role in regulating calcium-mediated muscle contraction through the interaction of actin monomers with myosin heavy chains. Troponin I prevents contraction in the absence of calcium through the inhibition of adenosine triphosphatase (ATPase) activity of the actin-myosin interaction. Troponin T is responsible for binding the troponin complex to tropomyosin.[23] In the early 1990s, serum measurements of troponin I and T were discovered to be highly sensitive and specific markers of myocardial injury.[24,25] Importantly, both troponin I and T targeted by standard assays are unique isoforms that are only expressed in the adult human heart.[26] Furthermore, the skeletal muscle does not express cardiac troponin during regenerative processes or in response to pathological stimuli, thus conferring an absolute specificity to the myocardium.[27]

Elevations of troponin I or T help define acute coronary syndrome (ACS) and predict short-term and long-term outcomes.[28] Although detectable levels of troponin are mostly studied in the context of coronary artery disease (CAD), their role as a marker of myocardial damage in other clinical conditions, such as heart failure, is increasingly recognized. Unlike cardiac enzymes such as creatinine kinase (CK) or CK-MB, the development of sensitive and specific assays measuring cardiac troponin I or T has provided more accurate measures of myocardial injury in heart failure.[29]

There are several processes, such as apoptosis and necrosis, in heart failure which may cause troponin elevation. Apoptosis is a form of cell death, characterized as isolated cells undergoing programmed cell death, but it is not clear whether it gives rise to detectable troponin levels.[30,31] In contrast, necrosis is a passive process involving groups of cells, precipitated by a focal injury such as reduced tissue perfusion, which can easily lead to troponin elevations.

Above the cellular level, pathophysiologic changes in heart failure can lead to troponin elevations. A hallmark of heart failure is reduced coronary reserve due to ventricular hypertrophy. At normal baseline ventricular function, this reduction in coronary reserve may have no noticeable affect, but during periods of stress it may become a critical factor because of the higher metabolic demands. It may be severe enough to induce myocyte necrosis, contributing to further decline in long-term function.[32] In addition, there are microcirculatory abnormalities of the coronary arteries due to endothelial dysfunction that may contribute to focal myocardial necrosis.

Another process that may lead to troponin elevation is the extensive remodeling of the myocardium—vascular and interstitial compartments. Morphological changes associated with remodeling include noncontiguous areas of cell death and foci of replacement fibrosis.[33–35] Hemodynamic changes associated with progressive heart failure may also increase troponin levels, with experimental evidence showing elevations in preload without ischemia, producing troponin, I degradation.[36] In addition, other experiments with cardiac muscle cells link myocardial wall stretch with myocyte functional injury and cell death.[37]

Most studies evaluating troponin elevations in clinical heart failure are small and have not exclusively been evaluated in ADHF. The first study demonstrating elevations in troponin levels in chronic heart failure was published by Missov *et al.* in 1997.[38] Cardiac troponin I was assayed in 35 subjects with NYHA functional class III or IV symptoms, 55 healthy blood donors, and 25 hospitalized control patients without known cardiac disease. Using highly-sensitive assays (lower detection limit of 3 pg/mL), heart failure patients had a mean troponin I level of 72.1 pg/mL as compared to control subjects with a mean of 25.4 pg/mL ($P < 0.01$). Although this study showed different levels between heart failure patients and controls, the absolute elevations were subtle. When standard troponin I assays with an upper reference limit of 0.1 ng/mL were used, only one patient (0.206 ng/mL) had a positive result that could have been considered a myocardial infarction (MI).

Detectable troponin T and I levels can occur in acute heart failure but not uniformly.[39] Detectable troponin levels in patients can range from 23% to 84% of those who present with heart failure, depending on the assay and the clinical scenario.[40,41] Those patients with undetectable levels have a significantly better prognosis than those with detectable levels.[42]

Several other studies have evaluated the prognostic role and clinical significance of elevated levels of troponin T or I in heart failure.[43–45] These studies include patients without clinical symptoms or signs of acute myocardial infarction (AMI), unstable angina, or acute myocarditis. Elevation in troponin T or I correlates with NYHA classification and can decrease significantly following medical treatment. It is predictive of death and rehospitalization for worsening heart failure. Persistent elevation is associated with worse prognosis, and it correlates with more frequent use of intravenous diuretics, nitrates, and inotropes.[46] Disease progression in troponin-positive patients also correlates with adverse remodeling evident as increased left ventricular (LV) diastolic diameter and lower ejection fraction (EF).[47]

Other evidence shows that troponin elevation correlates with hemodynamic markers often cited as poor prognostic signs.[48] Detectable troponin levels correlate with elevated BNP levels, elevated PCWP and lower cardiac index. In a study of 238 patients referred for transplant evaluation, patients with detectable troponin levels and BNP > 485 pg/mL, had a 12-fold increased risk of death as compared to those with undetectable troponin I levels and BNP < 485 pg/mL.

Although the evidence so far shows that troponin levels cannot be used exclusively as an indicator of acute heart failure, it does add significant prognostic information. Continued elevation of troponin levels appears to be associated with ongoing myocyte injury that is unmitigated by treatment of heart failure. Therefore, future goals of therapy may involve measurement of troponin levels as an indication of the severity of ongoing myocyte injury and as an important prognostic marker in acute heart failure.

Inflammatory Markers

Data accumulated in the past decade support an important role of inflammation in the pathogenesis of human heart failure. This concept was initially suggested by Levine *et al.*, who demonstrated the presence of elevated levels of the proinflammatory cytokine, tumor necrosis factor-alpha (TNF-α), in patients with chronic heart failure as compared to healthy controls.[49] Since that time, multiple lines of evidence have expanded our understanding of the relationship between inflammatory activation and heart failure. TNF is known to be elevated in a variety of conditions associated with LV dysfunction, including sepsis, myocarditis, and cardiac allograft rejection.[50–54] Physiologically relevant levels of TNF stimulate apoptosis in cultured myocytes,[55] and infusion of TNF into normal animals or humans leads to decreases in LV function and adverse remodeling characteristic of the heart failure phenotype.[56,57] Additionally, the failing heart has been shown to produce large quantities of TNF, whereas the normal heart does not.[58] Transgenic mouse models of TNF overproduction lend further support to the role of TNF in heart failure, as mice that overexpress TNF develop a phenotype of dilated cardiomyopathy.[59,60] On this background of basic research, multiple studies have demonstrated elevations in TNF in a variety of different populations with clinical heart failure, with higher concentrations in patients with more severe disease.[61–63] Additionally, it has been demonstrated that TNF elevation is an independent marker of poorer prognosis in patients with chronic heart failure.[64] Levels of the soluble TNF receptors have also been shown to modulate TNF activity and have prognostic importance in heart failure.[65] Although the majority of data on inflammatory stress in heart failure have focused on TNF, several other inflammatory markers that could serve as biomarkers do exist. The most consistent of these has been interleukin-6 (IL-6), a proinflammatory cytokine, which has been shown to be elevated in patients with acute MI and mild to moderate chronic heart failure.[66] Elevation of IL-6 has been shown to be an independent predictor of mortality in patients with chronic heart failure in some studies[64,67] but not in others.[63] As with TNF, the soluble receptor for IL-6 modulates IL-6 activity.[64]

Inflammation in acute heart failure

Despite the increasing evidence regarding the role of inflammation in heart failure, virtually all previous studies have focused on patients with chronic stable heart failure. Data on inflammatory cytokines in acute heart failure are significantly less robust. C-reactive protein (CRP), an acute phase reactant (produced in the liver in response to IL-6 and other inflammatory cytokines) and a measure of systemic inflammatory activity, has been shown to be associated with increased risk in a variety of acute cardiovascular disorders including unstable angina and MI.[68,69] Given the role of inflammation in the pathophysiology of heart failure, high-sensitivity CRP (hsCRP) seems ideally suited for use as a biomarker of inflammatory stress in decompensated heart failure. CRP has recently been shown to be associated with allograft failure after cardiac transplantation.[70] Despite being readily available in clinical laboratories, there is little existing data evaluating CRP in heart failure populations.[71,72] A few studies have examined the role of proinflammatory markers in acute heart failure. Sato *et al.* evaluated cytokines in eight patients with decompensated heart failure and demonstrated elevation in CRP, IL-6 and IL-4, all of which improved after successful heart failure treatment.[73] At least one small cohort study evaluating the role of CRP in risk stratification of patients hospitalized with heart failure found that elevated hsCRP on admission was associated with greater symptom severity and was an independent predictor of rehospitalization and mortality.[74] A recently published study evaluating inflammatory cytokines and other biomarkers in 30 patients presenting with acute pulmonary edema found elevations of inflammatory markers such as IL-6, TNF-α, and CRP that were significantly reduced by 60-day follow-up (Figure 10.5).[75] This study was notable in that it included patients with clinical heart failure in the setting of both impaired and preserved systolic function.

The hypothesis—that changes in the inflammatory milieu may precipitate or contribute to heart failure decompensation—is attractive but untested. The implications of this hypothesis for clinical care are 3-fold. First, elevation of circulating inflammatory markers may identify patients at higher risk, and thus may be a useful part of risk stratification in decompensated heart failure when combined with other clinical data. Second, lack of improvement of inflammatory cytokine levels after acute treatment may identify patients at particularly high risk for short-term events who could be candidates for more aggressive intervention or more intense follow-up. Finally, evidence that inflammation contributes to the transition of heart failure from a compensated to a decompensated clinical syndrome would suggest the possibility of direct therapeutic intervention

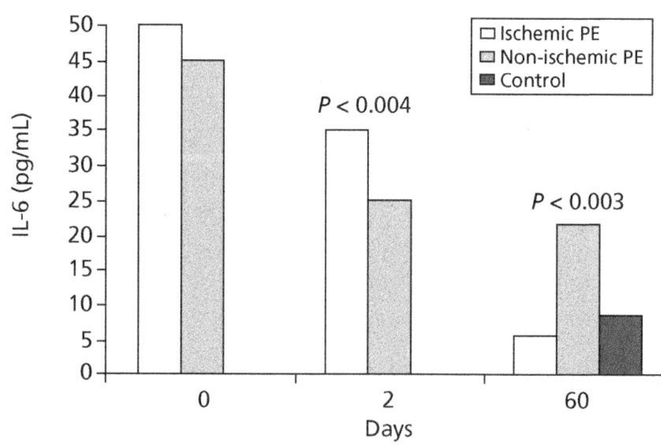

Figure 10.5. *Interleukin-6 levels in acute heart failure (Adapted with permission, from Milo* et al.[75]*)*

Abbreviations: IL-6 = interleukin-6; PE = pulmonary edema.

with antiinflammatory therapy in the subset of decompensated heart failure patients with evidence of inflammatory activation. All these hypotheses are untested, suggesting that much work is still required to define the potential role of inflammatory markers in ADHF.

Novel Biomarkers

The sequencing of the human genome was a major step in understanding human biology and will undoubtedly bring rapid advances in the understanding of cardiovascular disease along with the emerging field of proteomics.[76,77] Although sequencing of the human genome revealed approximately 30 000 genes, significantly fewer than expected, this still leaves a daunting task for the proteomics field, considering that there are probably 6 to 7 times as many distinct proteins.[78] However, as new technology emerges, investigations of the proteome will bring a plethora of novel biomarkers and patterns of proteins that will be used in cardiovascular disease and acute heart failure.

It will be difficult to understand the complexity of acute heart failure by measuring a single biomarker. Efforts to discover disease fingerprints based on protein markers or changes in patterns of proteins are increasing throughout medicine, and especially in cardiology.[79] Although previous work focused on investigating biomarkers singly—or now with genomic technology identifying a candidate biomarker—other technologies giving an unbiased evaluation of patterns of proteins in different disease states may be more useful. In other diseases, such as ovarian cancer, systematic approaches to defining protein fingerprints appear promising, using protein mass spectra. However, further studies are still needed to validate the results and determine the clinical utility.[80]

There are a number of techniques for evaluating serum or plasma to discover novel biomarkers and investigate multiple biomarkers in the same sample. Mass spectroscopy offers the most promise for providing comprehensive profiles of proteins in biological samples. Because of the small sample volumes used and the available high-throughput systems, this approach is highly suited for biomarker discovery.[81] However, to translate discoveries of important biomarkers in acute heart failure into clinical practice, other techniques will likely be needed. By combining important proteins or a biomarker into a platform where multiple markers can be assayed at the same time, a greater profile of biomarkers can be used clinically. With protein microarrays, technology exists to analyze a number of proteins on the same platform or chip, but decisions remain on which ones to include.[82]

The limitations of incorporating these systems include the current limitations of biostatistical analysis of multiple variables and the costs for widespread use. There are several key requirements for biomarkers to transition from basic discovery into clinical practice. Ideally, the technical accuracy of the biomarker will have high sensitivity, specificity, and reproducibility across a spectrum of patients and clinical laboratories. Second, a novel biomarker must relate to the pathophysiology of acute heart failure, so that changes in its level are linked to the clinical status of the patient. Finally, incorporation of multiple markers must be synergistic in guiding clinical care.

Until proteomic techniques such as mass spectroscopy or microarrays are widespread, novel biomarkers will likely parallel areas of research in heart failure such as vascular biology, oxidative stress, inflammation, or thrombosis. The limitation of these biomarkers to potential clinical importance depends on the stability of the biomarker measured, the technical qualities of the assay, and the role of the biomarker in clinical decision-making.

There are several examples of biomarkers that illustrate the promise and pitfalls of novel biomarkers. Norepinephrine levels are an important predictor in mortality, but performance of these assays is limited because of sample and timing requirements.[83] With advances in technology and stability of assay platforms, there may be other neurohormones, such as adrenomedullin, that may be more clinically useful in heart failure.[84]

An understanding of vascular biology has led to important discoveries in oncology and cardiovascular disease. Angiogenesis, which has been primarily of interest in the treatment of ischemic heart disease, may also be important in heart failure. Studies evaluating angiopoietins and vascular endothelial growth factors (VEGF), known primarily for their role in angiogenesis, may be important because tissue ischemia associated with acute heart failure may be a stimulus for production of these factors.[85,86]

Other areas of interest include the role of thrombosis and oxidative stress in acute heart failure. Platelet activity and markers of coagulation have been investigated in chronic heart failure and this work will extend into acute heart failure.[87,88] Oxidative stress has also been recognized as a potential mechanism in ischemic heart disease and heart failure.[89] Homocysteine levels have been associated with vascular disease and increased levels have been associated with the development of heart failure in adults without prior MI.[90] Other markers of oxidative stress, such as urinary 15-$F2_t$-isoprostane, correlate with plasma BNP and IL-6 levels and the highest levels are found in those with ADHF.[91]

Conclusion and Future Directions

Has the optimal biomarker for heart failure been identified? Ideally, the biomarker for heart failure would be easily and rapidly measured and reproducible across laboratories at low cost. To be clinically useful in the setting of acute heart failure, such a marker would have to show a high diagnostic value across a variety of different patient presentations, provide significant prognostic information above and beyond that obtained from standard clinical data, and allow titration of therapies in a way that could be shown to result in improved clinical outcomes.[92] Clearly, no currently available marker fulfills all these criteria, which may be too much to ask from a single measurement. Although the natriuretic peptides appear to have significant utility in heart failure diagnosis and management, their optimal use continues to be defined by ongoing studies. Future research will focus increasingly on a multi-marker strategy evaluating several different pathophysiologic systems simultaneously. Such an approach has been shown to be effective in patients with ACS.[93,94] Evolving proteomic approaches will accelerate the pace of discovery for candidate biomarkers in heart failure and other cardiovascular disorders. Careful investigation is needed to define the optimal strategy for adopting new biomarkers into clinical practice. Enthusiasm for biomarkers in diagnosis and treatment must be grounded in sound clinical judgment. Overreliance on biomarker measurements in diagnosis and prognosis may create as many problems as it solves. As has been pointed out by several investigators, the use of biomarkers to guide therapy can only be as effective as the therapies themselves.[17,95] Despite these cautions, the role of circulating biomarkers in heart failure seems likely to continue to expand, potentially improving diagnosis, triage, risk stratification, and treatment for patients with ADHF.

References

1. Klinge R, Hystad M, Kjekshus J, *et al.* An experimental study of cardiac natriuretic peptides as markers of development of congestive heart failure. Scand J Clin Lab Invest 1998; 58: 683–691.
2. Borgeson DD, Grantham JA, Williamson E, *et al.* Differential regulation of circulating atrial natriuretic peptide and brain natriuretic peptide by endogenous endothelin during the progression of experimental heart failure. J Am Coll Cardiol 1997; 29: 8169.
3. Stingo AJ, Clavell AL, Heublein DM, *et al.* Presence of C-type natriuretic peptide in cultured human endothelial-cells and plasma. Am J Physiol 1992; 263: H1318–H1321.
4. Tsutamoto T, Wada A, Maeda K, *et al.* Attenuation of compensation of endogenous cardiac natriuretic peptide system in chronic heart failure: prognostic role of plasma brain natriuretic peptide concentration in patients with chronic symptomatic left ventricular dysfunction. Circulation 1997; 96: 509–516.
5. Maeda K, Tsutamoto T, Wada A, Hisanaga T, Kinoshita M. Plasma brain natriuretic peptide as a biochemical marker of high left ventricular end-diastolic pressure in patients with symptomatic left ventricular dysfunction. Am Heart J 1998; 135: 825–832.
6. Yasue H, Yoshimura M, Sumida H, *et al.* Localization and mechanism of secretion of B-type natriuretic peptide in comparison with those of A-type natriuretic peptide in normal subjects and patients with heart-failure. Circulation 1994; 90: 195–203.

7. McNairy M, Gardetto N, Clopton P, *et al.* Stability of B-type natriuretic peptide levels during exercise in patients with congestive heart failure: implications for outpatient monitoring with B-type natriuretic peptide. Am Heart J 2002; 143: 406–411.
8. Nakagawa O, Ogawa Y, Itoh H, *et al.* Rapid transcriptional activation and early mRNA turnover of brain natriuretic peptide in cardiocyte hypertrophy: evidence for brain natriuretic peptide as an "emergency" cardiac hormone against ventricular overload. J Clin Invest 1995; 96: 1280–1287.
9. Muders F, Kromer EP, Griese DP, *et al.* Evaluation of plasma natriuretic peptides as markers for left ventricular dysfunction. Am Heart J 1997; 134: 442–449.
10. ProBrain Natriuretic Peptide (Roche Diagnostics, Inc.: Indianapolis, IN, 2002) (Package Insert).
11. Triage BNP (Biosite, Inc.: San Diego, CA, 2002) (Package Insert).
12. Dao Q, Krishnaswamy P, Kazanegra R, *et al.* Utility of B-type natriuretic peptide in the diagnosis of congestive heart failure in an urgent-care setting. J Am Coll Cardiol 2001; 37: 379–385.
13. Maisel AS, Krishnaswamy P, Nowak RM, *et al.* Rapid measurement of B-type natriuretic peptide in the emergency diagnosis of heart failure. N Engl J Med 2002; 347: 161–167.
14. Lainchbury JG, Campbell E, Frampton CM, *et al.* Brain natriuretic peptide and n-terminal brain natriuretic peptide in the diagnosis of heart failure in patients with acute shortness of breath. J Am Coll Cardiol 2003; 42: 728–735.
15. McCullough PA, Nowak RM, McCord J, *et al.* B-type natriuretic peptide and clinical judgment in emergency diagnosis of heart failure: analysis from Breathing Not Properly (BNP) Multinational Study. Circulation 2002; 106: 416–422.
16. Mueller C, Scholer A, Laule-Kilian K, *et al.* Use of B-type natriuretic peptide in the evaluation and management of acute dyspnea. N Engl J Med 2004; 350: 647–654.
17. Mark DB, Felker GM. B-type natriuretic peptide - a biomarker for all seasons? N Engl J Med 2004; 350: 718–720.
18. Cheng V, Kazanagra R, Garcia A, *et al.* A rapid bedside test for B-type peptide predicts treatment outcomes in patients admitted for decompensated heart failure: a pilot study. J Am Coll Cardiol 2001; 37: 386–391.
19. Bettencourt P, Ferreira S, Azevedo A, Ferreira A. Preliminary data on the potential usefulness of B-type natriuretic peptide levels in predicting outcome after hospital discharge in patients with heart failure. Am J Med 2002; 113: 215–219.
20. Kazanegra R, Cheng V, Garcia A, *et al.* A rapid test for B-type natriuretic peptide correlates with falling wedge pressures in patients treated for decompensated heart failure: a pilot study. J Card Fail 2001; 7: 21–29.
21. Stevenson LW. Tailored therapy to hemodynamic goals for advanced heart failure. Eur J Heart Fail 1999; 1: 251–257.
22. Sodian R, Loebe M, Schmitt C, *et al.* Decreased plasma concentration of brain natriuretic peptide as a potential indicator of cardiac recovery in patients supported by mechanical circulatory assist systems. J Am Coll Cardiol 2001; 38: 1942–1949.
23. Ricchiuti V, Zhang J, Apple FS. Cardiac troponin I and T alterations in hearts with severe left ventricular remodeling. Clin Chem 1997; 43: 990–995.
24. Adams JE IIIrd, Bodor GS, Davila-Roman VG, *et al.* Cardiac troponin I: a marker with high specificity for cardiac injury. Circulation 1993; 88: 101–106.
25. Katus HA, Remppis A, Neumann FJ, *et al.* Diagnostic efficiency of troponin T measurements in acute myocardial infarction. Circulation 1991; 83: 902–912.
26. Wu AH, Ford L. Release of cardiac troponin in acute coronary syndromes: ischemia or necrosis? Clin Chim Acta 1999; 284: 161–174.
27. Adams JE IIIrd, Bodor GS, Davila-Roman VG, *et al.* Cardiac troponin I: a marker with high specificity for cardiac injury. Circulation 1993; 88: 101–106.
28. Myocardial infarction redefined—a consensus document of The Joint European Society of Cardiology/American College of Cardiology Committee for the redefinition of myocardial infarction. Eur Heart J 2000; 21: 1502–1513.
29. Crowley LV. Creatine phosphokinase activity in myocardial infarction, heart failure, and following various diagnostic and therapeutic procedures. Clin Chem 1968; 14: 1185–1196.
30. Narula J, Haider N, Virmani R, *et al.* Apoptosis in myocytes in end-stage heart failure. N Engl J Med 1996; 335: 1182–1189.
31. Olivetti G, Abbi R, Quaini F, *et al.* Apoptosis in the failing human heart. N Engl J Med 1997; 336: 1131–1141.
32. Vatner SF, Hittinger L. Coronary vascular mechanisms involved in decompensation from hypertrophy to heart failure. J Am Coll Cardiol 1993; 22: 34A–40A.
33. Schaper J, Froede R, Hein S, *et al.* Impairment of the myocardial ultrastructure and changes of the cytoskeleton in dilated cardiomyopathy. Circulation 1991; 83: 504–514.
34. Beltrami CA, Finato N, Rocco M, *et al.* Structural basis of end-stage failure in ischemic cardiomyopathy in humans. Circulation 1994; 89: 151–163.

35. Colucci WS. Molecular and cellular mechanisms of myocardial failure. Am J Cardiol 1997; 80: 15L–25L.
36. Feng J, Schaus BJ, Fallavollita JA, Lee TC, Canty JM Jr. Preload induces troponin I degradation independently of myocardial ischemia. Circulation 2001; 103: 2035–2037.
37. Cheng W, Li B, Kajstura J, *et al*. Stretch-induced programmed myocyte cell death. J Clin Invest 1995; 96: 2247–2259.
38. Missov E, Calzolari C, Pau B. Circulating cardiac troponin I in severe congestive heart failure. Circulation 1997; 96: 2953–2958.
39. La Vecchia L, Mezzena G, Ometto R, *et al*. Detectable serum troponin I in patients with heart failure of nonmyocardial ischemic origin. Am J Cardiol 1997; 80: 88–90.
40. Del Carlo CH, Pereira-Barretto AC, Cassaro-Strunz C, Latorre MR, Ramires JA. Serial measure of cardiac troponin T levels for prediction of clinical events in decompensated heart failure. J Card Fail 2004; 10: 43–48.
41. La Vecchia L, Mezzena G, Ometto R, *et al*. Detectable serum troponin I in patients with heart failure of nonmyocardial ischemic origin. Am J Cardiol 1997; 80: 88–90.
42. Perna ER, Macin SM, Parras JI, *et al*. Cardiac troponin T levels are associated with poor short- and long-term prognosis in patients with acute cardiogenic pulmonary edema. Am Heart J 2002; 143: 814–820.
43. Horwich TB, Patel J, MacLellan WR, Fonarow GC. Cardiac troponin I is associated with impaired hemodynamics, progressive left ventricular dysfunction, and increased mortality rates in advanced heart failure. Circulation 2003; 108: 833–838.
44. Sato Y, Yamada T, Taniguchi R, *et al*. Persistently increased serum concentrations of cardiac troponin T in patients with idiopathic dilated cardiomyopathy are predictive of adverse outcomes. Circulation 2001; 103: 369–374.
45. Setsuta K, Seino Y, Takahashi N, *et al*. Clinical significance of elevated levels of cardiac troponin T in patients with chronic heart failure. Am J Cardiol 1999; 84: 608–611, A9.
46. Sato Y, Yamada T, Taniguchi R, *et al*. Persistently increased serum concentrations of cardiac troponin T in patients with idiopathic dilated cardiomyopathy are predictive of adverse outcomes. Circulation 2001; 103: 369–374.
47. Sato Y, Yamada T, Taniguchi R, *et al*. Persistently increased serum concentrations of cardiac troponin T in patients with idiopathic dilated cardiomyopathy are predictive of adverse outcomes. Circulation 2001; 103: 369–374.
48. Horwich TB, Patel J, MacLellan WR, Fonarow GC. Cardiac troponin I is associated with impaired hemodynamics, progressive left ventricular dysfunction, and increased mortality rates in advanced heart failure. Circulation 2003; 108: 833–838.
49. Levine B, Kalman J, Mayer L, Fillit HM, Packer M. Elevated circulating levels of tumor necrosis factor in severe chronic heart failure. N Engl J Med 1990; 323: 236–241.
50. Tracey KJ, Beutler B, Lowry SF, *et al*. Shock and tissue injury induced by recombinant human cachectin. Science 1986; 234: 470–474.
51. Parrillo JE, Parker MM, Natanson C, *et al*. Septic shock in humans. Advances in the understanding of pathogenesis, cardiovascular dysfunction, and therapy. Ann Intern Med 1990; 113: 227–242.
52. Tracey KJ, Fong Y, Hesse DG, *et al*. Anticachectin/TNF monoclonal antibodies prevent septic shock during lethal bacteraemia. Nature 1987; 330: 662–664.
53. Arbustini E, Grasso M, Diegoli M, *et al*. Expression of tumor necrosis factor in human acute cardiac rejection: an immunohistochemical and immunoblotting study. Am J Pathol 1991; 139: 709–715.
54. Smith SC, Allen PM. Neutralization of endogenous tumor necrosis factor ameliorates the severity of myosin-induced myocarditis. Circ Res 1992; 70: 856–863.
55. Krown KA, Page MT, Nguyen C, *et al*. Tumor necrosis factor alpha-induced apoptosis in cardiac myocytes: involvement of the sphingolipid signaling cascade in cardiac cell death. J Clin Invest 1996; 98: 2854–2865.
56. Suffredini AF, Fromm RE, Parker MM, *et al*. The cardiovascular response of normal humans to the administration of endotoxin. N Engl J Med 1989; 321: 280–287.
57. Pagani FD, Baker LS, Hsi C, *et al*. Left ventricular systolic and diastolic dysfunction after infusion of tumor necrosis factor-alpha in conscious dogs. J Clin Invest 1992; 90: 389–398.
58. Torre-Amione G, Kapadia S, Lee J, *et al*. Tumor necrosis factor-alpha and tumor necrosis factor receptors in the failing human heart. Circulation 1996; 93: 704–711.
59. Feldman AM, Combes A, Wagner D, *et al*. The role of tumor necrosis factor in the pathophysiology of heart failure. J Am Coll Cardiol 2000; 35: 537–544.
60. Kubota T, McTiernan CF, Frye CS, *et al*. Dilated cardiomyopathy in transgenic mice with cardiac-specific overexpression of tumor necrosis factor-alpha. Circ Res 1997; 81: 627–635.

61. McMurray J, Abdullah I, Dargie HJ, Shapiro D. Increased concentrations of tumour necrosis factor in "cachectic" patients with severe chronic heart failure. Br Heart J 1991; 66: 356–358.
62. Dutka DP, Elborn JS, Delamere F, Shale DJ, Morris GK. Tumour necrosis factor alpha in severe congestive cardiac failure. Br Heart J 1993; 70: 141–143.
63. Torre-Amione G, Kapadia S, Benedict C, *et al.* Proinflammatory cytokine levels in patients with depressed left ventricular ejection fraction: a report from the Studies of Left Ventricular Dysfunction (SOLVD). J Am Coll Cardiol 1996; 27: 1201–1206.
64. Deswal A, Peterson MJ, Feldman AM, *et al.* Cytokines and cytokine receptors in advanced heart failure: an analysis of the cytokine database from the Vesnarinone Trial (VEST). Circulation 2001; 103: 2055–2059.
65. Rauchhaus M, Doehner W, Francis DP, *et al.* Plasma cytokine parameters and mortality in patients with chronic heart failure. Circulation 2000; 102: 3060–3067.
66. Munger MA, Johnson B, Amber IJ, Callahan KS, Gilbert EM. Circulating concentrations of proinflammatory cytokines in mild or moderate heart failure secondary to ischemic or idiopathic dilated cardiomyopathy. Am J Cardiol 1996; 77: 723–727.
67. Tsutamoto T, Hisanaga T, Wada A, *et al.* Interleukin-6 spillover in the peripheral circulation increases with the severity of heart failure, and the high plasma level of interleukin-6 is an important prognostic predictor in patients with congestive heart failure. J Am Coll Cardiol 1998; 31: 391–398.
68. Liuzzo G, Biasucci LM, Gallimore JR, *et al.* The prognostic value of C-reactive protein and serum amyloid a protein in severe unstable angina. N Engl J Med 1994; 331: 417–424.
69. Ridker PM, Rifai N, Pfeffer MA, *et al.* Inflammation, pravastatin, and the risk of coronary events after myocardial infarction in patients with average cholesterol levels. Cholesterol and Recurrent Events (CARE) Investigators. Circulation 1998; 98: 839–844.
70. Eisenberg MS, Chen HJ, Warshofsky MK, *et al.* Elevated levels of plasma C-reactive protein are associated with decreased graft survival in cardiac transplant recipients. Circulation 2000; 102: 2100–2104.
71. Kaneko K, Kanda T, Yamauchi Y, *et al.* C-Reactive protein in dilated cardiomyopathy. Cardiology 1999; 91: 215–219.
72. Steele IC, Nugent AM, Maguire S, *et al.* Cytokine profile in chronic cardiac failure. Eur J Clin Invest 1996; 26: 1018–1022.
73. Sato Y, Takatsu Y, Kataoka K, *et al.* Serial circulating concentrations of C-reactive protein, interleukin (IL)-4, and IL-6 in patients with acute left heart decompensation. Clin Cardiol 1999; 22: 811–813.
74. Alonso-Martinez JL, Llorente-Diez B, Echegaray-Agara M, *et al.* C-reactive protein as a predictor of improvement and readmission in heart failure. Eur J Heart Fail 2002; 4: 331–336.
75. Milo O, Cotter G, Kaluski E, *et al.* Comparison of inflammatory and neurohormonal activation in cardiogenic pulmonary edema secondary to ischemic versus nonischemic causes. Am J Cardiol 2003; 92: 222–226.
76. Lander ES, Linton LM, Birren B, *et al.* Initial sequencing and analysis of the human genome. Nature 2001; 409: 860–921.
77. Venter JC, Adams MD, Myers EW, *et al.* The sequence of the human genome. Science 2001; 291: 1304–1351.
78. Loscalzo J. Proteomics in cardiovascular biology and medicine. Circulation 2003; 108: 380–383.
79. Granger CB, Van Eyk JE, Mockrin SC, Anderson NL. National Heart, Lung, and Blood Institute Clinical Proteomics Working Group report. Circulation 2004; 109: 1697–1703.
80. Petricoin EF, Ardekani AM, Hitt BA, *et al.* Use of proteomic patterns in serum to identify ovarian cancer. Lancet 2002; 359: 572–577.
81. Aebersold R, Mann M. Mass spectrometry-based proteomics. Nature 2003; 422: 198–207.
82. Hanash S. Disease proteomics. Nature 2003; 422: 226–232.
83. Anand IS, Fisher LD, Chiang YT, *et al.* Changes in brain natriuretic peptide and norepinephrine over time and mortality and morbidity in the Valsartan Heart Failure Trial (Val-HeFT). Circulation 2003; 107: 1278–1283.
84. Richards AM, Doughty R, Nicholls MG, *et al.* Plasma N-terminal pro-brain natriuretic peptide and adrenomedullin: prognostic utility and prediction of benefit from carvedilol in chronic ischemic left ventricular dysfunction. Australia-New Zealand Heart Failure Group. J Am Coll Cardiol 2001; 37: 1781–1787.
85. Chong AY, Caine GJ, Freestone B, Blann AD, Lip GY. Plasma angiopoietin-1, angiopoietin-2, and angiopoietin receptor tie-2 levels in congestive heart failure. J Am Coll Cardiol 2004; 43: 423–428.
86. Chin BS, Chung NA, Gibbs CR, Blann AD, Lip GY. Vascular endothelial growth factor and soluble P-selectin in acute and chronic congestive heart failure. Am J Cardiol 2002; 90: 1258–1260.

87. Gibbs CR, Blann AD, Watson RD, Lip GY. Abnormalities of hemorheological, endothelial, and platelet function in patients with chronic heart failure in sinus rhythm: effects of angiotensin-converting enzyme inhibitor and beta-blocker therapy. Circulation 2001; 103: 1746–1751.
88. Chin BS, Chung NA, Gibbs CR, Blann AD, Lip GY. Vascular endothelial growth factor and soluble P-selectin in acute and chronic congestive heart failure. Am J Cardiol 2002; 90: 1258–1260.
89. Keith M, Geranmayegan A, Sole MJ, *et al.* Increased oxidative stress in patients with congestive heart failure. J Am Coll Cardiol 1998; 31: 1352–1356.
90. Vasan RS, Beiser A, D'Agostino RB, *et al.* Plasma homocysteine and risk for congestive heart failure in adults without prior myocardial infarction. JAMA 2003; 289: 1251–1257.
91. Nonaka-Sarukawa M, Yamamoto K, Aoki H, *et al.* Increased urinary 15-F2t-isoprostane concentrations in patients with non-ischaemic congestive heart failure: a marker of oxidative stress. Heart 2003; 89: 871–874.
92. Bozkurt B, Mann DL. Use of biomarkers in the management of heart failure: are we there yet? Circulation 2003; 107: 1231–1233.
93. Newby LK, Storrow AB, Gibler WB, *et al.* Bedside multimarker testing for risk stratification in chest pain units: the chest pain evaluation by creatine kinase-MB, myoglobin, and troponin I (CHECKMATE) study. Circulation 2001; 103: 1832–1837.
94. Sabatine MS, Morrow DA, de Lemos JA, *et al.* Multimarker approach to risk stratification in non-ST elevation acute coronary syndromes: simultaneous assessment of troponin I, C-reactive protein, and B-type natriuretic peptide. Circulation 2002; 105: 1760–1763.
95. Packer M. Should B-type natriuretic peptide be measured routinely to guide the diagnosis and management of chronic heart failure? Circulation 2003; 108: 2950–2953.

CHAPTER 11

Noninvasive diagnostic evaluation of the acute heart failure patient with systolic dysfunction: focus on the electrocardiogram and chest x-ray

Jason N Katz, Robert C Kowal, Mark H Drazner

Introduction

There are approximately 5 million people in the United States with chronic heart failure (CHF) and nearly 550 000 new cases are diagnosed annually.[1] Despite advances in therapeutics since the Framingham study in 1971,[2] the mortality associated with CHF remains quite high, with 5-year survival rates less than 50%.[2–4] In addition, the annual expenditure on CHF approaches $38 billion in the United States alone.[5]

Early identification, and thus early treatment, of the heart failure patient will likely ease the burden of this disease, from both a medical and an economic perspective. However, despite the availability of several clinical scales,[2,6–7] assays of neurohormonal activation such as the natriuretic peptides, and two-dimensional echocardiography, diagnosis of acute heart failure remains difficult and there is, in fact, no current "gold standard."[8]

Herein, we will discuss diagnostic tests available to physicians which may assist them in making this sometimes challenging diagnosis. We will focus on using noninvasive diagnostic tests to answer common clinical questions such as whether a patient's symptoms are secondary to heart failure or another illness and what the etiology of the decompensated heart failure is.

Decompensated Congestive Heart Failure: Role of Chest X-ray and Electrocardiogram

Because the physical examination, transthoracic echocardiography (TTE), and assays of the natriuretic peptides are covered elsewhere in this book, we will focus on the role of the chest x-ray and electrocardiogram in the evaluation of patients with CHF.

The chest x-ray

The chest roentgenogram can assist the physician in evaluating for the presence of high-circulating blood volume (pulmonary vascular congestion) and pulmonary edema—both of which should prove useful in the diagnostic evaluation of the patient with decompensated CHF.

An assessment of pulmonary blood volume may be possible by chest x-ray interpretation. If it is increased, or if frank pulmonary edema is present, these findings are supportive, though not diagnostic, of decompensated CHF. Increased pulmonary blood volume can be identified radiographically by the presence of either vascular redistribution or interstitial edema.[9] Vascular redistribution is said to be present when veins in the upper pulmonary lobes are larger and more numerous than those in the lower lobes of the lung. Interstitial edema, on the other hand, can be described by the loss of definition of the pulmonary vascular markings in association with septal lines (Kerley's B lines),[10] perivascular or peribronchial cuffing, and hilar haze. The most sensitive finding for interstitial edema appears to be hilar haze, while septal lines are more specific but occur infrequently (Figure 11.1).[9]

Vascular redistribution appears to be a difficult diagnosis for the clinician, as demonstrated by only fair to moderate interobserver agreement. The finding of pulmonary vascular congestion has been shown to have a sensitivity of 53% and specificity of 63% for detecting an abnormal left ventricular ejection fraction (LVEF).[10] Of note, patient position, observer experience, and film quality are several variables which can impair the reliability of findings of vascular congestion in the evaluation of the patient with suspected decompensated CHF.

In addition, patients with CHF may have no pulmonary congestion radiographically, even in the presence of high pulmonary capillary wedge

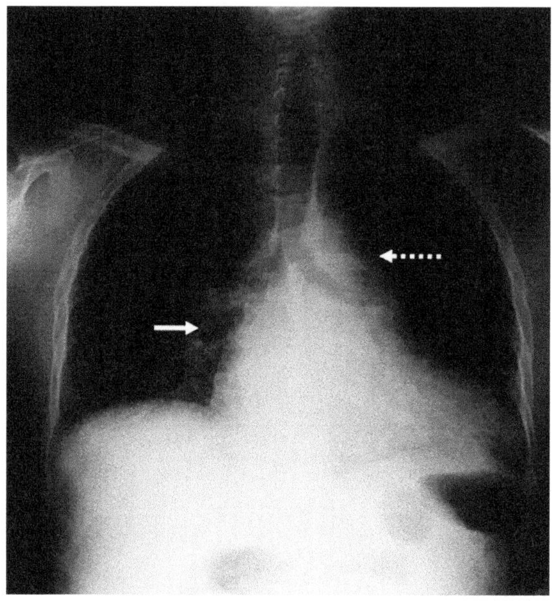

Figure 11.1B. *Progression of volume overload pattern with persistence of hilar haze (dashed arrow) and new evidence of peribronchiolar cuffing (solid arrow) (Image courtesy of Michael Landay, MD.)*

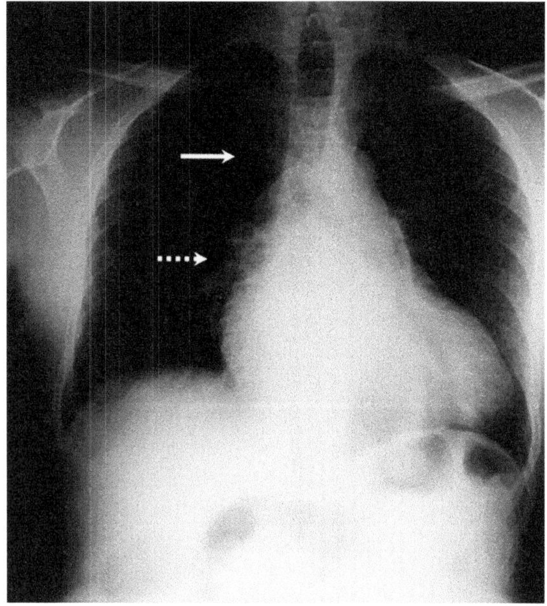

Figure 11.1A. *First in a series of chest radiographs showing early volume overload with pulmonary vascular redistribution (solid arrow) and hilar haze (dashed arrow) (Image courtesy of Michael Landay, MD.)*

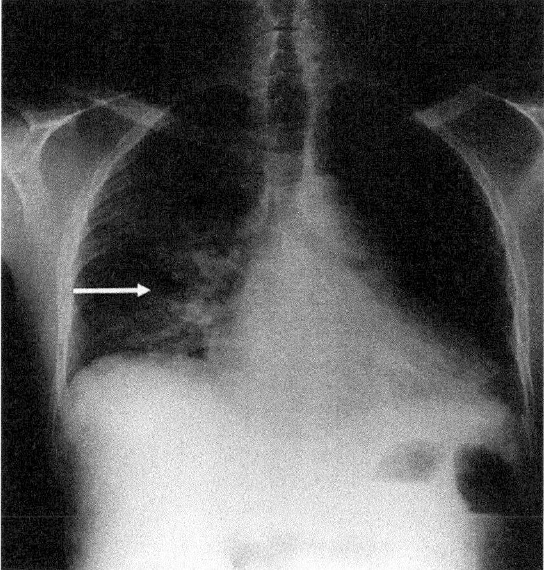

Figure 11.1C. *Chest radiograph now showing overt pulmonary edema with alveolar filling pattern (solid arrow) (Image courtesy of Michael Landay, MD.)*

pressures (PCWPs).[11] This is contrary to previous reports that have suggested that PCWP may directly translate into specific and predictable radiographic findings.[12]

Should the chest roentgenogram indicate the presence of pulmonary edema, the distinction between cardiogenic and noncardiogenic causes represents the next challenge for the clinician. Besides cardiac systolic dysfunction, pulmonary edema may result from acute myocardial ischemia with diastolic dysfunction (so-called flash pulmonary edema), valvular heart disease, iatrogenic volume overload, renal failure, or capillary leak syndromes such as the acute respiratory distress syndrome (ARDS).

Identifying mimics of congestive heart failure

In addition to being useful in identifying the patient with decompensated CHF, the chest x-ray may also be used to evaluate other potential causes of the patient's symptoms which might mimic heart failure. The presence of pneumonia might be suggested by interstitial or alveolar infiltrates. Cavitary disease, mass lesions, and intrathoracic lymphadenopathy could indicate the presence of neoplastic disease. Interstitial lung diseases may present with diffuse nodular or reticulonodular radiographic findings. Unilateral pleural disease may represent pulmonary manifestations of infectious, neoplastic, thromboembolic, or collagen vascular disorders. Amiodarone, a drug commonly used in this patient population, may precipitate pulmonary fibrosis (Figure 11.2). This consideration should be in the differential diagnosis of any patient on amiodarone with worsening dyspnea. In the presence of a low hematocrit or hemoptysis, pulmonary hemorrhage should be considered. Detection of calcium in the mitral valve or pericardium may alert the physician to the presence of mitral stenosis or constrictive pericarditis. Venous thromboembolic disease can both mimic and result in decompensated CHF. The radiological manifestations of pulmonary embolism include focal oligemia (Westermark's sign) and peripheral infarction (Hampton's hump), though none of these findings are particularly sensitive or specific for this diagnosis (Figure 11.3). The presence of a

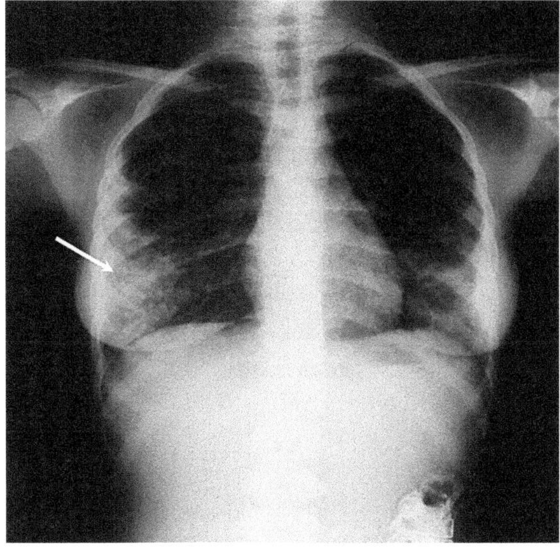

Figure 11.2. *Amiodarone pulmonary toxicity can mimic decompensated congestive heart failure with both alveolar and interstitial (arrow) infiltrates on chest x-ray (Image courtesy of Michael Landay, MD.)*

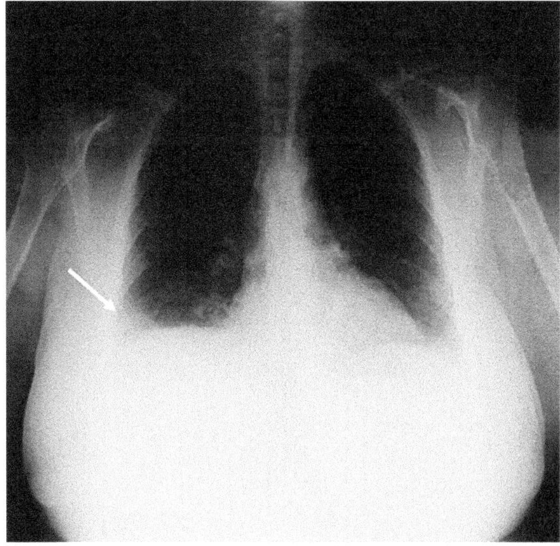

Figure 11.3. *Chest radiograph of patient with acute pulmonary embolism. Solid arrow depicts peripheral wedge-shaped infarct also known as Hampton's hump. Thromboembolic disease can mimic congestive heart failure (CHF) radiographically and may lead to loss of clinical stability in patients with CHF, resulting in decompensation (Image courtesy of Michael Landay, MD.)*

pericardial effusion can be suspected by an enlarged cardiac silhouette in the shape of a water bottle (Figure 11.4).

Of note, many of the above mimics of heart failure (such as pneumonia or pulmonary embolism) may also represent the condition leading to the loss of clinical stability and onset of decompensated heart failure.

The electrocardiogram

While no electrocardiographic findings are diagnostic for the presence of decompensated CHF, the ECG is recommended in the evaluation of all patients with suspected cardiac failure.[13] It is useful for the physician in both determining the etiology of decompensation as well as suggesting alternative causes of symptoms in the dyspneic patient.

A resting sinus tachycardia is often seen in decompensated heart failure. However, sinus tachycardia could suggest systemic infection in the presence of fever, or venous thromboembolic disease in the presence of asymmetric leg swelling. Sinus tachycardia may also be a manifestation of high-output heart failure states such as that seen with severe anemia, hyperthyroidism, beriberi, carcinoid, or in the presence of systemic arteriovenous fistulas. Other electrocardiographic manifestations of pulmonary thromboembolic disease include multifocal atrial tachycardia and right-heart strain patterns (right axis deviation or $S_1Q_3T_3$). The ECG should also be used by physicians to determine whether acute myocardial injury secondary to ischemia or infarction is present. The presence of ST-segment elevation or new left bundle branch block (LBBB) should make the clinician suspect acute infarction, while diffuse ST-segment elevation with associated PR-segment depression might lead to a diagnosis of acute pericarditis. ST-segment depression and T-wave inversions may suggest active myocardial ischemia. Low-voltage QRS complexes can occur in severe hypothyroidism or with an infiltrative process such as amyloidosis. Low voltage QRS complexes in conjunction with electrical alternans may also be present in the setting of a pericardial effusion and cardiac tamponade, another potential mimic of decompensated CHF.

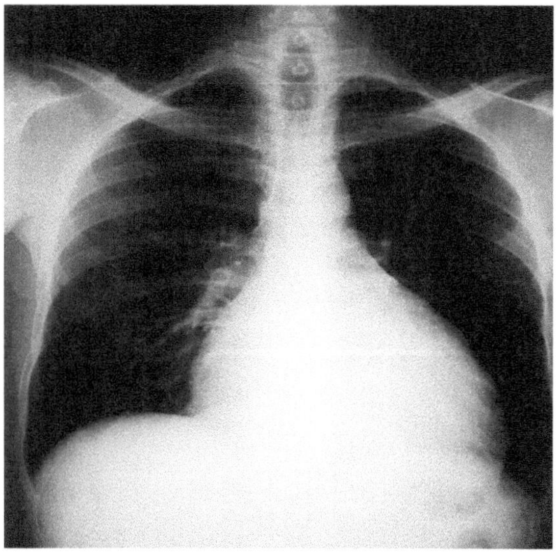

(A)

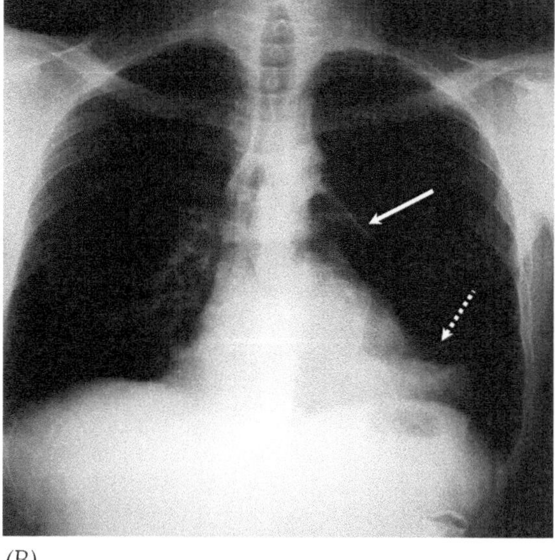

(B)

Figure 11.4. *The presence of a large pericardial effusion can often be detected radiographically (A) but can be confused with the cardiomegaly of CHF. Following pericardiocentesis (B), the outline of the pericardium (solid arrow) and an air-fluid level within the pericardium (dashed arrow) are seen and the heart size is now much reduced (Image courtesy of Michael Landay, MD.)*

Cardiac arrhythmias can also precipitate decompensated CHF. These include tachyarrhythmias, bradyarrhythmias, and atrioventricular block. Sinus bradycardia might suggest a superimposed infiltrative process or hypothyroidism. Atrioventricular block is often related to the underlying myocardial pathology but may be exacerbated by pharmacologic agents. Tachyarrhythmias, particularly ventricular tachycardia, are observed due to underlying chamber dysfunction, fibrosis and conduction delay. The acute onset of atrial fibrillation is a common precipitant of decompensated CHF due to the combined effects of a rapid and irregular ventricular response superimposed on a loss of atrial synchrony. In addition, tachyarrhythmias or bradyarrhythmias can be associated with digoxin toxicity. Finally, careful attention to the morphology of the P wave may identify an atrial tachycardia that is casually viewed as a sinus tachycardia (Figure 11.5).

Pacemaker malfunction may contribute to decompensation of CHF. More recently, evidence has emerged that right ventricular (RV) pacing may exacerbate CHF by inducing ventricular dyssynchrony. This is particularly relevant in patients with implantable cardioverter defibrillators (ICDs) and biventricular pacers with loss of LV lead capture. The change from biventricular to RV pacing on the surface ECG can be subtle (Figure 11.6). It is our practice to exclude pacemaker malfunction (whether it be a RV or biventricular pacemaker) in all paced patients with decompensated CHF.

Evaluation of the Patient with Suspected New Heart Failure

Patients who present for the first time with CHF represent a unique subgroup of those with acute heart failure. In this section we will focus on the role of the ECG and chest x-ray in evaluating such patients, recognizing that definitive assessment often includes echocardiography, cardiac magnetic resonance imaging (MRI), or cardiac catheterization. Nevertheless, the ECG and chest x-ray are often available to the physician before these other tests are completed and may provide important initial clues to the diagnosis.

The electrocardiogram

There have been many studies assessing the role of the 12-lead ECG for evaluating the dyspneic patient suspected of having acute heart failure. A common goal of such studies is to use the ECG to identify the etiology of LV dysfunction.

Is systolic dysfunction present?

A normal resting ECG is highly unusual in a patient with LV systolic dysfunction.[14–17] Because a normal resting ECG has approximately 95% positive predictive value for preserved left ventricular ejection fraction (LVEF),[18–19] a normal ECG should lead one to question a diagnosis of CHF due to systolic dysfunction. Other studies have found that electrocardiographic variables such as left ventricular hypertrophy (LVH) and left atrial abnormalities are significantly more common in patients with systolic dysfunction, though none of these findings had high positive or negative predictive values.[15,20–21] In addition, the presence of pathologic Q-waves does not appear to correlate with LVEF,[22] though the absence of anterior Q-waves has been incorporated into a prediction rule by Silver *et al.* to suggest preservation of systolic function following myocardial infarction (MI).[23]

A small study by Askenazi *et al.* in 1978 evaluated the QRS complex in ECGs of patients with angiographically-documented coronary artery disease (CAD), to determine if any clinical features of this complex correlated with LVEF. Based upon their analysis, the sum of the amplitudes of the R-waves in the 8 unipolar leads, or ΣR, correlated linearly with LVEF.[22] However, to our knowledge, no further studies have since validated these findings.

Ischemic or nonischemic cardiomyopathy?

Another common use of the ECG that has been well studied is whether or not the resting ECG can distinguish patients with nonischemic from ischemic cardiomyopathy. Historically, physicians have used the presence of pathologic Q-waves on the standard 12-lead ECG as indirect evidence for past infarction and hence obstructive coronary disease. However, even early case reports have demonstrated the poor specificity of this electrocardiographic finding.[24] While some argue that

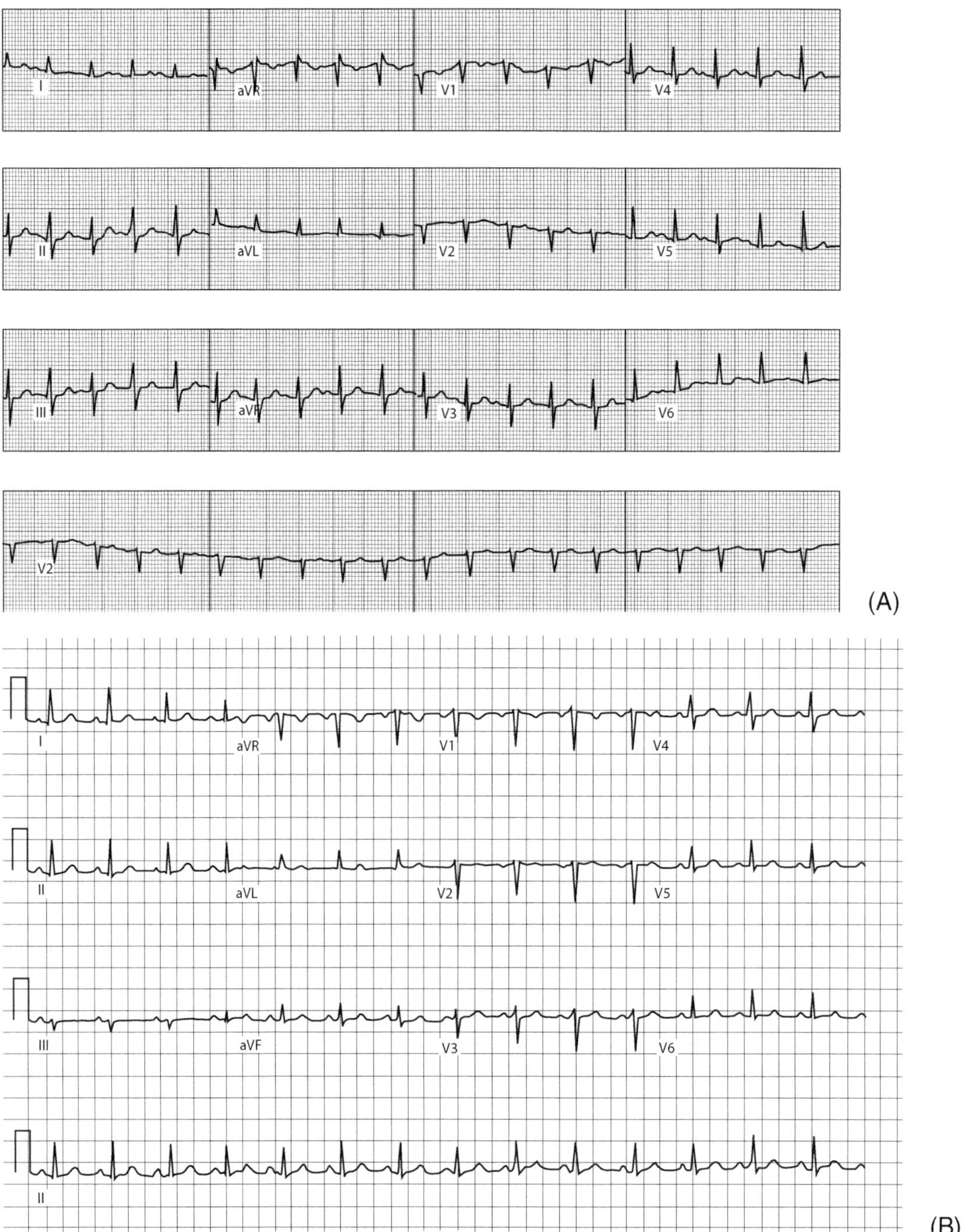

Figure 11.5. *Atrial tachycardia can mimic sinus tachycardia and provoke heart failure decompensation. (A) The presenting electrocardiogram (ECG) of a decompensated patient. Ventricular rate is 118 beats per minute. (B) ECG following ablation of the focus of atrial tachycardia at the mid-crista terminalis. Note the flatter P waves in leads II, III, F and V1, and the longer PR interval (A) prior to ablation, suggesting an ectopic atrial mechanism. Ventricular rate is 85 beats per minute.*

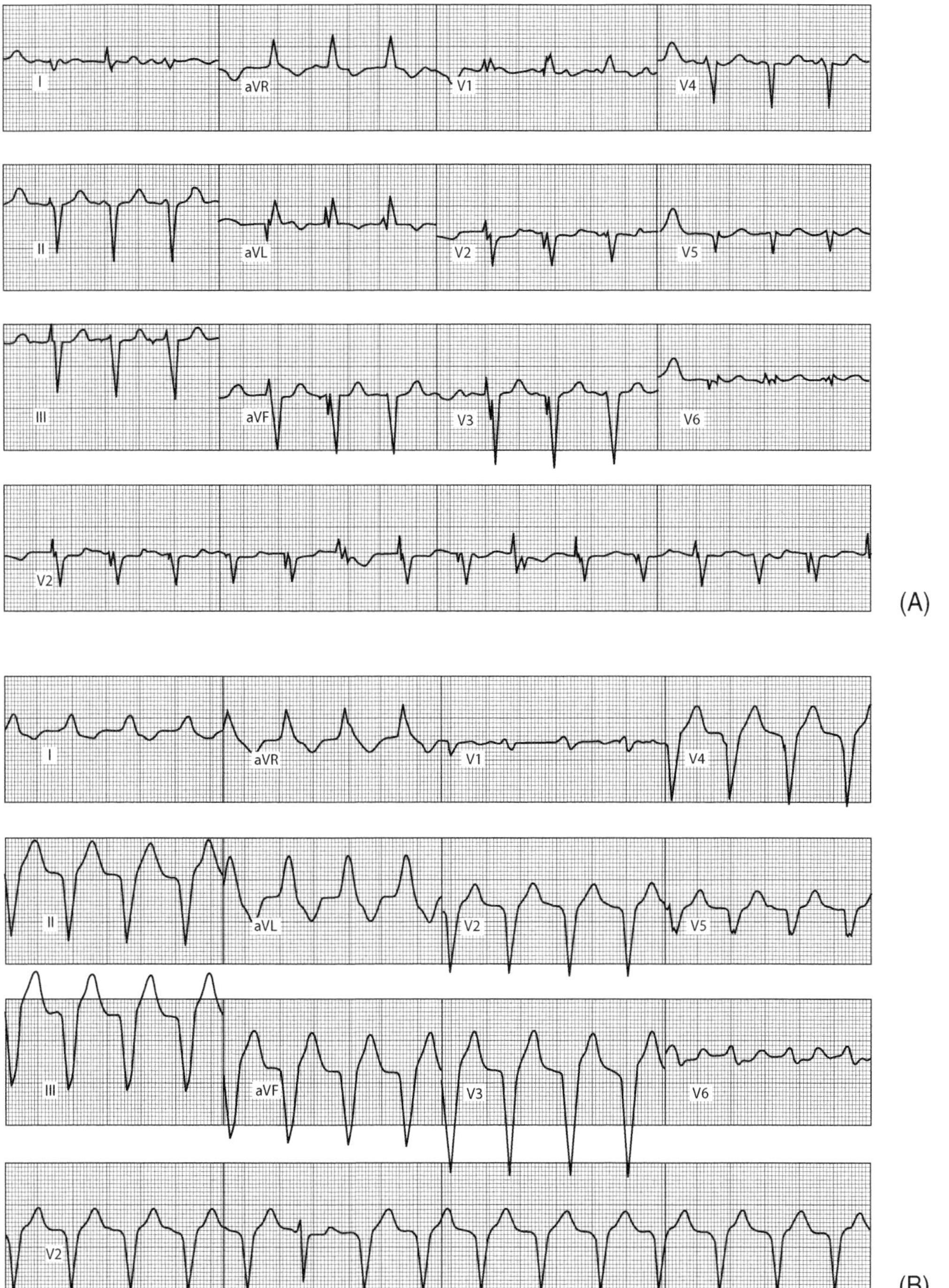

Figure 11.6. *The electrocardiogram (ECG) during biventricular (A) and right ventricular (RV) pacing (B). In patients treated with biventricular pacing, loss of left ventricular capture can provoke heart failure decompensation due to unopposed RV stimulation. The ECG findings may be subtle and include lengthening of the QRS duration with RV pacing and a change in electrical axis often best observed in leads I and V1.*

Q-waves are suggestive of an ischemic etiology,[25] angiographic and necropsy data have unequivocally demonstrated that the Q-wave infarct pattern provides insufficient evidence for a diagnosis of LV dysfunction due to CAD and can, in fact, be seen in the ECGs of patients with nonischemic cardiomyopathy.[26]

Other electrocardiographic variables have been studied in an attempt to identify patients with or without ischemic cardiomyopathy. Most studies have failed to find any criteria predictive of significant CAD,[27] though a LBBB has been found more commonly in patients with nonischemic cardiomyopathy.[27–28] A LBBB may also be an independent risk factor for adverse outcomes, conferring a 36% increase in all-cause mortality at 1 year, and a 35% increased risk of sudden cardiac death.[28]

While no studies have identified significant predictors of ischemic etiology from the ECG of patients with LV dysfunction, criteria have been identified which are more suggestive of a nonischemic etiology. Besides the presence of LBBB, Momiyama *et al.* found that nonischemic dilated cardiomyopathy can be characterized by a high RV_6 voltage and high voltage ratios of the R-wave in V_6 to the maximal R-wave in any of the inferior limb leads (RV_6/R_{max}). This index also correlated with the severity of systolic dysfunction.[29] To our knowledge, however, this finding has not been confirmed by others.

Other etiologies of cardiomyopathy

The ECG may demonstrate patterns suggestive of a specific diagnosis in patients with nonischemic cardiomyopathy. For instance, low limb lead voltages on the surface ECG with a pseudoinfarction pattern (loss of precordial R-wave progression or q waves) can suggest infiltrative diseases such as amyloidosis or sarcoidosis, especially when juxtaposed with an echocardiogram showing increased wall thickness. Tachyarrhythmias, specifically supraventricular and re-entrant tachycardias, may be seen in patients with tachycardia-mediated cardiomyopathy, and resting sinus tachycardia might be present in the initial ECG of patients with cardiomyopathy due to untreated thyrotoxicosis.

The chest x-ray: is ventricular dilation and systolic dysfunction present?

Besides assisting the physician in the evaluation of pulmonary vascular congestion or in identifying other medical conditions that are the cause of the patient's dyspnea, the chest x-ray may be used to identify ventricular dilatation. Radiographic cardiomegaly best correlates with the sum of the LV end-diastolic volume, the LV wall thickness, and the left atrial size,[9] and is the only consistent finding on chest x-ray in patients with end-stage CHF.[30–31] There are several ways for the physician to assess cardiomegaly, including the cardiothoracic ratio (CTR) and the relative cardiac volume. The concept of the CTR was popularized by Danzer in 1919, while evaluating the relationship of the heart to the thorax for diagnostic purposes. He identified that the ratio between the size of the heart and chest was quite constant, except when pathological processes such as heart failure existed. Danzer defined the cardiothoracic ratio by "dividing the transverse diameter of the heart by that of the thorax at a given level."[32] By testing some 500 cases, he described cardiomegaly as a CTR greater than 50%. This concept has changed fairly little in the modern era, and is still the most often used method for assessing radiographic cardiomegaly.

Unfortunately, more recent studies of the CTR have shown that it is inaccurate in its assessment of ventricular dilatation and, more importantly, appears to correlate poorly with cardiac systolic function. The diagnostic accuracy of the CTR for the presence of ventricular dilatation has been shown to be as low as 47%,[33] and sensitivity seems to improve only when the LV chamber volume increases to proportions greater than 66% of normal.[34] In addition, the correlation between CTR and LVEF appears poor. The CTR could not predict LVEF in patients with definite acute MI,[10] and had only weak negative correlation with the LVEF in chronic, stable CHF patients in the Digitalis Investigation Group (DIG) Trial and Veterans Affairs Cooperative Vasodilator-Heart Failure Trial (V-HeFT) databases.[35–36] Interestingly, however, the CTR was shown to be an independent predictor of survival in both of the V-HeFT trials.

The relative inadequacy of the CTR as a surrogate marker of LV chamber enlargement and systolic function has led to a search for other radiographic findings for these purposes. One such finding is that of the "plain heart volume," a measurement that takes into account the dimension of heart depth as assessed on the lateral radiograph. Theoretically, the plain heart volume reflects the sum of the volumes of all four cardiac chambers, including their mass, the pericardium, and the contents of the pericardial sac. While some have shown improved accuracy with this method,[33] most studies have suggested that this more cumbersome method does little to improve upon the findings of the CTR, and is equally poor in its correlation with LVEF.[9,31]

While the absence of radiographic cardiomegaly is thought to be inconsistent with a diagnosis of CHF and systolic dysfunction, the determination of cardiomegaly by various techniques correlates poorly with both actual cardiac chamber dilatation and ventricular function. In the end, a subjective assessment of radiographic LV size seems to be as sensitive as any other method.[34]

Other noninvasive tests to differentiate ischemic and nonischemic cardiomyopathy

As described with the ECG, a frequent part of the evaluation of a patient with new onset heart failure is whether or not the patient has underlying CAD. The American College of Cardiology (ACC)/ American Heart Association (AHA) guidelines for the diagnostic evaluation of the acute or chronic heart failure patient recommend invasive coronary angiography for those with CHF and either suspected CAD, scintigraphic evidence of reversible myocardial ischemia, or systolic dysfunction with unexplained cause despite noninvasive testing.[13,37] The following is a brief discussion of the various noninvasive tests besides the ECG which are available to the clinician for differentiating ischemic from nonischemic causes of heart failure.

Dobutamine stress echocardiography

The current ACC/AHA heart failure guidelines suggest that direct cardiac catheterization is the only method by which to absolutely rule out the presence of CAD with certainty.[37] However, as many as 30 to 50% of all patients with heart failure will not have CAD, and will therefore undergo unnecessary catheterization.

Early evidence suggested that the identification of regional as opposed to global wall motion abnormalities by two-dimensional echocardiography, could identify patients with LV dysfunction and CAD.[38] However, more recent studies have found that such segmental wall motion disturbances cannot be used to differentiate ischemic from nonischemic etiologies of heart failure. In fact, both regional wall motion abnormalities and global hypokinesis are equally likely to occur in either type of cardiomyopathy.[39–40]

With this in mind, investigators have sought to add dobutamine infusion to traditional TTE with the hopes of improving the diagnostic yield for assessment and identification of CAD. Dobutamine induces myocardial ischemia in patients with obstructive coronary disease by increasing LV contractility, chronotropy, wall stress, and, therefore, myocardial oxygen demand beyond that which can be met by supply. In several studies utilizing dobutamine stress echocardiography, this noninvasive test has been found to have a sensitivity ranging from 64% to 96% and specificity from 66% to 96% for the detection of ischemic cardiomyopathy—comparable with traditional exercise techniques for the noninvasive evaluation of CAD.[41–44] It should be noted, however, that optimal results were obtained at high-dose infusions of dobutamine (30–40 mcg/kg/min). At lower doses, inotropic contractile reserve may be retained despite significant coronary stenoses, likely indicating the presence of hibernating myocardium.[45]

Radionuclide imaging

Like traditional two-dimensional echocardiography, early studies of dipyridamole thallium-201 scintigraphy suggested a role for this imaging technique in the differentiation of ischemic and nonischemic etiologies of heart failure.[46–48] Thallium-201 is a potassium analogue and its ultimate distribution, following intravenous administration, is primarily intracellular. As a result, its initial distribution in the myocardium is directly related to regional myocardial blood flow.

Investigators have shown that rather large, heterogeneous, and extensive perfusion defects by thallium scintigraphy result in relatively high sensitivity but low specificity for ischemic cardiomyopathy.[46–49] However, others have argued that in the absence of such large and severe perfusion defects, thallium scintigraphy cannot reliably differentiate LV dysfunction due to CAD from nonischemic dilated cardiomyopathy.[50–51] In general, thallium scintigraphy appears to be more sensitive but less specific than dobutamine stress echocardiography for both the identification of CAD and myocardial viability.[52]

Positron emission tomography

Positron emission tomography (PET) characterizes the relative distributions of blood flow and glucose utilization. The application of PET to patients with LV dysfunction has resulted in high sensitivity, specificity, and diagnostic accuracy for the differentiation of ischemic and nonischemic cardiomyopathy in most studies.[53–54] However, a more recent study by Boffa *et al.* in 2000, demonstrated that while basal perfusion imaging with an N^{13}-ammonia tracer can clearly distinguish the two groups, glucose metabolism imaging resulted in significant overlap.[55]

PET imaging is often used to evaluate, identify, and characterize myocardial hibernation,[56–57] and in fact is considered by many to be the "gold standard" for this purpose. However, PET imaging is not without its limitations, perhaps most importantly expense and limited availability.

Computed tomography: electron beam and multidetector spiral computed tomography

Coronary calcium has been found to be closely associated with the presence of mural atheromatous plaque. A noninvasive means for establishing the presence of this coronary calcium might provide sufficient evidence for the presence of significant CAD. Electron-beam computed tomography (EBCT) has recently received a great deal of interest due to its reported ability to both identify and quantitate calcification of the coronary vessels. A 1996 consensus statement from the AHA declared EBCT to be "accurate for the prediction of angiographic stenosis."[58]

EBCT uses a fourth-generation computed tomography (CT) imaging process that utilizes a beam of electrons, generated from a stationary source, to obtain images rapidly and of high resolution.[59] Coronary artery calcification is then quantified, traditionally with a score developed by Agatston *et al.*[60] in which the area of a calcified plaque is multiplied by an estimated coefficient based on the peak density of the calcified lesion.

Several studies comparing coronary calcification by EBCT with conventional coronary angiography have shown that EBCT has high sensitivity and negative predictive value, with modest specificity for the presence of obstructive CAD.[60–62] In a recent meta-analysis, EBCT was found to have a pooled sensitivity of 92.3% and pooled specificity of 51.2% for identifying angiographically-significant coronary stenoses.[63] While no consistent coronary calcium cutpoints have been used to identify the presence or absence of CAD, receiver operating characteristic (ROC) curve analyses have shown that a range of "optimal" scores may be determined by the treating physician which can render the test either highly specific or highly sensitive, depending on the goals of the study and the specific clinical scenario.[64]

Not surprisingly, investigators have more recently begun to use this noninvasive technique in attempts to differentiate ischemic from nonischemic cardiomyopathy in patients with CHF. EBCT has already demonstrated better sensitivity, specificity, and accuracy than two-dimensional echocardiography, and appears to be a highly sensitive means of distinguishing angiographically-proven ischemic cardiomyopathy from nonischemic dilated cardiomyopathy.[65] In addition, EBCT calcium scores generally track with the amount of angiographic CAD, with the highest scores seen in those patients with 3-vessel disease by angiography.[66] The specificity of EBCT has only been modest in current studies of ischemic cardiomyopathy, ranging from 81% to 83%.[65–66] This may not be of concern for the heart failure clinician, however, if the goal of such a study is merely to rule out the presence of CAD in an attempt to prevent unnecessary cardiac catheterizations.

Multidetector computed tomography (MDCT) is another rapidly emerging noninvasive technique for assessment of CAD. Several small studies have documented the ability of MDCT to detect coronary atherosclerotic plaques in vivo.[67–70] A more recent investigation of patients with noncalcified atherosclerotic plaques, however, underscores the limitations of this technique with current technology for reliably detecting and quantifying these plaques throughout the coronary tree, despite its increased spatial and temporal resolution.[71]

Cardiac magnetic resonance imaging

Cardiac magnetic resonance (CMR) imaging can provide accurate, reproducible, three-dimensional high-resolution images, is not limited by acoustic windows, and is emerging rapidly for evaluation of cardiac size and function. Furthermore, with the use of ultrafast imaging and gadolinium contrast, CMR perfusion studies are being performed to identify obstructive coronary disease as well as to determine etiology of heart failure.[72]

In several studies of MRI for the detection of CAD, sensitivity has ranged from 38% to 90% with specificity ranging from 88% to 97%.[73–74] Cardiac MRI also has been found to accurately identify healed infarction, by demonstrating hyperenhancement in patients with a documented history of MI. This hyper-enhancement also correlated with the distribution of angiographically-proven obstructive coronary stenosis.[75]

Based upon preliminary studies of CMR for the detection of CAD, several investigators have attempted to use this imaging tool for the differentiation of heart failure patients with ischemic cardiomyopathy from those with nonischemic etiologies. A recent study, utilizing gadolinium-enhanced CMR, found that this technique had a high negative predictive value for excluding ischemic cardiomyopathy, but only modest positive predictive value.[76] Other investigators have used dobutamine infusions and utilized CMR to identify dobutamine-induced wall motion abnormalities suggestive of ischemia and hence significant CAD. These very small studies have found that CMR improves upon the sensitivity and specificity of traditional dobutamine stress echocardiography,[77] and appears to be a highly sensitive tool for the detection and localization of myocardial ischemia.[78]

References

1. American Heart Association. Heart Disease and Stroke Statistics—2004 Update (American Heart Association: Dallas, TX, 2003).
2. McKee PA, Castelli WP, McNamara PM, Kannel WB. The natural history of congestive heart failure: the Framingham study. N Engl J Med 1971; 285: 1441–1446.
3. Senni M, Tribouilloy CM, Rodeheffer RJ, *et al.* Congestive heart failure in the community: a study of all incident cases in Olmsted County, Minnesota, in 1991. Circulation 1998; 98: 2282–2289.
4. Mosterd A, Hoes AW, de Bruyne MC, *et al.* Prevalence of heart failure and left ventricular dysfunction in the general population. The Rotterdam Study. Eur Heart J 1999; 20: 447–455.
5. O'Connell JB. The economic burden of heart failure. Clin Cardiol 2000; 23: III6–III10.
6. Harlan WR, Oberman A, Grimm R, Rosati RA. Chronic congestive heart failure in coronary artery disease: clinical criteria. Ann Intern Med 1977; 86: 133–138.
7. Carlson KJ, Lee DC, Goroll AH, Leahy M, Johnson RA. An analysis of physicians' reasons for prescribing long-term digitalis therapy in outpatients. J Chron Dis 1985; 38: 733–739.
8. Marantz PR, Tobin JN, Wassertheil-Smoller S, *et al.* The relationship between left ventricular systolic function and congestive heart failure diagnosed by clinical criteria. Circulation 1988; 77: 607–612.
9. Badgett RG, Mulrow CD, Otto PM, Ramirez G. How well can the chest radiograph diagnose left ventricular dysfunction? J Gen Intern Med 1996; 11: 625–634.
10. Madsen EB, Gilpin E, Slutsky RA, *et al.* Usefulness of the chest x-ray for predicting abnormal left ventricular function after acute myocardial infarction. Am Heart J 1984; 108: 1431–1436.
11. Chakko S, Woska D, Martinez H, *et al.* Clinical, radiographic, and hemodynamic correlations in chronic congestive heart failure: conflicting results may lead to inappropriate care. Am J Med 1991; 990: 353–359.
12. Givertz MM, Colucci WS, Braunwald E. Clinical aspects of heart failure: high-output failure; pulmonary edema. In: Braunwald E, Zipes DP, Libby P (eds) Heart Disease: A Textbook of Cardiovascular Medicine, 6th edition (WB Saunders Company: Philadelphia, PA, 2001), 534–561.
13. Guidelines for the evaluation and management of heart failure. Report of the American College of Cardiology/American Heart Association Task Force on Practice Guidelines. Committee on Evaluation and

Management of Heart Failure. J Am Coll Cardiol 1995; 26: 1376–1398.

14. Davie AP, Francis CM, Love MP, *et al.* Value of the electrocardiogram in identifying heart failure due to left ventricular systolic dysfunction. BMJ 1996; 312: 222.
15. Gillespie ND, McNeill G, Pringle T, *et al.* Cross-sectional study of contribution of clinical assessment and simple cardiac investigations to diagnosis of left ventricular systolic dysfunction in patients admitted with acute dyspnoea. BMJ 1997; 314: 936–940.
16. Cleland JG, Habib F. Assessment and diagnosis of heart failure. J Intern Med 1996; 239: 317–325.
17. The Task Force on Heart Failure of the European Society of Cardiology. Guidelines for the diagnosis of heart failure. Eur Heart J 1995; 16: 741–751.
18. Christian TF, Miller TD, Chareonthaitawee P, *et al.* Prevalence of normal resting left ventricular function with normal rest electrocardiograms. Am J Cardiol 1997; 79: 1295–1298.
19. O'Keefe JH Jr., Zinsmeister AR, Gibbons RJ. Value of normal electrocardiographic findings in predicting left ventricular function in patients with chest pain and suspected coronary artery disease. Am J Med 1989; 86: 658–662.
20. Thomas JT, Kelley RF, Thomas SJ, *et al.* Utility of history, physical examination, electrocardiogram, and chest radiograph for differentiating normal from decreased systolic function in patients with heart failure. Am J Med 2002; 112: 437–445.
21. Houghton AR, Sparrow NJ, Toms E, Cowley AJ. Should general practitioners use the electrocardiogram to select patients with suspected heart failure for echocardiography? Int J Cardiol 1997; 62: 31–36.
22. Askenazi, J, Parisi AF, Cohn PF, Freedman WB, Braunwald E. Value of the QRS complex in assessing left ventricular ejection fraction. Am J Cardiol 1978; 41: 494–499.
23. Silver MT, Rose GA, Paul SD, *et al.* A clinical rule to predict preserved left ventricular ejection fraction in patients after myocardial infarction. Ann Intern Med 1994; 121: 750–756.
24. Tavel M, Fisch C. Abnormal Q waves simulating myocardial infarction in diffuse myocardial diseases. Am Heart J 1964; 68: 534–537.
25. Feld H, Priest S, Denson M. Importance of pathologic Q waves in patients with dilated cardiomyopathies. Am J Med 1993; 94: 546–548.
26. Gau GT, Goodwin JF, Oakley CM, *et al.* Q waves and coronary arteriography in cardiomyopathy. Br Heart J 1972; 34: 1034–1041.
27. Pirwitz MJ, Lange RA, Landau C, *et al.* Utility of the 12-lead electrocardiogram in identifying underlying coronary artery disease in patients with depressed left ventricular systolic function. Am J Cardiol 1996; 77: 1289–1292.
28. Baldasseroni S, Opasich C, Gorini M, *et al.*, Italian Network on Congestive Heart Failure Investigators. Left bundle-branch block is associated with increased 1-year sudden and total mortality rate in 5517 outpatients with congestive heart failure: a report from the Italian Network on Congestive Heart Failure. Am Heart J 2002; 143: 398–405.
29. Momiyama Y, Mitamura H, Kimura M. ECG differentiation of idiopathic dilated cardiomyopathy from coronary artery disease with left ventricular dysfunction. J Electrocardiol 1995; 28: 231–236.
30. Mahdyoon H, Klein R, Eyler W, Lakier JB, Chakko SC, Gheorghiade M. Radiographic pulmonary congestion in end-stage congestive heart failure. Am J Cardiol 1989; 63: 625–627.
31. Harlan WR, Oberman A, Grimm R, Rosati RA. Chronic congestive heart failure in coronary artery disease: clinical criteria. Ann Intern Med 1977; 86: 133–138.
32. Danzer, CS. The cardiothoracic ratio: an index of cardiac enlargement. Am J Med Sci 1919; 157: 513–521.
33. Chikos PM, Figley MM, Fisher L. Correlation between chest film and angiographic assessment of left ventricular size. AJR Am J Roentgenol 1977; 128: 367–373.
34. Rose CP, Stolberg HO. The limited utility of the plain chest film in the assessment of left ventricular structure and function. Invest Radiol 1982; 17: 139–144.
35. Philbin EF, Garg R, Danisa K, *et al.* The relationship between cardiothoracic ratio and left ventricular ejection fraction in congestive heart failure. Digitalis Investigation Group. Arch Intern Med 1998; 158: 501–506.
36. Cohn JN, Johnson GR, Shabetai R, *et al.* Ejection fraction, peak exercise oxygen consumption, cardiothoracic ratio, ventricular arrhythmias, and plasma norepinephrine as determinants of prognosis in heart failure. The V-HeFT VA Cooperative Studies Group. Circulation 1993; 87: VI5–VI16.
37. Scanlon PJ, Faxon DP, Audet AM, *et al.* ACC/AHA guidelines for coronary angiography: a report of the American College of Cardiology/American Heart Association Task Force on practice guidelines. (Committee on Coronary Angiography). Developed in collaboration with the Society for Cardiac Angiography and Interventions. J Am Coll Cardiol 1999; 33: 1756–1816.
38. Chen YZ, Sherrid MV, Dwyer EM Jr. Value of two-dimensional echocardiography in evaluating coronary

artery disease: a randomized blinded analysis. J Am Coll Cardiol 1985; 5: 911–917.

39. Wallis DE, O'Connell JB, Henkin RE, Costanzo-Nordin MR, Scanlon PJ. Segmental wall motion abnormalities in dilated cardiomyopathy: a common finding and good prognostic sign. J Am Coll Cardiol 1984; 4: 674–679.
40. Diaz RA, Nihoyannopoulos P, Athanassopoulos G, Oakley CM. Usefulness of echocardiography to differentiate dilated cardiomyopathy from coronary-induced congestive heart failure. Am J Cardiol 1991; 68: 1224–1227.
41. Sharp SM, Sawada SG, Segar DS, *et al.* Dobutamine stress echocardiography: detection of coronary artery disease in patients with dilated cardiomyopathy. J Am Coll Cardiol 1994; 24: 934–939.
42. Mazeika PK, Nadazdin A, Oakley CM. Dobutamine stress echocardiography for detection and assessment of coronary artery disease. J Am Coll Cardiol 1992; 19: 1203–1211.
43. Marcovitz PA, Armstrong WF. Accuracy of dobutamine stress echocardiography in detecting coronary artery disease. Am J Cardiol 1992; 69: 1269–1273.
44. Vigna C, Russo A, De Rito V, *et al.* Regional wall motion analysis by dobutamine stress echocardiography to distinguish between ischemic and nonischemic dilated cardiomyopathy. Am Heart J 1996; 131: 537–543.
45. Bonow RO. The hibernating myocardium: implications for management of congestive heart failure. Am J Cardiol 1995; 75: 17A–25A.
46. Iskandrian AS, Hakki A, Kane S. Resting thallium-201 myocardial perfusion patterns in patients with severe left ventricular dysfunction: differences between patients with primary cardiomyopathy, chronic coronary artery disease, or acute myocardial infarction. Am Heart J 1985; 111: 760–767.
47. Eichorn EJ, Kosinski EJ, Lewis SM, *et al.* Usefulness of dipyridamole-thallium-201 perfusion scanning for distinguishing ischemic from nonischemic cardiomyopathy. Am J Cardiol 1988; 62: 945–951.
48. Tauberg SG, Orie JE, Bartlett BE, Cottington EM, Flores AR. Usefulness of thallium-201 for distinction of ischemic from idiopathic dilated cardiomyopathy. Am J Cardiol 1993; 71: 674–680.
49. Chikamori T, Doi YL, Yonezawa Y, *et al.* Value of dipyridamole thallium-201 imaging in noninvasive differentiation of idiopathic dilated cardiomyopathy from coronary artery disease with left ventricular dysfunction. Am J Cardiol 1992; 69: 650–653.
50. Greenberg JM, Murphy JH, Okada RD, *et al.* Value and limitations of radionuclide angiography in determining the cause of reduced left ventricular ejection fraction: comparison of idiopathic dilated cardiomyopathy and coronary artery disease. Am J Cardiol 1985; 55: 541–544.
51. Glamann DB, Lange RA, Corbett JR, Hillis LD. Utility of various radionuclide techniques for distinguishing ischemic from nonischemic dilated cardiomyopathy. Arch Intern Med 1992; 152: 769–772.
52. Allman KC, Shaw LJ, Hachamovitch R, Udelson JE. Myocardial viability testing and impact of revascularization on prognosis in patients with coronary artery disease and left ventricular dysfunction: a meta-analysis. J Am Coll Cardiol 2002; 39: 1151–1158.
53. Eisenberg JD, Sobel BE, Geltman EM. Differentiation of ischemic from nonischemic cardiomyopathy with positron emission tomography. Am J Cardiol 1987; 59: 1410–1414.
54. Mody FV, Brunken RC, Stevenson LW, *et al.* Differentiating cardiomyopathy of coronary artery disease from nonischemic dilated cardiomyopathy utilizing positron emission tomography. J Am Coll Cardiol 1991; 17: 373–383.
55. Boffa GM, Zanco P, Della Valentina P, *et al.* Positron emission tomography is a useful tool in differentiating idiopathic from ischemic dilated cardiomyopathy. Int J Cardiol 2000; 74: 67–74.
56. Tillisch J, Brunken R, Marshall R, *et al.* Reversibility of cardiac wall-motion abnormalities predicted by positron tomography. N Engl J Med 1986; 314: 884–888.
57. Maes A, Flameng W, Nuyts J, *et al.* Histological alterations in chronically hypoperfused myocardium: correlation with PET findings. Circulation 1994; 90: 735–745.
58. Wexler L, Brundage B, Crouse J, *et al.* Coronary artery calcification: pathophysiology, epidemiology, imaging methods, and clinical implications: a statement for health professionals from the American Heart Association. Writing Group. Circulation 1996; 94: 1175–1192.
59. Salazar HP, Raggi P. Usefulness of electron-beam computed tomography. Am J Cardiol 2002; 89: 17B–23B.
60. Agatston AS, Janowitz WR, Hildner FJ, *et al.* Quantification of coronary artery calcium using ultrafast computed tomography. J Am Coll Cardiol 1990; 15: 827–832.
61. Budoff MJ, Georgiou D, Brody A, *et al.* Ultrafast computed tomography as a diagnostic modality in the detection of coronary artery disease: a multicenter study. Circulation 1996; 93: 898–904.
62. Haberl R, Becker A, Leber A, *et al.* Correlation of coronary calcification and angiographically documented

stenoses in patients with suspected coronary artery disease: results of 1 765 patients. J Am Coll Cardiol 2001; 37: 451–457.
63. Nallanmothu BK, Saint S, Bielak LF, *et al*. Electron-beam computed tomography in the diagnosis of coronary artery disease: a meta-analysis. Arch Intern Med 2001; 161: 833–838.
64. Rumberger JA, Sheedy PF, Breen JF, Schwartz RS. Electron beam computed tomographic coronary calcium score cutpoints and severity of associated angiographic lumen stenosis. J Am Coll Cardiol 1997; 29: 1542–1548.
65. Le T, Ko JY, Kim HT, Akinwale P, Budoff MJ. Comparison of echocardiography and electron beam tomography in differentiating the etiology of heart failure. Clin Cardiol 2000; 23: 417–420.
66. Budoff MJ, Shavelle DM, Lamont DH, *et al*. Usefulness of electron beam computed tomography scanning for distinguishing ischemic from nonischemic cardiomyopathy. J Am Coll Cardiol 1998; 32: 1173–1178.
67. Becker CR, Knez A, Ohnesorge B, Schoepf UJ, Reiser MF. Imaging of noncalcified coronary plaques using helical CT with retrospective ECG gating. AJR Am J Roentgenol 2000; 175: 423–424.
68. Schroeder S, Kopp AF, Baumbach A, *et al*. Noninvasive detection and evaluation of atherosclerotic coronary plaques with multislice computed tomography. J Am Coll Cardiol 2001; 37: 1430–1435.
69. Leber AW, Knez A, White CW, *et al*. Composition of coronary atherosclerotic plaques in patients with acute myocardial infarction and stable angina pectoris determined by contrast-enhanced multislice computed tomography. Am J Cardiol 2003; 91: 714–718.
70. Nikolaou K, Sagmeister S, Knez A, *et al*. Multidetector-row computed tomography of the coronary arteries: predictive value and quantitative assessment of non-calcified vessel-wall changes. Eur Radiol 2003; 13: 2505–2512.
71. Achenbach, S, Moselewski F, Ropers D, *et al*. Detection of calcified and noncalcified coronary atherosclerotic plaque by contrast-enhanced, submillimeter multidetector spiral computed tomography: a segment-based comparison with intravascular ultrasound. Circulation 2004; 109: 14–17.
72. Prasad S, Pennell DJ. Magnetic resonance imaging in the assessment of patients with heart failure. J Nuc Cardiol 2002; 9: 60S–70S.
73. Manning WJ, Li W, Edelman RR. A preliminary report comparing magnetic resonance coronary angiography with conventional angiography. N Engl J Med 1993; 328: 828–832.
74. Achenbach S, Ropers D, Matthias R, *et al*. Noninvasive coronary angiography by magnetic resonance imaging, electron-beam computed tomography, and multislice computed tomography. Am J Cardiol 2001; 88: 70E–73E.
75. Wu E, Judd RM, Vargas JD, *et al*. Visualisation of presence, location, and transmural extent of healed Q-wave and non-Q-wave myocardial infarction. Lancet 2001; 357: 21–28.
76. McCrohon JA, Moon JC, Prasad SK, *et al*. Differentiation of heart failure related to dilated cardiomyopathy and coronary artery disease using gadolinium-enhanced cardiovascular magnetic resonance. Circulation 2003; 108: 54–59.
77. Nagel E, Lehmkuhl HB, Bocksch W, *et al*. Noninvasive diagnosis of ischemic-induced wall motion abnormalities with the use of high-dose dobutamine stress MRI: comparison with dobutamine stress echocardiography. Circulation 1999; 99: 763–770.
78. Van Rugge FP, van der Wall EE, Spanjersberg SJ, *et al*. Magnetic resonance imaging during dobutamine stress for detection and localization of coronary artery disease: quantitative wall motion analysis using a modification of the centerline method. Circulation 1994; 90: 127–138.

CHAPTER 12

Noninvasive hemodynamic monitoring of the acute heart failure patient

Clyde Yancy

Decompensated Heart Failure: A Hemodynamic Malady

Acute decompensated heart failure (ADHF) has become one of the most pressing clinical problems in the management of patients with heart failure. The ability to effectively manage ADHF is hampered by a number of important limitations: uncertainty regarding diagnosis, lack of sufficient evidence-based treatment strategies, and limited tools to assess the response to therapy. This chapter profiles the role that non-invasive assessment of hemodynamics may have in overcoming these limitations and how it may lead to better management of ADHF.

Multiple pathophysiological mechanisms are believed to contribute to the development and progression of heart failure. These mechanisms include: the neurohormonal process which activates the renin-angiotensin-aldosterone system (RAAS), sympathetic nervous system, arginine vasopressin, endothelin, and natriuretic peptides;[1] the inflammatory process which activates free oxygen radicals and proinflammatory cytokines; the myocardial process which stimulates myocardial remodeling and leads to left ventricular hypertrophy (LVH), extracellular matrix turnover, and loss of functional myocytes; and the compensatory hemodynamic process which results in peripheral voasoconstriction, reduced cardiac output, and left or right atrial hypertension. While all four processes are thought to play a contributory role, it is believed that changes in both the RAAS and the activity of the sympathetic nervous system are primary factors in the progression of chronic heart failure, while changes in the hemodynamic response are primary factors in the development of ADHF.

Understanding and measuring these hemodynamic factors are central to the assessment, prognosis, and treatment of any patient with ADHF. The four determinants of cardiac output are the rate of the pump (heart rate), the volume of blood available to pump (preload), the pumping strength (contractility), and the force the heart must overcome to pump (afterload). Left or right atrial pressure overload is due to either frank volume excess or changes in ventricular compliance or both. ADHF can be viewed primarily as a hemodynamic disorder characterized by elevated atrial and ventricular filling pressures and possibly decreased cardiac output. These alterations lead to elevated venous pressures and decreased tissue perfusion, which in turn produce the fundamental symptoms of heart failure including swelling, dyspnea, fatigue, listlessness, and ultimately a decrease in exercise capacity. Elevated venous pressures lead to left or right atrial hypertension, which results in edema or dyspnea while increased peripheral resistance and reduced cardiac output lead to fatigue and reduced exercise capacity.[2]

Pharmacologic interventions for ADHF must be targeted at both neurohormonal and hemodynamic perturbations. Diuretics, digoxin, vasodilators, RAAS inhibitors, beta-blockers, and devices all improve the natural course of heart failure while diuretics, vasodilators, RAAS inhibitors, natriuretic peptides, and inotropic agents, along with certain mechanical interventions, all improve hemodynamic interrelationships in patients with acute decompensated failure.[3] To alleviate symptoms and improve patient well-being, acute pharmacological intervention for ADHF is targeted at underlying hemodynamic alterations. The selection of appropriate therapy for ADHF may, therefore, involve a more hemodynamically-oriented treatment strategy than is otherwise observed during titration of therapies for chronic heart failure.

Invasive hemodynamics

Clinical measurements of cardiac hemodynamics have been available since the 1970s. The standard approach has been the utilization of diagnostic catheters introduced percutaneously into the right-sided circulation. Pressure is measured by observation of fluctuations in transducers that are in-line with fluid-filled systems, and cardiac output is measured by one or more indicator dilution techniques including the Fick method, Green Dye method, or Thermodilution method. Of these, the use of a flow-directed, thermodilution catheter—also known as the Swan–Ganz catheter—represents the most widely applied technique.[4] In the United States, it is estimated that at least 2 million pulmonary artery (PA) catheter monitoring procedures are performed annually, most often in perioperative cardiac and vascular surgical patients, as well as patients with decompensated heart failure, multi-organ failure, and trauma.

Some studies have shown an improvement in outcomes with PA catheter-guided therapy,[5–10] while others have challenged the utility, safety, and economics of the PA catheter and suggested that it does not improve outcomes but does increase complications and cost.[11–14] Recently, there has been considerable debate about whether the benefits of PA catheter justify the risks associated with invasive monitoring. Physicians who utilize PA catheter monitoring in patients hospitalized with heart failure maintain that the information is helpful in their management decisions for an individual patient. The strongest advocates for such a strategy are those involved in critical care settings. However, due to the lack of proven benefit of the PA catheter in prospective trials and the cost and risk associated with the procedure, many physicians treating patients hospitalized with heart failure have reduced or eliminated their utilization of invasive hemodynamic monitoring and rely instead upon bedside observations and clinical empiricism to guide therapy.

Hemodynamic assessment

Symptoms, physical findings that include the vital signs, and laboratory findings, such as blood tests and chest radiographs, are imprecise measures of hemodynamic function. Unfortunately, without a PA catheter, they are the only data that many clinicians have at their disposal when making important decisions about the care of patients with heart failure. Stevenson *et al.*[15] described symptomatic heart failure as a hemodynamic disease, suggesting patient presentations as one of four possible hemodynamic profiles (Figure 12.1).

Classifying patients into one of the four clinical profiles of heart failure, based on physical examination and common clinical signs and symptoms for congestion and perfusion, has important implica-

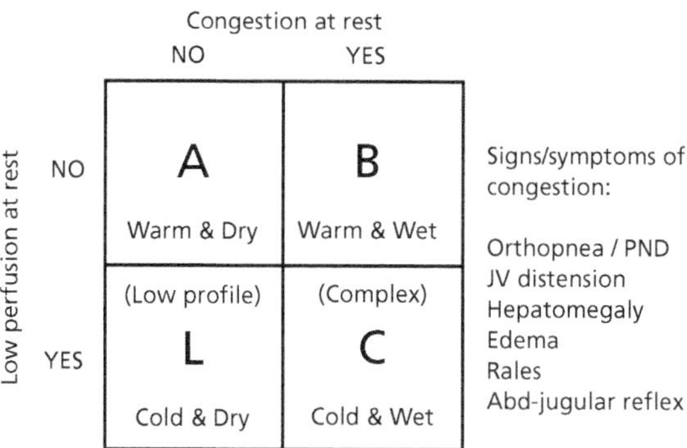

Figure 12.1. *Clinical profiles in heart failure (With permission from Stevenson.*[15]*)*

Abbreviations: PND = *paroxysmal nocturnal dyspnea;* JV = *jugular vein;* ACE = *angiotensin converting enzyme*

tions for prognosis and proper selection of therapy.[16]

Classical signs and symptoms of venous congestion, such as pulmonary and peripheral edema, are often primary diagnostic factors in hospital admittance and acute implementation of diuretic treatment, which is clearly appropriate. However, determining whether a patient is "warm and wet," "cold and wet," or somewhere in between can be a difficult clinical task, even for the most skilled practitioner. Reliance on physical examination skills such as jugular venous distention (JVD) or pulmonary rales is straightforward but relatively insensitive, and the ability to accurately judge a patient's clinical or hemodynamic status from the history and physical examination is inadequate. Studies evaluating the ability of clinicians to accurately assess preload based on an examination of the jugular venous pressure (JVP) indicate that clinicians are only correct about 50% of the time, especially when relying upon clinical judgment or skills through an interview and an examination to assess whether or not patients are "wet or dry" or "warm or cold."[17,18] Stevenson reported a sensitivity of 58% for clinical signs indicative of elevated pulmonary capillary wedge pressures (PCWPs).[19] Jonas reported only a 30% correct estimation of cardiac index by physical examination when compared to the less invasive lithium dilution method.[20] These shortcomings in the clinical assessment may relegate treatment decisions to empiric judgments or frank therapeutic misadventures.

Introducing a New Paradigm

In theory, a noninvasive way to monitor hemodynamics would provide exceptional clinical value because data similar to invasive hemodynamic monitoring methods could be obtained with much lower cost and no risk. While noninvasive hemodynamic monitoring can be used in patients who previously required an invasive procedure, the greatest impact may be on patients and care environments where invasive hemodynamic monitoring was neither possible nor worth the risk or cost. Heart failure is a condition in which awareness of hemodynamics plays an important role in the assessment, diagnosis, prognosis, and treatment.

Impedance cardiography technology: history and method

Impedance cardiography (ICG) is a continuous, noninvasive method to obtain hemodynamic data (cardiac output, left ventricular preload, afterload, and contractility) and assess thoracic fluid status. ICG is also referred to as thoracic electrical bioimpedance (TEB) or electrical impedance plethysmography (EIP), and has been researched since the 1940s.

Given the importance of hemodynamic considerations in heart failure treatment, ICG is a technology that permits economical, noninvasive monitoring of hemodynamic parameters in either the hospital or outpatient setting. The technology is based on Ohm's law, and applies a low amplitude, high frequency alternating electrical current to the thorax and measures the corresponding voltage in order to detect changes in thoracic impedance. The premise of ICG is based on an assumption that the thorax represents a cylinder in a cylinder. The inner cylinder is assumed to be fluid filled while the outer cylinder is composed of air. The resistance to propagation of an electrical impulse across this system then becomes a function of the dynamic changes in fluid volume within the inner cylinder. Four dual sensors are placed on either side of the neck and thorax (Figure 12.2).

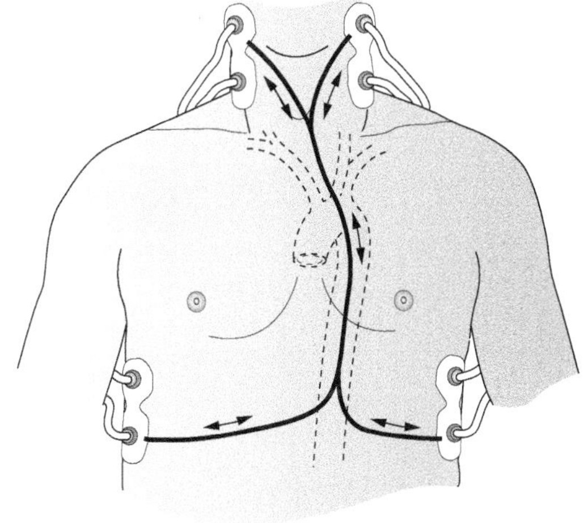

Figure 12.2. *Impedance cardiography method (With permission from CardioDynamics, Inc.[26])*

The outer sensors transmit the alternating electrical current, and the inner sensors determine the thoracic impedance. There are two primary components of impedance: (1) base impedance, which depends on thoracic blood and plasma volume, chest skeletal muscle, cardiac muscle, lung tissue, chest wall fat and air; and (2) dynamic impedance, which is caused by changing blood volume and velocity in the thoracic aorta. Biological tissues, such as muscle, bone, fat, blood and plasma, all have different electrical properties. Of these tissues, blood is the most electrically conductive. Since arterial blood flow is pulsatile and arterial vessel walls are compliant, pulsatile changes in blood volume occur in the thoracic arterial system, predominantly in the aorta, as a result of ventricular function. This change in blood volume results in a change in the electrical conductivity and thus the impedance of the thorax to electrical current. To calculate stroke volume and cardiac output, an algorithm is applied to the measured dynamic beat-to-beat changes in impedance that are processed. Fiducial points are determined from the electrocardiography (ECG) and ICG waveforms (Figure 12.3). The application of these fiducial points to measured and calculated ICG parameters is shown in Table 12.1.

Of great interest to many heart failure physicians is the parameter of thoracic fluid content (TFC), which is represented as the inverse of baseline impedance. As conductivity in the chest increases (impedance decreases), TFC increases. Since baseline impedance is dependent on the total thoracic tissue content, TFC is dependent on the total thoracic tissue content. Because fluid (both intravascular and extravascular) is the most conductive and variable component of thoracic tissue, changes in TFC primarily occur because of changes in fluid.[21] A baseline TFC must be established for each individual patient, and intra-patient directional changes in TFC will be indicative of directional changes in thoracic fluid.[22,23] Ultimately, it is assumed that some derivation of thoracic fluid content will be representative of volume status. This premise remains under active investigation.

Like many medical technologies, ICG has evolved from earlier experimental platforms to a commercially viable device today. In the 1960s, Kubicek *et al.* were commissioned by the National Aeronautics and Space Administration (NASA) to develop a noninvasive method of determining cardiac output (CO). A 5-year program led to the development of the Minnesota Impedance Cardiograph (MIC), an electronic system for measuring impedance changes across the thorax and a new equation for stroke volume (SV). In the 1980s, Sramek developed a less cumbersome ICG device with a revised SV equation by using a truncated cone rather than a cylindrical model of the chest. In 1986, Bernstein modified the Sramek equation to increase accuracy for the determination of the thorax volume. In the mid-1990s, proprietary adjustments were made to the Bernstein–Sramek equation and led to a more accurate ICG monitor (Z MARC®, Impedance Modulating AoRtic Compliance; BioZ; CardioDynamics; San Diego, CA).

Since that time, several additional ICG systems

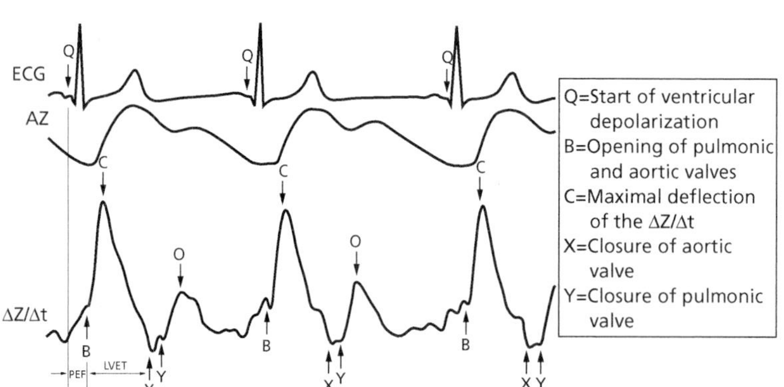

Figure 12.3. *Fiducial points derived from electrocardiography and impedance cardiography waveforms*

Table 12.1. *Impedance cardiography parameters*

Parameter	Measurement or calculation	Units
Flow		
Stroke volume (SV)	VI × LVET x VEPT (Z MARC® Algorithm)	mL/beat
Stroke index (SI)	SV/BSA	mL/beat/m^2
Cardiac output (CO)	SV × HR	L/min
Cardiac index (CI)	CO/BSA	L/min/m^2
Resistance		
Systemic vascular resistance (SVR)	[(MAP – CVP)/CO] × 80	dyne × s × cm^{-5}
Systemic vascular resistance index (SVRI)	[(MAP – CVP)/CI] × 80	dyne × s × cm^{-5} × m^2
Contractility		
Pre-ejection period (PEP)	ECG Q wave to aortic valve opening	ms
Left ventricular ejection time (LVET)	Aortic valve opening to closing	ms
Systolic time ratio (STR)	PEP/LVET	No units
Velocity index (VI)	First time derivative max/baseline impedance	/1000/s
Acceleration index (ACI)	Second time derivative max/baseline impedance	/100/s^2
Left cardiac work index (LCWI)	(MAP – PCWP) × CI × 0.0144	kg/min/m^2
Fluid Status		
Thoracic fluid content (TFC)	1 / baseline impedance	/kOhm

Abbreviations: BSA = body surface area; cm = centimeter; CVP = central venous pressure; ECG = electrocardiography; HR = heart rate; ICG = impedance cardiography; kg = kilogram; kOhm = kilo ohm; L = liter; m = meter; MAP = mean arterial pressure; mL = milliliter; ms = millisecond; min = minute; PCWP = pulmonary capillary wedge pressure (estimated value of 10 mm Hg); s = seconds; VEPT = volume of electrically participating tissue; VI = velocity index; Z MARC = impedance modulating aortic compliance.

have received US Food and Drug Administration 510(k) clearance. The development of these newer platforms, now supported with a reasonable database attesting to both accuracy and clinical utility, has led to widespread use for clinical assessment, diagnosis, prognosis, and treatment decisions. To date, ICG is widely utilized in patient management applications, a majority of which involve patients with moderate to severe ventricular dysfunction.[24] The known ICG device manufacturers include Cardiodynamics (BioZ® System), Hemosapiens (HOTMAN® System), Noninvasive Medical Technologies (IQ™ System), and SORBA (Steorra™ System). Of these, the BioZ system is most widely utilized and most of the validation and application studies involve this system. The revised algorithm in this system has been compared to prior versions and appears to be a significant improvement.[25]

Limitations of impedance cardiography

To ensure accurate calculation of stroke volume, a patient's height must be between 4 and 7 feet tall, and weight between 67 and 341 pounds. Severe aortic regurgitation, advanced sepsis, presence of an intraaortic balloon pump (IABP), or extreme tachycardia (heart rate > 250 bpm) represent clinical limitations and may invalidate ICG measurements.[26]

Validation studies

Physicians and providers depend on evidence-based validation studies before utilizing a new monitoring modality to make treatment decisions. Previous generations of ICG have shown inconsistent performance[27,28] and did not meet the threshold required to make clinical decisions. However, initial and ongoing research indicates that the current generation of ICG devices has achieved acceptable levels of accuracy compared to invasive hemodynamic methods. The first point of consideration in the evaluation of the latest generation of ICG is whether intra-day measurements are reproducible and whether inter-day measurements show expected variability in stable ambulatory patients. In stable cardiac rehabilitation patients, Verhoeve *et al.*[29] reported high intra-day correlation and expected inter-day correlation for ICG hemodynamic parameters. Greenberg *et al.*[30] reported acceptable and expectedly higher intra-day and inter-day variability in heart failure patients. Expected inter-day measurements are important as they provide a basis to evaluate whether changes in hemodynamics are occurring within natural variability or because of disease status or therapeutic intervention.

The latest-generation ICG devices accurately determine cardiac output and cardiac index compared to traditional invasive methods of thermodilution and direct Fick across a variety of patient types, including patients with chronic and acutely decompensated heart failure (Table 12.2).

Van de Water's study (Table 12.2) also demonstrated that ICG's standard deviation from the average thermodilution cardiac output (1.09 L/min) was comparable to individual thermodilution calculations compared to each other (1.03 L/min),

Table 12.2. *Validation studies comparing refined impedance cardiography to standard methods of cardiac output estimation*

Author (year)	Population	Parameter	Comparison	*R* Value	Bias	Precision
Albert (2003)[63]	Heart failure in intensive care unit (n = 33)	Cardiac output	ICG–TD	0.89	–0.46	1.38
Drazner (2002)[34]	Heart failure in catheterization laboratory (n = 59)	Cardiac output	ICG-Fick TD-Fick ICG-TD	0.73 0.81 0.76	0.74 0.75 0.03	1.1 0.95 1.1
Ziegler (1999)[64]	Mechanically ventilated (n = 52)	Cardiac output	ICG-TD	0.89	NR	NR
Sageman (2002)[65]	Post-CABG (n = 20)	Cardiac index	ICG-TD	0.92	0.07	0.40
Van de Water (2003)[25]	Post-CABG (n = 53)	Cardiac output	ICG-TD	0.81	–0.17	1.09
Yung (2004)[66]	Pulmonary hypertension (n = 42)	Cardiac output	ICG-Fick TD-Fick ICG-TD	0.84 0.89 0.80	–0.24 0.19 –0.43	0.87 0.76 1.01

Abbreviations: Bias calculation = ICG – reference measurement; CABG = coronary artery bypass graft surgery; Fick = direct Fick method; ICG = impedance cardiography; n = number of patients; NR = not reported; r value = Pearson's correlation coefficient; TD = bolus thermodilution method.

indicating good agreement to a method that, although commonly used in clinical practice, is far from perfect. Drazner *et al.* demonstrated that the correlation of ICG to Fick-derived cardiac output measurements is similar to the correlation of thermodilution to Fick-derived methods. Thus, the clinical "gold standard" of thermodilution-derived cardiac output measures is no more precise than ICG.[32]

Clinical application

Given its demonstrated validity compared to invasive methods, ICG is a potentially less costly alternative to PA catheter monitoring. Some authors have suggested that ICG may offer enough similar information as the PA catheter to reduce the need for a percentage of invasive procedures without the requisite costs and risks, and estimated that when ICG is utilized in place of a PA catheter, cost savings are between $600 and $3088 per patient.[31,32] A pilot study by Silver *et al.*[33] demonstrated a 71% reduction in PA catheter placement with the availability of noninvasive ICG.

A significant percentage of heart failure patients who are hospitalized are not treated in the cardiac care unit (CCU) and do not have measurements made of hemodynamic parameters. Moreover, patients with ADHF are often treated with parenterally-administered vasoactive therapies in a telemetry unit or step down unit without the capability to measure concurrent hemodynamics. These patients may benefit from the use of ICG, which can easily be performed in the sub-acute setting. It should be noted that ICG does not have a comparable parameter for the diagnostic determination of pulmonary artery wedge pressure (PAWP). The ICG parameter of thoracic fluid content has shown poor correlation to a single measurement of wedge pressure.[34] In a case report, ICG tracked well with changes in wedge pressure in ADHF[35] and multiple reports substantiate its ability to track changes in intravascular and extravascular volume and to be more immediate and sensitive than can be apparent clinically or with diagnostic x-ray or weight monitoring.[36–38]

ICG has demonstrated diagnostic and prognostic value in emergent and chronic heart failure. It has been shown to aid in the diagnosis of cardiac vs. non-cardiac causes of dyspnea[39,40] and systolic dysfunction vs. preserved systolic function in patients with elevated B-type natriuretic peptide (BNP) levels.[41] The same study showed that, when considered together, ICG and BNP levels measured in the emergency department had 75% prognostic accuracy for readmission or death within 90 days. Changes in ICG cardiac index and systolic time ratio have shown good correlation with changes in ejection fraction (EF) measured by echocardiography, potentially allowing inexpensive and more frequent assessments of changes in ventricular function.[42]

Additional studies in the acute setting have demonstrated that ICG values measured in the emergency department may predict length of stay and hospital charges when other vital signs do not[43] and have the ability to change the real-time diagnosis and treatment decisions in dyspneic patients.[44] In the chronic setting, changes in ICG parameters have been associated with improved functional measures of New York Heart Association (NYHA) class and 6-minute walk and quality of life measures such as visual analog scale and Minnesota Living with Heart Failure Questionnaire.[45] Zewail *et al.* assessed the relationships between systolic time ratio and BNP levels and mortality in heart failure transplant candidates. Systolic time ratio measurements correlated to NYHA class and mortality. Patients with elevated systolic time ratio had over a 3-fold higher risk for mortality than those with normal systolic time ratio, indicating a potential role for these measurements in the risk stratification and management.[46]

Other authors have reported on the clinical utility of ICG in prospective heart failure treatment,[47] including its use for titrating neurohormonal agents,[48] optimizing atrioventricular (AV) sequential pacemakers,[49–51] guide inotropic therapy,[52,53] and monitoring changes in hemodynamic status with neurohormonal therapy.[54–56] Table 12.3 summarizes diagnostic and treatment applications of ICG in patients with heart failure.

ICG has also shown value in the management of drug-resistant hypertension, which is often a factor in the development of heart failure and which also exists as a comorbid condition in many heart failure

Table 12.3. *Summary of impedance cardiography applications in heart failure*

Assessment and diagnostic applications
Establish baseline hemodynamics.
Trend changes to gauge level of hemodynamic decompensation.
Determine whether symptoms due to hemodynamic deterioration.
Aid in differentiation of systolic vs. diastolic dysfunction.
Prognostic applications
Emergency department values predictive of length of stay and hospital charges.
Changes associated with changes in functional and quality of life measures.
Abnormal values associated with mortality.
Treatment applications
Determine stability for initiation and uptitration of beta-blocker and angiotensin-converting enzyme (ACE) inhibitor therapy.
Assist in selection of drug agents and dosing.
Measure response to adjustments in therapy.
Determine need and optimal selection and dosing of intravenous therapy (dobutamine, milrinone, nesiritide).
Optimize left ventricular assist device (LVAD) settings and wean patients from LVAD support.
Determine optimal pacemaker settings in patients with atrioventricular sequential pacemakers.
Detect hemodynamic changes due to compensation, medication, and diet compliance.
Provide an adjunct to post-transplant myocardial biopsies.

Adapted from Yancy and Abraham.[58]

patients. In a randomized study of 104 drug-resistant hypertensive patients, patients randomized to the ICG-guided treatment arm achieved a 70% greater (56% vs. 33%) rate of blood pressure control (< 140/90 mm Hg) than patients in the control group treated by specialists.[57]

Given the current body of evidence and experience of clinicians using ICG for diagnostic, prognostic, and therapeutic decision-making, Strobeck and Silver have proposed ICG as a tool to help quantify the heart failure clinical profiles popularized by Stevenson (Figure 12.1). Their proposed model (Figure 12.4) uses ICG cardiac index to indicate perfusion status, changes in thoracic fluid content to indicate changes in congestion status, and systemic vascular resistance (SVR) to indicate the degree of relative vasoconstriction or vasodilation.

Variations of this conceptual model have been incorporated into algorithms utilizing ICG to guide specific treatment decisions in heart failure.[58–61] This model, albeit intriguing, has not been validated in rigorous clinical trials. In patients with chronic heart failure, there are several proven pharmacologic treatment options, including neurohormonal antagonists, diuretics, digoxin, and aldosterone antagonists. In the category of neurohormonal antagonists, ICG-derived cardiac index and SVR index can help determine how current therapy is impacting the patient from a hemodynamic perspective. When considering diuretic therapy, a focus on the change in TFC can provide a sensitive and independent evaluation of thoracic fluid response. Measures of contractility such as acceleration index and measures of flow such as cardiac index may be

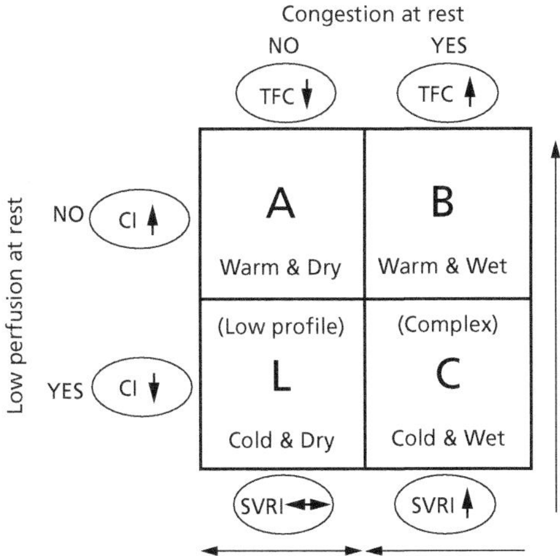

Figure 12.4. *Model for clinical profiles in heart failure utilizing impedance cardiography hemodynamic measurements.*

Abbreviations: CI = *cardiac index; TFC = thoracic fluid content; SVRI = systemic vascular resistance index*

useful as indicators for initiation of parental therapies. ICG parameter responsiveness may provide a mechanism for evaluating therapeutic responsiveness. Quantitative evaluation of hemodynamic indices and the adequacy of tissue perfusion should play a primary role in the decision to initiate additional therapies (e.g., intravenous vasodilators, natriuretic peptides, or inotropic agents) and to determine patient disposition upon hospitalization.

Conclusion

Most reported clinical research trials conducted on ICG are from single centers. Results from two major multicenter clinical trials are expected in 2005, the Prospective Evaluation and Identification of Decompensation by Impedance Cardiography Test (PREDICT) study in chronic heart failure and the Bioimpedance Cardiography (BIG) substudy of the Evaluation Study of Congestive Heart Failure and Pulmonary Artery Catheterization Effectiveness (ESCAPE) trials in ADHF. The PREDICT study will evaluate the association of serial ICG measurements to all-cause mortality and hospitalization or emergency department visits due to heart failure. The ESCAPE trial is designed to test outcomes of catheter-guided therapy as compared to outcomes of therapy guided by clinical assessment alone in hospitalized heart failure patients,[62] and the BIG substudy of ESCAPE will examine the diagnostic and prognostic role of ICG hemodynamics collected in a blinded fashion in both arms.

While it has been suggested that targeting hemodynamics can in fact improve outcomes in patients with decompensated advanced heart failure, this fundamental premise of hemodynamic monitoring, either invasive or noninvasive, remains unproven. Further studies will define the benefit of hemodynamic monitoring while refining the role of hemodynamic assessment by ICG.

References

1. Braunwald E. Disorders of the heart. In: Braunwald E, Fauci AS, Kasper DL, *et al.* (eds) *Harrison's Principles of Internal Medicine, Self-Assessment and Board Review*, 15th edition (New York, McGraw-Hill, 2001), 1309–1329.
2. Weber KT, Janicki JS, Campbell CT, Replogle R. Pathophysiology of acute and chronic cardiac failure. *Am J Cardiol* 1987; 60: 3C–9C.
3. Hunt SA, Baker DW, Chin MH, *et al.* ACC/AHA guidelines for the evaluation and management of chronic heart failure in the adult: executive summary: a report of the American College of Cardiology/American Heart Association Task Force on Practice Guidelines (Committee to revise the 1995 Guidelines for the Evaluation and Management of Heart Failure). *J Am Coll Cardiol* 2001; 36: 2101–2113.
4. Swan HJ, Ganz W, Forrester J, *et al.* Catheterization of the heart in man with use of a flow-directed balloon-tipped catheter. *N Engl J Med* 1970; 283: 447–451.
5. Rivers E, Nguyen B, Havstad S, *et al.*, Early Goal-Directed Therapy Collaborative Group. Early goal-directed therapy in the treatment of severe sepsis and septic shock. *N Engl J Med* 2001; 345: 1368–1377.
6. Ivanov RI, Allen J, Sandham JD, Calvin JE. Pulmonary artery catheterization: a narrative and systematic critique of randomized controlled trials and recommendations for the future. *New Horiz* 1997; 5: 268–276.
7. Steimle AE, Stevenson LW, Chelimsky-Fallick C, *et al.* Sustained hemodynamic efficacy of therapy tailored to

reduce filling pressures in survivors with advanced heart failure. *Circulation* 1997; 96: 1165–1172.
8. Hamilton MA, Stevenson LW, Child JS, *et al.* Sustained reduction in valvular regurgitation and atrial volumes with tailored vasodilator therapy in advanced congestive heart failure secondary to dilated (ischemic or idiopathic) cardiomyopathy. *Am J Cardiol* 1991; 67: 259–263.
9. Stevenson LW, Steimle AE, Fonarow G, *et al.* Improvement in exercise capacity of candidates awaiting heart transplantation. *J Am Coll Cardiol* 1995; 25: 163–170.
10. Fonarow GC, Stevenson LW, Walden JA, *et al.* Impact of a comprehensive heart failure management program on hospital readmission and functional status for patients with advanced heart failure. *J Am Coll Cardiol* 1997; 30: 725–732.
11. Connors AF Jr., Speroff T, Dawson NV, *et al.*, SUPPORT Investigators. The effectiveness of right heart catheterization in the initial care of critically ill patients. *JAMA* 1996; 276: 889–897.
12. Sandham JD, Hull RD, Grant RF, *et al.* A randomized controlled trial of the use of pulmonary-artery catheters in high-risk surgical patients. *New Eng J Med* 2003; 348: 5–14.
13. Richard C, Warszawski J, Anguel N, *et al.* Early use of the pulmonary artery catheter and outcomes in patients with shock and acute respiratory distress syndrome: a randomized controlled trial. *JAMA* 2003; 290: 2713–2721.
14. Polanczyk CA, Rohde LE, Goldman L, *et al.* Right heart catheterization and cardiac complications in patients undergoing noncardiac surgery: an observational study. JAMA 2001; 286: 309–314.
15. Stevenson LW. Tailored therapy to hemodynamic goals for advanced heart failure. Eur J Heart Fail 1999; 1: 251–257.
16. Shah MR, Hasselblad V, Stinnett SS, *et al.* Hemodynamic profiles of advanced heart failure: association with clinical characteristics and long-term outcomes. J Card Fail 2001; 7: 105–113.
17. Speroff T, Connors AF Jr., Dawson NV. Lens model analysis of hemodynamic status in the critically ill. Med Decis Making 1989; 9: 243–252.
18. Eisenberg PR, Jaffe AS, Schuster DP. Clinical evaluation compared to pulmonary artery catheterization in the hemodynamic assessment of critically ill patients. Crit Care Med 1984; 12: 549–553.
19. Stevenson LW, Perloff JK. The limited reliability of physical signs for estimating hemodynamics in chronic heart failure. JAMA 1989; 261: 884–888.
20. Jonas M, Bruce R, Knight J. Clinical assessment of cardiac output (CO) vs. Lidco indicator kelution (ID) measurement: are clinical estimates of cardiac output and oxygen delivery reliable enough to manage critically ill patients? Crit Care Med 2003; 30: A68 (Abstract).
21. Luepker R, Michael J, Warbasse JR, *et al.* Transthoracic electrical impedance: quantitative evaluation of a noninvasive measure of thoracic fluid volume. Am Heart J 1973; 85: 83–93.
22. Taler S, Textor S, Augustine J, *et al.* Volume control in treatment of resistant hypertension: dissociation between cardiopulmonary volume, ANP and declining GFR. J Am Soc Nephrol 2001; 12: 1492a (Abstract).
23. Brodin LA, Jogestrand, T, Larsen, FF, Tedner B, Walldius G. Effects of furosemide and slow-release furosemide on thoracic fluid volumes. Clin Cardiol 1986; 9: 561–564.
24. Official correspondence from the CardioDynamics International Corporation, June 2004.
25. Van de Water JM, Miller TW, Vogel RL, Mount BE, Dalton ML. Impedance cardiography: the next vital sign technology? Chest 2003; 123: 2028–2033.
26. CardioDynamics, Inc. BioZ® System Operator's Manual (CardioDynamics International Corporation: San Diego, 2002).
27. Belardinelli R, Ciampani N, Costantini C, Blandini A, Purcaro A. Comparison of impedance cardiography with thermodilution and direct Fick methods for noninvasive measurement of stroke volume and cardiac output during incremental exercise in patients with ischemic cardiomyopathy. Am J Cardiol 1996; 77: 1293–1301.
28. Marik PE, Penndelton JE, Smith R. A comparison of hemodynamic parameters derived from transthoracic electrical bioimpedance with those parameters obtained by thermodilution and ventricular angiography. Crit Care Med 1997; 25: 1545–1550.
29. Verhoeve PE, Cadwell CA, Tsadok S. Reproducibility of noninvasive bioimpedance measurements of cardiac function. J Card Fail 1998: 4: 53 (Abstract).
30. Greenberg BH, Hermann DD, Pranulis MF, Lazio L, Cloutier D. Reproducibility of impedance cardiography hemodynamic measures in clinically stable heart failure patients. Congest Heart Fail 2000; 6: 19–26.
31. Becker K Jr. Resolved: a pulmonary artery catheter should be used in the management of the critically ill patient. Con J Cardiothorac Vasc Anesth 1998; 12; 13–16.
32. Hendrickson K. Cost-effectiveness of noninvasive hemodynamic monitoring. AACN Clinical Issues 1999; 10: 419–426.

33. Silver M, Cianci, P, Brennan S, Longeran-Thomas, H, Ahmad F. Evaluation of impedance cardiography as an alternative to pulmonary artery catheterization in critically ill patients. J Card Fail 2004; 10: 17–21.
34. Drazner M, Thompson B, Rosenberg P, *et al.* Comparison of impedance cardiography with invasive hemodynamic measurements in patients with heart failure secondary to ischemic or nonischemic cardiomyopathy. Am J Cardiol 2002; 89: 993–995.
35. Ventura HO, Pranulis MF, Young C, Smart FW. Impedance cardiography: a bridge between research and clinical practice in the treatment of heart failure. Congest Heart Fail 2000; 6: 94–102.
36. Van de Water JM, Mount BE, Barela JR, Schuster R, Leacock FS. Monitoring the chest with impedance. Chest 1973; 64: 597–603.
37. Peacock WF IV, Albert NM, Kies P, White RD, Emerman CL. Bioimpedance monitoring: better than chest x-ray for predicting abnormal pulmonary fluid? Congest Heart Fail 2000; 6: 86–89.
38. Taler SJ, Augustine J, Textor SC. A hemodynamic approach to resistant hypertension. Congest Heart Fail 2000; 6: 90–93.
39. Marrocco A, Eskin B, Nashed AH, *et al.* Noninvasive bioimpedance monitoring differentiates cardiogenic from pulmonary causes of acute dyspnea in the emergency department. Acad Emerg Med 1998; 5: 476–477.
30. Springfield CL, Sebat F, Johnson D, Lengle S, Sebat C. Utility of impedance cardiography to determine cardiac vs. noncardiac cause of dyspnea in the emergency department. Congest Heart Fail 2004; 10: 14–16.
41. Kazanegra R, Barcarse E, Chen A, *et al.* Plasma levels of B–type natriuretic peptide (BNP) and non-invasive cardiac index in diagnosing congestive heart failure in the emergency department. J Card Fail 2002; 8: S84 (Abstract).
42. Parrott CW, Burnham KM, Quale C, Lewis DL. Comparison of changes in ejection fraction to changes in impedance cardiography cardiac index and systolic time ratio. Congest Heart Fail 2004; 10: 11–13.
43. Milzman D, Samaddar R, Napoli A, *et al.* The predictive value of noninvasive impedance cardiography in determining patient outcome in acute heart failure: a prospective blinded study. Ann Emerg Med 2000; 36: S4–S5.
44. Peacock F, Summers R, Emerman C. Emergent dyspnea impedance cardiography-aided assessment changes therapy: the ED IMPACT trial. Ann Emerg Med 2003; 42: S82 (Abstract).
45. Vijayaraghavan K, Crum S, Cherukuri, S, Barnett-Avery L. Association of impedance cardiography parameters with changes in functional and quality-of-life measures in patients with chronic heart failure. Congest Heart Fail 2004; 10: 22–27.
46. Zewail A, Broom C, Eastwood C, *et al.* J Card Fail 2003; 9: S105 (Abstract).
47. Rosenberg P, Yancy CW. Noninvasive assessment of hemodynamics: an emphasis on impedance cardiography. Curr Opin Cardiol 2000; 15: 151–155.
48. Strobeck JE, Silver MA, Ventura H. Impedance cardiography: noninvasive measurement of cardiac stroke volume and thoracic fluid content. Congest Heart Fail 2000; 6: 56–59.
49. Hayes DL, Hayes SN, Hyberger LK, *et al.* Atrioventricular interval optimization after biventricular pacing: echo/doppler vs. impedance plethysmography. Pacing Clin Electrophysiol 2000; 23: 590 (Abstract).
50. Tse HF, Yu C, Park E, Lau CP. Impedance cardiography for atrioventricular interval optimization during permanent left ventricular pacing. Pacing Clin Electrophysiol 2003; 26: 189–191.
51. Santos JF, Parreira L, Madeira J, *et al.* Noninvasive hemodynamic monitorization for AV interval optimization in patients with ventricular resynchronization therapy. Rev Port Cardiol 2003; 22: 1091–1098.
52. Lasater M. Managing inotrope therapy noninvasively. AACN Clinical Issues 1999; 10: 406–413.
53. Littmann L, Lasater M. Cost-effectiveness of noninvasive hemodynamic monitoring as a screening tool prior to initiation of inotrope infusion. J Cardiovasc Manag 1999; 10: 29–30.
54. Mulki G, Pisano C Silver M. Safety and efficacy of intermittent, short-term, outpatient nesiritide infusions for the treatment of decompensated heart failure. J Card Fail 2003; 9: S68 (Abstract).
55. Squires J, Vora K. Results from a pilot study to determine the feasibility in transitioning outpatient CHF patients from intermittent intravenous inotrope therapy to nesiritide. J Card Fail 2003: 9: S90 (Abstract).
56. Summers RL, Parrott CW, Quale C, Lewis DL. Use of noninvasive hemodynamics to aid decision making in the initiation and titration of neurohormonal agents. Congest Heart Fail 2004; 10: 28–31.
57. Taler SJ, Textor SC, Augustine JE. Resistant hypertension: comparing hemodynamic management to specialist care. Hypertension 2002; 39: 982–988.
58. Yancy C, Abraham WT. Noninvasive hemodynamic monitoring in heart failure: utilization of impedance cardiography. Congest Heart Fail 2003; 9: 241–250.
59. Strobeck J, Silver M. Beyond the four quadrants: the

critical and emerging role of impedance cardiography in heart failure. Congest Heart Fail 2004; 10: 1–6.

60. Silver M, Pisano C, Cianci P. Outpatient management of heart failure: program development and experience in clinical practice. In: Post Graduate Institute for Medicine (Advocate Christ Medical Center: Oak Lawn, IL, 2003).
61. Belott P. Bioimpedance in the pacemaker clinic. AACN Clinical Issues 1999; 10: 414–418.
62. Shah MR, O'Connor CM, Sopko G, *et al*. Evaluation Study of Congestive Heart Failure and Pulmonary Artery Catheterization Effectiveness (ESCAPE): design and rationale. Am Heart J 2001; 141: 528–535.
63. Albert N, Hail M, Li J *et al*. Equivalence of bioimpedance and TD in measuring CO/CI in patients with advanced, decompensated chronic heart failure hosp. in critical care. J Am Coll Cardiol 2003; 41: 211A (Abstract).
64. Ziegler D, Grotti L, Krucke G. Comparison of cardiac output measurements by TEB vs. intermittent bolus thermodilution in mechanical ventilated patients. Chest 1999; 116: 281S (Abstract).
65. Sageman WS, Riffenburgh RH, Spiess BD. Equivalence of bioimpedance and thermodilution in measuring cardiac index after cardiac surgery. J Cardiothorac Vasc Anesth 2002; 16: 8–14.
66. Yung GL, Fedullo PF, Kinninger K, Johnson W, Channick RN. Comparison of impedance cardiography to direct Fick and thermodilution cardiac output determination in pulmonary arterial hypertension. Congest Heart Fail 2004; 10: 7–10.

Part III

Comorbidities in the Acute Heart Failure Patient

CHAPTER 13

Arrhythmias in acute heart failure

William G Stevenson

Introduction

Arrhythmias often accompany acute heart failure (AHF). New-onset atrial fibrillation or flutter, or a cardiac arrest terminated by successful resuscitation, may precipitate or aggravate heart failure. Alternatively, these arrhythmias can be precipitated by AHF. Occasionally chronic tachycardia causes a potentially reversible tachycardia-induced cardiomyopathy.[1,2]

Supraventricular Tachycardias

Atrial fibrillation

The prevalence of atrial fibrillation increases with the severity of heart failure, from 7% in patients with mild heart failure to more than 40% in those with advanced heart failure.[3] Heart failure likely promotes atrial fibrosis and electrophysiologic changes that promote the development of atrial fibrillation.[4–6] Atrial fibrillation is commonly associated with heart failure exacerbation or the onset of acute heart failure.[7–9] Potential adverse effects may occur by loss of atrioventricular (AV) synchrony, rapid or slow ventricular rate responses, and variability in time for cardiac filling.[10–12] When atrial fibrillation is the major factor causing AHF, it is usually of recent onset and associated with a rapid ventricular response.

Several considerations guide management of patients with atrial fibrillation during AHF.[13] When atrial fibrillation is known to be chronic and persistent, it is unlikely to be the major exacerbating factor, and ensuring adequate rate control is the primary focus. A rapid rate, exceeding 100 bpm often reflects elevated sympathetic tone that is improved by treating the heart failure and any other exacerbating factors.

When new-onset atrial fibrillation occurs with a heart failure exacerbation, restoration of sinus rhythm, in addition to rate control, should be considered.[13] If the new onset of fibrillation precipitates hemodynamic deterioration or pulmonary edema, and immediate rate control cannot be achieved, prompt electrical cardioversion is warranted. Pharmacologic attempts to restore sinus rhythm are less effective and require time to implement, delaying restoration of normal rhythm. If electrical cardioversion fails to restore sinus rhythm, treatment is directed at controlling the ventricular rate while measures are undertaken to treat the heart failure and any other precipitating factors that might contribute to failure to maintain sinus rhythm. Administration of ibutilide followed by another attempt at electrical cardioversion can be considered.[14] This approach facilitated cardioversion in one series of patients with stable persistent fibrillation, but can be considered for those with AHF with appropriate monitoring for possible torsade de pointes.[14]

If urgent cardioversion is not required, but

restoration of sinus rhythm is desired, the timing of cardioversion depends on the severity of the hemodynamic impairment, and management to reduce the risk of thromboembolism. For patients who are not systemically anticoagulated, anticoagulation should be initiated with an intravenous agent provided that there are no contraindications. Those patients who have had < 24 to 48 hours of atrial fibrillation can be cardioverted to sinus rhythm with a very low risk of embolization, but systemic anticoagulation should be continued for a minimum of 3 weeks.[13] Patients with > 24 to 48 hours of fibrillation without systemic anticoagulation are at greater risk for thromboemboli. Cardioversion is best performed either after anticoagulation for a minimum of 3 weeks or after a transesophageal echocardiogram (TEE) has shown no left atrial thrombus.[15] Anticoagulation should be continued for a minimum of 3 weeks after cardioversion. Continuing chronic anticoagulation long term is a reasonable consideration even if sinus rhythm persists. Heart failure or depressed left ventricular (LV) function are markers of increased risk of thromboemboli and recurrent atrial fibrillation is common and can be asymptomatic.[13,16]

Sinus rhythm versus rate control

Deciding whether or not to attempt to restore and maintain sinus rhythm requires careful consideration.[3,17] Although heart failure patients with atrial fibrillation have a worse mortality than those who maintain sinus rhythm, whether or not fibrillation is detrimental or simply a marker of more severe disease is debated.[10,18–25] Several randomized trials have failed to show a benefit for the strategy of attempting to maintain sinus rhythm with antiarrhythmic drug therapy, but they did demonstrate that attempts to maintain sinus rhythm increase hospitalizations.[25–28] The majority of patients enrolled in these trials, however, did not have heart failure. In addition, the relatively low efficacy of antiarrhythmic drug therapy combined with their toxicities may offset the benefit in some of these patients.[21,25,29]

The approach should be individualized. We favor attempts to maintain sinus rhythm after a first episode of atrial fibrillation, for symptomatic paroxysms of atrial fibrillation, or when atrial fibrillation precipitates heart failure exacerbations. When the ventricular rate in fibrillation is difficult to control, attempting to maintain sinus rhythm before considering ablation of the AV junction with ventricular pacing is also reasonable. A rate-control approach is favored when atrial fibrillation is long-standing and asymptomatic.

Due to their safety, beta-blockers should be the initial agent employed. Angiotensin-converting enzyme (ACE) inhibitors may also reduce the likelihood of atrial fibrillation development, possibly through beneficial effects on heart failure and atrial remodeling.[30] When beta-blockers are ineffective, amiodarone (which is not specifically approved for this indication), dofetilide, and sotalol are the major antiarrhythmic drug options for attempting to maintain sinus rhythm in the long term. Amiodarone is more effective than sotalol and class I antiarrhythmic drugs.[31,32] However, careful monitoring is required for bradyarrhythmias and noncardiac toxicities. Drug interactions require decreases in warfarin and digoxin doses. Dofetilide and sotalol are options when amiodarone toxicities are of major concern, provided that renal function is preserved and that the risk of inducing torsade de pointes is acceptable.[33]

Catheter ablation with electrical isolation of regions of the left atrium around the pulmonary veins has increasingly been used for treatment of atrial fibrillation, largely in patients with little or mild heart disease and in a small number of patients with heart failure.[29,34] Although it potentially avoids long-term toxicities of antiarrhythmic drugs, success is less likely in patients with heart failure and in those with persistent rather than paroxysmal atrial fibrillation. With continued improvement, this technique may become a more viable option for selected heart failure patients.

Rate control

Acute rate control can be potentially achieved with intravenous administration of diltiazem, verapamil, beta-blockers, amiodarone, or digoxin.[35,36] Intravenous diltiazem has a faster onset of action than amiodarone, but also a greater incidence of hypotension.[35] Intravenous verapamil has similar effect to diltiazem. Beta-blockers also have negative inotropic effects. Although it does not have negative inotropic effects, digoxin has a delayed onset of action of typically > 20 minutes and blunted efficacy when sympathetic tone is elevated.

The goal of rate control during chronic therapy is maintenance of a ventricular rate < 80 bpm at rest and less than 100 bpm with gentle walking. Adequate rate control is extremely important, as persistent rapid rates can cause heart failure or aggravate existing heart failure.[1,12] Combinations of rate-controlling agents are often required.[36] Beta-blockers are the first line of therapy.[36,37] Digoxin can also help control the ventricular rate, but efficacy is limited when sympathetic tone is high.[36–38] Calcium channel blockers, diltiazem and verapamil, may be used if the combination of beta-blockers and digoxin are ineffective. Amiodarone is also effective for controlling heart rate in atrial fibrillation, but it is a last resort due to its noncardiac toxicities.[19]

Catheter ablation of the AV junction with permanent ventricular pacing is useful when adequate rate control cannot be achieved pharmacologically.[39–42] The rate is controlled and regularized. Although the atrial contribution to ventricular filling is not restored, symptoms improve and recurrent hospitalizations may be reduced, although exercise time and maximum oxygen uptake are not improved. In some patients, left ventricular ejection fraction (LVEF) improves. Occasionally, patients experience a deterioration in heart failure, probably due to the change in ventricular activation sequence if right ventricular (RV) pacing is employed.[43] Those with severely depressed ventricular function and severe mitral regurgitation are at greatest risk. Biventricular pacing (LV and RV pacing) rather than RV apical pacing alone should be considered in patients with depressed ventricular function; further studies will hopefully clarify optimal pacing methods.[44,45] Torsade de pointes, which has occurred after ablation, slows the heart rate and appears to be more likely in patients with depressed ventricular function or heart failure.[46–48] Pacing at ≥ 80 bpm to 90 bpm for the initial 1 to 3 months after ablation likely reduces this risk.[48]

Atrial Flutter and Paroxysmal Tachycardias

Atrial flutter is characterized by an organized atrial rhythm that is typically at a rate of 240 bpm to 300 bpm, but can be much slower in the presence of antiarrhythmic drug therapy or atrial disease. Acute management is similar to that for atrial fibrillation.[13] Rate control is often more difficult to achieve, and restoration of sinus rhythm is often warranted. Patients with atrial flutter and heart failure also commonly have episodes of atrial fibrillation and a risk of thromboembolism.[13,49–52] Electrical cardioversion is more often successful than for fibrillation, and pharmacologic cardioversion with intravenous administration of ibutilide is also a reasonable option for some patients.[53,54]

When atrial flutter is recurrent and requires long-term prophylactic therapy, catheter ablation should be considered.[55] Antiarrhythmic drug therapy is less effective than ablation, and has a risk of slowing the flutter rate and accelerating the ventricular rate. Catheter ablation of the isthmus between the tricuspid valve annulus and inferior vena cava abolishes the most common type of atrial flutter with minimal procedural risk.[55,56] After catheter ablation, atrial arrhythmia in the form of fibrillation continues to be a problem in > 20% of patients.[52,55,56] When atrial flutter develops during chronic drug therapy for atrial fibrillation, ablation of the flutter may allow maintenance of sinus rhythm if chronic drug therapy for prevention of atrial fibrillation is continued.[57]

Paroxysmal supraventricular tachycardias (PSVTs) due to atrial tachycardia, AV nodal reentry, or AV reentry using an accessory pathway occasionally precipitate heart failure in a patient with underlying heart disease. Management is as per guidelines.[58] If severe hemodynamic impairment is present, cardioversion should be performed. Otherwise, administration of an AV nodal blocking agent will often either terminate tachycardia or produce AV nodal blockade with persistent atrial tachycardia, establishing origin of the tachycardia in the atrium (most likely a reentrant atrial tachycardia or atrial flutter). Many of these supraventricular tachycardias (SVTs) can be controlled with a beta-adrenergic blocker.[58] If a beta-blocker is ineffective or not tolerated, calcium channel blockers, sotalol, amiodarone, or catheter ablation can be considered for prophylaxis.

Ventricular Arrhythmias During Acute Heart Failure

Ventricular arrhythmias during an AHF exacerbation may be due to the presence of a chronic arrhythmia substrate, such as an area of scar causing reentrant ventricular tachycardia (VT), or alternatively may indicate an acute process such as acute myocardial infarction (AMI) or myocarditis (Table 13.1).[59–61] Aggravating or precipitating factors, including hyperkalemia or hypokalemia, myocardial ischemia, and drug toxicities, should be sought and treated (Table 13.1).[62]

The electrocardiographic features of the arrhythmia are often helpful in suggesting potential causes (Figure 13.1). Monomorphic VT usually indicates a structural abnormality, such as an old area of MI or scar. Polymorphic VTs can be due to acute myocardial ischemia or torsade de pointes. In one series, 42% of cardiac arrests in advanced heart failure were attributed to potentially correctable factors, including pulmonary edema precipitating ventricular fibrillation (VF) (9 patients) or a bradyarrhythmia (2 patients), torsade de pointes from a drug (10 patients), or VT attributed to hypokalemia (1 patient).[63] Following correction of the arrhythmia, treatment aimed at the precipitating cause may not prevent sudden death, which occurred in 32% of this patient group within 1 year. Registry data from the Antiarrhythmics Versus Implantable Defibrillators (AVID) trial, also found a high overall mortality among patients with a secondary cause of cardiac arrest and depressed LV function.[64] Thus, a secondary cardiac arrest may be a marker for susceptibility to arrhythmias even when a potential correctable factor can be identified and treated. Implantable cardioverter defibrillators (ICDs) are an important consideration in these patients, although it is not known whether they improve survival after a secondary cardiac arrest.

Table 13.1. *Treatable or reversible causes of arrhythmias in acute heart failure*

Cause of arrhythmias	Type of arrhythmias
Acute MI	VT/VF, AV block, sinus bradycardia
Thromboemboli	
Stroke	Bradyarrhythmias, rarely torsade de pointes
Coronary emboli	Ischemic arrhythmias (bradyarrhythmias, rarely torsade de pointes)
Pulmonary emboli	Bradyarrhythmias, PEA, atrial fibrillation
Hyperkalemia	Bradyarrhythmia, sinusoidal VT
Hypokalemia	Torsade de pointes, ventricular ectopy
Drug-induced arrhythmias	Torsade de pointes with QT prolongation Ventricular flutter (sodium channel blockade) Bradyarrhythmias (beta-blockers, calcium channel blockers, amiodarone, other antiarrhythmics)
Respiratory insufficiency, pulmonary edema, sleep apnea	Bradyarrhythmias, ventricular ectopic activity

Abbreviations: AV, atrioventricular; MI, myocardial infarction; PEA, pulseless electrical activity; VF, ventricular fibrillation; VT, ventricular tachycardia.

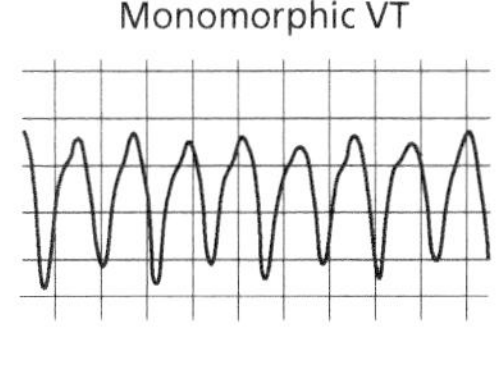

Polymorphic VT

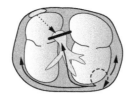

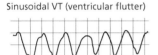

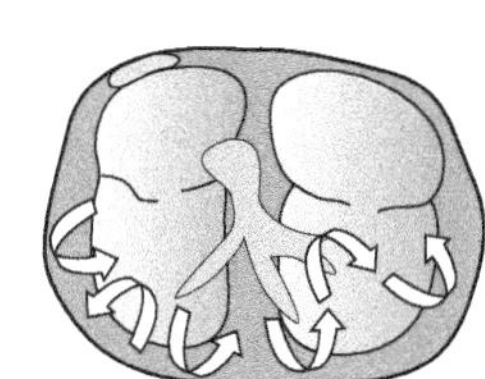

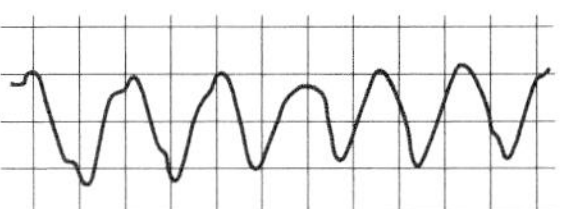

Figure 13.1. *Electrocardiographic types of ventricular tachycardia (VT). From the top are examples of sustained monomorphic VT, polymorphic VT, and sinusoidal VT. Sinusoidal VT was due to hyperkalemia. Diagrams at the right indicate the mechanism of production of the QRS complex for monomorphic and polymorphic VTs. Monomorphic VT indicates repetitive similar activation of the ventricle from beat to beat. Polymorphic VT indicates continuously changing ventricular activation.*

Sustained monomorphic ventricular tachycardia

Monomorphic VT has a uniform QRS configuration from beat to beat, indicating repetitive depolarization of the ventricles in the same sequence (Figure 13.1). A structural focus is usually present, most commonly an area of scar or infarction (Table 13.2). Distinguishing VT from SVT with aberrant conduction is the major diagnostic concern. Dissociation of atrial and ventricular electrical activity, with the atrial rate slower than the ventricular rate, reliably indicates VT. QRS morphology criteria for distinguishing VT from SVT with aberrancy are often unreliable in patients with heart failure.[65] A tachycardia QRS morphology identical to that of sinus rhythm, usually, but not always, indicates SVT.[65,66]

A diagnosis of VT should be assumed for regular wide QRS tachycardia, even if it is hemodynamically tolerated, and management should follow current guidelines.[58] Immediate cardioversion is warranted for wide QRS tachycardias that

Table 13.2. *Diagnostic considerations in monomorphic ventricular tachycardia*

Supraventricular tachycardia with aberrancy vs. ventricular tachycardia
- assume ventricular tachycardia until proven otherwise
- QRS morphology discriminators can be unreliable
- atrioventricular dissociation is the most reliable finding
- cardiac arrest is occasionally caused by a rapid supraventricular tachycardia

Left bundle branch block ventricular tachycardia (dominant S-wave in V1)
- arrhythmogenic right ventricular dysplasia
- bundle branch reentry
- idiopathic right ventricular outflow tract ventricular tachycardia—when incessant can cause tachycardia-induced cardiomyopathy

produce hypotension or are accompanied by severe symptoms of pulmonary edema or angina. When the arrhythmia is hemodynamically tolerated, administration of adenosine may terminate an SVT, or create an AV block, exposing the arrhythmia as atrial tachycardia or atrial flutter, but it will not generally affect VT.[58] Intravenous administration of amiodarone has become the most commonly employed initial pharmacological option for attempted termination.[67,68] Intravenous administration of lidocaine or procainamide can be considered, but they are less effective. Lidocaine is hemodynamically well tolerated. Procainamide is a potent vasodilator that can contribute to hypotension. Administration of multiple antiarrhythmic drugs should be avoided; proarrhythmia with incessant VT can occur. A low threshold for anesthesia and cardioversion is appropriate and they should be immediately available at all times. Intravenous administration of verapamil or diltiazem can produce hemodynamic collapse during VT and is contraindicated, with the uncommon exception of idiopathic VT that is known to be responsive to a calcium channel blocker.

Following restoration of a stable sinus rhythm, the type and significance of underlying heart disease should be assessed including the presence of coronary artery disease (CAD) and prior MI. When the diagnosis of VT is in doubt, an electrophysiologic study should be performed. VT is inducible in the electrophysiology laboratory in > 90% of patients who have had spontaneous sustained monomorphic VT due either to CAD or nonischemic cardiomyopathies. An old MI is the most common cause of sustained monomorphic VT, but areas of scar causing monomorphic VT are also encountered in nonischemic cardiomyopathies, particularly those due to cardiac involvement with sarcoidosis or Chagas' disease.[69–72]

The QRS configuration of VT can suggest its likely origin and often the underlying heart disease.[73] A very wide QRS complex (exceeding 200 ms) (Figure 13.1) likely indicates slow conduction through the myocardium caused by severe myocardial disease, hyperkalemia, or antiarrhythmic drug toxicity.[74,75] VT that has a left bundle branch block (LBBB)-like configuration in lead V1, with a dominant S-wave suggests that activation originates in the right ventricle or interventricular septum. Arrhythmogenic RV dysplasia, cardiac sarcoidosis, idiopathic RV outflow tract VT, and bundle branch reentry VT are possible etiologies. VT that has a dominant R-wave in V1 generally originates from the left ventricle.

Following termination of VT and restoration of hemodynamic stability, further arrhythmia management is determined by the underlying heart disease, prognosis from the standpoint of heart failure, and risk of arrhythmia recurrence. Sustained monomorphic VT is usually associated with an arrhythmia substrate with a high recurrence risk, even if precipitating factors are identified and treated, and despite antiarrhythmic drug therapy.[76–78] Even though the initial episode may be hemodynamically tolerated, subsequent episodes can cause cardiac arrest or exacerbate heart failure in patients with severe ventricular dysfunction.[76–78] Placement of an ICD should be considered for most patients. If VT is incessant or very frequent, it must be brought under control before ICD implantation, otherwise the patient is subject to frequent ICD therapies.

An ICD is not appropriate for patients with end-stage, New York Heart Association (NYHA) class IV heart failure who have a poor prognosis from the standpoint of their ventricular dysfunction, unless they are candidates for cardiac transplantation or support from a left ventricular assist device (LVAD). An ICD is usually not necessary for those with idiopathic VT causing tachycardia-induced cardiomyopathy that can be expected to improve or resolve after successful treatment of the VT.

Polymorphic ventricular tachycardia and ventricular fibrillation

Polymorphic VT has a continually changing QRS configuration indicating a changing sequence of ventricular depolarization (Figure 13.1). A fixed structural substrate, such as a region of scar, is not required. Sustained polymorphic VT usually degenerates to VF. Reversible triggers, such as myocardial ischemia, hypokalemia, or drug toxicity, are common causes and important considerations (Table 13.3).[79–81] Rare cases of polymorphic VT are due to LV epicardial pacing for cardiac

Table 13.3. *Polymorphic ventricular tachycardia*

Acute myocardial ischemia

Torsade de pointes
- QT prolongation is almost always present prior to VT
- Initiation of VT is usually pause-dependent
- Common precipitating factors:
  - hypokalemia
  - hypomagnesemia
  - hypocalcemia
  - bradycardia
  - Drugs (partial list)
    - sotalol
    - dofetilide
    - quinidine
    - ibutilide
    - procainamide (n-acetylprocainamide)
    - amiodarone (rare, often associated with bradycardia)
    - erythromycin
    - haloperidol

Abbreviations: VT, ventricular tachycardia.

resynchronization therapy, possibly due to a pacing-induced increase in dispersion of refractoriness.[82,83] Reprogramming of the device for pacing from the right ventricle may restore stability.

Following defibrillation, prompt assessment should consider the possibility of MI or ischemia and QT prolongation that may indicate torsade de pointes. If VF recurs, administration of intravenous magnesium and amiodarone should be considered.[67,84,85]

Occasionally a rapid SVT precipitates VF.[86,87] If this mechanism is suspected, an electrophysiologic study should be performed as this arrhythmia will likely cause inappropriate shocks from the ICD and is better treated with ablation or antiarrhythmic therapy.

Torsade de pointes

Polymorphic VT associated with prolongation of the QT interval is referred to as torsade de pointes and can be due to any cause of QT-interval prolongation including hypokalemia, bradycardia, or drugs such as sotalol, dofetilide, ibutilide, quinidine, acetylprocainamide-n, haloperidol, and erythromycin.[88] More extensive, updated lists are available at www.torsades.org. Although amiodarone prolongs the QT interval, torsade de pointes is rare, possibly due to blocking of other currents involved in initiating the arrhythmia.[89–91] Some cases have been associated with marked slowing of heart rate induced by the amiodarone.[92] The electrophysiologic remodeling of heart failure likely increases susceptibility.[93] Women are more susceptible than men.[94]

Administration of 1 g of magnesium sulfate ($MgSO_4$) intravenously will often suppress episodes, even when serum Mg is in the normal range. Administration of a second dose and continuous infusion should be considered if runs of VT or ventricular ectopic activity persist. Usually, torsade de pointes is "pause-dependent," initiated by a slowing of heart rate or a pause that follows a premature beat, further prolonging the QT interval. Overdrive pacing (typically starting at a rate of 100 bpm to 120 bpm) often suppresses episodes. An increase in heart rate produced by administration of isoproterenol can also be effective. Offending agents should be discontinued and hypokalemia and hypomagnesemia corrected.

Although the precipitating factor for torsade de pointes can usually be corrected, patients with advanced heart failure may remain at high risk for recurrence.[91] Amiodarone is not protective and may be contraindicated in this population.[91] Implantation of an ICD that also prevents bradycardias that promote torsade de pointes is a reasonable consideration for some patients.

Electrical storm

Frequent or incessant, sustained VT is referred to as an electrical storm.[62,95] An electrical storm can be a harbinger of heart failure deterioration and a marker for increased mortality from heart failure. Aggravating factors should be addressed. Reducing sympathetic tone with beta-adrenergic blockade, left stellate ganglion block, or administration of intravenous amiodarone has been useful. In some patients, intraaortic balloon counterpulsation restores stability.[96] In a small number of patients with recurrent VF triggered by identifiable, monomorphic premature ventricular contractions

(PVCs) early after MI, catheter ablation of the PVCs has effectively prevented recurrent arrhythmia.[97]

Ventricular ectopic activity and nonsustained ventricular tachycardia

Ventricular ectopic activity and nonsustained VT of 3 or more beats in duration are observed in two-thirds of patients with chronic heart failure and are markers for increased severity of disease.[98,99] During an exacerbation of heart failure, however, emergence of ventricular arrhythmias should prompt an evaluation for possible precipitating or aggravating factors, including myocardial ischemia, hypokalemia, or hypoxemia, as may occur during sleep apnea or impending respiratory arrest.[100] Nonsustained VT is typically < 6 beats in duration.[98] Fast, long runs of nonsustained VT and polymorphic VT should raise concern for possible myocardial ischemia or torsade de pointes.

Bradyarrhythmias

Bradyarrhythmias during AHF should prompt an immediate search for possible aggravating factors including hyperkalemia, myocardial ischemia, and hypoxemia or hypoventilation during respiratory decompensation or sleep apnea.[101] Other bradyarrhythmias are due to conduction system disease that is part of the underlying cardiac disease.[102]

Antiarrhythmic Drugs in Heart Failure

The potential benefits of antiarrhythmic drug therapy must be carefully balanced against the risks. Toxicities are common and potentially increased by diminished excretion, drug interactions, and concomitant electrolyte abnormalities (Table 13.4). Antiarrhythmic drug-induced proarrhythmia can take the form of slower, but more frequent or incessant, monomorphic VT.[74] Drugs that prolong the QT interval can cause torsade de pointes.[74,94] Antiarrhythmic drugs may cause bradyarrhythmias as well.

Class I sodium channel blocking drugs (quinidine, procainamide, disopyramide, flecainide, propafenone, and mexiletine) should be avoided, but are occasionally useful to control recurrent arrhythmias. These drugs have negative inotropic effects and several have been shown to increase mortality when administered chronically to patients with prior MI, or patients resuscitated from a cardiac arrest.[74,103]

Class III drugs (dofetilide, sotalol, amiodarone, and ibutilide) prolong action potential duration and thereby the QT interval. Dofetilide and sotalol are potassium channel blockers that prolong action potential duration and consequently the QT interval. Sotalol also has nonselective beta-blocking activity. Both drugs are excreted via the kidney and can accumulate during renal failure. Torsade de pointes is the major toxicity, occurring in 3% to 5% of patients. Therapy should be initiated only during continuous in-hospital electrocardiographic monitoring and renal insufficiency is a contraindication. Both drugs can reduce atrial fibrillation or episodes of VT causing ICD therapies.

Ibutilide, which is available only for intravenous administration for acute termination of atrial fibrillation or flutter, is a class III drug that blocks a repolarizing potassium current and also delays inactivation of the inward sodium current.[53,104] Ibutilide has a renal route of excretion. In patients without heart failure, efficacy of termination of recent onset atrial fibrillation is in the range of 30%; efficacy of termination of atrial flutter is 60% to 80%.[53,104] Torsade de pointes occurs in 2% to 11% of patients.[105,106]

Amiodarone

Amiodarone blocks cardiac sodium, potassium, and calcium currents and has sympatholytic effects. Amiodarone is a major option for acute and chronic antiarrhythmic drug therapy in patients with heart failure, largely because it has broad efficacy against ventricular and supraventricular arrhythmias and is relatively safe from a cardiac standpoint during chronic therapy.[31,107] Amiodarone has a small benefit or neutral effect on mortality in patients with heart failure but noncardiac toxicities limit usefulness and ICDs have superior efficacy to prevent sudden death in high-risk patients.[107,108]

Table 13.4. *Antiarrhythmic drugs*

Drug	Uses	ROA	Excretion	Proarrhythmia/Precautions
Beta-blockers	AF, AFL (control heart rate) VT, VT storm ≈	PO IV		Bradyarrhythmias, hypotension Aggravation of heart failure
Verapamil/Diltiazem Ca blocker	Rate control AF, AFL MFAT	PO IV		Bradyarrhythmias Negative inotropic effects
Amiodarone (Class I, II, III, IV)	AF, AFL, VT	IV	Liver	Hypotension, bradyarrhythmias, phlebitis
Amiodarone	Same	PO	Liver	Bradyarrhythmias, rare torsade de pointes Multiple noncardiac toxicities: liver, thyroid, lung Negative inotropic effect with large initial doses
Dofetilide (Class III – IKr blocker)	AF, AFL, VT in ICD patients	PO	Kidney	QT increase, torsade de pointes VT > 3% No negative impact on mortality when initiated in hospital with precautions for QT prolongation
Sotalol (Class III – IKr + beta-blocker)	AF, AFL, VT in ICD patients	PO	Kidney	QT increase, torsade de pointes Nonselective beta-blockade—negative inotropic effect
Quinidine (Class I + IKr block)	AF, AFL, VT	PO, IM, IV	Kidney, Liver	QT prolongation, torsade de pointes Diarrhea, nausea in > 20%
Procainamide (Class I + IKr block)	AF, AFL, VT	PO, IV	Liver (kidney – NAPA)	QT prolongation if NAPA accumulates Drug-induced SLE during long-term therapy
Disopyramide (Class I + IKr)	AF, AFL, VT	PO		QT prolongation Marked negative inotropic—contraindicated in heart failure Anticholinergic side effects
Flecainide (Class I)	AF, AFL	PO		VT proarrhythmia, AF slowing with rapid response—contraindicated in heart failure
Propafenone (Class I + beta and Ca block)	AF, AFL, VT	PO	Liver, active metabolites	VT proarrhythmia, AF slowing with rapid response, bradyarrhythmias—contraindicated in heart failure
Lidocaine	VT	IV	Liver	Confusion, nausea
Mexiletine	VT	PO		Similar to lidocaine

Abbreviations: AF, atrial fibrillation; AFL, atrial flutter; Ca, calcium; ICD, implantible cardioventer defibrillator; IKr, rapid delayed rectifier K current; IM, intramuscular; IV, intravenous; MFAT, multifocal atrial tachycardia; NAPA, n-acetylprocainamide; PO, per os (by mouth); ROA, route of administration; SLE, systemic lupus erythematosus; VT, ventricular tachycardia.

Intravenous amiodarone has antiadrenergic effects without prolongation of action potential duration. Adverse effects include hypotension due to vasodilation and negative inotropic effect and bradyarrhythmias. Administration through a peripheral vein for more than a day commonly produces phlebitis; administration through a central intravenous catheter is required for prolonged therapy. Proarrhythmia is uncommon, but torsade de pointes, bradyarrhythmias, and incessant VT can occur.[90]

During chronic oral therapy, amiodarone slows heart rate, depresses AV node conduction, and prolongs refractoriness in the atrium and ventricle, producing QT prolongation.[109] Bradyarrhythmias are the major cardiac risk, occurring in up to a third of patients.[32] Torsade de pointes and proarrhythmia are uncommon, but can occur.[91] Large loading doses (> 600 mg to 1200 mg daily) can exacerbate heart failure.[110] Amiodarone therapy can also aggravate heart failure if bradycardia results in chronic RV pacing from a pacemaker or defibrillator, producing dyschronous cardiac activation.[111]

Amiodarone-induced pulmonary toxicity occurs at a rate of approximately 1% per year of therapy and can mimic or exacerbate heart failure.[112] It can present as acute pneumonitis or the insidious development of interstitial fibrosis.[113] Right heart catheterization may be required to assess the possibility of pulmonary vascular congestion, and a chest CT scan to assess interstitial fibrosis can be helpful in assessing the possibility of pulmonary toxicity rather than heart failure.[114] With any suspicion of pulmonary toxicity, amiodarone should be immediately discontinued. Hyperthyroidism or hypothyroidism develops in up to 18% of patients and can precipitate heart failure decompensation.[115]

Conclusion

Arrhythmias can precipitate or aggravate AHF. In addition, heart failure exacerbations often precipitate ventricular or atrial arrhythmias. The prompt recognition and treatment of arrhythmias are important aspects of managing the patient with AHF.

References

1. Shinbane JS, Wood MA, Jensen DN, *et al.* Tachycardia-induced cardiomyopathy: a review of animal models and clinical studies. J Am Coll Cardiol 1997; 29: 709–715.
2. Umana E, Solares CA, Alpert MA. Tachycardia-induced cardiomyopathy. Am J Med 2003; 114: 51–55.
3. Maisel WH, Stevenson LW. Atrial fibrillation in heart failure: epidemiology, pathophysiology, and rationale for therapy. Am J Cardiol 2003; 91: 2D–8D.
4. Verheule S, Wilson E, Everett T, *et al.* Alterations in atrial electrophysiology and tissue structure in a canine model of chronic atrial dilatation due to mitral regurgitation. Circulation 2003; 107: 2615–2622.
5. Sanders P, Morton JB, Davidson NC, *et al.* Electrical remodeling of the atria in congestive heart failure: electrophysiological and electroanatomic mapping in humans. Circulation 2003; 108: 1461–1468.
6. Cardin S, Li D, Thorin-Trescases N, *et al.* Evolution of the atrial fibrillation substrate in experimental congestive heart failure: angiotensin-dependent and -independent pathways. Cardiovasc Res 2003; 60: 315–325.
7. Rathore SS, Berger AK, Weinfurt KP, *et al.* Acute myocardial infarction complicated by atrial fibrillation in the elderly: prevalence and outcomes. Circulation 2000; 101: 969–974.
8. Wong CK, White HD, Wilcox RG, *et al.* Significance of atrial fibrillation during acute myocardial infarction, and its current management: insights from the GUSTO-3 trial. Card Electrophysiol Rev 2003; 7: 201–207.
9. Tsuyuki RT, McKelvie RS, Arnold JM, *et al.* Acute precipitants of congestive heart failure exacerbations. Arch Intern Med 2001; 161: 2337–2342.
10. Wasmund SL, Li JM, Page RL, *et al.* Effect of atrial fibrillation and an irregular ventricular response on sympathetic nerve activity in human subjects. Circulation 2003; 107: 2011–2015.
11. Kay GN, Ellenbogen KA, Giudici M, *et al.* The Ablate and Pace Trial: a prospective study of catheter ablation of the AV conduction system and permanent pacemaker implantation for treatment of atrial fibrillation. APT Investigators. J Interv Card Electrophysiol 1998; 2: 121–135.
12. Khand AU, Rankin AC, Kaye GC, Cleland JG. Systematic review of the management of atrial fibrillation in patients with heart failure. Eur Heart J 2000; 21: 614–632.

13. Fuster V, Ryden LE, Asinger RW, *et al.* ACC/AHA/ESC guidelines for the management of patients with atrial fibrillation: executive summary: a report of the American College of Cardiology/American Heart Association Task Force on Practice Guidelines and the European Society of Cardiology Committee for Practice Guidelines and Policy Conferences (Committee to Develop Guidelines for the Management of Patients With Atrial Fibrillation) developed in collaboration with the North American Society of Pacing and Electrophysiology. J Am Coll Cardiol 2001; 38: 1231–1265.
14. Oral H, Souza JJ, Michaud GF, *et al.* Facilitating transthoracic cardioversion of atrial fibrillation with ibutilide pretreatment. N Engl J Med 1999; 340: 1849–1854.
15. Klein AL, Murray RD, Grimm RA. Role of transesophageal echocardiography-guided cardioversion of patients with atrial fibrillation. J Am Coll Cardiol 2001; 37: 691–704.
16. Rockson SG, Albers GW. Comparing the guidelines: anticoagulation therapy to optimize stroke prevention in patients with atrial fibrillation. J Am Coll Cardiol 2004; 43: 929–935.
17. Snow V, Weiss KB, LeFevre M, *et al.* Management of newly detected atrial fibrillation: a clinical practice guideline from the American Academy of Family Physicians and the American College of Physicians. Ann Intern Med 2003; 139: 1009–1017.
18. Pedersen OD, Brendorp B, Elming H, *et al.* Does conversion and prevention of atrial fibrillation enhance survival in patients with left ventricular dysfunction? Evidence from the Danish Investigations of Arrhythmia and Mortality ON Dofetilide/(DIAMOND) Study. Card Electrophysiol Rev 2003; 7: 220–224.
19. Deedwania PC, Singh BN, Ellenbogen K, *et al.* Spontaneous conversion and maintenance of sinus rhythm by amiodarone in patients with heart failure and atrial fibrillation: observations from the veterans affairs congestive heart failure survival trial of antiarrhythmic therapy (CHF-STAT). The Department of Veterans Affairs CHF-STAT Investigators. Circulation 1998; 98: 2574–2579.
20. Crijns HJ, Tjeerdsma G, de Kam PJ, *et al.* Prognostic value of the presence and development of atrial fibrillation in patients with advanced chronic heart failure. Eur Heart J 2000; 21: 1238–1245.
21. Steinberg JS, Sadaniantz A, Kron J, *et al.* Analysis of cause-specific mortality in the Atrial Fibrillation Follow-up Investigation of Rhythm Management (AFFIRM) study. Circulation 2004; 109: 1973–1980.
22. Wang TJ, Larson MG, Levy D, *et al.* Temporal relations of atrial fibrillation and congestive heart failure and their joint influence on mortality: the Framingham Heart Study. Circulation 2003; 107: 2920–2925.
23. Wyse DG, Love JC, Yao Q, *et al.* Atrial fibrillation: a risk factor for increased mortality—an AVID registry analysis. J Interv Card Electrophysiol 2001; 5: 267–273.
24. Pratt CM, Singh SN, Al-Khalidi HR, *et al.* The efficacy of azimilide in the treatment of atrial fibrillation in the presence of left ventricular systolic dysfunction: results from the Azimilide Postinfarct Survival Evaluation (ALIVE) trial. J Am Coll Cardiol 2004; 43: 1211–1216.
25. Corley SD, Epstein AE, DiMarco JP, *et al.* Relationships between sinus rhythm, treatment, and survival in the Atrial Fibrillation Follow-Up Investigation of Rhythm Management (AFFIRM) Study. Circulation 2004; 109: 1509–1513.
26. Opolski G, Torbicki A, Kosior D, *et al.* Rhythm control versus rate control in patients with persistent atrial fibrillation. Results of the HOT CAFE Polish Study. Kardiol Pol 2003; 59: 1–16; discussion 15–16.
27. Wyse DG, Waldo AL, DiMarco JP, *et al.* A comparison of rate control and rhythm control in patients with atrial fibrillation. N Engl J Med 2002; 347: 1825–1833.
28. Van Gelder IC, Hagens VE, Bosker HA, *et al.* A comparison of rate control and rhythm control in patients with recurrent persistent atrial fibrillation. N Engl J Med 2002; 347: 1834–1840.
29. Pappone C, Rosanio S, Augello G, *et al.* Mortality, morbidity, and quality of life after circumferential pulmonary vein ablation for atrial fibrillation: outcomes from a controlled nonrandomized long-term study. J Am Coll Cardiol 2003; 42: 185–197.
30. Vermes E, Tardif JC, Bourassa MG, *et al.* Enalapril decreases the incidence of atrial fibrillation in patients with left ventricular dysfunction: insight from the Studies Of Left Ventricular Dysfunction (SOLVD) trials. Circulation 2003; 107: 2926–2931.
31. Roy D, Talajic M, Dorian P, *et al.* Amiodarone to prevent recurrence of atrial fibrillation. Canadian Trial of Atrial Fibrillation Investigators. N Engl J Med 2000; 342: 913–920.
32. Weinfeld MS, Drazner MH, Stevenson WG, Stevenson LW. Early outcome of initiating amiodarone for atrial fibrillation in advanced heart failure. J Heart Lung Transplant 2000; 19: 638–643.
33. Pedersen OD, Bagger H, Keller N, *et al.* Efficacy of dofetilide in the treatment of atrial fibrillation-flutter

in patients with reduced left ventricular function: a Danish Investigations of Arrhythmia and Mortality On Dofetilide (DIAMOND) substudy. Circulation 2001; 104: 292–296.

34. Chen MS, Marrouche NF, Khaykin Y, *et al.* Pulmonary vein isolation for the treatment of atrial fibrillation in patients with impaired systolic function. J Am Coll Cardiol 2004; 43: 1004–1009.
35. Delle Karth G, Geppert A, Neunteufl T, *et al.* Amiodarone versus diltiazem for rate control in critically ill patients with atrial tachyarrhythmias. Crit Care Med 2001; 29: 1149–1153.
36. Olshansky B, Rosenfeld LE, Warner AL, *et al.* The Atrial Fibrillation Follow-up Investigation of Rhythm Management (AFFIRM) study: approaches to control rate in atrial fibrillation. J Am Coll Cardiol 2004; 43: 1201–1208.
37. Khand AU, Rankin AC, Martin W, *et al.* Carvedilol alone or in combination with digoxin for the management of atrial fibrillation in patients with heart failure? J Am Coll Cardiol 2003; 42: 1944–1951.
38. Dec GW. Digoxin remains useful in the management of chronic heart failure. Med Clin North Am 2003; 87: 317–337.
39. Brignole M, Menozzi C, Gianfranchi L, *et al.* Assessment of atrioventricular junction ablation and VVIR pacemaker versus pharmacological treatment in patients with heart failure and chronic atrial fibrillation: a randomized, controlled study. Circulation 1998; 98: 953–960.
40. Proclemer A, Della Bella P, Tondo C, *et al.* Radiofrequency ablation of atrioventricular junction and pacemaker implantation versus modulation of atrioventricular conduction in drug refractory atrial fibrillation. Am J Cardiol 1999; 83: 1437–1442.
41. Kay GN, Ellenbogen KA, Giudici M, *et al.* The Ablate and Pace Trial: a prospective study of catheter ablation of the AV conduction system and permanent pacemaker implantation for treatment of atrial fibrillation. APT Investigators. J Interv Card Electrophysiol 1998; 2: 121–135.
42. Lemery R, Brugada P, Cheriex E, Wellens HJ. Reversibility of tachycardia-induced left ventricular dysfunction after closed-chest catheter ablation of the atrioventricular junction for intractable atrial fibrillation. Am J Cardiol 1987; 60: 1406–1408.
43. Vanderheyden M, Goethals M, Anguera I, *et al.* Hemodynamic deterioration following radiofrequency ablation of the atrioventricular conduction system. Pacing Clin Electrophysiol 1997; 20: 2422–2428.
44. Garrigue S, Bordachar P, Reuter S, *et al.* Comparison of permanent left ventricular and biventricular pacing in patients with heart failure and chronic atrial fibrillation: a prospective hemodynamic study. Card Electrophysiol Rev 2003; 7: 315–324.
45. Simantirakis EN, Vardakis KE, Kochiadakis GE, *et al.* Left ventricular mechanics during right ventricular apical or left ventricular-based pacing in patients with chronic atrial fibrillation after atrioventricular junction ablation. J Am Coll Cardiol 2004; 43: 1013–1018.
46. Geelen P, Brugada J, Andries E, Brugada P. Ventricular fibrillation and sudden death after radiofrequency catheter ablation of the atrioventricular junction. Pacing Clin Electrophysiol 1997; 20: 343–348.
47. Nowinski K, Gadler F, Jensen-Urstad M, Bergfeldt L. Transient proarrhythmic state following atrioventricular junction radiofrequency ablation: pathophysiologic mechanisms and recommendations for management. Am J Med 2002; 113: 596–602.
48. Ozcan C, Jahangir A, Friedman PA, *et al.* Sudden death after radiofrequency ablation of the atrioventricular node in patients with atrial fibrillation. J Am Coll Cardiol 2002; 40: 105–110.
49. Elhendy A, Gentile F, Khandheria BK, *et al.* Thromboembolic complications after electrical cardioversion in patients with atrial flutter. Am J Med 2001; 111:433–438.
50. Corrado G, Sgalambro A, Mantero A, *et al.* Thromboembolic risk in atrial flutter. The FLASIEC (FLutter Atriale Societa Italiana di Ecografia Cardiovascolare) multicentre study. Eur Heart J 2001; 22: 1042–1051.
51. Schmidt H, von der Recke G, Illien S, *et al.* Prevalence of left atrial chamber and appendage thrombi in patients with atrial flutter and its clinical significance. J Am Coll Cardiol 2001; 38: 778–784.
52. Bertaglia E, Zoppo F, Bonso A, *et al.* Long term follow-up of radiofrequency catheter ablation of atrial flutter: clinical course and predictors of atrial fibrillation occurrence. Heart 2004; 90: 59–63.
53. VanderLugt JT, Mattioni T, Denker S, *et al.* Efficacy and safety of ibutilide fumarate for the conversion of atrial arrhythmias after cardiac surgery. Circulation 1999; 100: 369–375.
54. Abi-Mansour P, Carberry PA, McCowan RJ, *et al.* Conversion efficacy and safety of repeated doses of ibutilide in patients with atrial flutter and atrial fibrillation. Study Investigators. Am Heart J 1998; 136: 632–642.
55. Natale A, Newby KH, Pisano E, *et al.* Prospective randomized comparison of antiarrhythmic therapy versus first-line radiofrequency ablation in patients

with atrial flutter. J Am Coll Cardiol 2000; 35: 1898–1904.

56. Paydak H, Kall JG, Burke MC, *et al.* Atrial fibrillation after radiofrequency ablation of type I atrial flutter: time to onset, determinants, and clinical course. Circulation 1998; 98: 315–322.
57. Reithmann C, Hoffmann E, Spitzlberger G, *et al.* Catheter ablation of atrial flutter due to amiodarone therapy for paroxysmal atrial fibrillation. Eur Heart J 2000; 21: 565–572.
58. Blomstrom-Lundqvist C, Scheinman MM, Aliot EM, *et al.* ACC/AHA/ESC guidelines for the management of patients with supraventricular arrhythmias—executive summary: a report of the American College of Cardiology/American Heart Association Task Force on Practice Guidelines and the European Society of Cardiology Committee for Practice Guidelines (Writing Committee to Develop Guidelines for the Management of Patients With Supraventricular Arrhythmias). Circulation 2003; 108: 1871–1909.
59. Tai YT, Lau CP, Fong PC, *et al.* Incessant automatic ventricular tachycardia complicating acute coxsackie B myocarditis. Cardiology 1992; 80: 339–344.
60. Cooper LT Jr., Berry GJ, Shabetai R. Idiopathic giant-cell myocarditis—natural history and treatment. Multicenter Giant Cell Myocarditis Study Group Investigators. N Engl J Med 1997; 336: 1860–1866.
61. Inoue S, Shinohara F, Sakai T, *et al.* Myocarditis and arrhythmia: a clinico-pathological study of conduction system based on serial section in 65 cases. Jpn Circ J 1989; 53: 49–57.
62. Exner DV, Pinski SL, Wyse DG, *et al.* Electrical storm presages nonsudden death: the Antiarrhythmics Versus Implantable Defibrillators (AVID) trial. Circulation 2001; 103: 2066–2071.
63. Stevenson WG, Middlekauff HR, Stevenson LW, *et al.* Significance of aborted cardiac arrest and sustained ventricular tachycardia in patients referred for treatment therapy of advanced heart failure. Am Heart J 1992; 124: 123–130.
64. Wyse DG, Friedman PL, Brodsky MA, *et al.* Life-threatening ventricular arrhythmias due to transient or correctable causes: high risk for death in follow-up. J Am Coll Cardiol 2001; 38: 1718–1724.
65. Alberca T, Almendral J, Sanz P, *et al.* Evaluation of the specificity of morphological electrocardiographic criteria for the differential diagnosis of wide QRS complex tachycardia in patients with intraventricular conduction defects. Circulation 1997; 96: 3527–3533.
66. Oreto G, Smeets JL, Rodriguez LM, *et al.* Wide complex tachycardia with atrioventricular dissociation and QRS morphology identical to that of sinus rhythm: a manifestation of bundle branch reentry. Heart 1996; 76: 541–547.
67. Levine JH, Massumi A, Scheinman MM, *et al.* Intravenous amiodarone for recurrent sustained hypotensive ventricular tachyarrhythmias. Intravenous Amiodarone Multicenter Trial Group. J Am Coll Cardiol 1996; 27: 67–75.
68. Kowey PR, Marinchak RA, Rials SJ, Bharucha DB. Intravenous antiarrhythmic therapy in the acute control of in-hospital destabilizing ventricular tachycardia and fibrillation. Am J Cardiol 1999; 84: 46R–51R.
69. Koplan BK, Soejima K, Epstein LM, Stevenson WG. Refractory ventricular tachycardia secondary to cardiac sarcoid: electrophysiologic characteristics, mapping and ablation. Submitted 2005.
70. Delacretaz E, Stevenson WG, Ellison KE, *et al.* Mapping and radiofrequency catheter ablation of the three types of sustained monomorphic ventricular tachycardia in nonischemic heart disease. J Cardiovasc Electrophysiol 2000; 11: 11–17.
71. Winters SL, Cohen M, Greenberg S, *et al.* Sustained ventricular tachycardia associated with sarcoidosis: assessment of the underlying cardiac anatomy and the prospective utility of programmed ventricular stimulation, drug therapy and an implantable antitachycardia device. J Am Coll Cardiol 1991; 18: 937–943.
72. Sosa E, Scanavacca M, d'Avila A. Transthoracic epicardial catheter ablation to treat recurrent ventricular tachycardia. Curr Cardiol Rep 2001; 3: 451–458.
73. Akhtar M. Clinical spectrum of ventricular tachycardia. Circulation 1990; 82: 1561–1573.
74. Friedman PL, Stevenson WG. Proarrhythmia. Am J Cardiol 1998; 82: 50N–58N.
75. Stevenson WG, Middlekauff HR, Saxon LA. Ventricular arrhythmias in heart failure. In: Zipes DP, Jalife J (eds) Cardiac Electrophysiology: From Cell to Bedside, 2nd edition (W.B. Saunders Co.: Philadelphia, PA, 1995), 848–863.
76. Sarter BH, Finkle JK, Gerszten RE, Buxton AE. What is the risk of sudden cardiac death in patients presenting with hemodynamically stable sustained ventricular tachycardia after myocardial infarction? J Am Coll Cardiol 1996; 28: 122–129.
77. Raitt MH, Renfroe EG, Epstein AE, *et al.* "Stable" ventricular tachycardia is not a benign rhythm: insights from the Antiarrhythmics Versus Implantable Defibrillators (AVID) registry. Circulation 2001; 103: 244–252.

78. Pinski SL, Yao Q, Epstein AE, *et al.* Determinants of outcome in patients with sustained ventricular tachyarrhythmias: the Antiarrhythmics Versus Implantable Defibrillators (AVID) study registry. Am Heart J 2000; 139: 804–813.
79. Rask-Madsen C, Jensen G, Kober L, *et al.* Age-related mortality, clinical heart failure, and ventricular fibrillation in 4259 Danish patients after acute myocardial infarction. Eur Heart J 1997; 18: 1426–1431.
80. Thompson CA, Yarzebski J, Goldberg RJ, *et al.* Changes over time in the incidence and case-fatality rates of primary ventricular fibrillation complicating acute myocardial infarction: perspectives from the Worcester Heart Attack Study. Am Heart J 2000; 139: 1014–1021.
81. Mazur A, Anderson ME, Bonney S, Roden DM. Pause-dependent polymorphic ventricular tachycardia during long-term treatment with dofetilide: a placebo-controlled, implantable cardioverter-defibrillator-based evaluation. J Am Coll Cardiol 2001; 37: 1100–1105.
82. Roithinger FX, Berger T, Hintringer F. Effect of epicardial or biventricular pacing to prolong QT interval and increase transmural dispersion of repolarization. Circulation 2003; 108: e27–e28; author reply e27–e28.
83. Medina-Ravell VA, Lankipalli RS, Yan GX, *et al.* Effect of epicardial or biventricular pacing to prolong QT interval and increase transmural dispersion of repolarization: does resynchronization therapy pose a risk for patients predisposed to long QT or torsade de pointes? Circulation 2003; 107: 740–746.
84. Dorian P, Cass D, Schwartz B, *et al.* Amiodarone as compared with lidocaine for shock-resistant ventricular fibrillation. N Engl J Med 2002; 346: 884–890.
85. Kudenchuk PJ, Cobb LA, Copass MK, *et al.* Amiodarone for resuscitation after out-of-hospital cardiac arrest due to ventricular fibrillation. N Engl J Med 1999; 341: 871–878.
86. Wang YS, Scheinman MM, Chien WW, *et al.* Patients with supraventricular tachycardia presenting with aborted sudden death: incidence, mechanism and long-term follow-up. J Am Coll Cardiol 1991; 18: 1711–1719.
87. Hays LJ, Lerman BB, DiMarco JP. Nonventricular arrhythmias as precursors of ventricular fibrillation in patients with out-of-hospital cardiac arrest. Am Heart J 1989; 118: 53–57.
88. Passman R, Kadish A. Polymorphic ventricular tachycardia, long Q-T syndrome, and torsades de pointes. Med Clin North Am 2001; 85: 321–341.
89. Schrickel J, Bielik H, Yang A, *et al.* Amiodarone-associated "torsade de pointes": relevance of concomitant cardiovascular medication in a patient with atrial fibrillation and structural heart disease. Z Kardiol 2003; 92: 889–892.
90. Tomcsanyi J, Merkely B, Tenczer J, *et al.* Early proarrhythmia during intravenous amiodarone treatment. Pacing Clin Electrophysiol 1999; 22: 968–970.
91. Middlekauff HR, Stevenson WG, Saxon LA, Stevenson LW. Amiodarone and torsades de pointes in patients with advanced heart failure. Am J Cardiol 1995; 76: 499–502.
92. Yamada S, Kuga K, Yamaguchi I. Torsade de pointes induced by intravenous and long-term oral amiodarone therapy in a patient with dilated cardiomyopathy. Jpn Circ J 2001; 65: 236–238.
93. Tomaselli GF, Rose J. Molecular aspects of arrhythmias associated with cardiomyopathies. Curr Opin Cardiol 2000; 15: 202–208.
94. Wolbrette DL. Risk of proarrhythmia with class III antiarrhythmic agents: sex-based differences and other issues. Am J Cardiol 2003; 91: 39D–44D.
95. Nademanee K, Taylor R, Bailey WE, *et al.* Treating electrical storm: sympathetic blockade versus advanced cardiac life support-guided therapy. Circulation 2000; 102: 742–747.
96. Fotopoulos GD, Mason MJ, Walker S, *et al.* Stabilisation of medically refractory ventricular arrhythmia by intra-aortic balloon counterpulsation. Heart 1999; 82: 96–100.
97. Bansch D, Oyang F, Antz M, *et al.* Successful catheter ablation of electrical storm after myocardial infarction. Circulation 2003; 108: 3011–3016.
98. Teerlink JR, Jalaluddin M, Anderson S, *et al.* Ambulatory ventricular arrhythmias in patients with heart failure do not specifically predict an increased risk of sudden death. PROMISE (Prospective Randomized Milrinone Survival Evaluation) Investigators. Circulation 2000; 101: 40–46.
99. Singh SN, Fisher SG, Carson PE, Fletcher RD. Prevalence and significance of nonsustained ventricular tachycardia in patients with premature ventricular contractions and heart failure treated with vasodilator therapy. Department of Veterans Affairs CHF STAT Investigators. J Am Coll Cardiol 1998; 32: 942–947.
100. Shamsuzzaman AS, Gersh BJ, Somers VK. Obstructive sleep apnea: implications for cardiac and vascular disease. JAMA 2003; 290: 1906–1914.
101. Roche F, Xuong AN, Court-Fortune I, *et al.* Relationship among the severity of sleep apnea syndrome, cardiac arrhythmias, and autonomic imbalance. Pacing Clin Electrophysiol 2003; 26: 669–677.

102. Iuliano S, Fisher SG, Karasik PE, *et al.* QRS duration and mortality in patients with congestive heart failure. Am Heart J 2002; 143: 1085–1091.
103. Kuck KH, Cappato R, Siebels J, Ruppel R. Randomized comparison of antiarrhythmic drug therapy with implantable defibrillators in patients resuscitated from cardiac arrest: the Cardiac Arrest Study Hamburg (CASH). Circulation 2000; 102: 748–754.
104. Volgman AS, Carberry PA, Stambler B, *et al.* Conversion efficacy and safety of intravenous ibutilide compared with intravenous procainamide in patients with atrial flutter or fibrillation. J Am Coll Cardiol 1998; 31: 1414–1419.
105. Hennersdorf MG, Perings SM, Zuhlke C, *et al.* Conversion of recent-onset atrial fibrillation or flutter with ibutilide after amiodarone has failed. Intensive Care Med 2002; 28: 925–929.
106. Bernard EO, Schmid ER, Schmidlin D, *et al.* Ibutilide versus amiodarone in atrial fibrillation: a double-blinded, randomized study. Crit Care Med 2003; 31: 1031–1034.
107. Amiodarone Trials Meta-Analysis Investigators. Effect of prophylactic amiodarone on mortality after acute myocardial infarction and in congestive heart failure: meta-analysis of individual data from 6500 patients in randomised trials. Lancet 1997; 350: 1417–1424.
108. The Antiarrhythmics versus Implantable Defibrillators (AVID) Investigators. A comparison of antiarrhythmic-drug therapy with implantable defibrillators in patients resuscitated from near-fatal ventricular arrhythmias. N Engl J Med 1997; 337: 1576–1583.
109. Massie BM, Fisher SG, Radford M, *et al.* Effect of amiodarone on clinical status and left ventricular function in patients with congestive heart failure. CHF-STAT Investigators [published erratum appears in Circulation 1996; 94: 2668]. Circulation 1996; 93: 2128–2134.
110. Gottlieb SS, Riggio DW, Lauria S, *et al.* High dose oral amiodarone loading exerts important hemodynamic actions in patients with congestive heart failure. J Am Coll Cardiol 1994; 23: 560–564.
111. Wilkoff BL, Cook JR, Epstein AE, *et al.* Dual-chamber pacing or ventricular backup pacing in patients with an implantable defibrillator: the Dual Chamber and VVI Implantable Defibrillator (DAVID) Trial. JAMA 2002; 288: 3115–3123.
112. Dusman RE, Stanton MS, Miles WM, *et al.* Clinical features of amiodarone-induced pulmonary toxicity. Circulation 1990; 82: 51–59.
113. Singh SN, Fisher SG, Deedwania PC, *et al.* Pulmonary effect of amiodarone in patients with heart failure. The Congestive Heart Failure-Survival Trial of Antiarrhythmic Therapy (CHF-STAT) Investigators (Veterans Affairs Cooperative Study No. 320). J Am Coll Cardiol 1997; 30: 514–517.
114. Siniakowicz RM, Narula D, Suster B, Steinberg JS. Diagnosis of amiodarone pulmonary toxicity with high-resolution computerized tomographic scan. J Cardiovasc Electrophysiol 2001; 12: 431–436.
115. Loh KC. Amiodarone-induced thyroid disorders: a clinical review. Postgrad Med J 2000; 76: 133–140.

CHAPTER 14

Mechanical complications of acute decompensated heart failure

William B Haynos, Ron M Oren

Introduction

Acute decompensated heart failure (ADHF) is a clinical syndrome characterized by a variety of signs and symptoms. These typically include features of volume overload such as dyspnea, abdominal pain or bloating, and extremity edema. In addition, features of low cardiac output, such as anxiety, sense of doom, and fatigue can be seen. Commonly, these features (volume overload and low cardiac output) coexist in an individual patient; however, one or the other may predominate.

The vast majority of patients with ADHF have stable cardiomyopathy and chronic heart failure symptoms, which worsen suddenly; typically as a result of a precipitating factor such as infection or diet non-compliance. The diagnostic and therapeutic approach in these patients is focused on identifying the inciting factor, treating volume overload, when present, and optimizing chronic management—both pharmacological and non-pharmacological. On occasion, however, ADHF can become complicated by several factors which, if left undiagnosed and untreated, can substantially worsen outcome. Identifying these complicating factors, which is crucial to a successful outcome, can be difficult. The presence of these complications can be subtle and, because the signs and symptoms are similar, the clinical presentation often mimics that of uncomplicated ADHF.

Many of these complicating factors share a common theme of a clear mechanical aspect to pathophysiology or therapy. In this chapter, we will discuss several mechanical issues that can complicate or mimic ADHF. Awareness of these issues is important as the appropriate diagnosis requires a high index of suspicion, and therapy often leads to rapid improvement in symptoms. These mechanical issues include: (1) mechanical complications following myocardial infarction (MI); (2) mechanical complications of pericardial disease; (3) pleural effusions; (4) ascites; and (5) central venous obstruction.

Myocardial Rupture Following Acute Myocardial Infarction

Myocardial rupture is a dreaded complication of acute MI, often resulting in sudden onset of heart failure, cardiogenic shock, or death. It is the second leading cause of in-hospital death in post-MI patients.[1] The most common mechanical complications that result from myocardial rupture are (1) free wall rupture (FWR) with subsequent hemopericardium; (2) ventricular septal rupture (VSR); and (3) papillary muscle rupture (PMR) with subsequent acute mitral regurgitation (MR). Depending on the area of involved myocardium and the size of the infarction, rupture may result in only one or any combination of these events.[2–4] We will discuss each of these complications in further detail.

Regardless of the mechanical complication that results, the pathogenesis of myocardial rupture is similar. In the first 24 hours after infarction, rupture results when hemorrhage occurs in necrotic tissue and dissects through the myocardium. In cases that occur later—within 3 to 5 days—rupture results after the affected myocardium becomes thin and aneurysmal and ultimately perforates under high wall stress.[1,5–7] The timing of myocardial rupture is biphasic, reflecting the pathogenesis. Most events occur either within the first 24 hours post-MI or between days 3 and 5.[1,8] Advanced age, female gender, first MI, sustained chest pain, and sustained hypertension have all been associated with increased risk for myocardial rupture.[2,9,10] A delay in hospitalization and immoderate in-hospital physical activity have also been implicated.[11]

Free wall rupture

Free wall rupture (FWR) is the most common of the three post-MI mechanical complications[10] and is frequently a catastrophic event. FWR is the second leading cause of in-hospital post-MI mortality after cardiogenic shock from pump failure.[1] It may be responsible for 15 to 20% of all in-hospital MI-related deaths, though this number varies considerably from study to study.[12–14]

The era of reperfusion has likely resulted in a lowering of the rate of FWR; however, this is somewhat controversial. While thrombolysis was initially associated with higher rates of FWR,[13] subsequent data have not shown this.[14] Primary angioplasty appears to reduce the risk of FWR when compared to thrombolysis.[15] Low or absent blood flow in the infarct-related artery before or after angioplasty confers a higher risk for FRW, suggesting that restoration of blood flow prevents this complication.[16,17]

FWR occurs more often in the left ventricle than the right ventricle[18] and occurs most frequently in anterior and inferoposterior MIs.[1,10,13] FWR results in direct communication between the ventricle and pericardial space. This often leads to hemopericardium with tamponade and immediate cardiovascular collapse. In some instances, however, hemopericardium may be contained, either due to pericardial adhesions or incomplete rupture. These cases may be associated with a more subtle, subacute clinical course.[1,19,20] A pseudoaneurysm, the walls of which are formed by organized thrombus and pericardium, may also develop and seal off an area of ruptured myocardium. FWR may be a clinically silent event in these patients and may go unrecognized for long periods.[21] Patients with pseudoaneurysms often present with thromboembolic events.

The clinical course of FWR varies with the degree of hemopericardium that results and the rapidity with which the myocardium tears. Most cases are dramatic and catastrophic. The first indication is often profound cardiogenic shock with electromechanical dissociation. Without immediate surgical repair, death is imminent; even with surgery, survival is very poor.[11] In patients who have a more subacute course, due to limited rupture or pseudoaneurysm, an episode of hemodynamic collapse managed with supportive measures may occur.[1,19] These patients may require repeat pericardiocentesis prior to surgical intervention.

FWR is often diagnosed at surgery and necropsy.[3,9] Premorbid diagnosis is primarily echocardiographic—the presence of large pericardial effusion in the setting of electromechanical dissociation being the most common finding.[17,22] In the case of subacute FWR, serial echocardiograms are useful in monitoring the size of pericardial effusion and evidence of tamponade.[1] Pseudoaneurysms are easily visualized by two-dimensional echocardiography. The classic finding is a large, thin-walled aneurismal area with a narrow neck.[23] Left ventriculography is also helpful in visualizing the aneurismal area. Invasive hemodynamic monitoring may show evidence of tamponade with equalization of diastolic pressures or a low cardiac output state from pump failure.[20]

Treatment of acute FWR requires immediate surgical debridement and prosthetic patch repair.[20] However, many patients die before surgery and those who do make it to the operating room have a high surgical mortality.[1,19] Some investigators have demonstrated long-term survival in patients with subacute FWR treated non-surgically. These patients received supportive care (inotropes, intraaortic balloon pump, or mechanical ventilation) followed by prolonged bedrest and blood pressure control with beta-blockers.[19,21]

Ventricular septal rupture

Though not as common as FWR, ventricular septal rupture (VSR) complicates 1% to 3% of all AMIs and is responsible for 5% of all AMI-related deaths.[8] Recent data indicate that the incidence of VSR may be on the decline in the era of reperfusion. However, mortality remains high.[24] In the era of reperfusion, the timing of VSR appears to be primarily within the first 24 hours.[24,25]

VSRs occur in both anterior and inferoposterior MIs. The predominance of location varies from study to study. Apical septal rupture results from anterior MIs. Inferobasal rupture results from inferior MIs and usually convey a worse prognosis.[4,8,25,26] Morphologically, VSRs have several variants. They may appear as large through-and-through holes communicating across the septum. They also often occur as complex serpiginous tracts across the necrotic myocardium.[2,4]

The mechanism of heart failure in patients with VSR is not clear and may not be related to the degree of left-to-right shunting that occurs.[8,9] Heart failure in these patients may be due to right ventricular (RV) failure, occurring as a result of infarction and overloading secondary to left-to-right shunting.[5,11]

Sudden hemodynamic decline in a post-MI patient with a new murmur should raise the suspicion of VSR. The murmur of VSR is classically harsh, loud, holosystolic, and best heard at the left lower sternal border. It is often difficult to distinguish from the murmur of MR. A thrill is evident in about half of patients.[7,8,26] Right heart catheterization will demonstrate evidence of left-to-right shunting with a "step-up" of oxygen saturation from the right atrium to the right ventricle. High right-sided pressures and bizarre V-waves in the pulmonary arterial tracing may also be present.[4,7,8,26] Echocardiography is very useful in rapidly diagnosing VSR with color Doppler demonstrating left-to-right shunting through the defect.[7,24] Though not routinely done, ventriculography may be helpful in localizing the defect.[8]

Medical treatment for VSR is uniformly associated with a dismal prognosis and should be aimed at stabilizing and supporting patients prior to surgical repair. Afterload reduction, both with parenteral vasodilators and intraaortic balloon pump, is helpful in reducing the degree of shunting.[7,8,26] Surgical treatment consists of VSR repair and reconstruction with prosthetic material. Previously, a delay of several weeks prior to surgery in stable patients had been advocated. However, the favorable outcomes seen in such patients probably reflected a selection bias, as only the most stable patients were able to tolerate delay.[4,7] Subsequent data have refuted such an approach and current guidelines recommend urgent surgical repair in all patients.[27] Cardiogenic shock and inferobasal VSR are associated with a high surgical mortality.[24] For those patients who do survive surgery, prognosis appears reasonably good.[4]

Papillary muscle rupture

Papillary muscle rupture (PMR) is responsible for 5% of AMI-related deaths.[28] It occurs predominantly in the setting of an inferior MI; this finding likely reflects that the blood supply of the posteromedial papillary muscle is supplied solely by the posterior descending artery. Both the left anterior descending and the left circumflex arteries, in contrast, supply the anterolateral papillary muscle. Unlike FWR and VSR, PMR does occur in the setting of a non-Q wave MI.[2,9,11,28,29]

Clinically, patients with PMR develop acute pulmonary edema, a new systolic murmur, and shock.[30] Classically the onset occurs within 2 to 7 days. However, data in the reperfusion era suggests an earlier time course.[29] Diagnosis is usually echocardiographic with visualization of a flail mitral valve leaflet and severe MR with color flow Doppler.[28,30,31] Emergent surgical repair or replacement of the mitral valve is indicated in all patients. As in VSR, medical therapy, consisting of afterload reduction and supportive care, should be aimed at stabilizing patients prior to surgery.[28] Operative mortality is high but long-term prognosis for those who do survive surgery is good.[32,33]

Mechanical Complications of Pericardial Disease

The pericardium is a complex structure that has many functions. It serves as a barrier protecting the heart from infection and other inflammatory processes. The relative inelasticity of the pericardium limits excessive acute chamber dilation in cases of volume overload. It has a ligamentous function preventing excessive cardiac movement. Multiple disease processes can affect the pericardium either with or without affecting the heart.[34] The various diseases of the pericardium may cause heart failure as a result of constrictive pericarditis or cardiac tamponade.

Constrictive pericarditis

Constrictive pericarditis is the end result of many pericardial disease processes with etiologies ranging from infectious and inflammatory, to post-surgical and irradiation.[35] Constriction occurs when a fibrosed, usually thickened pericardium forms a rigid case around the heart. The result is reduced filling, elevated intracardiac pressures, and decreased cardiac output. Pericardial constriction may result acutely, subacutely, or many years after exposure to the etiologic agent.[35–37]

Patients usually present with symptoms of heart failure and have evidence of systemic venous congestion with jugular venous distension and peripheral edema; hepatomegaly with liver failure and ascites occurs as the disease progresses.[36–38] Classically described findings include Kussmaul's sign, a paradoxical increase in jugular venous pressure (JVP) with inspiration, and a pericardial "knock" in early diastole produced by sudden cessation of cardiac filling.[35,39] Right heart catheterization shows elevated filling pressures and equalization of diastolic pressures. The classic "dip and plateau" or "square root" pattern seen in right atrial, RV, and left ventricular (LV) tracing patterns reflects the rapid early diastolic filling and abrupt cessation of flow in mid-diastole.[36,38,40] Echocardiography is useful in diagnosis. Two-dimensional and M-mode imaging may show a diastolic septal "bounce" reflecting an abrupt change in pressure gradient across the septum.[35] Evidence of pericardial thickening may be seen and is perhaps better detected with transesophageal echocardiography (TEE). Doppler echocardiography plays an important role in diagnosis. The hallmark finding is respiratory variation in transmitral flow with decreased flow velocity during inspiration and increased flow velocity during expiration. The opposite pattern of flow may be observed across the tricuspid valve.[41–43] Cine computed tomography (CT) and magnetic resonance imaging (MRI) can detect pericardial thickening with high accuracy.[44–46] However, recent data indicate that the absence of pericardial thickening does not exclude the diagnosis of constrictive pericarditis.[47]

Differentiating constrictive pericarditis from restrictive cardiomyopathy is often a diagnostic challenge as they share many clinical and hemodynamic similarities. An RV systolic pressure ≤ 50 mm Hg, a difference between RV end-diastolic pressure and LV end-diastolic pressure of ≤ 5 mm Hg, and a ratio of RV end-diastolic pressure to RV systolic pressure $\geq 1{:}3$ have traditionally been described to favor a diagnosis of constriction over restriction.[48] However, the presence of discordant respiratory change in LV and RV pressures during inspiration—a reflection of ventricular interdependence—has been shown to be a more accurate hemodynamic finding in differentiating between the two entities.[40] Doppler echocardiography is very useful in differentiating constriction from restriction. The presence of respiratory change in RV and LV inflow velocities strongly favors constriction.[41,42] Tissue Doppler, a more recently developed technique, has shown promise in distinguishing between the two entities echocardiographically.[49] When diagnosis remains unclear, endomyocardial biopsy may be useful in demonstrating histological evidence of disease entities that can cause restrictive cardiomyopathy.[50]

Without surgical intervention, constrictive pericarditis has a slow, progressive course and carries a poor prognosis. Medical treatment is aimed at controlling volume overload and palliating symptoms.[37] Pericardectomy is associated with a good prognosis for most patients. Age, New York Heart Association (NYHA) class, and cardiac involvement are predictors of poor outcomes. Patients with irradiation pericarditis have considerably worse outcomes post-operatively.[35,51–53]

Cardiac tamponade

Cardiac tamponade is a dramatic, often catastrophic event that occurs when intrapericardial fluid compresses the heart, restricting filling in all chambers and reducing cardiac output.[36] Pericardial effusions may accumulate chronically, usually from an inflammatory process. In these cases, the pericardium has the ability to stretch over time and may accommodate several liters of fluid before tamponade occurs. Hemopericardium is a rapid process that typically results from trauma, usually surgical. Fluid accumulates before the pericardium is able to adapt and tamponade may occur with relatively little fluid in the intrapericardial space. Regardless of the timeframe, when fluid accumulation outstrips the capacity of the pericardium to distend, the intrapericardial pressure–volume curve becomes steep and small increases in volume result in large increases in pressure. Tamponade occurs when intrapericardial pressure exceeds intracardiac pressures.[54]

Clinically, tamponade often presents as cardiogenic shock. Patients are hypotensive, cyanotic, and tachypneic. Conscious patients may report a history consistent with acute pericarditis. The diagnosis should be considered in hemodynamically unstable patients with recent cardiac surgery or chest trauma and in patients with conditions predisposing them to pericarditis (malignancy, collagen vascular disease, renal insufficiency, or infection).[55]

On physical examination, patients are almost always tachycardic and often have signs of shock, including hypotension and cool, cyanotic extremities. Signs of venous congestion, most notably jugular venous distension, are apparent. Classically, one sees a steep x-descent and a blunted y-descent in the jugular venous pulsations. Cardiac examination usually reveals muffled heart sounds. When tamponade occurs as a result of acute pericarditis, a friction rub may be heard. An important physical finding is pulsus paradoxus, defined as an inspiratory drop in systolic pressure of > 10 mm Hg. An enlarged cardiac silhouette on chest x-ray may indicate the presence of pericardial effusion.[54,55]

Transthoracic echocardiography (TTE) is essential in diagnosing tamponade. Two-dimensional imaging will demonstrate the presence and location of pericardial effusion. Signs of tamponade include early diastolic collapse of the right ventricle and right atrial collapse. Failure of the inferior vena cava to collapse by > 50% with inspiration is also suggestive of tamponade. Doppler echocardiography will show a decrease in transmitral E wave of > 25% with inspiration. Right heart catheterization will show equalization of diastolic pressures. The right atrial pressure tracing mimics the steep x-descent and blunted y-descent of the jugular venous pulsations. Cardiac catheterization may be useful in monitoring hemodynamic response to pericardiocentesis and is useful in diagnosing constrictive-effusive pericarditis after pericardiocentesis.[37]

Treatment of tamponade requires pericardiocentesis. Medical therapy is aimed at supporting patients, usually with inotropes and intravenous fluids, prior to drainage of the effusion. Pericardiocentesis is usually performed through a subxiphoid approach and traditionally has been performed in the cardiac catheterization lab with hemodynamic monitoring. Echocardiographically-guided pericardiocentesis has proven to be safe and effective when compared to blind needle insertion. The use of an intrapericardial catheter for prolonged drainage has been shown to reduce the rate of fluid accumulation. Surgical drainage with creation of a pleuropericardial window for ongoing drainage of large effusions is safe and effective.[37,54,56]

Pleural Effusion

The development of abnormal fluid collections within the pleural space, called pleural effusions, can complicate ADHF in several ways. First, the worsening heart failure state can directly cause pleural effusion. Heart failure is a common cause of pleural effusion and such effusions are commonly seen (up to 70%) at some point in heart failure patients.[57] Second, a pleural effusion can develop, in a patient with stable heart failure, from one of several other comorbid illnesses. Diagnosing the presence of pleural effusion and understanding its cause are important to the successful treatment of ADHF.

The pleural space, which occurs between the visceral pleura (covering the lungs) and the parietal pleura (lining the chest wall) is, under normal circumstances, only a potential space coated by a thin layer of fluid. The fluid is produced by the visceral pleura at an astounding rate of 5 to 10 liters per day.

Normally, the pleural fluid does not accumulate because the fluid is absorbed through stomas in the parietal pleura which connect to lymphatics.[58] The rate of absorption normally equals the production rate.

An increased accumulation of pleural fluid can occur when the normal forces controlling fluid production and resorption are disrupted. Pleural fluid may increase either by increased production or decreased reabsorption. The vessels of the visceral pleura are part of the pulmonary circulation. Fluid production, therefore, can be increased when pulmonary pressures increase and hydrostatic forces are increased. Not surprisingly, in heart failure patients, the presence of pleural effusions is correlated with elevation of left heart filling pressures.[59,60] By altering vessel permeability, pleural inflammation can increase fluid production. Several processes may decrease fluid resorption and include obstruction of central lymphatic channels (with subsequent back pressure increase in pleural lymph pressure) or obstruction of lymph vessels on the pleural surface. The former may be the result of central mass or prior cardiothoracic surgery; the latter is usually a result of tumor cells.

Often much pleural fluid can accumulate before acute symptoms develop. Patients with substantial pleural fluid develop rest dyspnea and occasionally chest pain. Lesser degrees of effusion may worsen pre-existing chronic heart failure symptoms such as exertional dyspnea, orthopnea, or paroxysmal nocturnal dyspnea. The findings of pleural effusion on physical examination are dullness to percussion and decreased breath sounds over the area of effusion. Lung tissue compressed by the effusion may result in bronchial breath sounds and egophony at the periphery of the effusion. In patients with ADHF, pleural effusion is seen most often when substantial total body volume is present. Thus patients have the concomitant signs and symptoms of volume overload. On occasion, a substantial effusion is seen in patients with ADHF in the absence of signs and symptoms of total body volume overload. In these cases, investigation of a second comorbid cause of the effusion (other than ADHF), such as pulmonary embolism or malignancy, should be seriously considered.

Diagnostic considerations in pleural effusion focus on identifying its presence and defining its underlying cause. The radiographic findings of pleural effusion are well described. On upright chest radiography, typical findings may include an apparent elevation of the hemidiaphragm. Blunting of the costophrenic angle occurs with 200 to 300 mL of excess pleural fluid.[61] As fluid accumulates in greater volumes, the degree of hemithorax opacification increases. Typically, the density is shaped as a concave meniscus. Supine chest radiography can miss substantial amounts of fluid as the fluid layers in the posterior thorax and cannot be seen well. Lateral decubitus studies, where free-flowing fluid layers in a gravity-dependent manner, can provide useful information and clarify the presence of pleural effusion when other radiographs are uncertain. Ultrasound can identify fluid collections and is useful to target the location for thoracentesis. Computerized tomography can define loculated effusions, clarify the extent of effusions, and define potential thoracic processes,[62–64] which may play a causative role in the effusion development. The effusions associated with ADHF are usually bilateral but are commonly (approximately 10% to 20%) seen only on the right hemithorax.[57,66] An isolated left-sided pleural effusion may be related solely to ADHF, but because of its rarity (3% to 7%),[67] it should prompt consideration of causes other than ADHF.

Thoracentesis, with sampling and analysis of the pleural fluid, is an important step to understanding the circumstances which allowed the effusion to develop. The gross appearance of pleural fluid may provide diagnostic clues. Fluid may be chylous, purulent, or bloody. The hematocrit of bloody fluid helps separate a traumatic sampling from true bloody effusions. Findings in ADHF-associated fluid are clear, serous fluid. Other findings should prompt consideration of other pathologic processes. Traditionally, the fluid is classified as transudative or exudative based on its chemical composition. The transudative fluid of ADHF is characterized by low protein (<3 g/dL), low pleural/serum protein ratio (<0.5), and low pleural/serum lactate dehydrogenase (LDH) ratio (<0.6).[68] While exudative fluid can be seen in ADHF, especially when effusion is longstanding,[65] such a finding should lead to consideration of other diagnoses.

Transudative pleural effusions are not always caused by ADHF. Other conditions that can produce transudative pleural effusions include hypoalbuminemic states such as nephrotic syndrome, cirrhosis, and malnutrition, which may produce changes in osmotic pressure and resultant pleural effusion. Also, intra-abdominal fluid can pass directly into the thoracic space, and thus ascites or peritoneal dialysis may be associated with transudative pleural fluid.

Therapeutic considerations in pleural effusion are important. An acutely dyspneic patient with ADHF, in whom a substantial pleural effusion exists, can be drastically improved and stabilized with fluid drainage by thoracentesis. In patients with lower levels of distress, pleural effusion from ADHF usually does not require drainage. The fluid commonly resolves as the heart failure status improves. In rare cases, the effusions persist despite euvolemia and contribute to exertional dyspnea. Pleurodesis has occasionally been used in these patients. Pleurodesis is the induction of mesothelial injury, either chemically or surgically, with resultant formation of scarring and resultant fusion of the visceral and parietal pleura. This obliterates the potential pleural space, making effusion development less likely. While pleurodesis has been extensively studied in the care of chronic malignant pleural effusions or pneumothorax, its use in those conditions remains controversial.[69,70] The role of pleurodesis in heart failure is much less studied. Small studies have suggested a benefit of this approach in non-malignant refractory pleural effusions.[71–73]

Ascites

Ascites occurs when abnormally large amounts of fluid collect within the abdominal cavity. Ascites can complicate heart failure, either as part of total body volume overload or by the development of cardiac-related hepatic dysfunction termed *cardiac ascites*. Understanding the presence and severity of ascites in ADHF is important for several reasons. First, the ascites may represent undiagnosed, significant, underlying hepatic disease, which may impact other aspects of ADHF care. For example, use of pharmacological agents with a hepatic metabolism must be considered more carefully. Second, candidacy for therapeutic procedures such as cardiac transplant will be affected. Third, patients with ascites and heart failure may develop spontaneous bacterial peritonitis, which precipitates ADHF. Finally, in patients with substantial clinical instability, treatment of ascites with paracentesis may result in more rapid improvement.

Pathologically, ADHF affects the liver in several ways.[74–76] Elevated right atrial pressures are rapidly transmitted to the hepatic veins. Grossly, the liver in ADHF is enlarged with congestion. The hepatic venules and sinusoids are engorged. When sinusoidal pressure is severely elevated, hemorrhage and focal hepatic cellular necrosis can result. Hepatic reticulin condenses, collagen content increases, and central veins develop sclerosis. With continued heart failure, bridge scarring results and a complex cirrhosis pattern results. Thrombosis can be seen in the sinusoids and propagate into hepatic veins. Portal vein thrombosis and fibrosis also occurs. Low cardiac output also affects the liver by reducing hepatic perfusion, which may result in hepatocellular necrosis. Hepatic hypoperfusion also results in reticulin collapse and collagen increases, which also contributes to the loss of normal hepatic structural architecture.

Ascites occurs after the interplay of several factors which are not completely understood. First, increased sinusoidal pressure (as occurs in ADHF) produces an increase in hepatic lymph flow, ultimately into the thoracic duct. The thoracic duct can accommodate a 5-fold to 10-fold increase in flow. As this hepatic lymph flow increases further, the thoracic duct capacity is reached and fluid weeps from the liver's surface into the peritoneum.[77] An additional mechanism may involve baroreflexes because afferent baroreceptors are located in the sinusoids. Elevated sinusoidal pressures may thereby negatively affect neurohumoral vasculature control and renal salt and water excretion.

A second important factor in ascites development is impaired renal salt excretion. The initiating mechanism of this abnormality is debated. The "overflow theory"[78] suggests that the inciting event is abnormal renal salt retention caused by liver dysfunction or perhaps portal hypertension. The exact manner in which the liver abnormality produces abnormal renal salt handling is unclear but humoral factors or baroreflex alterations have been proposed as potential causes. The salt retention results in plasma volume expansion and ascites develops. The "underflow theory"[79] suggests that excessive peritoneal lymph fluid leads to a decrease in plasma volume and subsequent activation of renal mechanisms to retain salt and water. Hypervolemia ensues. The "arterial vasodilation theory" incorporates elements of both of these theories and suggests that a circulating factor (nitric oxide has been implicated)[80] causes peripheral vasodilation which subsequently stimulates renal salt and water retention.

The presence of ascites is most commonly diagnosed by physical examination. Classic findings include a tense abdomen, a palpable fluid wave, and "shifting dullness." These findings require substantial amounts of fluid and can be masked by a variety of factors, including obesity. Ultrasound examination of the abdomen can detect very small amounts of ascitic fluid. The etiology of ascites most often requires a sampling and analysis of ascitic fluid. For example, cellular analysis or culture can assist in the diagnosis of malignant ascites or spontaneous bacterial peritonitis. Chemical analysis is perhaps most helpful with the calculation of the serum–ascites albumin gradient (SAAG). This classification has now replaced the characterization of fluid as either exudative or transudative. Ascites caused by cirrhosis or chronic hepatic congestion from cardiac disease will be associated with a high (>1.1 g/dL) SAAG.[81]

Treatment of ascites complicating ADHF is largely similar to treatment of volume overloaded ADHF without ascites. The mainstays of treatment include dietary salt and water restriction and diuretics. However, important differences exist which require attention when ascites complicates ADHF. For example, excessive diuresis may produce or exacerbate hepatorenal syndrome[82] or hepatic encephalopathy.[83] In addition, large-volume paracentesis as a therapeutic strategy should not be overlooked. Removal of 4 to 6 liters of ascitic fluid via paracentesis can be a highly effective means to rapidly improve the unstable patient with ADHF, ascites, and volume overload. Salt-poor albumin is commonly administered intravenously as the paracentesis is performed. One study suggested that this approach is better tolerated than is pharmacological diuresis[84] and another study suggested a shorter length of hospital stay.[85] Risks such as depletion of proteins or development of spontaneous bacterial peritonitis do not seem to be increased with this approach.[86]

Superior Vena Cava Syndrome

Several of the signs and symptoms of ADHF can occur following thrombosis of one or more major thoracic veins. Thrombosis of the superior vena cava (SVC) syndrome is most likely to cause diagnostic confusion with ADHF. Occlusion of the SVC or other veins, such as the subclavian vein, may occur slowly and insidiously or may occur as an acute exacerbation. The SVC is well collateralized so the effect of substantial thrombus may be blunted. The azygos vein is particularly important in this regard. While typically the diagnosis of SVC obstruction is clear, as when facial edema and plethora are predominant, on occasion symptoms may mimic those seen in ADHF. Commonly, for example, patients experience cough, dyspnea, chest pain, and a vague bloating sensation. On physical examination, JVP is elevated and lung sounds are abnormal.[87]

Central venous thrombosis usually results from external compression by a thoracic tumor, usually lung cancers.[88] The central veins are easily compressed because of their thin-walled nature and the low intraluminal pressure. Nonmalignant processes, such as mediastinal fibrosis, may also result in SVC syndrome. The use of pacemaker and implantable cardioverter defibrillators is rarely associated with central vein thrombosis. However, with the increasing use of these therapies along with the use of central veinous catheters, the prevalence of this complication would be expected to increase.

SVC thrombosis can be diagnosed radiographically. Chest radiography typically demonstrates mediastinal widening. A pleural effusion may be seen. CT or MRI is useful for delineating the size and extent of the thrombotic process and the source of external SVC compression. Venography may be useful but, given the utility of other imaging techniques, is often unnecessary.

Therapy of SVC syndrome depends on the underlying cause, severity, and rapidity of symptom development. Anticoagulation can be used. Lytic therapy is considered when the thrombotic process is acute.[89] Catheter-based dilation procedures and surgery can improve the course of focal obstructions.[89] When the cause of SVC is external compression from malignancy, radiation or chemotherapy of the underlying condition is employed.

References

1. Purcaro A, Costantini C, Ciampani N, *et al.* Diagnostic criteria and management of subacute ventricular free wall rupture complicating acute myocardial infarction. Am J Cardiol 1997; 80: 397–405.
2. Figueras J, Cortadellas J, Soler-Soler J. Comparison of ventricular septal and left ventricular free wall rupture in acute myocardial infarction. Am J Cardiol 1998; 81: 495–497.
3. Mann JM, Roberts WC. Fatal rupture of both left ventricular free and ventricular septum (double rupture) during acute myocardial infarction: analysis of seven patients studied at necropsy. Am J Cardiol 1987; 60: 722–724.
4. Held AC, Cole PL, Lipton B, *et al.* Rupture of the interventricular septum complicating acute myocardial infarction: a multicenter analysis of clinical findings and outcome. Am Heart J 1988; 116: 1330–1336.
5. Becker AE, van Mantgem JP. Cardiac tamponade: a study of 50 hearts. Eur J Cardiol 1975; 3: 349–358.
6. Nakatsuchi Y, Minamino T, Fujii K, Negoro, S. Clinicopathological characterization of cardiac free wall rupture in patients with acute myocardial infarction: difference between early and late phase rupture. Int J Cardiol 1994; 47: S33–S38.
7. Birnbaum Y, Fishbein MC, Blanche C, Siegel RJ. Ventricular septal rupture after acute myocardial infarction. N Engl J Med 2002; 347: 1426–1432.
8. Radford MJ, Johnson RA, Daggett WM Jr., *et al.* Ventricular septal rupture: a review of clinical and physiologic features and an analysis of survival. Circulation 1981; 64: 545–553.
9. Feneley MP, Chang VP, O'Rourke MF. Myocardial rupture after acute myocardial infarction; ten year review. Br Heart J 1983; 49: 550–556.
10. Dellborg M, Held P, Swedberg K, Vedin A. Rupture of the myocardium, occurrence and risk factors. Br Heart J 1985; 54: 11–16.
11. Figueras J, Cortadellas J, Calvo F, Soler-Soler J. Relevance of delayed hospital admission on development of cardiac rupture during acute myocardial infarction, study in 225 patients with free wall, septal, or papillary muscle rupture. J Am Coll Cardiol 1998; 32: 135–139.
12. Stevenson WG, Linssen GC, Havenith MG, Brugada P, Wellens HJ. The spectrum of death after myocardial infarction: a necropsy study. Am Heart J 1989; 118: 1182–1188.
13. Becker RC, Gore JM, Lambrew C, *et al.* A composite view of cardiac rupture in the United States National Registry of Myocardial Infarction. J Am Coll Cardiol 1996; 27: 1321–1326.
14. Becker RC, Hochman JS, Cannon CP, *et al.* Fatal cardiac rupture among patients treated with thrombolytic agents and adjunctive thrombin antagonists: observations from the Thrombolysis and Thrombin Inhibition in Myocardial Infarction 9 Study. J Am Coll Cardiol 1999; 33: 479–487.
15. Moreno R, Lopez-Sendon J, Garcia E, *et al.* Primary angioplasty reduces the risk of left ventricular free wall rupture compared with thrombolysis in patients with acute myocardial infarction. J Am Coll Cardiol 2002; 39: 598–603.
16. Morishima I, Sone T, Mokuno S, *et al.* Clinical significance of no-reflow phenomenon observed on angiography after successful treatment of acute myocardial infarction with percutaneous transluminal coronary angioplasty. Am Heart J 1995; 30: 239–243.
17. Moreno R, Lopez de Sa E, Lopez-Sendon JL, *et al.* Frequency of left ventricular free-wall rupture in patients with acute myocardial infarction treated with primary angioplasty. Am J Cardiol 2000; 85: 757–760.
18. Reddy S, Roberts WC. Frequency of rupture of the left ventricular free wall or ventricular septum among necropsy cases of fatal acute myocardial infarction since introduction of coronary care units. Am J Cardiol 1989; 63: 906–911.
19. Figueras J, Cortadellas J, Evangelista A, Soler-Soler J. Medical management of selected patients with left ventricular free wall rupture during acute myocardial infarction. J Am Coll Cardiol 1997; 29: 512–518.
20. Pappas PJ, Cernaianu AC, Baldino WA, Cilley JH Jr., DelRossi AJ. Ventricular free-wall rupture after myocardial infarction, treatment and outcome. Chest 1991; 99: 892–895.
21. Figueras J, Cortadellas J, Domingo E, Soler-Soler J. Survival following self-limited ventricular free wall

rupture during myocardial infarction: management differences between patients with or without pseudoaneurysm formation. Intl J Cardiol 2001; 79: 103–111.

22. Slater J, Brown RJ, Antonelli TA, *et al.* Cardiogenic shock due to cardiac free-wall rupture or tamponade after acute myocardial infarction: a report from the SHOCK Trial Registry. SHould we emergently revascularize Occluded Coronaries for cardiogenic shocK? J Am Coll Cardiol 2000; 36: 1117–1122.
23. Gatewood RP Jr., Nanda NC. Differentiation of left ventricular aneurysm from true aneurysm with two-dimensional echocardiography. Am J Cardiol 1980; 46: 869–878.
24. Crenshaw BS, Granger CB, Birnbaum Y *et al.* Risk factors, angiographic patterns, and outcomes in patients with ventricular septal defect complicating acute myocardial infarction. GUSTO-I (Global Utilization of Streptokinase and TPA for Occluded Coronary Arteries) Trial Investigators. Circulation 2000; 101: 27–32.
25. Menon V, Webb JG, Hillis LD, *et al.* Outcome and profile of ventricular rupture with cardiogenic shock after myocardial infarction: a report from the SHOCK Trial Registry. SHould we emergently revascularize Occluded Coronaries for cardiogenic shocK? J Am Coll Cardiol 2000; 36: 1110–1116.
26. Lemery R, Smith HC, Giuliani ER, Gersh BJ. Prognosis in rupture of the ventricular septum after acute myocardial infarction and role of early surgical intervention. Am J Cardiol 1992; 70: 147–151.
27. Ryan TJ, Antman EM, Brooks NH, *et al.* 1999 Update: ACC/AHA guidelines for the management of patients with acute myocardial infarction, a report of the American College of Cardiology/American Heart Association Task Force on Practice Guidelines (Committee on Management of Acute Myocardial Infarction). J Am Coll Cardiol 1999; 34: 890–911.
28. Reeder GS. Identification and treatment of complications of myocardial infarction. Mayo Clin Proc 1995; 70: 880–884.
29. Thompson CR, Buller CE, Sleeper LA, *et al.* Cardiogenic shock due to acute severe mitral regurgitation complicating acute myocardial infarction: a report from the SHOCK Trial Registry. SHould we emergently revascularize Occluded Coronaries for cardiogenic shocK? J Am Coll Cardiol 2000; 36: 1104–1109.
30. Verma R, Freeman I. Images in clinical medicine. Rupture of papillary muscle during acute myocardial infarction. N Engl J Med 1999; 341: 247.
31. Smyllie JH, Sutherland GR, Geuskens R, *et al.* Doppler color flow mapping in the diagnosis of ventricular septal rupture and acute mitral regurgitation after myocardial infarction. J Am Coll Cardiol 1990; 15: 1449–1455.
32. Kishon Y, Oh JK, Schaff HV, *et al.* Mitral valve operation in postinfarction rupture of a papillary muscle: immediate results and long-term follow-up of 22 patients. Mayo Clin Proc 1992; 67: 1023–1030.
33. Pretre R, Ye Q, Grunenfelder J, *et al.* Operative results of "repair" of ventricular rupture after acute myocardial infarction. Am J Cardiol 1999; 84: 785–788.
34. Spodick DH. Macrophysiology, microphysiology, and anatomy of the pericardium: a synopsis. Am Heart J 1992; 124: 1046–1051.
35. Myers RB, Spodick DH. Constrictive pericarditis: clinical and pathophysiologic characteristics. Am Heart J 1999; 138: 219–232.
36. Spodick DH. The normal and diseased pericardium: current concepts of pericardial physiology, diagnosis and treatment. J Am Coll Cardiol 1983; 1: 240–251.
37. Topol EJ, Klein AL, Scalia EM. Diseases of the pericardium, restrictive cardiomyopathy, and diastolic dysfunction. In: Topol EJ (ed.) Comprehensive Cardiovascular Medicine (Lippincott-Raven Publishers: Philadelphia, PA, 1998), 669–733.
38. Yurchak PM, Deshpande V. Case record of the Massachusetts General Hospital, weekly clinicopathological exercises, Case 2–2003: a 60-year-old man with mild congestive heart failure of uncertain cause. N Engl J Med 2003; 348: 243–249.
39. Nicholson WJ, Cobbs BN Jr., Franch RH, Crawley IS. Early diastolic sound of constrictive pericarditis. Am J Cardiol 1980; 45: 378–382.
40. Hurrell DG, Nishimura RA, Higano ST, *et al.* Value of dynamic respiratory changes in left and right ventricular pressures for the diagnosis of constrictive pericarditis. Circulation 1996; 93: 2007–2013.
41. Hatle LK, Appleton CP, Popp RL. Differentiation of constrictive pericarditis and restrictive cardiomyopathy by Doppler echocardiography. Circulation 1989; 79: 357–370.
42. Oh JK, Hatle LK, Seward JB, *et al.* Diagnostic role of Doppler echocardiography in constrictive pericarditis. J Am Coll Cardiol 1994; 23: 154–162.
43. Klein AL, Cohen GI, Pietrolungo JF, *et al.* Differentiation of constrictive pericarditis from restrictive cardiomyopathy by Doppler transesophageal echocardiographic measurements of respiratory variations in pulmonary venous flow. J Am Coll Cardiol 1993; 22: 1935–1943.
44. Oren RM, Grover-McKay M, Stanford W, Weiss RM. Accurate preoperative diagnosis of pericardial con-

striction using cine computed tomography. J Am Coll Cardiol 1993; 22: 832–838.
45. Hartnell GG, Hughes LA, Ko JP, Cohen MC. Magnetic resonance imaging of pericardial constriction: comparison of cine MR angiography and spin-echo techniques. Clin Radiol 1996; 51: 268–272.
46. Kojima S, Yamada N, Goto Y. Diagnosis of constrictive pericarditis by tagged cine magnetic resonance imaging. N Engl J Med 1999; 341: 373–374.
47. Talreja DR, Edwards WD, Danielson GK, *et al.* Constrictive pericarditis in 26 patients with histologically normal pericardial thickness. Circulation 2003; 108: 1852–1857.
48. Vaitkus PT, Kussmaul WG. Constrictive pericarditis versus restrictive cardiomyopathy: a reappraisal and update of diagnostic criteria. Am Heart J 1991; 122: 1431–1441.
49. Rajagopalan N, Garcia MJ, Rodriguez L, *et al.* Comparison of new Doppler echocardiographic methods to differentiate constrictive pericardial heart disease and restrictive cardiomyopathy. Am J Cardiol 2001; 87: 86–94.
50. Schoenfeld MH, Supple EW, Dec GW Jr., Fallen JT, Palacius IF. Restrictive cardiomyopathy versus constrictive pericarditis: role of endomyocardial biopsy in avoiding unnecessary thoracotomy. Circulation 1987; 75: 1012–1017.
51. Bashi VV, John S, Ravikumar E, *et al.* Early and late results of pericardiectomy in 118 cases of constrictive pericarditis. Thorax 1988; 43: 637–641.
52. McCaughan BC, Schaff HV, Piehler JM, *et al.* Early and late results of pericardiectomy for constrictive pericarditis. J Thorac Cardiovasc Surg 1985; 89: 340–350.
53. Ling LH, Oh JK, Schaff HV. Constrictive pericarditis in the modern era: evolving clinical spectrum and impact on outcome after pericardiectomy. Circulation 1999; 100: 1380–1386.
54. Spodick, DM. Acute cardiac tamponade. N Engl J Med 2003; 349: 684–690.
55. Spodick, DH. Pericardial diseases. In: Braunwald E, Zipes DP, Libby P (eds) Heart Disease: A Textbook of Cardiovascular Medicine. Volume 2, 6th edition (W.B. Saunders: Philadelphia, PA, 2001), 1823–1876.
56. Tsang TS, Oh JK, Seward JB. Diagnosis and management of cardiac tamponade in the era of echocardiography. Clin Cardiol 1999; 22: 446–452.
57. Peterman TA, Brothers SK. Pleural effusions in congestive heart failure and in pericardial disease. N Engl J Med 1983; 309: 313–318.
58. Wang NS. The performed stomas connecting the pleural cavity and the lymphatics in the parietal pleura. Am Rev Respir Dis 1975; 111: 12–20.
59. Weiner-Kronish J, Broaddus V, Goldstien R, *et al.* Pulmonary hypertension and right atrial hypertension in the absence of left heart failure are not associated with pleural effusion. Am Rev Respir Dis 1986; 133: A130.
60. Broaddus V, Weiner-Kronish J, Jerome E, *et al.* Pleural effusions in volume overloaded pulmonary edema. Physiologist 1986; 29: 104–112.
61. Levin DL, Klein JS. Imaging techniques for pleural space infections. Semin Respir Infect 1999; 14: 31–38.
62. Muller NL. Imaging of the pleura. Radiology 1993; 186: 297–309.
63. McLoud TC. CT and MR in pleural disease. Clin Chest Med 1998; 19: 261–276.
64. McLoud TC, Flower CD. Imaging the pleura: sonography, CT, and MR imaging. AJR Am J Roentgenol 1991; 156: 1145–1153.
65. Chakko SC, Caldwell SH, Sforza PP. Treatment of congestive heart failure, its effect on pleural fluid chemistry. Chest 1989; 95: 798–802.
66. Weiss JM, Spodick DH. Laterality of pleural effusions in chronic congestive heart failure. Am J Cardiol 1984; 53: 951–957.
67. Edwards JE, Race GA, Scheifley CH. Hydrothorax in congestive heart failure. Am J Med 1957; 22: 83–89.
68. Light RW, MacGregor MI, Luchsinger PC, Ball WC Jr. Pleural effusions: the diagnostic separation of transudates and exudates. Ann Intern Med 1972; 77: 507–513.
69. Petrou M, Kaplan D, Goldstraw P. Management of recurrent malignant pleural effusions: the contemporary role of talc pleurodesis and pleuroperitoneal shunting. Cancer 1995; 75: 801–805.
70. Rodriguez-Panadero F, Antony VB. Pleurodesis: state of the art. Eur Respir J 1997; 10: 1648–1654.
71. Vargas FS, Milanez JR, Filomeno LT, *et al.* Intrapleural talc for the prevention of recurrence in benign or undiagnosed pleural effusions. Chest 1994; 106: 1771–1775.
72. Aelony Y, King R, Boutin C. Thoracoscopic talc poudrage pleurodesis for chronic recurrent pleural effusions. Ann Intern Med 1991; 115: 778–782.
73. Webb WR, Ozmen V, Moulder PV, Shabahang B, Breaux J. Iodized talc pleurodesis for the treatment of pleural effusions. J Thorac Cardiovasc Surg 1992; 103: 881–885.
74. Klatt EC, Koss MN, Young TS, Mccauley L, Martin SE. Hepatic hyalin globules associated with passive congestion. Arch Pathol Lab Med 1988; 112: 510–513.

75. Kubo SH, Walter BA, John DH, Clark M, Cody RJ. Liver function abnormalities in chronic heart failure: influence of systemic hemodynamics. Arch Intern Med 1987; 147: 1227–1230.
76. Lefkowitch JH, Mendez L. Morphologic features of hepatic injury in cardiac disease and shock. J Hepatol 1986; 2: 313–327.
77. Ring-Larsen H, Henriksen JH. Pathogenesis of ascites formation and hepatorenal syndrome; humoral and hemodynamic factors. Semin Liver Dis 1986; 6: 341–352.
78. Lieberman F, Denidson E, Reynolds T. The relationship between plasma volume, portal hypertension, ascites and renal sodium retention in cirrhosis: the overflow theory of ascites formation. Ann NY Acad Sci 1970: 70; 202–210.
79. Sherlock S, Shaldon S. The etiology and management of ascites in patients with hepatic cirrhosis: a review. Gut 1963; 4: 95–105.
80. Matsumoto A, Ogura K, Hirata Y, *et al.* Increased nitric oxide in the exhaled air of patients with decompensated liver cirrhosis. Ann Intern Med 1995; 123: 110–113.
81. Runyon BA, Montano AA, Akriviadis EA, *et al.* The serum-ascites albumin gradient is superior to exudate-transudate concept in the differential diagnosis of ascites. Ann Intern Med 1992; 117: 215–220.
82. Bichet DG, Van Putten VJ, Schrier RW. Potential role of increased sympathetic activity in impaired sodium and water excretion in cirrhosis. N Engl J Med 1982; 307: 1552–1557.
83. Sherlock S, Summerskill WH, White LP. Portal-systemic encephalopathy, neurological complications of liver disease. Lancet 1954; 267: 454–457.
84. Gines JP, Arroyo V, Quintero E, *et al.* Comparison of paracentesis and diuretics in the treatment of cirrhotics with tense ascites: results of a randomized study. Gastroenterology 1987; 93: 234–241.
85. Salerno F, Badalamenti S, Incerti P, *et al.* Repeated paracentesis and intravenous albumin infusion to treat "tense" ascites in cirrhotic patients, a safe alternative therapy. J Hepatol 1987; 5: 102–108.
86. Sola R, Andreu M, Coll S, *et al.* Spontaneous bacterial peritonitis in cirrhotic patients treated using paracentesis or diuretics: results of a randomized study. Hepatology 1995; 21: 340–344.
87. Lochridge SK, Knibbe WP, Doty DB. Obstruction of the superior vena cava. Surgery 1979; 85: 14–24.
88. Parish JM, Marschke RF Jr., Dines DE, Lee RE. Etiologic considerations in the superior vena cava syndrome. Mayo Clin Proc 1981; 56: 407–413.
89. Machleder HI, Evaluation of a new treatment strategy for Paget–Schroetter syndrome: spontaneous thrombosis of the axillary-subclavian vein. J Vasc Surg 1993; 17: 305–317.

CHAPTER 15

Cardiogenic shock

Gadi Cotter, Olga Milo-Cotter, Edo Kaluski

Introduction

Cardiogenic shock is a syndrome of extreme cardiovascular forward failure manifesting as low blood pressure, low perfusion of vital organs (such as the central nervous system, heart, and kidneys), and signs of increased filling pressure of the left ventricle (though not always overt pulmonary congestion[1]). It occurs mainly in the setting of a major acute coronary syndrome (ACS), although it may be the final pathway of end-stage cardiomyopathies.

The main shortcoming of cardiogenic shock research is the lack of an agreed-upon definition. This has caused a significant variation in the perceived incidence of this syndrome, leading to large variability in the reported etiology, pathogenesis, response to treatment, and outcome. Therefore, this chapter presents a broader view of cardiogenic shock, encompassing the different prevailing opinions in the literature while focusing on our view of the subject.

In general, cardiogenic shock occurs in approximately 6% to 7% of patients with acute ST elevation myocardial infarction (STEMI)[2–8] and 2.5% of patients with ACS without ST segment elevation.[9] Although in recent years a trend was reported toward decreased mortality over the years,[10] probably due to the increased rate of earlier diagnosis and improved revascularization of patients with cardiogenic shock complicating ACS, it remains a lethal condition with early (in-hospital or 1-month) mortality of > 45% even in the most recent reports.[2,3,5,6,9,11–21] Therefore, a better understanding of the definition, pathophysiology, clinical characteristics, and diagnosis is needed in order to develop improved treatments.

Definition

The definition of cardiogenic shock varies greatly among different institutions and research groups. All definitions include two main criteria: reduced systolic blood pressure and signs of peripheral hypoperfusion. Most authorities also require a measure of high filling pressure of the left ventricle. However, the required severity of these signs varies between experts and is highly dependent on the clinical setting. For example, there is no accepted definition for patients with end-stage cardiomyopathies developing cardiogenic shock. In such patients, low systolic blood pressure is common even in the compensated state, as are decreased peripheral perfusion and increased left ventricular (LV) filling pressures. Therefore, in these patients some authorities recommend the use of blood pressure decrease instead of absolute blood pressure for the definition of shock. However, such criteria were not assessed prospectively.

In patients with ACS, systolic blood pressure < 90 mm Hg, the need for hemodynamic support to maintain such blood pressure, or a decrease of systolic blood pressure by > 30 mm Hg are regarded as key signs for the diagnosis of cardiogenic shock.[5,6,11,12,14–21] Since, in many patients, transient blood pressure decreases occur during ACS, carrying less prognostic significance, we have suggested[22,23] a more restrictive approach in which cardiogenic shock is diagnosed only if low systolic blood pressure (< 100 mm Hg) persists despite maximal revascularization and substantial support by vasopressors for at least an hour. Such an approach is supported by a recent manuscript[24] showing significantly lower mortality in patients with cardiogenic shock responding to vasopressor support.

The definition of peripheral hypoperfusion is even less clear. Some authorities[25] have suggested cool, poorly-perfused extremities, decreased urine output, or acutely diminished central nervous system function, although this definition lacks objectivity and therefore can be interpreted differentially by different physicians. To overcome this lack of objectivity, it was suggested that blood lactate level be used as a marker of reduced peripheral perfusion. Lactate was shown in previous studies to correlate with adverse outcome in patients with large MIs requiring vasopressor support,[26] but studies on the value of this marker are limited and no cut-off measures have been established. Signs of increased LV filling pressure are required by most (although not all) authorities. These usually include an increased wedge pressure to > 15 mm Hg to 20 mm Hg in the face of reduced cardiac output (CO) during invasive hemodynamic monitoring.[3] Other options for diagnosis of increased LV pressure such as chest x-ray findings or increased B-type natriuretic peptide (BNP) levels were not examined previously.

Recently, with the advent of early percutaneous revascularization in patients with cardiogenic shock, leading to some reduction in morbidity and mortality,[11,16,17,21,27] we have suggested that the diagnosis of cardiogenic shock should be restricted to patients not responding within a short period of time to percutaneous revascularization.[22,23] This definition is now being examined in phase II of the SHOCK-2 (SHould we emergently revascularize Occluded Coronaries for cardiogenic shocK?) study.

Etiology, Characteristics, and Incidence

In broad terms, there are four main etiologies of cardiogenic shock: end-stage cardiomyopathies, mechanical cardiac dysfunction, post-coronary artery bypass grafting (CABG), and acute ischemic cardiac events. Post-CABG shock will not be reviewed in the present chapter.

Cardiogenic shock complicating cardiomyopathies

Cardiogenic shock may develop in patients with either acute cardiomyopathies (such as fulminant or post-partum cardiomyopathy) or as the final event in patients with different types of chronic cardiomyopathies, of which ischemic cardiomyopathy is probably the most common. Regrettably, the data and exact incidence of these syndromes are not reported in detail in the literature. Almost 1 000 000 patients are admitted with acute heart failure to hospitals in the United States each year. Since the in-hospital mortality for these patients is approximately 4%, of which 50% is due to progressive cardiac failure, one can assume that many patients with acute heart failure develop syndromes of severe forward cardiovascular failure accompanied by low blood pressure and decreased peripheral perfusion. However, specific data on the incidence and characteristics of such patients are lacking. Moreover, existing data on status 1 cardiac transplantation candidates are significantly biased due to the restrictive eligibility criteria for cardiac transplantation. In a series of 10 patients with cardiogenic shock treated by intravenous levosimendan in Vienna, Austria, only 4 out of the 10 patients had a recent ischemic event. Two patients developed shock after CABG and 4 patients had cardiomyopathies. The mean age was 72 years and hemodynamic measures were similar to those suggested for the diagnosis of cardiogenic shock during an ACS.[28] Nanas *et al.* have described a group of patients with severe acute heart failure who could not be weaned off intravenous dobutamine. The mean admission blood pressure was 99/67 mm Hg and the mean age was 62. Eighty-eight percent were males and about half had ischemic etiology. Hemodynamic measurements demonstrated a wedge pressure of 29 mm Hg, cardiac index (CI) of 2.2 L/min/m^2 and right ventricular (RV) pressure of 68/45 mm Hg. Mean creatinine levels were 1.7 mg/dL. Again, although demonstrative, these studies were small and exact characterization of patients with cardiogenic shock due to end-stage cardiomyopathies is lacking.

Mechanical cardiac dysfunction

Mechanical cardiac dysfunction occurs as the result of failure (either severe regurgitation or stenosis) of cardiac valves, especially the mitral and aortic valves, or due to rupture of the heart, mostly LV free wall rupture leading to tamponade, or rupture of the intraventricular septum leading to acute ventricular septal defect (VSD). Most such acute mechanical complications leading to cardiogenic shock occur during an acute ischemic event, although as opposed to ischemic events leading to cardiogenic shock, the ischemic events causing such mechanical complications are usually milder and therefore cardiogenic shock occurring in these circumstances is usually a surprising event. Other etiologies include end-stage primary valvular diseases (such as rheumatic, degenerative, and myxomatous valvular diseases), degeneration or malfunction of artificial cardiac valves, and complications of bacterial endocarditis.

Mitral regurgitation (MR) leading to cardiogenic shock in the setting of an acute myocardial infarction (AMI) is a relatively common event. In the largest series reported to date, Thompson *et al.*[29] examined the SHOCK study registry and found severe MR (as defined by the individual investigators) in 98 patients, approximately 9% of the overall registry and study population. Patients with severe MR were more likely to be female and have more inferior and posterior MIs. The MIs were less likely to be ST elevation MIs and there was a trend towards a smaller peak creatine kinase (CK); both of these indicators imply a smaller MI. On the other hand, despite similar wedge pressure and cardiac index (CI), as well as higher echocardiographic ejection fraction (EF), the severe MR group had more pulmonary edema on chest x-ray, required more mechanical ventilation, more inotropic and intraaortic balloon pump (IABP) support and more right heart catheterization. Hence, cardiogenic shock due to severe MR should be suspected in patients with relatively smaller MIs, especially inferior and posterior, who present with severe shock accompanied by pulmonary edema.

Cardiac free wall rupture in the setting of an AMI is a rare but usually distinct catastrophic event. Slater *et al.*[30] examining the SHOCK study registry reported its incidence as 2.7% of the cohort. The relative rarity of rupture and tamponade leading to cardiogenic shock did not allow for accurate statistics. However, patients with rupture had a milder history of cardiac disease; fewer had previous MIs and a history of heart failure. There was a trend towards later development of shock in patients with tamponade and less pulmonary edema. On coronary angiography, the culprit artery in patients with rupture and tamponade was more often the left anterior descending (LAD) and circumflex. Interestingly, there was no correlation between the administration of thrombolytics and rupture (as reported in other studies).

Finally, acute VSD is a rare and notoriously difficult to diagnose cause of cardiogenic shock. Reporting from the SHOCK trial and registry, Menon *et al.*[31] described 55 patients with acute VSD and cardiogenic shock (approximately 5% incidence). Patients with VSD were more likely to be female. Despite higher LVEF, the VSD patients had higher heart rates, more signs of peripheral hypoperfusion, and more need for inotropic amines and IABP. During right heart catheterization the most notable finding was higher pressure in both the right ventricle and atrium (as compared to patients without VSD). On coronary angiography, most patients had 1- and 2-vessel disease (as opposed to 3-vessel disease in the overall SHOCK study and registry) and the right coronary artery (RCA) was more often the culprit.

Therefore, mechanical cardiac dysfunction is a relatively common cause of cardiogenic shock both in patients with ACS and in those without such an event. In the SHOCK registry, overall, 17% of patients had either severe MR or rupture or VSD as their main etiology for cardiogenic shock. Hence, early echocardiographic evaluation is of crucial importance in the immediate evaluation of patients with cardiogenic shock.

Cardiogenic shock in the setting of an acute ischemic event

Cardiogenic shock occurs in approximately 2.5% of patients with non-ST elevation ACS (2.1% of patients without MI and 2.9% of patients with MI).[9] The incidence of cardiogenic shock in patients with STEMI differs in different studies. However, in recent series it is reported to occur in 6% to 7% of patients.[2–4,6–8]

In general, as compared to ACS patients who do not develop cardiogenic shock, patients with cardiogenic shock are older (mean age 65 years), they have a more extensive history of cardiovascular risk factors (such as diabetes mellitus and hypertension) as well as a higher rate of previous MI (approximately one-third) and heart failure (20%), but fewer are current smokers.[2,9] The extent of the acute ischemia in patients with cardiogenic shock is larger by electrocardiogram (EKG), cardiac enzymes, and echocardiographically as compared to patients with ACS without cardiogenic shock. On coronary angiography, most patients are found to have 3-vessel disease.[27,32,33] The results of percutaneous coronary interventions (PCIs) in these patients are less satisfactory, with TIMI III flow achieved in only approximately half the patients[17,23,27,32,33] and myocardial blush grade (MBG) of II/III is achieved in only one-third.[32,33]

As compared to patients who develop cardiogenic shock during an acute STEMI, patients with non-ST elevation ACS who develop cardiogenic shock are older and have more extensive background diseases (such as renal failure and peripheral vascular disease [PVD]). They also have more cardiac history of prior MIs, heart failure, and CABG.[34] Patients developing cardiogenic shock during non-ST elevation ACS have smaller infarct size by peak CK, but more extensive coronary disease.[34]

Finally, approximately 3% to 4% of patients who develop cardiogenic shock during an AMI have predominantly RV infarction.[35] Patients who develop cardiogenic shock due to RV infarction are younger, are less likely to have had previous MIs or CABG, and on coronary angiography are less likely to have multivessel disease. As expected, fewer had an anterior MI and the culprit artery was the RCA in 96% of the patients. Interestingly, the hemodynamic findings during right heart catheterization were very similar to those of patients with predominantly LV failure, with the exception of systolic pulmonary pressure, which was lower in patients with RV infarction.

Hemodynamic Measures and the Concept of Cardiac Power

The main goals in hemodynamic monitoring of patients with cardiogenic shock are assistance in optimization of fluid balance and measurement of cardiac power and vascular resistance to facilitate the diagnosis of cardiogenic shock.

Cardiac power

The concept of cardiac power is more than a century old, but in light of more recent conceptual and experimental advances in heart failure research, its relevance has become of paramount importance. An understanding of the relationship between flow and pressure in the circulation has long been known to involve the concept of hydraulic power.[36–38] The concept of energy and power is also inherent in E. H. Starling's *The Linacre Lecture on the Law of the Heart*.[39] In physics, "power" is "energy per unit time." In the context of cardiology, cardiac power output (CPO) is the rate at which the heart imparts hydraulic energy into the arterial system to maintain the circulation of blood. Without this energy, the circulation would come to a standstill. CPO is equal to the product of flow output and aortic pressure. Based on data emerging in the past two decades, the concept of cardiac hydraulic energy and power output is beginning to shed new light on how to directly evaluate cardiac function, which clearly influences the functional capacity and prognosis of patients with heart failure.

Earlier in vivo studies on CPO focused on the frequency components of the variable derived from the product of instantaneous flow velocity and pressure in the great arteries.[40–43] However, in daily clinical practice, although it is feasible to measure instantaneous flow or velocity in the ascending aorta or main pulmonary artery, this requires more sophisticated and costly equipment, which is not readily available. Therefore, just as the steady component of flow output from the heart, commonly known as cardiac output (CO), is the variable most commonly used in clinical practice, the steady component of power output is also the variable most commonly adopted clinically. It is the amount of hydraulic energy required to produce steady flow in the circulation, whereas the higher frequency components produce the pulsations. Hence, CPO is calculated as the product of mean arterial pressure (MAP) and CO measured simultaneously, after correcting for a constant of 0.0022, and its units are watts, (CPO = MAP × CO × 0.0022).

If CPO is the entity solely responsible for maintaining continuous blood flow in the circulation, then the highest CPO that can be produced by the heart must represent the peak function of the heart, and the difference between this value and the resting baseline value represents the reserve function of the heart.[44,45]

Each heart has its own ceiling peak pumping performance, above which it is physically impossible to exceed. This value would alter only if the intrinsic condition of the heart is altered, such as after an AMI or after successful relevant cardiac surgery. When compared, these maximal levels of individual cardiac function are direct and objective indicators of how relatively effective or impaired the hearts are as fluid pumps. They provide a means of grading the degree of functional impairment in heart failure along the scales below the norm, and conversely, the degree of superiority in function of athletic hearts (Figure 15.1).[46]

In a recent manuscript,[47] Cotter *et al.* evaluated the hemodynamic findings in 100 consecutive patients admitted to the intensive coronary unit (ICU) for hemodynamic instability, of which 11 had cardiogenic shock. The results of this study demonstrated that measurement of CO and wedge pressure was not instrumental in the diagnosis of cardiogenic shock due to significant overlaps in patients with acute heart failure and vasodilative shock. However, the measurement of CPO and systemic vascular resistance (SVR) was of greater value. Specifically, when CPO and SVR were plotted as a two-dimensional graph (Figure 15.2), a

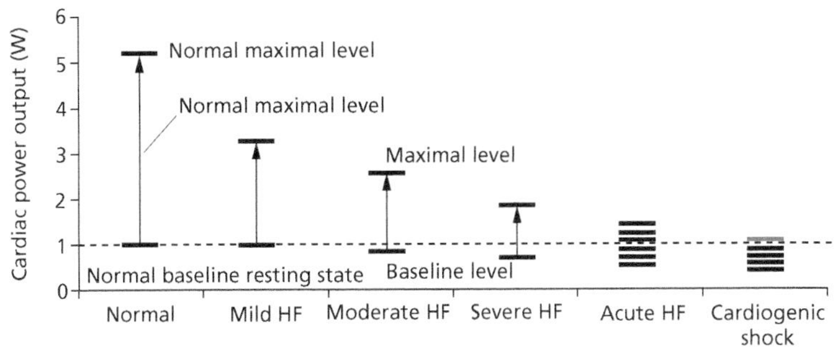

Figure 15.1. *Cardiac power at rest and cardiac power reserve in normal and patients with chronic heart failure (With permission from Cotter* et al.[89]*)*

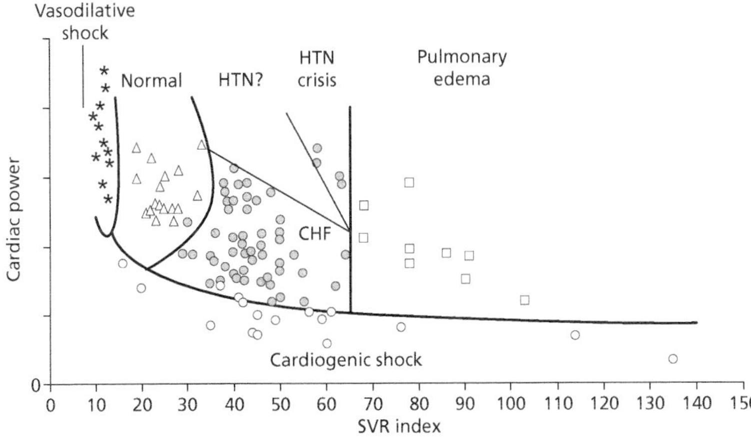

Figure 15.2. *Cardiac power and SVR in patients with hemodynamic instability due to cardiogenic shock, vasodilative shock, hypertensive crisis, pulmonary edema and acute systolic heart failure (With permission from Cotter* et al.[47]*)*

Abbreviations: CHF = *congestive heart failure;* HTN = *hypertension;* SVR = *systemic vascular resistance*

specific area in the graph determined by a mathematically calculated line could be drawn separating cardiogenic shock patients from those with heart failure exacerbation, pulmonary edema, and vasodilative shock. The most important feature required for this separation was that patients with cardiogenic shock have significant decreases in cardiac power (i.e., severely impaired LV contractility) combined with inappropriately low to normal SVR. Although the data available are not sufficient for formal statistical analysis, both from a practical point of view and as a marker of poor outcome CPO values < 0.6 watt, and especially < 0.5 watt, should be regarded as an ominous sign for the existence of cardiogenic shock.

Inappropriately low increase in systemic vascular resistance

The common wisdom regarding the hemodynamics of cardiogenic shock, as compared to acute and chronic heart failure, assumed that SVR should be increased. This assumption was maintained for two decades despite mounting evidence to the contrary. Already in the early 1960s Smith *et al.*[48] observed that SVR is not increased in most cardiogenic shock patients. This observation was confirmed by Mennon *et al.*, who observed an SVR of 1350 to 1400 dynes/s/cm^5 in the SHOCK study and registry data,[49] a value within the upper level of normal. Lim *et al.*[12] recently reported hemodynamic changes throughout the course of hospitalization in patients with cardiogenic shock. They have observed that in approximately one half of the patients, CI increased throughout the admission, despite no significant change in blood pressure (i.e., SVR decreased). These patients had the same outcome as those with lower CI. The reasons for this inappropriately low SVR are not clear. Recently, it has been suggested that inflammatory mechanisms involving the nitric oxide (NO) pathway may be responsible for some of this apparent inadequate response.

Pathophysiology and the New Paradigm of Cardiogenic Shock

Traditionally, cardiogenic shock was believed to be caused solely by insufficient cardiac contractility. Indeed, cardiogenic shock occurs in the overwhelming majority of cases when cardiac function is severely depressed either by a significant mechanical failure, severe cardiomyopathy (acute or chronic), or a large ischemic insult. However, this classic paradigm was recently questioned by Hochman[50] in light of new observations implying that inappropriate vasoconstriction in conjunction with inflammatory activation and perhaps overproduction of NO might play a crucial role in the pathogenesis or amplification of the cardiogenic shock syndrome.

A vicious cycle of severely decreased cardiac contractility and inadequate vasoconstriction

Early studies have demonstrated that in the setting of an acute ischemic event, cardiogenic shock will occur when the ischemic damage affects at least 40% of the myocardium.[51] In support of the major role of decreased cardiac contractility in cardiogenic shock, in a recent analysis of the shock registry data,[52] Fincke *et al.* found that in patients who had hemodynamic monitoring by Swan–Ganz catheter, admission CPO was the strongest independent predictor of in-hospital mortality (Figure 15.3). However, in most patients with cardiogenic shock, the severe decrease in cardiac contractility is not met by an appropriate increase in vascular resistance. Since blood pressure, and

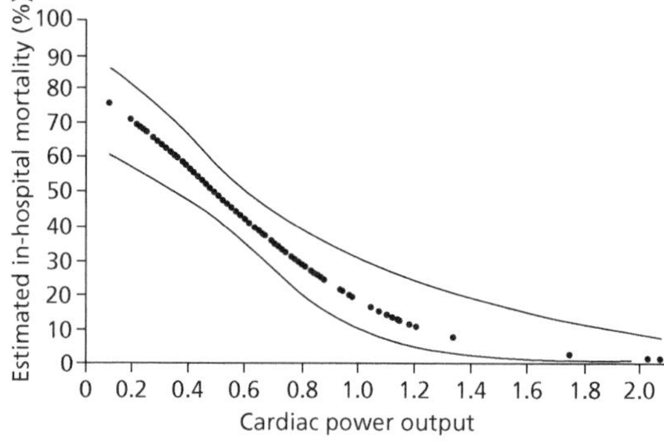

Figure 15.3. *Unadjusted estimated in-hospital mortality by cardiac power output in 189 patients in the SHOCK registry (With permission from Fincke* et al.[52])

hence perfusion pressure, is the product of the cardiac contractility and vascular resistance, failure to vasoconstrict in the presence of very low contractility translates into a significant reduction in both blood pressure and peripheral perfusion. Therefore, significant forward failure, the main symptom of the shock syndrome, is caused not only by decreased cardiac contractility but also by a failure of most patients to mount significant vasoconstriction.

This decreased perfusion pressure affects many vital organs, including the coronary arteries. Since patients developing cardiogenic shock have, in most cases, severe diffuse coronary artery disease (CAD), the perfusion of the myocardium in large coronary territories is not autoregulated and is highly dependent on aortic root pressure. This decreased myocardial perfusion leads to diffuse ischemia, causing both a further decrease in myocardial contractility as well as an increase in left ventricular end diastolic pressure (LVEDP), leading to pulmonary congestion and hypoxia. Furthermore, the decreased peripheral perfusion and hypoxia also lead to significant metabolic acidosis, respiratory failure (worsening hypoxia), renal failure (worsening acidosis), and hepatic failure. Therefore, the combination of ischemia, hypoxia, and acidosis induces a vicious cycle by which decreased myocardial contractility leads to further reduction in myocardial contractility, culminating in a state of deepening shock, multiorgan failure and, if untreated, death.

In recent years, it has become apparent that in addition to the severe decrease in cardiac contractility, other factors also contribute to the development of the shock syndrome.

Inflammatory activation in cardiogenic shock

Inflammatory activation is common in patients sustaining an AMI, however, the role of this inflammatory response in cardiogenic shock has been investigated in only a few studies. Hochman *et al.*[50] observed in the SHOCK study and registry that symptoms and signs of inflammatory response, such as fever, leukocytosis, and low SVR, are common in patients with cardiogenic shock, even when cultures remain negative and overt infection is not confirmed. de Werra *et al.*[53] observed an increase in some inflammatory mediators in patients with cardiogenic shock; however, this increase was smaller than in patients with sepsis. Interleukin-6 (IL-6) was most prominent among these mediators. Geppert *et al.*[54] have assessed IL-6 levels in 51 patients with cardiogenic shock, 26 patients with septic shock, and 11 non-critically ill controls. They observed that overall IL-6 levels were significantly increased in patients with cardiogenic shock, but not to the same extent as in patients with septic shock. However, in patients with cardiogenic shock who had higher levels of IL-6 (>200 pg/mL), the rate of multiorgan failure was significantly higher. In a separate study (Geppert *et al.*, personal communication), the same authors found a significant correlation between IL-6 increase and mortality. Hence, a systemic inflammatory response syndrome is common in patients with cardiogenic shock, usually without any underlying infection. The role of this inflammatory response in the shock syndrome is unknown, although IL-6 related inflammatory activation was shown to cause both decreased myocardial contractility and vascular resistance, both of which are crucial in the genesis of the shock syndrome. Further studies are required in order to determine whether this inflammatory activation plays an important part in the genesis, or perhaps amplification, of the shock syndrome or is the result of severe hypoperfusion.

Nitric oxide

NO (nitric oxide) is a regulatory molecule crucial in cardiovascular function, neuronal signaling, and host-defense reactions. NO is synthesized by nitric oxide synthase (NOS). There are three kinds of NOS. Two constitutive isoforms are designated eNOS (endothelial) and nNOS (neuronal). The third isoform, originally isolated from macrophages, is now designated iNOS (inducible) because its expression is induced in many cell types after exposure to inflammatory mediators (i.e., bacterial lipopolysaccharide, tumor necrosis factor-α, and interleukin-1), and such expression may lead to toxic fluxes of NO. eNOS in the vascular endothelium produces low levels of NO in a pulsatile manner, triggered by the beat-to-beat shear-force of flowing blood. This NO imposes a vasorelaxant "tone," offsetting the vasoconstrictory action of the norepinephrine released by sympathetic nerves. NO also inhibits platelet adhesion, mediates angiogenesis and attenuates proliferation of vascular smooth muscle.

All three NOS isoforms can be expressed in the heart. eNOS is constitutively expressed in endothelial and endocardial cells and, at a much lower concentration, in cardiac myocytes, while nNOS is found in nerve fibers and cardiac myocytes. Under normal circumstances, intracardiac NO is produced cyclically, with an abrupt increase during early diastolic filling that is associated with increased chamber stretch (preload).[55] NO derived from both eNOS, located in the sarcolemmal caveolae, and nNOS, located mainly in the sarcoplasmic reticulum of cardiac myocytes, has been implicated in the modulation of excitation–contraction coupling, via regulation of calcium ion (Ca^{2+}) influx through sarcolemmal L-type channels and release and re-uptake of Ca^{2+} by the sarcoplastic reticulum.[56,57] It is likely that NO will prove to be a fundamental autoregulatory molecule that tunes intra-myocyte Ca^{2+} cycling, contractile force generation, and oxygen (O_2) consumption to physiological demands. Stimulation by cytokines and perhaps other factors can cause iNOS expression and rapid, high-level NO synthesis in multiple cardiac cell types, including infiltrating inflammatory cells, endothelial cells, and cardiac myocytes. High-output NO from iNOS is a potent myocardial depressant factor,[58] disrupting Ca^{2+} cycling and suppressing mitochondrial respiration. In addition, iNOS-derived NO potently attenuates inotropic, chronotropic, and dromotropic responses of the heart to β-adrenoceptor stimulation.[59]

During ischemia and reperfusion, numerous studies support the view that eNOS-derived NO[60,61] or low levels of administered NO[60] afford protection against ischemia–reperfusion injury. Indeed, NO appears to mediate myocardial preconditioning,[62] the phenomenon that brief ischemic stimuli render the heart resistant to subsequent more severe ischemic episodes. Nonetheless, several findings implicate *larger* quantities of NO, typically iNOS-derived and produced in a setting of accelerated superoxide and peroxynitrite ($ONOO^-$) synthesis, as a major contributor to cardiac reperfusion injury. Indeed, in a few animal models it was demonstrated that NO production during ischemia–reperfusion is deleterious.[63,64] In an experimental model, iNOS knockout mice were shown to survive MI better than controls.[65] The exact mechanism of this deleterious effect of high levels of NO is not known. However, some studies have demonstrated that high levels of NO affect myocardial contractility directly by an uncoupling of calcium metabolism,[66,67] and may have an effect on responsiveness to catecholamines,[68] mitochondrial function in the nonischemic myocardium,[69] as well as effects on glucose metabolism[63] and systemic vasodilatatory response. Hence, high production of NO during ischemia (probably by iNOS) may act as an important mediator of myocardial stunning, leading to decreased myocardial contractility, as well as systemic vasodilatation, both fundamental to the genesis of cardiogenic shock. In two preliminary studies, Cotter *et al.*[22,23] observed improved outcome in patients with severe cardiogenic shock treated by NOS inhibitors.

Why do some patients develop cardiogenic shock while others don't?

The clinician treating patients with AMI is often perplexed by the observation that for the same apparent infarct size by echocardiography and cardiac enzymes some patients develop hemodynamic instability and shock, while others do not. There are a few possible reasons for this apparent paradox. First, it seems that some of the methods used to evaluate the severity of decrease in myocardial contractility inflicted by the acute coronary event (such as echocardiographic EF and cardiac enzymes) are only crude measures. By measuring cardiac power, better quantification can be obtained of the degree of myocardial dysfunction. Consistent use of cardiac power to evaluate myocardial contractility in hemodynamically unstable patients may prove valuable for the assessment of patients with apparent large infarctions. Second, if inflammatory activation and iNOS induction play a significant role in the pathogenesis or amplification of the shock syndrome, then natural variability of response between individual patients due to genetic or other factors may be important in the determination of the risk to develop cardiogenic shock, and early measurement of such parameters (such as IL-6) may prove valuable for the evaluation of patients with large MIs.

Diagnosis and Differential Diagnosis

Since the definition of cardiogenic shock is not based on strict objective criteria, it remains largely subjective and relies heavily on the experience of the treating physician. During an ACS, blood pressure fluctuations (significant increases as well as decreases) are common and in many cases transient due to the effect of fluctuating autonomic tone (sympathetic and parasympathetic) or transient arrhythmias. Every decrease in systolic blood pressure to the vicinity of 100 mm Hg should be regarded as an ominous sign of impending shock and should be fully evaluated.

The first step in the evaluation of low or decreasing blood pressure during an acute coronary event is to rule out significant arrhythmias and silent ischemia by full EKG and arrhythmia monitoring. In the setting of multiple antiaggregant and anticoagulant treatments, the possibility of overt or concealed hemorrhage leading to severe intravascular depletion should be explored meticulously. Retroperitoneal bleeding in this setting can sometimes be asymptomatic but massive, leading to significant hemodynamic deterioration. Therefore, this diagnosis should be entertained early in the course of the work-up. Concomitantly, a possible metabolic cause for the lower blood pressure should be sought by immediate laboratory re-evaluation, including full blood count (mainly to rule out a decrease in hemoglobin hinting at concealed bleeding or new leukocytosis as a sign of infection), extended chemistry to rule out severe hyperglycemia, unexpected evolving renal or liver failure, significant electrolyte imbalance and blood gases to rule out unexpected carbon dioxide (CO_2) retention. Any such laboratory finding should be immediately worked up, and appropriate treatment should be implemented. While initiating specific treatment, a full echocardiographic evaluation should be performed. This evaluation should include estimation of LVEF since reduced EF, especially to <30%, is an ominous sign in patients with hemodynamic instability during an ACS. Careful assessment of all cardiac segments and valves for both regurgitant and previously undiagnosed stenotic lesions, as well as a meticulous search for VSD and ventricular free wall rupture are essential. Some of these possible mechanical complications are difficult to diagnose, especially if LV contractility is significantly impaired. Therefore, it has been our policy to lower the threshold for transesophageal echocardiography (TEE) in any doubt or uncertainty.

Once recurrent ischemia, arrhythmias, bleeding, metabolic imbalance, and mechanical causes have been ruled out, the patient's response to treatment should be closely followed for approximately 1 hour. In some patients, administration of fluids and low doses of dopamine can lead to blood pressure stabilization and an increase in systolic blood pressure to >110 mm Hg. Although the diagnosis of cardiogenic shock may be uncertain in these patients, they should still be followed closely. If no other cause for the transient hemodynamic instability is detected, these patients should be treated as if they have cardiogenic shock, especially if significant LV dysfunction is detected by echocardiography. Likewise, patients not responding to fluid administration and low doses of dopamine, and in whom no precipitating factor for the hemodynamic instability can be detected, should be diagnosed as having cardiogenic shock. Concomitantly to initiating treatment, right heart catheterization should be performed to rule out concealed VSD, and a Swan–Ganz catheter should be placed for continuous hemodynamic monitoring. Measures of decreased cardiac power (<0.5 to 0.6 watt) in the presence of relatively low SVR (<2500 dynes/s/cm^5 and especially <2000 dynes/s/cm^5) and wedge pressure >15 mm Hg to 20 mm Hg are supportive of the diagnosis of cardiogenic shock.

Differentiating cardiogenic from septic shock

Although, theoretically, septic shock manifests as a severe inflammatory syndrome accompanied by low vascular resistance and relatively preserved cardiac contractility, recent findings of significant inflammation and reduced or normal vascular resistance in most patients with cardiogenic shock makes a differential diagnosis less obvious. The distinction between septic and cardiogenic shock is especially problematic in patients developing shock > 24 hours after an AMI while in the ICU. This distinction is also difficult in elderly patients presenting with signs of both acute ischemia and hemodynamic deterioration, when the ischemia could be the result of hemodynamic and metabolic impairment caused by sepsis rather than a primary cause of the shock syndrome.

Important features implying septic rather than cardiogenic etiology of the shock syndrome include clinical signs of localized infection by physical or radiological examination or findings of localized pus, high fever, and leukocytosis within the first few hours of admission before the development of overt shock. On hemodynamic monitoring, signs of acute myocardial ischemia and low SVR in the face of relatively preserved CPO (Figure 15.2) are also indicative of septic rather than cardiogenic shock. Recently, Geppert *et al.*[70] evaluated measurement of C-reactive protein (CRP) and procalcitonin for the differentiation between septic and cardiogenic shock. The results of their study are promising, showing that precalcitonin levels of <10 ng/dL, and to a lesser extent CRP levels <20 ng/mL, are relatively specific for the diagnosis of cardiogenic rather than septic shock. These results need confirmation in larger prospective studies.

Despite these findings, in many cases the exact clinical diagnosis remains difficult, and empirical treatment for both sepsis (with broad-spectrum antibiotics) and major ischemia (with maximal hemodynamic support, IABP, and coronary catheterization) must be applied in parallel. It is crucial that cultures of blood, urine, sputum, and any suspected organs are obtained several times before the administration of antibiotics. If these cultures remain sterile after 48 to 72 hours, the need for continuous antibiotic treatment should be critically re-assessed after repeated clinical assessment of any new symptoms and signs of localized infection, as well as the patient's overall clinical status.

Risk Stratification

Since the diagnosis of cardiogenic shock remains largely subjective and dependent on the physician's perception of the patient's hemodynamic and clinical status, risk stratification of the patient is of crucial significance. Accurate risk stratification enables a better understanding of the severity of the shock syndrome and hence clearer determination of the patient's prognosis and the appropriate aggressiveness of treatment.

Recent studies have suggested that four major factors determine the severity of the shock syndrome: (1) the patient's baseline characteristics (especially age, previous history of diabetes mellitus, hypertension, and renal failure, as well as extensive CAD by angiography); (2) time from the initial ischemia to development of shock; (3) severity of decrease in cardiac contractility (as measured by admission CPO or echocardiography); and (4) response to initial treatment (including response to inotropic amines as well as TIMI flow and myocardial perfusion after PCI).

Baseline characteristics

Elderly patients with cardiogenic shock, especially those more than 75 years old, have a worse outcome. In the SHOCK registry, Dzavik *et al.*[71] observed a 30-day mortality of 76% in patients >75 years vs. 55% in those <75 years. These data have been confirmed by virtually all studies of cardiogenic shock.[13,26] In the SHOCK registry data, diabetic patients who develop cardiogenic shock have more background diseases such as prior MI, heart failure, hypertension, PVD and renal failure.[72] In the same study diabetes mellitus was an independent risk factor for mortality (odds ratio, 1.47; 95% confidence interval, 1.1–1.96). This finding was confirmed by other studies.[9,14,18] In additional studies, hypertension was found to be an independent predictor of mortality.[52] Finally, renal failure, both chronic and acute, is correlated with unfavorable outcome in patients with cardiogenic shock. Koreny *et al.*[73] demonstrated that peak serum creatinine of > 3 mg/dL and acute renal failure manifesting as oliguria, or increase in serum creatinine by >0.5 mg/dL, or >50% above baseline, were associated with a significant increase in

30-day mortality. Patients who developed acute renal failure during admission were older and were more likely to have diabetes mellitus and more severe shock, explaining, at least in part, the association between renal failure and adverse outcome. The negative prognostic impact of renal failure in patients with cardiogenic shock was confirmed in other studies.[13] Other factors, such as gender, were not consistently shown to affect outcome.[74]

Timing of onset of shock after the acute ischemic event

In the SHOCK study and registry, most patients (approximately 75%) developed cardiogenic shock within the first 24 hours of admission.[75] Patients who developed late shock had less chest pain and fewer ST elevations on EKG at admission, fewer had inferior or right MI, more had renal failure and more developed recurrent ischemia after admission. The mortality of patients developing early shock (within 24 hours from admission) was lower when compared to those developing later shock (63% to 70% vs. 54% to 59%). In a subanalysis of the Trandolapril Cardiac Evaluation (TRACE) study,[2] early shock (within 48 hours of admission) was associated with better outcome as compared to late shock (45% vs. 80% mortality, $P < 0.05$). Hence, the impact of the timing of shock on outcome after the ACS is not known and may be related to selection bias of surviving patients.

Severity of cardiac contractility decrease

Decreased cardiac contractility is the primary insult leading to cardiogenic shock. Cardiac power is a hemodynamic measure of cardiac contractility. In a recent manuscript,[52] Fincke *et al.* analyzed the relationship between CPO and outcome in 189 hemodynamically-monitored patients enrolled in the SHOCK registry. Multivariate analysis has shown that the three independent predictors of in-hospital mortality are age, history of hypertension, and CPO; CPO was strongly correlated with in-hospital mortality (Figure 15.3).

Echocardiographic assessment of cardiac contractility (by LVEF) was also correlated with outcome in patients with cardiogenic shock.[13,18,76] In the SHOCK registry[76] survival was 24% in patients with LVEF < 28% vs. 56% in patients with LVEF ≥ 28%. Moreover, LVEF and the severity of MR were the only echocardiographic predictors of outcome. However, in our recent analysis[52] after assessment of CPO, LVEF was no longer an independent predictor of outcome in patients with cardiogenic shock. Therefore, echocardiographic assessment should be performed immediately in patients who develop hemodynamic instability during ACS, to rule out mechanical complications and to obtain a preliminary assessment of the severity of LV dysfunction and degree of MR. However, this assessment should be followed by early hemodynamic monitoring for better risk stratification of the severity of the LV dysfunction and for monitoring the patient's status and response to treatment.

Coronary angiography and response to treatment

Patients developing cardiogenic shock during an ACS have more extensive CAD, especially more 2-vessel and 3-vessel disease. The extent of this disease is also a strong predictor of outcome. In the SHOCK study,[27,77] 3-vessel disease was a strong predictor of death at 1 year ($P = 0.002$). This observation was also collaborated by findings of the SHOCK registry[32] as well as other recent series.[17] RCA as the culprit artery is associated with better outcome while saphenous vein graft culprit was associated with more adverse outcome.[32,77]

Percutaneous coronary interventions (PCIs) aimed at reperfusion of the ischemic myocardium are an important treatment measure in patients with cardiogenic shock.[78] Early and successful revascularization is important in the outcome of patients with cardiogenic shock. First, a few studies have suggested that early reperfusion is associated with better outcome. Webb *et al.*,[27] reporting from the SHOCK study, described a direct correlation between increasing time from SHOCK to PCI and increased mortality ($P = 0.019$). These results were also corroborated by a recent registry in Germany[17] as well as a single-center study in North Carolina.[7] Second, a few studies have demonstrated a strong correlation between the results of the revascularization procedure and patient outcome. Angiographic success, mainly measured as TIMI flow grade, after PCI was found to be one of the strongest predictors of outcome in cardiogenic shock. This finding was reported in the SHOCK study,[17,77] the SHOCK registry,[32] a very recent registry from Poland,[11] and a large registry from Germany.[17] Overall, these studies encompass over 3000 patients. Although no formal meta-analysis of these results was performed, it seems that in all these large registries, PCI results are the second strongest predictor of outcome after age. In a small recent cohort, Tarantini *et al.*[33] examined the role of myocardial blush grade (MBG) in the risk stratification of patients with cardiogenic shock. Patients with a worse MBG grade (0/1) had a higher mortality as compared to those with a better MBG grade (2/3). In a multivariate analysis, MBG grade and age, but not TIMI flow grade, were the only predictors of death. Therefore, lower angiographic PCI success in patients with cardiogenic shock, either by lower TIMI flow grade or MBG, is correlated with increased mortality. On the other hand, in all studies examining the angiographic results in patients with cardiogenic shock, better angiographic results were correlated with less disease severity by baseline characteristics as well as measures of the size of the ischemic insult, implying that successful angiographic results may be correlated with less adverse outcome in patients with cardiogenic shock due to their common association with less severe disease. The results of the SHOCK study, demonstrating that early revascularization is important in the outcome of cardiogenic shock,[3] adds weight to the possibility that success of revascularization is a significant determinant of outcome in these patients.

The response to supportive treatment as manifested by blood pressure increase and hemodynamic stabilization is also an important predictor of outcome in cardiogenic shock. In a small study, Tarantini *et al.*[70] examined the outcome of patients who had a positive response to vasopressors versus those who did not respond. They found a significant difference in in-hospital mortality (20% vs. 68%, $P = 0.02$). Similarly in the SHOCK study,[27] lower blood pressure in response to treatment was a significant predictor of mortality.

In conclusion, in patients developing cardiogenic shock during an ACS, mortality is correlated with more severe baseline characteristics (older age, diabetes mellitus, hypertension, renal failure, and diffuse CAD), earlier development of shock, more extensive ischemic damage as measured by lower LVEF and hemodynamic cardiac power, and less response to therapy both by angiography (lower TIMI flow or myocardial blush) and blood pressure increase on supportive measures.

Treatment and Course

Although the exact definition of cardiogenic shock is controversial, leading to some uncertainty regarding the diagnosis, an aggressive approach should be implemented early in patients with significant ischemic events associated with low blood pressure, pulmonary congestion, and signs of peripheral hypoperfusion.

These patients should be immediately evaluated to rule out noncardiac causes of instability, such as massive hemorrhage, sepsis, or metabolic imbalance, as well as treatable cardiac causes, including arrhythmias or mechanical complications while supportive treatment is being initiated.

The initial supportive treatment should address the main components of clinical instability. Patients with significant congestion leading to hypoxia should be treated with diuretics and noninvasive mechanical ventilation. Since hypoxia is one of the major precipitants involved in the amplification of the vicious cycle leading to cardiogenic shock, it should be treated aggressively. If after a short follow-up, the oxygen saturation does not improve or deteriorates further, especially <90%, immediate tracheal intubation and mechanical ventilation should be implemented. Any other precipitating factors such as severe hyperglycemia, anemia, intravascular depletion, or arrhythmia have to be addressed and treated to minimize any aggravating effect on the overall clinical condition of the patient.

None of the intravenous treatments currently used for cardiogenic shock was shown to improve the outcome of these patients. Nonetheless, intravenous treatment aimed at increasing blood pressure and improving peripheral perfusion should be initiated. It is our practice to use, as first-line treatment, intravenous dopamine in doses of 3 to 5 μg/kg/min uptitrated to achieve a systolic blood pressure of 90 mm Hg to 100 mm Hg while avoiding tachycardia and under intensive monitoring for tachyarrhythmias. The main advantages of dopamine at the recommend doses include a vasoconstricting effect, improvement of renal perfusion and minimal effect on myocardial oxygen consumption. Other authorities, especially in Europe, prefer norepinephrine and epinephrine to dopamine as the pressor of choice in cardiogenic shock. Regretfully, since no comparative studies have examined these drugs in the past, no solid recommendations can be made regarding the type to be used. Other possible treatments at this stage include fluid administration, especially in patients without clinical and radiographic signs of pulmonary congestion, and administration of other inotropic amines, such as dobutamine or milrinone. Recently, a small preliminary study demonstrated that levosimendan, a new inotropic amine acting through a few distinct mechanisms including calcium sensitization, may improve CI and stroke work index in patients with cardiogenic shock.[79] Since levosimendan was shown in previous studies to have no pro-arrhythmic effects and no effect on myocardial oxygen consumption, this drug may become an attractive alternative in the hemodynamic support of patients with cardiogenic shock.

While attempting to restore hemodynamic stability and exploring all possible precipitating causes for it, preparations should be made for the initiation of an invasive treatment strategy including coronary angiography and revascularization supported by the use of IABP. Although patients responding to treatment with vasopressors have a better prognosis, the prognosis of the responding patients remains dismal with a 20% mortality.[19] Hence, all patients displaying hemodynamic instability during the course of ACS should be treated invasively. This approach is supported by the results of the SHOCK study,[3,78] which demonstrated improved outcome at 1-year follow-up in patients with cardiogenic shock treated by immediate revascularization. The American College of Cardiology/American Heart Association class I recommendation for this approach is only for patients younger than 75 years of age. However, the SHOCK study results[80] and significant data in recently published manuscripts support implementation of an invasive approach in the elderly as well.[5,15,50,71]

The exact revascularization options used in patients with cardiogenic shock are highly debated. First, which method of revascularization should be used and what extent of revascularization should be performed? Current recommendations[50] suggest that PCI is the preferred method of revascularization for suitable 1- to 2-vessel disease, especially when treatment of some secondary lesions could be deferred to a second (staged) procedure. CABG is the preferred revascularization modality for 3-vessel disease or left main disease, especially when contemplating simultaneous revascularization of non-culprit coronaries due to the potential harmful effect of inducing no-reflow by PCI in non-culprit vessels, leading to further deterioration in myocardial contractility. Although CABG can be performed up to 18 hours after the onset of MI, some concerns regarding the time delay associated with this procedure, as well as some potential myocardial damage during the operation and reperfusion, have led a few authorities to recommend immediate revascularization of the infarct-related artery by PCI in all possible cases and referral for CABG only of patients who cannot be revascularized by PCI. A second debate surrounds the method of PCI and adjunctive therapy. Recent uncontrolled studies suggest that the use of stents[16,21] and adjunctive therapy with intravenous glycoprotein IIb/IIIa antagonists[9,21] are beneficial in the treatment of cardiogenic shock. However, this strategy was never examined in a prospective study. Even less is reported on the effect of drug-eluting stents on the outcome of cardiogenic shock, although in a recent series from the Serruys group,[14] cardiogenic shock occurred in 13% of consecutive patients with AMI treated with Cypher stents, of which 5 (42%) have died. This number is comparable to the overall reported mortality.

IABP is used by most authorities during the initial treatment of patients with cardiogenic shock. IABP has the advantage of improving peripheral perfusion while increasing diastolic flow in the coronary arteries and hence potentially reducing ischemia. In our practice, IABP is implemented early in parallel with the coronary angiography. This practice is supported by many observational studies,[18,20,81] although no prospective evaluation has been published to date. Again, despite a lack of prospective controlled data, we recommend that IABP treatment be maintained for at least 24 hours and removed only after significant hemodynamic stability is attained as determined by stable systolic blood pressure > 110 mm Hg accompanied by reasonable urine output when IABP augmentation is reduced to 1:3 for a few hours.

Maintaining reasonable oxygenation and peripheral perfusion after the revascularization procedure is a challenging obstacle in the treatment of patients with cardiogenic shock. Patients who develop cardiogenic shock have both a severe ACS and diffuse CAD. Therefore, in most, some degree of diastolic dysfunction exists, requiring higher filling pressures in order to optimize myocardial contractility. On the other hand, higher filling pressure may induce pulmonary congestion, leading to reduced oxygenation and systemic hypoxia, which is especially deleterious in patients with shock. Although higher doses of inotropic amines increase blood pressure and peripheral perfusion, such doses inevitably increase myocardial oxygen consumption in the face of major ischemia, potentially increasing the ischemic damage. They are also arrhythmogenic. Unfortunately, although many authorities have recommended using invasively-determined CO and wedge pressures as guidance to treatment titration in patients with cardiogenic shock, no cut-off values were ever determined and no study has shown utility for this method in improving the outcome of patients in shock. Hence, the best guidance for determining fluid balance and inotropic treatment in these patients is the combination of urine output and systemic oxygenation. It is our practice to initiate fluid treatment by the administration of 100 mL/h of normal saline accompanied by some intravenous diuretics. Inotropic support should include intravenous dopamine in doses up to 7 to 10 μg/kg/min or equivalent doses of norepinephrine or epinephrine (0.2 to 0.3 μg/kg/min). Some authorities use combination therapy including some of these agents at lower doses. Again, since no prospective studies were performed on this issue, no firm recommendations can be made at the present time. These treatments are titrated to achieve a urine output of at least 50 to 100 mL/h while maintaining systemic oxygen saturation >90% to 95%. If this goal cannot be achieved due to increasing desaturation, tracheal intubation and full mechanical ventilation should be implemented immediately, thus enabling increased fluid administration.

The course of patients with cardiogenic shock is almost without exception fluctuating and complicated. It is very common to observe periods of hemodynamic stability interspersed with periods of resumed and sometimes deepening shock. Due to the severity of both the hemodynamic compromise and the initial ischemic event, as well as the intensity and invasiveness of treatment, many patients who are initially diagnosed as having only cardiogenic shock may develop infectious, hemorrhagic, metabolic, or mechanical complications, leading to further deterioration in their clinical condition or sometimes simply slower resolution of the shock syndrome. Therefore, we recommend that during the course of hemodynamic instability, full laboratory and echocardiographic evaluation be performed twice daily in order to rule out such complications. Any new complications should be addressed immediately.

Some patients with cardiogenic shock develop progressive hemodynamic instability that finally culminates in multiorgan failure and death. The exact proportion of patients developing this downward spiraling course is not known, although most of the 50% of patients with cardiogenic shock dying during the first few days die due to progressive heart failure. Since no specific treatment has been developed for patients with cardiogenic shock, the only option for treating patients who remain in shock despite revascularization is continuous supportive treatment with IABP, inotropic amines, fluids, and mechanical ventilation, in the hope of a spontaneous recovery. In extreme cases, especially when cardiogenic shock occurs in younger patients with relatively few background diseases, support by mechanical assist devices is implemented as a bridge to possible cardiac transplantation.[82–85] However, this approach is limited by the relative paucity of potential organs and the restrictive nature of the criteria for cardiac transplantation. Hence, some authorities have suggested using new and simpler mechanical assist devices, some of which are implemented without surgery[79] as a bridge to recovery rather than transplant. The efficacy of this approach needs to be validated in large prospective studies. Other treatment modalities suggested for the treatment of refractory cardiogenic shock include hypothermia,[86] use of vasopressin as a pressor not increasing oxygen demand by the myocardium, and NO synthase inhibitors.[22,23] If, as suggested previously, NO plays an important part in the pathogenesis or amplification of the shock syndrome in patients with large acute coronary events, then short-term blockage of its production may have theoretical beneficial effect in patients with cardiogenic shock. In two preliminary studies, Cotter *et al.* observed a beneficial hemodynamic effect of the nitric oxide synthase inhibitor, L-NMMA, in patients with refractory shock[22] that led to some reduction in mortality in a small nonblinded comparative study.[23] In the currently presented preliminary results of SHOCK-2 phase II study, L-NMMA at doses of 0.15 mg/kg, 0.5 mg/kg, 1 mg/kg, and 1.5 mg/kg boluses and 5-hour drip were compared to placebo in a double-blind prospective study of 79 patients with low blood pressure after PCI for an ACS. The study has demonstrated an increase in SVR by L-NMMA and a trend towards lower mortality in the high dose (1 mg/kg and 1.5 mg/kg) L-NMMA arms as compared to the lower doses. The results of the study were difficult to interpret due to inclusion of many patients who responded to conventional treatment (low pressor requirement and high systolic BP at randomization) as well as a significantly lower effect of L-NMMA treatment in the first patients randomized in the study (learning curve). These encouraging results will be followed by a large prospective randomized study of L-NMMA in cardiogenic shock (TRIUMPH) that will be initiated in 2005.

Conclusion

Despite some progress achieved in the treatment of cardiogenic shock in the past two decades, the mortality of cardiogenic shock remains very high. In the most recent series, 1-month or in-hospital mortality was reported to be 40% to 65% (Table 15.1). Since the diagnosis of cardiogenic shock is based on subjective criteria, variation of disease severity in the different studies may account for some of the variability in the reported mortality. One of the limitations of the present analysis is that the largest series of cardiogenic shock patients reported during this period, including 9465 patients in the National Registry of Myocardial Infarction (NRMI), was published only as an abstract[8]. In this series, despite a comparable rate of cardiogenic shock (6–7% of the overall MI population), mortality was only 41% as compared to 58% in the rest of the studies reported (Table 15.1).

In recent years, some investigators have suggested that cardiogenic shock mortality is decreasing progressively. Such a trend was observed by some investigators,[10,17] but not others.[88] In a recent registry (Figure 15.4), Babaev *et al.*[8] have shown a continuous decrease in cardiogenic shock mortality. However, despite the relatively high number of patients enrolled, the overall mortality seems lower than in a recent manuscript (Table 15.1) and it is possible that these trends represent a drift in the definition of cardiogenic shock rather than a real decrease in mortality. Interestingly, the results from Babaev *et al.* suggest that a decrease in mortality indeed occurred from 1997 to 1998. However, mortality has remained constant since then. Such a time trend could explain the observation of Menon *et al.*[88] of no improvement in mortality between the period from 1990 to 1993 and 1995 to 1997. One could speculate that increasing use of stents and intravenous glycoprotein IIb/IIIa inhibitors, which were shown in small studies to be associated with improved outcome in patients with cardiogenic shock, could explain this apparent improved outcome.

Therefore, the exact mortality of patients with cardiogenic shock is not known. Estimations vary between 40% and 60%. Furthermore, although a trend towards decreased mortality in recent years was observed by most authors, this finding should be examined in well-designed prospective studies.

Table 15.1. *Mortality of patients with cardiogenic shock in studies reporting of patients diagnosed 1995–2002.*

Author	No. of patients with cardiogenic shock	Mortality % (1-month or in-hospital)	Years of recruitment
Antoniucci *et al.*[87]	77	29	1/1999–7/2001
Babaev *et al.*[8]	9465	41	1995–2001
Chan *et al.*[21]	96	44	1/1993–6/2000
Dauerman *et al.*[16]	583	59	4/1999–6/2001
Dens *et al.*[18]	132	55	12/1994–8/2000
Hasdai *et al.*[4]	237	66	11/1995–1/1997
Himbert *et al.*[6]	51	76	1988–1998
Hochman *et al.*[20]	958	60	4/1993–8/1999
Hochman *et al.*,[3]Conservative arm	150	47	4/1993–11/1998
Hochman *et al.*,[3] Invasive arm	152	56	4/1993–11/1998
Koreny *et al.*[73]	118	65	1/1993–3/2000
Karcz *et al.*[11]	41	49	2/2001–6/2002
Lesage *et al.*[13]	157	51	1/1996–12/2001
Lim *et al.*[12]	62	65	1/1999–12/2000
Menon *et al.*[88]	695	62	10/1995–1/1997
Prasad *et al.*[15]	61	47	4/1999–6/2001
Saia *et al.*[14]	12	42	4/2002–10/2002
Tarantini *et al.*[19]	32	53	5/1995–3/2001
Tarantini *et al.*[33]	41	58	10/1996–10/2002
Zeymer *et al.*[17]	1333	46	7/1994–3/2001
Overall	13 368	50.4	
Overall, excluding Babaev *et al.*[8]	4888	58	

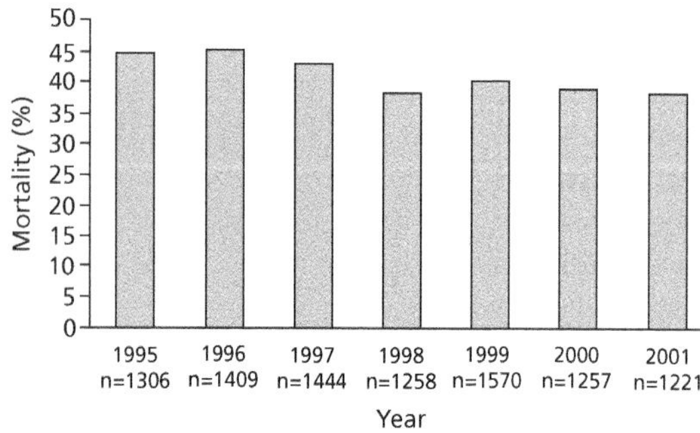

Figure 15.4. *Unadjusted estimated in-hospital mortality of cardiogenic shock patients in the National Registry of Myocardial Infarction (NRMI) registry (With permission from J. Hochman, personal communication.)*

An important issue when examining the outcome of patients with cardiogenic shock is the functional class of patients surviving the initial catastrophic event. In the SHOCK-1 study, most patients surviving the initial hospitalization survived to 1-year follow-up and surprisingly, most were in a relatively preserved functional class. This, however, may not be the case at the present time: if, indeed, more patients survive the acute event, presumably patients who have larger coronary events and hence more significant cardiac dysfunction. Unfortunately, no study has examined the long-term outcome of patients surviving cardiogenic shock in the recent decade and hence data on this issue are incomplete.

References

1. Menon V, White H, LeJemtel T, *et al.* The clinical profile of patients with suspected cardiogenic shock due to predominant left ventricular failure: a report from the SHOCK Trial Registry. SHould we emergently revascularize Occluded Coronaries for cardiogenic shocK? J Am Coll Cardiol 2000; 36: 1071–1076.
2. Lindholm MG, Kober L, Boesgaard S, Torp-Pedersen C, Aldershvile J. Trandolapril Cardiac Evaluation study group. Cardiogenic shock complicating acute myocardial infarction; prognostic impact of early and late shock development. Eur Heart J 2003; 24: 258–265.
3. Hochman JS, Sleeper LA, Webb JG, *et al.* Early revascularization in acute myocardial infarction complicated by cardiogenic shock. SHOCK Investigators. Should we emergently revascularize occluded coronaries for cardiogenic shocK?. N Engl J Med 1999; 341: 625–634.
4. Hasdai D, Holmes DR Jr., Topol EJ, *et al.* Frequency and clinical outcome of cardiogenic shock during acute myocardial infarction among patients receiving reteplase or alteplase. Results from GUSTO-III. Global Use of Strategies to Open Occluded Coronary Arteries. Eur Heart J 1999; 20: 128–135.
5. Tedesco JV, Williams BA, Wright RS, *et al*; Coronary Care Unit Group. Baseline comorbidities and treatment strategy in elderly patients are associated with outcome of cardiogenic shock in a community-based population. Am Heart J 2003; 146: 472–478.
6. Himbert D, Golmard JL, Juliard JM, Feldman LJ, Steg PG. Impact of smoking on the incidence and survival of cardiogenic shock complicating acute myocardial infarction treated with reperfusion therapy. Am J Cardiol 2002; 89: 73–75.
7. Brodie BR, Stuckey TD, Muncy DB, *et al.* Importance of time-to-reperfusion in patients with acute myocardial infarction with and without cardiogenic shock treated with primary percutaneous coronary intervention. Am Heart J 2003; 145: 708–715.
8. Babaev A, Every N, Frederick P, *et al.* Trends in revascularization and mortality in patients with cardiogenic shock complicating acute myocardial infarction: observations from the National Registry of Myocardial Infarction. Circulation 2002; 106: A1811 (Abstract).
9. Hasdai D, Harrington RA, Hochman JS, *et al.* Platelet glycoprotein IIb/IIIa blockade and outcome of cardiogenic shock complicating acute coronary syndromes without persistent ST-segment elevation. J Am Coll Cardiol 2000; 36: 685–692.
10. Carnendran L, Abboud R, Sleeper LA, *et al.* Trends in cardiogenic shock: report from the SHOCK Study. SHould we emergently revascularize Occluded Coronaries for cardiogenic shocK? Eur Heart J 2001; 22: 472–478.
11. Karcz M, Bekta P, Kepka C, *et al.* Acute myocardial infarction complicated by cardiogenic shock: in-hospital and mid-term results of invasive treatment in the National Institute of Cardiology, Warsaw-Anin. Kardiol Pol 2003; 58: 366–374.
12. Lim N, Dubois MJ, De Backer D, Vincent JL. Do all nonsurvivors of cardiogenic shock die with a low cardiac index? Chest 2003; 124: 1885–1891.
13. Lesage A, Ramakers M, Daubin C, *et al.* Complicated acute myocardial infarction requiring mechanical ventilation in the intensive care unit: prognostic factors of clinical outcome in a series of 157 patients. Crit Care Med 2004; 32: 100–105.
14. Saia F, Lemos PA, Lee CH, *et al.* Sirolimus-eluting stent implantation in ST-elevation acute myocardial infarction: a clinical and angiographic study. Circulation 2003; 108: 1927–1929.
15. Prasad A, Lennon RJ, Rihal CS, Berger PB, Holmes DR Jr. Outcomes of elderly patients with cardiogenic shock treated with early percutaneous revascularization. Am Heart J 2004; 147: 1066–1070.
16. Dauerman HL, Goldberg RJ, White K, *et al.*, Global Registry of Acute Coronary Events. GRACE Investigators. Revascularization, stenting, and outcomes of patients with acute myocardial infarction complicated by cardiogenic shock. Am J Cardiol 2002; 90: 838–842.
17. Zeymer U, Vogt A, Zahn R, *et al.*, The Arbeitsgemeinschaft Leitende Kardiologische Krankenhausärzte (ALKK). Predictors of in-hospital mortality in 1333 patients with acute myocardial infarction complicated by cardiogenic shock treated with primary percutaneous coronary intervention (PCI); Results of the primary PCI registry of the Arbeitsgemeinschaft Leitende Kardiologische Krankenhausärzte (ALKK). Eur Heart J 2004; 25: 322–328.
18. Dens J, Dubois C, Ector H, Desmet W, Janssens S. Survival of patients treated with intra-aortic balloon counterpulsation for cardiogenic shock in a tertiary centre: variables correlated with death. Eur J Emerg Med 2003; 10: 213–218.
19. Tarantini G, Ramondo A, Isabella G, *et al.* Pressure response to vasopressors and mortality after direct angioplasty for cardiogenic shock. Int J Cardiol 2004; 94: 197–202.
20. Hochman JS, Buller CE, Sleeper LA, *et al.* Cardiogenic shock complicating acute myocardial

infarction—etiologies, management and outcome: a report from the SHOCK Trial Registry. SHould we emergently revascularize Occluded Coronaries for cardiogenic shocK? J Am Coll Cardiol 2000; 36: 1063–1070.

21. Chan AW, Chew DP, Bhatt DL, *et al.* Long-term mortality benefit with the combination of stents and abciximab for cardiogenic shock complicating acute myocardial infarction. Am J Cardiol 2002; 89: 132–136.
22. Cotter G, Kaluski E, Blatt A, *et al.* L-NMMA (a nitric oxide synthase inhibitor) is effective in the treatment of cardiogenic shock. Circulation 2000; 101: 1358–1361.
23. Cotter G, Kaluski E, Milo O, *et al.* LINCS: L-NAME (a NO synthase inhibitor) in the treatment of refractory cardiogenic shock: a prospective randomized study. Eur Heart J 2003; 24: 1287–1295.
24. Potapov EV, Weng Y, Hausmann H, *et al.* New approach in treatment of acute cardiogenic shock requiring mechanical circulatory support. Ann Thorac Surg 2003; 76: 2112–2114.
25. Holmes DR Jr. Cardiogenic shock: a lethal complication of acute myocardial infarction. Rev Cardiovasc Med 2003; 4: 131–135.
26. Schreiber W, Herkner H, Koreny M, *et al.* Predictors of survival in unselected patients with acute myocardial infarction requiring continuous catecholamine support. Resuscitation 2002; 55: 269–276.
27. Webb JG, Lowe AM, Sanborn TA, *et al.*, SHOCK Investigators. Percutaneous coronary intervention for cardiogenic shock in the SHOCK trial. J Am Coll Cardiol 2003; 42: 1380–1386.
28. Nanas JN, Tsagalou EP, Kanakakis J, *et al.* Long-term intermittent dobutamine infusion, combined with oral amiodarone for end-stage heart failure: a randomized double-blind study. Chest 2004; 125: 1198–1204.
29. Thompson CR, Buller CE, Sleeper LA, *et al.* Cardiogenic shock due to acute severe mitral regurgitation complicating acute myocardial infarction: a report from the SHOCK Trial Registry. SHould we use emergently revascularize Occluded Coronaries for cardiogenic shocK? J Am Coll Cardiol 2000; 36: 1104–1109.
30. Slater J, Brown RJ, Antonelli TA, *et al.* Cardiogenic shock due to cardiac free-wall rupture or tamponade after acute myocardial infarction: a report from the SHOCK Trial Registry. SHould we emergently revascularize Occluded Coronaries for cardiogenic shocK? J Am Coll Cardiol 2000; 36: 1117–1122.
31. Menon V, Webb JG, Hillis LD, *et al.* Outcome and profile of ventricular septal rupture with cardiogenic shock after myocardial infarction: a report from the SHOCK Trial Registry. SHould we emergently revascularize Occluded Coronaries for cardiogenic shocK? J Am Coll Cardiol 2000; 36: 1110–1116.
32. Wong SC, Sanborn T, Sleeper LA, *et al.* Angiographic findings and clinical correlates in patients with cardiogenic shock complicating acute myocardial infarction: a report from the SHOCK Trial Registry. SHould we emergently revascularize Occluded Coronaries for cardiogenic shocK? J Am Coll Cardiol 2000; 36: 1077–1083.
33. Tarantini G, Ramondo A, Napodano M, *et al.* Myocardial perfusion grade and survival after percutaneous transluminal coronary angioplasty in patients with cardiogenic shock. Am J Cardiol 2004; 93: 1081–1085.
34. Jacobs AK, French JK, Col J, *et al.* Cardiogenic shock with non-ST-segment elevation myocardial infarction: a report from the SHOCK Trial Registry. SHould we emergently revascularize Occluded Coronaries for cardiogenic shocK? J Am Coll Cardiol 2000; 36: 1091–1096.
35. Jacobs AK, Leopold JA, Bates E, *et al.* Cardiogenic shock caused by right ventricular infarction: a report from the SHOCK registry. J Am Coll Cardiol 2003; 41: 1273–1279.
36. Frank O. Zur Dynamic des Herzmuskels (On the dynamics of the heart muscle). Zeitschrift für Biologie 1895; 32: 370–374.
37. Evans CL. The velocity factor in cardiac work. J Physiol 1918; 62: 6–12.
38. Katz LN. Observations on the external work of the isolated turtle heart. Am J Physiol 1932; 99: 579–597.
39. Starling EH. The Linacre Lecture on the Law of the Heart (Longmans, Green & Co.: London, 1918), 1–27.
40. Milnor WR, Bergel DH, Bargainer JD. Hydraulic power associated with pulmonary blood flow and its relation to heart rate. Circ Res 1966; 19: 467–480.
41. Tan LB, Schultz DL, Sdougos HP, Rajagopalan B, Lee G J. Separate contribution of ventricular pumping and load impedance on ventricular power output. Med Hypotheses 1981; 7: 1067–1077.
42. Firth BG, Tan LB, Rajagopalan B, Schultz DL, Lee Ge J. Assessment of myocardial performance in ischaemic heart disease from changes in left ventricular power output produced by graded-dose isoprenaline infusion. Cardiovasc Res 1981; 15: 351–364.
43. Sdougos HP, Schultz DL, Tan LB, *et al.* The effects of peripheral impedance and inotropic state on the power output of the left ventricle in dogs. Circ Res 1982; 50: 74–85

44. Tan LB. Clinical and research implications of new concepts in the assessment of cardiac pumping performance in heart failure. Cardiovasc Res 1987; 21: 615–622.
45. Tan LB. Evaluation of cardiac dysfunction, cardiac reserve and inotropic response. Postgrad Med J 1991; 67: S10–S20.
46. Delle Karth G, Buberl A, Geppert A, *et al.* Hemodynamic effects of a continuous infusion of levosimendan in critically ill patients with cardiogenic shock requiring catecholamines. Acta Anaesthesiol Scand 2003; 47: 1251–1256.
47. Cotter G, Moshkovitz Y, Kaluski E, *et al.* The role of cardiac power and systemic vascular resistance in the pathophysiology and diagnosis of patients with acute congestive heart failure. Eur J Heart Fail 2003; 5: 443–451.
48. Smith HJ, Oriol A, Morch J, McGregor M. Hemodynamic studies in cardiogenic shock: Treatment with isoproterenol and metaraminol. Circulation 1967; 35: 1084–1091.
49. Menon V, Slater JN, White HD, *et al.* Acute myocardial infarction complicated by systemic hypoperfusion without hypotension: report of the SHOCK trial registry. Am J Med 2000; 108: 374–380.
50. Hochman JS. Cardiogenic shock complicating acute myocardial infarction: expanding the paradigm. Circulation 2002; 107: 2998–3002.
51. Alonso DR, Scheidt S, Post M, Killip T. Pathophysiology of cardiogenic shock: quantification of myocardial necrosis, clinical, pathologic and electrocardiographic correlations. Circulation 1973; 48: 588–596.
52. Fincke R, Hochman JS, Lowe AM, *et al.*, SHOCK Investigators. Cardiac power is the strongest hemodynamic correlate of mortality in cardiogenic shock: a report from the SHOCK trial registry. J Am Coll Cardiol 2004; 44: 340–348.
53. de Werra I, Jaccard C, Corradin SB, *et al.* Cytokines, nitrite/nitrate, soluble tumor necrosis factor receptors, and procalcitonin concentrations: comparisons in patients with septic shock, cardiogenic shock, and bacterial pneumonia. Crit Care Med 1997; 25: 607–613.
54. Geppert A, Steiner A, Zorn G, *et al.* Multiple organ failure in patients with cardiogenic shock is associated with high plasma levels of interleukin-6. Crit Care Med 2002; 30: 1987–1994.
55. Pinsky DJ, Patton S, Mesaros S, *et al.* Mechanical transduction of nitric oxide synthesis in the beating heart. Circ Res 1997; 81: 372–379.
56. Campbell DL, Stamler JS, Strauss HC. Redox modulation of L-type calcium channels in ferret ventricular myocytes: dual mechanism regulation by nitric oxide and S-nitrosothiols. J Gen Physiol 1996; 108: 277–293.
57. Xu L, Eu JP, Meissner G, Stamler JS. Activation of the cardiac calcium release channel (ryanodine receptor) by poly-S-nitrosylation. Science 1998; 279: 234–237.
58. Werdan K, Muller U, Reithmann C, Pfeifer A, Hallstrom S, Koidl B, Schlag G. Mechanisms in acute septic cardiomyopathy: evidence from isolated myocytes. Basic Res Cardiol 1991; 86: 411–421.
59. Hare JM, Colucci WS. Role of nitric oxide in the regulation of myocardial function. Prog Cardiovasc Dis 1995; 38: 155–166.
60. Hannan RL, John MC, Kouretas PC, *et al.* Deletion of endothelial nitric oxide synthase exacerbates myocardial stunning in an isolated mouse heart model. J Surg Res 2000; 93: 127–132.
61. Czarnowska E, Kurzelewski M, Beresewicz A, Karczmarewicz E. The role of endogenous nitric oxide in inhibition of ischemia/reperfusion-induced cardiomyocyte apoptosis. Folia Histochem Cytobiol 2001; 39: 179–180.
62. Csonka C, Szilvassy Z, Fulop F, *et al.* Classic preconditioning decreases the harmful accumulation of nitric oxide during ischemia and reperfusion in rat hearts. Circulation 1999; 100: 2260–2266.
63. Depré C, Vanoverschelde JL, Goudemant JF, Mottet I, Hue L. Protection against ischemic injury by nonvasoactive concentrations of nitric oxide synthase inhibitors in the perfused rabbit heart. Circulation 1995; 92: 1911–1918.
64. Schulz R, Wambolt R. Inhibition of nitric oxide synthesis protects the isolated working rabbit heart from ischemia–reperfusion injury. Cardiovasc Res 1995; 30: 432–439.
65. Sam F, Sawyer DB, Xie Z, *et al.* Mice lacking inducible nitric oxide synthase have improved left ventricular contractile function and reduced apoptotic cell death late after myocardial infarction. Circ Res 2001; 89: 351–356.
66. Flesch M, Kilter H, Cremers B, *et al.* Acute effects of nitric oxide and cyclic GMP on human myocardial contractility. J Pharmacol Exp Ther 1997; 281: 1340–1349.
67. Kojda G, Kottenberg K, Nix P, *et al.* Low increase in cGMP induced by organic nitrates and nitrovasodilators improves contractile response of rat ventricular myocytes. Circ Res 1996; 78: 91–101.
68. Ziolo MT, Maier LS, Piacentino V IIIrd, *et al.* Myocyte nitric oxide synthase 2 contributes to blunted beta-adrenergic response in failing human hearts by decreasing Ca^{2+} transients. Circulation 2004; 109: 1886–1891.

69. Li W, Jue T, Edwards J, Wang X, Hintze TH. Changes in NO bioavailability regulate cardiac O_2 consumption: control by intramitochondrial SOD2 and intracellular myoglobin. Am J Physiol Heart Circ Physiol 2004; 286: H47–H54.
70. Geppert A, Steiner A, Delle-Karth G, Heinz G, Huber K. Usefulness of procalcitonin for diagnosing complicating sepsis in patients with cardiogenic shock. Intensive Care Med 2003; 29: 1384–1389.
71. Dzavik V, Sleeper LA, Cocke TP, *et al.*, SHOCK Investigators. Early revascularization is associated with improved survival in elderly patients with acute myocardial infarction complicated by cardiogenic shock: a report from the SHOCK Trial Registry. Eur Heart J 2003; 24: 828–837.
72. Shindler DM, Palmeri ST, Antonelli TA, *et al.* Diabetes mellitus in cardiogenic shock complicating acute myocardial infarction: a report from the SHOCK Trial Registry. SHould we emergently revascularize Occluded Coronaries for cardiogenic shocK? J Am Coll Cardiol 2000; 36: 1097–1103.
73. Koreny M, Karth GD, Geppert A, *et al.* Prognosis of patients who develop acute renal failure during the first 24 hours of cardiogenic shock after myocardial infarction. Am J Med 2002; 112: 115–119.
74. Wong SC, Sleeper LA, Monrad ES, *et al.*, SHOCK Investigators. Absence of gender differences in clinical outcomes in patients with cardiogenic shock complicating acute myocardial infarction. A report from the SHOCK Trial Registry. J Am Coll Cardiol 2001; 38: 1395–1401.
75. Webb JG, Sleeper LA, Buller CE, *et al.* Implications of the timing of onset of cardiogenic shock after acute myocardial infarction: a report from the SHOCK Trial Registry. SHould we emergently revascularize Occluded Coronaries for cardiogenic shocK? J Am Coll Cardiol 2000; 36: 1084–1090.
76. Picard MH, Davidoff R, Sleeper LA, *et al.*, SHOCK Trial. SHould we emergently revascularize Occluded Coronaries for cardiogenic shocK? Echocardiographic predictors of survival and response to early revascularization in cardiogenic shock. Circulation 2003; 107: 279–284.
77. Sanborn TA, Sleeper LA, Webb JG, *et al.*, SHOCK Investigators. Correlates of one-year survival in patients with cardiogenic shock complicating acute myocardial infarction: angiographic findings from the SHOCK trial. J Am Coll Cardiol 2003; 42: 1373–1379.
78. Hochman JS, Sleeper LA, White HD, *et al.*, SHOCK Investigators. Should we emergently revascularize Occluded Coronaries for cardiogenic shocK? One-year survival following early revascularization for cardiogenic shock. JAMA 2001; 285: 190–192.
79. Thiele H, Lauer B, Hambrecht R, *et al.* Reversal of cardiogenic shock by percutaneous left atrial-to-femoral arterial bypass assistance. Circulation 2001; 104: 2917–2922.
80. Wollert KC, Drexler H. Carvedilol prospective randomized cumulative survival (COPERNICUS) trial: carvedilol as the sun and center of the beta-blocker world? Circulation 2002; 106: 2164–2166.
81. Chen EW, Canto JG, Parsons LS, *et al.*, Investigators in the National Registry of Myocardial Infarction 2. Relation between hospital intra-aortic balloon counterpulsation volume and mortality in acute myocardial infarction complicated by cardiogenic shock. Circulation 2003; 108: 951–957.
82. Wernly JA. Ischemia, reperfusion, and the role of surgery in the treatment of cardiogenic shock secondary to acute myocardial infarction: an interpretative review. J Surg Res 2004; 117: 6–21.
83. Castells E, Calbet JM, Saura E, *et al.* Acute myocardial infarction with cardiogenic shock: treatment with mechanical circulatory assistance and heart transplantation. Transplant Proc 2003; 35: 1940–1941.
84. Magliato KE, Kleisli T, Soukiasian HJ, *et al.* Biventricular support in patients with profound cardiogenic shock: a single center experience. ASAIO J 2003; 49: 475–479.
85. Potapov EV, Weng Y, Hausmann H, *et al.* New approach in treatment of acute cardiogenic shock requiring mechanical circulatory support. Ann Thorac Surg 2003; 76: 2112–2114.
86. Rizik DG, Villegas BJ, Bouhasin A. Benefits of endovascular hypothermia on myocardial preservation in the setting of cardiogenic shock. J Invasive Cardiol 2003; 15: 525–526.
87. Antoniucci D, Valenti R, Migliorini A, *et al.* Abciximab therapy improves survival in patients with acute myocardial infarction complicated by early cardiogenic shock undergoing coronary artery stent implantation. Am J Cardiol 2002; 90: 353–357.
88. Menon V, Hochman JS, Stebbins A, *et al.* Lack of progress in cardiogenic shock: lessons from the GUSTO trials. Eur Heart J 2000; 21: 1928–1936.
89. Cotter G, Williams SG, Vered Z, Tan LB. Role of cardiac power in heart failure. Curr Opin Cardiol 2003; 18: 215–222.

CHAPTER 16

Hypertension in acute decompensated heart failure

Alan B Miller, Jun R Chiong

Introduction

Acute decompensated heart failure (ADHF) accounts for the bulk of the direct costs of heart failure. Heart failure hospitalizations in the United States total approximately 1 million patients with an estimated cost of approximately $23 billion.[1] While guidelines exist for the treatment of chronic congestive heart failure (CHF) through the American College of Cardiology (ACC) and the American Heart Association (AHA),[2] similar guidelines for ADHF are not available.

A registry to document information including demographics, clinical presentation, therapeutic interventions and outcomes data has been provided by the Acute Decompensated Heart Failure National Registry (ADHERE™).[3] Based on information from the ADHERE™ registry, most of the patients hospitalized with acute decompensation are older with a median age of 75 years and 54% demonstrate an ejection fraction (EF) calculated at < 40%. Only 2% of patients admitted had systolic blood pressures below 90 mm Hg and half of the hospitalized patients had systolic blood pressures greater than 140 mm Hg. The vast majority of patients who present with this syndrome have congestion and exhibit severe dyspnea as their primary symptom.

Hospitalization for heart failure can be categorized into three broad areas: (1) patients with new-onset heart failure that is usually precipitated by specific factors such as acute myocardial infarction (MI) or the result of the progression of relatively symptomatic left ventricular (LV) dysfunction; (2) patients who have chronic CHF as a baseline and develop acute decompensation; (3) patients categorized as Stage D in the new AHA/ACC guidelines who have severely impaired LV systolic dysfunction and who have frequent episodes of decompensation.

Hypertension and Heart Failure

Most patients with heart failure have antecedents to arterial hypertension.[4] Not only is hypertension an important coexisting disorder, but it also contributes pathogenetically to the development of systolic and diastolic heart failure. As well as being a major risk factor for ischemic heart disease, hypertension can also lead directly to the development of chronic heart failure by afterload-induced cardiac hypertrophy causing left ventricular hypertrophy (LVH), impaired myocyte contractility, ventricular chamber remodeling, and eventually systolic and diastolic dysfunction.[5–7]

Demographics

Patients presenting with acute pulmonary edema are more likely to be older, hypertensive, and have preserved left ventricular ejection fraction (LVEF) as compared with patients with other presentations of decompensated heart failure.[8] Early investigations of patients with chronic heart failure, such as the Framingham study,[9] cited hypertension as the most frequent comorbidity. About 15% of participants in SOLVD had diastolic blood pressures above 90 mm Hg at enrollment.[10] In a population-based, epidemiological study in Olmstead County, Minnesota, about 50% of patients presenting with new-onset heart failure had hypertension.[11] In a more recent study, patients were noted to have systolic blood pressures of ≥ 140 mm Hg when they presented with acute pulmonary edema[3] and often had markedly elevated pressures with a mean systolic blood pressure of 194 mm Hg.[12]

However, in clinical trials, hypertension is cited less frequently as a comorbidity and underlying etiology of heart failure. Recent randomized trials have probably underestimated the contribution of hypertension to the development and progression of chronic heart failure. Of note is the fact that CHF symptoms are rare in hypertensive individuals whose blood pressure is well controlled and who have not sustained a MI.[13]

Hypertension and Systolic Dysfunction

In hypertensive patients, heart failure occurs as a result of impaired inotropism. Myocardial and coronary mechanisms may be involved. In the myocardial mechanism, increased load gives rise to a hypertrophy-dilatation effect. The pathological time course of hypertensive heart disease involves two stages.

Initially, concentric hypertrophy of the left ventricle compensates pressure overload and normalizes systolic wall stress, and thus cardiac function is maintained. However, this adaptive hypertrophy is accompanied by structural modifications of the cardiac muscle, including alterations in gene expression, loss of cardiomyocytes, defective vascular development, and fibrosis. Thus, the compensatory response is inexorably followed by a transition to cardiac failure and progressive contractile dysfunction.[14]

In the second stage, diseased coronary vasculature due to arteriosclerosis or microangiopathy leads to increased coronary resistance and impaired oxygen supply, bringing about severe myocardial ischemia or even infarction, resulting in heart failure. Transient myocardial ischemia is one of the causes of flash pulmonary edema, which prompts the performance of coronary angiography. In both cases, blood pressure falls as systolic chronic heart failure develops such that the contribution to hypertension to the heart failure syndrome may be underappreciated.

The mechanism by which increased LV mass leads to depressed LVEF remains ill defined. MI is traditionally viewed as an obligatory event in the transition to depressed systolic function,[15] and it is an important risk factor, as it occurs in 16% of those who developed depressed LVEF as compared with 3% of those who did not.[16] However, there must be other operative mechanisms, because increased LV mass remains associated with the development of depressed LVEF in subjects free of clinically manifest coronary heart disease including MI. In a review of major long-term hypertension treatment trials, the prevention of disease progression, LVH and CHF were assessed.[13] The incidence of LVH in treated subjects was 35% less, representing a reduction in LVH with active antihypertensive treatment. The development of CHF was reported in 12 major trials and there was a 52% reduction in risk of development of CHF in the treated subjects.[17]

Systemic Vascular Resistance and Pulmonary Edema

Acute pulmonary edema is a frequently encountered and familiar entity. It is a consequence of acute heart failure (AHF) and is a clinical syndrome within the broad category of CHF exacerbation. It is defined as an acute increase in pulmonary interstitial and airspace water, and is characterized by the sudden onset of severe dyspnea and signs of pulmonary congestion. It is also accompanied by a sudden reduction in stroke volume which increases sympathetic nervous system activity in an attempt to maintain systemic arterial pressure.

The syndrome of AHF is usually precipitated by some event leading to an immediate diminution in the capacity of the heart to pump blood. The left atrial pressure rises acutely with no time for an increase of total body water and sodium content. The fluid in the lungs arises from a redistribution of fluid within the body. The sudden decrease in stroke volume causes an increase in systemic vascular resistance (SVR), which in turn further reduces stroke volume, finally leading to pulmonary edema.[18]

Hypertension as a favorable prognostic indicator

In contrast, low systolic blood pressure was the strongest predictor of subsequent mortality of the precipitants of acute pulmonary edema.[19] Patients with an systolic blood pressure of ≥ 160 mm Hg had a total mortality of 42.6%, whereas those with an systolic blood pressure of < 160 mm Hg had a mortality of 73.9%. Patients with an initial diastolic blood pressure > 100 mm Hg had a mortality of 38.9% and those with initial diastolic blood pressure of ≤ 100 mm Hg had a mortality of 60.4%.

Severe systolic LV dysfunction due to arterial hypertension has a favorable long-term prognosis with improvement of EF and functional improvement after treatment with ACE inhibitors, beta-blockers, and calcium antagonists.[20]

Upregulation of vasoconstrictor neurohormones

In the past, ADHF was often viewed as merely a disorder of volume overload and low cardiac output as patients presenting with pulmonary congestion have a variety of hemodynamic abnormalities. The vast majority of these individuals has a marked increase in LV filling pressures which impacts myocardial oxygen supply/demand, increases myocardial wall stress, precipitates myocardial ischemia, worsens mitral regurgitation and increases the risk of ventricular arrhythmias.

It is now well appreciated that structural changes in the myocardium are mediated not only by the mechanical stress of pressure overload but also by various neurohormonal substances that exert trophic effects on myocytes and non-myocytes in the heart.[21] Neurohormonal activation which is usually present in patients with chronic heart failure or patients who develop an acute infarction is further augmented, which plays a major role in the pathophysiology of the syndrome as well as the marked increase in blood pressure manifested by the majority of these patients. In many instances in the emergency room setting it is difficult to determine if a patient has developed a hypertensive emergency and then subsequently has developed ADHF manifested by pulmonary edema or has developed pulmonary edema with subsequent significant vasoconstriction triggered by neurohormonal activation.

In previous studies, it was demonstrated that acute pulmonary edema results from a rapidly deteriorating cycle of events in which patients with reduced baseline systolic and diastolic reserve are faced with an acute increase in SVR and hence, afterload.[22–25] This leads to an acute decompensated state, leading to decreased peripheral perfusion, neurohormonal activation, decreasing LV function, and increasing vascular resistance. The result of this vicious cycle is an increase in left ventricular end-diastolic pressure (LVEDP) that is transmitted backwards to the pulmonary vasculature, causing an acute increase in pulmonary capillary wedge pressure (PCWP) and the transudation of fluid from the intravascular compartment to the lung interstitium and alveoli, leading in turn to the full-blown syndrome of acute cardiogenic pulmonary edema.

Some patients, most of whom had prior a history of hypertension, develop a sustained hypertensive response upon recovery from heart failure. Improved ventricular performance in response to vasodilator therapy in some patients with a history of hypertension may lead to a restitution of the baseline hypertensive pathophysiology. If unchecked, this would establish a vicious cycle where the recurrent hypertension would result in new episodes of heart failure, each less amenable to correction as treatment strategies are exhausted.[26]

Hypertension and Diastolic Heart Failure

Elevated systolic arterial blood pressure impairs diastolic performance. This is dramatically apparent in patients who develop flash pulmonary edema in association with marked increases in systolic blood pressure > 200 mm Hg.[27] The presence of a markedly elevated blood pressure during an episode of CHF favors a diagnosis of diastolic heart failure.[28,29] A failing left ventricle with systolic dysfunction is more likely to result in a normal or low blood pressure.[30]

It is a clinical paradox that patients hospitalized with CHF may later be noted to have normal systolic function, as evidenced by a preserved EF. It has been proposed that a normal LVEF within 72 hours after an episode of pulmonary congestion indicates that the patient had heart failure due to diastolic rather than systolic dysfunction.[31] These investigators have suggested a diagnosis of diastolic heart failure in patients who present with heart failure symptoms and markedly elevated blood pressure, particularly if the symptoms improve with treatment directed at lowering blood pressure, the underlying cause of diastolic dysfunction.[31]

In a landmark study by Gandhi *et al.*, acute pulmonary edema in association with hypertension is not due to transient systolic dysfunction, but rather is due to isolated diastolic dysfunction.[32] The LVEF and the extent of regional wall motion measured during the acute episode of hypertensive pulmonary edema were similar to those measured after resolution of the congestion, when the blood pressure was controlled. Even in patients with systolic dysfunction (EF < 50%), the LVEF measured during the acute episode was similar to that measured after therapy, suggesting that diastolic dysfunction may also be an important contributor to acute hypertensive pulmonary edema in patients with baseline systolic dysfunction.

Coronary artery disease and pulmonary edema

Ischemia may play an important role in such patients either as a trigger of acute pulmonary edema, or in the form of subendocardial ischemia resulting from elevated end-diastolic pressures.[33] The majority of patients with flash pulmonary edema were found to have preserved systolic function (PSF).[12,19,34,35] Patients exhibiting this phenomenon are generally elderly and have severe coronary artery disease (CAD), typically with one occluded vessel and a severely stenosed coronary artery supplying collateral flow.[33] Patients with PSF and LVH are particularly susceptible to this type of episode because of their reduced ventricular distensibility, in which small changes in ventricular volume status lead to large changes in filling pressures. Such patients have a narrow range of LV filling pressures that are high enough to sustain both LV filling and adequate cardiac output, but low enough to prevent pulmonary edema. This abnormal diastolic pressure–volume relationship may also explain why these patients frequently improve quickly with diuresis and lowering arterial pressure.[27] Although rarely sought, this can be thought of as an angina equivalent or painless myocardial ischemia without infarction.

Clinical Syndromes of Acute Decompensated Heart Failure

Acute CHF can be classified into four major clinical syndromes: (1) acute pulmonary edema; (2) cardiogenic shock; (3) hypertensive crisis; and (4) exacerbated systolic heart failure.

Patients with hypertensive crisis have clinical signs and symptoms of AHF accompanied by high blood pressure (mean arterial pressure of > 130 mm Hg). The diagnosis of these clinical syndromes of acute heart failure may be difficult, due to an overlap in symptoms and signs among the different syndromes as well as lack of objective criteria for their diagnosis. In a study by Cotter *et al.*, the number of hypertensive crises was small and were considered together with the exacerbated systolic heart failure group (Figure 16.1).[24]

Cardiac power as an index of cardiac contractility

Measurement of invasive hemodynamic variables, including cardiac index (CI) and PCWP have been used in patients with acute decompensated and chronic compensated heart failure for more than two decades. In a recent hemodynamic study, Cotter *et al.* suggested the use of cardiac power as an index of cardiac contractility. This is calculated based on the classical physical rule of fluids, i.e., *power* = *flow* × *pressure*, hence cardiac power index (Cpi) is the product of simultaneously measured

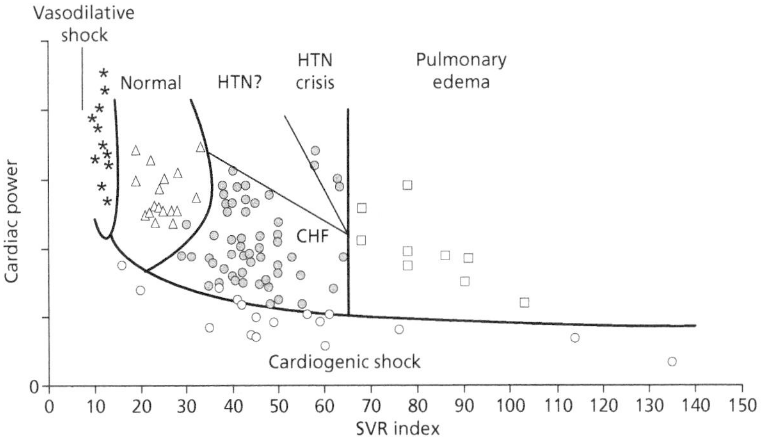

Figure 16.1. *Diagnostic graph for classification of the hemodynamic status of patients with different syndromes of acute CHF (Adapted, with permission, from Cotter et al.*[24]*)*

Abbreviations: CHF = *congestive heart failure;* HTN = *hypertension;* SVR = *systemic vascular resistance*

mean arterial blood pressure and cardiovascular flow: *Cpi = mean arterial pressure [MAP]* $\times$ *CI* $\times$ 0.0022. The units are watts/m^2.[24] In three separate studies,[36–38] Cpi increased during exercise and was the most reliable predictor of outcome in patients with chronic CHF, stronger than oxygen (O_2) consumption and echocardiographic EF.

Therapeutic Strategies

Advances in the understanding of the pathophysiology of ADHF and recent clinical trials have provided new insights into successful treatment strategies to rapidly reverse ADHF.[39] These therapeutic goals in patients presenting with ADHF are to reverse acute hemodynamic abnormalities, rapidly relieve symptoms, and initiate treatments that will decrease disease progression and improve survival.

The initial assessment of patients with AHF includes immediate bedside evaluation of left and right atrial filling pressures, LV filling pressure and function, assessment of organ perfusion, and identification of precipitating factors.

Regardless of its cause, the standard immediate treatment of AHF is to place the patient in an upright position and give oxygen. Intravenous morphine, usually accompanied by an antiemetic, and intravenous diuretics, are administered. This treatment is effective as observed by numerous physicians over many years. But there is little evidence in the form of controlled or randomized trials to support the use of this therapy.

Diuretics

Episodes of acute pulmonary edema are frequently associated with poorly controlled hypertension or dietary indiscretion and often respond quickly to diuretics and control of blood pressure. ADHF patients are frequently treated successfully by emergency department physicians and primary care providers, and may be under-represented in specialty heart failure practices. Diuretics remain the most popular choice of treatment for heart failure and are undoubtedly successful at relieving breathlessness and edema when overt fluid overload is present. Placebo-controlled studies have shown that diuretics effectively relieve symptoms[40,41] and a high incidence of recurrent symptoms happens when diuretics have been withdrawn.[42,43]

Loop diuretics such as furosemide and torsemide may exert their effect partly by being vasodilators. There is a concomitant decrease in stroke volume, increase in SVR, and pronounced neurohormonal activation. Increases in the renin-angiotensin-aldosterone activation and sympathetic activation can be seen after a single intravenous dose of furosemide.[44] Subjects who received high doses of furosemide compared to low doses, combined with intravenous vasodilators, were more likely to require mechanical ventilation.[22] As CHF involves complex autonomic and neurohormonal responses characterized by sympathetic overactivity, parasympathetic withdrawal, and the activation of renin-angiotensin-aldosterone and vasopressin systems, use of intravenous diuretics alone led to further increases in SVR and further deleterious neurohormonal activation,[45] an effect expected to be harmful.[46,47]

Vasodilators in heart failure

It has become apparent that in most cases ADHF is characterized hemodynamically by a marked increase in SVR, elevated right and left filling pressures, and decreased cardiac output.[32,39,48] The main benefit of therapy that improves hemodynamics is relief of symptoms. Direct vasodilators have been shown to cause a sustained reduction in LV pressures, with resulting clinical improvement and reduced mortality even in the absence of favorable neurohumoral effects.[49] Trials comparing direct vasodilators and ACE inhibitors have clearly shown that ACE inhibitors result in better overall survival, due to a reduction in sudden death. Progressive heart failure rates were equivalent with both agents.[50] The results of these trials have been interpreted as indicating that the mechanism of benefit of ACE inhibitors in heart failure may be entirely independent of their hemodynamic effects.

Angiotensin-converting enzyme inhibitors

Angiotensin-converting enzyme (ACE) inhibitors have revolutionized the clinical approach to patients with CHF. There is overwhelming evidence that ACE inhibitors satisfy all the goals of effective treatment for patients with heart failure because of LV systolic dysfunction. ACE inhibition delays the appearance of symptoms,[51,52] delays the worsening of symptoms,[53,54] and improves symptoms when they are moderate or severe.[55] They also reduce the risk of recurrent hospital admission from all causes with the greatest benefit being on hospital admission for heart failure.[51,56]

Every large, long term-trial of ACE inhibition in patients with LV dysfunction has reported a trend towards a reduction in MI. Ramipril and perindopril have shown risk reduction in MI in patients who are at risk but without LV systolic dysfunction.[57,58] In patients with LV dysfunction after an acute MI, ACE inhibition was of greater benefit to patients with a history of arterial hypertension.[59]

Nitrates

It became apparent that in most cases of ADHF, a marked increase in SVR is superimposed on insufficient systolic and diastolic myocardial functional reserve.[32,39] The emphasis has shifted from diuretic monotherapy to intravenous vasodilators.[48] This more physiologic approach has been shown to relieve symptoms more rapidly, and reduce patient morbidity, length of stay, and rehospitalization.[60,61]

Nitrates cause balanced vasodilatation of both venous and arterial sides of the circulation, thereby reducing LV preload and afterload, without impairing tissue perfusion.[62] Nitrates are well tolerated in acute MI. Clinically significant hypotension occurs in less than 4% of patients but responds to dose reduction and fluid replacement.[63] There have been two head-to-head comparisons of intravenous furosemide and nitrates in ADHF. In the first, subjects received a short infusion of sodium nitroprusside followed by 200 mg of furosemide, when hemodynamic conditions had returned to baseline. Nitrate infusion caused a greater reduction in LV filling pressure than furosemide and also increased cardiac output, which was unchanged after furosemide. The second study was a randomized study comparing intravenous furosemide with isosorbide dinitrate infusion in patients with decompensated heart failure due to acute MI. With furosemide, LV filling pressure fell progressively by 17% over 90 minutes, SVR increased by 7%, and cardiac output fell by 12%. By contrast, isosorbide dinitrate caused balanced vasodilatation, with 30% reduction in LV preload and a 13% fall in afterload, with no significant change in cardiac output.[62]

Nitrates have a better hemodynamic profile than loop diuretics, and also have a useful anti-ischemic effect. Nitrate preparations are widely available, simple to administer, and allow rapid dose titration to the desired hemodynamic goals. However, their use is limited in that administration requires frequent monitoring in a cardiac care unit setting with nurses well trained in its use and staffed to perform frequent dose titration to achieve meaningful symptomatic response. Like loop diuretics, there have only been a few small clinical trials that evaluated the use of nitrates for this purpose. The effect of nitrates on neurohormonal activation has not been well studied.

Natriuretic peptide regulation in heart failure

The renin-angiotensin-aldosterone system (RAAS) is counterbalanced by the release of natriuretic peptides. Atrial (A-type) natriuretic peptide (ANP) and brain (B-type) natriuretic peptide (BNP) are vasoactive peptides produced chiefly by atrial myocytes and ventricular myocytes, respectively, in normal humans.[64] Both are released in response to chamber wall dilatation and have important natriuretic and vasodilatory effects.[64–68] Plasma ANP and BNP are increased in heart failure patients and correlate with atrial filling pressures and disease severity.[64,65,69] In addition to vasodilator effects, ANP and BNP have been shown to suppress renin release and decrease angiotensin II and aldosterone production.[70] In severe heart failure, the vasodilatory effect of natriuretic peptides are blunted.[66,71]

Nesiritide

Until recently, the pathogenesis of ADHF leading to pulmonary edema was believed to result from fluid accumulation in the lungs because of systemic volume overload.[32] However, decompensation of heart failure and pulmonary edema may occur rapidly, developing over a few hours or even minutes. Therefore, net fluid accumulation cannot be the sole mechanism of pulmonary edema.

Nesiritide is synthetic recombinant human BNP that has novel venous, arterial, and coronary vasodilatory properties, reducing preload and afterload, increasing cardiac output without direct inotropic effects. The drug improves echocardiographic indices of diastolic function and improves symptoms in patients with ADHF.[72] In addition, nesiritide has been observed to increase glomerular filtration fraction, suppress the renin-angiotensin-aldosterone axis, and cause natriuresis in AHF patients.

In a study by Colucci *et al.*, the infusion of nesiritide in patients admitted with decompensated heart failure resulted in improvements in hemodynamic function with rapid and sustained improvement in clinical status. Nesiritide caused a dose-related decrease in PCWP. This effect was associated with a decrease in SVR and an increase in CI. Since nesiritide exerts no direct, positive inotropic action on the myocardium, the increase in cardiac output presumably reflects a reduction in LV afterload. These effects are evident in both groups receiving nesiritide at infusion rates of 0.015 μg/kg/min and 0.030 μg/kg/min. The drop in blood pressure is not associated with reflex tachycardia or an increase in norepinephrine.[73]

The Vasodilation in the Management of Acute CHF (VMAC) trial demonstrated the efficacy of nesiritide when added to standard care in comparison with placebo and nitroglycerin. This randomized trial enrolled severely ill patients with ADHF, dyspnea at rest, and many clinically important comorbidities, including acute coronary syndromes, atrial and ventricular arrhythmias, and renal insufficiency. In this study, nesiritide significantly reduced PCWP more than standard care plus nitroglycerin or placebo, and these effects were sustained for at least 24 hours.[74]

Use of other therapies

After reversal of acute decompensation, comprehensive neurohormonal blockade with ACE inhibitors, beta-blockers, and aldosterone antagonists can then be initiated or the dose adjusted to further reduce disability, hospitalizations, and death from heart failure.[2] Patients with acute pulmonary edema who have significant obstructive coronary disease or renal artery disease should receive some form of revascularization (Figure 16.2).[75,76]

Conclusion

Severe pulmonary edema in acute LV failure represents a critical situation that demands prompt resolution. Hemodynamically, systemic arterial pressure is often elevated and cardiac output may be decreased to such an extent that SVR is increased. LVEDP and PCWP are strikingly increased, leading to transudation. During acute pulmonary edema, the patient and relatives are in a state of considerable distress. In such circumstances, obtaining consent, let alone informed consent, is nearly impossible. The acute situation demands treatment, and that is what the public expects. The treatment of hypertension in AHF has not changed for many years, partly because of the difficulties of undertaking trials, and a poor understanding of the pathophysiology of this

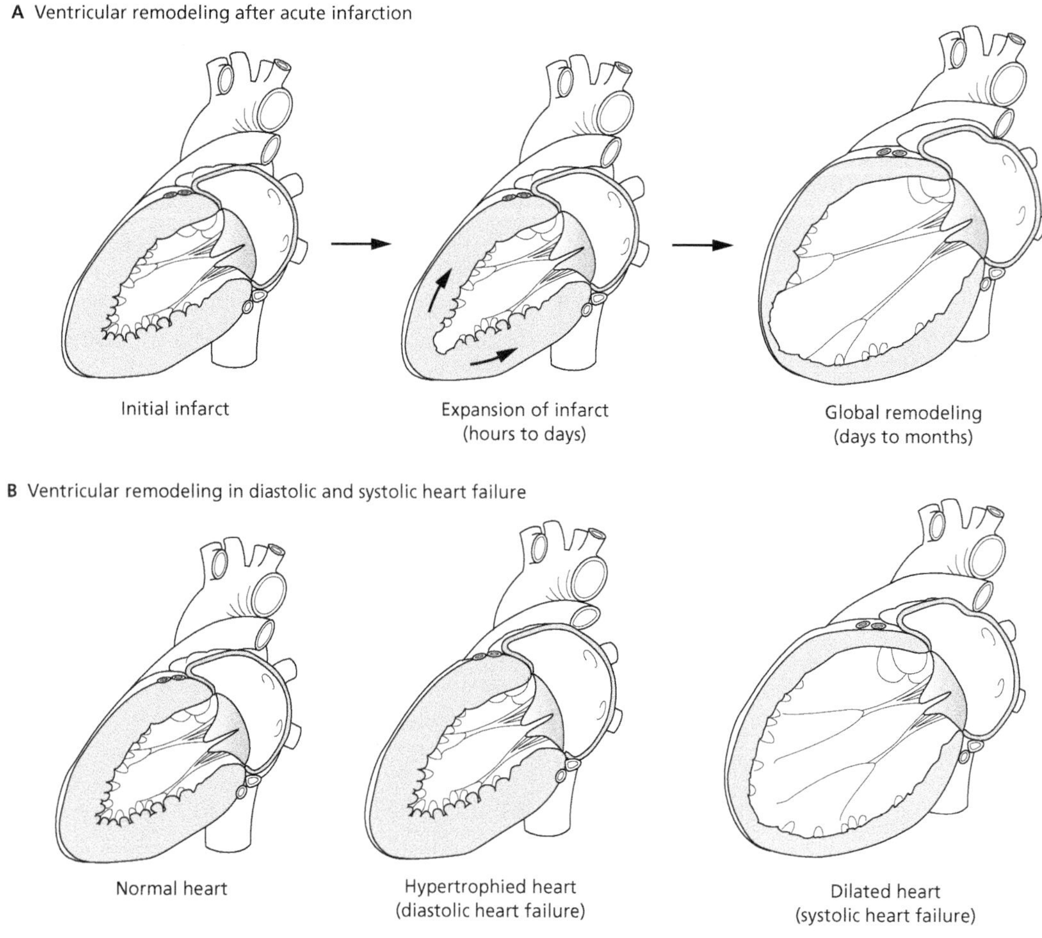

Figure 16.2. *Ventricular remodeling (With permission from Jessup and Brozena.[77])*

heterogeneous group of patients. Now that we have a better understanding of the neurohormonal concepts in heart failure and the predominance of elevated systolic blood pressure in patients presenting with ADHF, further studies are necessary to establish the clinical impact of lowering blood pressure in this population.

References

1. American Heart Association. Heart Disease and Stroke Statistics—2002 Update (Dallas, TX: American Heart Association, 2001).
2. Hunt SA, Baker DW, Chin MH, *et al.*, American College of Cardiology/American Heart Association. ACC/AHA guidelines for the evaluation and management of chronic heart failure in the adult: executive summary: a report of the American College of Cardiology/American Heart Association Task Force on Practice Guidelines (Committee to revise the 1995 Guidelines for the Evaluation and Management of Heart Failure). J Am Coll Cardiol 2001; 38: 2101–2113.
3. ADHERE™: Acute Decompensated Heart Failure National Registry. Available at: http://www.adhereregistry.com. Accessed July 13, 2004.
4. Kannel WB, Belanger AJ. Epidemiology of heart failure. Am Heart J 1991; 121: 951–957.
5. McKee PA, Castelli WP, McNamara PM, Kannel WB. The natural history of congestive heart failure: the Framingham study. N Engl J Med 1971; 285: 1441–1446.
6. Topol EJ, Traill TA, Fortuin NJ. Hypertensive hypertrophic cardiomyopathy of the elderly. N Engl J Med 1985; 312: 277–283.

7. Bonow RO, Udelson JE. Left ventricular diastolic dysfunction as a cause of congestive heart failure: mechanisms and management. Ann Intern Med 1992; 117: 502–510.
8. Felker GM, Adams KF Jr., Konstam MA, O'Connor CM, Gheorghiade M. The problem of decompensated heart failure: nomenclature, classification, and risk stratification. Am Heart J 2003; 145: S18–S25.
9. Levy D, Larson MG, Vasan RS, Kannel WB, Ho KK. The progression from hypertension to congestive heart failure. JAMA 1996; 275: 1557–1562.
10. Kostis JB. The effect of enalapril on mortal and morbid events in patients with hypertension and left ventricular dysfunction. Am J Hypertens 1995; 8: 909–914.
11. Senni M, Tribouilloy CM, Rodeheffer RJ, *et al.* Congestive heart failure in the community: trends in incidence and survival in a 10-year period. Arch Intern Med 1999; 159: 29–34.
12. Kramer K, Kirkman P, Kitzman D, Little WC. Flash pulmonary edema: association with hypertension and reoccurrence despite coronary revascularization. Am Heart J 2000; 140: 451–455.
13. Moser M, Hebert PR. Prevention of disease progression, left ventricular hypertrophy and congestive heart failure in hypertension treatment trials. J Am Coll Cardiol 1996; 27: 1214–1218.
14. Diez J, Fortuno MA, Ravassa S. Apoptosis in hypertensive heart disease. Curr Opin Cardiol 1998; 13: 317–325.
15. Dahlof B, Devereux RB, Kjeldsen SE, *et al.*, LIFE Study Group. Cardiovascular morbidity and mortality in the Losartan Intervention For Endpoint reduction in hypertension study (LIFE): a randomised trial against atenolol. Lancet 2002; 359: 995–1003.
16. Drazner MH, Rame JE, Marino EK, *et al.* Increased left ventricular mass is a risk factor for the development of a depressed left ventricular ejection fraction within five years: the Cardiovascular Health Study. J Am Coll Cardiol 2004; 43: 2207–2215.
17. Moser M, Herbert PR. Prevention of disease progression, left ventricular hypertrophy and congestive heart failure in hypertension treatment trials. J Am Coll Cardiol 1996; 27: 1214–1218.
18. Colucci WS, Braunwald E. Pathophysiology of Heart Failure. In: Braunwald E, Zipes DP, Libby P (eds) Heart Disease: A Textbook of Cardiovascular Medicine, 6th edition (W.B. Saunders Company: Philadelphia, PA, 2001), 503–533.
19. Goldberger JJ, Peled HB, Stroh JA, Cohen MN, Frishman WH. Prognostic factors in acute pulmonary edema. Arch Intern Med 1986; 146: 489–493.
20. Anguita M, Castillo JC, Ramirez A, *et al.* Heart failure caused by severe systolic ventricular dysfunction of hypertensive origin: long-term clinical and functional course. Rev Esp Cardiol 2000; 53: 927–931.
21. Johnson DB, Dell'Italia LJ. Cardiac hypertrophy and failure in hypertension. Curr Opin Nephrol Hypertens 1996; 5: 186–191.
22. Cotter G, Metzkor E, Kaluski E, *et al.* Randomised trial of high-dose isosorbide dinitrate plus low-dose furosemide versus high-dose furosemide plus low-dose isosorbide dinitrate in severe pulmonary edema. Lancet 1998; 351: 389–393.
23. Sharon A, Shpirer I, Kaluski E, *et al.* High-dose intravenous isosorbide-dinitrate is safer and better than Bi-PAP ventilation combined with conventional treatment for severe pulmonary edema. J Am Coll Cardiol 2000; 36: 832–837.
24. Cotter G, Moshkovitz Y, Kaluski E, *et al.* The role of cardiac power and systemic vascular resistance in the pathophysiology and diagnosis of patients with acute congestive heart failure. Eur J Heart Fail 2003; 5: 443–451.
25. Cotter G, Williams SG, Vered Z, Tan LB. Role of cardiac power in heart failure. Curr Opin Cardiol 2003; 18: 215–222.
26. Levine TB, Levine AB, Kathawala M, Narins B, Kaminski P. Paradoxical hypertension after reversal of heart failure in patients treated with intensive vasodilator therapy. Am J Hypertens 1998; 11: 1041–1047.
27. Zampaglione B, Pascale C, Marchisio M, Cavallo-Perin P. Hypertensive urgencies and emergencies: prevalence and clinical presentation. Hypertension 1996; 27: 144–147.
28. Badgett RG, Lucey CR, Mulrow CD. Can the clinical examination diagnose left-sided heart failure in adults? JAMA 1997; 277: 1712–1719.
29. Ghali JK, Kadakia S, Cooper RS, Liao YL. Bedside diagnosis of preserved versus impaired left ventricular systolic function in heart failure. Am J Cardiol 1991; 67: 1002–1006.
30. Eagle KA, Quertermous T, Singer DE, *et al.* Left ventricular ejection fraction: physician estimates compared with gated blood pool scan measurements. Arch Intern Med 1988; 148: 882–885.
31. Vasan RS, Levy D. Defining diastolic heart failure: a call for standardized diagnostic criteria. Circulation 2000; 101: 2118–2121.
32. Gandhi SK, Powers JC, Nomeir AM, *et al.* The pathogenesis of acute pulmonary edema associated with hypertension. N Engl J Med 2001; 344: 17–22.
33. Clark LT, Garfein OB, Dwyer EM Jr. Acute pulmonary edema due to ischemic heart disease without

accompanying myocardial infarction: natural history and clinical profile. Am J Med 1983; 75: 332–336.
34. Dodek A, Kassebaum DG, Bristow JD. Pulmonary edema in coronary-artery disease without cardiomegaly: paradox of the stiff heart. N Engl J Med 1972; 286: 1347–1350.
35. Chin MH, Goldman L. Correlates of major complications or death in patients admitted to the hospital with congestive heart failure. Arch Intern Med 1996; 156: 1814–1820.
36. Marmor A, Schneeweiss A. Prognostic value of noninvasively obtained left ventricular contractile reserve in patients with severe heart failure. J Am Coll Cardiol 1997; 29: 422–428.
37. Williams SG, Cooke GA, Wright DJ, *et al.* Peak exercise cardiac power output; a direct indicator of cardiac function strongly predictive of prognosis in chronic heart failure. Eur Heart J 2001; 22: 1496–1503.
38. Cohen-Solal A, Tabet JY, Logeart D, Bourgoin P, Tokmakova M, Dahan M. A non-invasively determined surrogate of cardiac power ("circulatory power") at peak exercise is a powerful prognostic factor in chronic heart failure. Eur Heart J 2002; 23: 806–814.
39. Nohria A, Lewis E, Stevenson LW. Medical management of advanced heart failure. JAMA 2002; 287: 628–640.
40. Sherman LG, Liang CS, Baumgardner S, Charuzi Y, Chardo F, Kim CS. Piretanide, a potent diuretic with potassium-sparing properties, for the treatment of congestive heart failure. Clin Pharmacol Ther 1986; 40: 587–594.
41. Patterson JH, Adams KF Jr., Applefeld MM, Corder CN, Masse BR. Oral torsemide in patients with chronic congestive heart failure: effects on body weight, edema, and electrolyte excretion. Torsemide Investigators Group. Pharmacotherapy 1994; 14: 514–521.
42. Walma EP, Hoes AW, van Dooren C, Prins A, van der Does E. Withdrawal of long-term diuretic medication in elderly patients: a double blind randomised trial. BMJ 1997; 315: 464–468.
43. Andrews R, Charlesworth A, Evans A, Cowley AJ. A double-blind, cross-over comparison of the effects of a loop diuretic and a dopamine receptor agonist as first line therapy in patients with mild congestive heart failure. Eur Heart J 1997; 18: 852–857.
44. Kubo SH, Clark M, Laragh JH, Borer JS, Cody RJ. Identification of normal neurohormonal activity in mild congestive heart failure and stimulating effect of upright posture and diuretics. Am J Cardiol 1987; 60: 1322–1328.
45. Neuberg GW, Miller AB, O'Connor CM, *et al.* Diuretic resistance predicts mortality in patients with advanced heart failure. Am Heart J 2002; 144: 31–38.
46. Francis GS, Siegel RM, Goldsmith SR, Olivari MT, Levine TB, Cohn JN. Acute vasoconstrictor response to intravenous furosemide in patients with chronic congestive heart failure: activation of the neurohumoral axis. Ann Intern Med 1985; 103: 1–6.
47. Bayliss J, Norell M, Canepa-Anson R, Sutton G, Poole-Wilson P. Untreated heart failure: clinical and neuroendocrine effects of introducing diuretics. Br Heart J 1987; 57: 17–22.
48. Fonarow GC. The treatment targets in acute decompensated heart failure. Rev Cardiovasc Med 2001; 2: 7–12.
49. Cohn JN, Archibald DG, Ziesche S, *et al.* Effect of vasodilator therapy on mortality in chronic congestive heart failure: results of a Veterans Administration Cooperative Study. N Engl J Med 1986; 314: 1547–1552.
50. Fonarow GC, Chelimsky-Fallick C, Stevenson LW, *et al.* Effect of direct vasodilation with hydralazine versus angiotensin-converting enzyme inhibition with captopril on mortality in advanced heart failure: the Hy-C trial. J Am Coll Cardiol 1992; 19: 842–850.
51. The SOLVD Investigators. Effect of enalapril on mortality and the development of heart failure in asymptomatic patients with reduced left ventricular ejection fractions. N Engl J Med 1992; 327: 685–691.
52. Pfeffer MA, Braunwald E, Moye LA, *et al.* Effect of captopril on mortality and morbidity in patients with left ventricular dysfunction after myocardial infarction: results of the survival and ventricular enlargement trial. The SAVE Investigators. N Engl J Med 1992; 327: 669–677.
53. Ball SG, Hall AS, Mackintosh AF, *et al.* Effect of ramipril and morbidity of survivors of acute myocardial infarction with clinical evidence of heart failure. Lancet 1993; 342: 821–828.
54. Kober L, Torp-Pedersen C, Carlsen JE, *et al.* A clinical trial of the angiotensin-converting-enzyme inhibitor trandolapril in patients with left ventricular dysfunction after myocardial infarction. Trandolapril Cardiac Evaluation (TRACE) Study Group. N Engl J Med 1995; 333: 1670–1676.
55. Narang R, Swedberg K, Cleland JG. What is the ideal study design for evaluation of treatment for heart failure? Insights from trials assessing the effect of ACE inhibitors on exercise capacity. Eur Heart J 1996; 17: 120–134.
56. The SOLVD Investigators. Effect of enalapril on survival in patients with reduced left ventricular ejection fractions and congestive heart failure. N Engl J Med 1991; 325: 293–302.

57. Yusuf S, Sleight P, Pogue J, Bosch J, Davies R, Dagenais G. Effects of an angiotensin-converting-enzyme inhibitor, ramipril, on cardiovascular events in high-risk patients. The Heart Outcomes Prevention Evaluation Study Investigators. N Engl J Med 2000; 342: 145–153.
58. Fox KM, EURopean trial On reduction of cardiac events with Perindopril in stable coronary Artery disease (EUROPA) Investigators. Efficacy of perindopril in reduction of cardiovascular events among patients with stable coronary artery disease: randomised, double-blind, placebo-controlled, multicentre trial (the EUROPA study). Lancet 2003; 362: 782–788.
59. Gustafsson F, Torp-Pedersen C, Kober L, Hildebrandt P. Effect of angiotensin converting enzyme inhibition after acute myocardial infarction in patients with arterial hypertension. TRACE Study Group, Trandolapril Cardiac Event. J Hypertens 1997; 15: 793–798.
60. Fonarow GC, Stevenson LW, Walden JA, *et al.* Impact of a comprehensive heart failure management program on hospital readmission and functional status of patients with advanced heart failure. J Am Coll Cardiol 1997; 30: 725–732.
61. Fonarow GC. Pharmacologic therapies for acutely decompensated heart failure. Rev Cardiovasc Med 2002; 3: S18–S27.
62. Nelson GI, Silke B, Ahuja RC, Hussain M, Taylor SH. Haemodynamic advantages of isosorbide dinitrate over frusemide in acute heart-failure following myocardial infarction. Lancet 1983; 1: 730–733.
63. Gruppo Italiano per lo Studio della Sopravvivenza nell'infarto Miocardico (GISSI-3). Effects of lisinopril and transdermal glyceryl trinitrate singly and together on 6-week mortality and ventricular function after acute myocardial infarction. Lancet 1994; 343: 1115–1122.
64. Burnett JC Jr., Kao PC, Hu DC, *et al.* Atrial natriuretic peptide elevation in congestive heart failure in the human. Science 1986; 231: 1145–1147.
65. Creager MA, Hirsch AT, Nabel EG, Cutler SS, Colucci WS, Dzau VJ. Responsiveness of atrial natriuretic factor to reduction in right atrial pressure in patients with chronic congestive heart failure. J Am Coll Cardiol 1988; 11: 1191–1198.
66. Cody RJ, Atlas SA, Laragh JH, *et al.* Atrial natriuretic factor in normal subjects and heart failure patients: plasma levels and renal, hormonal, and hemodynamic responses to peptide infusion. J Clin Invest 1986; 78: 1362–1374.
67. Grantham JA, Borgeson DD, Burnett JC Jr. BNP: pathophysiological and potential therapeutic roles in acute congestive heart failure. Am J Physiol 1997; 272: R1077–R1083.
68. Mukoyama M, Nakao K, Hosoda K, *et al.* Brain natriuretic peptide as a novel cardiac hormone in humans: evidence for an exquisite dual natriuretic peptide system, atrial natriuretic peptide and brain natriuretic peptide. J Clin Invest 1991; 87: 1402–1412.
69. Kazanegra R, Cheng V, Garcia A, *et al.* A rapid test for B-type natriuretic peptide correlates with falling wedge pressures in patients treated for decompensated heart failure: a pilot study. J Card Fail 2001; 7: 21–29.
70. Franco-Saenz R, Somani P, Mulrow PJ. Effect of atrial natriuretic peptide (8–33-Met ANP) in patients with hypertension. Am J Hypertens 1992; 5: 266–275.
71. Hirooka Y, Takeshita A, Imaizumi T, *et al.* Attenuated forearm vasodilative response to intra-arterial atrial natriuretic peptide in patients with heart failure. Circulation 1990; 82: 147–153.
72. Diaz T, Alderman J. Nesiritide for the treatment of diastolic dysfunction. Congest Heart Fail 2004; 10: 154–157.
73. Colucci WS, Elkayam U, Horton DP, *et al.* Intravenous nesiritide, a natriuretic peptide, in the treatment of decompensated congestive heart failure. Nesiritide Study Group. N Engl J Med 2000; 343: 246–253.
74. Publication Committee for the VMAC Investigators (Vasodilatation in the Management of Acute CHF). Intravenous nesiritide vs. nitroglycerin for treatment of decompensated congestive heart failure: a randomized controlled trial. JAMA 2002; 287: 1531–1540.
75. Kelly J. Flash pulmonary oedema: think of coronary artery disease first. Lancet 2001; 358: 1646–1647.
76. Walker F, Walker DA, Nielsen M. Flash pulmonary oedema. Lancet 2001; 358: 556.
77. Jessup M, Brozena S. Heart failure. N Engl J Med 2003; 348: 2007–2018.

CHAPTER 17

Psychiatric and psychosocial risks in acutely decompensated chronic heart failure patients

Wei Jiang, Christopher M O'Connor, Ranga R Krishnan

Introduction

Chronic heart failure is the end stage of many diseases of the heart and has a major negative impact on the American public. While mortality from coronary artery disease (CAD) is declining, the incidence of chronic heart failure is increasing. More than 50% of these cases are a result of CAD or ischemic heart disease (IHD). As of 1999, out of 4.8 million people in the United States living with chronic heart failure, 49% were men and 51% were women.[1] Approximately 550 000 new cases of heart failure are diagnosed annually. Experts expect this number to continue to rise as the population ages and as increasing numbers of people survive acute myocardial infarctions (AMIs).[2] As a major cause of morbidity and mortality, chronic heart failure is deadly as well as prevalent. Chronic heart failure is now the leading cause for hospitalization in patients > 65 years of age and it is the most costly cardiovascular disease in the United States. Chronic heart failure costs represent the largest single Medicare expenditure, as well as the most common discharge diagnosis for Medicare beneficiaries. In 1998, approximately 1 million chronic heart failure admissions totaled over $7 billion in Medicare spending, with an estimated total cost for chronic heart failure care exceeding $20 billion.[3]

Many advances in the treatment of chronic heart failure, such as angiotensin-converting enzyme (ACE) inhibitors, beta-blockers, and aldosterone receptor antagonist, have improved survival rates.[4] In addition, disease management programs involving patient education, nurse follow-up, and home visits targeting medication compliance have been able to reduce readmissions.[5–8] In spite of these efforts, 1-year mortality for patients with chronic heart failure approaches 10% for men and 20% for women, while 5-year mortality reaches more than 50% for both men and women.[1,9] Readmission rates are as high as 25% to 50% within 3 to 6 months after discharge.[1,10–12] Recent investigations seeking the roles of psychological factors in chronic heart failure have increased our understanding of the clinical implications of specific psychological factors in the progression of chronic heart failure. Despite this evidence and the importance of psychological factors in the outcome of chronic heart failure patients, these factors are often overlooked in clinical practice. This phenomenon may have several potential explanations including: (1) research findings about the negative link between psychosocial factors and chronic heart failure outcomes has not been adequately disseminated; (2) physicians or other health care providers in the non-psychiatric setting are not familiar with the measurement and interpretation of psychosocial factors; (3) many health care providers are concerned with the safety of using psychotropic medications in the chronic heart failure population; and

(4) the time available to focus on psychosocial factors in these patients is highly limited due to managed health care.

This chapter explores the roles of psychosocial factors and their potential mechanisms in chronic heart failure patients by reviewing results from the literature and scientific insights into psychological risks such as depression, anxiety, delirium, and social support in patients with acute decompensated heart failure (ADHF). Our aim is to increase the recognition of the clinical impact of psychological risks in acutely ill chronic heart failure patients.

Depression

Perhaps the most frequently explored psychological factor in patients with cardiac disease is depression. Most studies, especially those using self-administered questionnaires, have used an inclusive approach, i.e., the studies did not necessarily exclude subjects who might have had symptoms of mania or hypomania in the past. According to the *Diagnostic and Statistical Manual*, 4th edition (DSM-IV),[13] the standard psychiatric diagnostic manual, those patients would be identified as having bipolar disorder.[12] Bipolar disorder, which is much less common than unipolar disorders, is easier to identify and treat. Bipolar disorder itself and symptoms of mania or hypomania have not been considered a risk factor for IHD and chronic heart failure. In contrast, unipolar depressive disorders are the most common psychiatric problems in patients with cardiac diseases or other medical illnesses.[14–16] Unipolar depressive disorders include major depression, minor depression, and dysthymia. Studies examining the role of depression in cardiac disease have usually identified patients who are at the threshold of depression, then further identified patients with major depression at a specific point during the study. Therefore, patients in those studies with recognizable depression, but not major depression, were likely to have dysthymia or subclinical depression.

Depression and the progression of ischemic heart disease

Because IHD is the cause of chronic heart failure in more than 50% of patients, it is worth discussing the impact of depression on IHD.[12,17] In terms of primary prevention, depression may well be considered a primary risk factor for the development of IHD. Many epidemiological studies have consistently demonstrated that depression is associated with a greater likelihood of MI or cardiac death in patients without IHD at the time of assessment for depression.[18–30] To provide a thorough overview, we have summarized findings from published studies that have enrolled at least 2500 subjects (Table 17.1).[19–22,28,33–35] Self-administered questionnaires or standardized psychiatric interviews were used to identify depression in each of these studies. Although the tools used to assess depression varied, the finding that depression was associated with increased cardiac mortality or other forms of CAD was consistent across almost all the studies. The longest cohort study in the literature, but not included in Table 17.1, examining the primary effects of depression on IHD development, by Ford *et al.*, followed approximately 1100 medical school graduates for a total of 37 years.[30] On average, these subjects were 26 years old (standard deviation [SD] 2) when depression was assessed and none of them had IHD. During the 37-year follow-up, the subjects who were considered to have clinical depression via psychiatric interview had twice the rate of MIs as those without depression.

Depression is also a secondary risk factor in terms of preventing further disease progression. Depression is very common in patients with IHD. The rate of major depressive disorder (MDD) in IHD patients is approximately 4 to 5 times higher than the rate for community-dwelling adults, who are reported to have MDD in 5% to 9% of women and 2% to 3% of men.[13] The prevalence of MDD ranges from 16% to 20% in patients with a recent MI (< 30 days),[31,36–38] and up to 23% in patients with stable CAD.[13] The prevalence of minor depression or subclinical depression is even higher than that of MDD.[32,39,40] Table 17.2 outlines the prevalence of MDD and other forms of depression in various cardiac populations.

Recently, a number of studies have examined the relationship of depression in patients who had documented IHD, including MI, coronary artery bypass graft (CABG) surgery, and stable or unstable angina.

Table 17.1. *Studies of the relationship between depression and ischemic heart disease development among individuals without evidence of ischemic heart disease*

Author (year)	Country	Age (yr)	No. of patients	Gender (M/F)	Measures	Follow-up (yr)	Events (n)	Types of events	Relative risk*
Appels (1993)[143]	Netherlands	39–65	3877	3877/0	Depression (Maastricht questionnaire)	4.5	59	MI (21 fatal; 38 non-fatal)	2.28 for non-fatal MI; no association with fatal MI.
Anda (1993)[19]	United States	45–77	2832	1345/1487	Depression affect, hopelessness (subscale of general well-being schedule)	12.4	189	Fatal MI	1.5, depression affect; 1.6, moderate hopelessness; 2.1, severe hopelessness
Aromaa (1994)[20]	Finland	40–64	8000	2420/2935	Depression (GHQ, PSE)	6.6	91	Fatal CAD	3.36
Everson (1996)[21]	Finland	42–60	2428	2428/0	Hopelessness	6	A. 87 B. 95	A. CV death B. MI	A. 2.52, moderate hopelessness; 3.9, high hopelessness B. 2.39, high hopelessness; increased but nonsignificant, moderate hopelessness
Wassertheil-Smoller (1996)[22]	United States	≥60	4367	2053/2314	Depression (CES-D)	4.5	A. 355 B. 321 C. 126	A. All deaths B. MI or stroke C. MI	A. 1.26 B. 1.18 C. 1.14 but not significant*
Mendes de Leon (1998)[24]	United States	65–99	2812	945/1446	Depression (CES-D)	9	A. 255 B. 391	A. CAD death B. Non-fatal MI, cardiac death	A and B: 1.03‡
Ariyo (2000)[25]	United States	≥65	4493	NA	Depression (CES-D)	6	A. B.	A. CAD incidence B. All-cause mortality	(every 5-point increase in CES-D scores) 1.29 (every 5-point increase in CES-D scores)
Ferketich (2000)[26]	United States		7893	2886/5007	Depression (CES-D)	10	A. 129/137 B. 187/187	A. CAD incidence M/F B. CAD death M/F	A. 1.71/1.73 (M/F) B. 2.34/0.74 (M/F) (95% CI, 0.4–1.48)
Penninx (2001)[27]	Netherlands	55–85	2397	1091/1306	Depression (DSM-III, CES-D)	4		Cardiac mortality	3.9, major depression by DSM-III 1.5 (95% CI, 0.9–2.6), minor depression (CES-D score ≥16 but not meeting DSM-III for major depression)

* Adjusted for multiple factors which vary across studies (in general age, conventional cardiovascular risk factors such as smoking, cholesterol, weight or body mass index, and physical conditions at study enrollment).

† Per 5-unit increase in CES-D score during follow-up versus baseline.

‡ Per unit increase in CES-D score.

Abbreviations: CAD = coronary artery disease; CES-D = Center for Epidemiologic Studies Depression; CI = confidence interval; CV = cardiovascular; DSM-III = *Diagnostic and Statistical Manual*, 3rd edition; F = female; GHQ = General Health Questionnaire; M = male; MI = myocardial infarction; PSE = Psychiatric State Examination.

Table 17.2. *Prevalence of depression in patients with cardiovascular disease*

Author (year)	Cardiovascular disease	No. of patients	Major depressive disorder (%)	Elevated depression symptoms/ minor depression* (%)
Frasure-Smith (1993, 1999)[31,39]	Myocardial infarction	222	16	17
Lespérance (2000)[34]	Unstable angina	430	15	26
Jiang (2001)[12]	Chronic heart failure	374	14	20
Hance (1996)[144]	Catheterization	200	17	17
Connerney (2001)[145]	Coronary artery bypass grafting	309	20	8

* This category does not include patients who met the diagnosis of major depressive disorder.

Results from these studies have shown that depression is associated with significantly increased rates of death and non-fatal cardiac events. In the post-MI patient population, studies have shown that the mortality rate at 6 months post-MI, is 3 to 5 times higher in patients who met the DSM-III or DSM-IV criteria for MDD or whose depressive symptoms were rated as moderate to severe using the Standard Instruments of Psychological Inventory, as compared to non-depressed patients.

Frasure-Smith *et al.*[32] followed a group of post-MI patients for a period of 18 months. They found that patients with Beck Depression Inventory (BDI) scores ≥ 10 have mortality rates that are 6.6 times higher than patients whose BDI scores were < 10. Even after controlling for conventional prognostic risk factors, such as age, severity of cardiac dysfunction, and history of MI, this increased risk remained and persisted for 2 years[35] and longer.[41]

Two recent studies from the United Kingdom, which used either BDI[40] or the Hospital Anxiety and Depression scale,[42] found that depression was significantly associated with a decline in quality of life during a 12-month follow-up in post-MI patients. However, depression was not associated with increased mortality. Failure to find a relationship between depression and mortality is likely the result of an inadequate assessment of depression in limited sample size. Carney *et al.*[43] found that depression was the best predictor of cardiac events (MI, CABG, or death) at 1 year, among other risk factors, such as smoking, severity of coronary stenosis, and left ventricular (LV) function.

The adverse association between depression and cardiac-related death lasted for > 20 years in patients with stable IHD.[29] The adverse association between depression and poor cardiac outcome was also found during a 12-month follow-up after admission for unstable angina.[34] It is important to note that the severity of depression in the majority of these studies is subclinical, using self-administered questionnaires.

Depression and chronic heart failure

Recently, a number of studies have focused on the impact of depression in patients with chronic heart failure. Not surprisingly, depression was common and it was associated with an increased risk of poor prognosis in these patients.

In studies assessing depression with self-administered questionnaires and standardized diagnostic psychiatric interviews, the point prevalence of MDD[13] has been reported in the range of 14% to 36.5%.[44,45] The variation in rate among studies likely reflects the different characteristics of patients studied and differences in establishing a diagnosis of MDD. Table 17.3 summarizes the results of studies examining depression in patients hospitalized with chronic heart failure.

The highest rate of MDD (36.5%) was noted in Koenig's study[45] involving 107 chronic heart failure patients aged 60 years or older who were

Table 17.3. *Depression and outcome of hospitalized chronic heart failure patients*

Author (year)	Type of study	No. of patients	NYHA class	Depression measure	Depression (%)	Outcome
Freedland (1991)[44]	Cross-sectional	60	2.6–2.9	Structured interview (DMS-III-R)	17.0	Death at 1 year 50 vs. 29, NS
Fraticelli (1996)[146]	Cross-sectional	50	≥II	GDS	68.0 (GDS ≥ 11)	N/A
Krumholz (1998)[136]	Longitudinal	292	N/A	CES-D	23.3 (CES-D > 16)	Cardiac events 53 vs. 47, NS
Koenig (1998)[45]	Cross-sectional	107	N/A	DSM-IV/CES-D	36.4/21.5	Death 29 vs. 20, NS
Havranek (1999)[147]	Cross-sectional	45	N/A	CES-D	24.4 (CES-D ≥ 16)	N/A
Jiang (2001)[12]	Longitudinal	357	≥II	BDI/DMS-IV	35.3 (BDI ≥ 10) 13.9 DMS-IV MDD	Mortality/ re-hospitalizations $P < 0.05$
Vaccarino (2001)[148]	Longitudinal	391	N/A	GDS	35 (GDS ≥ 6 < 8) 33.5 (GDS ≥ 8 < 11) 9 (GDS ≥ 11)	Functional decline or death 31 vs. 43 vs. 49 vs. 60 $P < 0.05$
Rozzini (2002)[149]	Longitudinal	86	≥III	GDS	45.3 (GDS ≥ 6)	Death 20.5 vs. 14.9, $P < 0.05$
Fulop (2003)[150]	Longitudinal	203	N/A	GDS	36 (GDS ≥ 10)	Medical encounters/ re-hospitalization days $P < 0.05$

Abbreviations: BDI = Beck Depression Inventory; CES-D = Center for Epidemiological Studies-Depression Scale; DSM-III = *Diagnostic and Statistical Manual*, 3rd edition; DSM-IV = *Diagnostic and Statistical Manual*, 4th edition; GDS = Geriatric Depression Scale; MDD = major depressive disorder; N/A = not available; NS = not significant; NYHA = New York Heart Association.

admitted to the general medicine, cardiology, or neurology service in a tertiary-care hospital and remained on the service for at least 3 days. Patients who were transferred to or from other services or nursing homes were excluded. All 107 patients underwent a standardized diagnostic psychiatric interview by the same psychiatrist. The higher rate of MDD depression in this study, as compared to other studies, is likely due to patients being more ill (to be included, patients had to be hospitalized for > 3 days) and all patients undergoing the standardized diagnostic psychiatric interview.

Jiang *et al.* defined the point prevalence of MDD to be 14% among patients whose BDI scores were ≥ 10 in a sample of 357 patients with New York Heart Association (NYHA) class II or greater.[12] All participants were first screened by the BDI self-administered questionnaire. The 126 patients who scored ≥ 10 on the BDI then underwent the standardized diagnostic psychiatric interview. Of those patients, 26 did not complete the interview; this probably had a major effect on the lower rate of MDD because those patients had higher BDI scores and higher mortality as compared to patients who underwent the standardized diagnostic psychiatric interview during follow-up. Freedland *et al.*[44] reported a 17% incidence of MDD in a sample of 60 chronic heart failure patients who were ≥ 70 years old. Despite the large variation of incidence in these studies, it is fair to say that the prevalence of MDD is indeed higher in patients with chronic heart failure, possibly 3 to 5 times higher than the prevalence in the general population.[13] In addition to MDD, a large proportion of patients with heart failure are considered to have subclinical or minor depression, as measured by self-administered questionnaires, such as the BDI or Center for Epidemiological Studies-Depression Scale (CES-D), at approximately 21.5% in both Koenig's study[45] and Jiang's study.[12]

Early studies investigating depression in patients with heart failure failed to show a relationship between depression and increased mortality or re-hospitalizations, possibly because of inadequate sample size or patient selection bias. In the study by Freedland *et al.*, the 1-year mortality rate was considerably higher for depressed patients (50%) than for non-depressed patients (29%). The statistical insignificance of the difference in mortality rates between depressed and nondepressed patients was thought to be related to the small sample size (total n = 60),[44] which yielded too few end-points. Although studies by Koenig and Krumholz showed a higher rate of mortality in depressed patients with chronic heart failure, the differences were not statistically significant. Again, the lack of significance is likely a result of low power or patient selection bias. In the Jiang *et al.* study, patients with major depression were 2 to 3 times more likely to die or be readmitted to the hospital during 1-year follow-up as compared to patients who were not depressed. This difference became significant within 3 months after the assessment for depression. More importantly, the adverse effects of depression on the prognosis in patients with heart failure were independent of traditional risk factors such as age, NYHA class, and baseline ejection fraction (EF) (Table 17.4).[12]

One could easily conclude that such a negative association between depression and chronic heart failure is just an extension of the relationship between depression and the outcome in IHD. The study by Jiang *et al.* reported that patients whose chronic heart failure etiology was IHD suffered a higher rate of death during 1-year follow-up than patients whose chronic heart failure was not related to IHD (21.0 vs. 10.0, $P = 0.003$). However, the etiology of heart failure (ischemic vs. nonischemic) did not alter the predictability of depression for poor prognosis (Table 17.4). Faris *et al.*[46] in particular followed a cohort of 396 patients with nonischemic heart failure for 3 to 84 months (average of 48 months) after identifying consecutively hospitalized patients from the hospital records. Of those patients, 21% satisfied the authors' criteria for clinical depression and 67% of those patients had NYHA class ≥ II. During the follow-up period, patients with depression had a 3-fold higher rate of death as compared to patients without depression. The re-hospitalization rate of depressed patients was also significantly higher. In addition, patients with depression were reported to have more symptoms ($P < 0.0001$), longer duration of symptoms ($P = 0.04$), lower exercise capacity ($P = 0.02$), poorer LV function ($P = 0.04$), higher rate of left bundle branch block

Table 17.4. *Odds of mortality and morbidity in patients with heart failure and major depressive disorder versus no depression*

	Odds ratio	95% Confidence interval	*P*-value
Univariate analysis			
Mortality at 1 year	2.23	1.04–4.77	0.038
Morbidity at 1 year	3.07	1.41–6.66	0.005
Multivariate analysis*			
Mortality at 1 year	2.18	0.97–4.92	0.059
Morbidity at 1 year	2.62	1.19–5.79	0.017
Multivariate analysis†			
Mortality at 1 year	2.12	0.94–4.81	0.072
Morbidity at 1 year	2.57	1.16–5.68	0.019

* Adjustment for age, New York Heart Association (NYHA) class, and baseline ejection fraction.
† Adjustment for age, NYHA class, baseline ejection fraction, and cause of heart failure.
(Adapted, with permission, from Jiang *et al.*[12])

(LBBB) ($P = 0.05$), and a higher rate of renal impairment ($P = 0.008$). Clearly, there is another mechanism at work.

The negative impact of depression on chronic heart failure consequently results in significantly increased costs for chronic heart failure care, as demonstrated by the findings in the recent study by Sullivan *et al.*[47] This study compared the cost difference between depressed and nondepressed patients by examining the cost of 1098 adult patients who were first hospitalized with a primary diagnosis of chronic heart failure between January 1, 1993, and December 31, 1997. Data were gathered from the computerized cost accounting system of a large staff-model health maintenance organization (HMO), the Group Health Cooperative (GHC) of Puget Sound, Washington. Depression was assumed based on documentation of antidepressant prescription with or without a diagnosis of depression (except for bupropion hydrochloride prescription for smoking cessation). Use and cost of all health care services covered by the GHC were calculated for the 2 years before and 1 year after each of the 1098 patient's index chronic heart failure hospitalization. A total of 426 patients (38.8%) in this sample received antidepressant prescriptions and only 26.8% received a diagnosis of depression. Patients who received antidepressant prescriptions, whether or not they received a diagnosis of depression, had stayed longer in the hospital during the index admission, visited their doctors more frequently, obtained a higher number of refills for medications, and spent greater sums of money for the treatment of their conditions. As the authors concluded, these increased costs were due to increased inpatient and outpatient medical utilization, not increased mental health utilization.[47]

Potential mechanisms for the adverse effects of depression in cardiac diseases

A number of potential mechanisms have been suggested as being responsible for the increased risk of IHD in patients with depression. Several promising hypotheses include increased activation of the hypothalamic-pituitary-adrenal axis, increased platelet aggregation, and abnormalities in the sympathetic-parasympathetic system. Greater cerebral spinal fluid concentration of corticotropin-releasing hormone,[48] reduced function of the glucocorticoid receptor,[49] and higher plasma cortical level post-dexamethasone suppression (World Health Organization Collaborative Study, 1987)[50] have all been demonstrated in patients with depressive disorders as compared to normal controls. Corticosteroids can induce hypertension, hypercholesterolemia, and glucose dysregulation. The sympatho-medullary system, whose principal hormones include epinephrine and norepinephrine (NE), is particularly active in patients suffering from depression. Elevated plasma levels of NE and its metabolites, such as vanillylmandelic acid, in the urine are found in depressed patients.[51,52] While being stressed (i.e., cold or orthostatically challenged), depressed or melancholic patients displayed a greater increase in plasma levels of NE than normal controls.[53,54] A hyperactive sympatho-medullary system contributes to the progression of IHD and chronic heart failure through the effects of catecholamines on the heart, vessels, and platelets.[55] High corticosteroids levels are associated with the mobilization of free fatty acids and hyperlipidemia along with impending endothelial inflammation and excessive clotting. All of these are risk factors for the development of IHD as well as poor prognosis of IHD.[56,57]

Diminished heart rate variability (HRV) is another known predictor of increased mortality in chronic heart failure and IHD.[58–60] Several studies have recently observed that decreased HRV occurs in patients with IHD and MDD.[61] Increased platelet aggregation, a recently discovered biological abnormality in depression, plays a crucial role in coronary occlusion. In one study, depressed patients without IHD showed a 41% increase in platelet activity in contrast to normal controls.[62,63] Reichborn-Kjennerud *et al.* found that platelet monoamine oxidase activity was significantly elevated in depressed patients, especially women.[63] Further, among patients with IHD, elevation of beta-thromboglobulin level, plasma platelet factor 4, and expression of platelet surface receptors for glycoprotein IIb/IIIa and P-selectin is related to depression.[64]

More recently, patients with MDD were found to have activation of their inflammatory response system.[65] Serum interleukin-6 (IL-6), IL-8, IL-6 receptor, IL-6 receptor antagonist, gp130, and prostaglandin E2 were all found to be higher in depressed patients than in normal controls, which may be related to a low plasma level of tryptophan.[66] Activation of the inflammatory process is one of the mechanisms of coronary plaque rupture and restenosis, resulting in increased cardiac events.[67,68] Behavioral and psychosocial factors have been implicated in the poorer prognosis of depression among patients with heart disease. Depression is associated with reduced physical exercise,[69–71] lower socioeconomic status,[72] poor social-support systems or failure to use social-support resources,[73–76] higher incidence of smoking, and poor adherence to secondary prevention recommendations such as medication management.[77–79]

Perhaps the most direct link found is the association between depression and mental stress-induced myocardial ischemia. Myocardial ischemia, an important measure of the clinical activity of IHD, occurs when the myocardium does not receive enough blood supply as a result of either coronary constriction, high demand, or both. Mental stress has been shown to be a trigger by inducing myocardial ischemia in a laboratory setting and during routine daily living. Mental stress-induced myocardial ischemia (MSIMI) has been found to predict future increased adverse cardiac events.[80–82] In a sample of 132 patients with IHD and a recent positive exercise test, MSIMI was found to be associated with increased cardiac events during a 5-year follow-up (odds ratio [OR], 2.8; 95% confidence interval [CI], 1.0–7.7; $P < 0.5$), independent of age, history of prior MI, and baseline cardiac function. However, the rate of adverse cardiac events was not associated with exercise-induced ischemia in that study (OR, 1.5; 95% CI, 0.6–3.9; $P = 0.39$). Sheps *et al.* demonstrated that mental stress-induced ischemia was associated with an almost 3-fold increase in mortality among IHD patients.[82]

In a recently published study, Jiang *et al.* examined the relationship between depression and myocardial ischemia during mental stress testing in a sample of 135 patients with stable IHD (Figure 17.1).[83] Depression was assessed using the CES-D. The mean CES-D score was 8.2 (SD, 7.4; range, 0–47) with a median of score 7. Logistic regression models using restricted cubic splines revealed a curvilinear relation between CES-D scores and the probability of ischemia triggered by mental stress and during daily life. For patients with CES-D scores ≤ 19 (81.5% of the study population), a 5-point increment in the CES-D score was associated with roughly a 2-fold increase in the likelihood of

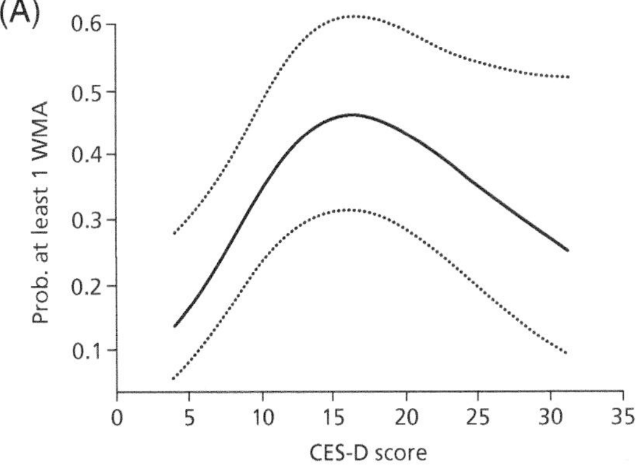

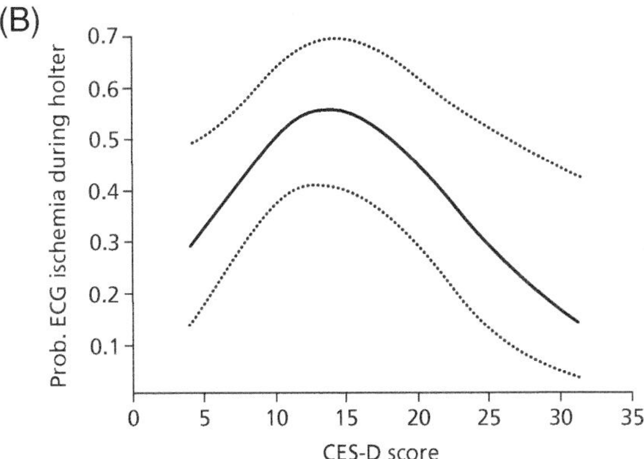

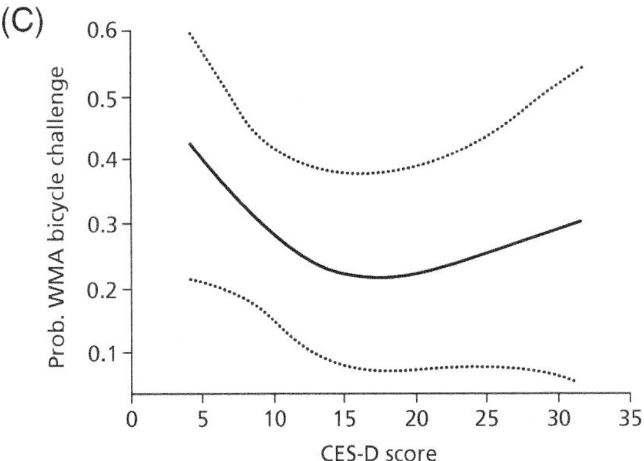

Figure 17.1. *Predicted probability of ischemia as function of the Center for Epidemiological Studies-Depression (CES-D) score for mental stress testing, daily living, and exercise testing. Solid line represents fitted probability of ischemia; dotted lines are 95% confidence limits. (A) Mental stress induced ischemia, (B) Daily ischemia, and (C) Exercise ischemia. (Adapted, with permission, from Jiang et al.*[83]*)*
Abbreviation: *WMA = wall motion abnormality*

MSIMI. For patients with CES-D scores > 19, the relationship between scores and ischemia during mental stress tended to be inverse but that portion of the sample size is very small (18.5%). Similar patterns were also observed for CES-D scores and ischemia during daily life. However, depression was not related to exercise-induced ischemia (Figure 17.1). These findings strongly indicate that myocardial ischemia may be a significant mechanism by which depression increases the risk of mortality and morbidity in patients with IHD.

The observed inverse association between higher levels of depressive symptoms (CES-D > 19) and ischemia was unexpected. The sample size was very low in the high CES-D subset (> 19) making the results susceptible to the effect of outliers that could manifest low ischemia. This would be compatible for reduced ischemia by all three measures. Nevertheless, the pattern of exercise-induced ischemic activity is almost in opposition to the pattern of mental stress-induced ischemic activity and ischemia during daily living (Figure 17.1). It is possible that the severely depressed patients did not try as hard emotionally because their systolic blood pressure response was characteristically lower, thought not statistically different, as compared to patients whose depressive symptoms were mild to moderate during mental stress testing. Because only 18.5% of the patients had CES-D scores > 19, these results need to be confirmed in a sample with greater representation among the more severely depressed patients.

The chief underlying mechanism in mental stress-induced myocardial ischemia is probably the transient micro-vasoconstriction of atherosclerotic coronary arteries. Using intracoronary Doppler, Yeung *et al.*[84] assessed the change in coronary blood flow during mental stress testing and endothelium-dependent vasodilatation in a group of IHD patients. Responses of the coronary arteries varied from 38% constriction to 29% dilation, with coronary blood flow ranging from a decrease of 48% to an increase of 42%. Compared to individuals without IHD, the coronary microcirculation of IHD patients was found to fail to dilate during mental stress testing,[85] a response likely mediated by alpha-adrenergic receptor activation. Furthermore, systemic vascular resistance (SVR) was found to increase significantly during mental stress, which is positively correlated with an increase in plasma epinephrine.[86] The findings of Jiang *et al.* indicate that mild to moderate depression increases the susceptibility of insufficient microcirculation of coronary as a response to negative emotional stress.[83]

In summary, depression plays a significant role in the prognosis of chronic heart failure. It puts chronic heart failure patients at high risk for death and increased morbidities. This risk cannot simply be accounted for by chronic heart failure with an ischemic cause. Promptly recognizing depression and providing effective treatment appears to be exceedingly imperative in this patient population.

Anxiety

Frequently, anxiety has been found to coexist with depression[87–89] especially in the elderly and medically ill populations. Symptoms of anxiety are seen in as many as 65% of older patients with depression,[90] and these symptoms are thought to be adversely associated with a high risk of IHD. In addition, depression and anxiety tend to share the same risk factors.[91] Despite the high comorbidity of anxiety and depression, anxiety is considered a discrete emotional experience, apart from depression. Characteristically, anxiety is defined as a future-oriented negative affective state with a component of fear, resulting from the perception of threat, typified by a perceived inability to predict, control, or obtain desired results in upcoming situations.[87] Although depression also possesses a high negative affective state, it uniquely features a very low level of positive affect, which distinguishes it from anxiety.[92] There is a paucity of literature on anxiety in individuals with chronic heart failure as well as the interaction between anxiety and depression in chronic heart failure patients. In patients with chronic heart failure, anxiety is thought to strongly correlate with dyspnea and can negatively affect cardiac output.[93]

Many investigators have sought to determine the mechanistic link between anxiety and IHD. Some studies have indicated that anxiety is associated with an increased level of plasma NE.[94,95] Electrophysiology studies have demonstrated that ventricular premature beats (VPBs) increase as a result of the stimulation of certain psychological stresses[96,97] and decrease with a reduction in sympathetic neural inputs.[98,99] This suggests a link between anxiety and electrical instability of the myocardium since VPBs have been identified as risk factors for myocardial electrical instability, and sudden cardiac death.[100,101] The most definitive finding is the association between anxiety and reduction in HRV.[102–105] HRV is a well-accepted indicator of cardiac autonomic modulation. Low or decreased HRV suggests excessive sympathetic or inadequate parasympathetic activity, and it is a powerful, independent predictor of mortality in patients with a recent MI.[106–109] Nevertheless, all the above associations indicating the potential mechanisms of anxiety and cardiac disease have also been observed in depression. For instance, depression is found to be significantly associated with a reduction in HRV for patients with and without IHD.[61,105,110–112]

Suggested by several large-scale, prospective epidemiological cohorts,[113–116] an association may exist between self-reported anxiety symptoms and the risk of developing IHD. Studies examining the association between anxiety and the prognosis of patients with established IHD also suggest that anxiety may be a risk factor for increased death as well as other non-fatal cardiac events. However, other studies either produced negative results[40] or suggested that the adverse prognosis of cardiac patients with high anxiety may be due to the presence of depression rather than anxiety itself.[117] Denollet and Brutsaert found that post-MI patients with an LVEF $\leq 50\%$ and a State and Trait Anxiety Inventory (STAI) score ≥ 48 had an increased mortality during an average 7.9-year follow-up as compared to patients with an STAI score < 48 (OR 3.7; $P = 0.04$). However, the adverse association between anxiety and mortality was not independent from Type D personality (patients with a distressed personality or the tendency to suppress negative emotions) when multiple regression analysis was performed.[41] Majani *et al.* compared the anxiety of 152 hospitalized, male, chronic heart failure patients who were not admitted for anxiety. They found no significant difference in the degree of either state anxiety or trait anxiety (as measured by the Cognitive Behavioral Assessment 2.0 Depression Scale) between patients with chronic heart failure and other medical conditions, although incidence of depression among chronic heart failure patients was significantly higher. The study did not examine prognostic effects of depression.[118]

To understand the role of anxiety in patients with chronic heart failure, we recently performed depression (BDI) and anxiety (STAI) assessments on a total of 291 hospitalized patients with chronic heart failure and then followed them for 1 year.[119] At 1-year follow-up, 15.7% of these patients were deceased. Table 17.5 outlines the demographic and clinical characteristics of the subjects.

Almost 30% of the patients studied might have been considered as having significant anxiety, because 29% of the patients had a state anxiety score ≥ 40 and 28% had a trait anxiety score ≥ 40.[120] Measurements of anxiety and depression were highly correlated. The R value for the scores of state anxiety against trait anxiety was 0.852 ($P < 0.0001$). The R value for state anxiety against depression scores was 0.518 and trait anxiety against depression was 0.585 ($P < 0.0001$). Patients who had died prior to 1-year follow-up had higher BDI scores than patients who were still alive ($P = 0.029$). Nevertheless, there was no difference in anxiety scores between patients who had died and those who were still alive ($P = 0.18$ and $P = 0.48$, respectively) (Table 17.6).

Cox proportional hazards regression model was used to examine the association of anxiety, depression, and several cardiac risk factors with mortality over time (Table 17.7). Age, NYHA class, chronic heart failure with ischemic cause, and depression were significantly associated with increased 1-year mortality among hospitalized chronic heart failure patients. The risk of depression for mortality persisted after adjusting for age, NYHA class, chronic heart failure with ischemic cause, left ventricular ejection fraction (LVEF), and anxiety. Notwithstanding the high correlation of anxiety and depression, anxiety played no negative role in the prognosis of patients with ADHF. It is interesting to note that the significance of the association between depression and increased mortality was attenuated in the model while state anxiety was included as a covariate (Table 17.8).

In another study that examined the role of anxiety in chronic heart failure, Reschke *et al.* found that both self-reported depression and anxiety were negatively correlated with performance on the 6-minute walk test ($R = -0.54$, $P < 0.0001$,

Table 17.5. *Baseline characteristics of patients hospitalized with chronic heart failure*

Characteristic	Data	Reason for index admission (%)	
Age (yr)	63±13	Chronic heart failure	39.9
Male gender (%)	64.2	Acute myocardial infarction	19.2
Race (White/Black/other) (%)	71.6/17.6/3.9	Ischemic heart disease	21.4
Married (%)	66.2	Arrhythmia	16.2
New York Heart Association Class II/III/IV (%)	52.8/38.8/8.5	Other	3.3
Left ventricular ejection fraction (%)	30.2±13.3		
Ischemic cause of chronic heart Failure (%)	53.1		
Beck depression inventory score	1.4±0.5		
State anxiety score	33.5±12.8		
Trait anxiety score	33.5±11.7		

(Adapted, with permission, from Jiang *et al.*[119])

Table 17.6. *Measures of anxiety and depression in deceased and living patients at 1 year*

Measure	Dead	Alive	*P*-value
State anxiety	36.2±15.1	32.9±12.4	0.18
Trait anxiety	34.7±13.0	33.2±11.4	0.48
Beck depression inventory score	11.5±8	8.3±7	0.03

(Adapted, with permission, from Jiang *et al.*[119])

Table 17.7. *Unadjusted Cox proportional analysis of anxiety, depression, and conventional cardiac risks with 1-year mortality*

Univariate analysis	Relative risk*	95% Confidence interval	*P*-value
State anxiety	1.017	0.996–1.039	0.115
Trait anxiety	1.010	0.985–1.035	0.441
Beck depression inventory score	1.041	1.010–1.073	0.009
Age	1.035	1.009–1.062	0.009
Left ventricular ejection fraction	1.010	0.987–1.032	0.405
New York Heart Association Class	1.774	1.169–2.693	0.007
Ischemic cause of congestive heart failure	2.602	1.315–5.149	0.006

* For each 1-unit increase in continuous variables.
(Adapted, with permission, from Jiang *et al.*[119])

Table 17.8. *Relation between anxiety and depression and 1-year mortality, adjusted for conventional cardiac risk factors*

	Relative risk*	95% Confidence interval	*P*-value
State anxiety model			
Beck depression inventory	1.036	0.998–1.075	0.0623
State anxiety	1.014	0.988–1.040	0.2967
Trait anxiety model			
Beck depression inventory	1.045	1.008–1.084	0.0158
Trait anxiety	1.001	0.971–1.031	0.9716

* For each 1-unit increase.
(Adapted, with permission, from Jiang *et al.*[119])

and $R = -0.36$, $P < 0.005$, respectively) in a group of outpatients with chronic heart failure.[42] Depression, however, was retained in a multiple regression analysis of the walk-test performance and was also found to be a stronger predictor than anxiety in functional impairment of daily activities in this sample.

While it is difficult to definitively determine the role of anxiety in chronic heart failure, current evidence suggests that when a patient with chronic heart failure presents with complaints of anxiety symptoms, depression needs to be assessed. Treatment with an antidepressant with anxiolytic effects for these patients may be more appropriate than conventional anxiolytic medications.

Delirium and Other Psychiatric Conditions

Delirium is a common mental disorder among hospitalized patients. It involves a transient alteration in the ability to attend and orient as well as a distortion in cognition. Existing literature reports that in the general hospital setting the diagnosis of delirium ranges from 14% to 56%.[121] Other literature suggests that 32% to 67% of patients with delirium go unrecognized during hospitalization.[121] Advanced age is probably considered the greatest risk factor for the development of delirium. Patients > 65 years old are the most frequently affected, with the highest reported risk occurring in patients > 85 years old.[121–123] The relationship between delirium and chronic heart failure has not been studied as much as the relationship between depression, anxiety, and chronic heart failure. Nevertheless, chronic heart failure has been reported to be a common factor associated with increased rate of delirium. Rockwood studied 80 elderly hospitalized patients (65 to 91 years old) and found that the rate of delirium was 25%.[124] Infection and chronic heart failure were found to be predominate causes for patients admitted with delirium. Moreover, Braekhus and Engedal examined 58 patients > 75 years, and found that 24% met a diagnosis of delirium. Of the 58 factors possibly associated with the onset of delirium, the authors identified drugs, cerebrovascular disease (CVD), and chronic heart failure as the factors most commonly associated with delirium.[125] The collected data strongly indicate that ADHF patients may have higher rates of delirium than patients hospitalized with other medical conditions.

Patients with delirium tend to have a higher rate of mortality either during the index admission or soon thereafter. Inouye *et al.* reported a 39% higher mortality in patients diagnosed with delirium at 1 year following the index admission than in age-matched patients who did not have delirium.[121] In many cases, even after recovery from delirium, the cognitive impairment that occurs often persists chronically, leading to permanent cognitive decline, decreased functional ability, extended hospitalization, and increased institutionalization.[126,127] The annual cost for delirium care has been estimated at more than $4 billion.[128] Although there is no report on mortality in chronic heart failure patients with delirium, based on findings of high mortality in acute chronic heart failure and chronic heart failure being a high risk for delirium development, it is reasonable to presume that the mortality rate is much higher in acute chronic heart failure patients with delirium than those without delirium.

Another commonly encountered psychiatric condition in hospitalized chronic heart failure patients is substance abuse. Several forms of substance abuse have etiologic roles in chronic heart failure.[129–131] However, literature discussing substance abuse in hospitalized chronic heart failure patients is scarce. In hospitalized chronic heart failure patients who show symptoms of delirium or autonomic instability, alcohol withdrawal should be considered. Cocaine or other stimulant abuse is also a concern, especially in young patients with MI. As a risk factor for MI and pulmonary disease, cigarette smoking indirectly contributes to the pathogenesis of ischemic chronic heart failure and chronic heart failure as a complication of pulmonary disease.

Psychosocial Support

Abundant literature, accumulated over the past several decades, strongly suggests that inadequate social support is a risk factor for increased mortality in IHD patients.[127,128,132–134] A number of more recent studies have demonstrated similar findings.[135–138] The term *social support* has been commonly used because inadequate support was found to be a risk factor for cardiac patients. We prefer the term *psychosocial support* to emphasize the perception of an individual with the social support he or she has, which may play a more critical role for the prognosis of cardiac disease.

Marital status, a significant component of psychosocial support, plays a significant role in the prognosis and compliance of patients with heart failure. Chin *et al.*[135] assessed the marital status among a group of 257 heart failure patients who survived hospital admission and followed them for 60 days. Approximately 50% of those patients were not married (i.e., divorced, widowed, never married, or not living as if married) at the time of the survey. During the 60-day follow-up period, as compared to their counterparts, the unmarried patients had a significantly higher rate of death or re-hospitalization. The adjusted hazard ratio (HR) was 2.1 and the 95% CI was 1.3–3.3. Single patients were more likely than non-single patients to be women (69% vs. 32%) and to report that they needed extra help after leaving the hospital that they could not obtain from family or friends (62% vs. 35%). A martial status of not married but living with someone did not seem to improve the poor outcome of patients with the "single" status. In another study of 600 hospitalized heart failure patients, Clary *et al.* found that > 60% of those patients were not married at the time of assessment.[139] One-year mortality was found to be significantly higher in the non-married heart failure patients as compared to the married ones. As compared to married patients, non-married heart failure patients tend to have poorer compliance for needed heart failure care.[137]

Among patients who are married, the effect of marital quality in heart failure prognosis should not be neglected. Coyne *et al.* evaluated marital quality including marital satisfaction, marital routine, and useful illness discussion among 189 patients with heart failure and their spouses.[138] Survival was then followed in those patients for up to 48 months. At the end of follow-up, 47.5% of male patients and 32% female patients were deceased. Cox proportional hazard regression analysis demonstrated low marital quality was significantly correlated with higher mortality in those heart failure patients and was independent of heart failure severity. Furthermore, female patients were more adversely affected by poor marital quality than male patients. Of the 8 female patients who were categorized in the poorest marital quality, 7 died within 2 years of initial assessment. Patients with poor marital quality and high NYHA class were at the greatest risk for dying (4-year survival = 41.9%), whereas patients with low NYHA class and high marital quality had the lowest risk of dying (4-year survival = 77.6%).

The important implication of perceived or subjective social support in cardiac patients has been well described. In a sample of 193 hospitalized elderly patients with IHD, negative life events were found to be associated with more than a 2-fold increase in the likelihood of depression. Whereas patients who considered themselves as having good social support, despite their true instrumental social support, were more likely to be protected from depression (OR, 0.79; 95% CI, 0.65–0.96).[74] Krumholz *et al.* demonstrated that lack of emotional support was a significant predictor of increased death or re-admission during the first year following the index admission. The OR for the association between lack of social support and death or re-admission was 2.4 with a 95% CI of 1.1–4.9. More important is that such an association was independent of instrumental support and social ties. The authors also found that the negative impact of the lack of emotional support on prognosis seemed to be much greater for female patients than for male patients.[136] Another group of researchers examined the association of active coping, seeking instrumental support, acceptance, denial, and behavioral disengagement with mortality in a total of 119 heart failure patients. Interestingly, behavioral disengagement and lack of acceptance were found to be predictors for poor prognosis but not the other factors, even when controlled for disease severity, gender, age.[140]

The underlying mechanism for the poor prognosis of patients with heart failure and IHD who lack social support remains unknown. It is possible that adequate social support is associated with effective adherence to medical therapy and lifestyle modification recommendations by the patient. However, lack of or inadequate instrumental support does not appear to have as significant a negative impact as the lack of perceived social support on the prognosis of heart failure. Social factors can influence psychological factors that interact with biological functioning through several pathways. For instance, emotional support may alleviate potentially damaging effects of negative emotional interactions on the neuroendocrine, inflammatory immune, and other bio-physiological regulatory systems.[141,142]

Conclusion

This chapter discussed several concerning psychiatric and psychosocial factors including depression, anxiety, delirium, substance abuse, inadequate social support, and emotional or perceived social support. Among these factors, depression, marital status of not married, and perceived social support appear to be significant risk factors for increased mortality and re-hospitalization in patients with heart failure. Further research on effective methods for modifying these risk factors may help decrease the high rates of morbidity and mortality in patients with chronic heart failure.

References

1. American Heart Association. Heart Disease and Stroke Statistics—2002 Update (American Heart Association: Dallas, TX, 2001).
2. MacMahon KM, Lip GY. Psychological factors in heart failure: a review of the literature. Arch Intern Med 2002; 162: 509–516.
3. Rich MW, Nease RF. Cost-effectiveness analysis in clinical practice: the case of heart failure. Arch Intern Med 1999; 159: 1690–1700.
4. Goldberg RJ, Meyer TE. Advances and stagnations in heart failure. Arch Intern Med 1997; 157: 17–19.
5. Rich MW, Beckham V, Wittenberg C, Leven CL, Freedland KE, Carney RM. A multidisciplinary intervention to prevent the readmission of elderly patients with congestive heart failure. N Engl J Med 1995; 333: 1190–1195.
6. Cline CM, Israelsson BY, Willenheimer RB, Broms K, Erhardt LR. Cost effective management programme for heart failure reduces hospitalisation. Heart 1998; 80: 442–446.
7. Stewart S, Vandenbroek AJ, Pearson S, Horowitz JD. Prolonged beneficial effects of a home-based intervention on unplanned readmissions and mortality among patients with congestive heart failure. Arch Intern Med 1999; 159: 257–261.
8. Rauh RA, Schwabauer NJ, Enger EL, Moran JF. A community hospital-based congestive heart failure program: impact on length of stay, admission and readmission rates, and cost. Am J Manag Care 1999; 5: 37–43.
9. Konstam MA, Dracup K, Baker D, *et al.* Heart failure: evaluation and care of patients with left ventricular dysfunction. J Card Fail 1995; 1: 183–187.
10. Gooding J, Jette AM. Hospital readmissions among the elderly. J Am Geriatr Soc 1985; 33: 595–601.
11. Vinson JM, Rich MW, Sperry JC, Shah AS, McNamara T. Early readmission of elderly patients with congestive heart failure. J Am Geriatr Soc 1990; 38: 1290–1295.
12. Jiang W, Alexander J, Christopher E, *et al.* Effect of depression on increased risk of mortality and rehospitalization in patients with congestive heart failure. Arch Intern Med 2001; 161: 1849–1856.
13. Diagnostic and Statistical Manual of Mental Disorders, 4th edition (American Psychiatric Association: Washington, DC, 1994).
14. Sartorius N, Ustun TB, Costa e Silva JA, *et al.* An international study of psychological problems in primary care. Preliminary report from the World Health Organization Collaborative Project on "Psychological Problems in General Health Care." Arch Gen Psychiatry 1993; 50: 819–824.
15. Weiller E, Lecrubier Y, Maier W, Ustun TB. The relevance of recurrent brief depression in primary care: a report from the WHO project on Psychological Problems in General Health Care conducted in 14 countries. Eur Arch Psychiatry Clin Neurosci 1994; 244: 182–189.
16. Simon GE, Goldberg D, Tiemens BG, Ustun TB. Outcomes of recognized and unrecognized depression in an international primary care study. Gen Hosp Psychiatry 1999; 21: 97–105.
17. Bourassa MG, Gurne O, Bangdiwala SI, *et al.* Natural history and patterns of current practice in heart failure. The Studies of Left Ventricular Dysfunction (SOLVD) Investigators. J Am Coll Cardiol 1993; 22: 14A–19A.
18. Hallstrom T, Lapidus L, Bengtsson C, Edstrom K. Psychosocial factors and risk of ischaemic heart

disease and death in women: a twelve-year follow-up of participants in the population study of women in Gothenburg, Sweden. J Psychosom Res 1986; 30: 451–459.
19. Anda R, Williamson D, Jones D, *et al.* Depressed affect, hopelessness, and the risk of ischemic heart disease in a cohort of U.S. adults. Epidemiology 1993; 4: 285–294.
20. Aromaa A, Raitasalo R, Reunanen A, *et al.* Depression and cardiovascular diseases. Acta Psychiatr Scand Suppl 1994; 377: 77–82.
21. Everson SA, Goldberg DE, Kaplan GA, *et al.* Hopelessness and risk of mortality and incidence of myocardial infarction and cancer. Psychosom Med 1996; 58: 113–121.
22. Wassertheil-Smoller S, Applegate WB, Berge K, *et al.* Change in depression as a precursor of cardiovascular events. SHEP Cooperative Research Group (Systolic Hypertension in the Elderly Project). Arch Intern Med 1996; 156: 553–561.
23. Pratt LA, Ford DE, Crum RM, Armenian HK, Gallo JJ, Eaton WW. Depression, psychotropic medication, and risk of myocardial infarction: prospective data from the Baltimore ECA follow-up. Circulation 1996; 94: 3123–3129.
24. Mendes de Leon CF, Krumholz HM, Seeman TS, *et al.* Depression and risk of coronary heart disease in elderly men and women: New Haven EPESE, 1982–1991. Established Populations for the Epidemiologic Studies of the Elderly. Arch Intern Med 1998; 158: 2341–2348.
25. Ariyo AA, Haan M, Tangen CM, *et al.* Depressive symptoms and risks of coronary heart disease and mortality in elderly Americans. Cardiovascular Health Study Collaborative Research Group. Circulation 2000; 102: 1773–1779.
26. Ferketich AK, Schwartzbaum JA, Frid DJ, Moeschberger ML. Depression as an antecedent to heart disease among women and men in the NHANES I study. National Health and Nutrition Examination Survey. Arch Intern Med 2000; 160: 1261–1268.
27. Penninx BW, Beekman AT, Honig A, *et al.* Depression and cardiac mortality: results from a community-based longitudinal study. Arch Gen Psychiatry 2001; 58: 221–227.
28. Appels A, Mulder P. Excess fatigue as a precursor of myocardial infarction. Eur Heart J 1988; 9: 758–764.
29. Barefoot JC, Schroll M. Symptoms of depression, acute myocardial infarction, and total mortality in a community sample. Circulation 1996; 93: 1976–1980.
30. Ford DE, Mead LA, Chang PP, Cooper-Patrick L, Wang NY, Klag MJ. Depression is a risk factor for coronary artery disease in men: the Precursors study. Arch Intern Med 1998; 158: 1422–1426.
31. Frasure-Smith N, Lespérance F, Talajic M, Depression following myocardial infarction. Impact on 6-month survival. JAMA 1993; 270: 1819–1825.
32. Frasure-Smith N, Lespérance F, Talajic M. Depression and 18-month prognosis after myocardial infarction. Circulation 1995; 91: 999–1005.
33. Barefoot JC, Helms MJ, Mark DB, *et al.* Depression and long-term mortality risk in patients with coronary artery disease. Am J Cardiol 1996; 78: 613–617.
34. Lespérance F, Frasure-Smith N, Juneau M, Theroux P. Depression and 1-year prognosis in unstable angina. Arch Intern Med 2000; 160: 1354–1360.
35. Irvine J, Basinski A, Baker B, *et al.* Depression and risk of sudden cardiac death after acute myocardial infarction: testing for the confounding effects of fatigue. Psychosom Med 1999; 61: 729–737.
36. Schleifer SJ, Macari-Hinson MM, Coyle DA, *et al.* The nature and course of depression following myocardial infarction. Arch Intern Med 1989; 149: 1785–1789.
37. Forrester AW, Lipsey JR, Teitelbaum ML, DePaulo JR, Andrzejewski PL. Depression following myocardial infarction. Int J Psychiatry Med 1992; 22: 33–46.
38. Shapiro PA, Lespérance F, Frasure-Smith N, *et al.* An open-label preliminary trial of sertraline for treatment of major depression after acute myocardial infarction (the SADHAT Trial). Sertraline Anti-Depressant Heart Attack Trial. Am Heart J 1999; 137: 1100–1116.
39. Frasure-Smith N, Lespérance F, Juneau M, Talajic M, Bourassa MG. Gender, depression, and one-year prognosis after myocardial infarction. Psychosom Med 1999; 61: 26–37.
40. Lane D, Carroll D, Ring C, Beevers DG, Lip GY. Mortality and quality of life 12 months after myocardial infarction: effects of depression and anxiety. Psychosom Med 2001; 63: 221–230.
41. Denollet J, Brutsaert DL. Personality, disease severity, and the risk of long-term cardiac events in patients with a decreased ejection fraction after myocardial infarction. Circulation 1998; 97: 167–173.
42. Reschke AH, Freedland KE, Carney RM. Effects of depression and anxiety on walk test performance in outpatients with congestive heart failure. Ann Behav Med 1999; 21: S176.
43. Carney RM, Rich MW, Freedland KE, *et al.* Major depressive disorder predicts cardiac events in

patients with coronary artery disease. Psychosom Med 1988; 50: 627–633.

44. Freedland KE, Carney RM, Krone RJ, *et al.* Psychological factors in silent myocardial ischemia. Psychosom Med 1991; 53: 13–24.
45. Koenig HG. Depression in hospitalized older patients with congestive heart failure. Gen Hosp Psychiatry 1998; 20: 29–43.
46. Faris R, Purcell H, Henein MY, Coats AJ. Clinical depression is common and significantly associated with reduced survival in patients with non-ischaemic heart failure. Eur J Heart Fail 2002; 4: 541–551.
47. Sullivan M, Simon G, Spertus J, Russo J. Depression-related costs in heart failure care. Arch Intern Med 2002; 162: 1860–1866.
48. Musselman DL, Evans DL, Nemeroff CB. The relationship of depression to cardiovascular disease: epidemiology, biology, and treatment. Arch Gen Psychiatry 1998; 55: 580–592.
49. Pariante CM, Miller AH. Glucocorticoid receptors in major depression: relevance to pathophysiology and treatment. Biol Psychiatry 2001; 49: 391–404.
50. The dexamethasone suppression test in depression. A World Health Organization Collaborative Study. Br J Psychiatry 1987; 150: 459–462.
51. Roy A, Linnoila M, Karoum F, Pichar D. Urinary-free cortisol in depressed patients and control: relationship to urinary indices of noradrenergic function. Psychol Med 1988; 18: 93–98.
52. Roy A, Pickar D, Dejong J, Karoum F, Linnoila M. Norepinephrine and its metabolites in cerebrospinal fluid, plasma and urine: relatioship to hypothalamic-pituitary-adrenal axis function in depression. Arch Gen Psychiatry 1988; 45: 849–857.
53. Roy A, Guthrie S, Pickar D, Linnoila M. Plasma norepinephrine responses to cold challenge in depressed patients and normal controls. Psychiatry Res 1987; 21: 161–168.
54. Roy A, Pickar D, Linnoila M, Potter WZ. Plasma norepinephrine level in affective disorders: relationship to melancholia. Arch Gen Psychiatry 1985; 42: 1181–1185.
55. Anfossi G, Trovati M. Role of catecholamines in platelet function: pathophysiological and clinical significance. Eur J Clin Invest 1996; 26: 353–370.
56. Malhotra S, Tesar GE, Franco K. The relationship between depression and cardiovascular disorders. Curr Psychiatry Rep 2000; 2: 241–246.
57. Gold PW, Chrousos GP. The endocrinology of melancholic and atypical depression: relation to neurocircuitry and somatic consequences. Proc Assoc Am Physicians 1999; 111: 22–34.
58. Klein E, Cnaani E, Harel T, Braun S, Ben-Haim SA. Altered heart rate variability in panic disorder patients. Biol Psychiatry 1995; 37: 18–24.
59. American College of Cardiology Cardiovascular Technology Assessment Committee. Heart rate variability for risk stratification of life-threatening arrhythmias. J Am Coll Cardiol 1993; 22: 948–950.
60. Cripps TR, Malik M, Farrell TG, Camm AJ. Prognostic value of reduced heart rate variability after myocardial infarction: clinical evaluation of a new analysis method. Br Heart J 1991; 65: 14–19.
61. Carney RM, Saunders RD, Freedland KE, *et al.* Association of depression with reduced heart rate variability in coronary artery disease. Am J Cardiol 1995; 76: 562–564.
62. Musselman DL, Tomer A, Manatunga AK, *et al.* Exaggerated platelet reactivity in major depression. Am J Psychiatry 1996; 153: 1313–1317.
63. Reichborn-Kjennerud T, Lingjaerde O, Oreland L. Platelet monoamine oxidase activity in patients with winter seasonal affective disorder. Psychiatry Res 1996; 62: 273–280.
64. Laghrissi-Thode F, Wagner WR, Pollock BG, Johnson PC, Finkel MS. Elevated platelet factor 4 and beta-thromboglobulin plasma levels in depressed patients with ischemic heart disease. Biol Psychiatry 1997; 42: 290–295.
65. Maes M, Ombelet W, De Jongh R, Kenis G, Bosmans E. The inflammatory response following delivery is amplified in women who previously suffered from major depression, suggesting that major depression is accompanied by a sensitization of the inflammatory response system. J Affect Disord 2001; 63: 85–92.
66. Song C, Lin A, Bonaccorso S, *et al.* The inflammatory response system and the availability of plasma tryptophan in patients with primary sleep disorders and major depression. J Affect Disord 1998; 49: 211–219.
67. Libby P. What have we learned about the biology of atherosclerosis? The role of inflammation. Am J Cardiol 2001; 88: 3J–6J.
68. Buffon A, Biasucci LM, Liuzzo G, D'Onofrio G, Crea F, Maseri A. Widespread coronary inflammation in unstable angina. N Engl J Med 2002; 347: 5–12.
69. Farmer ME, Locke BZ, Moscicki EK, Dannenberg AL, Larson DB, Radloff LS. Physical activity and depressive symptoms: the NHANES I Epidemiologic Follow-up Study. Am J Epidemiol 1988; 128: 1340–1351.
70. Weyerer S. Physical inactivity and depression in the community: evidence from the Upper Bavarian Field Study. Int J Sports Med 1992; 13: 492–496.

71. Siegler HC, Blumenthal JA, Barefoot JC, *et al.* Personality factors differentially predict exercise behavior in men and women. Women's Health 1997; 3: 61–70.
72. Adler NE, Boyce T, Chesney MA, *et al.* Socioeconomic status and health: the challenge of the gradient. Am Psychol 1994; 49: 15–24.
73. Horsten M, Mittleman MA, Wamala SP, Schenck-Gustafsson K, Orth-Gomer K. Depressive symptoms and lack of social integration in relation to prognosis of CHD in middle-aged women. The Stockholm Female Coronary Risk Study. Eur Heart J 2000; 21: 1072–1080.
74. Krishnan KR, George LK, Pieper CF, *et al.* Depression and social support in elderly patients with cardiac disease. Am Heart J 1998; 136: 491–495.
75. Glassman AH, Helzer JE, Covey LS. Smoking, smoking cessation and major depression. JAMA 1990; 264: 1546–1549.
76. Anda RF, Williamson DF, Escobedo LG, Mast EE, Giovino GA, Remington PL. Depression and the dynamics of smoking: a national perspective. JAMA 1990; 264: 1541–1545.
77. Carney RM, Freedland KE, Eisen SA, Rich MW, Jaffe AS. Major depression and medication adherence in elderly patients with coronary artery disease. Health Psychol 1995; 14: 88–90.
78. Blumenthal JA, Williams RS, Wallace AG, *et al.* Physiological and psychological variables predict compliance to prescribed exercise therapy in patients recovering from myocardial infarction. Psychosom Med 1982; 44: 519–527.
79. Ziegelstein RC, Fauerbach JA, Stevens SS, Romanelli J, Richter DP, Bush DE. Patients with depression are less likely to follow recommendations to reduce cardiac risk during recovery from a myocardial infarction. Arch Intern Med 2000; 160: 1818–1823.
80. Jiang W, Babyak M, Krantz DS, *et al.* Mental stress-induced myocardial ischemia and cardiac events. JAMA 1996; 275: 1651–1656.
81. Krantz DS, Santiago HT, Kop WJ, Bairey Merz CN, Rozanski A, Gottdiener JS. Prognostic value of mental stress testing in coronary artery disease. Am J Cardiol 1999; 84: 1292–1297.
82. Sheps DS, McMahon RP, Becker L, *et al.* Mental stress-induced ischemia and all-cause mortality in patients with coronary artery disease: results from the Psychophysiological Investigations of Myocardial Ischemia study. Circulation 2002; 105: 1780–1784.
83. Jiang W, Babyak MA, Rozanski A, *et al.* Depression and increased myocardial ischemic activity in patients with ischemic heart disease. Am Heart J 2003; 146: 55–61.
84. Yeung AC, Vekshtein VI, Krantz DS, *et al.* The effect of atherosclerosis on the vasomotor response of coronary arteries to mental stress. N Engl J Med 1991; 325: 1551–1556.
85. Dakak N, Quyyumi AA, Eisenhofer G, Goldstein DS, Cannon RO 3rd. Sympathetically mediated effects of mental stress on the cardiac microcirculation of patients with coronary artery disease. Am J Cardiol 1995; 76: 125–130.
86. Goldberg AD, Becker LC, Bonsall R, *et al.* Ischemic, hemodynamic, and neurohormonal responses to mental and exercise stress: experience from the Psychophysiological Investigations of Myocardial Ischemia (PIMI) study. Circulation 1996; 94: 2402–2409.
87. Barlow DH. Anxiety and Its Disorders (The Guilford Press: New York, 1988).
88. Clark LA. The anxiety and depression disorders: descriptive psychopathology and differential diagnosis. In: Kendall OC, Watson D (eds.) Anxiety and Depression: Distinctive and Overlapping Features (Academic Press: New York, 1989), 83–129.
89. Breier A, Charney DS, Heninger GR. Major depression in patients with agoraphobia and panic disorder. Arch Gen Psychiatry 1984; 41: 1129–1135.
90. Conwell Y. Suicide in elderly patients. In: Schneider LS, Reynolds CT, Lebowitz BD (eds) Diagnosis and Treatment of Depression in Late Life (American Psychiatric Press, Inc.: Washington, DC, 1996), 397–418.
91. Beekman AT, de Beurs E, van Balkom AJ, Deeg DJ, van Dyck R, van Tilburg W. Anxiety and depression in later life: co-occurrence and communality of risk factors. Am J Psychiatry 2000; 157: 89–95.
92. Clark LA, Watson D. Tripartite model of anxiety and depression: psychometric evidence and taxonomic implications. J Abnorm Psychol 1991; 100: 316–336.
93. Tavazzi L, Zotti AM, Mazzuero G. Acute pulmonary edema provoked by psychologic stress: report of two cases. Cardiology 1987; 74: 229–235.
94. Starkman MN, Cameron OG, Ness RM, Zelnik T. Peripheral catecholamine levels and symptoms of anxiety: studies in patients with and without pheochromocytoma. Psychosom Med 1990; 52: 129–142.
95. Sevy S, Papadimtriou GN, Surmont DW, Goldman S, Mendewicz J. Noradrenergic function in generalized anxiety disorder, major depressive disorder, and healthy subjects. Biol Psychiatry 1989; 25: 141–152.
96. Taggart P, Gibbons D, Somerville W. Some effects of motor-car driving on the normal and abnormal heart. Br Med J 1969; 4: 130–134.

97. Taggart P, Carruthers M, Somerville W. Electrocardiogram, plasma catecholamines, and lipids, and their modification by oxyprenolol when speaking before an audience. Lancet 1973; 2: 341–346.
98. Benson H, Alexander S, Feldman CL. Decreased premature ventricular contractions through use of the relaxation response in patients with stable ischaemic heart-disease. Lancet 1975; 1: 380–382.
99. Weiss T, Engel BT. Operant conditioning of heart rate in patients with premature ventricular contractions. Psychosom Med 1971; 33: 301–321.
100. Lown B, Ruberman W. The concept of precoronary care. Mod Concepts Cardiovasc Dis 1970; 39: 97–102.
101. Lown B, Graboys TB. Management of patients with malignant ventricular arrhythmias. Am J Cardiol 1977; 39: 910–918.
102. Tulen JH, Bruijn JA, de Man KJ, van der Velden E, Pepplinkhuizen L, Man in't Veld AJ. Anxiety and autonomic regulation in major depressive disorder: an exploratory study. J Affect Disord 1996: 40: 61–71.
103. Yeragani VK, Pohl R, Berger R, *et al.* Decreased heart rate variability in panic disorder patients: a study of power-spectral analysis of heart rate. Psychiatry Res 1993: 46: 89–103.
104. Thayer JF, Friedman BH, Borkovec TD. Autonomic characteristics of generalized anxiety disorder and worry. Biol Psychiatry 1996: 39: 255–266.
105. Watkins LL, Grossman P, Krishnan R, Blumenthal JA. Anxiety reduces baroreflex cardiac control in older adults with major depression. Psychosom Med 1999; 61: 334–340.
106. Kleiger RE, Miller JP, Bigger JT Jr., Moss AJ. Decreased heart rate variability and its association with increased mortality after acute myocardial infarction. Am J Cardiol 1987: 59: 256–262.
107. Bigger JT, Fleiss JL, Rolnitzky LM, Steinman RC. The ability of several short-term measures of RR variability to predict mortality after myocardial infarction. Circulation 1993: 88: 927–934.
108. Rich MW, Saini JS, Kleiger RE, Carney RM, teVelde A, Freedland KE. Correlation of heart rate variability with clinical and angiographic variables and late mortality after coronary angiography. Am J Cardiol 1988; 62: 714–717.
109. Jiang W, Hathaway WR, McNulty S, Larsen RL, Zhang Y, O'Connor CM. Diminished autonomic tone and prognosis in patients with advanced heart failure. Am J Cardiol 1997; 80: 808–811.
110. Pitzalis MV, Iacoviello M, Todarello O, *et al.* Depression but not anxiety influences the autonomic control of heart rate after myocardial infarction. Am Heart J 2001; 141: 765–771.
111. Hughes JW, Stoney CM. Depressed mood is related to high-frequency heart rate variability during stressors. Psychosom Med 2000; 62: 796–803.
112. Krittayaphong R, Cascio WE, Light KC, *et al.* Heart rate variability in patients with coronary artery disease: differences in patients with higher and lower depression scores. Psychosom Med 1997; 59: 231–235.
113. Haines AP, Imeson JD, Meade TW. Phobic anxiety and ischaemic heart disease. Br Med J (Clin Res Ed) 1987; 295: 297–299.
114. Kawachi I, Colditz GA, Ascherio A, *et al.* Prospective study of phobic anxiety and risk of coronary heart disease in men. Circulation 1994; 89: 1992–1997.
115. Kawachi I, Sparrow D, Vokonas PS, Weiss ST. Symptoms of anxiety and risk of coronary heart disease. The Normative Aging Study. Circulation 1994; 90: 2225–2229.
116. Eaker ED, Pinsky J, Castelli WP. Myocardial infarction and coronary death among women: psychosocial predictors from a 20-year follow-up of women in the Framingham Study. Am J Epidemiol 1992; 135: 854–864.
117. Frasure-Smith N, Lespérance F. Depression and other psychological risks following myocardial infarction. Arch Gen Psychiatry 2003; 60: 627–636.
118. Majani G, Pierobon A, Giardini A, *et al.* Relationship between psychological profile and cardiological variables in chronic heart failure: the role of patient subjectivity. Eur Heart J 1999; 20: 1579–1586.
119. Jiang W, Kuchibhatla M, Cuffe MS, *et al.* Prognostic value of anxiety and depression in patients with chronic heart failure. Circulation 2004; 110: 3452–3456.
120. Spielberger CD, Gorsuch RL, Lushene R, *et al.* Manual for the State-Trait Anxiety Inventory (Consulting Psychologists Press: Palo Alto, CA, 1983).
121. Inouye SK. The dilemma of delirium: clinical and research controversies regarding diagnosis and evaluation of delirium in hospitalized elderly medical patients. Am J Med 1994; 97: 278–288.
122. Cole MG, Primeau FJ. Prognosis of delirium in elderly hospital patients. CMAJ 1993; 149: 41–46.
123. Inouye SK. Predisposing and precipitating factors for delirium in hospitalized older patients. Dement Geriatr Cogn Disord 1999; 10: 393–400.
124. Rockwood K. Acute confusion in elderly medical

patients. J Am Geriatr Soc 1989; 37: 150–154.
125. Braekhus A, Engedal K. [Delirium (acute confusion) among elderly patients after admission to a medical department]. Tidsskr Nor Laegeforen 1994; 114: 2613–2615.
126. Levkoff S, Cleary P, Liptzin B, Evans DA. Epidemiology of delirium: an overview of research issues and findings. Int Psychogeriatr 1991; 3: 149–167.
127. Berkman LF, Leo-Summers L, Horwitz RI. Emotional support and survival after myocardial infarction: a prospective, population-based study of the elderly. Ann Intern Med 1992; 117: 1003–1009.
128. Farmer IP, Meyer PS, Ramsey DJ, *et al.* Higher levels of social support predict greater survival following acute myocardial infarction: the Corpus Christi Heart Project. Behav Med 1996; 22: 59–66.
129. Waldenstrom A. Alcohol and congestive heart failure. Alcohol Clin Exp Res 1998; 22: 315S–317S.
130. Leone A. Cigarette smoking and health of the heart. J R Soc Health 1995; 115: 354–355.
131. Fernandez-Sola J, Estruch R, Nicolas JM, *et al.* Comparison of alcoholic cardiomyopathy in women versus men. Am J Cardiol 1997; 80: 481–485.
132. Oxman TE, Freeman DH Jr., Manheimer ED. Lack of social participation or religious strength and comfort as risk factors for death after cardiac surgery in the elderly. Psychosom Med 1995; 57: 5–15.
133. Vogt TM, Mullooly JP, Ernst D, Pope CR, Hollis JF. Social networks as predictors of ischemic heart disease, cancer, stroke and hypertension: incidence, survival and mortality. J Clin Epidemiol 1992; 45: 659–666.
134. Woloshin S, Schwartz LM, Tosteson AN, *et al.* Perceived adequacy of tangible social support and health outcomes in patients with coronary artery disease. J Gen Intern Med 1997; 12: 613–618.
135. Chin MH, Goldman L. Correlates of early hospital readmission or death in patients with congestive heart failure. Am J Cardiol 1997; 79: 1640–1644.
136. Krumholz HM, Butler J, Miller J, *et al.* Prognostic importance of emotional support for elderly patients hospitalized with heart failure. Circulation 1998: 97: 958–964.
137. Evangelista LS, Berg J, Dracup K. Relationship between psychosocial variables and compliance in patients with heart failure. Heart Lung 2001; 30: 294–301.
138. Coyne JC, Rohrbaugh MJ, Shoham V, Sonnega JS, Nicklas JM, Cranford JA. Prognostic importance of marital quality for survival of congestive heart failure. Am J Cardiol 2001; 88: 526–529.
139. Clary GL, Davenport C, Biracree D, *et al.* Effects of antidepressant medication on mortality in patients with CHF based on ethnicity, gender, and marital status. 49th Annual Meeting, Consultation-Liaison Psychiatry: Human & Scientific; November 21–24, 2002 (Abstract).
140. Carver CS, Scheier MF, Weintraub JK. Assessing coping strategies: a theoretically based approach. J Pers Soc Psychol 1989; 56: 267–283.
141. Cohen S. Psychosocial models of the role of social support in the etiology of physical disease. Health Psychol 1988; 7: 269–297.
142. Seeman TE, Berkman LF, Blazer DG, Rowe JW. Social ties and support and neuroendocrine function. Ann Behav Med 1994; 16: 95–106.
143. Appels A, Schouten E. Exhausted awakening as a risk factor for coronary heart disease. Psychother Psychosom Med Psychol 1993; 43: 166–170.
144. Hance M, Carney RM, Freedland KE, Skala J. Depression in patients with coronary heart disease: a 12-month follow-up. Gen Hosp Psychiatry 1996; 18: 61–65.
145. Connerney I, Shapiro PA, McLaughlin JS, Bagiella E, Sloan RP. Relation between depression after coronary artery bypass surgery and 12-month outcome: a prospective study. Lancet 2001; 358: 1766–1771.
146. Fraticelli A, Gesuita R, Vespa A, Paciaroni E. Congestive heart failure in the elderly requiring hospital admission. Arch Gerontol Geriatr 1996; 23: 225–238.
147. Havranek EP, Ware MG, Lowes BD. Prevalence of depression in congestive heart failure. Am J Cardiol 1999; 84: 348–350, A9.
148. Vaccarino V, Kasl SV, Abramson J, Krumholz HM. Depressive symptoms and risk of functional decline and death in patients with heart failure. J Am Coll Cardiol 2001; 38: 199–205.
149. Rozzini R, Sabatini T, Frisoni GB, Trabucchi M. Depression and major outcomes in older patients with heart failure. Arch Intern Med 2002; 162: 362–364.
150. Fulop G, Strain JJ, Stettin G. Congestive heart failure and depression in older adults: clinical course and health services use 6 months after hospitalization. Psychosomatics 2003; 44: 367–373.

CHAPTER 18

Anemia in acute and chronic heart failure

G Michael Felker, Kirkwood F Adams, Jr

Introduction

Improved survival after acute myocardial infarction (AMI), combined with the aging of the population, has resulted in rapid growth in the number of patients living with chronic heart failure. With this increase in the prevalence of chronic heart failure has come a concomitant increase in the number of hospitalizations for decompensated heart failure, with approximately 1 million hospitalizations yearly in the United States. This growing prevalence of acute heart failure (AHF) has been accompanied by significant morbidity and mortality, with estimates of the risk of death or rehospitalization within 60 days as high as 60%. Despite the enormity of this problem, the development of new therapies for AHF has lagged behind that of comparable cardiovascular disorders such as MI. This has led to the search for novel therapeutic targets in both acute and chronic heart failure.

Anemia has been demonstrated to be a common comorbid condition in patients with chronic heart failure, and observational studies have suggested that anemia is associated with adverse outcomes across a wide spectrum of heart failure severity. Data on the importance of anemia in AHF are much less robust, although theoretical considerations suggest that anemia could exacerbate the hemodynamic stress associated with AHF exacerbations.

This chapter outlines the available data on anemia in acute and chronic heart failure, and assesses the potential of anemia as a therapeutic target.

Prevalence of Anemia in Acute and Chronic Heart Failure

Published estimates of the prevalence of anemia in patients with heart failure vary widely, ranging from 4% to 55%.[1–7] Reasons for this wide variation include differences in the definition of anemia, study methods used, and heart failure population studied. The most commonly employed definitions of anemia are those of the World Health Organization (hemoglobin < 13 g/dL in men or < 12 g/dL in women) and the National Kidney Foundation (hemoglobin ≤ 12.5 g/dL in men and post-menopausal women, or hemoglobin ≤ 11 g/dL in pre-menopausal women). Other studies have used International Classification of Diseases, Ninth Revision (ICD-9) codes for a diagnosis of anemia without defining specific hemoglobin levels. In general, the prevalence of anemia is greater in less selected populations, such as claims data, and lower in highly-selected populations, such as patients enrolled in clinical trials.

Anemia appears to be more common in older patients and patients with more severe disease, with a reported prevalence in patients with New York Heart Association (NYHA) class IV as high as 79%.[3] Additionally, patients hospitalized with AHF exacerbations tend to have a significantly higher prevalence of anemia than outpatient populations. The prevalence of anemia in selected heart failure studies is shown in Table 18.1.

Mechanistic Interactions between Anemia and Heart Failure

Although anemia is common in heart failure, controversy remains about whether its high prevalence in heart failure patients is directly related to heart failure itself or other comorbid conditions. In general, anemia is common in patients with chronic medical disorders, including heart failure. Both heart failure and anemia are diseases of the elderly.[8] Multiple comorbid conditions are common in heart failure patients, particularly renal insufficiency, which is closely associated with the development of anemia.[9,10] This raises the question of whether the high prevalence of anemia in heart failure patients is due to a direct effect or simply overlapping patient populations. Multiple potential mechanistic links between heart failure and anemia do exist. These include hemodilution, renal dysfunction, proinflammatory cytokines, malnutrition due to right-sided heart failure, decreased perfusion to the bone marrow, and drug therapy, such as angiotensin-converting enzyme (ACE) inhibitors. Realistically, it is likely that several of these mechanisms are active simultaneously, and that anemia in heart failure is the result of a complex interaction between cardiac performance, neurohormonal and inflammatory activation, renal function, and bone marrow responsiveness. This interplay has been termed the "cardio-renal-anemia syndrome."[11] A conceptual model for these interactions is shown in Figure 18.1. Notably, all these mechanisms could be

Table 18.1. *Prevalence of anemia in selected heart failure studies*

Study	Population	No. of patients	Definition of anemia	Prevalence (%)
Al-Ahmad[1]	LV dysfunction ± symptoms, clinical trial	6563	Hct < 0.35	4
Tanner[4]	Tertiary-care HF clinic	193	Hb < 12	15
Ezekowitz[5]	New HF diagnosis, claims data	12 065	MD defined (ICD-9 codes)	17
Mozaffarian[2]	Severe chronic HF, clinical trial	1130	Hb < 37.6	20
Horwich[6]	Heart transplant referrals, single center	1061	Hb < 13 (men) Hb < 12 (women)	30
Kosiborod[7]	Medicare patients, claims data	2281	Hct ≤ 0.37	48
Felker[38]	ADHF, clinical trial	949	Hb < 13 (men) Hb < 12 (women)	49
Silverberg[3]	Chronic HF, single center trial	142	Hb < 12	55

Abbreviations: ADHF = acute decompensated heart failure; Hb = hemoglobin; Hct = hematocrit; HF = heart failure; ICD-9 = International Classification of Diseases, Ninth Revision; LV = left ventricular; MD = medical doctor.
With permission from Felker *et al.*[71]

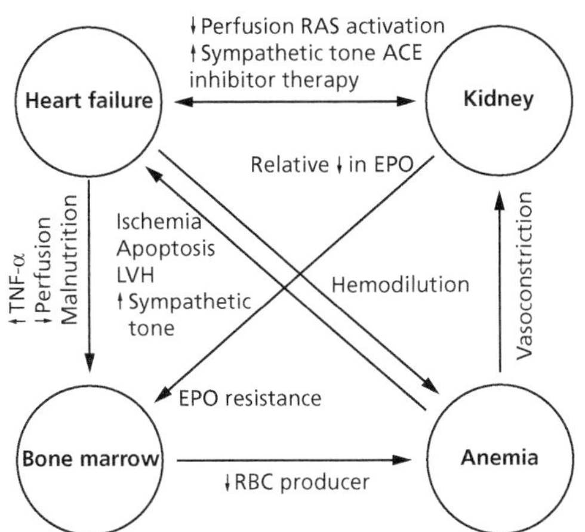

Figure 18.1. *Conceptual model of pathogenesis of anemia in patients with heart failure (With permission from Felker* et al.[71])

potentially operative in both acute and chronic heart failure.

Expansion of plasma volume is a characteristic of the heart failure syndrome. Therefore, some anemia may be dilutional rather than due to a true decrease in red blood cell mass.[12] In a recently published study of 37 heart failure patients by Androne *et al.*, true anemia (i.e., a decrease in red blood cell mass) was present in 54% of patients and hemodilution was present in 46%.[13] Notably, in this study, both hemodilution and true anemia were associated with adverse survival, with the worst survival rates seen in patients with hemodilution. Given that AHF hospitalization is usually accompanied by significant volume overload, it would be expected that hemodilution may play an even larger role in AHF.

Renal insufficiency is common in heart failure, with a prevalence from 30–50%, depending on the definition used and the population studied.[9,14] In patients with advanced renal disease, progressive renal dysfunction leads to a decrease in circulating levels of erythropoietin, with a subsequent decrease in bone marrow erythrocyte production and hemoglobin levels. It is well established that anemia in patients with end-stage renal disease (ESRD) is associated with a variety of adverse cardiac consequences, including the development of left ventricular hypertrophy (LVH), left ventricular (LV) dilation, and frank clinical heart failure.[15,16]

As shown in Figure 18.1, there is a complex interaction between renal insufficiency, erythropoietin production, and heart failure. Indeed, despite the high prevalence of renal dysfunction, circulating levels of erythropoietin are generally normal to elevated in heart failure, with a correlation between the degree of erythropoietin elevation and worsening functional class.[12] Increased renal production of erythropoietin may be driven by worsening cardiac performance and subsequent renal hypoperfusion and hypoxia, which is a powerful stimulus for erythropoietin production. In light of this elevation of erythropoietin levels in advanced heart failure, the high prevalence of anemia in this population is particularly notable.

Anemia in heart failure may be a state of relative resistance to the effects of erythropoietin, with persistent anemia despite high normal or frankly elevated erythropoietin levels. Several potential explanations for erythropoietin resistance in heart failure have been proposed, including the influence of proinflammatory cytokines and malnutrition.

Heart failure is known to be a state of persistent inflammatory activation, and higher levels of circulating proinflammatory cytokines are known to be associated with greater disease severity and worsened clinical outcomes.[17–19] Proinflammatory cytokines, such as tumor necrosis factor-alpha (TNF-α) and interleukin-6 (IL-6), also have direct effects on the bone marrow and are implicated in the mechanism of anemia of chronic disease.[20] Elevated levels of circulating proinflammatory cytokines lead to decreased erythropoietin production and resistance to the effects of erythropoietin on bone marrow production of red blood cells. Given that both proinflammatory cytokine activation and anemia are more pronounced in patients with more severe heart failure, it is attractive to hypothesize that inflammatory activation is a major contributor to anemia in this population. Recently presented data confirm the association between elevated circulating inflammatory markers and anemia, with significantly higher levels of TNF-α and TNF soluble receptors 1 and 2 in patients with anemia and heart failure.[21] Although data on inflammatory activation in AHF is more limited, some studies suggest that it may be even more pronounced. This suggests that this link may play a significant role in this disorder.[22]

Other potential mechanisms may involve regulation of erythropoietin secretion from the kidney, either from the heart failure syndrome itself or from pharmacologic treatment. Autonomic dysfunction, known to be present in heart failure, may result in impaired renal production of erythropoietin even in the setting of significant stimuli for erythrocyte production.[23,24] Therapy with ACE inhibitors is a mainstay in heart failure therapy, with clearly documented improvements in long-term survival.[25–27] Some data have suggested, however, that ACE-inhibitor therapy may reduce hemoglobin concentration in patients with heart failure. Therapeutic doses of ACE inhibitors have been shown to decrease renal secretion of erythropoietin in patients with hypertension,[28] renal insufficiency,[29] polycythemia,[30] and chronic heart failure.[31] The mechanistic role that these factors may play in the development of anemia in patients with heart failure is not clear.

Although many studies have identified a high prevalence of anemia in patients with heart failure, few have carefully examined the relationship between the burden of comorbidity and the prevalence of anemia. Hussein *et al.* recently presented data on the attributable cause of anemia from a retrospective cohort study of 699 consecutive outpatient visits to a heart failure clinic.[32] An explanation for anemia other than heart failure was identified in 98% of the study patients, with the most common causes being renal insufficiency (defined as creatinine clearance < 60 mL/min/m^2) and iron, folate, or B_{12} deficiency. Although limited by its retrospective design, this study suggests that mechanisms other than heart failure may be responsible for anemia in a significant proportion of heart failure patients. A prospective, ongoing study including both specialty and community sites, the STudy of AneMia IN AHeart Failure Population (STAMINA-HFP) registry, is evaluating the prevalence, etiologies, and mechanisms of anemia in a broad population of heart failure patients.[33]

Anemia and Outcomes in Acute and Chronic Heart Failure

A variety of observational studies have found that lower hemoglobin or hematocrit is associated with adverse clinical outcomes in heart failure (Table 18.2). This relationship persists whether considering hemoglobin concentration as a continuous variable or anemia as a categorical variable. Anemia has been shown to be a risk factor for new cardiovascular events in the general population.[34] Data from the Framingham Study found that lower hematocrit was a significant risk factor for the development of symptomatic heart failure.[35] Data from a large single-center cohort of patients, with primarily NHYA class IV symptoms referred for cardiac transplantation, identified an association between lower hemoglobin and impaired hemodynamics, lower functional capacity, and decreased long-term survival.[6] These findings persisted when patients were subdivided into a variety of subgroups based on gender, heart failure etiology, and age. Notably, this study identified a substantially increased risk even in patients with relatively mild anemia (hemoglobin < 12.6 g/dL for men or hemoglobin < 11.6 g/dL for women).

Anemia also contributes to the exercise intolerance that is a major comorbidity in chronic heart failure. A recently published study of 93 men with heart failure found that hemoglobin was a significant independent predictor of maximal exercise tolerance as measured by peak oxygen consumption, even after controlling for ejection fraction (EF), age, and renal function.[36] Not all studies have supported the association between anemia and adverse outcomes in heart failure. A study by Kalra *et al.* of 552 patients with new-onset heart failure found a significant incidence of anemia in this cohort (18% with hemoglobin < 11.5 g/dL) but no association between baseline hemoglobin and survival after adjustment for other variables.[37] The authors concluded that anemia early in the disease course was likely due to factors other than heart failure and was therefore unlikely to be associated with prognosis.

Most published studies have evaluated anemia in patients with chronic heart failure. The largest

Table 18.2. *Association between anemia and outcomes in selected heart failure studies*

Study	Population	Outcome	Adjusted HR/OR	Unit change
Al-Ahmad[1]	LV dysfunction ± symptoms, clinical trial	Mortality	1.027	1% Hct
Ezekowitz[5]	New HF diagnosis, claims data	Mortality	1.34	Anemic vs. not
Horwich[6]	Heart transplant referrals, single center	Mortality	1.13	1 g/dL Hb
Kosiborod[7]	Medicare patients, claims data	Mortality	1.02	1% Hct
Mozaffarian[2]	Severe chronic HF, clinical trial	Mortality	1.03	1% Hct
Felker[38]	ADHF, clinical trial	Death or rehospitalization	1.12	1 g/dL Hb

Abbreviations: Hb = hemoglobin; Hct = hematocrit; HF = heart failure; HR = hazard ratio; LV = left ventricular; OR = odds ratio.
With permission from Felker *et al.*[71]

study to address this question in patients hospitalized with AHF was a substudy of the Outcomes of a Prospective Trial of Intravenous Milrinone for Exacerbations of Chronic Heart Failure (OPTIME-CHF) trial.[38] The OPTIME-CHF study was a blinded, randomized, controlled trial of intravenous milrinone vs. placebo in 949 patients with AHF. A retrospective analysis of this study found a high prevalence of anemia in AHF patients (49%). Additionally, this study found hemoglobin level at randomization (within 48 hours of presentation) to be independently associated with adverse outcomes, with a 12% increased risk of death or rehospitalization at 60 days for every decrease of 1 g/dL of hemoglobin (Figure 18.2).

When taken as a whole, the observational data appear to suggest a relationship between anemia and outcomes in patients with heart failure. However, such studies must be interpreted with caution due to their retrospective design, and should not be construed as demonstrating a causative, mechanistic link between anemia, heart failure, and outcomes. Whether such a link exists is not clear from the currently available data.

Multiple theoretical reasons have been postulated to explain the observed association between anemia and outcomes in patients with heart failure. The presence of anemia may simply be a marker for greater severity of heart failure or greater burden of comorbidity. A recently presented study using data from the National Heart Failure Project found that while lower hematocrit

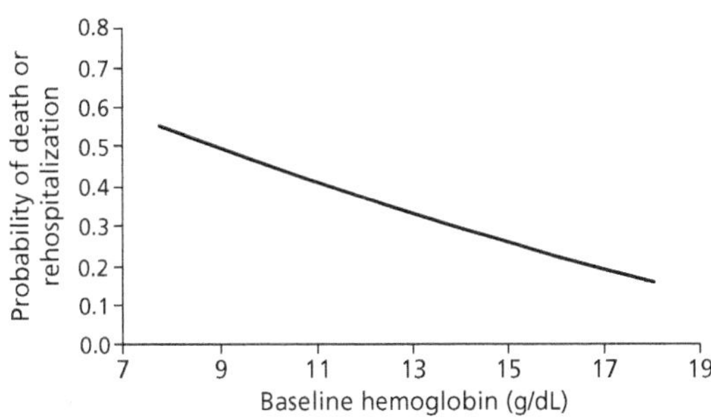

Figure 18.2. *Relationship between serum hemoglobin and risk of death or rehospitalization in patients with acute decompensated heart failure enrolled in the OPTIME-CHF trial*

levels were associated with higher mortality, this association was related to a greater severity of illness and burden of comorbidity, and that hematocrit was not independently associated with 1-year mortality.[39]

Patients with anemia are more likely to have concomitant renal insufficiency, which has been shown to be a powerful predictor of worsened outcomes in heart failure.[9,14] Multiple studies, however, have demonstrated an independent effect of anemia even after controlling for renal function,[1,5–7] suggesting that lower hemoglobin is not simply a surrogate for renal disease. Patients with greater severity of heart failure may have more volume retention and therefore increased prevalence of anemia due to hemodilution. Horwich *et al.*, however, reported that hemoglobin was a predictor of adverse outcome even after adjustment for volume overload as measured by invasive hemodynamic monitoring.[6] Alternatively, anemia may contribute directly to the pathophysiologic state in heart failure. Anemia results in decreased oxygen carrying capacity, which may be compensated for in the normal heart by increasing heart rate and stroke volume, resulting in an increase in cardiac output and maintenance of tissue oxygen delivery.[40] These adaptive responses may be limited, however, in patients with coronary artery disease (CAD) or heart failure.[41] Subsequent myocardial or tissue hypoxia may result in increased sympathetic activity, neurohormonal activation, and cytokine release, leading to a vicious cycle of heart failure progression.

Treatment studies

The association between anemia and adverse clinical outcomes in heart failure has led to substantial interest in anemia as a potential therapeutic target. Potential treatments for anemia include the use of red blood cell transfusions and treatment with erythropoietin analogs to increase red blood cell production. The impact of red blood cell transfusion on cardiovascular disease is controversial. Although a "transfusion threshold" of maintaining the hematocrit > 30% in patients with cardiovascular disease has been commonly accepted, this concept has been based primarily on expert opinion rather than on clinical trials.[42] In addition to the potential risk of infectious transmission, concerns have been raised about the potential immunosuppressive effects of blood transfusion.[43] A randomized controlled trial of a restrictive (7 g/dL) vs. liberal (10 g/dL) transfusion strategy in critically ill patients (26% of whom had cardiovascular disease) reported no significant difference in 30-day mortality, although there was a trend towards reduced mortality in the restrictive transfusion arm.[44] In contrast, a retrospective review of Medicare claims data in elderly patients with AMI found that transfusion in patients with admission hematocrit < 30% was associated with improved 30-day mortality rates.[45] Given the risks and costs of red blood cell transfusion and its uncertain benefit, it does not appear that transfusion represents a viable therapeutic strategy for the routine treatment of anemia in heart failure.

Recombinant human erythropoietin (rHuEPO) has become a mainstay in the treatment of anemia in patients with ESRD. In addition to well-documented improvements in quality of life and survival, data from patients with ESRD have suggested that rHuEPO treatment leads to an improvement in a variety of measures of cardiac performance, including reduced LVH and improved EF and cardiac output.[46–48] A randomized trial has shown that rHuEPO can be used in a critical care setting to reduce the need for RBC transfusion in critically ill patients.[49] The results from three small studies have been published which directly examine the effect of rHuEPO therapy on clinical outcomes in patients with heart failure. In an uncontrolled study, Silverberg *et al.* demonstrated an improvement in EF, functional class, and hospitalization after treatment with erythropoietin and intravenous iron in a group of 26 patients with NYHA class III–IV heart failure.[3] In this study, the dose of rHuEPO was adjusted to maintain a hemoglobin level of 12 g/dL. The same group of investigators subsequently conducted a small randomized trial of rHuEPO and intravenous iron in 32 patients with class III–IV heart failure, which demonstrated that treatment of anemia in this patient population resulted in improved functional class and a decrease in the need for hospitalization.[50] Several aspects of these studies suggest the need for caution in interpreting the results.

Both studies examined a very small number of patients. The initial study was not randomized and had no control group. Additionally, the randomized trial was significantly limited by its lack of a placebo control and the fact that neither patients nor investigators were blinded to treatment assignment. Given the subjectivity of functional class assessment and the criteria for diuretic dosing or heart failure hospitalization, these endpoints must be interpreted very cautiously in the setting of an unblinded study.

A recent randomized, single-blind, placebo-controlled study by Mancini *et al.* evaluated the effect of 3 months of erythropoietin treatment on exercise capacity in 26 patients with anemia and NYHA class III–IV heart failure.[51] This study demonstrated significant improvement in peak oxygen consumption (VO_2max) with erythropoietin (EPO) treatment (from 11 ± 0.8 to 12.7 ± 2.8 in the rHuEPO-treated patients [$P < 0.05$] vs. no significant change in the control patients). A significant correlation was observed between elevations in hemoglobin with rHuEPO treatment and increase VO_2. Notably, the improvement in exercise performance with rHuEPO treatment was observed whether the anemia was found to be from decreased red blood cell mass or from hemodilution. Although this study was randomized, placebo-controlled, single-blinded, and had an objective endpoint (VO_2max), the small sample size suggests the need for larger confirmatory studies before these results can be widely accepted.

All three of these studies used rHuEPO in a regimen similar to the one used in patients with ESRD. Newer erythropoietin analogs have been developed (such as darbepoetin alpha) which have a longer half-life and require less frequent administration, potentially making them more attractive for heart failure therapy. An ongoing phase II study of darbepoetin alpha in patients with heart failure and anemia will provide important preliminary data on the potential efficacy of this agent in the heart failure population.

At present there are no data on the use of treatments aimed at anemia in the setting of AHF. Given the high morbidity and mortality associated with hospitalization for AHF as well as the potential mechanistic rationale for the effectiveness of anemia therapy in this setting, this patient population represents a potential target for anemia therapy. Additionally, patients hospitalized for heart failure may represent an ideal population for screening for trials of anemia therapy, which could be initiated in the acute setting and transferred to chronic heart failure care.

Another area of ongoing investigation deals with the direct effects of rHuEPO on the heart. Erythropoietin receptors are present in a variety of tissues, including the heart, and erythropoietin appears to have antiinflammatory and antiapoptotic properties.[52] Recently published studies have demonstrated that treatment with rHuEPO favorably attenuated ischemia–reperfusion injury in a mouse model.[53,54] Whether these findings will have physiologic relevance in humans remains unknown, but they do suggest an additional potential mechanism for beneficial effects of erythropoietin treatment for heart failure in humans.

Potential risks of anemia treatment

As with all therapies, potential benefits must be balanced against potential risks, and concern does exist about possible adverse effects of anemia treatment in heart failure. In large part, these concerns are based on the results of a large randomized trial, the Normal Hematocrit Treatment Trial, which demonstrated a nonsignificant increase in mortality in hemodialysis patients with clinical heart disease (heart failure or ischemic heart disease) who were treated with erythropoietin to a goal hematocrit of 42% as opposed to 30%.[55] This trial was terminated prematurely when the Data Safety Monitoring Committee concluded that the trial would be unable to reach its pre-stated endpoint of demonstrating improved outcomes in the higher hematocrit group. Although not statistically significant, the relative risk of death or nonfatal MI in the high hematocrit group was 1.3 (95% confidence interval [CI] 0.9–1.9). Paradoxically, however, higher hematocrit values in this study were associated with a decreased mortality rate within each study group, suggesting that the higher hematocrit per se was not responsible for the increased mortality. These issues have led to significant controversy in interpreting these results.[56]

Other smaller studies have not replicated the results of the Normal Hematocrit Treatment Trial. Data from the Canadian Multicenter Study, which evaluated 146 patients with asymptomatic LVH or LV dilatation, found no evidence of improvement in echocardiographic parameters but did show improvements in quality of life with normalization of hemoglobin (target > 13.5 g/dL).[57] There was no difference in rates of thrombosis between the two groups, but there was a greater need for antihypertensive therapy in the high hemoglobin group. The Spanish Cooperative Quality of Life study group performed an uncontrolled trial in ESRD patients without heart failure and found that normalization of hematocrit was associated with improved quality of life and functional status.[58]

Several mechanisms could theoretically result in harmful effects from increasing hemoglobin in heart failure patients. Erythropoietin therapy is associated with worsening hypertension in 20% to 30% of patients on hemodialysis.[59] Additionally, erythropoietin use may be associated with increased risk of thrombosis, especially of vascular access grafts.[60–63] These effects may be due to increased platelet activation, increased blood viscosity, or effects on the levels of C and S proteins.[64–66] Finally, erythropoietin therapy may be associated with endothelial activation and the release of endothelin, a circulating peptide that has been shown to be associated with adverse outcomes in heart failure.[67,68]

Given that higher hemoglobin levels increase the potential risks associated erythropoietin therapy, caution seems well justified until more definitive data on the potential clinical benefits of anemia therapy in heart failure patients are available. Many important questions remain unanswered, including the optimal hemoglobin target and the appropriate rate of rise of hemoglobin. Importantly, the ultimate benefit of a therapy is related to the relative balance of risks and benefits in a given patient population. Thrombolytic therapy, for example, carries a finite risk of intracranial hemorrhage, but this risk is outweighed by the clinical benefits in appropriately selected patients with acute ST elevation MI. Such a balance of risks and benefits can only be established in appropriately designed, randomized controlled trials. Such studies, several of which are ongoing, will provide a substantially greater understanding of the balance between the risks and benefits of pharmacologic treatment of anemia in patients with heart failure.

Current Recommendations and Future Directions

At present, there are insufficient data to make a general recommendation for aggressive treatment of anemia in patients with heart failure. A diagnostic evaluation for potentially reversible causes of anemia, such as iron deficiency or occult blood loss, and subsequent treatment, if identified, is appropriate in all patients. Although pilot data on the treatment of anemic heart failure patients with erythropoietin analogs are promising, the studies published thus far have been significantly limited by very small sample size, lack of blinding, and the use of subjective endpoints. Based on currently available data, treatment of mild anemia with erythropoietin analogs cannot be considered a proven therapy for heart failure. The results of larger, more carefully controlled clinical trials are required before such treatment can be considered a viable therapy. The history of drug development in heart failure is notable for many therapies that appeared promising in small, early studies, such as chronic inotropic therapy or TNF-α blockade, only to be proven neutral or harmful when evaluated in large, carefully controlled trials.[69,70] Therefore, it is crucial that appropriate caution be exercised until data from prospective, blinded, controlled trials of adequate size are available. Many such studies are currently being planned or are under way, including prospective studies addressing the prevalence and incidence of anemia in heart failure populations,[33] the mechanisms of anemia in heart failure, and the effect of anemia treatment on quality of life, exercise tolerance, morbidity, mortality, and costs. Given the history of drug development in heart failure, a mixture of optimism and caution would appear to be the appropriate approach towards anemia therapy in heart failure at present.

Conclusion

Anemia is increasingly recognized as an important comorbid condition in patients with heart failure. Although the exact mechanism is not well defined, it appears that anemia in heart failure patients is the result of a complex interaction of cardiac performance, renal homeostasis, bone marrow responsiveness, and concomitant drug therapy. Multiple observational studies have confirmed the substantial prevalence of anemia in a variety of heart failure populations. Observational data have also suggested a significant independent association of lower hemoglobin levels with adverse clinical outcomes (Table 18.3). Although preliminary and limited, several pilot studies have also demonstrated the potential for therapies targeted at anemia to impact clinical outcomes in heart failure. Given the potential risks of worsening hypertension and thrombosis, larger carefully controlled studies are required before such therapy can be widely accepted. Such studies must also address important questions about mechanisms and the cost–benefit ratio of this type of therapy. Given the therapeutic ceiling that seems to have been reached with current modalities of neurohormonal modulation, anemia may represent an important novel target for addressing the substantial morbidity and mortality associated with the ongoing heart failure epidemic.

References

1. Al-Ahmad A, Rand WM, Manjunath G, *et al.* Reduced kidney function and anemia as risk factors for mortality in patients with left ventricular dysfunction. J Am Coll Cardiol 2001; 38: 955–962.
2. Mozaffarian D, Nye R, Levy WC. Anemia predicts mortality in severe heart failure: The Prospective Randomized Amlodipine Survival Evaluation (PRAISE). J Am Coll Cardiol 2003; 41: 1933–1939.
3. Silverberg DS, Wexler D, Blum M, *et al.* The use of subcutaneous erythropoietin and intravenous iron for the treatment of the anemia of severe, resistant congestive heart failure improves cardiac and renal function and functional cardiac class, and markedly reduces hospitalizations. J Am Coll Cardiol 2000; 35: 1737–1744.
4. Tanner H, Moschovitis G, Kuster GM, *et al.* The prevalence of anemia in chronic heart failure. Int J Cardiol 2002; 86: 115–121.
5. Ezekowitz JA, McAlister FA, Armstrong PW. Anemia is common in heart failure and is associated with poor outcomes: insights from a cohort of 12 065 patients with new-onset heart failure. Circulation 2003; 107: 223–225.
6. Horwich TB, Fonarow GC, Hamilton MA, MacLellan WR, Borenstein J. Anemia is associated with worse symptoms, greater impairment in functional capacity and a significant increase in mortality in patients with advanced heart failure. J Am Coll Cardiol 2002; 39: 1780–1786.
7. Kosiborod M, Smith GL, Radford MJ, Foody JM, Krumholz HM. The prognostic importance of anemia

Table 18.3. *Potential benefits and potential risks of anemia therapy with erythropoietin analogs in patients with heart failure*

Potential benefits	Potential risks
Improved oxygen delivery	Increased thrombosis
Improved exercise tolerance	Platelet activation
Attenuate adverse remodeling	Hypertension
Antiapoptotic	Endothelial activation
? Improved quality of life	
? Decrease in hospitalizations	
? Improved survival	

"?" Denotes potential benefits that have not yet been demonstrated in adequately powered clinical trials.
With permission from Felker *et al.*[71]

in patients with heart failure. Am J Med 2003; 114: 112–119.
8. Joosten E, Pelemans W, Hiele M, Noyen J, Verhaeghe R, Boogaerts MA. Prevalence and causes of anaemia in a geriatric hospitalized population. Gerontology 1992; 38: 111–117.
9. Dries DL, Exner DV, Domanski MJ, Greenberg B, Stevenson LW. The prognostic implications of renal insufficiency in asymptomatic and symptomatic patients with left ventricular systolic dysfunction. J Am Coll Cardiol 2000; 35: 681–689.
10. Hillege HL, Girbes AR, de Kam PJ, *et al.* Renal function, neurohormonal activation, and survival in patients with chronic heart failure. Circulation 2000; 102: 203–210.
11. Silverberg D. Outcomes of anaemia management in renal insufficiency and cardiac disease. Nephrol Dial Transplant 2003; 18: II7–II12.
12. Volpe M, Tritto C, Testa U, *et al.* Blood levels of erythropoietin in congestive heart failure and correlation with clinical, hemodynamic, and hormonal profiles. Am J Cardiol 1994; 74: 468–473.
13. Androne AS, Katz SD, Lund L, *et al.* Hemodilution is common in patients with advanced heart failure. Circulation 2003; 107: 226–229.
14. Mahon NG, Blackstone EH, Francis GS, Starling RC III, Young JB, Lauer MS. The prognostic value of estimated creatinine clearance alongside functional capacity in ambulatory patients with chronic congestive heart failure. J Am Coll Cardiol 2002; 40: 1106–1113.
15. Foley RN, Parfrey PS, Harnett JD, Kent GM, Murray DC, Barre PE. The impact of anemia on cardiomyopathy, morbidity, and mortality in end-stage renal disease. Am J Kidney Dis 1996; 28: 53–61.
16. Harnett JD, Kent GM, Foley RN, Parfrey PS. Cardiac function and hematocrit level. Am J Kidney Dis 1995; 25: S3–S7.
17. Levine B, Kalman J, Mayer L, Fillit HM, Packer M. Elevated circulating levels of tumor necrosis factor in severe chronic heart failure. N Engl J Med 1990; 323: 236–241.
18. Deswal A, Peterson MJ, Feldman AM, Young JB, White BG, Mann DL. Cytokines and cytokine receptors in advanced heart failure: an analysis of the cytokine database from the Vesnarinone Trial (VEST). Circulation 2001; 103: 2055–2059.
19. Torre-Amione G, Kapadia S, Benedict C, Oral H, Young JB, Mann DL. Proinflammatory cytokine levels in patients with depressed left ventricular ejection fraction: a report from the Studies of Left Ventricular Dysfunction (SOLVD). J Am Coll Cardiol 1996; 27: 1201–1206.
20. Voulgari PV, Kolios G, Papadopoulos GK, Katsaraki A, Seferiadis K, Drosos AA. Role of cytokines in the pathogenesis of anemia of chronic disease in rheumatoid arthritis. Clin Immunol 1999; 92: 153–160.
21. Bolger AP, Haehling S, Doehner W, Poole-Wilson PA, Coats AJ, Anker SD. Anemia and inflammation in chronic heart failure. J Card Fail 2003; 9: 33 (Abstract).
22. Milo O, Cotter G, Kaluski E, *et al.* Comparison of inflammatory and neurohormonal activation in cardiogenic pulmonary edema secondary to ischemic versus nonischemic causes. Am J Cardiol 2003; 92: 222–226.
23. Krum H, Bigger JT Jr., Goldsmith RL, Packer M. Effect of long-term digoxin therapy on autonomic function in patients with chronic heart failure. J Am Coll Cardiol 1995; 25: 289–294.
24. Obayashi K, Ando Y, Terazaki H, *et al.* Mechanism of anemia associated with autonomic dysfunction in rats. Auton Neurosci 2000; 82: 123–129.
25. Cohn JN, Johnson G, Ziesche S, *et al.* A comparison of enalapril with hydralazine-isosorbide dinitrate in the treatment of chronic congestive heart failure. N Engl J Med 1991; 325: 303–310.
26. The CONSENSUS Trial Study Group. Effects of enalapril on mortality in severe congestive heart failure. Results of the Cooperative North Scandinavian Enalapril Survival Study (CONSENSUS). N Engl J Med 1987; 316: 1429–1435.
27. The SOLVD Investigators. Effect of enalapril on survival in patients with reduced left ventricular ejection fractions and congestive heart failure. N Engl J Med 1991; 325: 293–302.
28. Griffing GT, Melby JC. Enalapril (MK-420) and the white cell count and haematocrit. Lancet 1982; 319: 1361.
29. Kamper AL, Nielsen OJ. Effect of enalapril on haemoglobin and serum erythropoietin in patients with chronic nephropathy. Scand J Clin Lab Invest 1990; 50: 611–618.
30. Plata R, Cornejo A, Arratia C, *et al.* Angiotensin-converting-enzyme inhibition therapy in altitude polycythaemia: a prospective randomised trial. Lancet 2002; 359: 663–666.
31. Fyhrquist F, Karppinen K, Honkanen T, Saijonmaa O, Rosenlof K. High serum erythropoietin levels are normalized during treatment of congestive heart failure with enalapril. J Intern Med 1989; 226: 257–260.
32. Hussein SJ, Jain R, Shlipak MG, Ansari M, Massie BM. Chronic heart failure is not an independent cause of anemia. J Card Fail 2003; 9: 19 (Abstract).
33. Adams KF, Patterson JH, Pina I, *et al.* Stamina-HFP (STudy of AneMia in a Heart Failure Population)

Registry: Rationale, Design, and Patient Characteristics. J Card Fail 2003; 9: 73 (Abstract).
34. Sarnak MJ, Tighiouart H, Manjunath G, *et al.* Anemia as a risk factor for cardiovascular disease in the Atherosclerosis Risk in Communities (ARIC) study. J Am Coll Cardiol 2002; 40: 27–33.
35. Kannel W. Epidemiology and prevention of cardiac failure: Framingham Study insights. Eur Heart J 1998; 8: 23–29.
36. Kalra PR, Bolger AP, Francis DP, *et al.* Effect of anemia on exercise tolerance in chronic heart failure in men. Am J Cardiol 2003; 91: 888–891.
37. Kalra PR, Collier T, Cowie MR, *et al.* Haemoglobin concentration and prognosis in new cases of heart failure. Lancet 2003; 362: 211–212.
38. Felker GM, Gattis WA, Leimberger JD, *et al.* Usefulness of anemia as a predictor of death and rehospitalization in patients with decompensated heart failure. Am J Cardiol 2003; 92: 625–628.
39. Kosiborod M, Curtis JP, Smith GL, Masoudi FA, Havranek EP, Krumholz HM. Anemia is not an independent predictor of mortality in patients with heart failure: results from the National Heart Failure Project. Circulation 2003; 108: IV-665–IV-666 (Abstract).
40. Weiskopf RB, Viele MK, Feiner J, *et al.* Human cardiovascular and metabolic response to acute, severe isovolemic anemia. JAMA 1998; 279: 217–221.
41. Levy PS, Kim SJ, Eckel PK, *et al.* Limit to cardiac compensation during acute isovolemic hemodilution: influence of coronary stenosis. Am J Physiol 1993; 265: H340–H349.
42. Welch HG, Meehan KR, Goodnough LT. Prudent strategies for elective red blood cell transfusion. Ann Intern Med 1992; 116: 393–402.
43. Goodnough LT, Brecher ME, Kanter MH, AuBuchon JP. Transfusion medicine. First of two parts—blood transfusion. N Engl J Med 1999; 340: 438–447.
44. Hebert PC, Wells G, Blajchman MA, *et al.* A multicenter, randomized, controlled clinical trial of transfusion requirements in critical care. Transfusion Requirements in Critical Care Investigators, Canadian Critical Care Trials Group. N Engl J Med 1999; 340: 409–417.
45. Wu CH, Raithore SS, Radford MJ, Krumholz HM. Blood transfusion in elderly patients with acute myocardial infarction. N Engl J Med 2001; 345: 1230–1236.
46. Low-Friedrich I, Grutzmacher P, Marz W, Bergmann M, Schoeppe W. Therapy with recombinant human erythropoietin reduces cardiac size and improves heart function in chronic hemodialysis patients. Am J Nephrol 1991; 11: 54–60.
47. Goldberg N, Lundin AP, Delano B, Friedman EA, Stein RA. Changes in left ventricular size, wall thickness, and function in anemic patients treated with recombinant human erythropoietin. Am Heart J 1992; 124: 424–427.
48. Linde T, Wikstrom B, Andersson LG, Danielson BG. Renal anemia treatment with recombinant human erythropoietin increases cardiac output in patients with ischemic heart disease. Scand J Urol Nephrol 1996; 30: 115–120.
49. Corwin HL, Gettinger A, Pearl RG, *et al.* Efficacy of recombinant human erythropoietin in critically ill patients: a randomized controlled trial. JAMA 2002; 288: 2827–2835.
50. Silverberg DS, Wexler D, Sheps D, *et al.* The effect of correction of mild anemia in severe, resistant congestive heart failure using subcutaneous erythropoietin and intravenous iron: a randomized controlled study. J Am Coll Cardiol 2001; 37: 1775–1780.
51. Mancini DM, Katz SD, Lang CC, LaManca J, Hudaihed A, Androne AS. Effect of erythropoietin on exercise capacity in patients with moderate to severe chronic heart failure. Circulation 2003; 107: 294–299.
52. Masuda S, Nagao M, Sasaki R. Erythropoietic, neurotrophic, and angiogenic functions of erythropoietin and regulation of erythropoietin production. Int J Hematol 1999; 70: 1–6.
53. Calvillo L, Latini R, Kajstura J, *et al.* Recombinant human erythropoietin protects the myocardium from ischemia–reperfusion injury and promotes beneficial remodeling. Proc Natl Acad Sci USA 2003; 100: 4802–4806.
54. Parsa CJ, Matsumoto A, Kim J, *et al.* A novel protective effect of erythropoietin in the infarcted heart. J Clin Invest 2003; 112: 999–1007.
55. Besarab A, Bolton WK, Browne JK, *et al.* The effects of normal as compared with low hematocrit values in patients with cardiac disease who are receiving hemodialysis and epoetin. N Engl J Med 1998; 339: 584–590.
56. Macdougall IC, Ritz E. The Normal Haematocrit Trial in dialysis patients with cardiac disease: are we any less confused about target hemoglobin? Nephrol Dial Transplant 1998; 13: 3030–3033.
57. Foley RN, Parfrey PS, Morgan J, *et al.* Effect of hemoglobin levels in hemodialysis patients with asymptomatic cardiomyopathy. Kidney Int 2000; 58: 1325–1335.
58. Moreno F, Sanz-Guajardo D, Lopez-Gomez JM, Jofre R, Valderrabano F. Increasing the hematocrit has a beneficial effect on quality of life and is safe in selected

hemodialysis patients. Spanish Cooperative Renal Patients Quality of Life Study Group of the Spanish Society of Nephrology. J Am Soc Nephrol 2000; 11: 335–342.

59. Mann JF. Hypertension and cardiovascular effects—long-term safety and potential long-term benefits of r-HuEPO. Nephrol Dial Transplant 1995; 10: 80–84.
60. Wolf RF, Gilmore LS, Friese P, Downs T, Burstein SA, Dale GL. Erythropoietin potentiates thrombus development in a canine arterio-venous shunt model. Thromb Haemost 1997; 77: 1020–1024.
61. Churchill DN, Muirhead N, Goldstein M, *et al.* Probability of thrombosis of vascular access among hemodialysis patients treated with recombinant human erythropoietin. J Am Soc Nephrol 1994; 4: 1809–1813.
62. Taylor JE, McLaren M, Henderson IS, Belch JJ, Stewart WK. Prothrombotic effect of erythropoietin in dialysis patients. Nephrol Dial Transplant 1992; 7: 235–239.
63. Muirhead N, Laupacis A, Wong C. Erythropoietin for anaemia in haemodialysis patients: results of a maintenance study (the Canadian Erythropoietin Study Group). Nephrol Dial Transplant 1992; 7: 811–816.
64. Tang WW, Stead RA, Goodkin DA. Effects of epoetin alfa on hemostasis in chronic renal failure. Am J Nephrol 1998; 18: 263–273.
65. Taylor JE, McLaren M, Henderson IS, Belch JJ, Stewart WK. Prothrombotic effect of erythropoietin in dialysis patients. Nephrol Dial Transplant 1992; 7: 235–239.
66. Macdougall IC, Davies ME, Hallett I, *et al.* Coagulation studies and fistula blood flow during erythropoietin therapy in haemodialysis patients. Nephrol Dial Transplant 1991; 6: 862–867.
67. Carlini RG, Dusso AS, Obialo CI, Alvarez UM, Rothstein M. Recombinant human erythropoietin (rHuEPO) increases endothelin-1 release by endothelial cells. Kidney Int 1993; 43: 1010–1014.
68. Pacher R, Stanek B, Hulsmann M, *et al.* Prognostic impact of big endothelin-1 plasma concentrations compared with invasive hemodynamic evaluation in severe heart failure. J Am Coll Cardiol 1996; 27: 633–641.
69. Felker GM, O'Connor CM. Inotropic therapy for heart failure: an evidence-based approach. Am Heart J 2001; 142: 393–401.
70. Louis A, Cleland JG, Crabbe S, *et al.* Clinical Trials Update: CAPRICORN, COPERNICUS, MIRACLE, STAF, RITZ-2, RECOVER and RENAISSANCE and cachexia and cholesterol in heart failure. Highlights of the Scientific Sessions of the American College of Cardiology, 2001. Eur J Heart Fail 2001; 3: 381–387.
71. Felker GM, Adams KF Jr., Gattis WA *et al.* Anemia as a risk factor and therapeutic target in heart failure J Am Coll Cardiol 2004; 44: 959–966.

Chapter 19

Acute pulmonary embolism

Victor F Tapson

Background and Incidence

Acute pulmonary embolism (PE) remains one of the most common yet vexing conditions in clinical medicine. Despite several centuries of clinical familiarity, acute PE remains one of the most common causes of unexpected death in hospitalized patients. The disease occurs when venous thrombosis, usually from the deep veins of the proximal legs, dislodges and migrates to the lungs, causing a potential spectrum of clinical consequences. Death, when death occurs, results from acute right ventricular failure. Deep venous thrombosis (DVT) and PE represent a continuum of the disease entity known as venous thromboembolism (VTE). Acute PE likely accounts for 100 000 to 200 000 deaths per year in the United States.[1,2] Although some patients dying from acute PE are already facing an underlying terminal illness, it still appears that acute PE is responsible for death in a considerable number of patients with an otherwise favorable prognosis. Autopsy studies have repeatedly documented the high frequency with which PE has gone unsuspected and thus, undetected.[3] While VTE is frequently associated with one or more specific risk factors, some patients present with idiopathic VTE with no underlying risk factors identified.[1,4–6] Because of the lack of specificity of symptoms and signs, DVT and PE are both frequently unsuspected clinically, leading to substantial diagnostic and therapeutic delays, and accounting for considerable morbidity and mortality.[1,2] Furthermore, DVT, and therefore PE, are often preventable, although prophylaxis continues to be dramatically underutilized.[4,7] The incidence of VTE is high in hospitalized patients, and both surgical and medical patients are at risk. While other substances such as malignant cells, fat droplets, air bubbles, and carbon dioxide may embolize to the lung, our discussion in this chapter is limited to pulmonary thromboembolism.

Pathophysiology

The German pathologist von Virchow described the insightful triad of stasis, hypercoagulability and venous injury more than 150 years ago. Risk factors based upon one or more of these are present in nearly all patients.[8] While idiopathic VTE is well-described, it likely involves an underlying prothrombotic state that is present but awaits characterization. Deep vein thrombi frequently originate in the calf veins and propagate proximally before embolizing. While emboli may occasionally originate directly from calf vein thrombi, more than 95% of thrombi that embolize to the lungs appear to dislodge from a proximal deep vein of the lower extremities (including and above the popliteal veins). Thrombosis developing in the axillary-subclavian veins because of the presence of a central venous catheter, particularly in patients with malignant disease, as well as in those with effort-induced upper extremity thrombosis may result in PE as well.

The implications of a particular embolic event depend upon the extent of obstruction of the cross-sectional area of the pulmonary arterial bed as well as upon the presence or absence of underlying cardiopulmonary disease.[9,10] In response to acute PE, hypoxemia develops, stimulating sympathetic tone with resulting systemic vasoconstriction, increased venous return, and a rise in stroke volume. In the setting of more massive emboli, cardiac output is reduced but may be sustained as the mean right atrial pressure increases. The increase in pulmonary vascular resistance impedes right ventricular outflow which reduces left ventricular preload. In the absence of underlying cardiopulmonary disease, occlusion of 25% to 30% of the vascular bed by emboli is associated with a rise in pulmonary artery pressure.[10] More than 50% obstruction of the pulmonary arterial bed is usually present before there is substantial elevation of the mean pulmonary artery pressure. When the extent of obstruction of the pulmonary circulation approaches 75%, the right ventricle must generate a systolic pressure in excess of 50 mm Hg and a mean pulmonary artery pressure of greater than 40 mm Hg to preserve pulmonary perfusion. A normal right ventricle is rarely able to achieve this and, hence, fails. Patients with underlying cardiopulmonary disease often experience a more substantial deterioration in cardiac output than normal individuals in the setting of massive PE. While supportive measures may sustain a patient with massive PE, subsequent increments in embolic burden are often fatal.

Clinical manifestations

Perhaps the most frustrating problem with acute VTE is the notorious lack of sensitivity and specificity of the history and physical examination for both acute DVT and PE.[11–13] The fact that large thrombi may be completely asymptomatic is evidenced by the occurrence of fatal PE in patients with no preceding leg pain or swelling. When erythema, warmth, pain, swelling, or tenderness is present, they are not diagnostic, but still merit further evaluation. Pain with dorsiflexion of the foot (Homan's sign) may be present in the setting of DVT, but it is neither sensitive nor specific. The most frequent symptom of acute PE is dyspnea which is commonly sudden in onset. Pleuritic chest pain and hemoptysis occur more often with pulmonary *infarction* due to smaller peripheral emboli. Palpitations, cough, anxiety, and lightheadedness are among the nonspecific symptoms of acute PE and may result from a number of other entities, contributing to the difficulty in making the diagnosis. Syncope or sudden death may occur with massive PE. Whenever unexplained dyspnea, syncope, hypotension, or hypoxemia, are present, PE should always be considered.[11–13] Tachypnea and tachycardia are the most common signs of PE but are also nonspecific. Other physical findings include fever, wheezing, rales, pleural rub, loud pulmonic component of the second heart sound, right-sided fourth heart sound, and right ventricular lift. Dyspnea, tachypnea, and hypoxemia in patients with concomitant cardiopulmonary disease (such as congestive heart failure, pneumonia, or chronic obstructive pulmonary disease) may be caused by the underlying disease or may be due to superimposed acute PE. Symptoms and signs consistent with PE (Tables 19.1 and 19.2) should be heeded particularly in the setting of risk factors for VTE such as concomitant malignancy, immobility, or the postoperative state.

Diagnosis

Generating a differential diagnosis in the setting of a clinical presentation consistent with either acute DVT or PE is aided by not only the specific symptoms and signs, but also by the presence of potential risk factors and knowledge of comorbid disease. When patients present with, for example, calf pain or swelling in the setting of prolonged immobilization, a diagnostic study should be pursued unless there is a clear, alternative explanation. In the setting of dyspnea or chest pain, the differential diagnosis may include a flare of asthma or chronic obstructive lung disease, pneumothorax, pneumonia, anxiety with hyperventilation, heart failure, angina or myocardial infarction (MI), musculoskeletal pain, rib fracture, pericarditis, pleuritis from collagen vascular disease, herpes zoster, intrathoracic cancer, or

Table 19.1. *Symptoms of acute pulmonary embolism*

Symptom	All patients (n = 383) (%)	Patients with no previous cardiopulmonary disease (n = 117) (%)
Dyspnea	78	73
Pleuritic chest pain	59	66
Cough	43	37
Leg pain	27	26
Hemoptysis	16	13
Palpitations	13	10
Wheezing	14	9
Angina-like pain	6	4

The symptoms listed above were based upon data from the PIOPED study[12,13] and adapted from tables presented in Stein, *Pulmonary Embolism*,[90] with permission.

Table 19.2. *Signs of acute pulmonary embolism*

Symptom	All patients (n = 383) (%)	Patients with no previous cardiopulmonary disease (n = 117) (%)
Tachypnea (20/min)	73	70
Crackles	55	51
Tachycardia (100/min)	30	30
Leg swelling	31	28
Loud P2	23	23
DVT	15	11
Wheezes	11	5
Diaphoresis	10	11
Temperature (≥ 38.5°C)	7	7
Pleural rub	4	3
Fourth heart sound	—	24
Third heart sound	5	3
Cyanosis	3	1
Homan's sign	3	4
Right ventricular lift	—	4

The clinical signs listed above were based upon data from the PIOPED study[12,13] and adapted from tables presented in Stein, *Pulmonary Embolism*,[90] with permission.
Abbreviations: P2 = pulmonic component of second heart sound; DVT = deep venous thrombosis.

occasionally, intraabdominal processes such as acute cholecystitis. The presence of obvious risk factors for VTE, such as prolonged immobility,[14] trauma,[15–17] recent surgery,[18] medical illness with reduced mobility,[19] cancer,[20,21] pregnancy,[22] MI,[23] recent prolonged travel,[24–26] or previous VTE in the setting of compatible symptoms and signs should prompt consideration of this entity. It is important to realize that acute PE can be superimposed upon another underlying cardiopulmonary disease, upon which new or worsening symptoms are sometimes blamed.

Laboratory tests

While hypoxemia is exceedingly common in acute PE, it is not universal. Some individuals, particularly young patients without underlying lung disease, may have a normal arterial oxygen tension (PaO_2) and even rarely a normal alveolar-arterial difference.[11,13] A sudden decrease in the PaO_2 or in the oxygen saturation in a patient unable to communicate an accurate history (e.g., a demented or mechanically ventilated patient) suggest the possibility of acute PE.

The diagnostic utility of plasma measurements of circulating D-dimer (a specific derivative of cross-linked fibrin) in patients with acute PE has been extensively evaluated.[27–30] A normal enzyme-linked immunosorbent assay (ELISA) appears sensitive in excluding PE, particularly when the clinical suspicion is relatively low. For example, when the D-dimer level cutoff is 500 μg/L or greater, the sensitivity for PE may be as high as 96% to 98% but the specificity is much lower. There are a number of D-dimer assays available and the sensitivity and specificity of these assays vary.[30] A positive D-dimer test means that DVT or PE is possible, but it is not proof. Similarly, while a negative D-dimer may strongly suggest that VTE is absent, a high clinical suspicion should not be ignored.

Clinical probability scores based upon simple clinical parameters have been utilized together with a negative D-dimer to help exclude PE. In a recent prospective clinical trial, the SimpliRed D-dimer test (a rapid red blood cell agglutination D-dimer assay) was used together with simple scoring parameters readily available in the emergency department.[28] Of the 437 patients with a negative D-dimer result and low clinical probability in this study, only one patient developed PE during follow-up (Table 19.3). Whether or not such scoring systems are used, D-dimer assays may prove

Table 19.3. *Determining pretest probability of acute pulmonary embolism using point system and D-dimer result*[28]

Variable	Points	Total score	Pretest probability‡
DVT symptoms/signs	3.0	< 2.0	Low
PE as more likely*	3.0	2.0 to 6.0	Moderate
HR > 100 bpm	1.5	< 6.0	High
Immobilization/surgery†	1.5		
Previous DVT or PE	1.5		
Hemoptysis	1.0		
Malignancy	1.0		

*PE as likely as or more likely than an alternative diagnosis. Physicians were told to use clinical information, along with chest radiography, electrocardiography, and laboratory tests.
†Immobilization surgery within the previous 4 weeks.
‡Of the 437 patients with a negative D-dimer result and low clinical probability, only 1 developed PE during follow-up. Thus, the negative predictive value for the combined strategy of using the clinical model with D-dimer testing in these patients was 99.5%.
Abbreviations: bpm = beats per minute; DVT = deep venous thrombosis; HR = heart rate; PE = pulmonary embolism.

increasingly useful in excluding acute DVT and PE, particularly when low clinical suspicion supports its absence.

Cardiac troponin-T and troponin-I levels have been found to be increased in acute PE.[32,33] This enzyme is specific for cardiac myocyte damage. In acute PE, the right ventricle appears to be the source of the enzyme elevation, particularly in more massive embolism in which myocyte injury due to right ventricular strain might be expected. Troponin levels cannot, however, be used like D-dimer testing; that is, they are not sensitive enough to rule out PE when clinical suspicion is relatively low, without additional diagnostic testing.

Electrocardiography

Although electrocardiographic abnormalities are present in the majority of patients with acute PE, they are nonspecific. ST-segment abnormalities, T-wave changes, and left or right axis deviation are common. Approximately one-third of patients with massive or submassive emboli have manifestations of acute cor pulmonale such as the $S_1Q_3T_3$ pattern, right bundle branch block, P-wave pulmonale, or right axis deviation. The utility of electrocardiography in suspected acute PE is best characterized by its ability to establish or exclude alternative diagnoses, such as pericarditis or acute MI.[13]

Chest radiography

As with electrocardiography, the chest radiograph is often abnormal but generally nonspecific in patients with acute PE. Frequent findings include atelectasis, pleural effusion, pulmonary infiltrates, and mild elevation of a hemidiaphragm.[13] Classic findings of pulmonary infarction such as Hampton's hump or decreased vascularity (Westermark's sign) are suggestive of the diagnosis, but are infrequent. A normal chest radiograph in the setting of severe dyspnea and hypoxemia without evidence of bronchospasm or anatomic cardiac shunt is strongly suggestive of PE. PE frequently coexists with underlying heart or lung disease. Because neither symptoms, signs, nor blood studies can prove the presence of DVT, and because neither symptoms, signs, laboratory tests, electrocardiography, nor radiographic findings are diagnostic of PE, when these entities are suspected, further evaluation with noninvasive or invasive testing is necessary.

Deep venous thrombosis: the radiographic approach

While venography has been the time-honored gold-standard technique for the diagnosis of acute DVT, its use has become extraordinarily uncommon.[34] The advent of ultrasound, a diagnostic test that is portable, noninvasive, and has a greater than 90% sensitivity in the setting of symptomatic DVT, has rendered venography infrequent. Similarly, another sensitive test, impedance plethysmography, is essentially never used. Magnetic resonance imaging (MRI) has proven extremely sensitive for both acute and chronic DVT,[34–36] although it is generally not necessary. It can be considered in the setting of suspected DVT, when ultrasound cannot be effectively utilized. A major limitation of ultrasound is its reduced sensitivity in the setting of asymptomatic DVT. Thus, it is not generally used as a screening test.

Pulmonary embolism: the radiographic approach

Ventilation-perfusion scanning

Historically, the ventilation-perfusion (VQ) scan had been the most common diagnostic test utilized when PE was suspected. Over the past decade, spiral (helical) computed tomography (CT) scanning has essentially replaced it at most centers. A normal lung perfusion scan rules out the diagnosis of PE with enough certainty that further diagnostic evaluation is almost never necessary.[37] Matching areas of decreased ventilation and perfusion in the presence of a normal chest radiograph generally represents a process other than PE. Low or intermediate probability (nondiagnostic) scans, however, are commonly found with PE, and in such situations further evaluation with pulmonary arteriography is often appropriate. In the Prospective Investigation of Pulmonary Embolism Diagnosis (PIOPED) trial, when the clinical suspicion of PE was considered very high, it was present in 96% of patients with high probability scans, 66% of patients with intermediate scans, and 40% of patients with low probability scans.[12] The diagnosis of PE should be rigorously pursued even when the lung scan is low or intermediate probability, if the clinical setting suggests the diagnosis.

Stable patients with suspected acute PE, nondiagnostic lung scans and adequate cardiopulmonary reserve may undergo noninvasive lower extremity testing in an attempt to diagnose DVT.[38] A positive compression ultrasound may present the opportunity to treat without further testing. If the ultrasound is negative, pulmonary angiography is an appropriate option. *Serial* noninvasive lower extremity testing in the setting of suspected PE should only be performed in centers where follow-up is guaranteed and validated protocols are utilized. MRI of the lower extremities may also be useful after a nondiagnostic lung scan, if the medical facility has experience with this technique.

Pulmonary arteriography

Pulmonary arteriography remains the accepted gold standard technique for the diagnosis of acute PE. It is an extremely sensitive, specific, and safe test.[39] Complications of pulmonary arteriography among 1111 patients suspected of PE in the PIOPED included death in 0.5% and major nonfatal complications in 1%.[12] Pulmonary arteriography is utilized when PE must be diagnosed or excluded, but preliminary testing has been nondiagnostic. In some centers, pulmonary arteriography can be performed at the bedside utilizing a pulmonary artery catheter and fluoroscopic guidance. However, it is being used less frequently as CT scanning has increasingly been employed.

Spiral computed tomography

Spiral (helical) CT scanning can be used for diagnosing both acute and chronic PE and is replacing VQ scanning at many centers. Some clinical trials have suggested very good sensitivity and specificity, but others have been less favorable. Retrospective reconstructions can be performed. A contrast bolus is required for imaging of the pulmonary vasculature. A major advantage of the VQ scan remains the near-infallible sensitivity of a normal perfusion scan.

In at least one early clinical trial, spiral CT has been associated with greater than 95% sensitivity and specificity.[40] More recent and larger trials have suggested a lower sensitivity.[41–48] A large, prospective Swiss study revealed a sensitivity of 70%, suggesting that a negative CT scan may not absolutely rule out smaller emboli.[49] Data from a large multicenter trial (PIOPED II) in the United States and Canada comparing CT (chest and legs) and VQ scanning is currently being analyzed. Spiral CT has the greatest sensitivity and specificity for emboli in the main, lobar, or segmental pulmonary arteries. For subsegmental emboli, spiral CT appears less accurate, although the importance of emboli of this size has been questioned. In published trials thus far, the outcome of selected patients with a negative CT in the setting of suspected PE appears to be good.[50] The use of thinner sections, as well as techniques such as multiplanar three-dimensional reformation, may enhance the usefulness of spiral CT for diagnosing PE. An advantage of spiral CT over VQ scanning and arteriography includes the ability to define nonvascular structures such as lymphadenopathy, lung tumors, emphysema, and other parenchymal abnormalities as well as pleural and pericardial disease.[51] Another advantage of spiral CT is the rapidity with which a study can be performed. Potential disadvantages of spiral CT include the fact that it is not portable at present, and that patients with significant renal insufficiency cannot be scanned without risk of renal failure.

Magnetic resonance imaging

As with DVT, MRI has been utilized to evaluate clinically suspected PE. At present, the excellent sensitivity and specificity for the diagnosis of DVT is the main advantage of MRI in this disease process.[41,52] Disadvantages include the potential difficulty in transporting and performing the technique in critically ill patients. Additional prospective investigations will determine the role of this modality in the evaluation of VTE.

Echocardiography in acute pulmonary embolism

The capability of the right ventricle to adequately function in acute PE is essential in survival. Echocardiography, which can often be obtained more rapidly than either lung scanning or pulmonary arteriography may reveal findings which strongly support hemodynamically significant PE.[53] Imaging or Doppler abnormalities of right ventricular size or function may suggest the diagnosis. Because patients with PE may have underlying cardiopulmonary disease, neither right ventricular dilation nor hypokinesis can be reliably used even as indirect evidence of PE in such settings. In the setting of documented acute PE, echocardiographic evidence of right ventricular dysfunction has been suggested as a means by which to determine the need for thrombolytic therapy.[54] Such cases need to be individualized and severe right ventricular dysfunction should lower the threshold for thrombolytic therapy once contraindications have been considered. Transesophageal echocardiography (TEE) has also been evaluated in the setting of acute PE, and while less convenient, may have potential advantages over the transthoracic approach. Intravascular ultrasound imaging has been shown in both the experimental and clinical setting to adequately image large emboli and may be performed at the bedside.[55] Published guidelines suggest that clinicians be afforded a certain degree of flexibility with regard to the diagnostic approach to suspected acute PE.[56]

Treatment

Therapeutic options for acute DVT and PE include anticoagulation with low molecular weight heparin (LMWH) or standard heparin, thrombolytic therapy, and inferior vena cava (IVC) filter placement. Massive PE is occasionally treated with surgical embolectomy. Each approach has specific indications as well as advantages and disadvantages.

Heparin and low molecular weight heparin

The primary anticoagulants used to treat acute DVT or PE include unfractionated heparin and LMWH. These anticoagulants exert a rapid antithrombotic effect by accelerating the action of antithrombin III, preventing thrombus extension. While they do not directly dissolve thrombus or emboli, they allow the fibrinolytic system to proceed unopposed and more readily reduce the size of the thromboembolic burden. While thrombus growth can be prevented, early recurrence can sometimes develop even in the setting of therapeutic anticoagulation. There are substantial advantages of LMWH preparations over unfractionated heparin.[57,58] Because of these advantages, use of the latter is becoming less common.

When DVT or PE are diagnosed or strongly suspected, anticoagulation should be instituted immediately unless contraindications are present. Confirmatory diagnostic testing should be arranged as soon as possible. When standard, unfractionated, intravenous heparin is initiated, the activated partial thromboplastin time (aPTT) should be followed at 6-hour intervals until it is consistently in the therapeutic range of 1.5 to 2.0 times control values. This range corresponds to a heparin level of 0.2 U/mL to 0.4 U/mL as measured by protamine sulfate titration. Achieving a therapeutic aPTT within 24 hours after the onset of treatment of PE has been shown to reduce the recurrence rate and it has become evident that the "traditional" heparin regimen consisting of a 5000-unit bolus and 1000 units/hour is inadequate in many patients. Heparin is administered as an intravenous bolus of 5000 units followed by a maintenance dose of at least 30 000 to 40 000 units per 24 hours by continuous infusion.[59] The lower dose is administered if the patient is considered at high risk for bleeding. This aggressive approach decreases the risk of subtherapeutic anticoagulation. It is possible that early initiation of warfarin, *without* heparin or LMWH may intensify hypercoagulability and increase the clot burden due to the short half-life of *anti*coagulation factors that are also inhibited by warfarin. Factor VII is the primary clotting factor affecting the prothrombin time and has a half-life of about 6 hours. Definitive anticoagulation requires the depletion of factor II (thrombin) which takes approximately 5 days. Thus, at least 5 days of intravenous heparin or LMWH is generally recommended. Heparin should be maintained at a therapeutic level until two consecutive therapeutic international normalized ratio (INR) values of 2.0 to 3.0 have been documented at least 24 hours apart.

The LMWH preparations have tremendous advantages over unfractionated heparin and have dramatically changed the treatment of thromboembolic disease. (Figure 19.1). Among the differences between these two substances is the greater bioavailability of the LMWHs and more predictable dosing.[57,58] The latter anticoagulants can be subcutaneously administered once or twice daily even at therapeutic doses and do not require monitoring of the aPTT. Intravenous LMWH is never required in VTE. In addition, LMWHs have a more profound effect in inhibiting clotting factor Xa relative to thrombin. The reduced frequency of heparin-induced thrombocytopenia with LMWH relative to unfractionated heparin is a very compelling reason to use LMWH instead of the latter whenever possible. Because of efficacy, safety, and convenience, compared with standard heparin, these drugs are replacing standard heparin in many settings. A number of clinical trials as well as meta-analyses have strongly suggested the efficacy and safety of LMWH for the treatment of established acute proximal DVT using recurrent symptomatic VTE as the primary outcome measure.[60–65] The incidence of DVT and recurrent bleeding in these trials indicate that LMWH preparations are at least as effective and as safe as unfractionated heparin. Meta-analytic data suggest that the use of LMWH reduces bleeding rates as well as mortality compared with unfractionated heparin for the treatment of established proximal DVT.[65]

Monitoring is not required with LMWHs except in certain circumstances. The best correlate with clinical effect appears to be the anti-factor Xa level. Appropriate patients include morbidly obese patients, very small patients (< 40 kg), pregnant patients, and those with renal insufficiency. Because these drugs are renally metabolized, monitoring is important, particularly when the creatinine clearance is less than 30 mL/min. Dosing recommendations for renal insufficiency (latter creatinine clearance) have been suggested for the most commonly used LMWH in the United States (enoxaparin). For prophylaxis indications, the usual 40 mg once-daily dose is reduced to 30 mg daily. For therapy, instead of 1 mg/kg every 12 hours, the same dose is administered once daily. With very severe renal insufficiency, and when there are significant fluctuations in renal function, standard heparin should be considered. There is

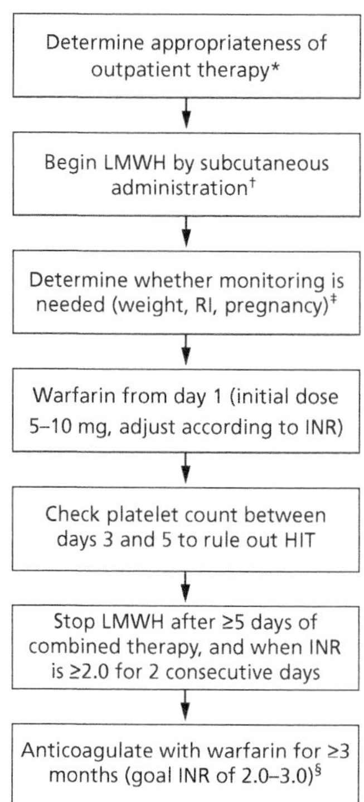

Figure 19.1. *Initiation of low molecular weight heparin for therapy of acute deep venous thrombosis or pulmonary embolism*

*Potential outpatients should be medically stable without severely symptomatic DVT. They should be compliant, capable of self-administration (or have a family member or visiting nurse for administration) and at low risk of bleeding, and reimbursement issues should be addressed.
†Enoxaparin (Lovenox) and tinzaparin (Innohep) are the 2 LMWHs that are FDA-approved for treatment of VTE. While LMWH preparations are sometimes used for patients presenting with PE in the United States, and while clinical trials support this use, the FDA-approvals read "established DVT with or without PE." Fondaparinux, a pentasaccharide, has also been approved for treatment of CVT and PE.
‡When enoxaparin is used in the setting of a (stable) creatinine clearance of < 30 mL/min, a dose of 1 mg/kg once-daily is appropriate.
§The duration of warfarin therapy should be at least 6 to 12 months in patients with idiopathic venous thromboembolism.
Abbreviations: DVT = deep venous thrombosis; HIT = heparin-induced thrombocytopenia; INR = international normalized ratio; LMWH = low molecular weight heparin; PE = pulmonary embolism; RI = renal insufficiency.

not clear agreement on a weight limit above which LMWH should not be used, but some feel that an upper limit of approximately 120 kg to 150 kg is reasonable, with intravenous standard heparin being used in larger patients. It is unnecessary to monitor other patients with anti-factor Xa levels.

Outpatient therapy for stable patients with proven DVT has become increasingly common. Two key clinical trials published in the *New England Journal of Medicine* in 1996 emphasized that therapy with LMWH could be safely initiated at home or continued at home after a brief hospitalization.[66,67] In the United States, at the present time, two LMWH preparations (enoxaparin and tinzaparin) have been approved by the United States Food and Drug Administration (US FDA) for use to treat patients presenting with DVT with or without acute PE. The most widely used LMWH, enoxaparin, is approved for both inpatient and outpatient use at a dose of 1 mg/kg subcutaneously every 12 hours, or at 1.5 mg/kg once-daily for inpatient use. The latter regimens were both proven effective in a large study of inpatients in which both doses proved as effective and as safe as unfractionated heparin. The American College of Chest Physicians has recently recommended LMWH over unfractionated heparin (grade 1A) in patients presenting with acute PE.[61,68] Finally, an "ultra-low molecular weight heparin," fondaparinux, has been studied in patients with acute DVT and PE and has proven effective for these indications.[68] This drug has been approved by the FDA for prophylaxis in specific orthopedic populations as well as for therapy of acute VTE. It should be noted that the prophylactic doses of these agents differ from the doses used for treating active disease. The characteristics of LMWHs compared with standard unfractionated heparin are shown in Table 19.4.

Proven proximal DVT or PE should be treated for 3 to 6 months. Treatment over a more extended interval is appropriate when significant risk factors persist, when thromboembolism is idiopathic, or when previous episodes of VTE have been documented.

Direct thrombin inhibitors

New antithrombotic agents are being investigated. Heparin and LMWH work indirectly, requiring

Table 19.4. *A comparison of low molecular weight heparin with unfractionated heparin*

Characteristic	UFH	LMWH
Mean molecular weight	12 000–15 000	4000–6000
Protein binding	Substantial	Minimal*
Anti-Xa activity	Substantial	Substantial
Anti-IIa activity	Substantial	Minimal
Administration (treatment)	Intravenous	Subcutaneous
Administration (prophylaxis)	Subcutaneous	Subcutaneous
Monitoring during treatment	aPTT every 6 hours	None in most settings†
Outpatient therapy	Difficult	Simplified
Incidence of HIT	3-5%	< 1%
Reversibility with protamine	Complete	Partial

*This implies significantly superior bioavailability of LMWH relative to UFH.
†LMWH requires monitoring in renal insufficiency (creatinine clearance < 30 mL/min), significant obesity (> 150 kg), very small patients (< 40 kg), and pregnant patients. Anti-Xa levels are followed and not the activated partial thromboplastin time.
Abbreviations: aPTT = activated partial thromboplastin time; HIT = heparin-induced thrombocytopenia; LMWH = low molecular weight heparin; UFH = unfractionated heparin.

antithrombin III as a cofactor. However, hirudin is a direct thrombin inhibitor which has several advantages over heparin, including efficacy against fibrin clot-bound thrombin. This drug, derived from the saliva of the medicinal leech (*Hirudo medicinalis*) does not require cofactors and is not inactivated by platelet factor 4 or plasma proteins. As with heparin, these direct thrombin inhibitors have very narrow therapeutic indices. Currently, ximelagatran, an oral direct thrombin inhibitor is being studied extensively in hopes of simplifying the treatment of acute VTE. It has proven effective for treatment of VTE compared with placebo after extended warfarin therapy.[69] Studies have been completed and are pending publication regarding the successful use of this drug compared with LMWH or warfarin in acute VTE.[70] While ximelagatran is associated with elevation of hepatic transaminases between approximately 8 weeks and 12 weeks, this is generally transient and reversible even with continued exposure to the drug. However, it is likely that liver function test monitoring, will be recommended, at least temporarily. The oral delivery, rapid onset, lack of significant drug and food interactions, and lack of need for INR monitoring are among the advantages over warfarin.

Bleeding is the major complication of anticoagulation. The rates of major bleeding in recent trials using heparin by continuous infusion or high-dose subcutaneous injection are less than 5%. Heparin-induced thrombocytopenia (defined as a platelet count less than 150 000 mm^3) typically develops 5 or more days after the initiation of heparin therapy, occurring in about 5% of patients.[71] The syndrome is caused by heparin-dependent IgG antibodies that activate platelets via their Fc receptors. If a patient is placed on heparin for VTE and the platelet count progressively decreases to 100 000/mm^3 or less, heparin therapy should be discontinued. The formation of heparin-dependent IgG antibodies and the risk of thrombocytopenia are lower with LMWH than with standard heparin.[71]

Argatroban and lepirudin are both FDA-approved for use in the setting of VTE with heparin-induced thrombocytopenia. The half-life of argatroban is 45 minutes, but it is prolonged in patients with hepatic dysfunction. Lepirudin is excreted by the kidneys so the dosage must be reduced in renal insufficiency. This drug has a short circulating half-life of 1.3 hours in patients with normal renal function but it may be as long as 2 days in patients with advanced renal failure. While there is no antidote for lepirudin at present, the short half-life in patients with normal renal function allows for rapid correction of prolonged aPTTs. A detailed discussion of heparin-induced thrombocytopenia is beyond the scope of this chapter.

Bleeding related to warfarin therapy increases with the intensity and duration of therapy. Warfarin-induced skin necrosis is a rare but serious complication mandating immediate cessation of the drug. It is related, at least in some patients, to protein C or S deficiency. Warfarin crosses the placenta and may cause fetal malformations if used during pregnancy.

Vena cava interruption

When anticoagulation is contraindicated, IVC filter placement can be performed to prevent lower extremity thrombi from embolizing to the lungs. The primary indications for filter placement include contraindications to anticoagulation, recurrent embolism while on adequate therapy, and significant bleeding complications during anticoagulation.[72] Filters are sometimes placed in the setting of massive PE when it is believed that any further emboli might be lethal, particularly if thrombolytic therapy is contraindicated. A number of filter designs exist but the Greenfield filter has been most widely used. Filters can be inserted via the jugular or femoral vein. These devices are effective and complications including insertion-related problems and migration are unusual. More recently, temporary filters are being placed in patients in whom the risk of bleeding appears to be short term. Most of these devices can be removed up to 2 weeks later, and some may remain in place even longer with subsequent removal.

Thrombolytic therapy

Rapid lysis of thromboemboli has clear beneficial implications. Thrombolytic agents activate plasminogen to form plasmin which then results in fibrinolysis as well as fibrinogenolysis. These agents can dramatically accelerate clot lysis in acute PE (and DVT) and such an approach was first documented more than several decades ago. Clinical trials have culminated in the approval of streptokinase, urokinase, and recombinant tissue-type plasminogen activator (tPA) for the treatment of massive PE.[73,74] While tenecteplase has been studied extensively in acute MI, and would be expected to be effective in VTE, far less data are available with this agent. The specific FDA-approved regimens are shown in Table 19.5.

For the past several decades, the clearly accepted recommendation for thrombolytic therapy has been PE with hemodynamic instability (hypotension). Patients with severely compromised oxygenation should also be considered for thrombolytic therapy. Although it may result in rapid improvement of right ventricular function in patients with acute PE, there has been controversy as to whether or not patients with echocardiographic right ventricular dysfunction but without hypotension should receive this form of treatment. Several large studies have suggested that such patients should be considered and a recent clinical trial offered further evidence of this. Results indicated a less frequent need for escalation of treatment when thrombolytic therapy was used in the setting of PE with right ventricular dysfunction.[75] The method of delivery of thrombolytic agents has also been investigated. While standard or low-dose intrapulmonary arterial thrombolytic infusions have been utilized in order to deliver a high concentration of drug in close proximity to the clot, intravenous therapy appears adequate in most cases.[76] More direct techniques, such as catheter-directed administration of intraembolic thrombolytic therapy have been utilized in small clinical studies but the data is inadequate to formulate recommendations.[77,78]

The use of thrombolytic therapy in patients with proximal occlusive DVT associated with significant swelling and symptoms is increasing. Catheter-directed techniques are often employed.[79] In DVT, such aggressive therapy with thrombolytics may reduce the frequency of postphlebitic syndrome.

The most concerning adverse effect associated with thrombolytic therapy is hemorrhage.[80,81] Lysis of hemostatic fibrin plugs as well as fibrinogenolysis can lead to bleeding complications which commonly occur at sites of invasive procedures such as pulmonary arteriography or arterial line placement. Invasive procedures should be minimized as much as possible. The most devastating complication associated with thrombolytic therapy is the development of intracranial hemorrhage, which occurs in less than 1% of patients. Retroperitoneal hemorrhage may result from a vascular puncture above the inguinal ligament and may be life-threatening. The primary contraindications to thrombolytic therapy include active bleeding, surgery within the previous 1 to 2 weeks (depending on the specific procedure), or previous intracranial surgery or pathology. When patients appear to be at extraordinary risk of rapid death from PE, cases should be individualized with regard to contraindications.

Table 19.5. *Thrombolytic therapy for acute pulmonary embolism: approved regimens*

Thrombolytic agent	Dosing
Streptokinase	250 000 U intravenously (loading dose over 30 minutes), then 100 000 U/h for 24 hours*
Urokinase	2000 U/lb intravenously (loading dose over 10 minutes), then 2000 U/lb/h for 12 to 24 hours
Tissue-type plasminogen activator	100 mg intravenously over 2 hours

*Streptokinase administered over 24 to 72 hours at this loading dose and rate has also been approved for use in patients with extensive deep venous thrombosis.

Management of unstable hemodynamics in massive PE

Massive PE should always be suspected in the setting of the sudden onset of hypotension or extreme hypoxemia. Electromechanical dissociation or sudden cardiac arrest should always make massive embolism a consideration. Once massive PE associated with hypotension or severe hypoxemia is suspected, supportive vasoactive treatment should be initiated immediately. Intravenous saline should be infused rapidly but cautiously since right ventricular function is often severely compromised. Dopamine or norepinephrine are acceptable choices of vasoactive therapy in massive PE and should be administered if the blood pressure is not rapidly restored.[82] Because death in this setting results from right ventricular failure, dobutamine has been recommended by some as a means by which to augment right ventricular output.[83] A vasopressor such as norepinephrine combined with dobutamine might offer optimal results and further exploration of such combined therapy might prove enlightening. Oxygen therapy is administered and thrombolytic therapy is considered as described above. Pulmonary embolectomy may be appropriate in patients with massive embolism who cannot receive thrombolytic therapy.

Prognosis

In the International Cooperative Pulmonary Embolism Registry of 2454 patients, all consecutive patients with a diagnosis of PE were included and PE was the principal cause of death.[84] The 3-month mortality was 17.5%. In the PIOPED, the mortality rate was approximately 15% but only 10% of deaths during the first year of follow-up were attributed to PE.[12] Mean 1-month mortality rates of treated and untreated PE have been estimated at 8% and 30% respectively.

While a small percentage of patients with acute PE will ultimately develop chronic dyspnea and hypoxemia due to chronic thromboembolic pulmonary hypertension, most patients who survive the acute episode have no long-term pulmonary sequelae. Chronic leg pain and swelling from DVT (postphlebitic syndrome) may, however, result in significant morbidity.

Prevention

Implementation of prophylaxis measures for VTE appear to be grossly underutilized.[4,7] A substantial reduction in the incidence of DVT can be achieved when patients who are at risk receive appropriate prophylaxis. For example, the risk of DVT after total hip or knee replacement is 50% or greater without prophylaxis. The superiority of LMWH over unfractionated heparin has been demonstrated in these settings, and extending the duration of prophylaxis to approximately 1 month after surgery further reduces the DVT rate in total hip replacement.[85,86] Unfractionated heparin is not recommended in total joint replacement.

In hospitalized general medical patients, anticoagulant prophylaxis should always be strongly considered as the rate of DVT, based upon a venographic endpoint, is as high as 15% in patients receiving placebo.[31] The rate of DVT, including proximal DVT, is statistically significantly lower when enoxaparin is administered as compared to placebo.[31] It appears that either LMWH (enoxaparin at 40 mg subcutaneously once daily) or subcutaneous heparin (5000 units every 8 hours) is adequate for medical patient prophylaxis.[87,88] Although 5000 units of heparin every 12 hours has been commonly used, there is less evidence to support this preventive regimen in medical patients. Intermittent pneumatic compression devices should be utilized when pharmacologic prophylaxis is contraindicated. Both methods combined would be reasonable in patients deemed to be at exceptionally high risk, but an additional reduction in risk in such patients has not been well substantiated. All patients admitted to the hospital should be assessed for the need for these prophylactic measures and all hospitals should strongly consider formulating their own written guidelines for each particular clinical setting, based upon the available medical literature.[89]

References

1. Anderson FA Jr., Wheeler HB. Venous thromboembolism. Risk factors and prophylaxis. Clin Chest Med 1995; 16: 235–251.

2. Dalen JE, Alpert JS. Natural history of pulmonary embolism. Prog Cardiovasc Dis 1975; 17: 259–270.
3. Lindblad B, Eriksson A, Bergqvist D. Autopsy-verified pulmonary embolism in a surgical department: analysis of the period from 1951 to 1988. Brit J Surg 1991; 78: 849–852.
4. Goldhaber SZ, Tapson VF., DVT FREE Steering Committee. A prospective registry of 5451 patients with ultrasound-confirmed deep vein thrombosis. Am J Cardiol 2004; 93: 259–262.
5. Coon WW. Risk factors in pulmonary embolism. Surg Gynecol Obstet 1976; 143: 385–390.
6. Kakkar VV, Howe CT, Nicolaides AN, Renney JT, Clarke MB. Deep vein thrombosis of the legs. Is there a "high risk" group? Am J Surg 1970; 120: 527–530.
7. Bratzler DW, Raskob, GE, Murray CK, Bumpus LJ, Piatt DS. Underuse of venous thromboembolism prophylaxis for general surgery patients: physician practices in the community hospital setting. Arch Intern Med 1998; 158: 1909–1912.
8. von Virchow R. Further investigation of blockages of the pulmonary artery and their consequences. Traube's Beiträge exp path u physiol 1846; 2: 21–31.
9. Goldhaber SZ. Pulmonary embolism. N Engl J Med 1998; 339: 93–104.
10. McIntyre KM, Sasahara AA. The ratio of pulmonary artery pressure to pulmonary vascular obstruction: index of preembolic cardiopulmonary status. Chest 1977; 71: 692–697.
11. Carson JL, Kelley MA, Duff A, *et al.* The clinical course of pulmonary embolism. N Engl J Med 1992; 326: 1240–1245.
12. The PIOPED Investigators. Value of the ventilation/perfusion scan in acute pulmonary embolism: results of the prospective investigation of pulmonary embolism diagnosis (PIOPED). JAMA 1990; 263: 2753–2759.
13. Stein PD, Terrin ML, Hales CA, *et al.* Clinical, laboratory, roentgenographic, and electrocardiographic findings in patients with acute pulmonary embolism and no pre-existing cardiac or pulmonary disease. Chest 1991; 100: 598–603.
14. Clason S. Three cases of pulmonary embolism following confinement, treated with heparin. Acta Med Scand 1941; 107: 131–135.
15. Fitts, WT Jr., Lehr HB, Bitner RL, Spelman JW. An analysis of 950 fatal injuries. Surgery 1964; 56: 663–668.
16. Lamb GC, Tomski MA, Kaufman J, Maiman DJ. Is chronic spinal cord injury associated with increased risk of venous thromboembolism? J Am Paraplegia Soc 1993; 16: 153–156.
17. Fisher M, Michele A, McCann W. Thrombophlebitis and pulmonary infarction associated with fractured hip. Clin Res 1963; 11: 407.
18. Clagett GP, Reisch JS. Prevention of venous thromboembolism in general surgical patients: results of a meta-analysis. Ann Surg 1988; 208: 227–240.
19. Samama MM, Cohen AT, Darmon JY, *et al.* A comparison of enoxaparin with placebo for the prevention of venous thromboembolism in acutely ill medical patients. Prophylaxis in Medical Patients with Enoxaparin Study Group. N Engl J Med 1999; 341: 793–800.
20. Pineo GF, Brain MC, Gallus AS, *et al.* Tumors, mucus production and hypercoagulability. Ann NY Acad Sci 1974; 230: 262–270.
21. Rickles FR, Edwards RL. Activation of blood coagulation in cancer: Trousseau's syndrome revisited. Blood 1983; 62: 14–31.
22. Toglia MR, Weg JG. Venous thromboembolism during pregnancy. N Engl J Med 1996; 335: 108–114.
23. Handley AJ, Emerson PA, Fleming PR. Heparin in the prevention of deep vein thrombosis after myocardial infarction. Br Med J 1972; 2: 436–438.
24. Kraaijenhagen RA, Haverkamp D, Koopman MM, *et al.* Travel and risk of venous thrombosis. Lancet 2000; 356: 1492–1493.
25. James PB. Jet "leg," pulmonary embolism, and hypoxia. Lancet 1996; 347: 1697.
26. Bagshaw M. Jet leg, pulmonary embolism, and hypoxia. Lancet 1996; 348: 415–416.
27. Bounameaux H, Cirafici P, de Moerloose P, *et al.* Measurement of D-dimer in plasma as diagnostic aid in suspected pulmonary embolism. Lancet 1991; 337: 196–200.
28. Wells PS, Anderson DR, Rodger M, *et al.* Excluding pulmonary embolism at the bedside without diagnostic imaging: management of patients with suspected pulmonary embolism presenting to the emergency department by using a simple clinical model and D-dimer. Ann Intern Med 2001; 135: 98–107.
29. Egermayer P, Town GI, Turner JG, *et al.* Usefulness of D-dimer, blood gas, and respiratory rate measurements for excluding pulmonary embolism. Thorax 1998; 53: 830–834.
30. Ahearn GS, Bounameaux H. The role of the D-dimer in the diagnosis of venous thromboembolism. Semin Respir Crit Care Med 2000; 21: 521–536.
31. Meyer T, Binder L, Hruska N, Luthe H, Buchwald AB. Cardiac troponin I elevation in acute pulmonary embolism is associated with right ventricular dysfunction. J Am Coll Cardiol 2000; 36: 1632–1636.

32. Douketis JD, Crowther MA, Stanton EB, Ginsberg JS. Elevated cardiac troponin levels in patients with submassive pulmonary embolism. Arch Intern Med 2002; 162: 79–81.
33. Tapson VF. Diagnosing and managing acute pulmonary embolism: role of cardiac troponins. Am Heart J 2003; 145: 751–753.
34. Burke B, Sostman HD, Carroll BA, Witty LA. The diagnostic approach to deep venous thrombosis: which technique? Clin Chest Med 1995; 16: 253–268.
35. Evans AJ, Tapson VF, Sostman HD, *et al.* The diagnosis of deep venous thrombosis: a prospective comparison of venography and magnetic resonance imaging. Chest 1992; 102: 120S (Abstract).
36. Witty LA, Tapson VF, Evans AJ, *et al.* MRI versus ultrasound: a radiologic and clinical evaluation of DVT. Am Rev Respir Dis 1993; 147: A998 (Abstract).
37. McNeil BJ, Hessel SJ, Branch WT, Bjork L, Adelstein SJ. Measures of clinical efficacy. III. The value of the lung scan in the evaluation of young patients with pleuritic chest pain. J Nucl Med 1976; 17: 163–169.
38. Hull RD, Raskob G, Ginsberg JS, *et al.* A noninvasive strategy for the treatment of patients with suspected pulmonary embolism. Arch Intern Med 1994; 154: 289–297.
39. Stein PD, Athanasoulis C, Alavi A, *et al.* Complications and validity of pulmonary angiography in acute pulmonary embolism. Circulation 1992; 85: 462–468.
40. Remy-Jardin M, Remy J, Wattinne L, Giraud F. Central pulmonary thromboembolism: diagnosis with spiral volumetric CT with the single-breath-hold technique—comparison with pulmonary angiography. Radiology 1992; 185: 381–387.
41. Sostman HD, Layish DT, Tapson VF, *et al.* Prospective comparison of helical CT and MR imaging in clinically suspected acute pulmonary embolism. J Magn Reson Imaging 1996; 6: 275–281.
42. van Rossum AB, Pattynama PM, Treurniat FE, *et al.* Spiral CT angiography for detection of pulmonary embolism: validation in 124 patients. Radiology 1995; 197(P): 303.
43. Goodman LR, Curtin JJ, Mewissen MW, *et al.* Detection of pulmonary embolism in patients with unresolved clinical and scintigraphic diagnosis: helical CT versus angiography. AJR Am J Roentgenol 1995; 164: 1369–1374.
44. Oser RF, Zuckerman DA, Gutierrez FR, Brink JA. Anatomic distribution of pulmonary emboli at pulmonary angiography: implications for cross-sectional imaging. Radiology 1996; 199: 31–35.
45. Teigen CL, Maus TP, Sheedy PF 2nd, Johnson CM, Stanson AW, Welch TJ. Pulmonary embolism: diagnosis with electron-beam CT. Radiology 1993; 188: 839–845.
46. Drucker, EA, Rivitz SM, Shepard JA, *et al.* Acute pulmonary embolism: assessment of helical CT for diagnosis. Radiology 1998; 209: 235–241.
47. van Rossum AB, Treurniat FE, Kieft GJ, Smith SJ, Schepers-Bok R. Role of spiral volumetric computed tomographic scanning in the assessment of patients with clinical suspicion of pulmonary embolism and an abnormal ventilation/perfusion lung scan. Thorax 1996; 51: 23–28.
48. Ferretti GR, Bosson J-L, Buffaz PD, *et al.* Acute pulmonary embolism: role of helical CT in 164 patients with intermediate probability at ventilation-perfusion scintigraphy and normal results at duplex US of the legs. Radiology 1997; 205: 453–458.
49. Perrier A, Howarth N, Didier D, *et al.* Performance of helical computed tomography in unselected outpatients with suspected pulmonary embolism. Ann Intern Med 2001; 135: 88–97.
50. Swensen SJ, Sheedy PF 2nd, Ryu JH, *et al.* Outcomes after withholding anticoagulation from patients with suspected acute pulmonary embolism and negative computed tomographic findings: a cohort study. Mayo Clin Proc 2002; 77: 130–138.
51. Garg K, Sieler H, Welsh CH, Johnson RJ, Russ PD. Clinical validity of helical CT being interpreted as negative for pulmonary embolism: implications for patient treatment. AJR Am J Roentgenol 1999; 172: 1627–1631.
52. Tapson VF. Pulmonary embolism—new diagnostic approaches. N Engl J Med 1997; 336: 1449–1451.
53. Come PC. Echocardiographic evaluation of pulmonary embolism and its response to therapeutic interventions. Chest 1992; 101: 151S–162S.
54. Goldhaber SZ, Haire WD, Feldstein ML, *et al.* Alteplase versus heparin in acute pulmonary embolism: randomised trial assessing right-ventricular function and pulmonary perfusion. Lancet 1993; 341: 507–511.
55. Tapson VF, Davidson CJ, Kisslo KB, Stack RS. Rapid visualization of massive pulmonary emboli utilizing intravascular ultrasound. Chest 1994; 105: 888–890.
56. Tapson VF, Carroll BA, Davidson BL, *et al.* The diagnostic approach to acute venous thromboembolism: clinical practice guideline. American Thoracic Society. Am J Respir Crit Care Med 1999; 160: 1043–1066.
57. Tapson VF, Hull RD. Management of venous thromboembolic disease: the impact of low-molecular-weight heparin. Clin Chest Med 1995; 16: 281–294.

58. Tapson VF. Treatment of acute deep venous thrombosis and pulmonary embolism: Use of low molecular weight heparin. Semin Respir Crit Care Med 2000; 21: 547–553.
59. Hull RD, Raskob GE, Rosenbloom D, *et al.* Optimal therapeutic level of heparin therapy in patients with venous thrombosis. Arch Intern Med 1992; 152: 1589–1595.
60. Merli G, Spiro T, Olsson CG, *et al.* Subcutaneous enoxaparin once or twice daily compared with intravenous unfractionated heparin for treatment of venous thromboembolic disease. Ann Intern Med 2001; 134: 191–202.
61. Simonneau G, Sors H, Charbonnier B, *et al.* A comparison of low-molecular-weight heparin with unfractionated heparin for acute pulmonary embolism. The THESEE Study Group. N Engl J Med 1997; 337: 663–669.
62. Lensing AW, Prins MH, Davidson BL, Hirsh J. Treatment of deep venous thrombosis with low-molecular-weight heparins. A meta-analysis. Arch Intern Med 1995; 155: 601–607.
63. Leizorovicz A, Simonneau G, Decousus H, Boissel JP. Comparison of efficacy and safety of low molecular weight heparins and unfractionated heparin in initial treatment of deep venous thrombosis: a meta-analysis. BMJ 1994; 309: 299–304.
64. Siragusa S, Cosmi B, Piovella F, Hirsh J, Ginsberg JS. Low-molecular-weight heparins and unfractionated heparin in the treatment of patients with acute venous thromboembolism: results of a meta-analysis. Am J Med 1996; 100: 269–277.
65. Dolovich LR, Ginsberg JS, Douketis JD, *et al.* A meta-analysis comparing low-molecular-weight heparins with unfractionated heparin in the treatment of venous thromboembolism: examining some unanswered questions regarding location of treatment, product type, and dosing frequency. Arch Intern Med 2000; 160: 181–188.
66. Levine M, Gent M, Hirsh J, *et al.* A comparison of low molecular-weight-heparin administered primarily at home with unfractionated heparin administered in the hospital for proximal deep-vein thrombosis. N Engl J Med 1996; 334: 677–681.
67. Koopman MM, Prandoni P, Piovella, F, *et al.* Treatment of venous thrombosis with intravenous unfractionated heparin administered in the hospital as compared with subcutaneous low-molecular-weight heparin administered at home. N Engl J Med 1996; 334: 682–687.
68. Buller HR, Davidson BL, Decousus H, *et al.*, Matisse Investigators. Subcutaneous fondaparinux versus intravenous unfractionated heparin in the initial treatment of pulmonary embolism. N Engl J Med 2003; 349: 1695–1702.
69. Schulman S, Wahlander K, Lundstrom T, Clason SB, Eriksson H., THRIVE III Investigators. Secondary prevention of venous thromboembolism with the oral direct thrombin inhibitor ximelagatran. N Engl J Med 2003; 349: 1713–1721.
70. Huisman M, *et al.* International Society of Thrombosis and Haemostasis. Birmingham, UK, 2003 (Abstract).
71. Warkentin TE, Levine MN, Hirsh J, *et al.* Heparin-induced thrombocytopenia in patients treated with low-molecular-weight heparin or unfractionated heparin. N Engl J Med 1995; 332: 1330–1335.
72. Becker DM, Philbrick JT, Selby JB. Inferior vena cava filters. Indications, safety, effectiveness. Arch Intern Med 1992; 152: 1985–1994.
73. Thrombolytic therapy in thrombosis: a National Institutes of Health consensus development conference. Ann Intern Med 1980; 93: 141–144.
74. Goldhaber SZ. Evolving concepts in thrombolytic therapy for pulmonary embolism. Chest 1992; 101: 183S–185S.
75. Konstantinides S, Geibel A, Heusel G, Heinrich F, Kasper W., Management Strategies and Prognosis of Pulmonary Embolism–3 Trial Investigators. Heparin plus alteplase compared with heparin alone in patients with submassive pulmonary embolism. N Engl J Med 2002; 347: 1143–1150.
76. Verstraete M, Miller GA, Bounameaux H, *et al.* Intravenous and intrapulmonary recombinant tissue-type plasminogen activator in the treatment of acute massive pulmonary embolism. Circulation 1988; 77: 353–360.
77. Tapson VF, Witty LA. Massive pulmonary embolism. Diagnostic and therapeutic strategies. Clin Chest Med 1995; 16: 329–340.
78. Tapson VF, Gurbel PA, Witty LA, Pieper KS, Stack RS. Pharmacomechanical thrombolysis of experimental pulmonary emboli: rapid low-dose intraembolic therapy. Chest 1994; 106: 1558–1562.
79. Semba CP, Dake MD. Iliofemoral deep venous thrombosis: aggressive therapy with catheter-directed thrombolysis. Radiology 1994; 191: 487–494.
80. Sane DC, Califf RM, Topol EJ, Stump DC, Mark DB, Greenberg CS. Bleeding during thrombolytic therapy for acute myocardial infarction: mechanisms and management. Ann Intern Med 1989; 111: 1010–1022.
81. Gore JM. Prevention of severe neurologic events in the thrombolytic era. Chest 1992; 101: 124S–130S.
82. Layish DT, Tapson VF. Pharmacologic hemodynamic support in massive pulmonary embolism. Chest 1997; 111: 218–224.

83. Jardin F, Genevray B, Brun-Ney D, Margairaz A. Dobutamine: a hemodynamic evaluation in pulmonary embolism shock. Crit Care Med 1985; 13: 1009–1012.
84. Goldhaber SZ, Visani L., The International Cooperative Pulmonary Embolism Registry. Chest 1995; 108: 302–304.
85. Bergqvist D, Benoni G, Bjorgell O, *et al.* Low-molecular-weight heparin (enoxaparin) as prophylaxis against venous thromboembolism after total hip replacement. N Engl J Med 1996; 335: 696–700.
86. Comp PC, Spiro T, Friedman, RJ, *et al.*, Enoxaparin Clinical Trial Group. Prolonged enoxaparin therapy to prevent venous thromboembolism after primary hip or knee replacement. J Bone Joint Surg Am 2001; 83-A: 336–345.
87. Lechler E, Schramm W, Flosbach CW. The venous thrombotic risk in non-surgical patients: epidemiological data and efficacy/safety profile of a low-molecular-weight heparin (enoxaparin). The Prime Study Group. Haemostasis 1996; 26: 49–56.
88. Kleber FX, Witt C, Vogel G, *et al.*, THE-PRINCE Study Group. Randomized comparison of enoxaparin with unfractionated heparin for the prevention of venous thromboembolism in medical patients with heart failure or severe respiratory disease. Am Heart J 2003; 145: 614–621.
89. Geerts WH, Heit JA, Clagett GP, *et al.* Prevention of venous thromboembolism. Chest 2001; 119: 132S–175S.
90. Stein PD (ed.) Pulmonary Embolism (Williams & Wilkins: Baltimore, MD, 1996).

CHAPTER 20

The role of myocardial ischemia in acute decompensated heart failure: diagnostic and management considerations

Jamieson M Bourque, Eric J Velazquez, Christopher M O'Connor

Introduction

As the most common causative agent, myocardial ischemia plays a significant role in the development of acute decompensated heart failure (ADHF).[1] Improvements in survival after myocardial infarction (MI) have enabled more patients to live long enough to develop left ventricular (LV) dysfunction. Moreover, the decreased perfusion that accompanies LV failure leads to a high prevalence of ischemic sequelae, creating an adverse positive feedback loop. Thus, myocardial ischemia must be a primary consideration when diagnosing and treating decompensated heart failure. It is essential that we identify ways to decrease ischemic burden to lessen the impact and reduce the prevalence of ADHF. This chapter describes the role of myocardial ischemia in ADHF, including epidemiologic, pathophysiologic, diagnostic, and treatment considerations.

Epidemiology

Ischemic heart disease (IHD) is closely tied to ADHF, with a high prevalence in this population. A recent large, national, multicenter observational registry, the Acute Decompensated Heart Failure National Registry (ADHERE™) examined 65 180 patients to better characterize the many epidemiologic facets of ADHF.[2] In this population, 58% of the patients had a history of coronary artery disease (CAD), one-third of whom (32%) had a prior MI. Other registries of patients with ADHF describe the same high prevalence of CAD. A systematic review of 13 multicenter heart failure trials found an IHD prevalence of 68%.[1] In the Epidémiologie de l'Insuffisance Cardiaque Avancée en Lorraine (EPICAL) study cohort, CAD was present in 46% of the 499 subjects with ADHF.[3]

As expected from the elevated rates of CAD, myocardial ischemia is a significant contributor to ADHF. The Italian Network on Congestive Heart Failure (IN-CHF) registry of 2701 outpatients followed by 133 cardiology centers was developed to examine the precipitating factors of ADHF. In this cohort, 8% of patients had decompensation requiring hospitalization. MI was the primary contributor to the decompensation in 5% of these patients.[4] In the ADHERE™ registry, 4% of patients admitted with ADHF had a MI or unstable angina. It should be noted, however, that these percentages reflect the primary admitting diagnosis in these registries.[2] Myocardial ischemia was very likely present in many more patients in a subclinical fashion or as a second or third diagnosis. A study by Michalsen *et al.* of 179 consecutive patients with ADHF found that 13.4% had myocardial ischemia as part of their presenting picture, and 49.3% of patients had ischemia in the IN-CHF registry.[4,5]

Another important potential ischemic complication is myocardial arrhythmia. In a study by Opasich *et al.* of 304 patients with decompensated heart failure undergoing transplant evaluation, 24% had arrhythmias as the etiology of their decompensation, more than half of which were ventricular tachyarrhythmias. Although there is an increased risk for lethal arrhythmias in patients with LV dysfunction, a significant proportion of these arrhythmias were likely due to the onset of myocardial ischemia.[6]

In addition to its contribution to the development of ADHF, myocardial ischemia is also closely related to prognosis in this population. In the Global Registry of Acute Coronary Events (GRACE), the presence of heart failure at admission increased in-hospital mortality 4-fold (12.0% vs. 2.9%; odds ratio [OR] 4.6; 95% confidence interval [CI], 3.85, 5.40). Moreover, this cohort had a 3-fold increase in 6-month mortality as well as higher rates of readmission.[7] In the EPICAL study, the mortality rate was high at 35%, and 81% of patients had a recurrent MI or hospitalization. The average time until readmission or death was 18 months.[3]

Given the close relationship between ADHF and ischemia as well as a higher prevalence of CAD in men and the elderly, one might expect a disparate incidence of ADHF in these populations. However, the connection between gender, age, and prognosis in decompensated heart failure has been unclear. In the Flolan International Randomized Survival Trial (FIRST) study of 471 patients with advanced symptomatic heart failure, the relative risk of death for men versus women in patients with a nonischemic etiology was 3.08 (95% CI, 1.56–6.09; $P = 0.001$), while the relative risk of death for men versus women was 1.64 (95% CI, 0.87–3.09; $P = 0.127$) for those with an ischemic etiology.[8] However, there was no difference in the rate of mortality or hospitalizations by gender in the IN-CHF cohort, despite a lower rate of ischemic etiology in women.[9] Thus, the role of gender remains to be determined. Older patients have a higher incidence in post-MI heart failure, but younger patients (< 55 years of age) have the highest relative increase in mortality with the development of heart failure.[7]

Patient Characteristics

The best information regarding the characteristics of patients with ischemic ADHF comes from the GRACE registry. The GRACE registry studied 13 307 patients who presented with a confirmed acute coronary syndrome (ACS) without prior history of heart failure or cardiogenic shock (Killip class IV).[7] Of these, 1778 patients developed heart failure (13%), an underestimation of the true incidence given their exclusions. The registry provides information on patients with ACS stratified by the presence of heart failure. Patients with heart failure (Killip class II or III) were older (72.5 years vs. 64.0 years) with a higher proportion of females and nonsmokers. The incidence of heart failure was similar among those with ST-elevation and non-ST-elevation MIs, but a higher proportion had anterior MIs (46.2% vs. 33.6%, $P < 0.0001$). Patients with heart failure were more likely to have comorbidities, including diabetes, hypertension, hyperlipidemia, renal disease, and atrial tachyarrhythmias. This cohort is not representative of the ischemic heart failure population as a whole, as those patients with chronic heart failure and cardiogenic shock were excluded.[7]

Pathophysiology

The pathophysiology of ADHF of ischemic origin is multifactorial, with structural, hemodynamic, neurohormonal, and genetic contributions. This complex interplay can be summarized as a positive feedback loop in which myocardial ischemia leads to progressive myocyte loss and thus worsening LV systolic and diastolic function. Progressive heart failure triggers a cascade of neurohormonal reactions, endothelial dysfunction, and genetic regulatory changes which promote ventricular remodeling and further failure. Left ventricular hypertrophy (LVH) and dilatation increase myocardial wall tension and oxygen demand, which lead to further myocardial ischemia, and the loop repeats itself.[10,11]

Myocyte loss can result from several mechanisms, including acute ischemia or infarction with vessel narrowing or occlusion from thrombosis or vasospasm. Myocyte destruction can also stem from chronic ischemia and excess catecholamine release.[12] The loss of functioning cells results in progressive left ventricular systolic dysfunction (LVSD) with myocardial stunning or hibernation, depending on the extent of the perfusion disruption.[13] These states involve contractile apparatus degradation, which can take months to reverse after reperfusion.[14,15] The affected areas become hypocontractile, worsening systolic dysfunction, decreasing forward flow, and increasing pulmonary and right-sided vascular congestion.

Other structural contributors to the acute heart failure (ADHF) state include left ventricular diastolic dysfunction and valvular disease. Diastolic LV dysfunction can result from reduced myocardial relaxation and augmented LV filling pressures from myocardial fibrosis and hypertrophy and calcium ion sequestration in the sarcoplasmic reticulum.[16] Ischemia can also cause acute valvular pathology, especially acute mitral regurgitation (MR), which can contribute to flash pulmonary edema and worsen forward flow.[17]

These structural changes trigger a neurohormonal and genetic cascade of factors, including endothelial dysfunction. The heart compensates for decreased forward flow by increasing peripheral vasoconstriction, blood volume, and myocardial contractility, all in an effort to maintain systemic blood pressure.[18] The sympathetic nervous system is activated in response to decreased tissue perfusion, and plasma norepinephrine levels are increased, which stimulate myocardial contractility and vasoconstriction. This increased catecholamine surge can increase cardiac output, but also worsens coronary ischemia.[19] Vasoconstriction occurs through increases in the renin-angiotensin-aldosterone system (RAAS) and vasopressin concentrations. These processes maintain blood pressure and redistribute blood flow to vital organs, but also increase the afterload against which the failing myocardium must pump.[18] Activation of this axis also increases blood volume, which worsens peripheral and pulmonary edema.[20]

Atrial natriuretic peptide (ANP) and brain natriuretic peptide (BNP) are involved in this process, with increased levels resulting from increased atrial stretch.[21,22] ANP appears to counter-regulate the neurohumoral response to heart failure, reducing ventricular remodeling and inhibiting crucial factors such as endothelin and norepinephrine.[23,24] Endothelial dysfunction also plays a critical role in the pathogenesis of heart failure, with secretion of nitric oxide, endothelin, cytokines, prostacyclin, and growth factors which regulate blood flow and myocardial structural changes.[11,25]

The result of these complex neurohumoral interactions is ventricular remodeling, which can increase myocardial wall tension and subsequently decrease blood flow to already underperfused areas. Myocyte death leads to ventricular wall fibrosis, and progressive dilation, hypertrophy, and scar tissue formation occurs.[10,26–28] One consequence of this remodeling process is an increase in cellular apoptosis as a result of altered genetic expression.[29] One analysis showed a 232-fold increase in apoptosis in myocardial samples from heart failure patients, represented by increased deoxyribonucleic acid (DNA) laddering. Interestingly, this increased apoptosis happens despite increased expression of B-cell leukemia/lymphoma 2 (BCL2), a proto-oncogene which appears to protect against the apoptotic process.[26] The extent of ventricular remodeling varies based on the amount of myocardial stunning and the size and nature of the infarct.[10]

Myocardial hypertrophy, increased wall tension from dilatation, and increased neurohumoral activation all increase the metabolic demands on the failing heart, reducing contractile function and forming hibernating myocardium. These processes also result in increased ischemia, completing the positive feedback loop.[10,30]

Diagnostic Workup

The diagnosis of ADHF with ischemic origin involves a multifactorial approach, using the history and physical examination, electrocardiogram, laboratory studies, and imaging modalities to characterize this state (Table 20.1).

Symptoms and signs

Heart failure typically manifests itself through 2 main classes of symptoms: (1) those due to fluid

Table 20.1. *Diagnostic workup of patients with acute ischemic heart failure*

Careful history and physical examination

Electrocardiography

Cardiac biomarkers

Imaging
- Nuclear perfusion imaging
- Echocardiography
- Cardiac magnetic resonance imaging

overload and (2) those from a reduction in cardiac output. Symptoms such as dyspnea on exertion, orthopnea, weakness, and fatigue are universal, regardless of the heart failure etiology. On the other hand, some symptoms may indicate heart failure with an ischemic etiology. Patients with exertional angina are likely to have IHD. However, a significant proportion of the patient population with nonischemic cardiomyopathy has typical angina (58% in the ischemic population versus 34% in the nonischemic, *P*-value not provided).[31] Thus, this sign cannot reliably predict an ischemic etiology. Moreover, many patients have anginal equivalents, including dyspnea on exertion. This respiratory difficulty can be confused with the dyspnea found in all forms of heart failure, complicating the diagnosis. Fatigue can be associated with the same difficulties. In the GRACE registry of patients with ACS, 13% of patients presented with symptomatic pulmonary edema, and an additional 5.6% developed these symptoms during their hospital course. This cohort excluded patients with chronic heart failure or cardiogenic shock, so this number is an under-approximation.[7]

Certain physical signs may help to indicate an ischemic etiology for the decompensated heart failure, predominately by providing for evidence of risk factors for atherosclerotic disease. Carotid, renal, or femoral bruits may indicate cerebrovascular disease and peripheral vascular disease, which are closely associated with IHD. Changes in blood pressure between the two arms may signify atherosclerotic stenoses. Findings of hyperlipidemia include xanthomas and arcus senilis. Many of the other physical findings are found in all forms of heart failure, as with symptoms. Papillary muscle dysfunction or rupture can lead to MR and a new holosystolic murmur best heard at the apex.

Electrocardiogram

Electrocardiogram (ECG) changes can distinguish heart failure from systolic dysfunction and help distinguish between ischemic and nonischemic cardiomyopathy. Patients with systolic heart failure have a high likelihood of ECG abnormalities (98% negative predictive value for a normal ECG).[32] Despite this, many findings are less common in patients with an ischemic etiology, including LVH (15.1% vs. 40.6%, $P < 0.001$) and left bundle branch block (LBBB) (1.8% vs. 23.4%, $P < 0.001$).[33] The ECG can be used to differentiate between ischemic and nonischemic cardiomyopathy, but there are significant limitations and diagnostic difficulties with this technique.

ST-segment elevation > 1 mm in 2 contiguous leads can localize areas of transmural ischemia and early infarction. Likewise, ST-segment depression signifies the presence of subendocardial ischemia, without the ability to localize based on lead-involvement.[33] LBBB can obscure the diagnosis of acute myocardial infarction (AMI) due to difficulties in ST-segment analysis. In this setting, ST-segment changes in the direction of the primary QRS vector or discordant changes (> 5 mm) away from the QRS vector suggest infarction.[34] ST-changes on the ECG in patients with ACS do not predict ADHF, as shown in the GRACE registry, in which patients with and without ADHF had equal incidences of these ECG abnormalities.[7]

After sufficient necrosis, QRS changes may occur, signifying decreased electrical forces in the infarcted tissue. Q waves can occur with both transmural and subendocardial lesions. However, in patients with LV dysfunction, Q waves are sometimes absent, even in the setting of a previous infarct. In one study, only 57% of patients with prior infarcts and LV dysfunction had Q waves. Their absence may be from ischemia or infarct in an area not adequately represented on a typical ECG, especially the circumflex territory. Moreover, some patients with non-ischemic cardiomyopathy do have Q waves. In these instances the LV dysfunction may be secondary to low-grade ischemia and myocardial stunning.[33] Thus, there is the potential for under-diagnosis of myocardial ischemia.

Laboratory markers

Myoglobin

Myoglobin is a small heme protein which is rapidly released from damaged tissue, including the myocardium. It increases in proportion to the myocardial muscle creatine kinase isoenzyme (CK-MB) and troponins in AMI and may be useful early in the course of ischemia due to its rapid elevations. However, it is not commonly used due to several significant limitations, including its varying levels from rapid release and degradation, its lack of myocardial specificity, and its impaired clearance in patients with renal insufficiency, a condition highly prevalent in ADHF.[35]

Creatine kinase—MB fraction

The MB-fraction of creatine kinase (CK-MB) is specific to the myocardium, avoiding the decreased specificity from concomitant musculoskeletal or neurologic disease.[36] Necrotic myocardium releases this marker into the bloodstream, with increased levels detectable 4 to 12 hours after injury and resolution within 36 to 48 hours with high sensitivity and specificity for MI (91% and 89% respectively).[37] This marker does not provide information on subacute infarction given its short half-life.[38] Patients with cardiogenic shock have higher levels and a longer plateau than other patients with infarction.[39]

Troponins

Serum troponins (T and I) have high sensitivity and specificity for MI (58% to 62% and 94% to 96% respectively).[37] However, they may also be elevated in patients with ischemic heart failure even in the absence of a true ACS.[40] Troponins also provide prognostic information. One prospective study of patients with ADHF showed an OR of 6.00 (95% CI, 1.04, 34.76) for death or 1-year readmission in patients with a persistently elevated troponin-T level > 0.020 ng/mL.[41] Moreover, LV function appears to deteriorate for patients with persistently elevated troponin-T or troponin-I levels.[42] Concomitant renal disease can complicate the diagnostic utility of troponins, with persistent elevations long after the ischemic event. However, elevated levels indicate that myocardial ischemia has occurred at some time, and concentrations above previously recorded levels represent new infarction.[43]

Other biochemical factors

Several other biochemical markers aid in the diagnosis and prognostication in ADHF of ischemic origin. BNP is a substance that mediates the deleterious reaction in heart failure, including increasing sodium excretion, reducing sympathetic activation, and inhibiting renin-angiotensin and endothelin.[44] In the setting of ACS, BNP levels correlate with increased mortality, worsening LV function, and additional risk of MI. The adjusted risk of death in one cohort had an OR of 3.8 to 5.8 for patients in higher quartiles of BNP level.[45] Serial measurements of BNP may help judge treatment efficacy and titrate therapy, as levels are sensitive to changes in cardiac hemodynamics.[46]

Imaging

Nuclear perfusion

Nuclear single-photon emission computed tomography (SPECT) imaging provides important diagnostic and prognostic information for patients with ADHF, helping to determine an ischemic versus nonischemic etiology. Rest-stress SPECT imaging has a sensitivity of 90% to 91% and specificity of 72% to 88% for the diagnosis of significant CAD, which would favor an ischemic cardiomyopathy. Additional testing such as assessment of wall motion and reversibility increase sensitivity but reduce specificity.[47]

SPECT imaging can also be used to assess myocardial viability, which provides prognostic information (improved outcomes with increased viability levels) and may aid in treatment. Thallium-201, the most common marker used, is a potassium analog that relies on cellular uptake through processes requiring an intact sarcolemmal membrane and adenosine triphosphate (ATP) stores. Through a rest or stress redistribution protocol, the marker is allowed to equilibrate, and the absence of redistribution indicates myocardial necrosis with a sensitivity of 68% and specificity 51%.[48,49] Technetium-99m is also used as a tracer, entering cells by passive electrochemical diffusion without redistribution.[50]

Echocardiography

Echocardiography is a highly versatile imaging modality which can identify LV dysfunction, IHD, and myocardial viability. Routine two-dimensional echocardiography has high sensitivity and specificity for the diagnosis of LV dysfunction (80% and 100% respectively).[51] Although regional wall motion abnormalities can be visualized with this technique and suggest an ischemic cardiomyopathy, they are not specific, occurring in as many as 50% to 60% of patients with dilated cardiomyopathy.[52] Stress testing with the addition of dobutamine can increase the ability to differentiate between ischemic and other forms of cardiomyopathy (80% sensitivity and 96% specificity) by assessing wall motion changes with increasing myocardial oxygen demand.[53]

Echocardiography can also identify additional structural lesions including LVH and atrial enlargement, complicating valvular abnormalities such as MR, and hemodynamic markers such as pulmonary capillary wedge pressure (PCWP).[54] Improvement in left ventricular ejection fraction (LVEF) with dobutamine also provides useful information regarding myocardial viability, with a sensitivity and specificity of 87% and 88% for functional gain after coronary artery bypass grafting (CABG).[55]

Magnetic resonance imaging

A relatively new and extremely versatile imaging modality is cardiac magnetic resonance imaging (MRI). This method can simultaneously evaluate cardiac structure, ventricular function, and myocardial perfusion and viability. More recent developments with cardiac MRI include the ability to identify atherosclerotic plaques.[56] The sensitivity and specificity of cardiac MRI for the identification of IHD are specific but less sensitive than other available modalities. In one study, dobutamine MRI had a sensitivity and specificity of 50% and 81% respectively, compared with 76% and 44% for radionuclide SPECT imaging.[48] Contrast-enhanced and dobutamine MRI can be used alone or in combination to help predict recovery of function in dysfunctional segments after revascularization.[57]

Treatment

There are many available treatments for ADHF of ischemic origin, both old and new, which play a critical role in the stabilization and acute treatment of this population. Numerous therapeutic modalities are available, from well-established therapies such as intravenous nitrates to complex devices and surgical therapies (Table 20.2). Strategies can be tailored to the individual patient to maximize benefit. Ongoing studies will provide novel treatments and further refine the role of existing modalities.

Table 20.2. *Summary of treatment modalities*

General measures to decrease myocardial oxygen demand

Intravenous therapies
- Nitrates
- Beta-blockers
- Antithrombin therapy
- Unfractionated and low molecular weight heparins

Oral agents
- Angiotensin-converting enzyme inhibitors/angiotensin receptor blockers
- Antiplatelet agents

Device therapy
- Automatic implantable cardioverter-defibrillators
- Cardiac resynchronization therapy
- Left ventricular assist devices

Revascularization
- Percutaneous coronary intervention/coronary artery bypass grafting
- Cardiac transplantation
- Systolic ventricular reduction and other surgeries

The management of patients with ADHF involves increasingly complex medical and surgical therapies, but patients can derive great benefit from some simple general considerations (Table 20.3).

Reduction of myocardial oxygen demand

The initial nonpharmacologic and nonsurgical therapies for patients with ADHF focus on reducing myocardial oxygen demand, which plays a critical role in promoting ischemic LV dysfunction. Patients with ADHF of ischemic origin should be prescribed strict bed rest, as activity increases myocardial oxygen demand and may cause destabilization through promotion of ischemia.

Acute dyspnea can cause significant anxiety, and increased adrenergic activation can be a significant source of myocardial oxygen demand through reflex-mediated tachycardia.[58] Morphine sulfate and anxiolytics can ease respiratory distress and adrenergic activation. In some instances, stress reduction techniques taught by trained providers may even provide additional benefit. Adequate oxygenation is also essential to reduce myocardial oxygen demand and thus ischemic LV dysfunction.

Treatment of associated conditions

Anemia

The role of the treatment of anemia in acute ischemic heart failure has been less clear. Anemia is associated with advanced heart failure, with increasing incidence as New York Heart Association (NYHA) functional class decreases, in part due to increased cytokine activation.[59] The decreased oxygen-carrying capacity of the blood leads to reflex tachycardia and decreased vascular resistance, which increases myocardial oxygen demand.[58] Anemia has been well-established as a risk factor for mortality in patients with severe heart failure, with each 1-point drop in hematocrit under 37 carrying an 11% increased risk of death among 407 patients with NYHA class IIIB or IV heart failure in the Prospective Randomized Amlodipine Survival Evaluation (PRAISE) trial.[60] However, the threshold for transfusion is not well defined and has not been studied in the ADHF setting. In the AMI population, one retrospective study of 78 974 hospitalized Medicare beneficiaries ≥ 65 years showed improved survival with transfusion to a hematocrit of 30.[61] Another cohort with cardiac disease had a trend towards increased mortality with hemoglobin levels < 9.5 g/dL, suggesting a target hematocrit of 30 for transfusion.[62] Further research is needed to determine if these thresholds are appropriate for patients with ADHF.

Table 20.3. *General treatment measures in the setting of acute heart failure of ischemic origin*

Maintain adequate oxygenation
Bed rest
Anxiolytics/stress reduction
Correct anemia
Manage volume status (? Swan–Ganz catheterization)

Arrhythmias

The presence of ventricular arrhythmias in acute ischemic heart failure is an adverse prognostic sign. Sustained ventricular tachycardia (VT) is associated with higher in-hospital mortality. Increased myocardial oxygen demand can increase ischemia. This arrhythmia can be treated with amiodarone, with improved outcomes in two meta-analyses.[63,64] However, the SCD-HeFT trial failed to find a benefit with long-term use of this antiarrhythmic agent. The class I agents and sotalol have been associated with proarrhythmia and worse outcomes.[65] Nonsustained ventricular tachycardia (NSVT) is found in 50% to 80% of patients with ischemic cardiomyopathy, and no treatment is recommended at this time. The Congestive Heart Failure: Survival Trial of Antiarrhythmic Therapy (CHF-STAT) trial found no improvement in outcomes in 674 patients with NSVT randomized to amiodarone or placebo. Ventricular fibrillation also causes an increased mortality in patients with ischemic heart failure, and this arrhythmia mandates cardioversion with post-conversion amiodarone therapy.[66]

Invasive monitoring

Patients with refractory ADHF have a complex interplay of hemodynamic processes which complicate their management, especially patients with conditions such as pulmonary hypertension and tricuspid regurgitation, in which jugular venous pressure is not an accurate measurement of LV function. Invasive pulmonary artery catheters (Swan–Ganz) can be used to measure central venous, right ventricular, pulmonary artery, and PCWPs, and thus indirectly estimate left atrial pressures. They can also provide mixed venous oxygen saturations and estimates of cardiac output and pulmonary and systemic vascular resistance (SVR) using thermodilution techniques. These parameters can be used to differentiate between forms of shock and pulmonary edema, as well as direct ventilator, fluid, and pharmacologic therapies, and provide estimates of prognosis in ADHF.[67] Contrary to the perceived benefit from this information, small observational studies have suggested increased mortality at 30 days and increased utilization of resources for patients with ADHF.[68] However, a multicenter randomized trial of 433 patients, the Evaluation Study of Congestive Heart Failure and Pulmonary Artery Catheterization Effectiveness (ESCAPE) trial, found a similar 30-day mortality and no difference in complication rates or clinical outcomes at 6 months.[69] The lack of benefit may stem from many reasons, but 1 limitation is that physicians interpreting Swan–Ganz data have significant and wide variations in interobserver variability, both in assessment of results and treatment recommendations.[70,71] As a consortium of societies jointly recommended in 1997, there is no indication for a moratorium on the use of Swan–Ganz catheters, and the decision should be made based on patient characteristics and circumstances.[72] Patients without complicating conditions, such as pulmonary hypertension, right ventricular failure, or severe lung disease, may have adequate assessment through central venous pressure monitoring.[72]

Behavioral modifications

After the acute episode of heart failure has been resolved, there are several issues which should be addressed prior to patient discharge. ADHERE™ registry data on Joint Commission on Accreditation of Healthcare Organizations (JCAHO) quality indicators indicated that only 30% of patients were given complete discharge instructions, including information on diet, daily weight monitoring, and assessment of recurrent symptoms. It is also critical that smoking cessation counseling be performed, and only 40% of eligible patients were counseled on the risks of smoking and importance of cessation.[2]

Another important discharge prescription for patients with ADHF is cardiac rehabilitation. Exercise training has been shown to reduce recurrent cardiac events in patients with LV dysfunction from ischemic causes.[73] One study of patients receiving 4 weeks of exercise training post-MI found that this rehabilitation decreased the risk of cardiac death by > 8 times for patients with a LVEF < 41% ($P = 0.04$).[74] In this study, the rehabilitation program consisted of 4 weeks of supervised 30-minute sessions of bicycle ergometry and calisthenics 5 times per week, followed by daily calisthenics and > 30 minutes of walking every other day.[74] The American Heart Association has established guidelines for exercise prescription in patients with heart failure.[75] Briefly, exercise training should occur 3 to 5 times per week to a goal of 55% to 90% maximum heart rate or 40% to 85% maximum oxygen consumption (VO_2) for 20 to 60 minutes duration. Suggested forms of exercise include walking, running or jogging, rowing, arm ergometry, swimming, and aerobics, among others.[76] For patients with heart failure, closer medical supervision as well as careful monitoring of blood pressure response to exercise and ECG for ventricular arrhythmias are appropriate.[75]

Pharmacologic Therapies

Intravenous therapies

Nitrates

Intravenous nitrates are an important therapy in patients with ADHF of ischemic origin, as they provide significant decreases in pulmonary arteriolar resistance and LV filling pressure, and thus lower mean right atrial pressure in ways that other afterload reducers, such as angiotensin-converting enzyme (ACE)-inhibitors, do not.[77] Nitrates reduce LV afterload, decrease MR, and thus lower myocardial oxygen demand, reducing myocardial ischemia.[78] These actions lead to a favorable increase in cardiac output with a lower fall in mean arterial pressure than with ACE inhibitors. In a randomized trial of 104 patients with severe pulmonary edema receiving either high-dose isosorbide dinitrate with low-dose furosemide or high-dose furosemide plus low-dose isosorbide dinitrate, the high-dose nitrates group had a 21% lower risk of death or recurrent MI ($P = 0.41$).[77]

Nitrate resistance is a limitation to therapy, however, with reduced bioactivity of nitric oxide and activation of the RAAS.[79] ACE inhibitors are useful adjuncts, as they may prevent nitrate tolerance by reducing hypersensitivity to vasoconstrictors and angiotensin II.[80] Nitrates are contraindicated in patients with a systolic blood pressure < 90 mm Hg or 30 mm Hg below baseline, marked bradycardia or tachycardia, hypertrophic cardiomyopathy, severe aortic stenosis, use of a phosphodiesterase (PDE) inhibitor for erectile dysfunction within the past 24 hours, or with suspected right ventricular infarction due to the risks of hemodynamic decompensation with these conditions.[81]

Beta-blockers

Beta-blockers have been well established as essential adjunctive therapy in patients post-MI with symptomatic LV dysfunction through subgroup analyses of the Survival and Ventricular Enlargement (SAVE), Studies of Left Ventricular Dysfunction (SOLVD), and Acute Infarction Ramipril Efficacy (AIRE) ACE inhibitor trials, with beta-blockers typically given at hospital discharge. Beta-blockers were associated with decreased progression to severe heart failure, decreased cardiovascular death, and reduced total mortality (hazard ratio [HR] 0.66; 95% CI, 0.48–0.90 in the AIRE study).[82–84] A randomized trial of carvedilol in patients with heart failure post-MI, the Carvedilol Post-Infarct Survival Control in Left Ventricular Dysfunction (CAPRICORN) trial, showed 3% absolute reductions in all-cause mortality and nonfatal MI.[85]

A frequent concern is that beta-blocker initiation during an episode of ADHF could worsen outcomes, and close supervision during initiation is essential. However, the data do not support this hypothesis of increased risk. Patients with advanced heart failure and euvolemia in the Carvedilol Prospective Randomized Cumulative Survival (COPERNICUS) trial who received carvedilol spent fewer days in the hospital and had a lower incidence of sudden death and cardiogenic shock ($P = 0.002$).[86] Moreover, the Initiation Management Predischarge: Process for Assessment of Carvedilol Therapy for Heart Failure (IMPACT-HF) trial studied pre-discharge versus post-discharge initiation of carvedilol (> 2 weeks) and found that the median length of stay was equivalent in the 2 groups (5 days) with equal percentages of adverse events. In addition, the rate of beta-blocker utilization at 60 days was higher in the early intervention group, indicating that early initiation of beta-blockers does not hurt long-term compliance.[87] American College of Cardiology (ACC) guidelines suggest that beta-blockers can be continued during acute exacerbations unless hypoperfusion and bradycardia are significant contributors. They lower the rate of chest pain, reduce reinfarction, alter remodeling, and have improved survival.[88]

Antithrombin therapy

Antithrombin agents are designed to prevent thrombus progression and stabilize atherosclerotic lesions, reducing the risk of further damage from myocardial ischemia causing the AHF decompensation. These drugs act in conjunction with the antiplatelet agents aspirin, clopidogrel, and glycoprotein IIb/IIIa (GP2B3A) inhibitors, providing additional anticoagulation and benefit. The two primary agents used are unfractionated heparin and the low-molecular-weight heparin (LMWH) enoxaparin. Enoxaparin has been shown to be more effective than unfractionated heparin in mild to moderate risk non-ST elevation MI. The Superior Yield of the New Strategy of Enoxaparin, Revascularization and Glycoprotein IIb/IIIa Inhibitors (SYNERGY) trial, however, examined patients with non-ST elevation ACS who were receiving aggressive evidence-based therapy. The overall study conclusion was that enoxaparin was non-inferior to unfractionated heparin. However, the subgroup of heart failure patients had more of a trend towards increased benefit with enoxaparin ($P = 0.020$ for death or non-fatal MI at 30 days).[89]

A meta-analysis by Yusef *et al.* of heparin versus enoxaparin found no significant differences in short-term mortality or recurrent MI, with increased major bleeding with LMWH versus placebo.[90] Thus, at this time, a trend towards increased improvement with LMWH versus unfractionated heparin is present, but these data are inconclusive and a potential risk of additional bleeding must be weighed against the possible benefits. Further study is needed to clarify this critical issue.

Oral medications

Angiotensin-converting enzyme inhibitors and angiotensin receptor antagonists

There are many proposed mechanisms for the benefit of ACE inhibitors in patients with heart failure post-MI. They are thought to reduce the remodeling that occurs shortly after MI, as angiotensin II plays a prominent role in the remodeling process.[91] Remodeling may impair the process of ischemic preconditioning, and thus ACE inhibitors aid this compensatory mechanism as well. In the hyperacute setting, they reduce myocardial ischemia by reversing angiotensin II-induced vasoconstriction and inotropy, prevent the depletion of high-energy phosphate stores, and enhance nitric oxide release through prevention of bradykinin release.[92] ACE inhibitors may even decrease hypercoagulability through endothelial release of tissue plasminogen activator (t-PA) and inhibitor decreases.[93] All these strategies lead to increased cardiac output for the failing ventricle and decreased recurrent MI rates.

In large part due to these factors, ACE inhibitors have been shown to be beneficial for patients with LV dysfunction in the immediate post-MI setting. The Trandolapril Cardiac Evaluation (TRACE) trial evaluated 1749 patients meeting these criteria and found a 7% absolute reduction in mortality rate (35% vs. 42%, $P = 0.001$), as well as reduced progression to severe heart failure.[94] In patients with ADHF symptoms, the Acute Infarction Ramipril Efficacy (AIRE) Study evaluated the effects of ramipril given from day 3 to day 10 post-MI and found a relative risk reduction in mortality of 27% (95% CI, 11–40%; $P = 0.002$), with a concomitant reduction in severe heart failure.[95] Further education is necessary to promote the use of this beneficial class of drugs. Only 73% of eligible patients with LV dysfunction were prescribed an ACE inhibitor in the ADHERE™ registry, and this number is likely lower in the post-MI setting.[2] Based on these results, an ACE inhibitor is a class I indication in the American College of Cardiology/American Heart Association (ACC/AHA) guidelines for patients with heart failure or LV dysfunction after an AMI.[96]

Due to the beneficial effects seen with inhibition of the RAAS by ACE inhibitors and the frequency of intolerance to these medicines from cough or angioedema, an alternative approach utilizing angiotensin I inhibition through angiotensin receptor blockers (ARBs) has been analyzed. Two studies have examined the role of ARBs in patients with LV dysfunction or heart failure in the setting of AMI.

The Optimal Trial in Myocardial Infarction with Angiotensin II Antagonist Losartan (OPTIMAAL) was a randomized, controlled trial of 5477 patients in which subjects receiving a target dose of 50 mg daily of losartan had a trend toward increased mortality over patients receiving captopril 50 mg 3 times daily.[97] In contrast to these findings, the Valsartan in Acute Myocardial Infarction Trial (VALIANT) found valsartan to be non-inferior to captopril in 14 703 randomized patients, although it did not show superiority (HR for mortality 1.00 (97.5% CI, 0.90–1.11).[98] Thus, current data are equivocal regarding the benefits of an ARB over ACE inhibitor, and an ACE inhibitor should be considered for first-line therapy in patients with decompensated heart failure in the AMI setting unless a contraindication or prior adverse reaction exists.

In the combination arm of VALIANT, valsartan and captopril together showed no increased effect over captopril alone (HR 0.98; 95% CI, 0.89–1.09) and had a higher incidence of discontinuation from adverse effects (8% relative risk index). These results differed from that of the Candesartan in Heart failure: Assessment of

Reduction in Mortality and Morbidity (CHARM)-Added trial, in which patients with stable LV dysfunction benefited from the combination ACE inhibitor and ARB therapy.[99] The lack of superiority of the combination treatment in this population may stem from the fact that the ACE inhibitor and ARB were titrated at the same time, but most likely result from the early timeframe post-MI.[100] Thus, combination therapy is not indicated in the ADHF setting post-MI.

Novel agents

Endothelin antagonists

Endothelin (ET) is a powerful vasoconstrictor peptide expressed in the myocardium where it increases myofilament sensitivity to calcium and modulates the hypertrophy that occurs from chronic pressure and volume overload in the heart failure state. Its levels correlate strongly with heart failure symptoms with levels 2 to 3 times higher than controls, and thus selective endothelin receptor antagonists (ERAs) have been designed and preliminarily studied.[101] Tezosentan is a dual ETa/ETb endothelin receptor antagonist that has been shown to reduce SVR and pulmonary vascular resistance (PVR), thus decreasing the PCWP and increasing cardiac output in several small studies of ADHF. The Randomized Intravenous Tezosentan (RITZ) studies include 4 trials of tezosentan in different populations. RITZ-4 examined the effects of 48 hours of intravenous tezosentan versus placebo in 193 patients with ADHF of ischemic origin.[102] No difference was found in the primary composite endpoint of death, worsening heart failure, or recurrent ischemia/infarction within 72 hours (24.2% vs. 28.9%; $P = 0.515$), with an increased incidence of symptomatic hypotension. However, tezosentan did not increase ischemia, and further studies are warranted using lower doses. This medication remains experimental at this time. Interestingly, animal studies have suggested that angiotensin II may stimulate endothelin synthesis, and thus ACE inhibitors may be exhibiting some of their benefit in heart failure by reducing endothelin levels.[103]

Nesiritide

Extensive research has focused on the natriuretic peptides and their role in heart failure. BNP levels are markedly elevated in heart failure and are useful both as diagnostic markers and as a therapeutic agent. Nesiritide is recombinant human BNP, and an infusion of this agent causes reduced PCWP and SVR, which leads to an increased cardiac index, with no increase in heart rate.[104] Nesiritide was compared against intravenous nitroglycerin and placebo in the Vasodilation in the Management of Acute Congestive Heart Failure (VMAC) trial and was found to provide a significant reduction in PCWP. It reduced dyspnea in a similar fashion as nitroglycerin. It has also been associated with a significant reduction in hospital readmission rate.[105]

Levosimendan

Levosimendan is a calcium sensitizer that increases the response of cardiac myocyte myofilaments to calcium, providing an inotropic effect. Most importantly, it appears to provide these effects without increasing oxygen consumption, and thus does not promote myocardial ischemia.[106] Cardiac filling pressures, PCWP, and right-sided pressures all decrease while stroke volume and cardiac index increase. The net result is a decrease in fatigue and dyspnea.[107] The effects of a levosimendan infusion in 504 patients with heart failure after an AMI were studied in the Randomized Study on Safety and Effectiveness of Levosimendan in Patients with Left Ventricular Failure After an Acute Myocardial Infarct (RUSSLAN) trial, with a 6-hour infusion providing a 40% risk reduction in the composite endpoint of death or worsening heart failure after 24 hours and at 14 days.[106] These results are very promising, and further confirmatory studies will hopefully promote this therapy from the investigational stage.

Drugs to avoid

Along with the many medications shown to be beneficial in ADHF of ischemic etiology, an equal number of drugs have been found to be harmful (Table 20.4).

Dobutamine

Inotropic agents have been a mainstay of therapy for decompensated heart failure due to their augmentation in cardiac output. Dobutamine is a

Table 20.4. *Drugs to avoid*

Dobutamine
Phosphodiesterase inhibitors (milrinone)
Calcium channel blockers
Nonsteroidal antiinflammatory drugs
Cyclooxygenase (COX)-2 inhibitors

beta-1 and beta-2 selective agonist that increases myocardial contractility, and it has been shown to improve symptoms for up to 30 days. For this reason, patients with decompensated heart failure have historically been given "dobutamine holidays."[108] However, published studies have shown no survival benefit, and 1 unpublished study was stopped early due to increased mortality in the dobutamine group. For this reason, dobutamine is only used when absolutely necessary to reduce intolerable symptoms for patients with ADHF.[109]

Phosphodiesterase inhibitors

Phosphodiesterase (PDE) inhibitors increase intracellular calcium concentrations and thus myocardial contractility through decreased cyclic adenosine monophosphate (cAMP) degradation. Inhibition of PDE in the peripheral tissues results in increased arterial and venous dilatation, and thus afterload reduction.[110] Milrinone has been shown to have the same beneficial symptomatic relief as dobutamine in ADHF.[111] However, OPTIME-CHF, a randomized trial of 949 patients admitted with ADHF of ischemic etiology found an increase in the combined endpoint of hospitalizations and mortality with intravenous infusion of milrinone versus placebo (42% vs. 36%, $P = 0.01$).[112] Vesnarinone, another PDE inhibitor, has been associated with a similar increase in mortality in patients with severe ischemic heart failure.[113]

Calcium channel blockers

Calcium channel blockers, which cause peripheral vasodilatation, were studied in heart failure for the potential benefits of afterload reduction. However, diltiazem has been associated with increased mortality in patients with ADHF in the Multicenter Diltiazem Postinfarction Trial (MDPIT) trial, and verapamil was shown to have no benefit in Danish Verapamil Infarction Trial (DAVIT) II.[114] The calcium channel blockers without negative inotropy, such as amlodipine, are safe for use but show no benefit in heart failure of ischemic etiology.[115]

Nonsteroidal antiinflammatory drugs

Nonsteroidal antiinflammatory drugs (NSAIDs) have been shown to increase the incidence of ADHF exacerbations approximately 10-fold in 2 cohort studies.[116,117] NSAIDs lead to systemic vasoconstriction and thus increase afterload, which depresses cardiac output. They can also lead to increased renal insufficiency and reduce diuretic effectiveness.[118] The combination of NSAIDs and aspirin, which is indicated for all ischemic cardiomyopathy patients, may reverse the beneficial effects of ACE inhibitors and thus reduce the survival benefits with this drug class.[119]

Cyclooxygenase-2 inhibitors

Selective cyclooxygenase-2 (COX-2) inhibitors have similar evidence indicating adverse effects on IHD and heart failure exacerbation. In the Vioxx Gastrointestinal Outcomes Research (VIGOR) study of rofecoxib and naproxen for rheumatoid arthritis, patients receiving rofecoxib had a 5-fold higher incidence of MI.[120] A possible mechanism for this elevated risk is a selective reduction in the levels of the protective molecule prostacyclin without a decrease in thromboxane A2, a procoagulant. The resulting imbalance can damage the endothelium.[121] Cox-2 inhibitors have also been shown to increase the incidence of decompensated heart failure in a large administrative database (adjusted relative risk 1.8 for rofecoxib).[122] New data are surfacing regarding the risk of cardiovascular events with valdecoxib, although a prior meta-analysis of 10 trials failed to show a significantly-increased risk. Further research is needed to fully elucidate the risk with this class of medications. In the meantime, it would be prudent to avoid the use of these agents unless absolutely necessary.[123]

Devices

Sudden death prevention

A major advance in the management of chronic ischemic heart failure has been the use of automatic implantable cardioverter-defibrillators (AICDs) to reduce arrhythmic sudden death. The Multicenter Automatic Defibrillator Trial (MADIT)-1 was the first trial to show a survival benefit of AICDs in patients with ischemic cardiomyopathy, but it had significant limitations that limited its applicability, including inducible NSVT as an entry criterion.[124] MADIT-II corrected for some of these deficiencies and expanded the indications for implantation.[125] This trial randomized 1232 patients with LVEF ≤ 30% and an MI > 30 days prior to enrollment to treatment with an ICD or conventional medical therapy. The trial was stopped early with an average follow-up of 20 months after an interim analysis revealed a significant reduction in all-cause mortality with an AICD (14.2% mortality vs. 19.8%; HR 0.69; 95% CI, 0.51–0.93; $P = 0.016$). This benefit was entirely due to a reduction in sudden death and was consistent across the subgroups analyzed, including age, EF, NYHA class, and QRS interval.[125] The ACC/AHA has incorporated this data into its guidelines, with a class IIA indication for patients with a prior MI and LVEF ≤ 30%, without CABG in the 3 months prior.

Management of progressive ischemia

Cardiac resynchronization therapy

Another important advance in decompensated heart failure device therapy is the use of cardiac resynchronization therapy with biventricular pacing. Patients with ischemic heart failure often have intraventricular conduction delays (IVCD) or LBBB (20% to 30% of symptomatic patients), which lead to dyssynchronous depolarization and contraction of the left and right ventricles. This dyssynchrony decreases the efficiency of ventricular contraction and can enhance functional MR by distortion of the normal ventricular geometry. An additional benefit of pacemaker placement is that beta-blocker therapy can be aggressively titrated without bradycardia.

The Multicenter InSync Randomized Clinical Evaluation (MIRACLE) study examined patients with decompensated heart failure, LVEF ≤ 35%, and QRS interval ≥ 130 ms, and found that patients utilizing cardiac resynchronization therapy had a 3-fold to 4-fold increase in 6-minute walk distance, improved LVEF and quality of life, and a lower rate of hospitalization at 6 months. There was no survival benefit. Similar benefits were found in a substudy of patients receiving a joint pacemaker-ICD.[126,127]

The first trial to show a survival benefit was the Comparison of Medical Therapy, Pacing, and Defibrillation in Chronic Heart Failure (COMPANION) trial, in which 1520 patients with NYHA class III or IV heart failure and a QRS interval ≥ 120 ms were randomized to a biventricular pacemaker with or without a defibrillator or medical therapy. The pacemaker group had a significant reduction in death or heart failure hospitalization (HR 0.81, $P = 0.014$), while the pacemaker-ICD group had a 36% relative risk reduction in all-cause mortality.[128] A meta-analysis of four major trials in cardiac resynchronization—MIRACLE, Multisite Stimulation in Cardiomyopathy (MUSTIC), and the unpublished InSync ICD and CONTAK CD® trials—revealed reduced mortality from progressive heart failure by 51% (OR 0.49; 95% CI, 0.25–0.93) and heart failure hospitalization by 29% at 3 to 6 months. The reduction in all-cause death was nonsignificant.[129]

Limitations of cardiac resynchronization therapy include difficulties in anterior lead placement, a small risk of dissection or perforation, and a lack of benefit in 30% of treated patients. The benefit does not appear to relate to the extent of QRS duration.[130]

Left ventricular assist devices

There are two primary forms of left ventricular assist devices (LVADs): (1) therapies viable only in the short-term, such as intraaortic balloon pumps (IABPs); and (2) longer-term LVADs. These latter devices can assist during acute and reversible decompensations in cardiac function, such as after CABG, or can serve as a bridge to transplantation. Moreover, there is promising ongoing research into use of these devices as destination therapy.

IABPs can be used in the acute setting to stabilize cardiogenic shock primarily from ischemia or worsening MR, and has an ACC/AHA class I indication for the same. The balloon is placed in the descending thoracic aorta and repeatedly inflates and deflates with the cardiac cycle, lowering afterload and increasing coronary blood flow. There is limited data supporting its efficacy. One study was performed in 1973 before the advent of lytics or percutaneous coronary intervention (PCI), revealing improved cardiac output and mental status with fewer arrhythmias. However, this remains a temporary therapy, with intensive monitoring required.[131]

Other devices include an extracorporeal pump that pneumatically pumps blood from the left ventricle to the systemic circulation with a 30% success rate and duration as long as 42 days. A benefit of this device is its pulsatile flow, which is more physiologic for the other organ systems. However, significant hemolysis mandates heparin use to prevent a generalized inflammatory response. This device can serve as bridge to transplantation as well as for post-transplantation temporary cardiac dysfunction. Axial flow pumps, on the other hand, use an LV screw to propel blood in a nonpulsatile fashion, which results in a low level of hemolysis but can promote end-organ dysfunction, especially renal. This device cannot be used in the setting of aortic insufficiency. These devices can provide up to 6 liters of flow based on the point of insertion. Extracorporeal membrane oxygenation (ECMO) can also be utilized, shunting blood from the venous system through the artificial membrane lung and back into the arterial system. This method is often used as bridge to a longer-term LVAD.[132]

The long-term devices in use are implanted sub-diaphragmatic, intraperitoneal or properitoneal for heart transplant candidates on maximal inotropic support with poor cardiac index (typically < 2.0 L/min) or an elevated PCWP. The Randomized Evaluation of Mechanical Assistance for the Treatment of Congestive Heart Failure (REMATCH) trial randomized patients to LVAD implantation or medical therapy. The LVAD cohort had a 2-fold improvement in survival (52% vs. 25%, $P = 0.002$) at 1 year. The benefit was limited to the 91 patients utilizing intravenous inotropes. The LVAD group had a higher incidence of neurologic complications, mechanical failure, and infection, the major cause of death. Despite the dismal survival at 2 years (23%), the potential exists for eventual destination therapy, especially as the study participants were older and had greater comorbidity than the transplant population. Current limitations include the necessity of external hardware and short battery life.[133] Experimental total artificial hearts have been developed but are limited in use because of significant complications, including infection, bleeding, and thromboembolism.[134]

Surgical therapy

Revascularization

A primary treatment for patients with ADHF of ischemic origin is myocardial revascularization (either PCI and stenting or CABG). In the GRACE registry, patients with ACS and heart failure had a lower 6-month mortality rate (adjusted hazard ratio 0.5; 95% CI, 0.37–0.68).[7] In the chronic heart failure population, revascularization of the myocardium has been associated with significant improvements in LV function, symptoms, and survival, but only in a fraction of patients. An analysis of 25 years of data from the Duke Databank for Cardiovascular Disease revealed a 5-year survival of 61% with CABG versus 37% with medical therapy ($P < 0.0001$).[135] Some patients derive no benefit, however, and patients with severe heart disease have higher surgical mortality rates.[136,137] Thus, it is critical to differentiate between those patients who are likely to improve and those without a significant likelihood of benefit.

Some areas of myocardium may lack sufficient oxygen to contract but retain viability and can regain function after restoration of perfusion. Rahimtoola first termed this hibernating myocardium.[138] Identification of this viable myocardium may aid in treatment allocation. Several imaging modalities provide information on myocardial viability, including nuclear SPECT, dobutamine echocardiography, positron emission tomography (PET), and cardiac MRI.[48,55,57] Many consider PET the preferred test due to its high sensitivity and specificity and its unique ability to quantitate blood flow noninvasively while independently measuring viability. A good alternative with low cost and high sensitivity is nuclear

SPECT imaging with radionuclide markers such as thallium, technetium, and 18-fluorodeoxyglucose (18-FDG).[139,140]

Myocardial viability has been shown to predict improvements in symptoms, EF, and short-term mortality.[141] Although studies have examined the effects of viability determination on long-term mortality, including a meta-analysis which suggests a benefit to viability-based treatment allocation decisions, a definitive conclusion has not been reached.[142,143] There is a referral bias in patients referred for myocardial viability imaging, and existing studies have been retrospective cohorts with few subjects and arbitrarily-defined levels of viability.[143–145] A trial of patients with ischemic cardiomyopathy, the Surgical Treatment for Ischemic Heart Failure (STICH) trial, is currently randomizing patients to CABG versus medical therapy, and a more definitive answer will be available in 5 to 7 years.[146]

Cardiac transplantation

Cardiac transplantation is the final treatment option for many patients with ischemic heart failure. Less than one-half of patients on the waiting list ever receive an organ, and many more are not listed due to age limitations, increased pulmonary valvular resistance, or comorbidities such as diabetes or chronic obstructive pulmonary disease (COPD).[147] Careful patient selection is imperative, as a study of cardiac transplantation in Germany showed that only patients with inotrope or LVAD dependence have a significant survival benefit from cardiac transplantation.[148] Despite increasing patient complexity, the mortality rates for patients on the United Network for Organ Sharing (UNOS) waiting list and patients undergoing transplantation have fallen dramatically with the increased use of pre-transplant LVADs and decreased contraindications (higher pre-transplantation panel reactive antibody concentrations and PVR allowed).[149] Even if patients survive the surgical procedure, many future complications remain, including allograft rejection, atypical infection, post-transplant lymphoproliferative disorders, and post-transplant vasculopathy.[149] Despite the many management issues surrounding this therapy, it remains the final treatment option for many patients with progressive heart failure. Work is under way to develop LVADs as a alternate destination therapy.

Other surgical interventions

Several other surgical interventions have been proposed with the goal to prevent adverse remodeling or restore the normal shape and function of the left ventricle in order to reduce myocardial wall stress and thus reduce ischemia.

The Dor procedure attempts to restore LV shape through reparation of aneurysms that occur post-MI, with a Dacron or pericardial flap used to cover the affected area. In one study of 495 patients undergoing the Dor procedure, there was a significant increase in LVEF (33% vs. 50%) without significant arrhythmia. The amount of scar increases the peri-procedural mortality but increases the magnitude of benefit. Patients with anterior MIs and large areas of regional akinesis benefit the most from this procedure.[150] It is contraindicated in patients with pulmonary hypertension or right ventricular failure.[151] A form of this systolic ventricular reduction surgery is being studied in the STICH trial in patients with anterior wall aneurysms and LV dysfunction. The results of this study should be available in 5 to 7 years.[146]

Two procedures that are no longer performed but which showed initial promise are the Batista procedure and cardiomyoplasty. The Batista procedure is a partial left ventriculectomy, in which a portion of the LV free wall between the papillary muscles is removed in an attempt to decrease myocardial stress. It is associated with an increase in LVEF but has a high recurrence of symptomatic heart failure, and is thus not commonly in use.[152]

Cardiomyoplasty, in which the latissimus dorsi is placed around the heart and paced during systole, is another procedure that improved surrogate outcomes such as LVEF, but has fallen out of favor after a randomized controlled trial failed to enroll sufficient patients and showed marginal clinical benefit.[153]

Future Directions

There are still many questions to be answered in the management of patients with ADHF of ischemic origin. We need to further characterize this population so that studies can be specifically tailored to address the unique issues these patients present. In the ADHERE™ registry, 51% of the patients had preserved systolic function, and there is a critical need for further study of this distinctive subgroup. Finally, we must identify strategies to increase the use of therapies determined to be beneficial, from smoking cessation counseling and beta-blocker use to implantation of cardiac resynchronization devices.

Summary

IHD is the most common etiology for heart failure, and ADHF often occurs as a result of myocardial ischemia and its sequelae.[1] A variety of biochemical and imaging techniques can be utilized to help identify ischemic etiology and provide additional prognostic information. There are many treatment modalities which can reduce the impact of myocardial ischemia in this condition, including medical therapy with aspirin, ACE inhibitors, diuretics, and statins, as well as revascularization and device treatments. Advances in diagnosis and treatment have dramatically reduced the impact of myocardial ischemia in decompensated heart failure, and we strive to continue these advances.

References

1. Gheorghiade M, Bonow RO. Chronic heart failure in the United States: a manifestation of coronary artery disease. Circulation 1998; 97: 282–289.
2. Fonarow GC. The Acute Decompensated Heart Failure National Registry (ADHERE™): opportunities to improve care of patients hospitalized with acute decompensated heart failure. Rev Cardiovasc Med 2003; 4 Suppl 7: S21–S30.
3. Zannad F, Briancon S, Juillière Y, *et al.* Incidence, clinical and etiologic features, and outcomes of advanced chronic heart failure: the EPICAL Study. Epidémiologie de l'Insuffisance Cardiaque Avancée en Lorraine. J Am Coll Cardiol 1999; 33: 734–742.
4. Opasich C, Rapezzi C, Lucci D, *et al.* Precipitating factors and decision-making processes of short-term worsening heart failure despite "optimal" treatment (from the IN-CHF Registry). Am J Cardiol 2001; 88: 382–387.
5. Michalsen A, Konig G, Thimme W. Preventable causative factors leading to hospital admission with decompensated heart failure. Heart 1998; 80: 437–441.
6. Opasich C, Febo O, Riccardi PG, *et al.* Concomitant factors of decompensation in chronic heart failure. Am J Cardiol 1996; 78: 354–357.
7. Steg PG, Dabbous OH, Feldman LJ, *et al.* Determinants and prognostic impact of heart failure complicating acute coronary syndromes: observations from the Global Registry of Acute Coronary Events (GRACE). Circulation 2004; 109: 494–499.
8. Adams KF, Jr., Sueta CA, Gheorghiade M, *et al.* Gender differences in survival in advanced heart failure. Insights from the FIRST study. Circulation 1999; 99: 1816–1821.
9. Opasich C, Tavazzi L, Lucci D, *et al.* Comparison of one-year outcome in women versus men with chronic congestive heart failure. Am J Cardiol 2000; 86: 353–357.
10. Sutton MG, Sharpe N. Left ventricular remodeling after myocardial infarction: pathophysiology and therapy. Circulation 2000; 101: 2981–2988.
11. Klein L, Gheorghiade M. Coronary artery disease and prevention of heart failure. Med Clin North Am 2004; 88: 1209–1235.
12. Tomai F, Crea F, Chiariello L, *et al.* Ischemic preconditioning in humans: models, mediators, and clinical relevance. Circulation 1999; 100: 559–563.
13. Braunwald E, Kloner RA. The stunned myocardium: prolonged, postischemic ventricular dysfunction. Circulation 1982; 66: 1146–1149.
14. Wijns W, Vatner SF, Camici PG. Hibernating myocardium. N Engl J Med 1998; 339: 173–181.
15. Arai AE, Grauer SE, Anselone CG, *et al.* Metabolic adaptation to a gradual reduction in myocardial blood flow. Circulation 1995; 92: 244–252.
16. Piccini JP, Klein L, Gheorghiade M, *et al.* New insights into diastolic heart failure: role of diabetes mellitus. Am J Med 2004; 116 Suppl 5A: 64S–75S.
17. Reeder GS. Identification and treatment of complications of myocardial infarction. Mayo Clin Proc 1995; 70: 880–884.
18. Francis GS, Goldsmith SR, Levine TB, *et al.* The neurohumoral axis in congestive heart failure. Ann Intern Med 1984; 101: 370–377.
19. Kaye DM, Lambert GW, Lefkovits J, *et al.* Neurochemical evidence of cardiac sympathetic activation and increased central nervous system norepinephrine turnover in severe congestive heart failure. J Am Coll Cardiol 1994; 23: 570–578.

20. Dzau VJ. Renal and circulatory mechanisms in congestive heart failure. Kidney Int 1987; 31: 1402–1415.
21. Anand IS, Fisher LD, Chiang YT, *et al.* Changes in brain natriuretic peptide and norepinephrine over time and mortality and morbidity in the Valsartan Heart Failure Trial (Val-HeFT). Circulation 2003; 107: 1278–1283.
22. Wei CM, Heublein DM, Perrella MA, *et al.* Natriuretic peptide system in human heart failure. Circulation 1993; 88: 1004–1009.
23. Brunner-La Rocca HP, Kaye DM, Woods RL, *et al.* Effects of intravenous brain natriuretic peptide on regional sympathetic activity in patients with chronic heart failure as compared with healthy control subjects. J Am Coll Cardiol 2001; 37: 1221–1227.
24. Hayashi M, Tsutamoto T, Wada A, *et al.* Intravenous atrial natriuretic peptide prevents left ventricular remodeling in patients with first anterior acute myocardial infarction. J Am Coll Cardiol 2001; 37: 1820–1826.
25. Bell DM, Johns TE, Lopez LM. Endothelial dysfunction: implications for therapy of cardiovascular diseases. Ann Pharmacother 1998; 32: 459–470.
26. Olivetti G, Abbi R, Quaini F, *et al.* Apoptosis in the failing human heart. N Engl J Med 1997; 336: 1131–1141.
27. Anversa P, Li P, Zhang X, *et al.* Ischaemic myocardial injury and ventricular remodelling. Cardiovasc Res 1993; 27: 145–157.
28. Bing OH. Hypothesis: apoptosis may be a mechanism for the transition to heart failure with chronic pressure overload. J Mol Cell Cardiol 1994; 26: 943–948.
29. Velazquez EJ, Pfeffer MA. Acute heart failure complicating acute coronary syndromes: a deadly intersection. Circulation 2004; 109: 440–442.
30. Rahimtoola SH. Concept and evaluation of hibernating myocardium. Annu Rev Med 1999; 50: 75–86.
31. Bart BA, Shaw LK, McCants CB, Jr., *et al.* Clinical determinants of mortality in patients with angiographically diagnosed ischemic or nonischemic cardiomyopathy. J Am Coll Cardiol 1997; 30: 1002–1008.
32. Davie AP, Francis CM, Love MP, *et al.* Value of the electrocardiogram in identifying heart failure due to left ventricular systolic dysfunction. Br Med J 1996; 312: 222.
33. Pirwitz MJ, Lange RA, Landau C, *et al.* Utility of the 12-lead electrocardiogram in identifying underlying coronary artery disease in patients with depressed left ventricular systolic function. Am J Cardiol 1996; 77: 1289–1292.
34. Sgarbossa EB, Pinski SL, Barbagelata A, *et al.* Electrocardiographic diagnosis of evolving acute myocardial infarction in the presence of left bundle-branch block. GUSTO-1 (Global Utilization of Streptokinase and Tissue Plasminogen Activator for Occluded Coronary Arteries) Investigators. N Engl J Med 1996; 334: 481–487.
35. Plebani M, Zaninotto M. Diagnostic strategies in myocardial infarction using myoglobin measurement. Eur Heart J 1998; 19 Suppl N: N12–N15.
36. Adams JE III, Abendschein DR, Jaffe AS. Biochemical markers of myocardial injury. Is MB creatine kinase the choice for the 1990s? Circulation 1993; 88: 750–763.
37. Zimmerman J, Fromm R, Meyer D, *et al.* Diagnostic marker cooperative study for the diagnosis of myocardial infarction. Circulation 1999; 99: 1671–1677.
38. Puleo PR, Guadagno PA, Roberts R, *et al.* Early diagnosis of acute myocardial infarction based on assay for subforms of creatine kinase-MB. Circulation 1990; 82: 759–764.
39. Gutovitz AL, Sobel BE, Roberts R. Progressive nature of myocardial injury in selected patients with cardiogenic shock. Am J Cardiol 1978; 41: 469–475.
40. Ishii J, Nomura M, Nakamura Y, *et al.* Risk stratification using a combination of cardiac troponin T and brain natriuretic peptide in patients hospitalized for worsening chronic heart failure. Am J Cardiol 2002; 89: 691–695.
41. Del Carlo CH, Pereira-Barretto AC, Cassaro-Strunz C, *et al.* Serial measure of cardiac troponin T levels for prediction of clinical events in decompensated heart failure. J Card Fail 2004; 10: 43–48.
42. Del Carlo CH, O'Connor CM. Cardiac troponins in congestive heart failure. Am Heart J 1999; 138: 646–653.
43. Freda BJ, Tang WH, Van Lente F, *et al.* Cardiac troponins in renal insufficiency: review and clinical implications. J Am Coll Cardiol 2002; 40: 2065–2071.
44. Baig MK, Mahon N, McKenna WJ, *et al.* The pathophysiology of advanced heart failure. Am Heart J 1998; 135: S216–S230.
45. Wang TJ, Larson MG, Levy D, *et al.* Plasma natriuretic peptide levels and the risk of cardiovascular events and death. N Engl J Med 2004; 350: 655–663.
46. Yoshimura M, Mizuno Y, Nakayama M, *et al.* B-type natriuretic peptide as a marker of the effects of

enalapril in patients with heart failure. Am J Med 2002; 112: 716–720.
47. O'Keefe JH Jr., Barnhart CS, Bateman TM. Comparison of stress echocardiography and stress myocardial perfusion scintigraphy for diagnosing coronary artery disease and assessing its severity. Am J Cardiol 1995; 75: 25D–34D.
48. Gunning MG, Anagnostopoulos C, Knight CJ, *et al.* Comparison of 201Tl, 99mTc-tetrofosmin, and dobutamine magnetic resonance imaging for identifying hibernating myocardium. Circulation 1998; 98: 1869–1874.
49. Pohost GM, Zir LM, Moore RH, *et al.* Differentiation of transiently ischemic from infarcted myocardium by serial imaging after a single dose of thallium-201. Circulation 1977; 55: 294–302.
50. Piwnica-Worms D, Kronauge JF, Chiu ML. Uptake and retention of hexakis (2-methoxyisobutyl isonitrile) technetium(I) in cultured chick myocardial cells. Mitochondrial and plasma membrane potential dependence. Circulation 1990; 82: 1826–1838.
51. Erbel R, Schweizer P, Krebs W, *et al.* Sensitivity and specificity of two-dimensional echocardiography in detection of impaired left ventricular function. Eur Heart J 1984; 5: 477–489.
52. Yamaguchi S, Tsuiki K, Hayasaka M, *et al.* Segmental wall motion abnormalities in dilated cardiomyopathy: hemodynamic characteristics and comparison with thallium-201 myocardial scintigraphy. Am Heart J 1987; 113: 1123–1128.
53. Vigna C, Russo A, De Rito V, *et al.* Regional wall motion analysis by dobutamine stess echocardiography to distinguish between ischemic and nonischemic dilated cardiomyopathy. Am Heart J 1996; 131: 537–543.
54. Pozzoli M, Capomolla S, Pinna G, *et al.* Doppler echocardiography reliably predicts pulmonary artery wedge pressure in patients with chronic heart failure with and without mitral regurgitation. J Am Coll Cardiol 1996; 27: 883–893.
55. Perrone-Filardi P, Pace L, Prastaro M, *et al.* Dobutamine echocardiography predicts improvement of hypoperfused dysfunctional myocardium after revascularization in patients with coronary artery disease. Circulation 1995; 91: 2556–2565.
56. Tan RS, Chen KK. Coronary artery disease: comprehensive evaluation by cardiovascular magnetic resonance imaging. Ann Acad Med Singapore 2004; 33: 437–443.
57. Kaandorp TA, Bax JJ, Schuijf JD, *et al.* Head-to-head comparison between contrast-enhanced magnetic resonance imaging and dobutamine magnetic resonance imaging in men with ischemic cardiomyopathy. Am J Cardiol 2004; 93: 1461–1464.
58. Deedwania PC, Carbajal EV. Role of myocardial oxygen demand in the pathogenesis of silent ischemia during daily life. Am J Cardiol 1992; 70: 19F–24F.
59. Horwich TB, Fonarow GC, Hamilton MA, *et al.* Anemia is associated with worse symptoms, greater impairment in functional capacity and a significant increase in mortality in patients with advanced heart failure. J Am Coll Cardiol 2002; 39: 1780–1786.
60. Mozaffarian D, Nye R, Levy WC. Anemia predicts mortality in severe heart failure: the prospective randomized amlodipine survival evaluation (PRAISE). J Am Coll Cardiol 2003; 41: 1933–1939.
61. Wu WC, Rathore SS, Wang Y, *et al.* Blood transfusion in elderly patients with acute myocardial infarction. N Engl J Med 2001; 345: 1230–1236.
62. Hebert PC, Wells G, Tweeddale M, *et al.* Does transfusion practice affect mortality in critically ill patients? Transfusion Requirements in Critical Care (TRICC) Investigators and the Canadian Critical Care Trials Group. Am J Respir Crit Care Med 1997; 155: 1618–1623.
63. Effect of prophylactic amiodarone on mortality after acute myocardial infarction and in congestive heart failure: meta-analysis of individual data from 6500 patients in randomised trials. Amiodarone Trials Meta-Analysis Investigators. Lancet 1997; 350: 1417–1424.
64. Sim I, McDonald KM, Lavori PW, *et al.* Quantitative overview of randomized trials of amiodarone to prevent sudden cardiac death. Circulation 1997; 96: 2823–2829.
65. Mont L, Cinca J, Blanch P, *et al.* Predisposing factors and prognostic value of sustained monomorphic ventricular tachycardia in the early phase of acute myocardial infarction. J Am Coll Cardiol 1996; 28: 1670–1676.
66. Newby KH, Thompson T, Stebbins A, *et al.* Sustained ventricular arrhythmias in patients receiving thrombolytic therapy: incidence and outcomes. The GUSTO Investigators. Circulation 1998; 98: 2567–2573.
67. Mueller HS, Chatterjee K, Davis KB, *et al.* ACC expert consensus document. Present use of bedside right heart catheterization in patients with cardiac disease. American College of Cardiology. J Am Coll Cardiol 1998; 32: 840–864.
68. Connors AF Jr., Speroff T, Dawson NV, *et al.* The effectiveness of right heart catheterization in the initial care of critically ill patients. SUPPORT Investigators. JAMA 1996; 276: 889–897.

69. Stiles, S. ESCAPE: Swan–Ganz cath for tailoring acute-HF therapy is safe but doesn't change outcomes. HeartWire. Available at: http://www.theheart.org/viewArticle.do?primaryKey=362209 Accessed February 18, 2004.
70. Komadina KH, Schenk DA, LaVeau P, *et al.* Interobserver variability in the interpretation of pulmonary artery catheter pressure tracings. Chest 1991; 100: 1647–1654.
71. Gnaegi A, Feihl F, Perret C. Intensive care physicians' insufficient knowledge of right-heart catheterization at the bedside: time to act? Crit Care Med 1997; 25: 213–220.
72. Pulmonary Artery Catheter Consensus conference: consensus statement. Crit Care Med 1997; 25: 910–925.
73. Belardinelli R, Georgiou D, Purcaro A. Low dose dobutamine echocardiography predicts improvement in functional capacity after exercise training in patients with ischemic cardiomyopathy: prognostic implication. J Am Coll Cardiol 1998; 31: 1027–1034.
74. Specchia G, De Servi S, Scire A, *et al.* Interaction between exercise training and ejection fraction in predicting prognosis after a first myocardial infarction. Circulation 1996; 94: 978–982.
75. Fletcher GF, Balady GJ, Amsterdam EA, *et al.* Exercise standards for testing and training: a statement for healthcare professionals from the American Heart Association. Circulation 2001; 104: 1694–1740.
76. Shephard RJ, Balady GJ. Exercise as cardiovascular therapy. Circulation 1999; 99: 963–972.
77. Packer M, Medina N, Yushak M, *et al.* Comparative effects of captopril and isosorbide dinitrate on pulmonary arteriolar resistance and right ventricular function in patients with severe left ventricular failure: results of a randomized crossover study. Am Heart J 1985; 109: 1293–1299.
78. Elkayam U, Roth A, Kumar A, *et al.* Hemodynamic and volumetric effects of venodilation with nitroglycerin in chronic mitral regurgitation. Am J Cardiol 1987; 60: 1106–1111.
79. Mangione NJ, Glasser SP. Phenomenon of nitrate tolerance. Am Heart J 1994; 128: 137–146.
80. Heitzer T, Just H, Brockhoff C, *et al.* Long-term nitroglycerin treatment is associated with supersensitivity to vasoconstrictors in men with stable coronary artery disease: prevention by concomitant treatment with captopril. J Am Coll Cardiol 1998; 31: 83–88.
81. Antman EM, Anbe DT, Armstrong PW, *et al.* ACC/AHA guidelines for the management of patients with ST-elevation myocardial infarction—executive summary. A report of the American College of Cardiology/American Heart Association Task Force on Practice Guidelines (Writing Committee to revise the 1999 guidelines for the management of patients with acute myocardial infarction). J Am Coll Cardiol 2004; 44: 671–719.
82. Vantrimpont P, Rouleau JL, Wun CC, *et al.* Additive beneficial effects of beta-blockers to angiotensin-converting enzyme inhibitors in the Survival and Ventricular Enlargement (SAVE) Study. SAVE Investigators. J Am Coll Cardiol 1997; 29: 229–236.
83. Spargias KS, Hall AS, Greenwood DC, *et al.* Beta blocker treatment and other prognostic variables in patients with clinical evidence of heart failure after acute myocardial infarction: evidence from the AIRE study. Heart 1999; 81: 25–32.
84. Exner DV, Dries DL, Waclawiw MA, *et al.* Beta-adrenergic blocking agent use and mortality in patients with asymptomatic and symptomatic left ventricular systolic dysfunction: a post hoc analysis of the Studies of Left Ventricular Dysfunction. J Am Coll Cardiol 1999; 33: 916–923.
85. Dargie HJ. Effect of carvedilol on outcome after myocardial infarction in patients with left-ventricular dysfunction: the CAPRICORN randomised trial. Lancet 2001; 357: 1385–1390.
86. Packer M, Coats AJ, Fowler MB, *et al.* Effect of carvedilol on survival in severe chronic heart failure. N Engl J Med 2001; 344: 1651–1658.
87. Gattis WA, O'Connor CM, Gallup DS, *et al.* Predischarge initiation of carvedilol in patients hospitalized for decompensated heart failure: results of the Initiation Management Predischarge: Process for Assessment of Carvedilol Therapy in Heart Failure (IMPACT-HF) trial. J Am Coll Cardiol 2004; 43: 1534–1541.
88. Roberts R, Rogers WJ, Mueller HS, *et al.* Immediate versus deferred beta-blockade following thrombolytic therapy in patients with acute myocardial infarction. Results of the Thrombolysis in Myocardial Infarction (TIMI) II-B Study. Circulation 1991; 83: 422–437.
89. Ferguson JJ, Califf RM, Antman EM, *et al.* Enoxaparin vs unfractionated heparin in high-risk patients with non-ST-segment elevation acute coronary syndromes managed with an intended early invasive strategy: primary results of the SYNERGY randomized trial. JAMA 2004; 292: 45–54.
90. Eikelboom JW, Anand SS, Malmberg K, *et al.* Unfractionated heparin and low-molecular-weight heparin in acute coronary syndrome without ST elevation: a meta-analysis. Lancet 2000; 355: 1936–1942.

91. Greenberg B, Quinones MA, Koilpillai C, *et al.* Effects of long-term enalapril therapy on cardiac structure and function in patients with left ventricular dysfunction. Results of the SOLVD echocardiography substudy. Circulation 1995; 91: 2573–2581.
92. Longobardi G, Ferrara N, Furgi G, *et al.* Improvement of myocardial blood flow to ischemic regions by angiotensin-converting enzyme inhibition. J Am Coll Cardiol 2000; 36: 1437–1438.
93. Minai K, Matsumoto T, Horie H, *et al.* Bradykinin stimulates the release of tissue plasminogen activator in human coronary circulation: effects of angiotensin-converting enzyme inhibitors. J Am Coll Cardiol 2001; 37: 1565–1570.
94. Kober L, Torp-Pedersen C, Carlsen JE, *et al.* A clinical trial of the angiotensin-converting-enzyme inhibitor trandolapril in patients with left ventricular dysfunction after myocardial infarction. Trandolapril Cardiac Evaluation (TRACE) Study Group. N Engl J Med 1995; 333: 1670–1676.
95. Effect of ramipril on mortality and morbidity of survivors of acute myocardial infarction with clinical evidence of heart failure. The Acute Infarction Ramipril Efficacy (AIRE) Study Investigators. Lancet 1993; 342: 821–828.
96. Ryan TJ, Antman EM, Brooks NH, *et al.* 1999 update: ACC/AHA guidelines for the management of patients with acute myocardial infarction. A report of the American College of Cardiology/American Heart Association Task Force on Practice Guidelines (Committee on Management of Acute Myocardial Infarction). J Am Coll Cardiol 1999; 34: 890–911.
97. Dickstein K, Kjekshus J. Effects of losartan and captopril on mortality and morbidity in high-risk patients after acute myocardial infarction: the OPTIMAAL randomised trial. Optimal Trial in Myocardial Infarction with Angiotensin II Antagonist Losartan. Lancet 2002; 360: 752–760.
98. Pfeffer MA, McMurray JJ, Velazquez EJ, *et al.* Valsartan, captopril, or both in myocardial infarction complicated by heart failure, left ventricular dysfunction, or both. N Engl J Med 2003; 349: 1893–1906.
99. McMurray JJ, Ostergren J, Swedberg K, *et al.* Effects of candesartan in patients with chronic heart failure and reduced left-ventricular systolic function taking angiotensin-converting-enzyme inhibitors: the CHARM-Added trial. Lancet 2003; 362: 767–771.
100. Demers C, McKelvie RS. Valsartan plus captopril did not improve survival more than captopril alone after myocardial infarction. ACP J Club 2004; 141: 3.
101. Levin ER. Endothelins. N Engl J Med 1995; 333: 356–363.
102. O'Connor CM, Gattis WA, Adams KF Jr., *et al.* Tezosentan in patients with acute heart failure and acute coronary syndromes: results of the Randomized Intravenous TeZosentan Study (RITZ-4). J Am Coll Cardiol 2003; 41: 1452–1457.
103. Clavell AL, Mattingly MT, Stevens TL, *et al.* Angiotensin converting enzyme inhibition modulates endogenous endothelin in chronic canine thoracic inferior vena caval constriction. J Clin Invest 1996; 97: 1286–1292.
104. Mills RM, LeJemtel TH, Horton DP, *et al.* Sustained hemodynamic effects of an infusion of nesiritide (human b-type natriuretic peptide) in heart failure: a randomized, double-blind, placebo-controlled clinical trial. Natrecor Study Group. J Am Coll Cardiol 1999; 34: 155–162.
105. Silver MA, Horton DP, Ghali JK, *et al.* Effect of nesiritide versus dobutamine on short-term outcomes in the treatment of patients with acutely decompensated heart failure. J Am Coll Cardiol 2002; 39: 798–803.
106. Moiseyev VS, Poder P, Andrejevs N, *et al.* Safety and efficacy of a novel calcium sensitizer, levosimendan, in patients with left ventricular failure due to an acute myocardial infarction: a randomized, placebo-controlled, double-blind study (RUSSLAN). Eur Heart J 2002; 23: 1422–1432.
107. Slawsky MT, Colucci WS, Gottlieb SS, *et al.* Acute hemodynamic and clinical effects of levosimendan in patients with severe heart failure. Study Investigators. Circulation 2000; 102: 2222–2227.
108. Oliva F, Latini R, Politi A, *et al.* Intermittent 6-month low-dose dobutamine infusion in severe heart failure: DICE multicenter trial. Am Heart J 1999; 138: 247–253.
109. Dies, F., Krell, M., Whitlow, P. Intermittent dobutamine in ambulatory outpatients with chronic cardiac failure. Circulation 1986; 74: 38 (Abstract).
110. Colucci WS, Wright RF, Jaski BE, *et al.* Milrinone and dobutamine in severe heart failure: differing hemodynamic effects and individual patient responsiveness. Circulation 1986; 73: III175–III183.
111. Yamani MH, Haji SA, Starling RC, *et al.* Comparison of dobutamine-based and milrinone-based therapy for advanced decompensated congestive heart failure: Hemodynamic efficacy, clinical outcome, and economic impact. Am Heart J 2001; 142: 998–1002.
112. Felker GM, Benza RL, Chandler AB, *et al.* Heart failure etiology and response to milrinone in decompensated heart failure: results from the OPTIME-CHF study. J Am Coll Cardiol 2003; 41: 997–1003.

113. Cohn JN, Goldstein SO, Greenberg BH, *et al.* A dose-dependent increase in mortality with vesnarinone among patients with severe heart failure. Vesnarinone Trial Investigators. N Engl J Med 1998; 339: 1810–1816.
114. Effect of verapamil on mortality and major events after acute myocardial infarction (the Danish Verapamil Infarction Trial II—DAVIT II). Am J Cardiol 1990; 66: 779–785.
115. O'Connor CM, Carson PE, Miller AB, *et al.* Effect of amlodipine on mode of death among patients with advanced heart failure in the PRAISE trial. Prospective Randomized Amlodipine Survival Evaluation. Am J Cardiol 1998; 82: 881–887.
116. Feenstra J, Heerdink ER, Grobbee DE, *et al.* Association of nonsteroidal anti-inflammatory drugs with first occurrence of heart failure and with relapsing heart failure: the Rotterdam Study. Arch Intern Med 2002; 162: 265–270.
117. Page J, Henry D. Consumption of NSAIDs and the development of congestive heart failure in elderly patients: an underrecognized public health problem. Arch Intern Med 2000; 160: 777–784.
118. Dzau VJ, Packer M, Lilly LS, *et al.* Prostaglandins in severe congestive heart failure. Relation to activation of the renin-angiotensin system and hyponatremia. N Engl J Med 1984; 310: 347–352.
119. Hall D, Zeitler H, Rudolph W. Counteraction of the vasodilator effects of enalapril by aspirin in severe heart failure. J Am Coll Cardiol 1992; 20: 1549–1555.
120. Bombardier C, Laine L, Reicin A, *et al.* Comparison of upper gastrointestinal toxicity of rofecoxib and naproxen in patients with rheumatoid arthritis. VIGOR Study Group. N Engl J Med 2000; 343: 1520–8, 2, 2 p following 1528.
121. Caughey GE, Cleland LG, Penglis PS, *et al.* Roles of cyclooxygenase (COX)-1 and COX-2 in prostanoid production by human endothelial cells: selective upregulation of prostacyclin synthesis by COX-2. J Immunol 2001; 167: 2831–2838.
122. Mamdani M, Juurlink DN, Lee DS, *et al.* Cyclooxygenase-2 inhibitors versus non-selective nonsteroidal anti-inflammatory drugs and congestive heart failure outcomes in elderly patients: a population-based cohort study. Lancet 2004; 363: 1751–1756.
123. White WB, Strand V, Roberts R, *et al.* Effects of the cyclooxygenase-2 specific inhibitor valdecoxib versus nonsteroidal antiinflammatory agents and placebo on cardiovascular thrombotic events in patients with arthritis. Am J Ther 2004; 11: 244–250.
124. Moss AJ, Hall WJ, Cannom DS, *et al.* Improved survival with an implanted defibrillator in patients with coronary disease at high risk for ventricular arrhythmia. Multicenter Automatic Defibrillator Implantation Trial Investigators. N Engl J Med 1996; 335: 1933–1940.
125. Moss AJ, Zareba W, Hall WJ, *et al.* Prophylactic implantation of a defibrillator in patients with myocardial infarction and reduced ejection fraction. N Engl J Med 2002; 346: 877–883.
126. Abraham WT, Fisher WG, Smith AL, *et al.* Cardiac resynchronization in chronic heart failure. N Engl J Med 2002; 346: 1845–1853.
127. Young JB, Abraham WT, Smith AL, *et al.* Combined cardiac resynchronization and implantable cardioversion defibrillation in advanced chronic heart failure: the MIRACLE ICD Trial. JAMA 2003; 289: 2685–2694.
128. Bristow MR, Saxon LA, Boehmer J, *et al.* Cardiac-resynchronization therapy with or without an implantable defibrillator in advanced chronic heart failure. N Engl J Med 2004; 350: 2140–2150.
129. St John Sutton MG, Plappert T, Abraham WT, *et al.* Effect of cardiac resynchronization therapy on left ventricular size and function in chronic heart failure. Circulation 2003; 107: 1985–1990.
130. Saxon LA, Ellenbogen KA. Resynchronization therapy for the treatment of heart failure. Circulation 2003; 108: 1044–1048.
131. Scheidt S, Wilner G, Mueller H, *et al.* Intra-aortic balloon counterpulsation in cardiogenic shock. Report of a co-operative clinical trial. N Engl J Med 1973; 288: 979–984.
132. Smedira NG, Moazami N, Golding CM, *et al.* Clinical experience with 202 adults receiving extracorporeal membrane oxygenation for cardiac failure: survival at five years. J Thorac Cardiovasc Surg 2001; 122: 92–102.
133. Rose EA, Gelijns AC, Moskowitz AJ, *et al.* Long-term mechanical left ventricular assistance for end-stage heart failure. N Engl J Med 2001; 345: 1435–1443.
134. Copeland JG, Smith RG, Arabia FA, *et al.* Cardiac replacement with a total artificial heart as a bridge to transplantation. N Engl J Med 2004; 351: 859–867.
135. O'Connor CM, Velazquez EJ, Gardner LH, *et al.* Comparison of coronary artery bypass grafting versus medical therapy on long-term outcome in patients with ischemic cardiomyopathy (a 25-year experience from the Duke Cardiovascular Disease Databank). Am J Cardiol 2002; 90: 101–107.
136. Lee KS, Marwick TH, Cook SA, *et al.* Prognosis of

patients with left ventricular dysfunction, with and without viable myocardium after myocardial infarction. Relative efficacy of medical therapy and revascularization. Circulation 1994; 90: 2687–2694.
137. vom DJ, Eitzman DT, al Aouar ZR, *et al.* Relation of regional function, perfusion, and metabolism in patients with advanced coronary artery disease undergoing surgical revascularization. Circulation 1994; 90: 2356–2366.
138. Rahimtoola SH. The hibernating myocardium. Am Heart J 1989; 117: 211–221.
139. Marin-Neto JA, Dilsizian V, Arrighi JA, *et al.* Thallium scintigraphy compared with 18F-fluorodeoxyglucose positron emission tomography for assessing myocardial viability in patients with moderate versus severe left ventricular dysfunction. Am J Cardiol 1998; 82: 1001–1007.
140. Dilsizian V, Bonow RO. Current diagnostic techniques of assessing myocardial viability in patients with hibernating and stunned myocardium. Circulation 1993; 87: 1–20.
141. Iskander S, Iskandrian AE. Prognostic utility of myocardial viability assessment. Am J Cardiol 1999; 83: 696–702, A7.
142. Allman KC, Shaw LJ, Hachamovitch R, *et al.* Myocardial viability testing and impact of revascularization on prognosis in patients with coronary artery disease and left ventricular dysfunction: a meta-analysis. J Am Coll Cardiol 2002; 39: 1151–1158.
143. Bourque JM, Hasselblad V, Velazquez EJ, *et al.* Revascularization in patients with coronary artery disease, left ventricular dysfunction, and viability: a meta-analysis. Am Heart J 2003; 146: 621–627.
144. Bourque JM, Velazquez EJ, Borges-Neto S, *et al.* Clinical characteristics and referral pattern of patients with left ventricular dysfunction and significant coronary artery disease undergoing radionuclide imaging. J Nucl Cardiol 2004; 11: 118–125.
145. Bourque JM, Velazquez EJ, Borges-Neto S, *et al.* Radionuclide viability testing: should it affect treatment strategy in patients with cardiomyopathy and significant coronary artery disease? Am Heart J 2003; 145: 758–767.
146. Joyce D, Loebe M, Noon GP, *et al.* Revascularization and ventricular restoration in patients with ischemic heart failure: the STICH trial. Curr Opin Cardiol 2003; 18: 454–457.
147. Westaby S. Coronary revascularization in ischemic cardiomyopathy. Surg Clin North Am 2004; 84: 179–199, x.
148. Deng MC, De Meester JM, Smits JM, *et al.* Effect of receiving a heart transplant: analysis of a national cohort entered on to a waiting list, stratified by heart failure severity. Comparative Outcome and Clinical Profiles in Transplantation (COCPIT) Study Group. Br Med J 2000; 321: 540–545.
149. Deng MC. Cardiac transplantation. Heart 2002; 87: 177–184.
150. Di Donato M, Sabatier M, Dor V, *et al.* Akinetic versus dyskinetic postinfarction scar: relation to surgical outcome in patients undergoing endoventricular circular patch plasty repair. J Am Coll Cardiol 1997; 29: 1569–1575.
151. Menicanti L, Di Donato M. The Dor procedure: what has changed after fifteen years of clinical practice? J Thorac Cardiovasc Surg 2002; 124: 886–890.
152. Stolf NA, Moreira LF, Bocchi EA, *et al.* Determinants of midterm outcome of partial left ventriculectomy in dilated cardiomyopathy. Ann Thorac Surg 1998; 66: 1585–1591.
153. Acker MA. Dynamic cardiomyoplasty: at the crossroads. Ann Thorac Surg 1999; 68: 750–755.

PART IV

Treatment Strategies

CHAPTER 21

Treatment of acute heart failure in patients with preserved systolic function

Marvin W Kronenberg

Introduction

Definition

There has been relatively little information about heart failure with normal (preserved) or relatively preserved left ventricular (LV) function. Although this condition is a common cause of heart failure, especially in the elderly,[1–5] it was poorly recognized until recently. Also, there has been disagreement about the most appropriate nomenclature for this condition. The terms *heart failure with normal ejection fraction* (HFNEF) and *diastolic heart failure* are the most commonly applied. This chapter uses HFNEF since it is a term that applies to a broad set of conditions (Table 21.1) and does not restrict our thinking to emphasizing LV diastolic dysfunction as the primary pathology. Indeed, when referring to HFNEF due to hypertensive-hypertrophic heart disease, abnormal systemic arterial stiffness interacting with excessive ventricular stiffness, may be the cause of worsening heart failure, further emphasizing the need for a broad term to describe this disorder.

Diagnosis

Patients with HFNEF may have (1) endocardial, myocardial, or pericardial disorders; or (2) valvular, pulmonary/right ventricular (RV) or metabolic disorders. The diagnosis of HFNEF currently rests on three basic findings: (1) clinical signs and symptoms of heart failure; (2) findings of preserved or relatively preserved LV systolic performance, as estimated by the left ventricular ejection fraction (LVEF); and (3) echocardiographic or catheterization data showing diastolic dysfunction. Findings 1 and 2 are essential for the diagnosis, and are supported by finding 3. Table 21.1 summarizes the wide variety of disorders that produce heart failure with preserved systolic function. Because LV dysfunction may lead to pulmonary hypertension and secondary RV dysfunction, there may be some overlap among the categories. However, because of this large, diverse group of conditions, it is of great importance to make as accurate a diagnosis as possible in order to provide the correct treatment. It is recognized that most of the therapeutic uncertainty will relate to the treatment of the myocardial dysfunction that leads to HFNEF, and much of the following discussion will focus on this aspect of HFNEF.

Case history

The following case history of a patient seen recently at our institution illustrates some of the common features of HFNEF. The patient was a 63-year-old woman with a past medical history of type 2 diabetes mellitus and hypertension. She felt well until October 2001, when she had the sudden onset of acute dyspnea waking her from sleep. There was no associated chest discomfort. Her blood pressure at an outside hospital was 136/108 mm Hg. Oxygen saturation was 73% using a non-rebreath-

Table 21.1 *Differential Diagnosis of Heart Failure with Preserved Left Ventricular Ejection Fraction*

I. Non-dilated LV
   A. LV Hypertrophy
      1. Aortic stenosis
      2. Hypertrophic cardiomyopathy
      3. Hypertensive hypertrophic cardiomyopathy
   B. Infiltrative cardiomyopathy (e.g. amyloidosis)
   C. Normal thickness LV
      1. Mitral valve obstruction
         a. mitral stenosis
         b. left atrial myxoma
      2. Pericardial disease
         a. pericardial tamponade
         b. pericardial constriction
      3. Ischemic heart disease
      4. Restrictive cardiomyopathy
         a. endocardial fibrosis
         b. myocardial fibrosis
         c. carcinoid
   D. Pulmonary hypertension, with secondary RV dysfunction (cor pulmonale)
      1. Pulmonary parenchymal disorders
      2. Pulmonary thromboembolic disorders
      3. Primary pulmonary hypertension
      4. Other pulmonary disorders (interstitial, vascular)
         a. connective tissue disorders
            1) systemic lupus erythematosus
            2) scleroderma
            3) dermatomyositis
         b. sarcoidosis
         c. asbestosis
         d. radiation-induced fibrosis
      5. Pulmonary veno-occlusive disease
   E. RV dysfunction, isolated
      1. Predominant RV infarction
      2. Carcinoid

II. Dilated LV
   A. Regurgitant valvular lesions
      1. Aortic regurgitation
      2. Mitral regurgitation
   B. High output heart failure
      1. Left-to-right shunts
      2. Anemia
      3. Thiamine deficiency (beriberi heart disease)
      4. Thyrotoxicosis

Abbreviations: LV = left ventricular; RV = right ventricular.

ing mask. An arterial blood gas showed a partial pressure of carbon dioxide (P_{CO_2}) of 70 torr, and the chest radiograph showed pulmonary edema. The patient was intubated and oxygenation improved. The initial electrocardiogram (ECG) was said to show sinus tachycardia and ischemic-appearing anterior T-wave inversion. She was transferred to our institution for further care. The patient's family history was significant for two aunts and a sister who had deep venous thromboses, and one brother who had post-operative pulmonary embolism.

Following transfer, the patient's blood pressure was 126/64 mm Hg, and her heart rate was 90 bpm and regular. The respiratory rate was 16, and she was afebrile. The jugular venous pressure was estimated at 6 cm of water at 40 degrees elevation (normal). The carotid upstroke was normal, and there were no carotid bruits. There were bibasilar pulmonary rales. The cardiac apical impulse was at the mid-clavicular line. There was no lift or thrill. The first and second heart sounds were normal. There was no murmur, rub, or gallop. The abdominal examination was normal, and the extremities were also normal.

The ECG (Figure 21.1) showed sinus rhythm, a prolonged QT interval and diffuse T-wave inversion strongly suggestive but not diagnostic of ischemia. Troponin-T was mildly elevated at 1.1 ng/mL. At catheterization shortly after arrival, LV pressure was 139/19 mm Hg. The left ventricle showed anterior, apical, and distal inferior hypokinesis, with preserved wall motion in only the anterobasal and inferobasal segments. The estimated LVEF was 35%. The coronary arteries were normal except for an approximate 70% lesion in the distal third of the left anterior descending (LAD) artery. This was not judged to be anatomically in the location to cause the more widespread hypokinesis noted on the ventriculogram. Tests of

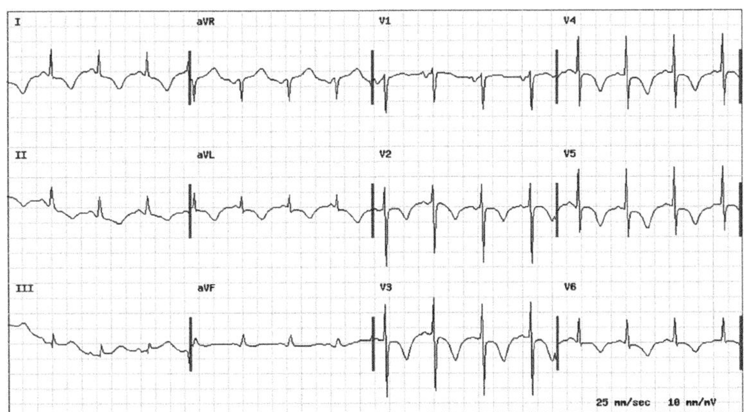

Figure 21.1. *Electrocardiogram after initial admission with pulmonary edema*

clotting demonstrated a slight elevation of the lupus anticoagulant.

Two days after admission, an echocardiogram showed normal LV wall thickness at 9 mm, plus normal LV and RV wall motion. The estimated LVEF had increased to 55%. The mitral Doppler evaluation showed a reversal of the early (E) and atrial filling (A) waves, consistent with diastolic dysfunction. There was focal thickening of the aortic valve, but no aortic stenosis, and the other valves were anatomically normal. An endomyocardial biopsy was subsequently performed and showed myocyte hypertrophy, patchy interstitial fibrosis, and no inflammatory infiltrate. Further clinical events included intermittent, symptomatic atrial fibrillation with a rapid ventricular rate, eventually necessitating treatment with amiodarone, and after some months, because of recurrences, atrioventricular node ablation plus a RV pacemaker.

Six months later, she did not take diuretics for 2 days and became severely dyspneic. On admission, her blood pressure was 170/78 mm Hg. The patient's heart rate was 78 bpm and regular. There were diffuse pulmonary rales and the pH was 7.12. Chest x-ray showed interstitial pulmonary edema (Figure 21.2). An ECG showed sinus rhythm without the prior severe T-wave inversion. The echocardiographic LVEF was 40% to 50%, with apical and distal inferior hypokinesis. She improved and was discharged on warfarin, amiodarone, metoprolol, losartan, furosemide, aspirin, and glipizide. She was readmitted 1 year later with recurrent pulmonary edema. A myocardial infarction (MI) was excluded. The echocardiographic LVEF was 40% and LV wall motion was normal.

In summary, this patient has several features of HFNEF, with some unusual and confusing features that prompted a more extensive evaluation (including an endomyocardial biopsy) than is usually necessary for the diagnosis. The main criteria for the diagnosis of HFNEF were fulfilled. There was acute heart failure (AHF) with normal LV dimensions. The initial EF was moderately depressed, but on all other echocardiograms the EF was normal. The LV diastolic pressure was moderately elevated, consistent with diastolic dysfunction. There were features

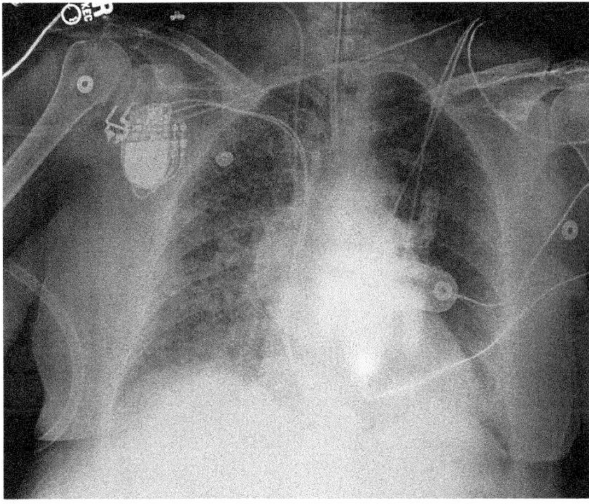

Figure 21.2. *Anteroposterior chest radiograph following readmission 6 months later with pulmonary edema*

commonly associated with HFNEF, with the presence of atrial fibrillation as a severe, complicating factor. While there was a history of hypertension, the LV wall thickness was surprisingly, and unusually, normal. It was difficult to explain the exact cause of her heart failure, and an endomyocardial biopsy was performed to aid in this evaluation. While there was coronary atherosclerosis, her physician concluded that this was not sufficient to cause the ischemic LV dysfunction present on her initial admission, and the tentative diagnosis of a hypercoagulable syndrome or excess myocardial fibrosis with poor LV compliance was proposed after an endomyocardial biopsy showed patchy fibrosis but failed to demonstrate myocarditis or an infiltrative disorder. She suffered the typical need for readmissions to the hospital in spite of her physician's best efforts at treatment. Eventually, her treatment was stabilized, and the patient has had no further episodes of symptomatic heart failure in the past 9 months.

Background

Incidence and prevalence of heart failure with normal ejection fraction

Several studies have estimated the prevalence of heart failure in communities, and a recent result from Olmstead County, MN, found that 2.2% of the randomly sampled population age ≥ 45 years had a validated diagnosis of heart failure.[6] Of these, 44% had an EF of 50% or greater. Fully 28% of the total population had some degree of diastolic dysfunction, and 5.6% of this group had moderate or severe diastolic dysfunction and normal EF (*isolated diastolic dysfunction*). Further, the presence of any degree of diastolic dysfunction was associated with increased mortality over a median follow-up interval of 3.5 years. Several clinical characteristics were associated with diastolic dysfunction, including age ≥ 65, LVEF ≤ 50%, hypertension, diabetes mellitus, coronary artery disease, MI, and a diagnosis of congestive heart failure of any type (all $P < 0.001$). Other work has shown that elderly and female patients, as well as those with hypertension are especially prone to HFNEF.[3,7] Among five prospective studies of HFNEF, the patients' ages ranged from 72 to 79 years, and the percentage of females ranged from 61 to 76%.[1,3,5,8,9]

Mortality and readmission to hospitals

There is little information about the acute mortality of HFNEF. One report found an in-hospital mortality of 4.2% among 619 patients admitted with this diagnosis,[5] which was similar to 5% mortality in another study.[1] In follow-up studies, Smith *et al.* found that readmissions to hospitals were similar in those with preserved or depressed LVEF, but others have found that readmissions trended lower.[9] Most research has shown that the long-term mortality of HFNEF is considerable, but less than in patients with LV dilation and reduced EF.[1,3,4]

Pathophysiology

The myocardium in pressure-overloaded ventricles demonstrates hypertrophy (left ventricular hypertrophy [LVH])[10] and increased extracellular matrix, especially collagen.[11] In dilated hearts with hypertrophy, there is strong evidence for abnormal calcium handling with delayed relaxation.[12] Similarly, in hypertrophic cardiomyopathy, as compared to normal, isolated trabeculae showed marked elevations in diastolic calcium concentration and tension as pacing frequency was increased, with incomplete relaxation and fusion of twitches, which resulted in reduced systolic tension development.[13] It was postulated that such abnormalities may explain, in part, why patients with hypertrophic cardiomyopathy poorly tolerate tachycardia. In a clinical study of patients with LVH (most of whom had HFNEF), Liu *et al.*[14] showed that the end-diastolic pressure was abnormally high, and electrical pacing reduced contractility at faster rates, as shown by the end-systolic pressure–volume (P–V) relation. These findings were thought to be due to abnormalities of calcium entry and reuptake, but no worsening of diastolic P–V relations occurred, in contrast to the previously cited studies in hypertrophic trabeculae.

In addition to abnormal calcium handling, there are additional myocyte abnormalities of myofilament regulatory proteins and abnormal energetics, plus changes in the cytoskeleton and abnormalities in the neurohormonal milieu which have been discussed in a recent review by Zile and Brutsaert.[15]

Several reviews have summarized the similarities and differences in heart failure with normal and reduced LVEF. Similarities include hypertrophy and increased LV mass, interstitial fibrosis, abnormal calcium handling, and slowed relaxation. However, there are also significant differences in LV volumes and chamber stiffness.[16] Both patients with HFNEF and dilated ventricles have LVH, but the type of hypertrophy differs. Usually, patients with HFNEF have concentric hypertrophy while patients with dilated ventricles have eccentric hypertrophy. The cause of this difference in hypertrophy is uncertain.

A recent clinical study compared the pathophysiology of HFNEF (LVEF ≥ 50%) and systolic heart failure.[17] In HFNEF patients, there was an increased mass/volume ratio consistent with concentric hypertrophy, but similar total body oxygen consumption during exercise and similar norepinephrine levels. The patients with HFNEF had less elevated B-type natriuretic peptide (BNP) and less disability as measured by quality of life methods.

In a catheterization study, there were abnormal pressure-derived indices of diastolic performance in 92% of patients, abnormal echocardiography-derived diastolic indices in 94% of patients, and at least one of the above in 100% of a sample of patients with HFNEF.[18] Thus, the diagnosis of HFNEF can be made on the basis of symptoms and signs of heart failure plus a normal LVEF. Recently, in the same patients (two-thirds of which were hypertensive men with an average age of 59 years), further analysis of diastolic P–V relations using micromanometer-tipped catheters showed prolonged isovolumic relaxation and abnormal diastolic P–V relations, as compared to normal subjects.[19]

It is important to emphasize the interaction of systemic vascular characteristics and LV mechanics in the pathogenesis of HFNEF. Recent studies have shown that patients with HFNEF have increased arterial elastance (stiffness) (e.g. reduced arterial compliance) compared to hypertensive patients without heart failure and compared to other control subjects.[20] In this study, ventricular systolic elastance, as judged by the end-systolic pressure–volume relationship, was also greater than normal in patients with HFNEF. Importantly, there was linkage of arterial and ventricular stiffening which produced a marked increase in LV diastolic pressure during isometric exercise (Figure 21.3), and it is possible that this is an

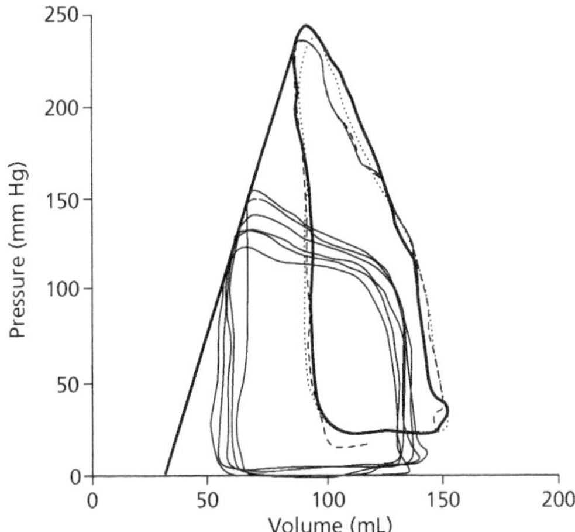

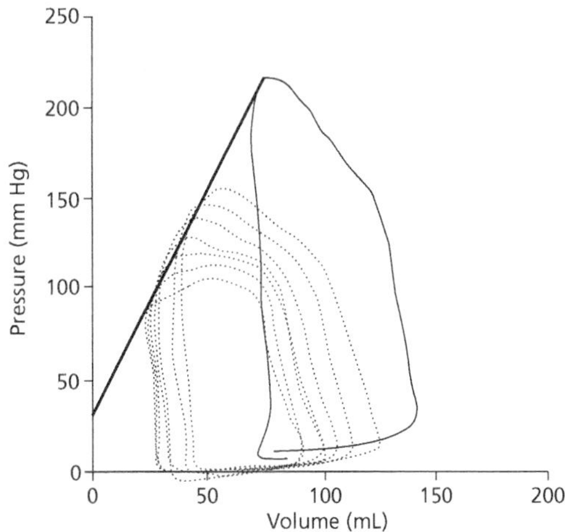

Figure 21.3. *Effect of isometric exercise on systemic arterial pressure and left ventricular (LV) pressure–volume (P–V) relations. The increase in systemic arterial pressure was associated with a marked increase in LV diastolic pressure, nearing or exceeding that associated with pulmonary edema. P–V relations before (dashed line) and after (dark solid line) sustained isometric handgrip in two patients with HFNEF. Baseline loops display elevated E_{es} and E_a, predicting the marked hypertensive response with loading. This was accompanied by increased end-diastolic pressure and prolonged relaxation, supporting a mechanism whereby ventricular-arterial stiffening could couple to diastolic function (With permission from Kawaguchi et al.[20])*

important mechanism in the pathogenesis of pulmonary edema in such patients. Others have observed reduced aortic distensibility in such patients.[21] Figure 21.4 demonstrates the classic concept of an abnormal diastolic pressure-volume relationship in HFNEF, but also shows new information demonstrating that the diastolic pressure–volume relationships of patients with HFNEF are sometimes

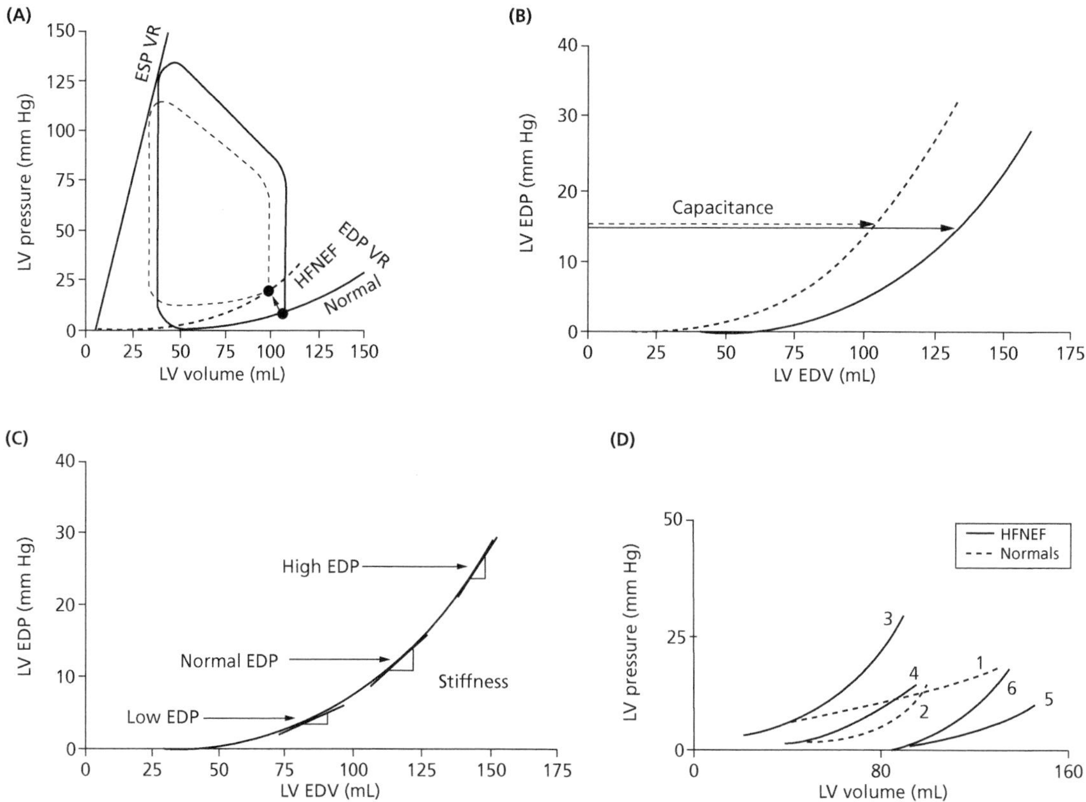

Figure 21.4. *Diagram of left ventricular (LV) pressure–volume (P–V) relations in the normal condition and in the condition of pure diastolic dysfunction with reduced LV compliance. (A) P–V representation of prevailing paradigm of heart failure with normal ejection fraction (HFNEF), showing elevated end-diastolic pressure–volume relationship (EDPVR) with no significant effect on end-systolic pressure–volume relationship (ESPVR). Respective end-diastolic pressure–volume point shown by filled circles. (B) When the entire EDPVR cannot be measured, an alternate means of indexing diastolic properties for purposes of comparing heart sizes is via capacitance, the volume at a specified filling pressure. (C) Left EDPVR is nonlinear, so that stiffness (the slope of the relationship, $\Delta P/\Delta V$) depends on filling pressure, as indicated by the tangent line at each level of end-diastolic pressure (EDP). EDV indicates end-diastolic volume. (D) LV diastolic pressure–volume relations in normal patients and in patients with HFNEF. Note that some patients with HFNEF have normal diastolic pressure-volume relations. End-diastolic P–V relations are re-plotted from Kawaguchi et al[20]; curves 4 and 5) and from Figure 3 of Liu et al.[14] (curves 2 and 6). EDPVRs of the HFNEF patients may be shifted to the left (curve 3), shifted to the right (curves 5 and 6), or may not be significantly different (curve 4) than those of normal patients (curves 1 and 2). Knowledge of patient age, sex, and body size would enhance ability to interpret the meaning of these differences (curves 1 and 3). With permission from Burkhoff* et al.[22]

similar to normal, supporting the hypothesis of abnormal vascular-ventricular interaction underlying heart failure in at least some of these patients, rather than abnormal LV properties alone.[22]

Evaluation and Treatment of Acute Heart Failure in Patients with Normal Ejection Fraction, Assuming no Prior Information is Available

Evaluation

An accurate history and physical examination are essential for understanding heart failure. It is important to assess the blood pressure accurately in both arms using a cuff sphygmomanometer. One should not rely on automated assessments, at least at first, keeping in mind that one must detect pulsus paradoxus if present, and detect pressure differences between the arms, if present. Further, a lack of pedal pulses in a patient with hypertension should suggest the possibility of coarctation of the aorta, although peripheral atherosclerosis is the more likely cause in the elderly. It is important to address the character of the carotid pulse contour, the level of estimated jugular venous pressure, the presence and extent of rales, the presence of signs of pulmonary disease, the cardiac examination, the presence of hepatomegaly, and the signs of circulatory volume overload.

By the history and physical examination, it should be possible to define a working clinical diagnosis, plus the reason for cardiovascular decompensation. Recently, investigators in the New York Heart Failure Registry addressed the reasons for hospitalization for HFNEF.[5] Cardiovascular or medical conditions and new events precipitating hospitalization were sought. The main factors precipitating hospitalization included severe hypertension, medical noncompliance, severe mitral or aortic regurgitation, renal insufficiency, and supraventricular tachyarrhythmias, with a smaller percentage of severe respiratory problems and aortic or mitral stenosis. Overall, 53% of patients had an identifiable factor (Figure 21.5). For the

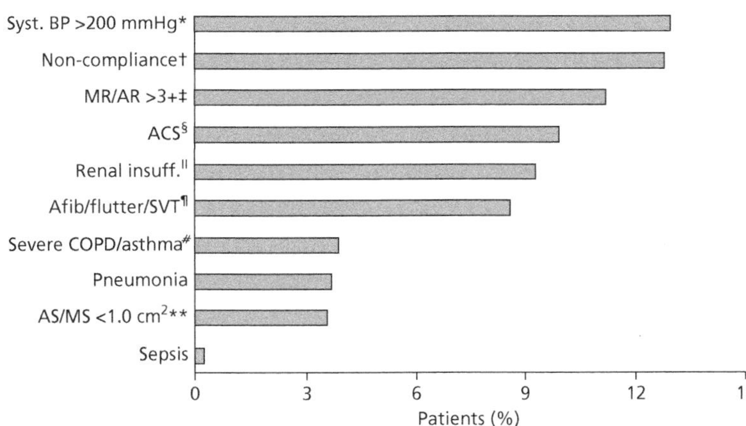

Figure 21.5. *Reasons for clinical decompensation in patients admitted with heart failure with normal ejection fraction. While 53% of patients had an identifiable reason for decompensation, the remainder did not. Cardiovascular or medical conditions and new events precipating hospitalization. Ranked by prevalence (With permission from Klapholz* et al.[5]*)*

*Syst. BP = systolic blood pressure upon presentation (emergency department)
†non-compliance = non-compliance with medication
‡MR/AR = mitral regurgitation/aortic regurgitation (severity scale from 1+ to 4+)
§ACS = acute coronary syndrome
‖baseline dialysis or creatinine >3 mg/dL
¶Afib/Flutter/SVT = atrial fibrillation or atrial flutter/supraventricular tachycardia ≤ 1 week duration or heart rate ≥ 130 bpm
#COPD = chronic obstructive pulmonary disease—severe was defined by pulmonary function tests or by the need for systemic steroid therapy
**AS/MS = aortic stenosis/mitral stenosis

remaining patients, the reason was classified as "an absence of functional reserve."

The initial tests should include an ECG, chest radiograph, complete blood count, electrolyte panel plus blood urea nitrogen (BUN), creatinine and glucose, cardiac enzyme evaluation if ischemic heart disease is suspected, and liver function tests including measurement of serum albumin if edema is extensive. Other specific tests, such as blood cultures depend on the differential diagnosis.

The second step in the evaluation of such a patient should include an imaging test, usually echocardiography. With this, an evaluation of the LVEF and parameters of diastolic filling can be made, in addition to an assessment of LV wall thickness, pericardial abnormalities, myocardial texture, endocardial characteristics, valvular anatomy, pulmonary artery systolic pressure, and right heart characteristics.

Keeping in mind the differential diagnosis of heart failure and with knowledge of the causes of heart failure, including the broad list of items in Table 21.1, a more exact diagnosis of the etiology of heart failure should now be possible. It must be emphasized that the clinical diagnosis of normal or depressed LVEF is prone to error. An imaging procedure is needed to correctly categorize HFNEF as opposed to heart failure with depressed LVEF, as was shown in a study of a consecutive series of patients who underwent radionuclide ventriculography.[23] This showed frequent errors in the clinical categorization of LVEF. While an imaging procedure such as echocardiography is essential, the timing is not crucial. Gandhi *et al.*[24] showed that LVEF and LV wall motion were highly comparable, with only rare exceptions, during the acute phase of admission for hypertensive pulmonary edema and 24 to 72 hours later when their patients were better compensated. This held true for patients with normal EF as well as subnormal EF. Our case study was somewhat exceptional, with an unusually depressed LVEF, probably due to ischemia, whereas subsequently the LVEF was ≥ 40%.

There has been considerable interest in using BNP for the diagnosis and follow-up evaluation of patients with possible or proven heart failure. This appears to be a useful test for the emergency department diagnosis of heart failure versus other conditions causing dyspnea,[25] but it should be noted that there is a marked overlap of values between heart failure with systolic dysfunction and HFNEF. Thus, this test will not be a useful discriminator for the type of heart failure. Further, while there is a highly significant statistical difference between decompensated heart failure and dyspnea due to noncardiac causes in patients with coexistent LV dysfunction, there is considerable overlap between these values, plus modest overlap with patients thought to have no congestive heart failure after further study.[26] The BNP level may be a good indicator of overall cardiac dysfunction, rather than of a specific condition. A recent study showed, by multivariate analysis, that diastolic dysfunction, LVEF, RVEF, mitral regurgitation, severity, age, and creatinine clearance were independent predictors of BNP levels, and that a combination of these factors provided the best fit for correlation to the BNP level.[27] The serial evaluation of BNP was useful in the chronic follow-up and the estimation of prognosis in heart failure patients with systolic dysfunction,[28] but at present there are no published prospective studies of patients with HFNEF.

Treatment

Much of the treatment of HFNEF is based on extrapolation from the treatment of patients with LV dilation and systolic dysfunction or the treatment of conditions such as hypertension or ischemic heart disease without heart failure. Acute treatment should be based on the basic principles of ventricular function, with acute modification of preload, afterload, heart rate, and rhythm. Positive inotropic drugs to stimulate contractility should be avoided.

Reducing preload

With heart failure due to LV pressure–volume overload, and a presumed elevation of the left ventricular end-diastolic pressure (LVEDP), an acute reduction in ventricular diastolic volume, thence pressure, is indicated. Diuretics and possibly morphine sulfate should be given intravenously for acute pulmonary edema. In addition to an eventual decrease in blood volume and filling pressure, there is a more immediate, slight venodilating effect[29,30] and a decrease in pulmonary blood volume.[29] The secondary effect of reducing the circulating blood volume is enhanced activation of the renin-angiotensin-aldosterone system, but the overall effect is beneficial.

It is especially useful to employ sublingual or intravenous nitroglycerin for its acute, reversible venodilating effects. This, with a sitting or inclined posture, will very promptly reduce end-diastolic volume, modestly reduce the systemic arterial pressure, and thus likely reduce myocardial oxygen demand, while improving subendocardial perfusion as the transmural LV gradient for coronary blood flow improves. In a study of patients with excess arterial stiffness, intravenous nitroglycerin especially improved arterial compliance and stroke volume, whereas in normal subjects there was more of a preload effect.[31] In patients with coronary artery disease, venodilation is also thought to reduce LV end-diastolic volume and pressure by reducing RV volume, leading to reduced ventricular interaction.[32] Other acute benefits from nitroglycerin include reduction in the LVEDP, as seen following the intracoronary injection of nitroglycerin or sodium nitroprusside, without systemic effects.[33] These studies were performed in patients with aortic stenosis and LVH. The long-term effects of systemic nitrate administration on ventricular performance are not known. There are potential beneficial short-term[34] and long-term effects of nitrates in dilated cardiomyopathy,[35] possibly mediated by endothelial and neuronal nitric oxide synthases (NOS),[36] but they may be counteracted by the cytotoxic effects of inducible NOS in heart failure.[37] There appear to be no data specifically applicable to HFNEF. Thus, there may be controversy about long-term benefits versus toxicity, but the short-term effects are very useful.

Reducing preload with nesiritide

Infusion of nesiritide causes profound natriuresis and reduces intracardiac filling pressures. Also, there is also a decrease in serum aldosterone, catecholamines, and endothelin-1 levels, without reducing the serum potassium or renal function.[38] There is little published experience in patients with HFNEF.

Reducing afterload with antihypertensive therapy

Normalizing the blood pressure is very important since hypertension is a common cause of HFNEF exacerbations. It is especially useful to keep in mind the concept of vascular-ventricular interaction, and that reducing the systemic arterial pressure should produce a prompt, marked hemodynamic benefit. The initial goal might be to reduce the blood pressure to 140/70 mm Hg, and lower if tolerated. The initial blood pressure was 200/100 mm Hg in a group of patients with HFNEF and pulmonary edema studied at Wake Forest University Baptist Medical Center.[24] All patients in this group were treated with furosemide and nitrates, and by 1 to 3 days later, at the time of follow-up echocardiography, the mean blood pressure was 139/64 mm Hg. At that time, most patients were receiving beta-adrenergic blocking drugs (58%) and angiotensin converting-enzyme inhibitors (76%), with 29% receiving calcium-channel blocking drugs. While nitrates, furosemide, and oxygen are excellent initial therapy, it will be necessary to initiate these additional drug classes for producing long-term effects. In addition, one must consider the responses to therapy, such that, if the blood pressure is not in excellent control in a short timeframe, such as 30 minutes after presentation in pulmonary edema, additional, fast-acting antihypertensive drugs should be given. Depending on the severity of the problem, intravenous sodium nitroprusside or labetalol might be considered. If less urgent, oral clonidine or sustained-release nifedipine might be considered, expecting that the blood pressure will come into the desired range within a short time. Obviously, if the clinical situation warrants, endotracheal intubation and ventilation may be needed to reduce the work of breathing.

Improving heart rate and rhythm

As noted above, supraventricular tachyarrhythmias are a common cause of decompensation requiring hospitalization. An ECG should lead to a correct diagnosis promptly. For atrioventricular (AV) nodal re-entrant tachycardia, intravenous adenosine should block the circus rhythm and stop the arrhythmia. For atrial tachyarrhythmias, such as atrial flutter, atrial fibrillation, or ectopic atrial tachycardia, it is important to slow AV conduction to the physiologic range. For this, intravenous diltiazem or a beta-adrenergic blocking drug should decrease AV conduction. While there are potentially deleterious short-term effects of these drugs on contractility in patients with dilated ventricles with reduced EF, this should not be an issue in HFNEF. With a reduction in intracardiac pressure, one predisposing factor should resolve. Further decisions about synchronized cardioversion, a long-term strategy of AV block, anticoagulation, or chronic antiarrhythmic therapy are the next steps toward successful rate or rhythm improvement. These will be affected by the underlying cardiopulmonary pathology and prognosis.

Improving vascular-ventricular interaction

There are no large clinical studies showing improved outcomes in HFNEF with calcium-channel blocking drugs such as verapamil. However, several lines of investigation have shown modest benefit from improving ventricular filling, reducing systemic arterial pressure, improving arterial compliance, and treating angina. Slower heart rates allow improved calcium re-uptake in the sarcoplasmic reticulum.[12,13,39] This effect should be expected to improve ventricular filling characteristics, and this has been demonstrated in patients with hypertrophic obstructive cardiomyopathy.[40] In addition, these investigators demonstrated improved exercise capacity in patients who showed improved LV filling. In healthy elderly subjects, verapamil reduced vascular and ventricular stiffness and improved exercise capacity.[41] Verapamil also has beneficial effects in angina, related to reducing the rate-pressure product. Finally, there may be less ST-segment depression at a given rate-pressure product, which has been interpreted as showing an improvement in subendocardial perfusion.[42]

Reducing myocardial ischemia and improving myocardial metabolism with beta-adrenergic blocking drugs

Using this class of drugs in patients with angina produces clear antiischemic effects. Slowing the heart rate reduces myocardial oxygen demand. In patients with coronary artery disease, atrial tachypacing can cause ischemia, with a sharp increase in LV diastolic pressure.[43] Therefore, reducing the heart rate with beta-adrenergic blocking drugs should reduce ischemia, reduce the LVEDP, and benefit LV filling. The benefits of slowing AV conduction in supraventricular tachycardia were discussed previously. There are further benefits at the molecular level from chronic treatment with beta-adrenergic blocking drugs in heart failure. These data come from studies in patients with dilated ventricles with reduced LVEF, rather than in HFNEF. In such excised hearts, LV volume was less than in patients not previously treated with beta-blocking drugs.[44] Further, trabeculae from these hearts showed improved contractility, and this was associated with improved function of calcium-release channels. This improvement in systolic function would be expected to improve diastolic calcium reuptake; and therefore, an improvement in diastolic performance, also. In other studies with metoprolol and carvedilol, Lowes *et al.* showed an improvement in the proteins associated with calcium reuptake and reduced the pulmonary capillary wedge pressure (PCWP). This change in pressure was likely due to improved ventricular compliance.[45]

Reducing ischemia in unstable coronary syndromes by medical treatment and cardiac surgery

Patients with HFNEF may rarely present with pulmonary edema due to severe myocardial ischemia or acute myocardial infarction (AMI). Many of the steps noted previously are part of the standard treatment of ischemia, but it is important to recognize myocardial ischemia with severe, rare complications such as transient papillary muscle dysfunction causing flash pulmonary edema. For ischemia, percutaneous revascularization or coronary bypass surgery may be needed. Other complications may also occur, including an infarct-related ventricular septal defect with persistent severe mitral regurgitation due to papillary muscle necrosis and possibly a flail mitral valve leaflet. Cardiac catheterization and prompt surgical intervention is indicated for the latter two conditions.[46,47]

Improving blood pressure and reducing cardiovascular events with angiotensin converting-enzyme inhibitors and angiotensin receptor-blocking drugs

Patients with atherosclerotic cardiovascular disease and diabetes with an additional risk factor (hypertension, elevated total cholesterol, reduced high density lipoprotein, cigarette smoking, or microalbuminuria) have all been shown to benefit from treatment with angiotensin-converting enzyme (ACE) inhibitors by having reduced rates of death, MI, and development of heart failure.[48] While this study of ramipril specifically excluded patients with heart failure, we may speculate without data that the same benefits apply to patients with HFNEF, many of whom belong in these disease categories. The recently published LIFE study compared treatment with the angiotensin receptor blocker (ARB), losartan, to atenolol in patients with hypertension and LVH. These investigators found similar reductions in blood pressure (by approximately 30/17 mm Hg) in both groups, but losartan caused a reduction in the combined endpoint of death, MI, or stroke because of a reduction in stroke rate.[49] Losartan treatment was also associated with a greater reduction in LVH by ECG criteria than was atenolol. Patients with heart failure were specifically excluded from this study, also.

The CHARM-Preserved trial is the only study to date to specifically assess treatment in HFNEF, using the ARB candesartan.[50] Qualifying patients had New York Heart Association (NYHA) class II to IV heart failure and LVEF ≥ 40%. Treatment with candesartan as compared to placebo was associated with a borderline-significant reduction in the combined endpoint of death or adjudicated rehospitalization, and confirmed by a reduction in total investigator-reported hospitalizations for heart failure. The death rate did not differ between the groups. CHARM studied patients with HFNEF of at least 4 weeks duration and a prior admission for heart failure. However, it is likely that beginning such therapy in the hospital setting is reasonable and would achieve similar results.

Avoiding positive inotropic drugs

A recent retrospective analysis of the ADHERE™ study (Acute Decompensated Heart Failure National Registry) disclosed that 10% of 47 000 patients were treated with positive inotropic drugs, and 15% (782) of these had preserved systolic function. Among the latter, in-hospital mortality was 19%, and this was significantly greater than patients with HFNEF not treated with positive inotropic drugs (2%) or patients with depressed systolic function treated with positive inotropic drugs (14%).[51] Apparently, this treatment occurred before an evaluation of LV function could be made. The investigators concluded that the use of positive inotropic drugs may be associated with adverse outcomes. The mechanisms leading to excess mortality were not stated, but the results argue for a relatively prompt echocardiographic evaluation if positive inotropic drugs are contemplated.

Potential complications in treating heart failure with normal ejection fraction

The importance of reducing LV preload and afterload have been emphasized. One must keep in mind the potential for extreme effects of such therapy, especially in patients with very stiff ventricles (reduced compliance), as may occur with severe degrees of LVH. By aggressive preload reduction, a noncompliant LV might become underfilled, leading to hypotension, reduced coronary perfusion, subendocardial ischemia, cerebral and renal hypoperfusion, with attendant complications. The only way to avoid such possible complications is for the physician to pay close attention serially to the results of each treatment. A plan for improving each situation should be kept in mind. For instance, stopping intravenous nitroglycerin or sodium nitroprusside, plus elevating the legs to improve LV preload should bring a prompt improvement as the drug effects resolve.

After the first hours of acute treatment, it is important to monitor the clinical progress of patients to avoid complications of overdiuresis or overtreatment with potent drugs. Thus, one should evaluate patients by determining daily weight and blood pressure, including an examination for orthostatic changes, heart rate and rhythm, serial examination of the jugular venous pressure, cardiac findings, such as a change in gallop rhythm, and laboratory investigation for pre-renal azotemia and hypokalemia. As time goes by, treating and assessing patients in the sitting position, rather than supine, are important here, as well as for all types of heart failure when hypotension is a possible result of treatment.

Importance of a correct diagnosis

In a condition such as HFNEF, which includes a wide variety of disorders, it is of maximal importance to make a clear diagnosis. There are numerous confounding conditions that may mimic HFNEF, including pulmonary disease, anemia, obesity, liver failure, renal failure, nephrotic syndrome, venous insufficiency, thyroid dysfunction, and drug-induced fluid retention due to calcium-channel blocking drugs, nonsteroidal anti-inflammatory drugs, and thiazolidinediones.[52] In addition, after excluding confounders, it is very important to clarify the type of HFNEF. Most of the previously described recommendations were made for hypothetical patients with myocardial problems, such as hypertensive-hypertrophic cardiomyopathy, and one must obviously have the correct clinical diagnosis in order to treat each patient knowledgeably. For instance, aggressive treatment with diuretics and nitrates could produce marked hypotension for a patient with pericardial tamponade or constriction. A patient with hypertrophic cardiomyopathy when over-diuresed might become hypotensive, and further treatment with positive inotropic drugs could add to the problem. Similarly, severe aortic stenosis, mitral stenosis, or infective endocarditis would all require different approaches. Thus, relatively prompt echocardiography is be an essential factor in ensuring correct treatment.

Other pitfalls

Disorders may frequently coexist. For instance, primary pulmonary hypertension might, by ventricular interaction, increase LV stiffness, raising the LV diastolic pressure. A recent patient in our institution had marked signs of right heart failure. At catheterization, the pulmonary artery pressure was 97/50 mm Hg, and the PCWP was surprisingly 28 mm Hg, in the absence of LVH or other causes of increased left-sided pressure. Following further diuresis, the pulmonary artery pressure declined to 84/47 mm Hg, and the wedge pressure declined to 14 mm Hg, without systemic hypotension or pre-renal azotemia. The findings were interpreted as being due to ventricular interaction in a patient with primary pulmonary hypertension.

Conclusion

There is little information about the treatment of AHF in HFNEF. The main principles include making an accurate diagnosis of the actual underlying disorder, understanding the precipitating cause of the acute decompensation, and using the principles of ventricular function to treat HFNEF optimally. Many of the same principles and drugs employed to treat heart failure with reduced EF will be applicable to HFNEF, but the more normal contractile state will allow the easier use of drugs with negative inotropic effects, and the avoidance of positive inotropic drugs.

References

1. Philbin EF, Rocco TA Jr., Lindenmuth NW, Ulrich K, Jenkins PL. Systolic versus diastolic heart failure in community practice: clinical features, outcomes, and the use of angiotensin-converting enzyme inhibitors. Am J Med 2000; 109: 605–613.
2. Vasan RS, Benjamin EJ, Levy D. Prevalence, clinical features and prognosis of diastolic heart failure: an epidemiologic perspective. J Am Coll Cardiol 1995; 26: 1565–1574.
3. Smith GL, Masoudi FA, Vaccarino V, Radford MJ, Krumholz HM. Outcomes in heart failure patients with preserved ejection fraction: mortality, readmission, and functional decline. J Am Coll Cardiol 2003; 41: 1510–1518.
4. Vasan RS, Larson MG, Benjamin EJ, *et al.* Congestive heart failure in subjects with normal versus reduced left ventricular ejection fraction: prevalence and mortality in a population based cohort. J Am Coll Cardiol 1999; 33: 1948–1955.
5. Klapholz M, Maurer M, Lowe AM, *et al.*, New York Heart Failure Consortium. Hospitalization for heart failure in the presence of a normal left ventricular ejection fraction: results of the New York Heart Failure Registry. J Am Coll Cardiol 2004; 43: 1432–1438.

6. Redfield MM, Jacobsen SJ, Burnett JC Jr., *et al.* Burden of systolic and diastolic ventricular dysfunction in the community: appreciating the scope of the heart failure epidemic. JAMA 2003; 289: 194–202.
7. Senni M, Tribouilloy CM, Rodeheffer RJ, *et al.* Congestive heart failure in the community: a study of all incident cases in Olmsted County, Minnesota, in 1991. Circulation 1998; 98: 2282–2289.
8. Chen HH, Lainchbury JG, Senni M, Bailey KR, Redfield MM. Diastolic heart failure in the community: clinical profile, natural history, therapy, and impact of proposed diagnostic criteria. J Card Fail 2002; 8: 279–287.
9. McDermott MM, Feinglass J, Lee PI, *et al.* Systolic function, readmission rates, and survival among consecutively hospitalized patients with congestive heart failure. Am Heart J 1997; 134: 728–736.
10. Pearlman ES, Weber, Janicki JS, Pietra GG, Fishman AP. Muscle fiber orientation and connective tissue content in the hypertrophied human heart. Lab Invest 1982; 46: 158–164.
11. Huysman JA, Vliegen HW, Van der Laarse A, Eulderink F. Changes in nonmyocyte tissue composition associated with pressure overload of hypertrophic human hearts. Pathol Res Practice 1989; 184: 577–581.
12. Gwathmey JK, Copelas L, MacKinnon R, *et al.* Abnormal intracellular calcium handling in myocardium from patients with end-stage heart failure. Circ Res 1987; 61: 70–76.
13. Gwathmey JK, Warren SE, Briggs GM, *et al.* Diastolic dysfunction in hypertrophic cardiomyopathy. Effect on active force generation during systole. J Clin Invest 1991; 87: 1023–1031.
14. Liu CP, Ting CT, Lawrence W, *et al.* Diminished contractile response to increased heart rate in intact human left ventricular hypertrophy. Systolic versus diastolic determinants. Circulation 1993; 88: 1893–1906.
15. Zile MR, Brutsaert DL. New concepts in diastolic dysfunction and diastolic heart failure: Part II: causal mechanisms and treatment. Circulation 2002; 105: 1503–1508.
16. Zile MR. Heart failure with preserved ejection fraction: is this diastolic heart failure? J Am Coll Cardiol 2003; 41: 1519–1522.
17. Kitzman DW, Little WC, Brubaker PH, *et al.* Pathophysiological characterization of isolated diastolic heart failure in comparison to systolic heart failure. JAMA 2002; 288: 2144–2150.
18. Zile MR, Gaasch WH, Carroll JD, *et al.* Heart failure with a normal ejection fraction: is measurement of diastolic function necessary to make the diagnosis of diastolic heart failure? Circulation 2001; 104: 779–782.
19. Zile MR, Baicu CF, Gaasch WH. Diastolic heart failure—abnormalities in active relaxation and passive stiffness of the left ventricle. N Engl J Med 2004; 350: 1953–1959.
20. Kawaguchi M, Hay I, Fetics B, Kass DA. Combined ventricular systolic and arterial stiffening in patients with heart failure and preserved ejection fraction: implications for systolic and diastolic reserve limitations. Circulation 2003; 107: 714–720.
21. Hundley WG, Kitzman DW, Morgan TM, *et al.* Cardiac cycle-dependent changes in aortic area and distensibility are reduced in older patients with isolated diastolic heart failure and correlate with exercise intolerance. J Am Coll Cardiol 2001; 38: 796–802.
22. Burkhoff D, Maurer MS, Packer M. Heart failure with a normal ejection fraction: is it really a disorder of diastolic function? Circulation 2003; 107: 656–658.
23. Marantz PR, Tobin JN, Wassertheil-Smoller S, *et al.* The relationship between left ventricular systolic function and congestive heart failure diagnosed by clinical criteria. Circulation 1988; 77: 607–612.
24. Gandhi SK, Powers JC, Nomeir AM, *et al.* The pathogenesis of acute pulmonary edema associated with hypertension. N Engl J Med 2001; 344: 17–22.
25. Maisel AS, McCord J, Nowak RM, *et al.*, Breathing Not Properly Multinational Study Investigators. Bedside B-Type natriuretic peptide in the emergency diagnosis of heart failure with reduced or preserved ejection fraction, results from the Breathing Not Properly Multinational Study. J Am Coll Cardiol 2003; 41: 2010–2017.
26. Maisel AS, Krishnaswamy P, Nowak RM, *et al.*, Breathing Not Properly Multinational Study Investigators. Rapid measurement of B-type natriuretic peptide in the emergency diagnosis of heart failure. N Engl J Med 2002; 347: 161–167.
27. Troughton RW, Prior DL, Pereira JJ, *et al.* Plasma B-type natriuretic peptide levels in systolic heart failure: importance of left ventricular diastolic function and right ventricular systolic function. J Am Coll Cardiol 2004; 43: 416–422.
28. Maeda K, Tsutamoto T, Wada A, *et al.* High levels of plasma brain natriuretic peptide and interleukin-6 after optimized treatment for heart failure are independent risk factors for morbidity and mortality in patients with congestive heart failure. J Am Coll Cardiol 2000; 36: 1587–1593.
29. Biddle TL, Yu PN. Effect of furosemide on hemodynamics and lung water in acute pulmonary edema secondary to myocardial infarction. Am J Cardiol 1979; 43: 86–90.

30. Jhund PS, Davie AP, McMurray JJ. Aspirin inhibits the acute venodilator response to furosemide in patients with chronic heart failure. J Am Coll Cardiol 2001; 37: 1234–1238.
31. Haber HL, Simek CL, Bergin JD, *et al.* Bolus intravenous nitroglycerin predominantly reduces afterload in patients with excessive arterial elastance. J Am Coll Cardiol 1993; 22: 251–257.
32. Ludbrook PA, Byrne JD, Kurnik PB, McKnight RC. Influence of reduction of preload and afterload by nitroglycerin on left ventricular diastolic pressure-volume relations and relaxation in man. Circulation 1977; 56: 937–943.
33. Matter CM, Mandinov L, Kaufmann PA, *et al.* Effect of NO donors on LV diastolic function in patients with severe pressure-overload hypertrophy. Circulation 1999; 99: 2396–2401.
34. Gray R, Chatterjee K, Vyden JK, *et al.* Hemodynamic and metabolic effects of isosorbide dinitrate in chronic congestive heart failure. Am Heart J 1975; 90: 346–352.
35. Elkayam U, Johnson JV, Shotan A, *et al.* Double-blind, placebo-controlled study to evaluate the effect of organic nitrates in patients with chronic heart failure treated with angiotensin-converting enzyme inhibition. Circulation 1999; 99: 2652–2657.
36. Heymes C, Vanderheyden M, Bronzwaer JG, Shah AM, Paulus WJ. Endomyocardial nitric oxide synthase and left ventricular preload reserve in dilated cardiomyopathy. Circulation 1999; 99: 3009–3016.
37. Drexler H. Nitric oxide synthases in the failing human heart: a doubled-edged sword? Circulation 1999; 99: 2972–2975.
38. Elkayam U, Akhter MW, Tummala P, Khan S, Singh H. Nesiritide: a new drug for the treatment of decompensated heart failure. J Cardiovasc Pharmacol Ther 2002; 7: 181–194.
39. Grossman W. Diastolic dysfunction in congestive heart failure. N Engl J Med 1991; 325: 1557–1564.
40. Bonow RO, Dilsizian V, Rosing DR, *et al.* Verapamil-induced improvement in left ventricular diastolic filling and increased exercise tolerance in patients with hypertrophic cardiomyopathy: short- and long-term effects. Circulation 1985; 72: 853–864.
41. Chen CH, Nakayama M, Talbot M, *et al.* Verapamil acutely reduces ventricular-vascular stiffening and improves aerobic exercise performance in elderly individuals. J Am Coll Cardiol 1999; 33: 1602–1609.
42. Brodsky SJ, Cutler SS, Weiner DA, *et al.* Treatment of stable angina of effort with verapamil: a double-blind, placebo-controlled randomized crossover study. Circulation 1982; 66: 569–574.
43. Aroesty JM, McKay RG, Heller GV, *et al.* Simultaneous assessment of left ventricular systolic and diastolic dysfunction during pacing-induced ischemia. Circulation 1985; 71: 889–900.
44. Reiken S, Wehrens XH, Vest JA, *et al.* Beta-blockers restore calcium release channel function and improve cardiac muscle performance in human heart failure. Circulation 2003; 107: 2459–2466.
45. Lowes BD, Gilbert EM, Abraham WT, *et al.* Myocardial gene expression in dilated cardiomyopathy treated with beta-blocking agents. N Engl J Med 2002; 346: 1357–1365.
46. Kishon Y, Oh JK, Schaff HV, *et al.* Mitral valve operation in postinfarction rupture of a papillary muscle: immediate results and long-term follow-up of 22 patients. Mayo Clin Proc 1992; 67: 1023–1030.
47. David TE. Operative management of postinfarction ventricular septal defect. Semin Thorac Cardiovasc Surg 1995; 7: 208–213.
48. Yusuf S, Sleight P, Pogue J, *et al.* Effects of an angiotensin-converting-enzyme inhibitor, ramipril, on cardiovascular events in high-risk patients. The Heart Outcomes Prevention Evaluation Study Investigators. N Engl J Med 2000; 342: 145–153.
49. Dahlof B, Devereux RB, Kjeldsen SE, *et al.*, LIFE Study Group. Cardiovascular morbidity and mortality in the Losartan Intervention For Endpoint reduction in hypertension study (LIFE): a randomised trial against atenolol. Lancet 2002; 359: 995–1003.
50. Yusuf S, Pfeffer MA, Swedberg K, *et al.* for the CHARM Investigators and Committees. Effects of candesartan in patients with chronic heart failure and preserved left-ventricular ejection fraction: the CHARM-Preserved Trial. Lancet 2003; 362: 777–781.
51. Adams KF Jr., DeMarco T, Berkowitz RL, Chang S for the ADHERE™ Scientific Advisory Committee and Investigators. Inotrope use and negative outcomes in treatment of acute heart failure in patients with preserved systolic function: data from the ADHERE™ database. Circulation 2003; 108: IV-695 (Abstract).
52. Massie BM. Natriuretic peptide measurements for the diagnosis of "nonsystolic" heart failure: good news and bad. J Am Coll Cardiol 2003; 41: 2018–2021.

CHAPTER 22

Inotropes and other new therapies for acute heart failure

G Michael Felker, Mihai Gheorghiade

Introduction

The aging of the population, in combination with improved survival after acute myocardial infarction (AMI), has resulted in a substantial increase in the number of patients living with chronic heart failure.[1] This increase in heart failure prevalence has led to a parallel rise in the number of hospitalizations for acute decompensated heart failure (ADHF), which account for 6.5 million hospital days annually in the United States.[2]

Almost 1 million patients per year are discharged with a diagnosis of heart failure as compared with an estimated 800 000 with AMI, and heart failure is the leading cause of hospital admission in the Medicare population in the United States.[3]

In addition to its high prevalence, hospitalization for decompensated heart failure is associated with extraordinarily high morbidity and mortality. Depending on the population studied, the risk of death or rehospitalization within 60 days after acute heart failure (AHF) hospitalization may be as high as 60%.[4–6]

Finally, hospitalization for AHF is a major determinant of health care costs, with the costs of inpatient care accounting for as much as 75% of the approximately $20 billion spent on heart failure annually in the United States.[7] The rapidly expanding population of patients with ADHF has resulted in a search for new therapies as well as a reexamination of old agents.

In this context, this chapter reviews the current understanding of the role of positive inotropic agents in the management of ADHF.

Goals of Therapy in Acute Heart Failure

Understanding the role of pharmacologic therapies for AHF requires an appreciation of the appropriate goals of therapy for this complex patient population. The term *acute heart failure* broadly defines a heterogeneous patient population—ranging from patients with myocardial ischemia and acute pulmonary edema to those with worsening of volume overload in the setting of chronic heart failure. Importantly, up to 40% of patients with ADHF may have preserved systolic function, which may require unique therapeutic approaches.[8]

Despite this heterogeneity, a few general statements regarding the goals of acute therapy apply to the great majority of patients with this condition. Patients hospitalized with ADHF are typically profoundly symptomatic, with symptoms that may include dyspnea at rest or with minimal exertion, severe fatigue, and peripheral edema.

Unlike chronic heart failure, where the association between central hemodynamics and symptoms is uncertain, symptoms in the setting of AHF exacerbation appear to be closely related to central hemodynamics.[9] Clearly, improvement of acute hemodynamic derangement and accompanying symptom relief is a major goal of AHF therapy. Additionally, however, hospitalization for heart failure portends a substantial future morbidity (primarily rehospitalization for heart failure) and mortality in the 6 months following the index hospitalization. Optimal therapy would, therefore, not only relieve symptoms, facilitate adequate diuresis, and maximize end-organ perfusion, but also limit the length of hospitalization, prevent rehospitalization, improve short-term mortality, and decrease costs.

Individual agents may accomplish some of these goals and not others. For example, loop diuretics are very effective at managing symptoms related to volume overload such as pulmonary congestion and peripheral edema, but do not favorably impact future clinical outcomes. Indeed, available data suggest that diuretic use may be associated with excess mortality.[10] In contrast, glycoprotein IIb/IIIa inhibitors in acute coronary syndromes improve outcomes without impacting short-term symptoms, and thrombolytic therapy for acute ST-elevation MI improves both symptoms and outcomes.

At present, most agents used in AHF management have focused on improvement in symptoms, and therapy that can favorably impact long-term outcomes has remained elusive. Whether a therapy can be developed that will both improve acute symptoms and impact longer-term outcomes in AHF patients remains an open question.

Inotropic Agents in Acute Heart Failure

A decrease in cardiac contractility is the central initiating hemodynamic event in the cycle that leads to the heart failure syndrome. Based on this model, increasing cardiac contractility has long been an attractive therapeutic target in the development of heart failure therapies. Despite the intellectual appeal of increasing cardiac contractility, therapeutic development focusing on this goal has been one of the major disappointments in cardiovascular medicine. Multiple clinical trials in chronic heart failure have consistently demonstrated increased mortality with inotropic agents, suggesting that these agents have no role in chronic heart failure management. A summary of the large placebo controlled trials of oral inotropic therapy in chronic heart failure is shown in Table 22.1.

In contrast to chronic heart failure, hemodynamic considerations may play a larger role in patients with ADHF. Given that much of the symptom complex of AHF is related to perturbations in central hemodynamics, it stands to reason that improvement in the underlying hemodynamic

Table 22.1. *Mortality in trials of chronic inotropic therapy*

Trial	Inotrope	NYHA class	Number of patients	Mortality vs. placebo
PROMISE[18]	Milrinone	III-IV	1088	28% increase in RR of death
VEST[42]	Vesnarinone	III-IV	3833	11% increase in RR of death
Xamoterol[43]	Xamoterol	III-IV	516	HR for death 2.5 (95% CI, 1.04–6.18)
PRIME II[44]	Ibopamine	III-IV	1906	HR for death 1.26 (95% CI, 1.04–1.53)
PICO[45]	Pimobendan	II-III	317	HR for death 1.8 (95% CI, 0.9–3.5)

Abbreviations: CI = confidence interval; HR = hazard ratio; NYHA = New York Heart Association; RR = relative risk, PROMISE=Prospective Randomized Milrinone Survival Evaluation, VEST=Vesnarinone Trial, PRIME II=Second Prospective Randomized Study of Ibopamine on Mortality and Efficacy, PICO=Pimobendan in Congestive Heart Failure.

defect would lead to clinical improvement in AHF. Despite the salutary effects of inotropic agents on acute hemodynamics, their potential risks (such as exacerbation of arrhythmias or myocardial ischemia) remain of substantial concern. Overall, the optimal balance of risks and benefits is uncertain, but the preponderance of data suggest that inotropes are not beneficial to most patients being hospitalized with ADHF.

Despite these concerns, inotropic agents continue to be widely used in the management of AHF. Although the exact reasons for this are unclear, it may be due to the acuity of illness, the intellectual attractiveness of increasing contractility, and the lack of other appealing therapeutic options in this population. At present, two indications for inotropic agents seem appropriate: (1) in the short-term management of ADHF accompanied by end-organ hypoperfusion or cardiogenic shock; and (2) as a "pharmacologic bridge" to definitive therapy such as revascularization or cardiac transplantation.

Mechanisms of action

Understanding the risk/benefit ratio of inotropic therapy in AHF requires an appreciation of the underlying mechanisms, including the potential benefits as well as the potential harm. Currently available inotropic agents increase contractility via a final common pathway of increasing intracellular levels of cyclic adenylate monophosphate (cAMP), resulting in increased contractile force due to increased calcium release from the sarcoplasmic reticulum.[11] Catecholamines (such as dobutamine) increase cAMP production via beta-adrenergic-mediated stimulation of adenylate cyclase, which stimulates cAMP production.[12] Phosphodiesterase (PDE) inhibitors (such as milrinone) selectively inhibit PDE III, the enzyme that catalyzes the breakdown of cAMP. In addition to its inotropic effect in the myocardium, PDE inhibition in vascular smooth muscle cells results in vasodilation. Milrinone is frequently referred to as an "inodilator" with both positive inotropic and vasodilatory effects. A comparison between the hemodynamic effects of milrinone and dobutamine is shown in Table 22.2.

Both dobutamine and milrinone may exacerbate malignant arrhythmias or myocardial ischemia. Dobutamine increases cardiac contractility at the expense of increasing myocardial oxygen demand, although the degree to which this occurs may be offset by improved coronary perfusion.[13] Additionally, adrenergic stimulation appears to have a direct toxic effect on the myocardium, as suggested by the well-proven clinical benefit of beta-blocker therapy.[14–16]

Other agents that increase cAMP levels (such as milrinone and other PDE inhibitors) also appear to precipitate arrhythmias and lead to progression of heart failure when given chronically.[17,18] Packer and colleagues demonstrated that left ventricular (LV) function after withdrawal of the oral inotrope amrinone deteriorated to below pretreatment levels, suggesting that inotropic therapy accelerated the deterioration of LV function.[19] Overall, the mechanism of both dobutamine and milrinone appears to favor short-term hemodynamic benefits at the expense of the acceleration of underlying disease progression.

Intravenous inotropes in acute decompensated heart failure

Intravenous inotropes are frequently used in inpatients with ADHF, although until recently the

Table 22.2. *Comparison of hemodynamic effects of dobutamine and milrinone*

Inotropic agent	CO	HR	MAP	SVR	PVR	MVO_2
Dobutamine	↑	↑	↔	↓	↓	↔↑
Milrinone	↑	↔↑	↓	↓↓	↓↓	↔

Abbreviations: CO = cardiac output; HR = heart rate; MAP = mean arterial pressure; MVO_2 = myocardial oxygen consumption; PVR = pulmonary vascular resistance; SVR = systemic vascular resistance; ↑ = increases; ↓ = decreases; ↔ = no change.

usefulness and safety of this approach had not been carefully evaluated in clinical trials. Proposed benefits of this approach include restoring perfusion to end-organs and thereby facilitating adequate diuresis, shortening the length of hospitalization, and allowing up-titration of chronic therapies such as angiotensin-converting enzyme (ACE) inhibitors. Retrospective data have been mixed, with some small studies suggesting clinical benefit.[20,21] In contrast, retrospective data from the Flolan International Randomized Survival Trial (FIRST) of epoprostenol suggested that the use of intravenous dobutamine in patients with ADHF was associated with adverse outcomes.[22]

In order to prospectively evaluate the role of inotropes in this population, the Outcomes of a Prospective Trial of Intravenous Milrinone for Exacerbations of Chronic Heart Failure (OPTIME-CHF) study was designed as the first randomized trial to assess the utility of an intravenous inotrope (milrinone) in patients admitted with ADHF.[23] This study randomized 951 patients, who were not felt to require inotropic support, to a 48- to 72-hour infusion of intravenous milrinone or placebo, with a primary endpoint of days hospitalized for cardiovascular causes or dead within 60 days of randomization. Important secondary endpoints were mortality, treatment failure, adverse events, ability to achieve target dose of ACE inhibitors, and quality of life. This study showed no benefit in the primary endpoint from treatment with milrinone (6 days vs. 7 days for placebo, $P = 0.71$). Other important secondary endpoints such as the composite of death or rehospitalization at 60 days, 60-day mortality, achieving target dosing of ACE inhibitors, and quality of life measurements were also neutral. Selected results from the OPTIME-CHF study are shown in Table 22.3. Randomization to milrinone therapy was associated with significantly more hypotension and arrhythmias than treatment with placebo. The results of OPTIME-CHF suggest that most patients with heart failure decompensation do not benefit from the routine addition of milrinone to standard medical care. Although decreasing the duration of hospitalization, and therefore costs, is a frequently suggested benefit of acute inotropic therapy, this was not borne out by the OPTIME-CHF results. Interpretation of the results from OPTIME-CHF requires careful notice of the population studied, in that patients felt by the treating physician to have a requirement for inotropic therapy were excluded from the study.

Such "inotrope requiring" patients are difficult to define, but usually include those with refractory hypotension in the setting of volume overload or end-organ impairment (primarily renal) due to hypoperfusion. Unfortunately, the dividing line between these "inotrope requiring" patients and the OPTIME-CHF population is difficult to define with precision, and physician judgment rather than randomized data will continue to play a large role in selecting patients with ADHF for inotropic therapy.

Subsequent analysis of the data from OPTIME-CHF has suggested the possibility that subgroups of patients could derive benefit from inotropic therapy, specifically patients with nonischemic cardiomyopathy.[24] Although the explanation for this

Table 22.3. *Results from the OPTIME-CHF study*

Primary or secondary endpoint	Milrinone (n = 477)	Placebo (n = 472)	*P*-value
Primary endpoint (days of cardiovascular hospitalization within 60 days)	12.3	12.5	0.71
60-day mortality	10.3%	8.9%	0.41
Death + rehospitalization at 60 days	35%	35%	0.92

Abbreviations: OPTIME-CHF = Outcomes of a Prospective Trial of Intravenous Milrinone for Exacerbations of Chronic Heart Failure.

difference based on heart failure etiology is uncertain, it may relate to less arrhythmogenesis from milrinone in the nonischemic cohort. Given the retrospective nature of this analysis, such data must be interpreted with caution. Given the risks of chronic inotropic therapy and the results of OPTIME-CHF, it is appropriate to limit the use of inotropic agents to AHF patients manifesting severe end-organ perfusion or shock who appear unlikely to be stabilized with standard medical therapy alone.

Intravenous inotropes: bridging to transplant or recovery

For patients with refractory heart failure who are candidates for cardiac transplantation, intravenous inotropes have been successfully used as a bridge to transplantation. In patients with treatable or reversible causes of AHF (such as stunned or hibernating myocardium after MI) who are refractory to conventional therapy, short-term use of intravenous inotropes is an appropriate bridge to definitive therapy (revascularization) or recovery. Given the history of chronic inotropic therapy in heart failure, questions remain about the safety and efficacy of longer-term inotropic use as a bridge to transplantation. Depending on blood type and body size, substantial in-hospital waiting time for cardiac transplant may occur, exposing patients to the risks of long-term inotropic use.

Despite these concerns, the use of intravenous inotropes to maintain clinical stability in hospitalized patients awaiting cardiac transplant remains a frequent indication in transplant centers around the world. In a highly-monitored inpatient setting, bridging to definitive therapy can usually be undertaken with a low risk of adverse events.[25,26] Patients with advanced heart failure awaiting cardiac transplantation who cannot be supported with inotropic therapy alone are considered for mechanical support with an intraaortic balloon pump or left ventricular assist device (LVAD).

As device technology improves, earlier use of mechanical assistance may become increasingly common in advanced heart failure patients awaiting transplantation. Mechanical support devices provide more complete circulatory support than inotropes, improving end-organ perfusion and functional status.[27] Additionally, the use of mechanical assist devices eliminates the risk associated with long-term inotrope use, albeit while introducing the risks associated with device implantation and maintenance. Some retrospective data does suggest that long-term post transplant outcomes are superior in patients who were bridged with LVAD rather than inotropic therapy.[28] At present, no satisfactory data exist to guide the choice of bridging strategies. In patients with expected prolonged waiting times, or those without sufficient clinical stability on inotropes alone, early LVAD implantation seems likely to become an increasingly favored option.

The Choice of Inotrope in Acute Heart Failure

If inotropic therapy is to be used in AHF, the best choice of inotropic agent remains uncertain. Both dobutamine and milrinone are frequently used for both treatment of acute exacerbations as well as pharmacologic bridging, but no randomized trials of significant power have been performed comparing the two agents for either indication. Retrospective data addressing this issue is mixed. In decompensated heart failure, data from the Cleveland Clinic Foundation suggest that dobutamine may be as efficacious as milrinone at a much lower cost.[29]

For bridging to cardiac transplantation, the choice of inotropic agent varies widely between centers, primarily based on physician preference. Nonrandomized data suggest that milrinone appears to be associated with a more stable clinical course and better outcomes that dobutamine.[25,26] A recent small randomized trial found no difference in clinical outcomes between bridging with dobutamine or milrinone, but the sample size was too small to rule out small to moderate differences in efficacy between the two agents.[30]

Concomitant Inotrope and Beta-blocker Therapy

Greater numbers of patients with ADHF are receiving chronic beta-blocker therapy, a fact that impacts the choice of inotropic therapy. Although high doses of beta-adrenergic agonists such as dobutamine may competitively overcome the effect of beta-blockers, this usually requires doses of dobutamine (15 to 20 mcg/kg/min) that result in substantial heart rate increases and increased myocardial oxygen demand. Because they work via a beta-adrenergic-independent mechanism, the effect of PDE inhibitors such as milrinone is not attenuated by beta-blockers, suggesting that milrinone may be more effective than dobutamine in the setting of beta-blocker therapy.[12] Indeed, some data suggest that the favorable hemodynamic response to milrinone may be accentuated by treatment with beta-blockade.[31,32] Intravenous milrinone therefore may be preferred in patients with acute decompensation who require inotropic support in the setting of chronic beta-blocker therapy.

New Inotropic Agents: Levosimendan

Several novel inotropic agents continue to be developed and studied. Levosimendan, an intravenous PDE inhibitor with significant calcium-sensitizing properties, is a promising agent that is currently being evaluated in advanced heart failure. Levosimendan acts through a calcium-dependent interaction with troponin C to increase sensitivity to intracellular calcium. Calcium sensitization may theoretically increase inotropy without the increase in myocardial oxygen demand or potential for arrhythmogenesis than is seen with other inotropic agents. Additionally, at pharmacologic doses levosimendan does not appear to have significant PDE inhibition.[33] Infusion of levosimendan results in hemodynamic effects similar to milrinone, including an increase in cardiac output and a decrease in pulmonary artery pressure and wedge pressure.[34]

Two large clinical trials of levosimendan have recently been published. In the Levosimendan Infusion versus Dobutamine (LIDO) trial, levosimendan demonstrated improved hemodynamics and lower mortality compared to dobutamine in patients with severe low output heart failure (Figure 22.1).[35] Additionally, in contrast to dobutamine, the hemodynamic effects of levosimendan were not attenuated by beta-blocker therapy (Figure 22.2). In the Randomized Study on Safety and Effectiveness of Levosimendan in Patients with Left Ventricular Failure after an Acute Myocardial Infarct (RUSSLAN) trial, low-dose levosimendan was shown to reduce mortality and worsening heart failure without an increase in hypotension or myocardial ischemia in patients with AHF and MI.[36] Despite these promising early results, more definitive studies will be needed before levosimendan can be considered a standard therapy for patients with severe AHF. Because the LIDO study did not have a placebo control, it is impossible to

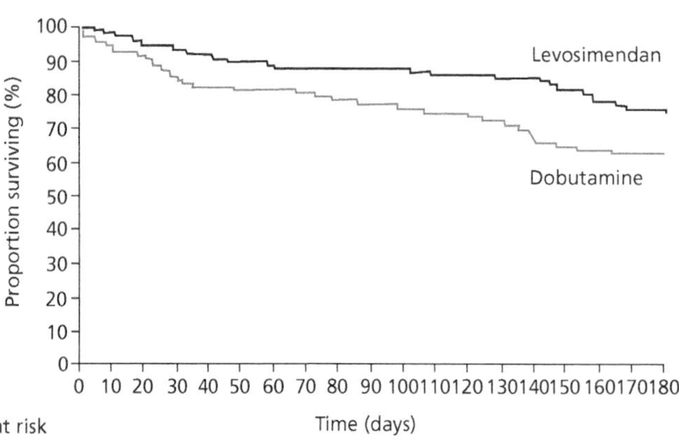

Figure 22.1. *Kaplan-Meier estimates (analysis of time to first event) of risk of death during first 180 days after randomization (based on the intention-to-treat analysis) (With permission from Follath* et al.[35])

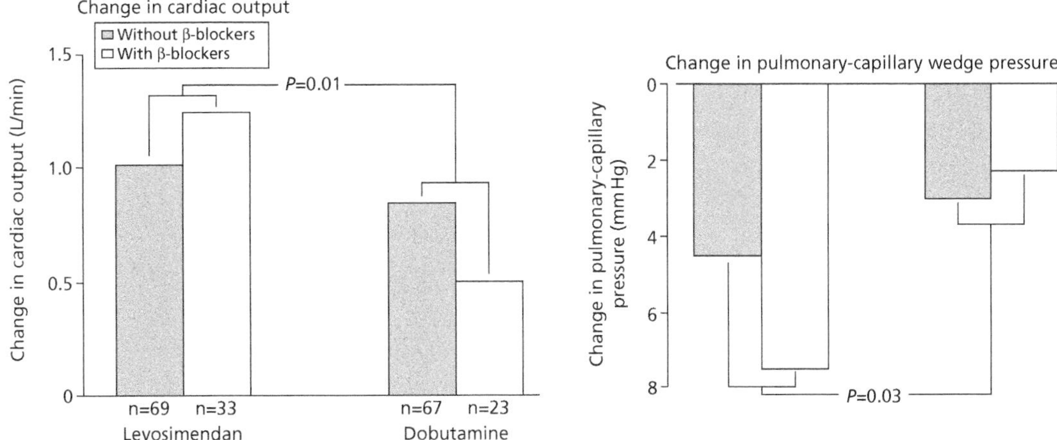

Figure 22.2. *Effect of concomitant beta-blockade on cardiac output and pulmonary capillary wedge pressure. Interaction test P-values based on ANCOVA with effects for treatment, subgroup, treatment group interaction, and baseline value as covariate (With permission from Follath* et al.[35])

determine whether the observed differences represented improved outcomes with levosimendan or simply the adverse effects of dobutamine therapy. A phase III clinical trial of levosimendan in decompensated heart failure, the Randomized Multicenter Evaluation of Intravenous Levosimendan Efficacy vs. Placebo in the Short-term Treatment of Acute Heart Failure (REVIVE) study, is currently ongoing and will provide an important comparison of levosimendan to placebo.

Inotropes as a Destination Therapy

Despite improvements in heart failure therapy, some patients remain highly symptomatic and severely debilitated by heart failure. In such patients, who are not candidates for revascularization, cardiac transplant, or other definitive therapy, chronic inotropic therapy is sometimes considered as a palliative intervention. The rationale, risks, and benefits of such an approach have been recently reviewed in detail.[37] Some anecdotal reports and small studies have suggested that in patients with refractory heart failure either chronic or intermittent inotrope infusions may result in decreased symptom severity and hospitalizations, with subsequent improvement in quality of life.[21,38] Other studies in a similar population have shown trends towards increased mortality with no effect on symptoms.[39] Clearly, some patients may be willing to "trade off" length of life for quality of life, but such issues are notoriously difficult to quantify (i.e., how much life for how much symptomatic relief?). A study by Stanek *et al.* found that patients with severe heart failure were generally more interested in symptomatic improvement than increased survival.[40] Given the significant limitations of the available data, such a course of therapy must be undertaken with a clear understanding by both patient and physician that such therapy is palliative, and may increase short-term mortality. In light of the substantial suffering of patients with truly refractory heart failure, however, the appropriate use of palliative therapies, including chronic inotropes, should be given careful consideration after informed discussion of the potential risks and benefits of such an approach.

Conclusion

ADHF is a clinical syndrome of substantial morbidity and rapidly increasing prevalence. Despite this fact, therapeutic development for this syndrome has lagged behind that of other comparable disorders. Short-term inotropic therapy may be indicated in selected patients with end-organ hypoperfusion or hypotension. Notably, available data from the ADHERE™ registry suggest that such patients represent a low percentage of the ADHF population, with only 2% of ADHF patients presenting with a systolic blood pressure < 90 mm Hg.[41] Data from the OPTIME study suggest that inotropic therapy is unlikely to be helpful in patients whose primary manifestation of heart failure is volume overload, and may be particularly harmful in the setting of ischemic heart disease.[24] Longer-term inotropes may be required in order to bridge patients to more definitive treatment such as revascularization or cardiac transplantation. Of the currently available agents, data suggest that dobutamine and milrinone are similar in terms of efficacy. Newer agents such as levosimendan are in development that may provide some of the benefits of current therapies without the associated risks. Given data on chronic inotropic therapy and increased mortality, the use of inotropes for any indication must be undertaken with careful consideration of the potential risks and benefits.

References

1. Bonneux L, Barendregt JJ, Meeter K, Bonsel GJ, van der Maas PJ. Estimating clinical morbidity due to ischemic heart disease and congestive heart failure: the future rise of heart failure. Am J Public Health 1994; 84: 20–28.
2. Ghali JK, Cooper R, Ford E. Trends in hospitalization rates for heart failure in the United States, 1973–1986. Evidence for increasing population prevalence. Arch Intern Med 1990; 150: 769–773.
3. American Heart Association. Heart Disease and Stroke Statistics—2001 Update (American Heart Association: Dallas, TX, 2000).
4. Krumholz HM, Parent EM, Tu N, *et al.* Readmission after hospitalization for congestive heart failure among medicare beneficiaries. Arch Intern Med 1997; 157: 99–104.
5. Rich MW, Beckham V, Wittenberg C, *et al.* A multidisciplinary intervention to prevent the readmission of elderly patients with congestive heart failure. N Engl J Med 1995; 333: 1190–1195.
6. McAlister FA, Lawson FM, Teo KK, Armstrong PW. A systemic review of randomized trials of disease management programs in heart failure. Am J Med 2001; 110: 378–384.
7. O'Connell JB. The economic burden of heart failure. Clin Cardiol 2000; 23III: 6–10.
8. Vasan RS, Benjamin EJ, Levy D. Prevalence, clinical features and prognosis of diastolic heart failure: an epidemiologic perspective. J Am Coll Cardiol 1995; 26: 1565–1574.
9. Steimle AE, Stevenson LW, Chelimsky-Fallick C, *et al.* Sustained hemodynamic efficacy of therapy tailored to reduce filling pressures in survivors with advanced heart failure. Circulation 1997; 96: 1165–1172.
10. Cooper HA, Dries DL, Davis CE, Shen YL, Domanski MJ. Diuretics and risk of arrhythmic death in patients with left ventricular dysfunction. Circulation 1999; 100: 1311–1315.
11. Silver PJ, Harris AL, Canniff PC, *et al.* Phosphodiesterase isozyme inhibition, activation of the cAMP system, and positive inotropy mediated by milrinone in isolated guinea pig cardiac muscle. J Cardiovasc Pharmacol 1989; 13: 530–540.
12. Lowes BD, Simon MA, Tsvetkova TO, Bristow MR. Inotropes in the beta-blocker era. Clin Cardiol 2000; 23: III-11–III-16.
13. Leier CV, Binkley PF. Parenteral inotropic support for advanced congestive heart failure. Prog Cardiovasc Dis 1998; 41: 207–224.
14. Packer M, Bristow MR, Cohn JN, *et al.* The effect of carvedilol on morbidity and mortality in patients with chronic heart failure. N Engl J Med 1996; 334: 1349–1355.
15. MERIT-HF Study Group. Effect of metoprolol CR/XL in chronic heart failure: Metoprolol CR/XL Randomised Intervention Trial in Congestive Heart Failure (MERIT-HF). Lancet 1999; 353: 2001–2007.
16. The CIBIS II Investigators. The Cardiac Insufficiency Bisoprolol Study II (CIBIS-II): a randomised trial. Lancet 1999; 353: 9–13.
17. DiBianco R, Shabetai R, Kostuk W, *et al.* A comparison of oral milrinone, digoxin, and their combination in the treatment of patients with chronic heart failure. N Engl J Med 1989; 320: 677–683.
18. Packer M, Carver JR, Rodeheffer RJ, *et al.* Effect of oral milrinone on mortality in severe chronic heart failure. N Engl J Med 1991; 325: 1468–1475.
19. Packer M, Medina N, Yushak M. Hemodynamic and clinical limitations of long-term inotropic therapy with amrinone in patients with severe chronic heart failure. Circulation 1984; 70: 1038–1047.
20. Karlsberg RP, DeWood MA, DeMaria AN, Berk MR,

Lasher KP. Comparative efficacy of short-term intravenous infusions of milrinone and dobutamine in acute congestive heart failure following acute myocardial infarction. Clin Cardiol 1996; 19: 21–30.

21. Oliva F, Latini R, Politi A, *et al.* Intermittent 6-month low dose dobutamine infusion in severe heart failure: DICE Multicenter Trial. Am Heart J 1999; 138: 247–253.
22. O'Connor CM, Gattis WA, Uretsky BF, *et al.* Continuous intravenous dobutamine is associated with an increased risk of death in patients with advanced heart failure: Insights from the Flolan International Randomized Survival Trial (FIRST). Am Heart J 2000; 138: 78–86.
23. Cuffe MS, Califf RM, Adams KF Jr., *et al.* Short-term intravenous milrinone for acute exacerbation of chronic heart failure: a randomized controlled trial. JAMA 2002; 287: 1541–1547.
24. Felker GM, Benza RL, Chandler AB, *et al.* Heart failure etiology and response to milrinone in decompensated heart failure: results from the OPTIME-CHF study. J Am Coll Cardiol 2003; 41: 997–1003.
25. Mehra MR, Ventura HO, Kapoor C, *et al.* Safety and clinical utility of long-term intravenous milrinone in advanced heart failure. Am J Cardiol 1997; 80: 61–64.
26. Higginbotham MB, Russell SD, Mehra MR, Ventura HO. Bridging patients to cardiac transplantation. Congest Heart Fail 2000; 238–242.
27. Goldstein DJ, Oz MC, Rose EA. Implantable left ventricular assist devices. N Engl J Med 1998; 339: 1522–1533.
28. Aaronson KD, Eppinger MJ, Dyke DB, Wright S, Pagani FD. Left ventricular assist device therapy improves utilization of donor hearts. J Am Coll Cardiol 2002; 39: 1247–1254.
29. Yamani MH, Haji SA, Starling RC, *et al.* Comparison of dobutamine-based and milrinone-based therapy for advanced decompensated congestive heart failure: Hemodynamic efficacy, clinical outcome, and economic impact. Am Heart J 2001; 142: 998–1002.
30. Aranda JM Jr., Schofield RS, Pauly DF, *et al.* Comparison of dobutamine versus milrinone therapy in hospitalized patients awaiting cardiac transplantation: a prospective, randomized trial. Am Heart J 2003; 145: 324–329.
31. Bohm M, Deutsch HJ, Hartmann D, Rosee KL, Stablein A. Improvement of postreceptor events by metoprolol treatment in patients with chronic heart failure. J Am Coll Cardiol 1997; 30: 992–996.
32. Travill CM, Pugh S, Noble MI. The inotropic and hemodynamic effects of intravenous milrinone when reflex adrenergic stimulation is suppressed by beta-adrenergic blockade. Clin Ther 1994; 16: 783–792.
33. Sonnenblick EH, LeJemtel TH, Frishman WH. Inotropic agents. In: Sonnenblick EH, Sica DA (eds) Cardiovascular Pharmacotherapeutics (McGraw-Hill: New York, 2003), 191–202.
34. Nieminen MS, Akkila J, Hasenfuss G, *et al.* Hemodynamic and neurohumoral effects of continuous infusion of levosimendan in patients with congestive heart failure. J Am Coll Cardiol 2000; 36: 1903–1912.
35. Follath F, Cleland JG, Just H, *et al.* Efficacy and safety of intravenous levosimendan compared with dobutamine in severe low-output heart failure (the LIDO study): a randomised double-blind trial. Lancet 2002; 360: 196–202.
36. Moiseyev VS, Poder P, Andrejevs N, *et al.* Safety and efficacy of a novel calcium sensitizer, levosimendan, in patients with left ventricular failure due to an acute myocardial infarction: a randomised, placebo-controlled, double-blind study (RUSSLAN). Eur Heart J 2002; 23: 1422–1432.
37. Mehra MR, Uber PA. The dilemma of late-stage heart failure: rationale for chronic parenteral inotropic support. Cardiol Clin 2001; 19: 627–636.
38. Marius-Nunez AL, Heaney L, Fernandez RN, *et al.* Intermittent inotropic therapy in an outpatient setting: A cost-effective therapeutic modality in patients with refractory heart failure. Am Heart J 1996; 132: 805–808.
39. Elis A, Bental T, Kimchi O, Ravid M, Lishner M. Intermittent dobutamine treatment in patients with chronic refractory congestive heart failure: a randomized, double-blind, placebo-controlled study. Clin Pharmacol Ther 1998; 63: 682–685.
40. Stanek EJ, Oates MB, McGhan WF, Denofrio D, Loh E. Preferences for treatment outcomes in patients with heart failure: Symptoms versus survival. J Card Fail 2000; 6: 225–232.
41. Scios Inc. ADHERE™ Acute Decompensated Heart Failure National Registry. Third Quarter 2003 National Benchmark Report. Available at: http://www.adhereregistry.com/national_BMR/Q3_2003_ADHERE_National_BMR.pdf. Accessed June 1, 2004.
42. Cohn JN, Goldstein SO, Greenberg BH, *et al.* A dose-dependent increase in mortality with vesnarinone among patients with severe heart failure. N Engl J Med 1998; 339: 1810–1816.
43. The Xamoterol in Severe Heart Failure Study Group. Xamoterol in severe heart failure. Lancet 1990; 336: 1–6.
44. Hampton JR, Van Veldhusisen DJ, Kleber FX, *et al.*

Randomized study of effect of ibopamine on survival in patients with advanced heart failure. Lancet 1997; 349: 971–977.

45. The Pimobendan in Congestive Heart Failure (PICO) Investigators. Effect of pimobendan on exercise capacity in patients with heart failure: Main results from the Pimobendan in Congestive Heart Failure (PICO) Trial. Heart 1996; 76: 223–231.

CHAPTER 23

Diuretics and newer therapies for sodium and edema management in decompensated heart failure

Robert J Cody

Introduction

Frequently, acute cardiac decompensation is the clinical expression of left ventricular (LV) dysfunction, occurring as the result of diverse etiologies. Even at advanced stages, many patients initially thought to require transplantation, due to acute decompensation, can continue to be managed with medical therapy. Many factors contribute to the progression of heart failure, from mild forms to the advanced or refractory condition. However, the precise characteristics which govern the rate of progression vary from patient to patient. As a result, the onset of decompensation or refractory presentation is difficult to predict and may be abrupt. In this regard, evidence of deterioration must be monitored carefully. For patients with chronic heart failure, fluid retention is typically considered the primary cause of abrupt decompensation, and surveys of hospital admissions support this observation. However, it is important to remember that fluid retention is just one of many factors that can result in abrupt decompensation (Table 23.1). The hallmark of acute cardiac decompensation is pulmonary edema, which results from excessive sodium retention, acute LV dysfunction, or mechanical disorders of the left ventricle. Sodium retention results from the inability of the body to excrete sodium at a rate commensurate with dietary sodium intake. In fact, the characteristics which are identified as the hallmark of acute cardiac decompensation are, for the most part, findings of excess sodium retention: pulmonary congestion, peripheral edema, increased jugular venous pressure (JVP), an S_3 gallop, and hepatomegaly or ascites. In addition to urgent care measures, the most common therapy for acute cardiac decompensation is the use of diuretics. This chapter will emphasize acute therapy with diuretics and the transition to a more stable chronic regimen.

Table 23.1. *Factors that may contribute to acute decompensation of chronic heart failure patients*

Pulmonary edema
Progressive or persistent severe fluid retention
Fatigue or weakness with minimal exertion or rest
Frequent nocturnal decompensation or dyspnea
New or recurrent angina
Progressive unexplained weight loss
Loss of independent function
Progressive renal failure

Decompensated Heart Failure and Edema

Clinical conditions

Acute pulmonary edema is often the result of the many presentations of coronary artery disease (CAD) and its complications. A patient may present with a massive myocardial infarction (MI), and subsequently develop papillary muscle dysfunction or a ventricular septal defect, which could contribute to worsening LV dysfunction and pulmonary edema. Also, a patient with previous LV dysfunction may have worsening LV function with myocardial ischemia, or infarction with resultant acute pulmonary edema. Although CAD is probably the most common etiology of acute cardiac decompensation with resultant pulmonary edema, other etiologies include aortic stenosis and diastolic dysfunction in hypertensive crisis.

Mechanisms

Cardiac decompensation is characterized by decreased LV systolic function, and in most cases, abnormal diastolic function. The resultant decrease in cardiac output and increased left ventricular end-diastolic pressure (LVEDP) set the stage for sodium retention. Decreased cardiac output and increased systemic resistance lead to decreased renal blood flow, and the magnitude of the renal blood flow reduction is correlated with decreased cardiac output.[1,2] Diminished renal blood flow is a stimulus for activation of neurohormonal vasoconstriction pathways, particularly the renin system,[3,4] which produces vasoconstriction and aldosterone secretion. Total body water, extracellular fluid, and plasma volume are increased as compared to controls.[5] When this is moderate to severe, impaired renal function and increased cardiac filling pressures occur. These hemodynamic responses become the basis for sodium retention.

The reduction of glomerular filtration rate (GFR) in heart failure is highly correlated with hemodynamic parameters, where the greatest reduction in cardiac output and renal blood flow are associated with the greatest reduction in GFR.[1,6] Renal blood flow and function tend to decrease with age in normal subjects and an age effect can be superimposed on the overall reduction in renal blood flow and function due to the heart failure process.[6] The resulting diminished delivery of sodium to the distal nephron at the level of the macula densa, becomes a potent stimulus for renin release.[7] Aldosterone further increases sodium retention at the distal nephron at the expense of potassium excretion. Although current therapy for heart failure may improve cardiac output and renal blood flow, no current oral therapy has uniformly improved GFR.

Neurohormonal factors that promote retention of sodium and water include aldosterone, vasopressin, angiotensin II, norepinephrine, and the vasoconstrictor prostaglandins. In contrast, prostacyclin, dopamine, and atrial natriuretic factor favor sodium excretion.[3,4] The effect of vasopressin is primarily the promotion of free water retention, rather than sodium retention, and this typically contributes to hyponatremia.

Pharmacokinetics of Diuretic Therapy

Response to diuretic administration for acute cardiac decompensation

The sites of diuretic action and their role in the edema of cardiac decompensation have been reviewed,[9,10] and there have been no substantial breakthroughs in new diuretic development or mechanisms. The hemodynamic response to diuretic therapy has been characterized primarily in the setting of pulmonary edema. The acute hemodynamic response revealed a vasodilator effect[11–13] and reduction of cardiac filling pressures.[11–14]

During acute decompensated heart failure (ADHF), changes in cardiac output varied from increased to no change to a significant reduction; and changes in hemodynamics could precede or lag the production of diuresis. Such evaluations were conducted in diverse patient populations and must be interpreted accordingly. It has been stated that the vasodilator effect could precede the occurrence of diuresis, but the supporting data for this effect are limited. Studies have reported either vasoconstriction,[15] or initial vasodilation followed by vasoconstriction[16] with acute or short-term follow-up. A review of the cited literature therefore reveals a fully divergent range of hemodynamic responses to diuretics, although the majority of acute studies demonstrate a reduction in cardiac filling pressures.[11–14]

Loop diuretics have been shown to decrease renal vasculature resistance and to increase total and cortical renal blood flow.[12,17,18] However, this may be related to the severity of heart failure.[19] It is difficult to isolate a single neurohormonal factor as being primarily responsible for the overall hemodynamic and regional hemodynamic response to diuretics. Acute diuretic therapy may increase renin and aldosterone.[15,16,19,20] Sympathetic nervous system activity also increases in response to diuretics.[19,20] The impact of neurohormonal activation is an attenuation of the otherwise favorable effects of diuretics.

Loop diuretics

As this chapter focuses on acute cardiac decompensation, the response to parenteral diuretic therapy will be emphasized (Table 23.2), without an extensive review of pharmacology. The term *loop diuretic* has evolved to encompass pharmacologic compounds which exert their primary action on the thick ascending loop of Henle. In order to reach the intraluminal site of action, these organic acids must first be secreted into the proximal tubule via the organic acid pathway. Once in the lumen, active reabsorption of chloride is inhibited in both the medullary and cortical portions of the loop of Henle. Decreased sodium reabsorption also occurs since the chloride ion is co-transported with sodium and potassium.

The three loop diuretics traditionally used in the United States to treat the edema of heart failure are furosemide, bumetanide, and torsemide. They are of equal efficacy but vary in pharmacokinetic properties.[9,21] Although ethacrynic acid is still available, it has a progressively diminishing role in edema management.[22–24] Despite equal efficacy among loop diuretics, clinicians often substitute one for the other, with the hope of improved efficacy. Although torsemide has a greater duration of action than its counterparts, in general, the strategy of changing from one loop diuretic to another is typically not effective. After oral administration, furosemide has 40% bioavailability, bumetanide 80%, and torsemide > 80%. Diminished diuresis and prolonged renal elimination of the drug may be expected in heart failure when renal dysfunction is evident. Torsemide has two active metabolites, which probably accounts for its longer elimination half-life of 3 hours.

Residual loop diuretic concentration is eliminated by nonrenal mechanisms including hepatic degradation and excretion. Because of the differences in bioavailability and potency, equivalent doses of bumetanide, furosemide, and torsemide, are 1 mg, 40 mg, and 20 mg, respectively. All three agents are extensively bound to plasma proteins and are rapidly secreted by the organic acid

Table 23.2. *Pharmacokinetics of intravenous diuretics: are there appreciable differences?*

Drug	Route	Onset	Peak	Duration	Dosage*
Loop diuretics					
Ethacrynic acid	IV	5 min	15–30 min	2 h	50–100 mg
Furosemide	IV	5 min	30 min	2 h	20–120 mg
Bumetanide	IV	5 min	30–45 min	2 h	0.5–1.0 mg
Torsemide	IV	5 min	15–30 min	4–6 h	20–100 mg
Thiazide diuretics					
Chlorothiazide	IV	15 min	30 min	2 h	250–500 mg

*Clinically-accepted dosages and intervals in heart failure which are not strictly determined by pharmacokinetics.
Abbreviations: IV = intravenous.

pathway of the proximal tubule. In chronic renal failure, competition for this pathway by exogenous and accumulated endogenous organic acids causes a lower peak concentration of the drug at its site of action. Therefore, a diminished diuresis and a prolonged renal elimination of the drug may be expected in heart failure when renal dysfunction is evident. The diuretic effect is apparent within 30 minutes after oral administration and peaks in 1 to 2 hours.[25–29] Bumetanide has a somewhat shorter duration of action than furosemide or torsemide. Torsemide, like other loop diuretics, must be secreted into the urine by the organic acid secretory system in the proximal tubule in order to be effective.[22] It produces a maximum sodium excretion rate within approximately the same time with either intravenous or oral administration. Although the pharmacokinetics of torsemide are linear, increases in doses above 50 mg do not appear to increase the maximum sodium excretion rate; however, it does increase the duration of the pharmacodynamic effect. One study has defined a ceiling dose of 100 mg of torsemide in patients with renal insufficiency and has recommended that repeated administration of torsemide is more effective than increasing the dose.[22] Results from another study showed that 20 mg of intravenous torsemide is approximately as effective as 40 mg of intravenous furosemide.[23] However, additional well-controlled trials of torsemide are necessary to determine whether it provides clinical benefit beyond current loop diuretics.

Thiazides and potassium-sparing diuretics

Thiazide diuretics are derivatives of the benzothiadiazine structure.[9,21] Like loop diuretics, they are organic acids and are highly protein bound. Since they cannot be filtered, they gain access to the tubular lumen via the organic acid secretory pathway of the proximal tubule. Chlorothiazide is the only thiazide available in a soluble form that permits intravenous administration. This formulation has recently been discontinued and limited stores remain. Its appreciable benefits, when combined with an intravenous loop diuretic, are now of primarily historical interest. Oral hydrochlorothiazide or metolazone are effective in most cases, but delayed gastric and small bowel absorption are common in the presence of severe edema. Despite this limitation, the combination of loop and thiazide diuretics appreciably augments diuresis. Experimental animal data demonstrate reactive hypertrophy of the distal nephron during long-term sodium depletion.[30] With distal nephron tubular hypertrophy, the blockade of sodium reabsorption produced by loop diuretics at the thick ascending limb is often attenuated. This adverse structural adaptation is overcome by the addition of a thiazide diuretic, which blocks sodium reabsorption at the distal nephron.

Although potassium-sparing diuretics uniformly act at the distal nephron and collecting duct, their effect is achieved by two different mechanisms.[9,21] Active sodium reabsorption in the distal tubule and the collecting duct occurs in exchange for potassium and hydrogen. One mechanism is mediated by aldosterone and may be antagonized by spironolactone, which is a competitive receptor antagonist. The effects of triamterene and amiloride are independent of mineralocorticoids, and they act by direct inhibition of sodium transport. Differing from spironolactone, these two drugs must first reach their site of action by means of glomerular filtration and the organic base secretory pathway of the proximal tubule. Overall these agents decrease sodium reabsorption, potassium excretion, and theoretically potentiate hyperkalemia, although the latter is uncommon in heart failure. Pharmacokinetic properties of the potassium-sparing diuretics help explain their differences in onset and duration of action. Onset of diuretic action occurs rapidly, within 2 to 4 hours, with amiloride and triamterene. This effect may persist for 24 hours despite early peak plasma concentrations and an elimination half-life of 6 to 9 hours. Following a single oral dose of spironolactone, peak serum concentrations of the parent drug are seen in 1 to 2 hours while the active metabolites peak in 2 to 4 hours.

Although spironolactone is traditionally considered a potassium-sparring diuretic, its greatest benefit is as an anti-aldosterone agent. The Randomized Aldactone Evaluation Study (RALES) demonstrated significant clinical and survival benefit, independent of a diuretic effect.

Survival included a significant reduction in sudden cardiac death, as compared to placebo.[31]

Practical Considerations

The cycle of sodium and water management in heart failure

When a patient can no longer be managed on an outpatient basis for persistent severe edema, weakness, fatigue, or dyspnea, or when acute decompensation occurs in an otherwise stable heart failure patient, hospitalization is warranted. A decision to pursue parenteral therapy should be initiated from the moment of admission, while diagnostic studies are pending (Table 23.3). This should include intravenous diuretics, electrolyte replacement, and intravenous inotropic support such as dobutamine.[8] When afterload reduction is desired, intravenous nitroprusside can be used. An alternative approach to vasodilation is the use of intravenous milrinone, which has both inotropic and direct vasodilator properties. Intravenous nitroglycerin is frequently used to treat ADHF, but it is important to remember that most patients demonstrate hemodynamic tachyphylaxis within the first 24 hours of administration, so that hemodynamics return towards baseline and are not significantly different from placebo. In view of the diverse causes of acute cardiac decompensation, the initial therapeutic intervention should be accompanied by appropriate diagnostic studies to identify the cause of the decompensation, to plan more tailored therapeutic interventions.

Optimizing intravenous diuretic response

Intravenous diuretic therapy may be used acutely in several clinical situations. In pulmonary edema, the obvious benefit of acute intravenous diuretic therapy is the rapid clearance of pulmonary congestion, likely mediated by natriuresis and diuresis,

Table 23.3. *Fluid management to minimize hospitalization frequency and duration*

Outpatient management	Inpatient management	
	At admission	*At discharge*
Identify target diuretic dosage Daily weights 2000 mg sodium intake limit 2-3 L fluid limit Phone check for patient status BNP measurement* Patient and family education regarding fluid retention	Identify contributing etiologies for decompensation Intensify diuretic therapy: ■ intravenous route ■ combination of diuretics Fluid restriction Dopamine? AVP antagonist? BNP administration? Additional supporting therapy	Treat, correct, or mitigate factors producing edema Reset oral diuretic regimen Resume or reset ACE inhibitor dosage Add thiazide diuretic if necessary Add spironolactone for survival benefit and electrolyte effects Patient and family education regarding fluid retention

*At the time of this writing, BNP measurement is not recommended for routine follow-up of all patients. However, for problematic management issues, for long-distance telemanagement, and for patients with significant chronic lung disease, the trend of BNP plasma levels provides very useful information for trends of fluid retention and pulmonary congestion.
Abbreviations: ACE = angiotensin-converting enzyme; AVP = arginine vasopressin; BNP = brain natruretic peptide.

a reduction of intravascular volume, and vasodilation. As subacute decompensation is a prelude to pulmonary edema, the goals of intravenous diuretic therapy are similar to the treatment of pulmonary edema. The primary goal of intravenous diuretic therapy is the elimination of edema. Concerns regarding adverse activation of neurohormonal activity and electrolyte depletion are of lesser importance, although potassium and magnesium (Mg) intake should be supplemented. For acute reversal of sodium retention and fluid overload, therapy with a loop diuretic is indicated. It should be given intravenously, to a ceiling dose that is twice the normal dose (e.g., furosemide at 80 mg; bumetanide at 2 mg; or torsemide at 40 mg), increased as necessary, and combined with other agents. A thiazide diuretic in combination with a loop diuretic is often very effective.[32–35] However, an oral thiazide diuretic, particularly metolazone, may require several days to achieve its maximal favorable response, due to delayed absorption. The ability to utilize intravenous chlorothiazide (Diuril) is often overlooked. Unlike hydrochlorothiazide, chlorothiazide can be given intravenously in a dose of 250 mg to 500 mg, which is equivalent to an oral hydrochlorothiazide dosage of 25 mg to 50 mg. When combined with a loop diuretic, intravenous chlorothiazide produces greater diuresis than the loop diuretic alone. This is discussed further in the section on resistance to diuretics.

Diuretic-induced electrolyte imbalance

Electrolyte abnormalities in congestive heart failure (CHF) are due to both the underlying pathophysiology and the concurrent administration of diuretic therapy.[21] The pathologic factors predisposing patients to electrolyte abnormalities include abnormal neurohormonal activation and marked reduction of renal blood flow and function. Angiotensin II impedes the excretion of a given sodium load by direct effects on the tubular cells of the nephron. The enhanced stimulation of aldosterone secretion due to angiotensin II results in potassium excretion and sodium retention at the distal nephron. This not only contributes to sodium retention but also results in total body potassium depletion and hypokalemia. Magnesium excretion is coupled with potassium excretion in the exchange for sodium. Hyponatremia is a hallmark of heart failure. Although hyponatremia is well-correlated with activation of the renin system (and a good surrogate of this activity), its occurrence is the result of enhanced arginine vasopressin (AVP) activity at the V_2 vasopressin receptor site of the distal nephron tubule. Activation of the V_2 receptor reduces free water clearance. This solute-free retention of water, combined with excessive dietary intake of sodium and water, results in hyponatremia, which is a common chronic occurrence in heart failure.[44,45] In addition to the imbalance produced by abnormal neurohormonal activation, electrolyte imbalance is sustained by the chronic renal insufficiency (CRI) that occurs in the majority of heart failure patients. Furthermore, diuretics produce hypokalemia, hyponatremia, hypocalcemia, hypomagnesemia, hyperuricemia, and metabolic alkalosis.[46,47] Hypokalemia is the most common electrolyte disturbance, mediated by direct tubular mechanisms and hypersecretion of aldosterone. Hypokalemia and hypomagnesemia may be associated with myalgias, leg cramps, and an increase in ventricular arrhythmias. Most patients require the concomitant use of potassium supplements to correct hypokalemia. Angiotensin-converting enzyme (ACE) inhibitors may also reduce potassium loss. Most commonly, diuretic-induced hypokalemia is associated with a metabolic alkalosis and a coexisting chloride deficit. Intravenous administration of potassium is recommended to correct moderate to severe potassium deficits, with or without the occurrence of cardiac arrhythmias. This route of administration is also useful when oral replacement is not feasible or not tolerated due to a decrease in gastrointestinal motility. Oral, slow-release potassium chloride preparations are employed in the chronic management of diuretic-induced hypokalemia. Currently there is no dosage form which is superior to another with respect to the ulcerative effect on the gastrointestinal mucosa. The dosage of potassium chloride (KCl) is adjusted on an individual basis and is dependent on the use of other medication, such as ACE inhibitors or concomitant diuretics. Generally, patients require between 40 mEq q.d. and 120 mEq q.d. to maintain potassium homeostasis, but requirements may be increased in the setting of acute diuretic administration.

Acute diuretic therapy also leads to hypomagnesemia.[48] Magnesium, primarily an intracellular ion, plays a pivotal role in mitochondrial function, oxidation-phosphorylation reaction, and neuromuscular transmission.[49] Potassium and magnesium have an interrelationship where magnesium is a cofactor in the appropriate function of the sodium-potassium adenosine triphosphatase (ATPase) pump. Therefore, hypokalemia may persist until the magnesium deficiency is corrected. Although normal serum magnesium concentrations range from 1.6 mEq/L to 2.0 mEq/L, only 1% of Mg is found in the extracellular compartment. The potential problem of magnesium deficiency in the heart failure population is the occurrence of lethal cardiac arrhythmias. Intravenous supplementation is essential in this situation. The administration of 2 g to 5 g (equivalent to 16 mEq to 40 mEq) of magnesium sulfate ($MgSO_4$) by slow intravenous infusion at 1 g/h, repeated in 12 hours if needed, will correct magnesium at a satisfactory rate.

Diuretic-resistant edema

Patients are considered to have "diuretic resistance" when they demonstrate progressive edema despite escalating oral or intravenous diuretic therapy.[9] In contrast to diuretic resistance, *diuretic adaptation* involves the activation of counterbalancing endogenous structural or functional mechanisms which tend to limit the clinical effects of diuretics.

The factors that contribute to diuretic resistance have been summarized in the literature.[35,36] Renal insufficiency can reduce tubular secretion of the diuretic as well as the filtered load of sodium. Therefore, patients with decreased renal function due to heart failure[1] or superimposed age,[1,6] frequently have a reduced response to diuretics. In addition, studies have demonstrated that indomethacin and other nonsteroidal antiinflammatory drugs (NSAIDs) reduced the maximal response to furosemide.[37] Mesenteric congestion may also limit the absorption and bioavailability of orally-administered medications.

Escalating the dosage of intravenous loop diuretics is the most common approach and the dosage should be rapidly doubled until the desired effect is produced. An ultra-high dose of loop diuretic may be effective.[38,39] However, the overall response to ultra-high doses is often unimpressive. Also, continuous intravenous infusion of furosemide after a loading dose has been shown to be as effective, if not more so, as intermittent bolus therapy in producing diuresis and natriuresis.

Another approach is based on the concept that a continuous infusion of loop diuretic may be more effective than intermittent bolus administration, in terms of net sodium excretion.[40,41] Careful metabolic studies have demonstrated a greater net sodium excretion using this approach, as compared to intermittent bolus administration, despite comparable amounts of bumetanide appearing in the urine.[41] In CRI, continuous intravenous bumetanide has been shown to produce a greater natriuresis than equivalent bolus intravenous doses. Continuous bumetanide produces lower peak levels and therefore may decrease toxicity of the diuretic in patients with impaired renal function.

In view of the structural hypertrophy of the distal nephron described earlier, an alternative and perhaps more physiologic treatment is the combination of a thiazide and a loop diuretic. Although precise dose limits are difficult to define when a patient achieves a requirement, for instance, of 240 mg of furosemide daily, addition of an intravenous (chlorothiazide) or oral thiazide diuretic will be more effective than further increases of the loop diuretic. The combination of loop diuretic and thiazide diuretic is more effective than ultra-high doses of a loop diuretic alone.

In severe acute decompensation, when response to parenteral diuretics is completely attenuated, or in patients requiring rapid fluid removal, acute ultrafiltration and hemodialysis can be utilized.[42,43]

When diuretics fail

In ADHF with edema, the failure of diuretics to adequately reduce edema and improve symptoms is a palpable risk. Some of the characteristics of the patient with diuretic failure include severe hypotension, renal impairment and hyponatremia.

Concomitant disorders such as diabetes and hypertensive nephrosclerosis further impair the effectiveness of diuretics. This profile is accelerated in the elderly, where reduction of glomerular filtration is a common side effect of the aging process, even in the absence of heart failure. In such circumstances mechanical intervention is necessary.

Ultrafiltration provides the most common and accessible form of sodium and water clearance in the setting of diuretic failure. It requires high flow vascular access and adequate systemic blood pressure to be effective. It can often be accomplished without adverse effects on baseline hemodynamics and renal function. Newer approaches to bedside fluid removal exist, but are sufficiently recent that standardized recommendations cannot be given. In the setting of electrolyte imbalance and insufficient clearance of metabolic catabolic products, hemodialysis is necessary.

To avoid the risk of diuretic failure, associated nephrotoxic agents should be identified and avoided. These include nephrotoxic antibiotics and antiinflammatory agents with known adverse renal effects. The most notorious among the latter is indomethacin. Agents that also produce interstitial nephritis should be identified and avoided. Paradoxically, long-term administration of loop diuretics in excessive doses may produce interstitial nephritis, and the discontinuance of such therapy may result in spontaneous recovery of diuresis.

Newer Approaches to Sodium and Edema Management

Vasopressin antagonists

Normal extracellular fluid volume and osmolality are maintained when serum sodium is regulated within a narrow range (136 mEq/L to 148 mEq/L). Such control is achieved by maintaining a balance between fluid intake, which is normally controlled by thirst, and renal water excretion, which is controlled primarily by AVP. Hyponatremia—defined by a decline in serum sodium concentration ($[Na^+]$) to < 136 mEq/L—develops when regulation of this balance is lost, either as a result of excessive fluid intake or, more commonly, by an impaired capacity for renal water excretion. Hyponatremia may also develop as a primary consequence of either renal or extrarenal sodium loss. Compounds that block AVP are associated with a water diuresis (aquaresis), by reversing the retention of solute-free water which is produced by high circulating levels of vasopressin in heart failure. Attempts to commercialize effective antagonists of vasopressin over the past two decades have meet with a variety of obstacles. These have included difficulties with chemical formulation, ineffective clinical trials, and the focus for such agents in heart failure patients with hyponatremia. However, the history of neurohormonal antagonists clearly demonstrates that neurohormonal activation produces adverse physiologic and clinical effects in the absence of excessively elevated circulating levels, and evidence suggests that vasopressin antagonists may play an important clinical role, even when serum sodium levels (the surrogate of vasopressin activation) are only mildly decreased.

Vasopressin regulates free water retention through the V_2 receptor, and mediates vascular constriction through the V_1a receptor, which also appears to adversely affect myocardial contractility. Currently, several vasopressin antagonists are undergoing clinical development, as either intravenous or oral therapy. Administration of these agents has been associated with substantial weight reduction, aquaresis, and correction of serum sodium levels. Tolvaptan, a selective V_2 antagonist, effectively normalizes serum sodium concentrations in hyponatremic heart failure patients. Tolvaptan is an orally active, once-daily V_2-receptor blocker, and its benefits have been recently described. In patients with hyponatremia, there was a decrease in body weight and normalization of serum sodium.[50] In patients with CHF with mild signs of congestion on chronic diuretic therapy, there was evidence of improved diuresis in the setting of baseline diuretic therapy. Another agent, conivaptan blocks both the V_1a and V_2 receptor. It is currently available for intravenous administration only and provides a favorable hemodynamic effect, in addition to improving free water clearance. The potential role of these agents has recently been reviewed.[51]

The future of this class of agents may bring particular benefit to the management of acute decompensation and edema of heart failure, where extensive edema and clinical compromise cannot be effectively managed by diuretics, due to the presence of profound hyponatremia. In that situation, one is left with the rather unsatisfactory option of slowly waiting for sodium correction by means of stringent fluid restriction. In the setting of acute decompensation, vasopressin antagonists offer considerable promise.

Additional approaches to augment diuresis in heart failure

Since the initial discovery and clinical assessment of natriuretic peptides over 20 years ago, the anticipation has been that pharmaceutical agents derived from these peptides would provide a physiologic approach to sodium and water management in edema-forming states. Unfortunately, although there have been many attempts at intravenous and oral formulations of natriuretic peptides, this has not been the case. In small controlled studies of heart failure, one may demonstrate a small but statistically significant increase of sodium excretion in response to natriuretic peptides. However, these agents do not mount a clinically significant diuresis in heart failure. From the time of initial characterization until the present, heart failure patients have shown a blunted response of sodium and water excretion, compared to normal subjects when exposed to either oral or intravenous administration of natriuretic peptides. In contrast, the direct vasodilator properties of the natriuretic peptides are retained in heart failure. Of the natriuretic peptides, the intravenous formulation of brain natriuretic peptide (BNP) produces a vasodilator effect that is statistically greater than nitroglycerin in comparative trials. Based on smaller studies, a small but significant increase in sodium excretion can be detected, as compared to placebo. However, the magnitude of the response is meager when compared to the response to a dose of loop diuretic, and certainly less that the augmentation that one identifies when a thiazide diuretic is added to a loop diuretic. Unfortunately, this meager response has been promoted to suggest that BNP is an effective diuretic agent in decompensated heart failure. As nesiritide is one of the most costly heart failure medications (on a per diem basis), its use is not justified to promote diuresis, particularly in the absence of more efficient and cost-effective options.

Dopamine is not a primary diuretic agent. However, empirical observation has suggested that low-dose dopamine (2 mg/kg to 3 mg/kg) may augment the renal response to diuretics. Well-controlled clinical studies suggest that dopamine does not augment the diuretic response to furosemide. Its use is a matter of clinical judgment and perspective. As a relatively low-cost agent, its empiric use has a negligible economic impact.

Similarly, a recurring question is whether dobutamine and milrinone can augment diuresis in the edematous patient with decompensated heart failure. A rationale for this concept can be developed based on the pathophysiology of decompensated heart failure. Many patients with advanced heart failure have impaired renal function due to hypoperfusion. In that setting, reduction of glomerular filtration produces proximal sodium and water retention and limits tubular transport of sodium to the loop of Henle, where loop diuretics are effective. It is thus rational to postulate that increasing cardiac output and cardiac decompression produces improved regional perfusions and responsiveness to diuretic therapy. Adequate controlled studies are nonexistent and this concept, while well founded, cannot be substantiated.

Conclusion

Diuretics remain the most poorly-characterized class of heart failure therapy. These agents are diverse, maximal doses are often exceeded, and guidelines for optimal combinations do not exist. The use of diuretics in acute cardiac decompensation remains a combination of science and art. The desired endpoint, in the absence of more objective changes, remains the relief of the symptoms related to edema: dyspnea and congestion. However, careful use of diuretics in appropriate combination with other more specific therapies of acute cardiac decompensation will produce clinical improvement without adverse consequences.

References

1. Cody RJ, Ljungman S, Covit AB, *et al.* Regulation of glomerular filtration rate in chronic congestive heart failure patients. Kidney Int 1988; 34: 361–367.
2. Leithe ME, Margorien RD, Hermiller JB, Unverferth DV, Leier CV. Relationship between central hemodynamics and regional blood flow in normal subjects and in patients with congestive heart failure. Circulation 1984; 69: 57–64.
3. Cody RJ, Neurohormonal influences in the pathogenesis of congestive heart failure. In: Weber K, Cardiology Clinics (eds) Heart Failure (W.B. Saunders Company: Philadelphia, PA, 1989), 73.
4. Francis GS, Goldsmith SR, Levine TB, Olivari MT, Cohn JN. The neurohormonal axis in congestive heart failure. Ann Intern Med 1984; 101: 370–377.
5. Anand IS, Ferrari R, Kalra GS, *et al.* Edema of cardiac origin: studies of body water and sodium, renal function, hemodynamic indexes, and plasma hormones in untreated congestive cardiac failure. Circulation 1989; 80: 299–305.
6. Cody RJ, Torre S, Clark M, Pondolfino K. Age-related hemodynamic, renal, and hormonal differences in patients with congestive heart failure. Arch Intern Med 1989; 149: 1023–1028.
7. Skott O, Briggs JP. Direct demonstration of macula densa-mediated renin secretion. Science 1987; 237: 1618–1620.
8. Leier CV. Cardiotonic Drugs (Marcell Dekker Inc.: New York, 1991).
9. Konstam MA, Cody RJ. Short-term use of intravenous milrinone for heart failure. Am J Cardiol 1995; 75: 822–826.
10. Wilcox CS. Diuretics. In: Brenner BM, Rector FC Jr. (eds) The Kidney, 4th edition, Volume II (W.B. Saunders Company: Philadelphia, PA, 1991), 2133.
11. Lal S, Murtagh JG, Pollock AM, Fletcher E, Binnion PF. Acute haemodynamic effects of frusemide in patients with normal and raised left atrial pressures. Br Heart J 1969; 31: 711–717.
12. Dikshit K, Vyden JK, Forrester JS, *et al.* Renal and extrarenal hemodynamic effects of furosemide in congestive heart failure after myocardial infarction. N Engl J Med 1973; 288: 1087–1090.
13. Magrini F, Niarchos AP. Hemodynamic effects of massive peripheral edema. Am Heart J 1983; 105: 90–97.
14. Stampfer M, Epstein SE, Beiser DG, Braunwald E. Hemodynamic effects of diuresis at rest and during intense upright exercise in patients with impaired cardiac function. Circulation 1968; 37: 900–911.
15. Francis GS, Siegel RM, Goldsmith SR, *et al.* Acute vasoconstrictor response to intravenous furosemide in patients with chronic congestive heart failure. Ann Intern Med 1985; 103: 1–6.
16. Ikram H, Chan W, Espiner EA, Nicholls MG. Haemodynamic and hormone responses to acute and chronic furosemide therapy in congestive heart failure. Clin Sci 1980; 59: 443–449.
17. Birtch AG, Zakheim RM, Jones LG, Barger AC. Redistribution of renal blood flow produced by furosemide and ethacrynic acid. Circ Res 1967; 21: 869–878.
18. Kilcoyne MM, Schmidt DH, Cannon PJ. Intrarenal blood flow in congestive heart failure. Circulation 1973; 47: 786–797.
19. Kubo SH, Clark M, Laragh JH, Borer JS, Cody RJ. Identification of normal neurohormonal activity in mild congestive heart failure and stimulating effect of upright posture and diuretics. Am J Cardiol 1987; 60: 1322–1328.
20. Bayliss J, Norell M, Canepa-Anson R, Sutton G, Poole-Wilson P. Untreated heart failure: Clinical and neuroendocrine effects of introducing diuresis. Br Heart J 1987; 57: 17–22.
21. Cody RJ, Pickworth KK. Approaches to diuretic therapy and electrolyte imbalance in congestive heart failure. In: Deedwania PC (ed.) Update in Congestive Heart Failure, Volume 12 (W.B. Saunders Company: Philadelphia, PA, 1994), 37.
22. Friedel HA, Buckley MM. Torsemide. A review of its pharmacological properties and therapeutic potential. Drugs 1991; 41: 81–103.
23. Brater DC, Leinfelder J, Anderson SA. Clinical pharmacology of torsemide, a new loop diuretic. Clin Pharmacol Ther 1987; 42: 187–192.
24. Cuvelier R, Pellegrin P, Lesne M, van Ypersele de Strihou C. Site of action of torsemide in man. Eur J Clin Pharmacol 1986; 31: 15–19.
25. Cook JA, Smith DE, Cornish LA, *et al.* Kinetics, dynamics, and bioavailability of bumetanide in healthy subjects and patients with congestive heart failure. Clin Pharmacol Ther 1988; 44: 487–500.
26. Cutler RE, Blair AD. Clinical pharmacokinetics of frusemide. Clin Pharmacokinet 1979; 4: 279–296.
27. Ward A, Heel RC. Bumetanide. A review of its pharmacodynamic and pharmacokinetic properties and therapeutic use. Drugs 1984; 28: 426–464.
28. Weiner IM, Mudge GH. Diuretics and other agents employed in the mobilization of edema fluid, In: Hardman JG, Limbird LE (eds) Goodman & Gilman's The Pharmacologic Basis of Therapeutics, 7th edition (MacMillan Publishing Co.: New York, 1985), 887.

29. Brater DC. Clinical pharmacology of loop diuretics. Drugs 1991; 41: 14–22.
30. Ellison DH, Velazquez H, Wright FS. Adaptation of the distal convoluted tubule of the rat. Structural and functional effects of dietary salt intake and chronic diuretic infusion. J Clin Invest 1989; 83: 113–126.
31. Pitt B, Zannad F, Remme WJ, *et al.*, Randomized Aldactone Evaluation Study Investigators. The effect of spironolactone on morbidity and mortality in patients with severe heart failure. N Engl J Med 1999; 341: 709–717.
32. Brater DC, Pressley RH, Anderson SA. Mechanisms of the synergistic combination of metolazone and bumetanide. J Pharmacol Exp Ther 1985; 233: 70–74.
33. Wollam GL, Tarazi RC, Bravo EL, Dunstan HP. Diuretic potency of combined hydrochlorothiazide and furosemide therapy in patients with azotemia. Am J Med 1982; 72: 929–938.
34. Oster JR, Epstein M, Smoller S. Combined therapy with thiazide-type and loop diuretic agents for resistant sodium retention. Ann Intern Med 1983; 99: 405–406.
35. Ellison DH. The physiologic basis of diuretic synergism: its role in treating diuretic resistance. Ann Intern Med 1991; 114: 886–894.
36. Brater DC. Resistance to loop diuretics. Why it happens and what to do about it. Drugs 1985; 30: 427–443.
37. Chennavasin P, Seiwell R, Brater DC. Pharmacokinetic-dynamic analysis of the indomethacin-furosemide interaction in man. J Pharmacol Exp Ther 1980; 215: 77–81.
38. Brater DC. Resistance to diuretics: emphasis on a pharmacological perspective. Drugs 1981; 22: 477–494.
39. Gerlag PG, van Meijel JJ. High-dose furosemide in the treatment of refractory congestive heart failure. Arch Intern Med 1988; 148: 286–291.
40. Copeland JG, Campbell DW, Plachetka JR, Salomon NW, Larson DF. Diuresis with continuous infusion of furosemide after cardiac surgery. Am J Surg 1983; 46: 796–799.
41. Rudy DW, Voelker JR, Greene PK, Esparza EA, Brater DC. Loop diuretics for chronic renal insufficiency: a continuous infusion is more efficacious than bolus therapy. Ann Intern Med 1991; 115: 360–366.
42. Agostoni PG, Marenzi GC, Pepi M, *et al.* Isolated ultrafiltration in moderate congestive heart failure. J Am Coll Cardiol 1993; 21: 424–431.
43. Rimondini A, Cipolla CM, Della Bella PD, *et al.* Hemofiltration as short-term treatment for refractory congestive heart failure. Am J Med 1987; 83: 43–48.
44. Schaer GL, Covit AB, Laragh JH, Cody RJ. Association of hyponatremia with increased renin activity in chronic congestive heart failure: impact of diuretic therapy. Am J Cardiol 1983; 51: 1635–1638.
45. Packer M, Medina N, Yushak M. Correction of dilutional hyponatremia in severe chronic heart failure by converting-enzyme inhibition. Ann Intern Med 1984; 100: 782–789.
46. Dorup I, Skajaa K, Clausen T, Kjeldsen K. Reduced concentrations of potassium, magnesium, and sodium-potassium pumps in human skeletal muscle during treatment with diuretics. Br Med J 1988; 296: 455–458.
47. Dyckner T, Wester PO. Plasma and skeletal muscle electrolytes in patients on long-term diuretic therapy for arterial hypertension and/or congestive heart failure. Acta Med Scand 1987; 222: 231–236.
48. Massry SG, Seelig MS. Hypomagnesemia and hypermagnesemia. Clin Nephrol 1977; 7: 147–153.
49. Flink EB. Magnesium deficiency. Etiology and clinical spectrum. Acta Med Scand Suppl 1981; 647: 125–137.
50. Lee CR, Watkins ML, Patterson JH, Gattis W, *et al.* Vasopressin: a new target for the treatment of heart failure. Am Heart J 2003; 146: 9–18.
51. Gheorghiade M, Niazi I, Ouyang J, Czerwiec, *et al.* Tolvaptan Investigators. Vasopressin V2-receptor blockade with tolvaptan in patients with chronic heart failure results from a double-blind, randomized trial. Circulation 2003; 107: 2690–2696.

CHAPTER 24

Contemporary aspects of intravenous vasodilator therapy with nesiritide or nitrates in acute heart failure

Kirkwood F Adams, Jr

Introduction

Intravenous vasodilators remain attractive to many cardiologists in the management of acute decompensated heart failure (ADHF), a growing and severe public health problem. Acute heart failure (AHF) is characterized by elevated left ventricular (LV) filling pressure and is well documented to be accompanied by a significant degree of systemic hypertension in many patients.[1] Elevated systemic pressure points to increased systemic vascular resistance (SVR) and increased filling pressure are a well-known consequence of congestion. The major direct effect of intravenous vasodilators, reduction in filling pressure and SVR, obviously counters these pathophysiological abnormalities.

Intravenous nitrate therapy, a traditional means of providing a vasodilator effect in patients with AHF, has been particularly embraced when AHF is accompanied by evidence of myocardial ischemia.[2] Recently, a new strategy for vasodilator therapy has emerged from clinical investigation—nesiritide, a peptide identical to human B-type natriuretic peptide (BNP). Nesiritide, from the family of hormones known as the natriuretic peptides, has been shown to reduce both SVR and pulmonary vascular resistance (PVR) with favorable clinical effects.[3–6] This chapter explores the roles of both of these drugs in the treatment of ADHF.

Nesiritide

The natriuretic peptide family

There are currently at least 4 known members of the structurally similar, but genetically distinct, natriuretic peptide hormone family: atrial natriuretic peptide (ANP), B-type natriuretic peptide (BNP), C-type natriuretic peptide (CNP), and dendroaspis natriuretic peptide (DNP) which remains controversial as a biologically active peptide in humans.[7–12] ANP is secreted primarily by cardiac atria in response to atrial distension. In contrast, BNP is secreted by both atrial and ventricular myocardium. But in states of systolic ventricular dysfunction, this peptide is predominately secreted by the left ventricle. Natriuretic peptides with biological activity are generated from larger precursor molecules which are biologically inert. These peptides interact with specific cellular receptors to mediate their biological effects. Experimental evidence indicates that natriuretic peptide receptor A (NPR-A) and natriuretic peptide receptor B (NPR-B) mediate the cellular and physiological actions of natriuretic hormones.

Physiologic effects of B-type natriuretic peptide

There are a number of significant physiological effects of the natriuretic peptides (Figure 24.1). BNP produces venous and arterial dilatation which leads to reduction in venous resistance and

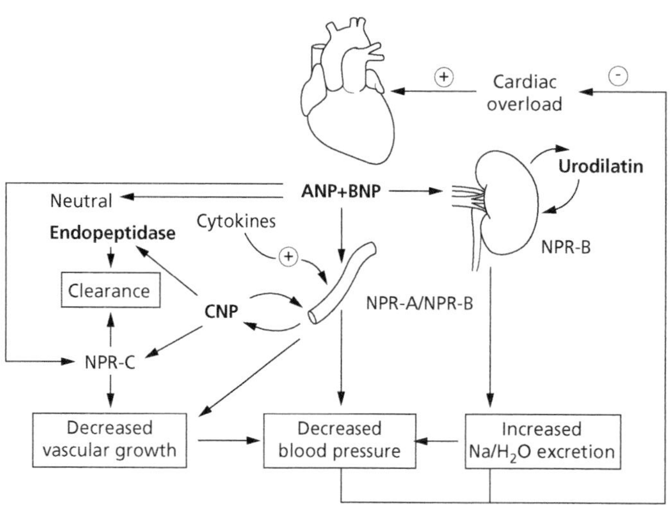

Figure 24.1. *Physiological effects of natriuretic peptides. Potential for favorable effects in patients with acute heart failure is evident (Adapted, with permission, from Wilkins* et al.[44]*)*

SVR.[13,14] BNP does not increase heart rate despite its actions to reduce preload and afterload.[14] BNP has a natriuretic effect which can produce a diuretic effect.[14–16] Changes in glomerular filtration rate (GFR) are variable but renal blood flow tends to be preserved even as volume loss occurs. Maintenance of renal function in the face of a diuretic effect may be related to the neurohormonal actions of BNP, which have been shown in some studies to limit activation of the renin-angiotensin-aldosterone system (RAAS) and endothelin system.[16,17] BNP does not appear to exert any inotropic effect, either positive or negative, on the myocardium.[18] Importantly, BNP may exert a favorable effect on myocardial oxygen supply and demand since it results in coronary vasodilation without increasing myocardial oxygen consumption.[19] Down-regulation of natriuretic receptor activity is known to reduce the physiologic actions of endogenous BNP in patients with heart failure. However, if sufficient exogenous BNP is administered (2-fold to 3-fold the maximum levels of endogenous BNP generally encountered) then substantial physiological effects occur.

B-type natriuretic peptide counterregulates pathogenic hormones

Although the therapeutic role of the neurohormonal modulating effects of BNP in AHF is uncertain, there is ample experimental evidence to indicate that this peptide antagonizes the effects of a number of toxic neurohormones that are activated in heart failure. Natriuretic peptides decrease renin release, inhibit the secretion of endothelin-1 in response to angiotensin II, and reduce the activity of the sympathetic nervous system under experimental conditions.[20–23] Data are emerging to suggest that neurohormonal antagonism by BNP may be observed in patients with heart failure. The production of aldosterone may decrease, sympathetic activity may be attenuated, and there may be a decline endothelin-1 after short-term infusion of BNP in patients with heart failure.[5,24–25]

Clinical effects of B-type natriuretic peptide in heart failure

Nesiritide, a peptide identical to human BNP and produced by recombinant technology, represents the currently available form of BNP for clinical use. This drug has been evaluated in patients with heart failure almost exclusively due to left ventricular systolic dysfunction (LVSD) with documented beneficial acute hemodynamic and neurohormonal effects.[26–29] These studies demonstrate dose-dependent reduction in filling pressure, SVR and PVR as well as increases in cardiac output (Figure 24.2).

In a randomized, double-blind, placebo-controlled study, Mills *et al.* examined the effects of

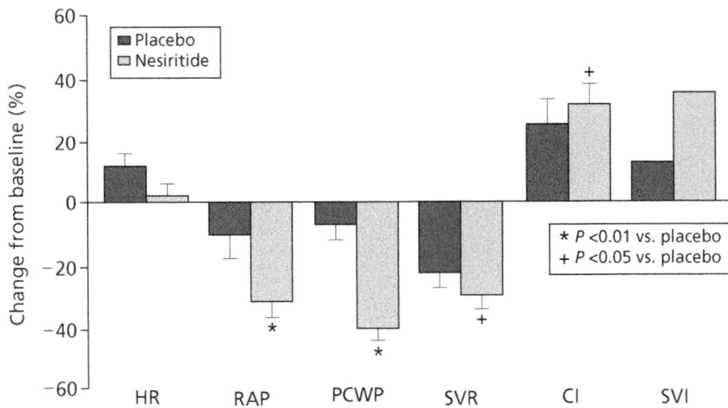

Abbreviations: CI = cardiac index; HR = heart rate; PCWP = pulmonary capillary wedge pressure; RAP = right atrial pressure; SVI = stroke volume index; SVR = systemic vascular resistance.

Figure 24.2. *Acute hemodynamic effects of nesiritide in patients with heart failure. Sixteen patients received a 4-hour continuous infusion of human B-type natriuretic peptide (hBNP) (0.025 μg/kg/min and 0.05 μg/kg/min) or placebo. Note at these doses compared to those used in the VMAC study, there is evidence of both reduction in filling pressure and systemic vascular resistance, the latter associated with an improvement in cardiac index.*[15]

a 24-hour infusion of nesiritide at 0.015 μg/kg/min, 0.03 μg/kg/min, or 0.06 μg/kg/min, preceded by a 0.25 μg/kg, 0.5 μg/kg, or 1.0 μg/kg bolus, respectively.[30] A total of 103 symptomatic patients were studied, most of whom had New York Heart Association (NYHA) class III (61%) or class IV (33%) heart failure with a low ejection fraction (EF) (= 35%) and a baseline mean pulmonary capillary wedge pressure (PCWP) of 29 mm Hg and a mean cardiac index (CI) of 1.9 L/min/m^2. The mean BNP levels at baseline were in the 800 pg/mL range in the nesiritide dose groups. Nesiritide produced a significant reduction in PCWP (27% to 39% decrease by 6 hours) as well as in mean right atrial pressure (RAP) and SVR. These changes were accompanied by a significant increase in CI and stroke volume index (SVI) with no significant effect on heart rate. Hemodynamic effects were evident at 1 hour and were sustained throughout the 24-hour infusion.

The study termed the *efficacy trial* was a randomized, double-blind, placebo-controlled, trial of 127 patients with prior moderate-to-severe heart failure due to LVSD who were hospitalized for worsening heart failure.[14] Evidence of hemodynamic compromise was require for study entry (baseline PCWP = 18 mm Hg, CI = 2.7 L/min/m^2) and systolic blood pressure had to be > 90 mm Hg. Patients were randomized to 1 of 3 treatment groups: (1) nesiritide 0.3 μg/kg intravenous bolus followed by 0.015 μg/kg/min infusion; (2) nesiritide 0.6 μg/kg intravenous bolus followed by 0.03 μg/kg/min infusion; or (3) placebo. Both doses of nesiritide resulted in significant hemodynamic and clinical improvements and urine output increased significantly. Hemodynamic responses, effects on clinical signs and symptoms of congestive heart failure, urine output, and diuretic requirements are shown in Table 24.1. In addition, the short-term treatment with nesiritide was associated with reduced plasma aldosterone levels ($P = 0.03$, comparison between the three groups).

Clinical studies of the renal effects in patients with heart failure related to LVSD show no consistent effect on GFR and renal blood flow.[31–34] The results on the effect of nesiritide on sodium excretion and urine output in these clinical studies have been more variable, with some results demonstrating enhanced urinary output and increased sodium excretion and others not. A number of hypotheses have been proposed to explain these variable effects including the dose of nesiritide employed, presence or absence of diuretic therapy, and the nature of the population studied. Despite the results of these small studies, clinical observation demonstrates that significant diuresis may occur with nesiritide, especially when given in combination with a loop diuretic. To avoid side effects related to fluid loss, careful attention to volume changes is important in these patients.

The lack of a proarrhythmic effect of nesiritide compared to dobutamine was demonstrated in a prospective randomized trial which studied 255

Table 24.1. *Efficacy trial: changes from baseline hemodynamics after 6 hours of therapy*

Hemodynamic measurement	Placebo*	Nesiritide*		*P*-value
		0.015 µg/kg/min	0.030 µg/kg/min	
Pulmonary capillary wedge pressure (mm Hg)	+2.0 ± 7.2	−6.0 ± 7.2†	−9.6 ± 6.2†	<0.001
Right atrial pressure (mm Hg)	−0.4 ± 4.6	−2.6 ± 4.4‡	−5.1 ± 4.7†	<0.001
Systemic vascular resistance (dyn/s/cm^5)	+161 ± 481	−247 ± 4.4†	−347 ± 499†	<0.001
Cardiac index (L/min/m^2)	−0.1 ± 0.47	+0.2 ± 0.49‡	+0.4 ± 0.69†	<0.001
Systolic blood pressure (mm Hg)	+0.3 ± 11	−4.4 ± 10.2	−9.3 ± 12.6†	<0.001

*Values are means + SD. *P*-values are for the comparison among all 3 groups, calculated with the omnibus F test.
†$P < 0.001$ for the pairwise comparison with placebo, by the F test.
‡$P < 0.05$ for the pairwise comparison with placebo, by the F test.

patients with decompensated heart failure who were treated with 1 of 2 doses of intravenous nesiritide (0.015 µg/kg/min or 0.03 µg/kg/min) or dobutamine (≥ 5 µg/kg/min).[35] Dobutamine significantly increased the mean number of ventricular tachycardic events per 24 hours, the repetitive ventricular beats per hour, and the number of premature ventricular beats per hour. In contrast, there was no change in these indicators of a proarrhythmic effect in the patients treated with nesiritide.

The Vasodilation in the Management of Acute Congestive Heart Failure (VMAC) study is critical to the understanding and evaluation of the role of nesiritide in patients hospitalized with decompensated heart failure.[36] This trial was conducted as a multicenter, randomized, double-blind study of 489 patients. The study compared the effects of nesiritide plus standard care, intravenous nitroglycerin plus standard care, and standard care alone in the management of patients previously treated for ADHF in the hospital setting. The trial had a complex design. Hemodynamic monitoring was part of the protocol, but it was performed at the discretion of the study investigator. For the first 3 hours after randomization, there was a placebo-controlled period which was followed by randomization into one of the two active treatment arms (while still double-blinded). VMAC used a different strategy for dosing nesiritide as compared to the efficacy trial. The drug was given as a larger bolus (2 µg/kg) and at a lower infusion rate (0.01 µg/kg/min). In the other active treatment arm of the study, intravenous nitroglycerin was titrated as clinically indicated to optimize its effects. Patients were enrolled in VMAC following an initial period of treatment which left them with dyspnea at rest or with minimal exertion (NYHA class IV symptoms) and evidence of elevated cardiac filling pressures (baseline PCWP = 20 mm Hg or clinical signs of congestion). Prior therapies included intravenous diuretics and, in some patients, administration of dopamine and dobutamine. The primary endpoints of the VMAC trial were change in PCWP (catheterized patients only) and dyspnea symptoms at 3 hours as compared to baseline.

There was hemodynamic and clinical evidence of benefit from nesiritide during the placebo-controlled period, which was more apparent with nesiritide than intravenous nitrates. When added to standard therapy, nesiritide significantly decreased PCWP as compared to both placebo and intravenous nitrates ($P < 0.001$) at the 3-hour time point. In contrast, nitroglycerin administration was not associated with a significant decline in filling pressures compared to placebo after 3 hours of treatment. Serial determinations of hemodynamics determined that nesiritide had sustained effects on filling pressure throughout 48 hours of treatment. This favorable effect on filling pressure occurred even though doses of the drug were not increased, suggesting no tolerance developed to the effects of the drug. The primary method of clinical assessment was through determination of a dyspnea score. Dyspnea was assessed using a patient self-assessment with a 7-point ordinal scale. By this measurement, dyspnea was significantly reduced with nesiritide ($P = 0.034$), but not with nitroglycerin as compared to placebo (standard therapy consisting mostly of diuretics) following 3 hours of therapy. There was no longer a placebo control by 24 hours of therapy. However, there was a trend for improvement in the other clinical assessment used in the trial—global clinical status—in patients taking nesiritide as compared to intravenous nitroglycerin (89 vs. 81% respectively, $P = 0.075$). Whether more aggressive up-titration of nitroglycerin could have improved its efficacy cannot be fully determined. However, this issue was examined in a subset of patients enrolled in the VMAC trial (Figure 24.3). At 1 site, nitroglycerin was titrated to 160 μg/min over 2 hours and filling pressures fell to a similar degree as compared to those treated with nesiritide.[37] However, there was rapid induction of tachyphylaxis to nitroglycerin when administered in this fashion and PCWP was noted to return toward baseline in several hours despite ongoing treatment with nitroglycerin.

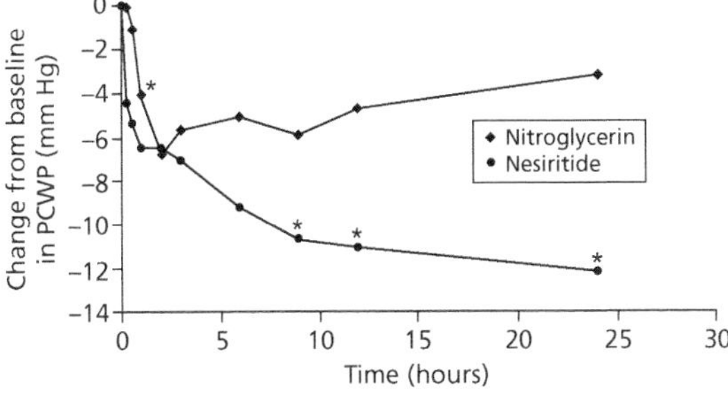

Figure 24.3. *Change in pulmonary capillary wedge pressure from baseline during 24 hours of intravenous infusion of nitroglycerin and nesiritide. Circles, nesiritide; diamonds, nitroglycerin.*

*$P < 0.05$ versus baseline.

Adverse effects

The potential side effects of nesiritide include hypotension and headache. The risk of hypotension appears to be dose dependent; in the VMAC study the occurrence of hypotension was less than in earlier trials which used higher doses of nesiritide. The incidence of symptomatic hypotension was similar in patients treated with nitroglycerin and nesiritide in the VMAC trial, while headache was significantly more common with nitroglycerin. Due to the longer effective half-life of nesiritide, hypotension with this agent may be of longer duration than that seen with nitroglycerin. In general, the risk of hypotension appears to be reduced in the presence of fluid overall. Correct assessment of fluid status will help to minimize the occurrence of this side effect. If rapid onset of hemodynamic effect is not needed, then the bolus dose of nesiritide can be omitted and this may lessen the risk of symptomatic hypotension.

To date, controlled trials of nesiritide have not been appropriately designed to determine the effect of this drug on morbidity and mortality in patients admitted with AHF. Published results of the combined analysis of the various studies that have been conducted to date have failed to produce convincing evidence of a long-term effect of this agent on mortality as compared to standard therapy or nitroglycerin. The preliminary results from a preliminary analysis of the Acute Decompensated Heart Failure National Registry (ADHERE™) data suggest that patients hospitalized with AHF who are treated with nesiritide have a similar outcome to those treated with nitroglycerin and a better outcome than those treated with inotropes.[38]

Nitroglycerin

Although recent clinical trial data to support the clinical efficacy of nitroglycerin in AHF treatment are lacking, clinical observation suggests that this drug may be effective in patients hospitalized for worsening heart failure.[39] Intravenous nitroglycerin may reduce LV filling pressure, which acts to reduce pulmonary congestion and may also reduce systemic afterload and pressure to increase stroke volume and cardiac output. Intravenous nitroglycerin may improve coronary blood flow; so it may be more effective in patients with decompensated heart failure due to acute ischemia or myocardial infarction (MI).

Studies of the efficacy of intravenous nitroglycerin in patients with heart failure and congestive symptoms are very limited.[39] Some of the best data in support of this therapy come from a trial of isosorbide dinitrate in patients with severe pulmonary congestion.[40] In this trial, 110 patients were randomized to treatment with: (1) repeated high-dose boluses of intravenous isosorbide dinitrate (3 mg every 5 minutes) plus a single 40-mg bolus of intravenous furosemide; or (2) repeated high-dose furosemide (80 mg every 15 minutes with continuous low-dose isosorbide dinitrate). These regimens were administered until oxygen saturation was > 96% or mean arterial blood pressure decreased by 30% or to < 90 mm Hg. The complications of AHF, including the need for mechanical ventilation as well as the likelihood of MI within 24 hours of admission, were reduced in the high-dose isosorbide dinitrate group versus the high-dose furosemide.

Dosing

Nitroglycerin may be given sublingually or intravenously to patients experiencing acute pulmonary edema. There are no well-established dosing regimens for nitroglycerin in patients with AHF. One reasonable approach is to give intravenous nitroglycerin at an initial dose of 5 μg/min, with subsequent titration of the infusion every 3 to 5 minutes. In the VMAC study, the median dose after 3 hours in the catheterized group was 13 μg/min (25th to 75th quartile range of 10 μg/min to 40 μg/min and in the noncatheterized group was 10 μg/min (25th to 75th quartile range of 10 μg/min to 20 μg/min).

Tolerance

Approximately 20% of patients with heart failure are resistant to any dose of nitroglycerin.[41,42] Patients who do not respond hemodynamically to high doses of intravenous nitroglycerin (> 200 μg) will not respond to further increases in dose. The rapid development of tolerance significantly limits the efficacy of nitroglycerin. Although high doses of nitroglycerin may produce rapid declines in filling pressure, tolerance occurs quickly with this method of administration. Tolerance develops to a lesser extent at lower doses, but hemodynamic benefit is likewise reduced. In the large majority of trials, nitrates were indistinguishable from placebo after 24 hours of continuous therapy, which was likely the result of nitrate tolerance. To prevent tolerance, a nitrate-free interval is recommended; however, the PCWP may become elevated during the nitrate-free interval, which would likely be undesirable during therapy for patients with AHF.

Adverse effects

The adverse effects of nitroglycerin therapy include headache and symptomatic hypotension. Hypotension is more likely when preload is low, which may occur as filling pressures decline in response to diuretic therapy. Symptomatic hypotension and headache respond to a reduction in dose but may require discontinuation of therapy. The serum half-life of nitroglycerin is approximately 3 minutes and pharmacodynamic effects closely parallel this. In most cases, the short half-life of the drug limits the duration of symptomatic hypotension.

Conclusion

Intravenous vasodilator therapy for patients admitted with AHF remains an area of active clinical investigation and significant evolution. Despite the availability of a wide variety of diuretic approaches and the substantial clinical improvement with these agents noted in many studies, the use of intravenous vasodilators is still deemed necessary in many patients admitted with ADHF. This therapy is utilized to more rapidly reduce filling pressures, especially in patients with severe pulmonary congestion, promote diuresis in patients who respond poorly to diuretic therapy, treat "low output" failure in patients with severe LVSD and poor organ perfusion, and provide more rapid relief of congestion and reduce the length of hospital stay in patients with severe volume overload.

The potential role of nesiritide in the management of patients admitted with AHF should be considered in the context of clinical trial results with other vasoactive agents traditionally considered the parenteral drugs of choice in this population. The recent OPTIME-CHF trial results show that inotropic therapy is not indicated for the management of the typical patient admitted to the hospital with ADHF.[43] Use of inotropic therapy may still be considered in patients with heart failure who have significant low-output failure or cardiogenic shock but the OPTIME-CHF results argue that these agents are not effective in patients with volume overload and preserved cardiac output. Data from the VMAC study demonstrate the safety of intravenous nitrates but do not provide convincing evidence for the efficacy of this agent in AHF. Results from trials of nitrate therapy in patients with severe congestion (acute pulmonary edema) are more encouraging but limitations have been noted. The development of tolerance to therapy appears to significantly limit the efficacy of nitroglycerin following the first few hours of treatment and may not be effectively overcome even with increasing doses. This tachyphylaxis may limit therapeutic response, especially when large hemodynamically-effective doses are administered to achieve rapid symptom relief in patients with ADHF. The role of nesiritide in the treatment of ADHF continues to be defined. The best agent for the treatment of ADHF remains to be defined.

References

1. Adams KF, Fonarow GC, Emerman CL, *et al.* Characteristics and outcomes of patients hospitalized for heart failure in the United States: Rationale, design, and preliminary observations from the first 100000 cases in the Acute Decompensated Heart Failure National Registry (ADHERE™). Am Heart J 2005; 149: 209–216.
2. Mackway-Jones, K. Towards evidence based emergency medicine: best BETs from the Manchester Royal Infirmary. Emerg Med J 2003; 1: 61.
3. Burger MR, Burger AJ. BNP in decompensated heart failure: diagnostic, prognostic and therapeutic potential. Curr Opin Investig Drugs 2001; 2: 929–935.
4. Hobbs RE, Mills RM, Young JB. An update on nesiritide for treatment of decompensated heart failure. Expert Opin Investig Drugs 2001; 10: 935–942.
5. Colucci WS. Nesiritide for the treatment of decompensated heart failure. J Card Fail 2001; 7: 92–100.
6. Brunner-La Rocca HP, Kiowski W, Ramsay D, Sutsch G. Therapeutic benefits of increasing natriuretic peptide levels. Cardiovasc Res 2001; 51: 510–520.
7. Chen HH, Burnett JC. Natriuretic peptides in the pathophysiology of congestive heart failure. Curr Cardiol Rep 2000; 2: 198–205.
8. Mattingly MT, Brandt RR, Heublein DM, Wei CM, Nir A, Burnett JC Jr. Presence of C-type natriuretic peptide in human kidney and urine. Kidney Int 1994; 46: 744–747.
9. Suzuki T, Yamazaki T,Yazaki Y. The role of the natriuretic peptides in the cardiovascular system. Cardiovasc Res 2001; 51: 489–494.
10. Silberbach M, Roberts CT Jr. Natriuretic peptide signaling: molecular and cellular pathways to growth regulation. Cell Signal 2001; 13: 221–231.
11. Kone BC. Molecular biology of natriuretic peptides and nitric oxide synthases. Cardiovasc Res 2001; 51: 429–441.
12. Richards AM, Lainchbury JG, Nicholls MG, Cameron AV, Yandle TG. Dendroaspis natriuretic peptide: endogenous or dubious? Lancet 2002; 359: 5–6.
13. Protter AA, Wallace AM, Ferraris VA, Weishaar RE. Relaxant effect of human brain natriuretic peptide on human artery and vein tissue. Am J Hypertens 1996; 9: 432–436.
14. Colucci WS, Elkayam U, Horton DP, *et al.* Intravenous nesiritide, a natriuretic peptide, in the treatment of decompensated congestive heart failure. Nesiritide Study Group. N Engl J Med 2000; 343: 246–253.
15. Abraham WT, Lowes BD, Ferguson DA, *et al.* Systemic hemodynamic, neurohormonal, and renal effects of a steady-state infusion of human brain natriuretic peptide in patients with hemodynamically decompensated heart failure. J Card Fail 1998; 4: 37–44.
16. Jensen KT, Carstens J, Pedersen EB. Effect of BNP on renal hemodynamics, tubular function and vasoactive hormones in humans. Am J Physiol 1998; 274: F63–F72.
17. La Villa G, Fronzaroli C, Lazzeri C, *et al.* Cardiovascular and renal effects of low dose brain natriuretic peptide infusion in man. J Clin Endocrinol Metab 1994; 78: 1166–1171.
18. Hirose M, Furukawa Y, Kurogouchi F, *et al.* C-type natriuretic peptide increases myocardial contractility

and sinus rate mediated by guanylyl cyclase-linked natriuretic peptide receptors in isolated, blood-perfused dog heart preparations. J Pharmacol Exp Ther 1998; 286: 70–76.

19. Okumura K, Yasue H, Fujii H, *et al.* Effects of brain (B-type) natriuretic peptide on coronary artery diameter and coronary hemodynamic variables in humans: comparison with effects on systemic hemodynamic variables. J Am Coll Cardiol 1995; 25: 342–348.
20. Akabane S, Matsushima Y, Matsuo H, *et al.* Effects of brain natriuretic peptide on renin secretion in normal and hypertonic saline-infused kidney. Eur J Pharmacol 1991; 198: 143–148.
21. Kohno M, Yokokawa K, Horio T, *et al.* Atrial and brain natriuretic peptides inhibit the endothelin–1 secretory response to angiotensin II in porcine aorta. Circ Res 1992; 70: 241–247
22. Abramson BL, Ando S, Notarius CF, Rongen GA, Floras JS. Effect of atrial natriuretic peptide on muscle sympathetic activity and its reflex control in human heart failure. Circulation 1999; 99: 1810–1815.
23. Wada A, Tsutamoto T, Matsuda Y, Kinoshita M, Cardiorenal and neurohumoral effects of endogenous atrial natriuretic peptide in dogs with severe congestive heart failure using a specific antagonist for guanylate cyclase-coupled receptors. Circulation 1994; 89: 2232–2240.
24. Brunner-La Rocca HP, Kaye DM, Woods RL, Hastings J, Esler MD. Effects of intravenous brain natriuretic peptide on regional sympathetic activity in patients with chronic heart failure as compared with healthy control subjects. J Am Coll Cardiol 2001; 37: 1221–1227.
25. Aronson D, Burger A. Effect of nesiritide on endothelin–1 levels in patients with decompensated congestive heart failure. J Am Coll Cardiol 2001; 37: 148A (Abstract).
26. Adams KF Jr., Mathur VS, Gheorghiade M. B-type natriuretic peptide: from bench to bedside. Am Heart J 2003; 145: S34–S46.
27. Hayashi M, Tsutamoto T, Wada A, *et al.* Intravenous atrial natriuretic peptide prevents left ventricular remodeling in patients with first acute anterior myocardial infarction. J Am Coll Cardiol 2001; 37: 1820–1826.
28. Hobbs RE, Miller LW, Bott-Silverman C, James KB, Rincon G, Grossbard EB. Hemodynamic effects of a single intravenous injection of synthetic human brain natriuretic peptide in patients with heart failure secondary to ischemic or idiopathic dilated cardiomyopathy. Am J Cardiol 1996; 78: 896–901.
29. Marcus LS, Hart D, Packer M, *et al.* Hemodynamic and renal excretory effects of human brain natriuretic peptide infusion in patients with congestive heart failure: a double-blind, placebo-controlled, randomized crossover trial. Circulation 1996; 94: 3184–3189.
30. Mills RM, LeJemtel TH, Horton DP, *et al.* Sustained hemodynamic effects of an infusion of nesiritide (human b-type natriuretic peptide) in heart failure: a randomized, double-blind, placebo-controlled clinical trial. Natrecor Study Group. J Am Coll Cardiol 1999; 34: 155–162.
31. Wang DJ, Dowling TC, *et al.* Nesiritide does not improve renal function in patients with chronic heart failure and worsening serum creatinine. Circulation 2004; 110: 1620–1625.
32. Lainchbury JG, Richards AM, Nicholls MG, *et al.* The effects of pathophysiological increments in brain natriuretic peptide in left ventricular systolic dysfunction. Hypertension 1997; 30: 398–404.
33. Abraham WT, Lowes BD, Ferguson DA, *et al.* Systemic hemodynamic, neurohormonal, and renal effects of a steady-state infusion of human brain natriuretic peptide in patients with hemodynamically decompensated heart failure. J Card Fail 1998; 4: 37–44.
34. Jensen KT, Eiskjaer H, Carstens J, Pedersen EB. Renal effects of brain natriuretic peptide in patients with congestive heart failure. Clin Sci (Lond) 1999; 96: 5–15.
35. Burger AJ, Aronson D, Horton DP, Burger MR. Comparison of the effects of dobutamine and nesiritide (B-type natriuretic peptide) on ventricular ectopy in acutely decompensated ischemic versus non-ischemic cardiomyopathy. Am J Cardiol 2003; 91: 1370–1372.
36. Publication Committee for the VMAC Investigators (Vasodilatation in the Management of Acute CHF). Intravenous nesiritide vs nitroglycerin for treatment of decompensated congestive heart failure: a randomized controlled trial. JAMA 2002; 287: 1531–1540.
37. Elkayam U, Akhter MW, Singh H, Khan S, Usman A. Comparison of effects on left ventricular filling pressure of intravenous nesiritide and high-dose nitroglycerin in patients with decompensated heart failure. Am J Cardiol 2004; 93: 237–240.
38. Abraham WT, Adams KF, Fonarow GC, *et al.* ADHERE™ Scientific Advisory Committee and Investigators. Comparison of in-hospital mortality in patients treated with nesiritide vs other parenteral vasoactive medications for acutely decompensated heart failure: an analysis from a large prospective registry database. J Card Fail 2003; 9: S81 (Abstract).

39. Elkayam U, Bitar F, Akhter MW, *et al.* Intravenous nitroglycerin in the treatment of decompensated heart failure: potential benefits and limitations. J Cardiovasc Pharmacol Ther 2004; 9: 227–241.
40. Cotter G, Metzkor E, Kaluski E, *et al.* Randomized trial of high-dose isosorbide dinitrate plus low-dose furosemide versus high-dose furosemide plus low-dose isosorbide dinitrate in severe pulmonary oedema. Lancet 1998; 351: 389–393.
41. Fung HL, Bauer JA. Mechanisms of nitrate tolerance. Cardiovasc Drugs Ther 1994; 8: 489–499.
42. Elkayam U. Nitrates in the treatment of congestive heart failure. Am J Cardiol 1996; 77: 41C–51C.
43. Cuffe MS, Califf RM, Adams KF Jr., *et al.* Outcomes of a Prospective Trial of Intravenous Milrinone for Exacerbations of Chronic Heart Failure (OPTIME-CHF) Investigators. Short-term intravenous milrinone for acute exacerbation of chronic heart failure: a randomized controlled trial. JAMA 2002; 287: 1541–1547.
44. Wilkins MR, Redondo J, Brown LA. The natriuretic-peptide family. Lancet 1997; 349: 1307–1310.

CHAPTER 25

Pacing therapy for acute decompensated heart failure

Aysha Arshad, Shahriar Iravanian, Jonathan S Steinberg

Introduction

Heart failure remains a major cardiovascular health problem, afflicting millions of people worldwide. Despite effective medical therapy, which has reduced the morbidity and mortality from this condition, many patients remain severely limited and continue to be at risk for sudden death. Deaths in patients who are less functionally limited tend to be arrhythmic in nature, while in patients with more advanced heart failure, deaths from progressive pump failure predominate.

A normal electrical activation sequence is essential for optimal pump function of the heart. Pathological involvement of the natural pacemaker and conduction pathways, including sinus node, atria, atrioventricular (AV) node, His bundle, bundle branches, and Purkinje fibers may cause derangement in the coordinated cardiac electrical activity, resulting in deterioration in cardiac performance. Pacing therapy can substitute, augment or bypass the diseased section of the conduction system and improve cardiac electrical and hemodynamic function. Pacing goals might include rate support, maintenance of AV synchrony, or reversal of ventricular dyssynchrony. Several studies have shown hemodynamic and clinical improvement from AV sequential pacing or biventricular (BV) pacing in subsets of patients with intractable heart failure (Figure 25.1). BV pacing is achieved by using

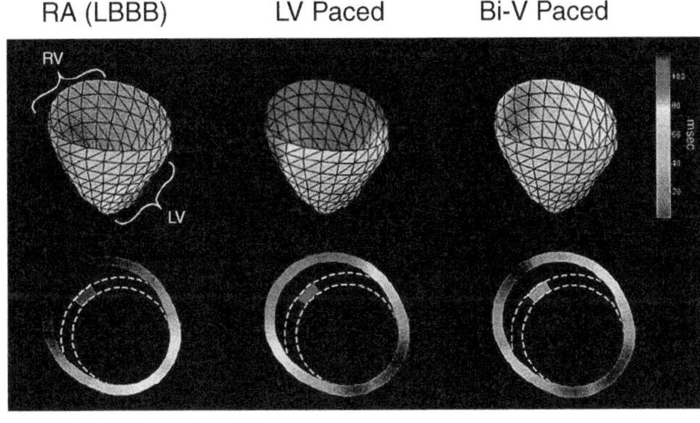

Figure 25.1. *Electrical response with different pacing modes. Top row: Electrical epicardial activation map of whole heart for three pacing modes. Activation time is color coded (blue early → red late). With right atrial (RA) pacing (left bundle branch block [LBBB]), electrical activation spreads from right to left, whereas LV pacing reversed the pattern but did not reduce conduction delay. Biventricular (BV) pacing, however, showed improved electrical synchrony. Bottom row: Short-axis slice demonstrating that activation time at the endocardial septum was similar to that at epicardial electrodes over the same region. (With permission from Leclercq* et al.[74]*). See color plate section.*

the coronary sinus to access the epicardial left ventricle via the cardiac veins.

The role of pacing in acute heart failure (AHF) is different from its role in chronic, compensated failure. Pacing is clearly indicated in the case of acute bradycardia or AV block accompanied by pulmonary edema or heart failure decompensation. Pacing is also approved for use in patients with chronic stable heart failure with intraventricular conduction delay (cardiac resynchronization therapy). This chapter describes the spectrum of pacing options for patients with acute decompensated heart failure (ADHF).

Atrioventricular and Ventricular Synchrony

Normal activation pattern and contribution to mechanical homeostasis

The normal cardiac activation sequence contributes significantly to its performance as a pump. An impulse originating in the sinus node must traverse the right atrium to reach the AV node. Although there are no anatomic data supporting the presence of internodal tracts that facilitate internodal conduction, preferential pathways of atrial conduction exist and are related to the spatial and geometric arrangements of myocardial fibers. The sinus node is situated at the upper part of the sulcus terminalis, to the right of the opening of the superior vena cava into the right atrium. Once initiated, the cardiac impulse spreads through the atrial myocardium to reach the AV node. The AV node is situated in the lower part of the atrial septum above the attachment of the septal cusp of the tricuspid valve. The cardiac impulse is conducted to the ventricles by the AV bundle. This descends behind the septal cusp of the tricuspid valve to reach the inferior border of the membranous part of the ventricular septum and then divides into the bundle branches. The AV node conduction time accounts for the majority of the transit time between the atrium and ventricle. AV conduction delay can vary greatly with changes in the patient's clinical state and autonomic tone. An optimal AV delay results in near complete emptying of the atria before ventricles contract and close the tricuspid and mitral valves.

The activation of ventricles begins from the His bundle, which divides after a short distance into the right and left bundle branches. The right bundle branch is a discrete conduction pathway that travels on the right side of the septum, does not supply any branch to it, and inserts at the endocardial surface of the right ventricle apex. In contrast, the left bundle branch almost immediately divides into multiple branches, which form two functional pathways, the anterior and posterior fascicles. These branches travel on the left side of the interventricular septum and provide a rich supply of Purkinje fibers to it. Both the left and right conduction systems continue in the ventricular free walls as a dense network of Purkinje fibers on the endocardial surface.

During normal conduction, the first area of the ventricles to be activated is the left side of the septum through the branches of the left bundle, followed in a few milliseconds by the right ventricular (RV) apex, which is activated through the right bundle branch. The activation wave in the free walls then propagates from the apex toward the base and from the endocardial surface toward the epicardial surface. In the septum, the activation propagates from the left toward the right. Such a normal activation sequence has electrophysiological consequences apparent on the surface electrocardiogram (ECG). The activation of the septum from left to right generates a small r wave in lead V_1 and, usually, a corresponding q wave in lateral leads (V_5, V_6, I, aVL). The near simultaneous activation of the two ventricles through the specialized conduction system results in a narrow QRS complex. In fact, a major contributor to the width of the normal QRS complex is the time it takes for the depolarization wave to travel from the endocardial to the epicardial surface.

In addition to defining the normal QRS complex, the activation pattern has important hemodynamic consequences. The activation of the septum from left to right means that the interventricular septum, even though anatomically shared between the two ventricles, functionally behaves as part of the left ventricle. Near simultaneous contraction of the ventricles and the apex to base activation sequence reduces the amount of back flow during systole and improves the pumping performance of the heart.

How Abnormal Pacemaker Function and Conduction Patterns May Contribute to Heart Failure

Sinus Bradycardia

Cardiac output is equal to the product of the heart rate and stroke volume (SV). In a normal heart a sudden decrease in heart rate can be almost completely compensated for by increase in stroke volume (for example, by the Frank–Starling mechanism). However, in a failing heart, which has already saturated the compensatory mechanisms, heart rate is a major determinant of cardiac output. Medications that are commonly used in the treatment of heart failure, including beta-blockers and many antiarrhythmic agents, often aggravate resting bradycardia and produce chronotropic incompetence. Bradycardia is capable of worsening heart failure state and functional status even if the bradycardia is not profound and not associated with arrhythmic symptoms.

There is also evidence that bradycardia may be a relatively important mechanism for sudden cardiac death in patients with advanced heart failure. To define the mechanisms of unexpected cardiac arrest in advanced heart failure, data were reviewed from electrocardiographic monitoring and from clinical and autopsy data in patients hospitalized for cardiac transplantation evaluation and management of advanced heart failure (mean EF of 0.18 ± 0.08) who were stable while on vasodilator and diuretic therapy. Luu and Stevenson found that 21 cardiac arrests occurred in 20 out of 216 patients during a 4-year period. The rhythm at the time of arrest was severe bradycardia or electromechanical dissociation in 13 patients (62%), whereas arrests in 21 patients (38%) occurred due to ventricular tachycardia or ventricular fibrillation.[1]

Intraatrial conduction delay

In individuals with normal diastolic function, the percentage of contribution to total LV filling occurring during atrial filling has been estimated as 13% to 36%.[2] Atrial contraction assists in the diastolic filling of the ventricle, and the increased ventricular volume may augment contractility by the Frank–Starling mechanism. The loss of the atrial contribution to filling can be deleterious to patients who have abnormal diastolic function, outflow obstruction, or both. The importance of atrial contraction in patients with heart failure is more controversial. Despite some reports to the contrary, most of the evidence accumulated on patients with heart failure with elevated filling pressures indicates that loss of the atrial contribution to filling is poorly tolerated. Tyberg *et al.* concluded that in the presence of an intact pericardium, atrial systole shifts the stroke-volume end-diastolic pressure relation because it alters the end-diastolic pressure-diameter relation, and improves left ventricular (LV) performance by increasing preload.[3] In a recent study, pacing modes were studied in 21 subjects with heart failure and conduction system disease.[4] Comparisons were made between pacing in atrial inhibited (AAI), ventricular inhibited (VVI), and dual-chamber (DDD) pacemaker modes. The pacing rate was kept constant in each patient and the order of testing was randomized. Compared with AAI pacing, there was no improvement in any hemodynamic parameter with DDD pacing from either RV site. Hemodynamic function worsened after VVI pacing from both RV sites, due to AV dyssynchrony. AAI pacing did not have associated adverse hemodynamics since AV synchrony and the atrial contribution to ventricular filling were maintained.

Conduction delay in the left atrium is more common than in the right atrium. A correlation between left atrial (LA) size and ECG LA enlargement is best seen in rheumatic and primary myocardial disease, but poorly seen in patients with coronary artery disease (CAD). Studies have demonstrated a prolonged P-wave duration on signal-averaged ECG to be an independent predictor of future atrial fibrillation (AF), common in heart failure, in susceptible populations.[5] Age-related atrial conduction delay also occurs and is detectable on signal-averaged ECG.[6] With increasing LA conduction delay, LA systole may occur substantially later than right atrial (RA) contraction causing RA/LA as well as LA/LV dyssynchrony and related hemodynamic consequences. This loss of the atrial contribution to filling can be especially deleterious to individuals with stiff noncompliant ventricles.

First degree atrioventricular block

Hemodynamic parameters may be markedly affected by AV conduction time. A marked prolongation of the AV conduction time (i.e., an AV interval > 0.3 s) causes AV dyssynchrony and reduces the ejection fraction (EF). When atrial and ventricular activation are synchronous, there is a detrimental effect on chamber filling and increased atrial pressures. Shortening a prolonged interval can diminish mitral regurgitation (MR), lengthen the time available for diastolic filling, and alter the filling pattern from one characterized principally by an early-filling wave to one with more physiologically balanced early and late (atrial) filling components. The latter pattern should also lower mean atrial pressures.[7]

This was shown in another study in which AV delay was varied broadly and in a highly controlled manner.[8] Although the relationship between percentage of improvement in dP/dt_{max} and AV delay displays a decrease at either extreme, there is a broad mid-region where the precise delay makes little difference.

Hemodynamic parameters during dual-chamber pacing can be affected by AV conduction time. Fifteen patients with severe LV systolic dysfunction were studied acutely during AV sequential pacing at various AV intervals (60, 100, 120, 140, 180, and 240 ms) with the use of combined Doppler velocity curves and pressures obtained by high fidelity manometer-tipped catheters and thermodilution cardiac output.[9] In patients with prolonged PR intervals > 200 ms, cardiac output was significantly increased when AV sequential pacing at the optimal AV interval to output was compared with that at the baseline state, because timing of mechanical atrial and ventricular synchrony was optimized. Dual-chamber pacing may improve acute hemodynamic variables in patients with dilated cardiomyopathy, mainly by optimizing the timing of mechanical atrial and ventricular synchrony.[9,10] Reestablishment of the optimal diastolic filling period and abolition of diastolic MR may also contribute to hemodynamic improvement.

This relationship is complex and may be affected by variables such as interatrial conduction time, level of hydration, afterload, degree of diastolic dysfunction, and interventricular conduction delay. This is even more important in the heart failure population where a small reduction in cardiac performance may adversely affect functional status.

Second and third degree atrioventricular block

Type I second degree AV block, which is relatively common, is due to intermittent failure of conduction through the AV node. It may be a manifestation of a pathologic process, precipitated by a variety of commonly used medications (e.g., beta-blockers, amiodarone), or physiologic at certain rates or during periods of enhanced vagal tone (e.g., sleep). Type I second degree AV block, especially when associated with a normal QRS duration, is generally benign but may cause symptoms due to varying RR intervals or lowered effective heart rate.

Type II second degree AV block results from failure of conduction in the specialized system below the AV node and is pathologic. It often occurs in association with complete, or third degree heart block, or heralds its occurrence. The presence of second degree AV block of any type may aggravate heart failure by reducing heart rate and thus cardiac output. There may be hemodynamic consequences to concomitant AV delay with varying intervals in type I, and in type II due to a loss of AV synchrony.

Complete AV block, third degree AV block, may be associated with consequences of a slow ventricular escape rate, AV dyssynchrony, loss of atrial contribution to filling, and a broad QRS escape rhythm. The risk of asystole, torsade de pointes, shock, syncope, cardiac arrest, or death is always present in this situation.

Short atrioventricular delay

The value of altering the AV interval has been investigated when applied to patients undergoing dual-chamber pacing. AV conduction delay may have acute hemodynamic effects, but shortening the AV conduction period may not prove beneficial. Gold *et al.* examined the effect of dual-chamber pacing with a short AV delay in a randomized study of 12 patients with chronic congestive heart failure (CHF) despite optimal medical therapy.[11] On the day after implantation of a dual-chamber pacemaker, invasive hemodynamic measurements were made at varying AV delays from 100 to 200 ms. Patients were then randomized to either DDD pacing or backup VVI at 40 bpm. After 4 to 6 weeks crossover to the other pacing mode was programmed. Hemodynamic measurements on the day after pacemaker implantation demonstrated no benefit of pacing with any AV delay compared with intrinsic conduction. No patient had an increase in EF nor did any patient improve in New York Heart Association (NYHA) class. It was concluded that dual-chamber pacing with a short AV delay does not improve hemodynamic and clinical status or EF in patients with CHF. Liebold *et al.* found that dual-chamber pacing with a short AV delay failed to improve hemodynamics in patients after coronary artery bypass grafting (CABG). AV delay in this study was shortened from 160 to 40 ms in DDD mode and from 100 to 40 ms in VDD mode.[12] Some reports suggest that a short AV delay may improve hemodynamics but only in patients with isolated pure MR.[13]

Wide QRS and Bundle Branch Block

There are two main types of electrical dyssynchrony: AV dyssynchrony and interventricular/intraventricular (IV) dyssynchrony. Ventricular dyssynchrony is any derangement in the normal activation pattern of the ventricles. It could present as the loss of coordination between the two ventricles (interventricular or BV dyssynchrony) or delayed and discoordinate activation within the left ventricle (intraventricular dyssynchrony). The conventional marker of possible ventricular dyssynchrony is widening of the QRS complex to more than 120 ms, usually manifest as a bundle branch block on the surface ECG. Left bundle branch block (LBBB) may result from the involvement of discrete specialized branches or the more distal ramifications of the conduction system and intraventricular conduction delay (IVCD) usually

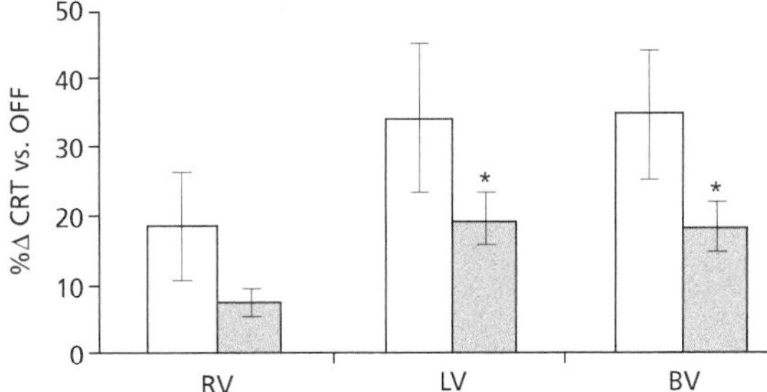

Figure 25.2. *Hemodynamic response with differential site pacing. Improvement in lateral and septal phase relationship (open bars) and peak positive LV pressure (shaded bars) displayed as the percent change from no pacing (OFF) for every cardiac resynchronization (CRT) mode (right ventricular [RV], left ventricular [LV], and biventricular [BV]). Lateral and septal phase relationship is an echocardiographic measure of synchrony. Data are presented as the mean value ± SEM. Number of patients = 16, *P < 0.001 in comparison to RV (With permission from Breithardt* et al.[73]*)*

results from diffuse involvement of the conduction system, including the free walls. The prevalence of intraventricular conduction delay of any kind in patients with dilated cadiomyopathy and heart failure is 12% to 40%.[14–17]

The presence of LBBB has been found to be an independent predictor of mortality in CHF. In a review of the Italian Congestive Heart Failure Registry, which included 5517 patients, the presence of LBBB (QRS > 140 ms) was associated with an increased 1-year mortality rate (hazard ratio [HR] 1.58, 95% confidence interval [CI] 1.21–2.06). In a multivariate analysis, QRS duration was associated with a significant increase in deaths even after adjustment for age, cardiac disease etiology, use of beta-blockers and angiotensin-converting enzyme (ACE) inhibitors.[18] Other studies have confirmed this finding.[18–20]

Deleterious effects of right ventricular pacing

Abnormal, ineffective, and delayed contraction of the ventricles is termed mechanical dyssynchrony (Figure 25.2). In view of the importance of a well-choreographed activation sequence on hemodynamics and systolic performance of the heart, mechanical dyssynchrony can result in a decrease in the stroke volume. Experimentally, it has been shown that mechanical dyssynchrony reduces the EF, time for aortic ejection, and LV dP/dt_{max}, and increases LV end-systolic and diastolic volumes. When ventricular pacing techniques were initially developed, the RV apex was selected preferentially because it was accessible and provided good pacing and sensing characteristics with an acceptable incidence of lead dislodgement. Consequently, pacing from the RV apex causes an abnormal activation pattern, which functionally mimics the electrophysiological properties of LBBB and has potentially the same hemodynamic effects. There are many potential reasons why RV pacing, in general, and RV apical pacing, in particular, may be suboptimal. RV pacing has been shown to produce paradoxical septal motion and to interfere with the normal functioning of the mitral apparatus, potentially causing mitral insufficiency. In addition, it affects diastolic function and reduces diastolic filling time.[21] Rosenqvist *et al.* evaluated the relative hemodynamic importance of a normal LV activation sequence compared to AV synchrony with respect to systolic and diastolic function.[22] Twelve patients with intact AV conduction and AV sequential pacemakers underwent radionuclide studies at rest and Doppler echocardiographic studies at rest and during submaximal exercise, comparing AAI to DDD and VVI. Studies at rest were performed at a constant heart rate between pacing modes, and the exercise study was performed at a constant heart rate and workload. Cardiac output was higher during AAI than during both DDD and VVI modes (6.2 ± 1 vs. 5.6 ± 1 and 5.3 ± 1 L/min, respectively, $P < 0.05$). Likewise, LVEF was higher during AAI ($55 \pm 12\%$ vs. $49 \pm 11\%$ vs. $51 \pm 13\%$, respectively, $P < 0.05$). VVI or DDD pacing was associated with a paradoxical septal motion pattern, resulting in a 25% impairment of regional septal EF. In addition, LV contraction duration was more homogeneous during AAI. They concluded that normal ventricular activation is a prerequisite for optimal LV function. Pacing systems allowing a normal ventricular activation pattern (AAI or DDD with a long AV delay) are preferred for patients who have intact AV conduction but require artificial pacing.[22]

Aurrichio *et al.* studied 27 patients with severe LV systolic dysfunction and LV conduction disorder who were implanted with endocardial pacing leads in the right atrium and right ventricle and epicardial lead on the LV, and instrumented with micromanometer catheters in the LV, aorta, and RV (Figure 25.3). Patients in normal sinus rhythm were stimulated in the RV, LV, or both ventricles simultaneously at preselected AV delays in a repeating 5-paced/15-nonpaced beat sequence. Maximum LV pressure derivative (dP/dt_{max}) and aortic pulse

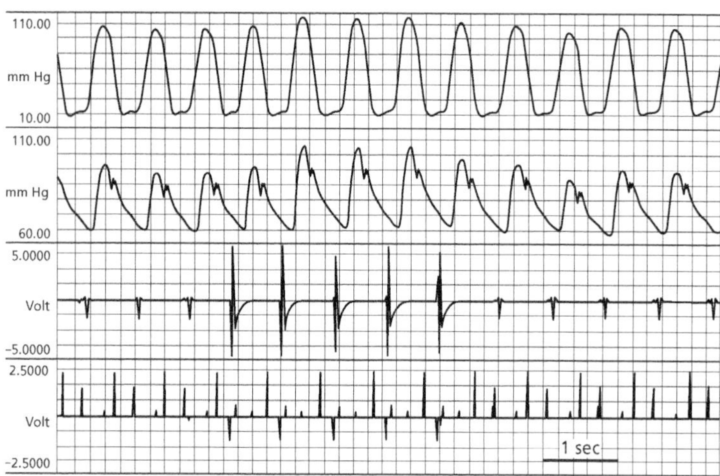

Figure 25.3. *Hemodynamic effect of left ventricular (LV) pacing. Simultaneous recording of LV pressure waveforms and electrograms during a transient LV pacing sequence in VDD mode. Immediate changes of LV pressure, LV positive dP/dt_{max}, and aortic pressure occur when pacing starts, as indicated by larger potentials in electrogram. (With permission from Auricchio* et al.[8]*)*

pressure (PP) changed immediately at pacing onset, increasing at a patient-specific optimal AV delay in 20 patients with wide surface QRS (180 ± 622 ms) and decreasing at short AV delays in 5 patients with narrower QRS (128 ± 612 ms, $P = 0.0001$). Overall, BV and LV pacing increased dP/dt_{max} and PP more than RV pacing ($P = 0.01$), whereas LV pacing increased dP/dt_{max} more than BV pacing ($P = 0.01$). They concluded CHF patients with sufficiently wide surface QRS benefit from atrial-synchronous ventricular pacing, LV stimulation is required for maximum acute benefit, and the maximum benefit at any site occurs with a patient-specific AV delay.[8]

Whether pacing is performed from the RV apex or RV outflow tract, hemodynamics are comparable. To assess the effects of pacing site and mode on acute hemodynamic function, Gold *et al.* evaluated subjects with heart failure and intrinsic conduction disease. Hemodynamic measurements were compared in AAI, VVI, and DDD modes with pacing from the RV apex or high septum. Compared with AAI pacing, there were no improvements in any hemodynamic parameter with DDD pacing from either RV site. Hemodynamic function worsened with VVI pacing from either RV site. Subgroup analysis of patients with dilated cardiomyopathy, with prolonged PR, with or without significant MR, failed to demonstrate an improvement with pacing.[11]

RV apical pacing causes dyssynchronous LV contraction, decreased LVEF, myocardial perfusion defects, mitral and tricuspid valvular insufficiency, altered diastolic function, diminution of diastolic filling time, and an increase in serum catecholamine concentrations.[11] There are important hemodynamic and physiological consequences to pacing in this mode. These effects have been observed in a host of recent studies manifesting as increases in heart failure hospitalization and occurrence of AF. This has also directly been observed in one randomized controlled trial. The MOde Selection Trial (MOST) suggested that the likelihood of heart failure hospitalization and occurrence of AF was associated not with pacing mode but with a pattern of > 40% of RV pacing (Figure 25.4).[23]

Multicenter Automatic Defibrillator Implantation Trial (MADIT) II evaluated the prophylactic benefit in CAD patients with a LVEF of < 30%, and reported that heart failure hospitalizations increased in those with implantable cardioverter defibrillator (ICD), although mortality was reduced.[24] In a MADIT II substudy, Steinberg *et al.* looked into the relationship of RV pacing and outcome.[25] They concluded that high utilization of RV pacing in post-infarction patients with severe LV dysfunction was associated with an increased risk of CHF and with ventricular tachycardia/fibrillation requiring ICD therapy. This clearly indicates that in patients with ICD, special programming features for pacing must be considered unless there is a demonstrable need for both anti-bradycardia and ventricular pacing.

Recently, the adverse consequences of RV pacing and a paced left bundle were also observed

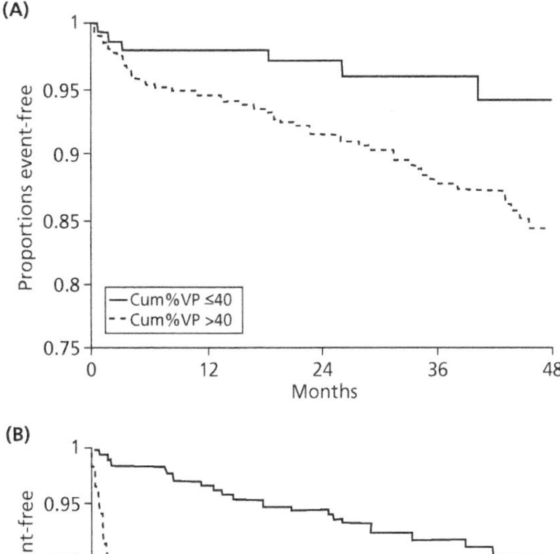

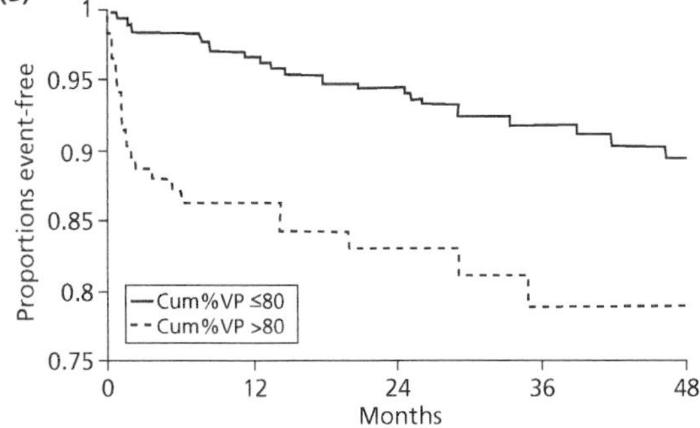

Figure 25.4. *Kaplan-Meier rates of freedom from first heart failure hospitalization by percent ventricular paced during the first 30 days in the MOST trial. (A) DDDR mode; (B) VVIR mode (With permission from Sweeney* et al.*[23])*

in a prospective trial. The Dual Chamber and VVI Implantable Defibrillator (DAVID) trial was a single-blind parallel group randomized clinical trial to determine the efficacy of dual-chamber pacing compared with backup ventricular pacing in patients with standard indications for ICD but without indications for anti-bradycardia pacing. It was concluded that dual-chamber pacing offered no advantage over ventricular backup pacing and may be detrimental by increasing the combined endpoint of death or hospitalization from heart failure (Figure 25.5). One-year survival free of the composite endpoint was 83.9% for patients treated with VVI-40 as compared with 73.3% for patients treated with DDDR-70 (HR 1.61, 95% CI 1.06–2.44).[26]

Atrial fibrillation

The most dramatic example of AV electrical dyssynchrony is AF, where complete loss of the atrial "kick" results in a fall in the stroke volume of approximately 20%.[26,27] In susceptible hearts, for example in hypertrophic hearts with diastolic relaxation abnormalities, the loss of atrial contribution to stroke volume may precipitate acute pulmonary edema. In a cohort of patients aged ≥ 65 years who had abnormal LV diastolic relaxation, studies suggested the presence of increased risk of both heart failure and AF, with the highest risks evident in those with the largest left atria.[28] It is not known whether AF itself contributes to mortality or whether it is a marker for more severe disease or comorbid conditions. Direct compromise of cardiac function as result of the adverse hemodynamic effects of AF, the increased risk of arterial thromboembolism, and the deleterious effects of antiarrhythmic therapy may all contribute. Furthermore, irregularity of the cardiac cycle can decrease cardiac output and elevate filling pressures.[29] A rapid ventricular rate may aggravate heart failure and occasionally cause cardiomyopathy.[30] Together AF and CHF create a vicious cycle—heart failure promotes AF and AF aggravates heart failure.[31]

Cardiac Resynchronization Therapy

The goal of cardiac resynchronization therapy (CRT) is to restore AV and IV synchrony. CRT is achieved by pacing via atrial and RV and LV leads. The RV lead is usually placed transvenously in the apical region of the right ventricle, whereas the LV lead is placed on the epicardial surface by transvenous passage through the coronary sinus.

With the advent of modern heart failure pharmacotherapy in the early 1990s, including ACE inhibitors and beta-blockers, it became clear that some patients would not improve significantly even after optimal medical therapy. Pacing therapy as an adjuvant modality was considered an attractive option in these patients. Initially, dual-chamber pacemakers were used in an attempt to compensate for abnormal AV delay, with negative or at best mixed success.[9–11] The failure of dual-chamber pacing to significantly improve hemodynamic status in the majority of patients with advanced heart failure focused the attention of researchers on the body of work related to the deleterious effects of RV pacing or intrinsic LBBB on the functional performance of the left ventricle.

As early as 1964, it was shown that pacing site affects cardiac output in an experimental dog model.[32] Further studies showed that RV pacing not only decreased cardiac output, it also negatively affected the LV relaxation and consequently precipitated diastolic dysfunction.[33,34] Widened QRS complex—not only because of acquired block secondary to RV pacing but from any etiology—is a specific, albeit not sensitive, indicator of decreased EF.[19] This effect is partly mediated by the loss of septal contribution in patients with LBBB.[35] In the early 1990s, BV pacing was proposed as a method to restore synchrony and improve LV pump function, especially in patients with drug-refractory heart failure and prolonged QRS complex. Early studies clearly demonstrated the acute hemodynamic benefits of CRT.

The introduction of coronary sinus leads, placed transvenously, changed the prospect for the use of BV pacing.[36] Rather than an acute or short-term intervention, it could be used on a long-term basis in patients with drug-refractory heart failure. Multiple clinical trials, mostly randomized, studied the effects of BV pacing on symptomatic improvement in heart failure.[37–48] Although the details differ, most of these studies followed a similar design. The inclusion criteria usually constituted refrac-

Table 25.1. *Current indications for cardiac resynchronization therapy in patients with chronic stable heart failure*

Chronic symptomatic heart failure (New York Heart Association class III or IV)
Optimum medical therapy
Ejection fraction ≤ 35%
QRS duration ≥ 120 ms
Left ventricular end-diastolic diameter ≥ 55 mm

From the meta-analysis by Bradley *et al.*,[50] with permission.

tory chronic heart failure (NYHA class III or IV) with widened QRS complexes (> 120 ms to 150 ms). The primary endpoints included improvement in the functional status measured using the NYHA scale, exercise tolerance measured as the peak oxygen consumption during exercise or 6-minute walking distance, and change in quality of life assessed using the Minnesota Living with Heart Failure Questionnaire (MLHFQ). In general, these trials confirmed that BV pacing improves functional status and quality of life. Subsequently, the United States Food and Drug Administration (FDA) approved the use of CRT (AV and BV). Table 25.1 lists the current guidelines for patient selection for CRT.[49] Systematic reviews of these studies have not only shown the beneficial effects of CRT on morbidity, they have also demonstrated a mortality benefit.[50–52]

Response to cardiac resynchronization therapy

Not all patients with heart failure and widened QRS respond favorably to CRT. The response rate to CRT has been consistently shown to be 75% to 80%.[53] It is difficult to predict which patient may benefit from CRT. Multiple studies have shown that the width of QRS complex, either at baseline or after pacing, is not a reliable indicator of response to CRT.[54–57].

One reason for the failure of CRT is placement of the LV lead in a segment that is not late in the mechanical activation sequence. Clearly, such placement is not optimal in reversing the underlying cause of dyssynchrony. In transvenous coronary sinus lead placement, the position of the LV lead is determined by anatomical and technical factors. The segment that is activated last is usually, but

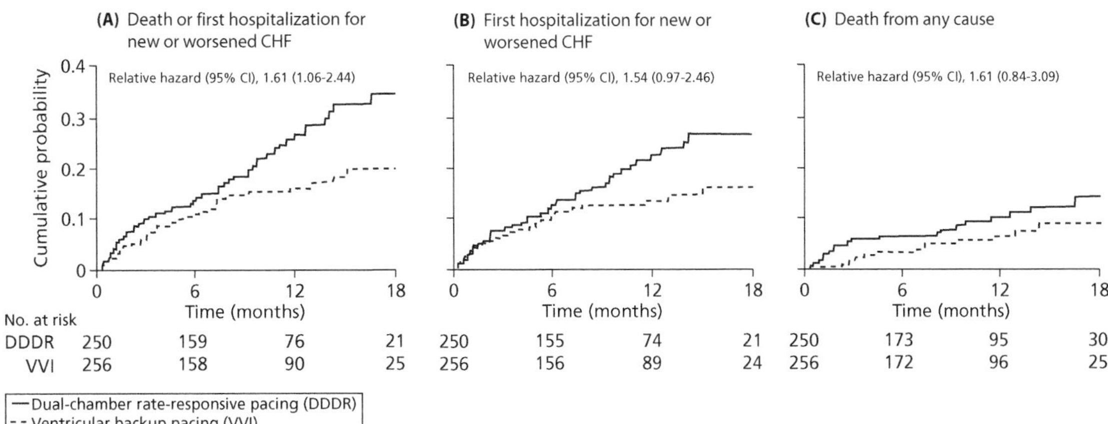

Figure 25.5. *Survival curves for the Dual Chamber and VVI Implantable Defibrillator (DAVID) Trial endpoints. (A) Survival to death or first hospitalization for congestive heart failure (CHF). Unadjusted P = 0.02; adjusted for sequential monitoring, P = 0.03. (B) Survival to first hospitalization for CHF. Patients are censored at death. Log-rank P = 0.07. (C) Survival to death from any cause. Log-rank P = 0.15. (With permission from Wilkoff* et al.[26]*)*

Table 25.2. *Overview of the major clinical trials of cardiac resynchronization therapy*

Trial	Patients	Primary endpoint	Main finding	Status
MUSTIC[75]	NYHA III, LVEF < 35%, QRS > 150 ms, sinus rhythm, on optimal medical therapy	Distance walked in 6 min	CRT resulted in a significant improvement in the distance walked in 6 min, $P < 0.001$	Published in 2001
PATH-CHF I[76]	NYHA III or IV, sinus rhythm, QRS ≥ 120 ms, on optimal medical therapy	Exercise capacity as measured by peak oxygen consumption and 6-min walking distance	LV pacing alone or in combination with RV pacing resulted in a significant improvement in peak oxygen consumption and 6-min walking distance	Published in 2002
PATH-CHF II[77]	NYHA II, III, or IV, LVEF ≤ 30%, QRS > 120 ms	Peak oxygen consumption, distance walked in 6 min, and QoL score	CRT resulted in no improvement in any of the primary endpoints in patients with QRS of 120-150 ms. CRT resulted in a significant improvement in peak oxygen consumption ($P < 0.001$), distance walked in 6 min ($P = 0.024$), and QoL score ($P = 0.004$)	Published in 2003
MIRACLE[78]	NYHA III or IV, LVEF ≤ 35%, QRS ≥ 130 ms, LVEDD* ≥ 55 mm, 6-min walking distance ≤ 450 m, optimal medical therapy	NYHA class, QoL score and distance walked in 6 min	CRT resulted in a significant improvement in NYHA class ($P < 0.001$), QoL score ($P = 0.001$), and distance walked in 6 min ($P = 0.005$)	Published in 2002
InSync ICD[79]	Approved indication for an ICD, LVEF < 35%, symptomatic CHF, LVEDD > 55 mm, QRS > 130 ms, on optimal medical therapy	Not specified	CRT-ICD was associated with a significant improvement in the distance walked in 6 min ($P < 0.001$) and QoL ($P < 0.001$)	Published in 2002
MIRACLE ICD[80]	Approved indication for an ICD, NYHA III or IV, LVEF ≤ 35%, QRS ≥ 130 ms, on optimal medical therapy	QoL, NYHA class, and distance walked in 6 min	CRT-ICD resulted in a significant improvement in QoL ($P = 0.02$), NYHA class ($P = 0.007$), but no significant improvement in distance walked in 6 min	Published in 2003

Table 25.2. *continued*

Trial	Patients	Primary Endpoint	Main Finding	Status
CONTAK CD[81]	Approved indication for an ICD, NYHA II, III or IV, LVEF ≤ 35%, QRS ≥ 120 ms	Progression of CHF, defined as all-cause mortality, hospitalization for CHF, and VT/VF requiring device intervention	CRT did not result in a significant reduction in the primary endpoint	Published in 2003
COMPANION[83]	NYHA III or IV, QRS ≥ 120 ms, LVEF ≤ 35%, hospitalization for the treatment of CHF within 12 months	Time to overall mortality or hospitalization for any cause	CRT resulted in a 19% relative risk reduction in overall mortality ($P = 0.014$) and CRT-ICD resulted in a 20% relative risk reduction in mortality ($P = 0.01$)	Published in 2004

Abbreviations: CHF = congestive heart failure; CRT = cardiac resynchronization therapy; ICD = implantable cardioverter defibrillator; LVEDD: left ventricular end diastolic dimension; LV = left ventricular; LVEF = left ventricular ejection fraction; NYHA = New York Heart Association; QoL = quality of life; RV = right ventricular.

not always, the posterolateral segment of the left ventricle; that is the reason coronary sinus lead placement is usually beneficial. However, a tissue Doppler image-guided targeted nontransvenous lead placement strategy should substantially improve the response rate.[58]

The effect of the underlying etiology of heart failure—ischemic versus nonischemic dilated cardiomyopathy—on response rate to CRT is controversial. It has been postulated that ischemic cardiomyopathy, by virtue of having fixed scars, would be less responsive to CRT. The results so far have been inconsistent, but mostly they have failed to show any preferential response in the dilated cardiomyopathy group.[59–60]

Cardiac resynchronization therapy in the acute setting

CRT was initially developed and studied in patients with chronic stable heart failure. Most randomized clinical trials to date have included only stable patients (Table 25.2). Consequently, CRT has been approved for use in this setting. Nevertheless, there is no theoretical reason why CRT would not be beneficial in AHF. In fact, early observational studies have shown an acute improvement in invasive hemodynamic measurements in patients. Foster *et al.* performed one of the earliest proof-of-concept studies.[61] This study demonstrated the link between restoration of synchrony and hemodynamic improvement. It documented the restoration of synchrony in the BV pacing mode by detection of fusion beats on surface ECG and correlation with epicardial activation maps, and demonstrated the beneficial effects of short duration BV pacing (10 min) in increasing cardiac output. Further studies confirmed these observations and demonstrated the beneficial effects of acute LV or BV pacing in increasing cardiac index,[62] decreasing pulmonary wedge pressure,[62,63] increasing systolic pressure,[63] increasing stroke work, and lowering end-systolic volumes.[64] A recent study has confirmed this result by showing improvement in the noninvasive

Doppler echocardiographic indices of cardiac performance after 1 month of CRT therapy.[65] Specifically, this study demonstrated an increase in aortic outflow velocity time integral and total transmitral filling time, both of which are measures of cardiac output, and a reduction in myocardial performance index, which is an indicator of ventricular ejection time and inversely proportional to dP/dt_{max}.

In addition, the acute beneficial effect of CRT on reversing functional MR has been documented.[66] Acute changes in functional MR severity between intrinsic conduction and CRT were quantified according to the proximal isovelocity surface area method by measuring the effective regurgitant orifice area. It was compared with the changes in the estimated maximal rate of LV systolic pressure rise and transmitral pressure gradients. CRT decreased the effective regurgitant orifice area from 25 ± 19 mm^2 to 13 ± 8 mm^2. The results support the hypothesis that an increase in transmitral pressure gradients, mediated by a rise in LV dP/dt_{max} due to more coordinated LV contraction may facilitate effective mitral valve closure.

Nevertheless, a beneficial acute hemodynamic impact in a chronic stable setting does not directly extrapolate to the ADHF setting. A case-control study of 21 patients with decompensated heart failure who were on inotropic support at the time of BV pacemaker implantation showed an improvement in the ability to wean from inotropic support. However, the study did not show any benefit in terms of length of hospitalization or mortality.[67] This result suggests that CRT in acute settings may have a role as a temporary stabilization strategy until a more long-term procedure can be performed. CRT has been proposed as a "bridge" modality in patients who are on the transplantation waiting list or as an alternative to left ventricular assist devices (LVADs).[68]

Indeed, anecdotal reports support the beneficial effect of CRT in patients awaiting cardiac transplantation. An analysis of a subgroup of patients from the Multicenter InSync Randomized Clinical Evaluation (MIRACLE) InSync® ICD and Comparison of Medical Therapy, Pacing and Defibrillation in Heart Failure (COMPANION) CONTAK® CD trials, who initially met the criteria for cardiac transplantation and had prolonged QRS duration, showed that after 6 months of active CRT management only 6% of the patients still met the transplantation criteria.[69] The reason for being moved off of the transplantation list was usually an improvement in functional class and, less often, an increase in maximum peak VO_2. The long-term effect of CRT and its effect on mortality in this situation are debatable, but it is possible that after CRT some patients may never need transplantation.

Temporary Pacing for Rate Support in Acute Heart Failure

Patients with heart failure are not only at a higher risk for a variety of derangements in the conduction system, but they are also more sensitive to the deleterious hemodynamic effects of such conduction abnormalities. Heart failure patients with degenerative or infiltrative conditions or acute ischemia can develop conduction block at the level of the sinus node (sick sinus syndrome), AV node, or in the IV conduction system. In addition, many of these patients are on beta-blockers or other medications with negative chronotropic or dromotropic effect. In such patients, even first-degree heart block, which is an innocuous rhythm in normal hearts, can worsen AV dyssynchrony and precipitate AHF.

In general, indications for the placement of a temporary or permanent pacemaker in patients with heart failure are similar to those for other patients. Class I indications include third-degree and advanced second-degree AV block, associated with any one of the following conditions: bradycardia with symptoms (including *heart failure*) presumed to be due to AV block, arrhythmias and other medical conditions that require drugs that result in symptomatic bradycardia, and documented periods of asystole greater than or equal to 3.0 seconds or escape rate less than 40 bpm in awake, symptom-free patients. Class II indications include asymptomatic third-degree AV block, type II second-degree AV block with a narrow QRS interval, type I second-degree AV block at intra-His or infra-His levels, or first-degree or second-degree AV block with symptoms similar to those of pacemaker syndrome.[49]

The main distinction between class I and class II recommendations is the presence of *symptoms*. Possible symptoms range from worsening of heart failure to frank pulmonary edema, chest pain, or even bradycardia-induced tachyarrhythmias such as torsade de pointes. Patients with heart failure are more sensitive to abnormalities of heart rate or rhythm and become symptomatic with a lesser degree of abnormality than patients without heart failure. Therefore, the threshold for pacemaker placement will be lower. The decision to place a temporary transvenous pacemaker versus a permanent pacemaker is dictated in part by the perceived duration of the abnormality (transient vs. permanent), and whether the patient can tolerate the procedure, especially in the case of AHF with pulmonary edema, and the acuity of the arrhythmic disturbance and clinical deterioration.

Temporary pacemakers are generally placed in the apex of the right ventricle and are set to VVI mode. Although it is possible to place a dual-chamber temporary pacemaker, the procedure is lengthy, complicated, and rarely attempted. Hence, temporary pacemakers result in a loss of AV and BV synchrony. In addition, VVI mode pacing is associated with a high incidence of pacemaker syndrome, defined as symptomatic hemodynamic abnormalities precipitated by a normal functioning ventricular pacemaker. The usual constellation of symptoms in pacemaker syndrome includes shortness of breath, feeling of pulsation in neck, drop in systolic blood pressure, near syncope and syncope, and nonspecific signs and symptoms.[70] Failing hearts are prone to worsen under these conditions.

In the Pacemaker Selection in the Elderly (PASE) trial, the presence of nonischemic cardiomyopathy was a predictor of the inability to tolerate the VVI mode.[71] The MOST trial showed a reduction in signs and symptoms of heart failure in DDD mode in comparison to VVI mode.[72] However, rate support takes precedence over such secondary effects and these short-term concerns should not preclude the placement of a temporary pacemaker. If the patient in heart failure fails to improve or worsens after temporary pacemaker, consideration should be given to changing to a dual-chamber or even a BV pacemaker. Whether or not a patient with heart failure should receive a BV pacemaker when a permanent pacemaker is indicated is still an unresolved issue.[73,74]

Conclusion

There are a variety of indications for pacing in patients with heart failure. Bradycardia and intrinsic conduction system disease can lead to ineffective filling and a decrease in cardiac output leading to heart failure. RV pacing, though traditionally used, may in fact contribute to electromechanical dyssynchrony. CRT can restore electromechanical synchrony.

References

1. Luu M, Stevenson WG, Stevenson LW, Baron K, Walden J. Diverse mechanisms of unexpected cardiac arrest in advanced heart failure. Circulation 1989; 80: 1675–1680.
2. Spencer KT, Mor-Avi V, Kirkpatrick J, *et al.* Normal values of left ventricular systolic and diastolic function derived from signal-averaged acoustic quantification waveforms: a multicenter study. J Am Soc Echocardiogr 2003; 16: 1244–1251.
3. Linderer T, Chatterjee K, Parmley WW, *et al.* Influence of atrial systole on the Frank–Starling relation and the end-diastolic pressure-diameter relation of the left ventricle. Circulation 1983; 67: 1045–1053.
4. Gold MR, Brockman R, Peters RW, Olsovsky MR, Shorofsky SR. Acute hemodynamic effects of right ventricular pacing site and pacing mode in patients with congestive heart failure secondary to either ischemic or idiopathic dilated cardiomyopathy. Am J Cardiol 2000; 85: 1106–1109.
5. Steinberg JS, Zelenkofske S, Wong SC, *et al.* Value of the P-wave signal-averaged ECG for predicting AF after cardiac surgery. Circulation 1993; 88: 2618–2622.
6. Babaev AA, Vloka ME, Sadurski R, Steinberg JS. Influence of age on atrial activation as measured by the P-wave signal-averaged electrocardiogram. Am J Cardiol 2000; 86: 692–695.
7. Kass DA, Chen CH, Curry C, *et al.* Improved left ventricular mechanics from acute VDD pacing in patients with dilated cardiomyopathy and ventricular conduction delay. Circulation 1999; 99: 1567–1573.

8. Auricchio A, Stellbrink C, Block M, *et al.* Effect of pacing chamber and atrioventricular delay on acute systolic function of paced patients with congestive heart failure. The Pacing Therapies for Congestive Heart Failure Study Group. The Guidant Congestive Heart Failure Research Group. Circulation 1999; 99: 2993–3001.
9. Nishimura RA, Hayes DL, Holmes DR Jr., Tajik AJ. Mechanism of hemodynamic improvement by dual-chamber pacing for severe left ventricular dysfunction: an acute Doppler and catheterization hemodynamic study. J Am Coll Cardiol 1995; 25: 281–288.
10. Brecker SJ, Xiao HB, Sparrow J, Gibson DG. Effects of dual-chamber pacing with short atrioventricular delay in dilated cardiomyopathy. Lancet 1992; 340: 1308–1312.
11. Gold MR, Feliciano Z, Gottlieb SS, Fisher ML. Dual-chamber pacing with a short atrioventricular delay in congestive heart failure: a randomized study. J Am Coll Cardiol 1995; 26: 967–973.
12. Liebold A, Haisch G, Rosada B, Kleine P. Internal atrial defibrillation—a new treatment of postoperative atrial fibrillation. Thorac Cardiovasc Surg 1998; 46: 323–326.
13. Rossi R, Muia N Jr., Turco V, Sgura FA, Molinari R, Modena MG. Short atrioventricular delay reduces the degree of mitral regurgitation in patients with a sequential dual-chamber pacemaker. Am J Cardiol 1997; 80: 901–905.
14. Lasser RP, Haft JI, Friedberg CK. Relationship of right bundle-branch block and marked left axis deviation (with left parietal or peri-infarction block) to complete heart block and syncope. Circulation 1968; 37: 429–437.
15. De Bacquer D, De Backer G, Kornitzer M. Prevalences of ECG findings in large population based samples of men and women. Heart 2000; 84: 625–633.
16. Hardarson T, Arnason A, Eliasson GJ, Palsson K, Eyjolfsson K, Sigfusson N. Left bundle branch block: prevalence, incidence, follow-up and outcome. Eur Heart J 1987; 8: 1075–1079.
17. Igarashi M, Shiina Y, Tanabe T, Handa S. Significance of electrocardiographic QRS width in patients with congestive heart failure: a marker for biventricular pacing. J Cardiol 2002; 40: 103–109.
18. Baldasseroni S, Opasich C, Gorini M, *et al.*, Italian Network on Congestive Heart Failure Investigators. Left bundle-branch block is associated with increased 1-year sudden and total mortality rate in 5517 outpatients with congestive heart failure: a report from the Italian network on congestive heart failure. Am Heart J 2002; 143: 398–405.
19. Murkofsky RL, Dangas G, Diamond JA, Mehta D, Schaffer A, Ambrose JA. A prolonged QRS duration on surface electrocardiogram is a specific indicator of left ventricular dysfunction. J Am Coll Cardiol 1998; 32: 476–482.
20. Shenkman HJ, Pampati V, Khandelwal AK, *et al.* Congestive heart failure and QRS duration, establishing prognosis study. Chest 2002; 122: 528–534.
21. Betocchi S, Piscione F, Villari B, *et al.* Effects of induced asynchrony on left ventricular diastolic function in patients with coronary artery disease. J Am Coll Cardiol 1993; 21: 1124–1131.
22. Rosenqvist M, Isaaz K, Botvinick EH, *et al.* Relative importance of activation sequence compared to atrioventricular synchrony in left ventricular function. Am J Cardiol 1991; 67: 148–156.
23. Sweeney MO, Hellkamp AS, Ellenbogen KA, *et al.* MOde Selection Trial Investigators. Adverse effect of ventricular pacing on heart failure and atrial fibrillation among patients with normal baseline QRS duration in a clinical trial of pacemaker therapy for sinus node dysfunction. Circulation 2003; 107: 2932–2937.
24. Moss AJ, Zareba W, Hall WJ, *et al.* Multicenter Automatic Defibrillator Implantation Trial II Investigators. Prophylactic implantation of a defibrillator in patients with myocardial infarction and reduced ejection fraction. N Engl J Med 2002; 346: 877–883.
25. Steinberg JS. Multicenter Automatic Defibrillator Implantation Trial II Substudy. Late breaking clinical trials session, NASPE 2003. 24th Annual Scientific Sessions, Washington, DC (Abstract).
26. Wilkoff BL, Cook JR, Epstein AE, *et al.* Dual Chamber and VVI Implantable Defibrillator Trial Investigators. Dual-chamber pacing or ventricular backup pacing in patients with an implantable defibrillator: the Dual Chamber and VVI Implantable Defibrillator (DAVID) Trial. JAMA 2002; 288: 3115–3123.
27. Clark DM, Plumb VJ, Epstein AE, Kay GN. Hemodynamic effects of an irregular sequence of ventricular cycle lengths during atrial fibrillation. J Am Coll Cardiol 1997; 30: 1039–1045.
28. Tsang TS, Barnes ME, Gersh BJ, Bailey KR, Seward JB. Risks for atrial fibrillation and congestive heart failure in patients ≥ 65 years of age with abnormal left ventricular diastolic relaxation. Am J Cardiol 2004; 93: 54–58.
29. Garrigue S, Bordachar P, Reuter S, *et al.* Comparison of permanent left ventricular and biventricular pacing in patients with heart failure and chronic atrial fibrillation: Prospective hemodynamic study. Heart 2002; 87: 529–534.

30. Anselme F, Boyle N, Josephson M. Incessant fascicular tachycardia: a cause of arrhythmia induced cardiomyopathy. Pacing Clin Electrophysiol 1998; 21: 760–763.
31. Stevenson WG, Stevenson LW. Atrial fibrillation in heart failure. N Engl J Med 1999; 341: 910–911.
32. Lister JW, Klotz DH, Jomain SL, Stuckey JH, Hoffman BF. Effect of pacemaker site on cardiac output and ventricular activation in dogs with complete heart block. Am J Cardiol 1964; 14: 494–503.
33. Zile MR, Blaustein AS, Shimizu G, Gaasch WH. Right ventricular pacing reduces the rate of left ventricular relaxation and filling. J Am Coll Cardiol 1987; 10: 702–709.
34. Aoyagi T, Iizuka M, Takahashi T, *et al.* Wall motion asynchrony prolongs time constant of left ventricular relaxation. Am J Physiol 1989; 257: H883–H890.
35. Grines C, Bashore T, Boudoulas H, *et al.* Functional abnormalities in isolated left-bundle branch-block—the effect of interventricular asynchrony. Circulation 1989; 79: 845–853.
36. Daubert JC, Ritter P, Le Breton H, *et al.* Permanent left ventricular pacing with transvenous leads inserted into the coronary veins. Pacing Clin Electrophysiol 1998; 21: 239–245.
37. Abraham WT, Young JB, Leon AR. Medtronic InSync® ICD Cardiac Resynchronization System (draft sponsor presentation). U.S. Food and Drug Administration Center for Devices and Radiological Health Circulatory System Devices Advisory Panel meeting. March 5, 2002; Gaithersburg, Md. Available at: http:\\www.fda.gov/ohrms/dockets/ac/02/briefing/3843b2.htm. Accessed June 18, 2002.
38. Gras D, Leclercq C, Tang AS, Bucknall C, Luttikhuis HO, Kirstein-Pedersen A. Cardiac resynchronization therapy in advanced heart failure the multicenter InSync clinical study. Eur J Heart Fail 2002; 4: 311–320.
39. Abraham WT. Rationale and design of a randomized clinical trial to assess the safety and efficacy of cardiac resynchronization therapy in patients with advanced heart failure: the Multicenter InSync Randomized Clinical Evaluation (MIRACLE). J Card Fail 2000; 6: 369–380.
40. Cazeau S, Leclercq C, Lavergne T, *et al.* Multisite Stimulation in Cardiomyopathies (MUSTIC) Study Investigators. Effects of multisite biventricular pacing in patients with heart failure and intraventricular conduction delay. N Engl J Med 2001; 344: 873–880.
41. Leclercq C, Walker S, Linde C, *et al.* Comparative effects of permanent biventricular and right-univentricular pacing in heart failure patients with chronic atrial fibrillation. Eur Heart J 2002; 23: 1780–1787.
42. Auricchio A, Stellbrink C, Sack S, *et al.* Pacing Therapies in Congestive Heart Failure (PATH-CHF) Study Group. Long-term clinical effect of hemodynamically optimized cardiac resynchronization therapy in patients with heart failure and ventricular conduction delay. J Am Coll Cardiol 2002; 39: 2026–2033.
43. Guidant Cardiac Resynchronization Therapy Defibrillator System Including the CONTAK CD® Pulse Generator and the EASYTRAK® Left Ventricular Coronary Venous Lead. Pre-market approval number P010012. Guidant Corporation, Indianapolis, IN. Available at: http://www.fda.gov/cdrh/pdf/P010012.html. Accessed April 24, 2003.
44. Young JB, Abraham WT, Smith AL, *et al.*, Multicenter InSync ICD Randomized Clinical Evaluation (MIRACLE ICD) Trial Investigators. Combined cardiac resynchronization and implantable cardioversion defibrillation in advanced chronic heart failure: the MIRACLE ICD Trial. JAMA 2003; 289: 2685–2694.
45. Stellbrink C, Aurricchio A, Butter C, *et al.* Pacing therapies in congestive heart failure II study. Am J Cardiol 200; 86: K138–K143.
46. Bristow MR, Saxon LA, Boehmer JP, *et al.* Cardiac resynchronization therapy (CRT) reduces hospitalizations, and CRT plus an implantable defibrillator reduces mortality in chronic heart failure: preliminary results of the COMPANION trial. Presented at: American College of Cardiology 2003 Scientific Sessions; 2003, Chicago IL.
47. Leclercq C, Kass DA. Retiming the failing heart: principles and current clinical status of cardiac resynchronization. J Am Coll Cardiol 2002; 39: 194–201.
48. Zardini M, Tritto M, Bargiggia G, *et al.* Analysis of clinical outcome and considerations on the selection of candidates to left ventricular resynchronization. Eur Heart J Supplements 2000; 2: J16–J22 (Abstract).
49. Gregoratos G, Abrams J, Epstein AE, *et al.* ACC/AHA/NASPE 2002 guideline update for implantation of cardiac pacemakers and antiarrhythmia devices: summary article: a report of the American College of Cardiology/American Heart Association Task Force on Practice Guidelines (ACC/AHA/NASPE Committee to Update the 1998 Pacemaker Guidelines). Circulation 2002; 106: 2145–2161.
50. Bradley DJ, Bradley EA, Baughman KL, *et al.* Cardiac resynchronization and death from progressive heart failure: a meta-analysis of randomized controlled trials. JAMA 2003; 289: 730–740.

51. Salukhe TV, Dimopoulos K, Francis D. Cardiac resynchronisation may reduce all-cause mortality: meta-analysis of preliminary COMPANION data with CONTAK-CD, InSync ICD, MIRACLE and MUSTIC. Int J Cardiol 2004; 93: 101–103.
52. Abraham WT. Cardiac resynchronization therapy: a review of clinical trials and criteria for identifying the appropriate patient. Rev Cardiovasc Med 2003; 4: S30–S37.
53. Adamson PB, Abraham WT. Cardiac resynchronization therapy for advanced heart failure. Curr Treat Options Cardiovasc Med 2003; 5: 301–309.
54. Pitzalis MV, Iacoviello M, Romito R, *et al.* Cardiac resynchronization therapy tailored by echocardiographic evaluation of ventricular asynchrony. J Am Coll Cardiol 2002; 40: 1615–1622.
55. Yu CM, Lin H, Zhang Q, Sanderson JE. High prevalence of left ventricular systolic and diastolic asynchrony in patients with congestive heart failure and normal QRS duration. Heart 2003; 89: 54–60.
56. Auricchio A, Yu CM. Beyond the measurement of QRS complex toward mechanical dyssynchrony: cardiac resynchronisation therapy in heart failure patients with a normal QRS duration. Heart 2004; 90: 479–481.
57. Sogaard P, Egeblad H, Kim WY, *et al.* Tissue Doppler imaging predicts improved systolic performance and reversed left ventricular remodeling during long-term cardiac resynchronization therapy. J Am Coll Cardiol 2002; 40: 723–730.
58. Steinberg JS, Maniar PB, Higgins SL, *et al.* Noninvasive assessment of the biventricular pacing system. Ann Noninvasive Electrocardiol 2004; 9: 58–70.
59. Mansourati J, Etienne Y, Gilard M, *et al.* Left ventricular-based pacing in patients with chronic heart failure: comparison of acute hemodynamic benefits according to underlying heart disease. Eur J Heart Fail 2000; 2: 195–199.
60. Molhoek SG, Bax JJ, van Erven L, *et al.* Comparison of benefits from cardiac resynchronization therapy in patients with ischemic cardiomyopathy versus idiopathic dilated cardiomyopathy. Am J Cardiol 2004; 93: 860–863.
61. Foster AH, Gold MR, McLaughlin JS. Acute hemodynamic effects of atrio-biventricular pacing in humans. Ann Thorac Surg 1995; 59: 294–300.
62. Leclercq C, Cazeau S, Le Breton H, *et al.* Acute hemodynamic effects of biventricular DDD pacing in patients with end-stage heart failure. J Am Coll Cardiol 1998; 32: 1825–1831.
63. Blanc JJ, Etienne Y, Gilard M, *et al.* Evaluation of different ventricular pacing sites in patients with severe heart failure: results of an acute hemodynamic study. Circulation 1997; 96: 3273–3277.
64. Kass DA, Chen CH, Curry C, *et al.* Improved left ventricular mechanics from acute VDD pacing in patients with dilated cardiomyopathy and ventricular conduction delay. Circulation 1999; 99: 1567–1573.
65. Breithardt OA, Stellbrink C, Franke A, *et al.*, Pacing Therapies for Congestive Heart Failure Study Group; Guidant Congestive Heart Failure Research Group. Acute effects of cardiac resynchronization therapy on left ventricular Doppler indices in patients with congestive heart failure. Am Heart J 2002; 143: 34–44.
66. Breithardt OA, Sinha AM, Schwammenthal E, *et al.* Acute effects of cardiac resynchronization therapy on functional mitral regurgitation in advanced systolic heart failure. J Am Coll Cardiol 2003; 41: 765–770.
67. Honeycutt DC Jr., Langberg J, Leon AR, Smith AL. Experience with cardiac resynchronization in heart failure patients requiring inotropic support. PACE 2003; 26: 1041 (Abstract).
68. Kaplinsky EJ, Pesce R, Favaloro M, Perrone SV. Biventricular resynchronization as an unusual bridge to transplantation: acute effects. Tex Heart Inst J 2001; 28: 326–327.
69. Greenberg JM, Leon AR, Book WM, *et al.* Benefits of cardiac resynchronization therapy in outpatients with indicators for heart transplantation. J Heart Lung Transplant 2003; 22: 1134–1140.
70. Lamas GA, Ellenbogen KA. Evidence base for pacemaker mode selection: from physiology to randomized trials. Circulation 2004; 109: 443–451.
71. Ellenbogen KA, Stambler BS, Orav EJ, *et al.* Clinical characteristics of patients intolerant to VVIR pacing. Am J Cardiol 2000; 86: 59–63.
72. Lamas GA, Lee KL, Sweeney MO, *et al.* Mode Selection Trial in Sinus-Node Dysfunction. Ventricular pacing or dual-chamber pacing for sinus-node dysfunction. N Engl J Med 2002; 346: 1854–1862.
73. Breithardt OA, Stellbrink C, Kramer AP, *et al.*, PATH-CHF Study Group, Pacing Therapies for Congestive Heart Failure. Echocardiographic quantification of left ventricular asynchrony predicts an acute hemodynamic benefit of cardiac resynchronization therapy. J Am Coll Cardiol 2002; 40: 536–545.
74. Leclercq C, Faris O, Tunin R, *et al.* Systolic improvement and mechanical resynchronization does not require electrical synchrony in the dilated failing heart with left bundle-branch block. Circulation 2002; 106: 1760–1763.

CHAPTER 26

Implantable cardioverter defibrillators and biventricular devices in acute heart failure

Sana M Al-Khatib

Introduction

Congestive heart failure (CHF) is a major public health problem which afflicts 5 million Americans.[1] A new diagnosis of CHF is made in 400 000 Americans each year.[1] CHF is the most common cardiovascular discharge diagnosis in elderly patients. With the aging of the American population, the prevalence of CHF is expected to increase markedly.

Management of patients with CHF has improved appreciably in the past decade. This improvement has resulted, in part, from the use of device therapy in patients with CHF. Not only has device therapy evolved rapidly in the past decade, but our understanding of its role in patients with CHF has grown substantially. The first part of this chapter addresses sudden cardiac death in CHF, and provides an overview of implantable cardioverter defibrillator (ICD) therapy in patients with CHF. The second part of the chapter tackles cardiac dyssynchrony and offers a detailed review of cardiac resynchronization therapy (CRT). It should be noted that because there have been no randomized clinical trials of ICD therapy and CRT in patients with acute heart failure (AHF), no recommendations could be made in relation to ICD or CRT use in patients with AHF. However, patients who seek medical attention for AHF can and should be considered for ICD or CRT implantation after their AHF is under control.

Causes of Death in Heart Failure

The two most common causes of death in patients with CHF are sudden cardiac death and progressive pump failure. Sudden cardiac death usually results from ventricular tachyarrhythmias, but it could also result from bradyarrhythmias. Progressive pump failure usually involves progressive end-organ hypoperfusion, hypotension, and electromechanical dissociation. The mode of death in patients with CHF seems to vary with the etiology of CHF. Patients with ischemic heart disease, for example, are more likely to die suddenly than patients with nonischemic cardiomyopathy.

Another important factor that affects the mode of death in patients with CHF is the severity of CHF symptoms as defined by the New York Heart Association (NYHA) functional class. Patients with NYHA class II and III symptoms are more likely to die suddenly, than to die from progressive pump failure. Patients with NYHA class IV symptoms are more likely to die of pump failure and less likely to die suddenly.[2] However, in absolute terms, the risk of sudden cardiac death is higher in patients with advanced CHF than in patients with less advanced CHF.

Risk stratification for sudden cardiac death in patients with CHF

In patients with CHF, the risk of sudden cardiac death is 6 to 9 times greater than in the general population.[1,3] Indeed, left ventricular (LV) dysfunction is the strongest predictor of sudden cardiac death.[4–6] While it is known that the risk for sudden cardiac death correlates with the severity of LV dysfunction, there is no clinical marker specific for sudden cardiac death in patients with LV dysfunction.[7] Thus, our ability to predict which patients with CHF will die suddenly is currently limited.

Several tests have been proposed to predict sudden cardiac death vulnerability in patients with LV dysfunction. However, to date, no individual test has been proven to have sufficient negative predictive value. While in risk stratifying patients with ischemic cardiomyopathy, the electrophysiology study (EPS) was the gold standard test for many years, in the Multicenter Unsustained Tachycardia Trial (MUSTT), its negative predictive value did not exceed 81%.[8] In the Multicenter Automatic Defibrillator Trial-II (MADIT-II), a positive EPS could not predict future occurrence of ventricular fibrillation (VF) and was only poorly predictive of future occurrence of ventricular tachycardia (VT). In MADIT-II, the two variables that predicted a higher risk of mortality were a history of atrial fibrillation and QRS width of ≤ 120 ms.[9] In patients with nonischemic cardiomyopathy, the value of EPS is worse. For these patients the EPS seems to have no predictive value.[10–13]

Other potentially effective noninvasive tests have been studied. While some studies have shown that a negative signal averaged ECG (SAECG) is a strong predictor of lack of future arrhythmic events, in a recent study, SAECG had a disappointingly low negative predictive value of 88%.[14–17] In the MUSTT trial, however, patients with an abnormal SAECG had significantly higher 5-year rates of arrhythmic death (28% vs. 17%; $P = 0.0001$) and all-cause mortality (43% vs. 35%; $P = 0.0001$) than patients with normal SAECG.[18] Although QT dispersion has been proposed as a helpful marker of increased sudden cardiac death vulnerability in survivors of myocardial infarction (MI), in the only prospective study of the predictive value of QT dispersion in post-MI patients, QT dispersion failed to predict subsequent death.[19]

Heart rate variability and baroreflex sensitivity were shown in the Autonomic Tone and Reflexes After Myocardial Infarction (ATRAMI) trial to have significant prognostic value independent of left ventricular ejection fraction (LVEF) and spontaneous ventricular arrhythmias. In that trial, the negative predictive value of heart rate variability and baroreflex sensitivity was approximately 97%.[20] However, the mean LVEF of patients enrolled in ATRAMI was 49%.[20] Thus, it is not known whether these tests are as predictive in patients with worse LV dysfunction.

One promising test is microvolt T-wave alternans (TWA). TWA is a change in T-wave amplitude, width, or shape that occurs with each alternate beat. This change is thought to reflect differences in action potential, which create dispersion of recovery. This dispersion can result in re-entrant ventricular arrhythmias.[21] Microvolt TWA was prospectively evaluated initially as a marker of vulnerability to arrhythmias in patients referred for a diagnostic EPS. It was found to be a significant independent predictor of ventricular arrhythmia, inducibility on EPS, and arrhythmic event occurrence during a 20-month follow-up period. In that study, the 20-month survival for alternans-negative patients was 94%.[22] Among patients with CHF, TWA was found to be superior to 6 other tests of arrhythmic risk at predicting arrhythmic events.[23] In patients with nonischemic cardiomyopathy, TWA successfully identified patients at an increased risk for ventricular arrhythmias.[24,25]

Prevention of sudden cardiac death in patients with congestive heart failure

Medications

Numerous studies have tested the ability of antiarrhythmic medications to prevent sudden cardiac death in patients with CHF or LV dysfunction. The results of these studies have been disappointing. In the Cardiac Arrhythmia Suppression Trial (CAST)-I and CAST-II trials, flecainide, encainide, and moricizine were proven to increase the mortality rate of patients with premature ventricular contractions following an acute myocardial infarction (AMI).[26–28] In survivors of cardiac arrest, propafenone was associated with a higher risk of death than metoprolol, amiodarone, and ICD.[29] In the Survival With Oral d-Sotalol (SWORD) trial, d-sotalol was associated with a high risk of death among post-infarct patients and reduced LV function.[30] However, the effect of d-sotalol on the survival of such patients is uncertain and needs to be investigated in future clinical trials. Although many studies have shown a significant reduction in sudden cardiac death with amiodarone, this reduction has not led to a reduction in all-cause mortality. Amiodarone had no effect on mortality in the European Myocardial Infarct Amiodarone Trial (EMIAT), the Canadian Amiodarone Myocardial Infarction Arrhythmia Trial (CAMIAT), the Survival Trial of Antiarrhythmic Therapy in Congestive Heart Failure (STAT-CHF), or the recently reported Sudden Cardiac Death in Heart Failure Trial (SCD-HeFT).[31–34] The latter trial examined the effect of amiodarone, ICD therapy, and placebo on the survival of patients with NYHA class II and III symptoms and an LVEF of ≤ 35%.[34] In the Danish Investigations of Arrhythmia and Mortality on Dofetilide (DIAMOND) and DIAMOND-CHF trials, dofetilide was shown not to increase the mortality of survivors of MI and patients with CHF.[35] In the Azimilide Postinfarct Survival Evaluation (ALIVE) trial, azimilide had no effect on the mortality of post-MI patients with an LVEF of 15% to 35% (hazard ratio [HR], 0.95; 95% confidence interval [CI], 0.71–1.27).[36]

Studies that tested the efficacy of non-antiarrhythmic medications at reducing the risk of sudden cardiac death have yielded promising results. Beta-blockers have been repeatedly proven to reduce all-cause mortality and sudden cardiac death in survivors of MI and patients with CHF.[37–40] In the Randomized Aldactone Evaluation Study (RALES) study, when spironolactone was compared with placebo in patients with severe heart failure and an LVEF of ≤ 35%, it was found to result in a significant reduction in sudden cardiac death (relative risk [RR], 0.71; 95% CI, 0.54–0.95; P = 0.02).[41] In the Eplerenone Post-Acute Myocardial Infarction Heart Failure Efficacy and Survival (EPHESUS) study, when eplerenone was compared with placebo in patients with AMI complicated by LV dysfunction and heart failure, it was found to result in a significant reduction in sudden cardiac death (RR, 0.79; 95% CI, 0.64–0.97; P = 0.03).[42] The mechanism by which these drugs cause a reduction in sudden cardiac death is uncertain.

Although studies of the effect of angiotensin-converting enzyme (ACE) inhibitors on sudden cardiac death have yielded conflicting results, the overall evidence suggests that ACE inhibitors have a salutary effect on sudden cardiac death.[43–45] The effect of angiotensin receptor blockers (ARBs) on the risk of sudden cardiac death is uncertain and needs to be investigated in future studies.

Whether lipid-lowering drugs have an antiarrhythmic effect is uncertain. At least in one substudy of the Antiarrhythmics Versus Implantable Defibrillators (AVID) trial, lipid-lowering therapy was associated with a significant reduction in the recurrence of ventricular arrhythmias in the subgroup of patients with coronary artery disease (CAD) and an ICD.[46] While these results suggest that lipid-lowering drugs have an antiarrhythmic effect, this hypothesis needs to be confirmed in future studies.

Implantable Cardioverter Defibrillator

Today, the ICD is the most efficacious therapy at reducing the risk of sudden cardiac death in different patient populations. The evidence that supports the use of ICD therapy in patients with CHF has grown rapidly in the past few years (Table 26.1). Although the AVID trial and the Canadian Implantable Defibrillators Study (CIDS) enrolled survivors of cardiac arrest or hemodynamically unstable VT, CHF or LV dysfunction were present in an appreciable number of patients in those two studies.[47,48] In a secondary analysis of the AVID trial, the survival of patients with an LVEF of ≤ 35% was not improved with ICD therapy. However, the survival of patients with an LVEF of 20% to 34% was significantly improved with ICD therapy as compared with antiarrhythmic medications. In the smaller subgroup of patients with an LVEF of < 20%, the same magnitude of survival difference was seen as that in the subgroup of patients with an LVEF of 20% to 34%, but the difference was not statistically significant.[49] In a secondary analysis of the CIDS trial, the CIDS

Table 26.1. *Overview of the major clinical trials of implantable cardioverter defibrillator therapy*

Trial	Patients	Primary endpoint	Main finding	Status
MADIT-I[51]	NYHA I, II, or III, prior MI, LVEF≤ 35%, NSVT,* nonsuppressible ventricular arrhythmia on EPS	Overall mortality	ICD resulted in a 56% relative risk reduction in mortality, $P = 0.009$	Published in 1996
AVID[47]	Near-fatal VT with syncope, or sustained VT with an LVEF ≤ 40% and symptoms of hemodynamic compromise	Overall mortality	ICD resulted in a 31% relative risk reduction in mortality, $P < 0.02$	Published in 1997
CABG-PATCH[53]	LVEF < 36%, abnormal SAECG, scheduled for CABG	Overall mortality	ICD had no effect on mortality	Published in 1997
MUSTT[8]	CAD, LVEF ≤ 40%, NSVT, inducible sustained VT on EPS	Cardiac arrest or death from arrhythmia	ICD resulted in a 76% relative risk reduction in the primary endpoint, $P < 0.001$	Published in 1999
CIDS[48]	Documented VF, out of hospital cardiac arrest requiring defibrillation, documented sustained VT causing syncope, sustained VT causing symptoms with an LVEF ≤ 35%, syncope with subsequent documentation of sustained VT or inducible VT on EPS	Overall mortality	ICD had no significant effect on mortality	Published in 2000
CASH[29]	Near-fatal cardiac arrest due to documented sustained ventricular arrhythmias	Overall mortality	ICD resulted in a 23% relative risk reduction in mortality, $P = 0.081$	Published in 2000
MADIT-II[52]	History of MI, LVEF ≤ 30%	Overall mortality	ICD resulted in a 31% relative risk reduction in mortality, $P = 0.016$	Published in 2002

Table 26.1. *continued*

Trial	Patients	Primary endpoint	Main finding	Status
DEFINITE[54]	Nonischemic cardiomyopathy, LVEF ≤ 35%, PVCs or NSVT	Overall mortality	ICD resulted in a 35% relative risk reduction in mortality, $P = 0.08$	Published in 2004
SCD-HeFT[34]	NYHA II and III, LVEF ≤ 35%	Overall mortality	ICD resulted in a 23% relative risk reduction in mortality, $P = 0.007$	Un-published

Abbreviations: CABG = coronary artery bypass grafting; CAD = coronary artery disease; EPS = electrophysiology study; ICD = implantable cardioverter defibrillator; LVEF = left ventricular ejection fraction; MI = myocardial infarction; NSVT = non-sustained ventricular tachycardia; NYHA = New York Heart Association; PVC = premature ventricular contraction; SAECG = signal averaged ECG; VF = ventricular fibrillation; VT = ventricular tachycardia.

investigators identified older age, LVEF of ≤ 35%, and NYHA class III or IV as factors with significant effect on survival. Patients who had all 3 risk factors had a significant improvement in survival with ICD therapy as compared with amiodarone.[50] Although these secondary analyses suggest that patients with LVEF of ≤ 35% do not derive survival benefit from an ICD, the results of these analyses should be interpreted with great caution. Because patients with a higher LVEF are less likely to have sudden cardiac death than patients with a lower EF, a greater number of patients with a higher EF or a longer follow-up time are required to accurately assess the effect of ICD therapy on the survival of such patients.

The MADIT-I study enrolled patients who had a MI ≤ 3 weeks before entry into the study, an LVEF of ≤ 35%, an episode of asymptomatic non-sustained ventricular tachycardia (NSVT) and inducible sustained VT on an EPS. The episode of NSVT had to be 3 to 30 beats long at a rate of 120 beats per minute (bpm) and unrelated to an AMI. Of the 196 patients enrolled, 101 patients received conventional medical therapy and 95 patients received an ICD. The mean duration of follow-up was 27 months, and the primary endpoint of the study was all-cause mortality. ICD therapy was significantly better than conventional medical therapy at reducing the risk of death ($P = 0.009$); ICD therapy was associated with a 54% relative risk reduction in all-cause mortality. Although patients who received an ICD were more likely to be treated with beta-blockers, there was no evidence from statistical modeling that this imbalance in beta-blocker use had any effect on the observed results.[51]

The MUSTT trial enrolled 704 patients with a history of CAD, an LVEF of ≤ 40%, asymptomatic NSVT and inducible sustained VT on EPS. Patients were randomized to antiarrhythmic therapy, including antiarrhythmic medications and ICD or no antiarrhythmic therapy. The median duration of follow-up was 39 months, and the primary endpoint of the study was cardiac arrest or death from an arrhythmia. The risk of the primary endpoint in patients who received an ICD was significantly lower than that in patients who did not receive an ICD ($P < 0.001$). Likewise, the risk of overall mortality was significantly reduced with ICD therapy ($P < 0.001$). Antiarrhythmic medications, however, did not result in a significant reduction in the risk of cardiac arrest or death from an arrhythmia.[8]

The MADIT-II study enrolled patients with a history of MI and an LVEF of ≤ 30%. Patients were not eligible for enrollment in this study if they had a MI within a month before entry into the study and if their most recent revascularization occurred within 3 months before entry into the study. Patients with NYHA class IV symptoms were excluded. Despite treating patients with optimal medical therapy, the ICD was associated with a 31% relative risk reduction in all-cause mortality. This finding was consistent across all the subgroups.[52]

Currently, it is not known whether the prophylactic implantation of an ICD at the time of revascularization or during the first few months after revascularization improves the survival of patients with ischemic cardiomyopathy. The MADIT-I and MADIT-II studies excluded patients who underwent revascularization within 2 to 3 months before entry into those studies.[51,52] The Coronary Artery Bypass Graft Patch (CABG-PATCH) trial was conducted specifically to determine if the prophylactic implantation of an ICD at the time of elective coronary artery bypass grafting (CABG) would improve the survival of patients with an LVEF of < 36% and an abnormal SAECG. CABG-PATCH enrolled 900 patients; 446 patients were randomized to the ICD arm and 454 patients were randomly assigned to the control arm. During a mean follow-up duration of 32 months, there was no significant difference in overall mortality between the two arms.[53]

Although most of the randomized clinical trials of ICD therapy were conducted in patients with ischemic cardiomyopathy, two recent studies have included patients with nonischemic cardiomyopathy. The Defibrillators in Non-ischemic Cardiomyopathy Treatment Evaluation (DEFINITE) trial enrolled patients with nonischemic cardiomyopathy, an LVEF of ≤ 35%, and premature ventricular complexes or NSVT. It showed that ICD therapy is associated with a strong trend toward improved survival (HR, 0.65; 95% CI, 0.40–1.06; $P = 0.08$) and a significant reduction in sudden cardiac death (HR, 0.20; 95% CI, 0.06–0.71; $P = 0.006$).[54] The second trial that included patients with nonischemic cardiomyopathy is the SCD-HeFT trial. SCD-HeFT examined the effect of amiodarone, placebo, and ICD therapy on the survival of patients with ischemic or nonischemic cardiomyopathy, if they had NYHA class II and III symptoms for at least 3 months and LVEF of ≤ 35%. Compared with placebo, ICD therapy was associated with a significant reduction in all-cause mortality (HR, 0.77; 95% CI, 0.62–0.96; $P = 0.007$). Amiodarone, however, did not result in a significant reduction in mortality (HR, 1.06; 95% CI, 0.86–1.30; $P = 0.529$).[34]

It should be noted that because patients with NYHA class IV symptoms were excluded from MADIT-I, MUSTT, MADIT-II, DEFINITE and SCD-HeFT, it is uncertain whether those patients would derive significant survival benefit from ICD therapy.[8,34,51,52,54]

Cardiac Dyssynchrony

About 30% of patients with moderate to severe CHF have interventricular and intraventricular conduction delays manifested by a widening of the QRS complex to ≤ 120 ms. These delays have been shown, in many studies, to be associated with worsened morbidity and mortality.[55–57] In an analysis of 5517 outpatients with CHF enrolled in the Italian Network on CHF Registry, left bundle branch block (LBBB) was a strong independent predictor of all-cause mortality and sudden cardiac death.[55]

Pathophysiology of cardiac dyssynchrony

Conduction delays have adverse effects on cardiac function that result from loss of intraventricular, atrioventricular, and interventricular synchrony. Loss of intraventricular synchrony results in increased myocardial stiffness, impaired systolic and diastolic functions, reduced diastolic filling time, prolonged mitral regurgitation duration, and an abnormal interventricular septal wall motion. LBBB affects myocardial activation appreciably as it causes the septum to contract first and the late-activated wall, typically the lateral wall, to contract last. The energy generated by this early septal activation is used to distend the late-activated wall. As such, this energy could not be used to generate sufficient pressure in the left ventricle to close the mitral valve. Because the mitral valve remains open, diastole is prolonged and systole is delayed.[58] Delayed contraction of the late-activated wall occurs in late systole. Some of the energy generated by the delayed contraction of the late-activated wall is wasted on trying to stretch the early-activated septum which is now beginning to relax. This results in the movement of the septum toward the right ventricle in mid to late systole. Stretching of the early-activated septum in late systole has adverse effects on LV function. Because blood tends to pool in the stretched septal area, it is not ejected. This results in a reduced cardiac output. Late stretching of the early activated septum can also result in non-uniform repolarization that could lead to re-entrant ventricular arrhythmias.[59–61]

Loss of atrioventricular synchrony results in reduced diastolic filling time. This, in turn, leads to increased pre-systolic mitral regurgitation and reduced cardiac output. Loss of interventricular synchrony alters ventricular interdependence and results in reduced LV filling. These hemodynamic changes exacerbate the symptoms of CHF.

Cardiac resynchronization therapy

CRT reverses the adverse effects of conduction delays by partial or total correction of intraventricular, atrioventricular, and interventricular dyssynchrony. Indeed, many studies have shown that CRT improves the hemodynamic parameters in patients with CHF and a wide QRS complex.[62–69] In a study by Kerwin *et al.*, biventricular pacing resulted in a significant improvement in LVEF; this improvement correlated significantly with improvement in interventricular synchrony.[64] In a study of patients with dilated cardiomyopathy and LBBB, Nelson *et al.* showed that LV and biventricular pacing resulted in a significant improvement in cardiac output and modest reduction in energy expenditure.[65] In another study of patients with CHF and QRS complex of > 120 ms, as compared with RV pacing, LV and biventricular pacing at short atrioventricular delays (80 ms to 120 ms) led to the greatest improvement in LV Doppler indices that included filling time, aortic velocity time and myocardial performance index.[68] In a study by Duncan *et al.*, atrio-biventricular pacing was assessed in 34 patients with an LVEF of < 35% and intraventricular conduction delay. Three months of atrio-biventricular pacing resulted in a significant reduction in total isovolumic time and LV cavity size.[69]

For CRT to be most effective, the atrioventricular delay should be optimized. In a study of 39 patients with CHF and ventricular conduction delay, LV and biventricular pacing led to a significant increase in systolic hemodynamics without a significant rise in the left ventricular end-diastolic pressure (LVEDP). When the LVEDP was reduced by shortening the AV delay, LV pressure, aortic pulse pressure, and atrioventricular mechanical latency decreased.[70]

Leclercq and coworkers conducted an acute hemodynamic study of biventricular pacing in patients with NYHA class III and IV heart failure symptoms and prolonged QRS complex. Using a Swan–Ganz catheter, they showed that biventricular pacing resulted in a significant decrease in the pulmonary capillary wedge pressure and a significant increase in the cardiac index.[71] Yu *et al.* used tissue Doppler echocardiography to evaluate 25 patients with NYHA class III and IV symptoms and a QRS width of > 140 ms after biventricular pacing for 3 months and when pacing was held for 1 month. They found that biventricular pacing not only reversed LV remodeling, but it also resulted in a significant improvement in EF, maximum rate of rise in ventricular pressure (dP/dt_{max}), myocardial performance index, mitral regurgitation, and LV end systolic and end diastolic volumes. The improvement in all these parameters led to a significant improvement in the 6-minute walk distance and quality-of-life score.[72]

Whether biventricular pacing affects autonomic nervous system function was uncertain until a study by Hamdan *et al.* showed that in patients with LVEF of < 35%, biventricular pacing or LV pacing alone improves sympathetic nerve activity.[73]

In one study, three-dimensional echocardiography was used to assess hemodynamic effects of biventricular pacing in 15 patients with CHF and LBBB. Biventricular pacing resulted in a significant reduction in LV end-diastolic volume, end-systolic volume, and mitral regurgitant fraction and a significant improvement in forward stroke volume and exercise capacity.[74]

Prospective studies of cardiac resynchronization therapy

Although numerous studies have proven the salutary effect of CRT on the hemodynamic parameters of patients with advanced CHF and a wide QRS complex, the clinical efficacy and safety of CRT have, until recently, been uncertain. The Multisite Stimulation in Cardiomyopathies (MUSTIC) study was one of the first studies to report on the clinical efficacy of CRT. This single-blind, randomized, controlled cross-over clinical trial enrolled patients with NYHA class III CHF symptoms, an LVEF of < 35%, an end-diastolic diameter of > 60 mm and a QRS complex of > 150 ms. It compared the responses of 48 patients during a 3-month period of inactive pacing and a 3-month period of atrio-biventricular pacing. It showed that active atrio-biventricular pacing resulted in a significant improvement in the exercise tolerance and quality of life of enrolled patients. Specifically, atrio-biventricular pacing led to a 23% increase in the mean distance walked in 6 minutes ($P < 0.001$), a 32% increase in the quality-of-life score ($P < 0.001$) and an 8% increase in peak oxygen uptake ($P < 0.03$). Although this study showed a significant reduction in the number of hospitalizations with atrio-biventricular pacing, due to its small sample size and short follow-up, no definitive conclusions could be derived regarding the effect of CRT on morbidity and mortality.[75]

The Pacing Therapies in Congestive Heart Failure (PATH-CHF) I trial was conducted in Europe and enrolled patients with NYHA class III and IV CHF symptoms, sinus rhythm, and a QRS width of > 120 ms. This single-blind study included 42 patients who received 2 dual-chamber pacemakers: 1 connected to a right atrial lead and a RV lead and the other connected to another right atrial lead and an epicardial LV lead. During surgical implantation of the LV lead, all patients underwent acute hemodynamic testing. Patients were randomized to 1 month of optimized univentricular or biventricular pacing followed by 1 month of no pacing. During the third month of the study, the patients crossed over to the other pacing mode. After 3 months, all patients were paced in the mode that provided the best response during intraoperative testing of acute hemodynamics. Patients were followed for 12 months, and the primary endpoints were functional capacity as measured by peak oxygen consumption and 6-minute walking distance. In this study, LV pacing alone or in combination with RV pacing resulted in a significant improvement in peak oxygen consumption, 6-minute walking distance, and quality of life.[76]

Subsequent to the PATH-CHF I trial, the PATH CHF II trial was conducted and enrolled patients with NYHA class II–IV CHF symptoms, an LVEF of ≤ 30%, peak oxygen consumption of < 18 mL/kg/min on maximum exercise testing, and a QRS width of ≤ 120 ms. All patients received either a pacemaker or an ICD, and the best site for ventricular pacing was determined by the patient's acute hemodynamic response to pacing. In the majority of patients, the best pacing mode was LV pacing. Patients were randomized to 3 months of active pacing (univentricular) or inactive pacing and were crossed over to 3 months of the therapy that they did not receive in the first 3 months. The order of the two pacing modes (active pacing and inactive pacing) was randomly assigned. This study showed that active pacing resulted in a significant improvement in NYHA class, quality of life score, distance walked in 6 minutes, and peak oxygen uptake.[77]

The Multicenter InSync Randomized Clinical Evaluation (MIRACLE) trial examined the effect of CRT on the NYHA functional class, quality of life, and the distance walked in 6 minutes in patients with NYHA class III and IV heart failure symptoms refractory to optimal medical therapy. Patients had to have an LVEF of ≤ 35%, a LV end-diastolic dimension of ≤ 55 mm, a QRS interval of ≥ 130 ms, and a 6-minute walking distance of ≤ 450 m. In this double-blind study, all patients underwent implantation of a CRT device; however, 228 patients were randomized to the CRT arm and 225 patients were randomized to the control arm (no pacing). All patients were followed for 6 months. Compared with patients in the control arm, patients in the CRT arm had a significant improvement in the NYHA functional class ($P < 0.001$), quality of life ($P = 0.001$), and the distance walked in 6 minutes ($P = 0.005$). Patients in the CRT arm also had a significant reduction in hospitalizations for CHF ($P < 0.05$) and the need for intravenous medications for the treatment of decompensated CHF ($P < 0.05$). This study showed no significant difference in mortality between the CRT arm and the control arm.[78]

The InSync ICD trial was a prospective, nonrandomized study that examined the efficacy of combined CRT and ICD in 84 patients with a conventional indication for an ICD, NYHA class II-IV CHF symptoms, an LVEF of < 35%, a LV end-diastolic diameter of 55 mm, and a QRS duration of > 130 ms. Within 3 months of follow-up, CRT resulted in a significant improvement in the distance walked in 6 minutes, quality of life, and NYHA class.[79]

The MIRACLE ICD trial explored the efficacy and safety of combined CRT and ICD therapy in 369 patients with NYHA class III and IV CHF symptoms refractory to optimized medical therapy, an LVEF of ≤ 35%, a QRS duration of ≤ 130 ms, and at high risk for life-threatening ventricular arrhythmias. In this randomized, double-blind, controlled trial, all patients underwent implantation of a device with CRT and ICD capabilities, but in 182 patients CRT was turned off and in 187 patients CRT was turned on. The primary endpoints of this study were identical to those of MIRACLE, and all patients were followed for 6 months. In this study, CRT resulted in a significant improvement in the NYHA functional class ($P = 0.007$) and quality-of-life score ($P = 0.02$) but not in the distance walked in 6 minutes ($P = 0.36$) or the rates of hospitalization ($P = 0.69$). CRT was associated with a significant increase in treadmill exercise duration and peak oxygen consumption. Although in MIRACLE, ICD CRT did not improve survival, CRT was not associated with an increase in the rate of arrhythmic events.[80]

In another trial, using the CONTAK CD® device, Higgins *et al.* examined the efficacy of the combination of CRT and ICD therapy. This randomized, double-blind, controlled study enrolled patients with NYHA class II to IV symptoms, an LVEF of ≤ 35%, a QRS width of ≤ 120 ms, and a conventional indication for ICD therapy. All patients (490) received a device with CRT and ICD capabilities, but CRT was programmed on only in 245 patients. The primary endpoint of this study was a composite endpoint of all-cause mortality, hospitalization for CHF, and ventricular arrhythmias requiring device therapy. Although a 15% reduction in the composite endpoint was observed with CRT, this reduction was statistically insignificant ($P = 0.35$). CRT was associated with a significant improvement in peak VO_2 and the distance walked in 6 minutes; however, CRT was not associated with a significant improvement in NYHA class and quality-of-life score.[81]

Although none of the randomized clinical trials of CRT discussed thus far found a significant improvement in survival with CRT, none of these studies had enough statistical power to show such an effect. Thus, the meta-analysis of the MUSTIC, MIRACLE, MIRACLE ICD, and CONTAK CD studies is noteworthy. This meta-analysis showed that CRT reduced death from progressive CHF by 51% (odds ratio [OR], 0.49; 95% CI, 0.25–0.93) and heart failure hospitalization by 29% (OR, 0.71; 95% CI, 0.53–0.96). CRT, however, was not associated with a significant reduction in all-cause mortality (OR, 0.77; 95% CI, 0.51–1.18).[82]

The Comparison of Medical Therapy, Pacing, and Defibrillation in Heart Failure (COMPANION) study was done to determine if CRT with or without an ICD would reduce the risk of death and hospitalization from any cause in patients with NYHA class III or IV CHF symptoms refractory to optimized medical therapy, an LVEF of ≤ 35%, a QRS width of ≤ 120 ms, a PR interval of > 150 ms, and a hospitalization for the treatment of CHF within 12 months from enrollment in the study. Patients had to be in sinus rhythm at enrollment and they had to have no clinical indication for a pacemaker or an ICD. Patients were randomized in a 1:2:2 ratio for optimal medical therapy alone, optimal medical therapy and CRT with a pacemaker, or optimal medical therapy and CRT with a pacemaker-defibrillator. In this study, both CRT with a pacemaker and CRT with a pacemaker-defibrillator resulted in a significant reduction of the primary endpoint (HR, 0.81, $P = 0.014$ and HR, 0.80, $P = 0.01$, respectively). CRT with a pacemaker reduced the risk of the secondary endpoint of all-cause mortality by 24% ($P = 0.059$), and CRT with a pacemaker-defibrillator reduced all-cause mortality by 36% ($P = 0.003$).[83]

Uncertainties about cardiac resynchronization therapy

Although our knowledge of CRT has been expanding rapidly, a lot remains to be learned. One critical question that has important implications for patient care is whether or not one can predict response to CRT. The aforementioned trials of CRT showed that up to one-third of patients treated with CRT show no clinically meaningful improvement in functional status or quality of life. So, it is important to learn more about responders and nonresponders to CRT. It has been proposed that the width of the QRS complex predicts response to CRT. However, the correlation between QRS width and acute hemodynamic response to CRT is modest at best, and studies of chronic response to CRT showed poor correlation between QRS width and response to CRT.[84–87]

In a comparison of responders and nonresponders to CRT, Reuter *et al.* identified a history of MI, a low cardiac output, and absence of significant mitral regurgitation as predictors of lack of response to CRT. They further showed that age, presence of chronic atrial fibrillation, electrical parameters, NYHA class, and LVEF were not significant predictors of response to CRT.[87] Another study examined the clinical efficacy of CRT as a function of the severity of ventricular conduction delay. That study showed significant improvements in peak VO_2, distance walked in 6 minutes, and quality-of-life score with CRT. However, these improvements were only observed in patients with a QRS width of > 150 ms. Patients with a QRS width between 120 ms and 150 ms derived no benefit from CRT.[77] These conflicting results suggest that the QRS width may not be a reliable surrogate for ventricular dyssynchrony. Thus, some echocardiographic parameters have been proposed as more reliable surrogates for ventricular dyssynchrony than QRS width. Although a few of these echocardiographic parameters seemed to predict acute hemodynamic improvement to CRT, more studies are needed to better define the full potential of these echocardiographic measures.[88,89]

Another important question relates to the efficacy of CRT in patients with chronic atrial fibrillation. Although a few studies attempted to answer this question, those studies were too small to convey a definitive answer. One study included 20 patients with NYHA functional class III or IV CHF symptoms, an LVEF of ≤ 35%, a history of prior AV nodal ablation, and RV pacing performed for chronic atrial fibrillation of at least 6 months' duration. In these patients, CRT led to a significant improvement in NYHA functional class, LVEF, and quality-of-life score.[90]

In a single-blind, randomized sub-study of the MUSTIC trial, CRT was tested in 37 patients with chronic atrial fibrillation and a slow ventricular response necessitating permanent ventricular pacing, a paced QRS width of ≤ 200 ms, NYHA class III CHF symptoms, and significant LV systolic dysfunction. Patient response was monitored during two 3-month treatment periods of conventional right-univentricular pacing and biventricular pacing. This study showed a significant increase in the distance walked in 6 minutes and a significant decrease in the rate of hospitalization for CHF with CRT.[91] Another study included 37 patients (22 patients in sinus rhythm and 15 patients in atrial fibrillation) with dilated cardiomyopathy, severe CHF symptoms refractory to medical therapy, and a QRS width of ≤ 120 ms. CRT led to a significant improvement in NYHA class and peak VO_2 in patients in sinus rhythm and those in atrial fibrillation.[92] Although these results are promising, they certainly need to be confirmed by future randomized clinical trials.

Additional uncertainties that need to be addressed in future studies include the role of CRT in patients with right bundle branch block (RBBB), the efficacy of CRT in patients with a narrow QRS complex, and the role of CRT in patients with mild CHF symptoms. Clinical trials of CRT either excluded patients with RBBB or included a small number of patients with RBBB. For example, only 10% of patients enrolled in the COMPANION trial had RBBB.[83] Whether CRT benefits patients with a narrow QRS complex is largely uncertain. However, 1 study of CRT that included 14 patients with a QRS complex of ≤ 120 ms and severe heart failure showed significant improvements in the NYHA functional class, LVEF, and the distance walked in 6 minutes. Interestingly, these improvements were similar between the group of patients with a narrow QRS complex and the group of patients with a wide QRS complex (> 120 ms).[93]

Another important question relates to the best implantation site for the LV lead. Because LBBB results in late activation of the lateral wall, it has been proposed that the lateral wall is the best site for LV lead placement. In the PATH-CHF II trial, left free wall pacing resulted in a significantly better LV systolic performance than anterior wall pacing.[94] These results, however, could not be reproduced by another study that examined the long-term efficacy of CRT based on different LV pacing sites. This study included 158 patients with a mean EF of 29% and a mean QRS width of 174 ms. CRT resulted in a significant improvement in exercise capacity and EF regardless of the LV pacing site.[95]

Whether CRT has any effect on the incidence of tachyarrhythmias is uncertain. At least 1 study of 32 patients enrolled in the Ventak CHF trial examined the effect of CRT on the need for tachyarrhythmia therapy. Patients completed two 3-month treatment periods of biventricular pacing and no pacing. While programmed to biventricular pacing, 16% of the patients had at least one tachyarrhythmic episode, and while programmed to no pacing 35% of the patients had at least one tachyarrhythmic episode ($P = 0.035$). Although these results are intriguing, larger studies are needed to define the effect of CRT on tachyarrhythmias.[96]

One additional question that needs to be addressed is the effect of chronic RV pacing on survival. The Dual Chamber and VVI Implantable Defibrillator (DAVID) trial was done to compare the efficacy of dual-chamber pacing at 70 bpm with that of backup RV pacing at 40 bpm. This single-blind, randomized clinical trial enrolled patients with an LVEF of ≤ 40%, an approved indication for an ICD, no indication for pacing, and no history of atrial arrhythmias. The majority of the enrolled patients had a history of CHF, and the mean LVEF was 27%. This study showed that dual-chamber pacing was associated with a slight increase in the composite endpoint of time to death or first hospitalization for CHF.[97] Although these results are of concern, more studies are needed to address this issue definitively.

Conclusion

There is no doubt that device therapy has an important role in the management of patients with CHF. In the arena of sudden cardiac death prevention, numerous randomized clinical trials have proven the efficacy of ICD therapy at reducing the risk of death. In the arena of cardiac dyssynchrony, numerous clinical trials have proven that CRT improves patient hemodynamics, functional capacity, quality of life, and outcomes. Undoubtedly, the number of patients with CHF who could benefit from ICD therapy or CRT is enormous. Thus, efforts should be directed at making these therapies affordable and widely available.

References

1. American Heart Association. Heart Disease and Stroke Statistics—2001 Update (American Heart Association: Dallas, TX, 2000).
2. Effect of metoprolol CR/XL in chronic heart failure: Metoprolol CR/XL Randomised Intervention Trial in Congestive Heart Failure (MERIT-HF). Lancet 1999; 353: 2001–2007.
3. Kannel WB, Ho K, Thom T. Changing epidemiological features of cardiac failure. Br Heart J 1994; 72: S3–S9.
4. Bigger JT, Fleiss JL, Kleiger, Miller JP, Rolnitzky LM. The relationship between ventricular arrhythmias, left ventricular dysfunction, and mortality in the 2 years after myocardial infarction. Circulation 1984; 69; 250–258.
5. Cupples LA, Gagnon DR, Kannel WB. Long- and short-term risk of sudden coronary death. Circulation 1992; 85: I11–I18.
6. Mukharji J, Rude RE, Poole WK, *et al.* Risk factors for sudden death after acute myocardial infarction: two-year follow-up. Am J Cardiol 1984; 54: 31–36.
7. Goldman S, Johnson G, Cohn JN, *et al.* Mechanism of death in heart failure. The Vasodilator-Heart Failure Trials. The V-HeFT VA Cooperative Studies Group. Circulation 1993; 87: VI24–VI31.
8. Buxton AE, Lee KL, Fisher JD, *et al.* A randomized study of the prevention of sudden death in patients with coronary artery disease. Multicenter Unsustained Tachycardia Trial Investigators. N Engl J Med 1999; 341: 1882–1890.
9. Moss AJ, Zareba W, Hall WJ, *et al.* Prophylactic implantation of a defibrillator in patients with myocardial infarction and reduced ejection fraction. N Engl J Med 2002; 346: 877–883.
10. Chen X, Shenasa M, Borggrefe M, *et al.* Role of programmed ventricular stimulation in patients with

idiopathic dilated cardiomyopathy and documented sustained ventricular tachyarrhythmias: inducibility and prognostic value in 102 patients. Eur Heart J 1994; 15: 76–82.

11. Turitto G, Ahuja RK, Caref EB, el-Sherif N. Risk stratification for arrhythmic events in patients with nonischemic dilated cardiomyopathy and nonsustained ventricular tachycardia: role of programmed ventricular stimulation and the signal-averaged electrocardiogram. J Am Coll Cardiol 1994; 24: 1523–1528.
12. Grimm W, Hoffmann J, Menz V, Luck K, Maisch B. Programmed ventricular stimulation for arrhythmia risk prediction in patients with idiopathic dilated cardiomyopathy and nonsustained ventricular tachycardia. J Am Coll Cardiol 1998; 32: 739–745.
13. Brilakis ES, Shen WK, Hammill SC, *et al.* Role of programmed ventricular stimulation and implantable cardioverter defibrillators in patients with idiopathic dilated cardiomyopathy and syncope. Pacing Clin Electrophysiol 2001; 24: 1623–1630.
14. Kuchar DL, Thorburn CW, Sammel NL. Late potentials detected after myocardial infarction: natural history and prognostic significance. Circulation 1986; 74: 1280–1289.
15. Kuchar DL, Thorburn CW, Sammel NL. Prediction of serious arrhythmic events after myocardial infarction: signal-averaged electrocardiogram, Holter monitoring and radionuclide ventriculography. J Am Coll Cardiol 1987; 9: 531–538.
16. Farrell TG, Bashir Y, Cripps T, *et al.* Risk stratification for arrhythmic events in postinfarction patients based on heart rate variability, ambulatory electrocardiographic variables and the signal-averaged electrocardiogram. J Am Coll Cardiol 1991; 18: 687–697.
17. Gold MR, Bloomfield DM, Anderson KP, *et al.* A comparison of T-wave alternans, signal-averaged electrocardiography and programmed ventricular stimulation for arrhythmia risk stratification. J Am Coll Cardiol 2000; 36: 2247–2253.
18. Gomes JA, Cain ME, Buxton AE, *et al.* Prediction of long-term outcomes by signal-averaged electrocardiography in patients with unsustained ventricular tachycardia, coronary artery disease, and left ventricular dysfunction. Circulation 2001; 104: 436–441.
19. Zabel M, Klingenheben T, Franz MR, Hohnloser SH. Assessment of QT dispersion for prediction of mortality or arrhythmic events after myocardial infarction: results of a prospective long-term follow-up study. Circulation 1998; 97: 2543–2550.
20. La Rovere MT, Bigger JT Jr., Marcus FI, Mortara A, Schwartz PJ. Baroreflex sensitivity and heart-rate variability in prediction of total cardiac mortality after myocardial infarction. ATRAMI (Autonomic Tone and Reflexes After Myocardial Infarction) Investigators. Lancet 1998; 351: 478–484.
21. Costantini O, Drabek C, Rosenbaum DS. Can sudden cardiac death be predicted from the T wave of the ECG? A critical examination of T wave alternans and QT interval dispersion. Pacing Clin Electrophysiol 2000; 23: 1407–1416.
22. Rosenbaum DS, Jackson LE, Smith JM, *et al.* Electrical alternans and vulnerability to ventricular arrhythmias. N Engl J Med 1994; 330: 235–241.
23. Klingenheben T, Zabel M, D'Agostino RB, Cohen RJ, Hohnloser SH. Predictive value of T-wave alternans for arrhythmic events in patients with congestive heart failure. Lancet 2000; 356: 651–652.
24. Adachi K, Ohnishi Y, Yokoyama M. Risk stratification for sudden cardiac death in dilated cardiomyopathy using microvolt-level T-wave alternans. Jpn Circ J 2001; 65: 76–80.
25. Hennersdorf MG, Perings C, Niebch V. T wave alternans as a risk predictor in patients with cardiomyopathy and mild-to-moderate heart disease. Pacing Clin Electrophysiol 2000; 23: 1386–1391.
26. The Cardiac Arrhythmia Suppression Trial (CAST) Investigators. Preliminary report: effect of encainide and flecainide on mortality in a randomized trial of arrhythmia suppression after myocardial infarction. N Engl J Med 1989; 321: 406–412.
27. Echt DS, Liebson PR, Mitchell LB, *et al.* Mortality and morbidity in patients receiving encainide, flecainide, or placebo. The Cardiac Arrhythmia Suppression Trial. N Engl J Med 1991; 324: 781–788.
28. The Cardiac Arrhythmia Suppression Trial II Investigators. Effect of the antiarrhythmic agent moricizine on survival after myocardial infarction. N Engl J Med 1992; 327: 227–233.
29. Kuck KH, Cappato R, Siebels J, Ruppel R. Randomized comparison of antiarrhythmic drug therapy with implantable defibrillators in patients resuscitated from cardiac arrest: the Cardiac Arrest Study Hamburg (CASH). Circulation 2000; 102: 748–754.
30. Waldo AL, Camm AJ, de Ruyter H, *et al.* Effect of d-sotalol on mortality in patients with left ventricular dysfunction after recent and remote myocardial infarction. The SWORD Investigators. Survival With Oral d-Sotalol. Lancet 1996; 348: 7–12.
31. Julian DG, Camm AJ, Frangin G, *et al.* Randomised trial of effect of amiodarone on mortality in patients with left ventricular dysfunction after recent myocardial infarction: EMIAT. European Myocardial Infarct Amiodarone Trial Investigators. Lancet 1997; 349: 667–674.

32. Cairns JA, Connolly SJ, Roberts R, Gent M. Randomised trial of outcome after myocardial infarction in patients with frequent or repetitive ventricular premature depolarisations: CAMIAT. Canadian Amiodarone Myocardial Infarction Arrhythmia Trial Investigators. Lancet 1997; 349: 675–682.
33. Singh SN, Fletcher RD, Fisher SG, *et al.* Amiodarone in patients with congestive heart failure and asymptomatic ventricular arrhythmia. Survival Trial of Antiarrhythmic Therapy in Congestive Heart Failure. N Engl J Med 1995; 333: 77–82.
34. Results from the Sudden Cardiac Death in Heart Failure Trial (SCD-HeFT). Presented at: American College of Cardiology 2004 Scientific Sessions, New Orleans, LA, March 2004.
35. Torp-Pedersen C, Moller M, Bloch-Thomsen PE, *et al.* Dofetilide in patients with congestive heart failure and left ventricular dysfunction. Danish Investigations of Arrhythmia and Mortality on Dofetilide Study Group. N Engl J Med 1999; 341: 857–865.
36. Pratt CM, Singh SN, Al-Khalidi HR, *et al.* ALIVE Investigators. The efficacy of azimilide in the treatment of atrial fibrillation in the presence of left ventricular systolic dysfunction: results from the Azimilide Postinfarct Survival Evaluation (ALIVE) trial. J Am Coll Cardiol 2004; 43: 1211–1216.
37. Timolol-induced reduction in mortality and reinfarction in patients surviving acute myocardial infarction. N Engl J Med 1981; 304: 801–807.
38. A randomized trial of propranolol in patients with acute myocardial infarction. I. Mortality results. JAMA 1982; 247: 1707–1714.
39. Hjalmarson A, Elmfeldt D, Herlitz J, *et al.* Effect on mortality of metoprolol in acute myocardial infarction: a double-blind randomised trial. Lancet 1981; 2: 823–827.
40. The Cardiac Insufficiency Bisoprolol Study II (CIBIS-II): a randomised trial. Lancet 1999; 353: 9–13.
41. Pitt B, Zannad F, Remme WJ, *et al.* The effect of spironolactone on morbidity and mortality in patients with severe heart failure. Randomized Aldactone Evaluation Study Investigators. N Engl J Med 1999; 341: 709–717.
42. Pitt B, Remme W, Zannad F, *et al.* Eplerenone Post-Acute Myocardial Infarction Heart Failure Efficacy and Survival Study Investigators. Eplerenone, a selective aldosterone blocker, in patients with left ventricular dysfunction after myocardial infarction. N Engl J Med 2003; 348: 1309–1321.
43. Singh SN, Karasik P, Hafley GE, *et al.* for the MUSTT Investigators. Multicenter UnSustained Tachycardia Trial. Electrophysiologic and clinical effects of angiotensin-converting enzyme inhibitors in patients with prior myocardial infarction, nonsustained ventricular tachycardia, and depressed left ventricular function. Am J Cardiol 2001; 87: 716–720.
44. Domanski MJ, Exner DV, Borkowf CB, *et al.* Effect of angiotensin converting enzyme inhibition on sudden cardiac death in patients following acute myocardial infarction. A meta-analysis of randomized clinical trials. J Am Coll Cardiol 1999; 33: 598–604.
45. Yusuf S, Sleight P, Pogue J, *et al.* Effects of an angiotensin-converting-enzyme inhibitor, ramipril, on cardiovascular events in high-risk patients. The Heart Outcomes Prevention Evaluation Study Investigators. N Engl J Med 2000; 342: 145–153.
46. Mitchell BL, Powell JL, Gillis AM, *et al.* Are lipid-lowering drugs also antiarrhythmic drugs? An analysis of the Antiarrhythmic versus Implantable Defibrillators (AVID) trial. J Am Coll Cardiol 2003; 42: 81–87.
47. The Antiarrhythmics versus Implantable Defibrillators (AVID) Investigators. A comparison of antiarrhythmic drug therapy with implantable defibrillators in patients resuscitated from near-fatal ventricular arrhythmias. N Engl J Med 1997; 337: 1576–1583.
48. Connolly SJ, Gent M, Roberts RS, *et al.* Canadian implantable defibrillator study (CIDS): a randomized trial of the implantable cardioverter defibrillator against amiodarone. Circulation 2000; 101: 1297–1302.
49. Domanski MJ, Sakseena S, Epstein AE, *et al.* Relative effectiveness of the implantable cardioverter-defibrillator and antiarrhythmic drugs in patients with varying degrees of left ventricular dysfunction who have survived malignant ventricular arrhythmias. AVID Investigators. Antiarrhythmics versus Implantable Defibrillators. J Am Coll Cardiol 1999; 34: 1090–1095.
50. Sheldon R, Connolly S, Krahn A, *et al.* Identification of patients most likely to benefit from implantable cardioverter-defibrillator therapy: the Canadian Implantable Defibrillator Study. Circulation 2000; 101: 1660–1664.
51. Moss AJ, Hall WJ, Cannom DS, *et al.* Improved survival with an implanted defibrillator in patients with coronary disease at high risk for ventricular arrhythmia. Multicenter Automatic Defibrillator Implantation Trial Investigators. N Engl J Med 1996; 335: 1933–1940.
52. Moss AJ, Zareba W, Hall WJ, *et al.* Multicenter Automatic Defibrillator Implantation Trial II Investigators. Prophylactic implantation of a defibrillator in patients with myocardial infarction and

reduced ejection fraction. N Engl J Med 2002; 346: 877–883.
53. Bigger JT, Jr. Prophylactic use of implanted cardiac defibrillators in patients at high risk for ventricular arrhythmias after coronary artery bypass graft surgery. Coronary Artery Bypass Graft (CABG) Patch trial Investigators. N Engl J Med 1997; 337: 1569–1575.
54. Kadish A, Dyer A, Daubert JP *et al.* Defibrillators in Non-ischemic Cardiomyopathy Treatment Evaluation (DEFINITE) Investigators. Prophylactic defibrillator implantation in patients with non-ischemic dilated cardiomyopathy. N Engl J Med 2004; 350: 2151–2158.
55. Baldasseroni S, Opasich C, Gorini M, *et al.* Italian Network on Congestive Heart Failure Investigators. Left bundle-branch block is associated with increased 1-year sudden and total mortality rate in 5517 outpatients with congestive heart failure: a report from the Italian network on congestive heart failure. Am Heart J 2002; 143: 398–405.
56. Iuliano S, Fisher SG, Karasik PE, Fletcher RD, Singh SN, Department of Veterans Affairs Survival Trial of Antiarrhythmic Therapy in Congestive Heart Failure. QRS duration and mortality in patients with congestive heart failure. Am Heart J 2002; 143: 1085–1091.
57. Shamim W, Francis DP, Yousufuddin M, *et al.* Intraventricular conduction delay: a prognostic marker in chronic heart failure. Int J Cardiol 1999; 70: 171–178.
58. Leclercq C, Faris O, Tunin R, *et al.* Systolic improvement and mechanical resynchronization does not require electrical synchrony in the dilated failing heart with left bundle-branch block. Circulation 2002; 106: 1760–1763.
59. Eckardt L, Kirchhof P, Breithardt G, Haverkamp W. Load-induced changes in repolarization: evidence from experimental and clinical data. Basic Res Cardiol 2001; 96: 369–380.
60. Taggart P, Sutton PM. Cardiac mechano-electric feedback in man: clinical relevance. Prog Biophys Mol Biol 1999; 71: 139–154.
61. Franz MR, Cima R, Wang D, Profitt D, Kurz R. Electrophysiological effects of myocardial stretch and mechanical determinants of stretch-activated arrhythmias. Circulation 1992; 86: 968–978.
62. Kass DA, Chen CH, Curry C, *et al.* Improved left ventricular mechanics from acute VDD pacing in patients with dilated cardiomyopathy and ventricular conduction delay. Circulation 1999; 99: 1567–1573.
63. Wyman BT, Hunter WC, Prinzen FW, McVeigh ER. Mapping propagation of mechanical activation in the paced heart with MRI tagging. Am J Physiol 1999; 276: H881–H891.
64. Kerwin WF, Botvinick EH, O'Connell JW, *et al.* Ventricular contraction abnormalities in dilated cardiomyopathy: effect of biventricular pacing to correct interventricular dyssynchrony. J Am Coll Cardiol 2000; 35: 1221–1227.
65. Nelson GS, Berger RD, Fetics BJ, *et al.* Left ventricular or biventricular pacing improves cardiac function at diminished energy cost in patients with dilated cardiomyopathy and left bundle-branch block. Circulation 2000; 102: 3053–3059.
66. Sogaard P, Egeblad H, Kim WY, *et al.* Tissue Doppler imaging predicts improved systolic performance and reversed left ventricular remodeling during long-term cardiac resynchronization therapy. J Am Coll Cardiol 2002; 40: 723–730.
67. Stellbrink C, Breithardt OA, Franke A, *et al.*, PATH-CHF (PAcing THerapies in Congestive Heart Failure) Investigators; CPI Guidant Congestive Heart Failure Research Group. Impact of cardiac resynchronization therapy using hemodynamically optimized pacing on left ventricular remodeling in patients with congestive heart failure and ventricular conduction disturbances. J Am Coll Cardiol 2001; 38: 1957–1965.
68. Breithardt OA, Stellbrink C, Franke A, *et al.*, Pacing Therapies for Congestive Heart Failure Study Group; Guidant Congestive Heart Failure Research Group. Acute effects of cardiac resynchronization therapy on left ventricular Doppler indices in patients with congestive heart failure. Am Heart J 2002; 143: 34–44.
69. Duncan A, Wait D, Gibson D, Daubert JC; MUSTIC (Multisite Stimulation in Cardiomyopathies) Trial. Left ventricular remodelling and haemodynamic effects of multisite biventricular pacing in patients with left ventricular systolic dysfunction and activation disturbances in sinus rhythm: sub-study of the MUSTIC (Multisite Stimulation in Cardiomyopathies) trial. Eur Heart J 2003; 24: 430–441.
70. Auricchio A, Ding J, Spinelli JC, *et al.* Cardiac resynchronization therapy restores optimal atrioventricular mechanical timing in heart failure patients with ventricular conduction delay. J Am Coll Cardiol 2002; 39: 1163–1169.
71. Leclercq C, Cazeau S, Le Breton H, *et al.* Acute hemodynamic effects of biventricular DDD pacing in patients with end-stage heart failure. J Am Coll Cardiol 1998; 32: 1825–1831.
72. Yu CM, Chau E, Sanderson JE, *et al.* Tissue Doppler echocardiographic evidence of reverse remodeling and improved synchronicity by simultaneously delaying regional contraction after biventricular pacing therapy in heart failure. Circulation 2002; 105: 438–445.

73. Hamdan MH, Zagrodzky JD, Joglar JA, *et al.* Biventricular pacing decreases sympathetic activity compared with right ventricular pacing in patients with depressed ejection fraction. Circulation 2000; 102: 1027–1032.
74. Kim WY, Sogaard P, Mortensen PT, *et al.* Three dimensional echocardiography documents haemodynamic improvement by biventricular pacing in patients with severe heart failure. Heart 2001; 85: 514–520.
75. Cazeau S, Leclercq C, Lavergne T, *et al.*, Multisite Stimulation in Cardiomyopathies (MUSTIC) Study Investigators. Effects of multisite biventricular pacing in patients with heart failure and intraventricular conduction delay. N Engl J Med 2001; 344: 873–880.
76. Auricchio A, Stellbrink C, Sack S, *et al.*, Pacing Therapies in Congestive Heart Failure (PATH-CHF) Study Group. Long-term clinical effect of hemodynamically optimized cardiac resynchronization therapy in patients with heart failure and ventricular conduction delay. J Am Coll Cardiol 2002; 39: 2026–2033.
77. Auricchio A, Stellbrink C, Butter C, *et al.*, Pacing Therapies in Congestive Heart Failure II Study Group; Guidant Heart Failure Research Group. Clinical efficacy of cardiac resynchronization therapy using left ventricular pacing in heart failure patients stratified by severity of ventricular conduction delay. J Am Coll Cardiol 2003; 42: 2109–2116.
78. Abraham WT, Fisher WG, Smith AL, *et al.*, MIRACLE Study Group. Multicenter InSync Randomized Clinical Evaluation. Cardiac resynchronization in chronic heart failure. N Engl J Med 2002; 346: 1845–1853.
79. Kuhlkamp V; InSync 7272 ICD World Wide Investigators. Initial experience with an implantable cardioverter-defibrillator incorporating cardiac resynchronization therapy. J Am Coll Cardiol 2002; 39: 790–797.
80. Young JB, Abraham WT, Smith AL, *et al.*, Multicenter InSync ICD Randomized Clinical Evaluation (MIRACLE ICD) Trial Investigators. Combined cardiac resynchronization and implantable cardioversion defibrillation in advanced chronic heart failure: the MIRACLE ICD Trial. JAMA 2003; 289: 2685–2694.
81. Higgins SL, Hummel JD, Niazi IK, *et al.* Cardiac resynchronization therapy for the treatment of heart failure in patients with intraventricular conduction delay and malignant ventricular tachyarrhythmias. J Am Coll Cardiol 2003; 42: 1454–1459.
82. Bradley DJ, Bradley EA, Baughman KL, *et al.* Cardiac resynchronization and death from progressive heart failure: a meta-analysis of randomized controlled trials. JAMA 2003; 289: 730–740.
83. Bristow MR, Saxon LA, Boehmer J, *et al.*, Comparison of Medical Therapy, Pacing, and Defibrillation in Heart Failure (COMPANION) Investigators. Cardiac-resynchronization therapy with or without an implantable defibrillator in advanced chronic heart failure. N Engl J Med 2004; 350: 2140–2150.
84. Nelson GS, Curry CW, Wyman BT, *et al.* Predictors of systolic augmentation from left ventricular preexcitation in patients with dilated cardiomyopathy and intraventricular conduction delay. Circulation 2000; 101: 2703–2709.
85. Pitzalis MV, Iacoviello M, Romito R, *et al.* Cardiac resynchronization therapy tailored by echocardiographic evaluation of ventricular asynchrony. J Am Coll Cardiol 2002; 40: 1615–1622.
86. Fauchier L, Marie O, Casset-Sernon D, *et al.* Interventricular and intraventricular dyssynchrony in idiopathic dilated cardiomyopathy: a prognostic study with Fourier phase analysis of radionuclide angioscintigraphy. J Am Coll Cardiol 2002; 40: 2022–2030.
87. Rueter S, Garrigue S, Barold SS, *et al.* Comparison of characteristics in responders versus nonresponders with biventricular pacing for drug-resistant congestive heart failure. Am J Cardiol 2002; 89: 346–350.
88. Gorcsan J 3rd, Kanzaki H, Bazaz R, Dohi K, Schwartzman D. Usefulness of echocardiographic tissue synchronization imaging to predict acute response to cardiac resynchronization therapy. Am J Cardiol 2004; 93: 1178–1181.
89. Breithardt OA, Stellbrink C, Kramer AP, *et al.*, PATH-CHF Study Group. Pacing Therapies for Congestive Heart Failure. Echocardiographic quantification of left ventricular asynchrony predicts an acute hemodynamic benefit of cardiac resynchronization therapy. J Am Coll Cardiol 2002; 40: 536–545.
90. Leon AR, Greenberg JM, Kanuru N, *et al.* Cardiac resynchronization in patients with congestive heart failure and chronic atrial fibrillation: effect of upgrading to biventricular pacing after chronic right ventricular pacing. J Am Coll Cardiol 2002; 39: 1258–1263.
91. Leclercq C, Walker S, Linde C, *et al.* Comparative effects of permanent biventricular and right-univentricular pacing in heart failure patients with chronic atrial fibrillation. Eur Heart J 2002; 23: 1780–1787.
92. Leclercq C, Victor F, Alonso C, *et al.* Comparative effects of permanent biventricular pacing for refractory heart failure in patients with stable sinus rhythm or chronic atrial fibrillation. Am J Cardiol 2000; 85: 1154–1156.
93. Achilli A, Sassara M, Ficili S, *et al.* Long-term effectiveness of cardiac resynchronization therapy in

patients with refractory heart failure and "narrow" QRS. J Am Coll Cardiol 2003; 42: 2117–2124.

94. Butter C, Auricchio A, Stellbrink C, *et al.*, Pacing Therapy for Chronic Heart Failure II Study Group. Effect of resynchronization therapy stimulation site on the systolic function of heart failure patients. Circulation 2001; 104: 3026–3029.
95. Gasparini M, Mantica M, Galimberti P, *et al.* Is the left ventricular lateral wall the best lead implantation site for cardiac resynchronization therapy? Pacing Clin Electrophysiol 2003; 26: 162–168.
96. Higgins SL, Yong P, Sheck D, *et al.* Biventricular pacing diminishes the need for implantable cardioverter defibrillator therapy. Ventak CHF Investigators. J Am Coll Cardiol 2000; 36: 824–827.
97. Wilkoff BL, Cook JR, Epstein AE, *et al.*, Dual Chamber and VVI Implantable Defibrillator Trial Investigators. Dual-chamber pacing or ventricular backup pacing in patients with an implantable defibrillator: the Dual Chamber and VVI Implantable Defibrillator (DAVID) trial. JAMA 2002; 288: 3115–3123.

Chapter 27

Intraaortic balloon pumps in acute heart failure

David Bragin-Sánchez, Patricia P Chang, E Magnus Ohman

Introduction

The intraaortic balloon pump (IABP) is the most commonly used method of mechanical cardiac support with more than a 100 000 insertions per year worldwide.[1–3] Its popularity is due primarily to widespread availability, simplicity of implantation and removal, and low cost, when compared with other mechanical circulatory support devices. IABP has been shown to hemodynamically stabilize and reduce mortality in patients with cardiogenic shock of various etiologies.[4–10] Moreover, the use of IABP does not significantly increase hospital costs and can be cost effective.[11–13] In this chapter, we will review the utility of IABP use among patients with congestive heart failure (CHF). Although the majority of recent data is derived from acute myocardial infarction (AMI) patients with CHF, we will attempt to extrapolate this information to patients with acute-on-chronic CHF. We will outline the physiological aspects of IABP and how it exerts the clinical benefits observed.

Historical Perspective

The Kantrowitz brothers laid down the theoretical groundwork for the development of the IABP in 1953 when they hypothesized that coronary blood flow could be improved by delaying the transmission of the pulse wave during diastole.[14] In 1961, Clauss *et al.* introduced the concept of counterpulsation, which could reduce work stress on the heart and permit improved tissue perfusion.[15] Moulopoulos demonstrated that IABP produced hemodynamic benefits in the failing canine heart in 1962.[16] In 1968, Adrian Kantrowitz heralded the modern day use of IABP in humans with cardiogenic shock and predicted many of its present-day uses.[17] This chapter reviews the modern-day use of IABP in the setting of acutely decompensated heart failure (ADHF), including the proper operation of this therapy and management of patients receiving it.

Review of the historic and present literature

In the history of IABP technology, indications and techniques of insertion have evolved over time. Initially IABP was strictly for surgical use and inserted through cutdown or transthoracic technique. Now, it is almost strictly a percutaneous technique.[1] Unfortunately, there is minimal randomized trial data on the use of IABP and much less information in its use among patients with CHF. A randomized trial of preoperative IABP in patients undergoing coronary artery bypass grafting (CABG) with left ventricular hypertrophy (LVH) and ejection fraction (EF) $< 40\%$ was associated with reduced mortality and improved hospital course.[18] The use of IABP in primary percutaneous interventions during AMI has also been studied in randomized trials and has not proven to reduce mortality or improve myocardial salvage.[19,20] A reason for this lack of data is the very nature of patients in whom IABP is used, namely critically ill patients in whom control group or placebo is not an alternative. In 1 center, IABP was used in a total of 1760 heart failure patients with 672 deaths or 38.2% mortality.[21]

In this chapter, we review the trends in use and indications of IABP over time. For this purpose, we performed a Medline search for articles published between 1950 and June 2004, in which IABP was used for one or multiple indications and its outcomes in terms of mortality were defined. Keywords used were "intraaortic balloon pump," "balloon counterpulsation," and "balloon pump." We grouped the studies by indication (Tables 27.1, 27.2, and 27.3). In a large population of critically ill patients with coronary artery disease (CAD) (2538 patients with AMI or unstable angina), the mortality after IABP use is reasonably low at 13% (Table 27.1). When IABP is primarily used as a bridge to transplant, the mortality has been quite

Table 27.1. *Intraaortic balloon pumps in patients with acute coronary syndromes*

Authors	Year	No. of patients	Mortality no. (%)
Hagemeijer *et al.*[23]	1977	25	5 (20)
Tobias *et al.*[24]	1979	60	37 (61)
Torchiana *et al.*[21]	1997	2453	292 (12)
Total		2538	334 (13)

Table 27.2. *Intraaortic balloon pumps in patients as a bridge to transplant*

Author	Year	Patients no.	Mortality no. (%)
Birovljev *et al.*[25]	1992	14	3 (23)
Lazar *et al.*[22]	1992	49	20 (41)
Masters *et al.*[26]	1996	13	2 (15)
Total		76	25 (33)

Table 27.3. *Use of intraaortic balloon pumps in cardiac surgery according to time of implantation*

		Postsurgical		Intrasurgical		Presurgical	
Authors	Year	Number of patients	Mortality no. (%)	Number of patients	Mortality no. (%)	Number of patients	Mortality no. (%)
Scanlon *et al.*[27]	1976	40	18 (45)				
Macoviak *et al.*[28]	1980	178	116 (65)				
Golding *et al.*[29]	1980	197	53 (27)				
Downing *et al.*[30]	1981	280	126 (45)				
Kafrouni[31]	1984	399	160 (40)				
McGeehin *et al.*[32]	1987	39	22 (56)				
Creswell *et al.*[33]	1992	76	47 (20)	353	14 (32)	240	47 (20)
Torchiana *et al.*[21]	1997	276	277 (14)	771	275 (36)	2038	277 (14)
Mueller *et al.*[34]	1998	24	13 (54)				
Arafa *et al.*[35]	2001	622	287 (45.1)				
Hausmann *et al.*[36]	2001	391	133 (34)				
Castelli *et al.*[37]	2001	105	38 (36)				
Meco *et al.*[38]	2002	116	67 (58)				
Total		2767	1177 (43)	1124	389 (35)	2278	324 (14)

high, at 33%, in this much smaller population (76 patients) (Table 27.2). This group is of particular interest as the population of patients with end-stage heart disease grows. When this group presents with an acute heart failure exacerbation verging on cardiogenic shock, there are few resources available to treat these patients and the threshold for initiation of mechanical support is much lower. Prolonged IABP use for up to 46 days has been reported[22] as a bridge to transplant or to another mechanical device.

The most extensively reported experience with IABP is in patients undergoing cardiac surgery, which has been mostly bypass surgery but also includes other types of cardiac surgery (Table 27.3). If the IABP was implanted postoperatively or intraoperatively, the mortality was relatively high at 43% or 35%, respectively. But if patients had the IABP implanted preoperatively because of anticipated high perioperative risk (advanced age, low EF, cardiogenic shock, emergent surgery), the mortality was much lower, at 14%, similar to the estimated mortality for IABP use for acute coronary syndrome (ACS). Thus, it appears that the mortality risk is greatest among patients in whom IABP is used as a bridge to transplant or as an intraoperative or postoperative procedure during cardiac surgery.

Indications

Cardiogenic shock is the most severe expression of acute cardiac failure. Many indications have been recognized by the American College of Cardiology, the American Heart Association, and the European Society of Cardiology (Table 27.4),[39–41] but most of these are based in the setting of acute coronary disease. Other indications have been suggested by clinical studies in surgical patients[4,33,42]

Table 27.4 *Indications for use of intraaortic balloon pump*

Cardiogenic shock in the setting of MI not reversed with pharmacologic therapy; stabilization before revascularization (class I)*
Acute MR or ventricular septal defect complicating MI (class I)*
Recurrent intractable arrhythmias with hemodynamic compromise (class I)*
Refractory post MI angina; stabilization before revascularization, such as PCI or CABG (class I)*
Severe ischemia despite maximum medical therapy or with hemodynamic compromise before or after coronary angiography (class IIa)*
Hemodynamic compromise, poor LV function or persistent ischemia in patients with large areas of myocardium at risk (class IIa)*
As an adjunct to high-risk CABG or if unable to wean from cardiopulmonary bypass after surgery
Prophylactic use in high-risk PCI
Stabilization of hemodynamically compromised severe aortic stenosis
Myocarditis or other reversible cause of heart failure with hemodynamic compromise
Acute decompensated heart failure which is not responsive to conventional medical therapy
Short-term bridge to transplant
In patients with successful PCI after thrombolysis or those with 3-vessel disease to prevent reocclusion (class IIb)*
In patients known to have large areas of myocardium at risk with or without ischemia (class IIb)*

*Adapted from American College of Cardiology and American Heart Association Guidelines.[41]
Abbreviations: ADHF = acute decompensated heart failure; CABG = coronary artery bypass grafting; LV = left ventricular; MI = myocardial infarction; MR = mitral regurgitation; PCI = percutaneous coronary intervention.

and by case series experience with heart failure patients.[3,4,43] Thus, the spectrum for the use of IABP has expanded to include ischemic heart disease, cardiomyopathies and advanced heart failure, valvular heart disease, and malignant arrhythmias.

The most widely accepted indication for IABP use is cardiogenic shock in the setting of AMI.[10,39,40] When myocardial blood supply is so severely compromised that extensive areas of myocardium are compromised, the mechanical pump function of the heart is acutely impaired. This acute dysfunction, or acute heart failure, causes end-organ hypoperfusion and hypotension. In the setting of AMI, the presence of cardiogenic shock is a poor prognostic indicator.[44] The standard of care for an acute ST elevation MI is percutaneous coronary intervention (PCI) when possible.[39,40] The most common use of IABP stems from this setting, as adjunctive therapy to a high-risk PCI procedure.[1,10] If emergent cardiac surgery is required, IABP implantation should be carried out if there is severe LV dysfunction.[1,5,39,40] Mechanical complications of MI such as, ventricular septal wall rupture or hemodynamically compromising mitral regurgitation (MR) have also been shown to respond to IABP as a temporary measure until surgery can be carried out to correct these defects.[1,8,10,39]

IABP use in high-risk cardiac surgery patients is well established,[1,2,10,12,33] as is the use in patients who cannot be weaned from cardiopulmonary bypass after cardiac surgery.[1,2,10,33] A new indication for IABP use is in off-pump cardiac surgery, which permits improved cardiac exposure for anastomoses placement with less hemodynamic instability.[45,46]

Ventricular tachycardia can be a complication or presentation of AMI. Refractory ventricular arrhythmias can be seen in acute ischemia or cardiomyopathy, as well as other predisposing arrhythmic conditions, such as Long QT syndrome, arrhythmogenic right ventricular dysplasia, Wolff–Parkinson–White syndrome, and Brugada syndrome. Ventricular arrhythmias compromise ventricular filling and reduce stroke volume and cardiac output. Ischemia can be a contributing factor to arrhythmia and is also worsened by the arrhythmia. IABP could reduce ischemia, improve ventricular filling, stroke volume, and cardiac output and lead to control of arrhythmia in a large majority of patients (86%).[47]

Myocarditis due to any cause, postpartum cardiomyopathy, and other cardiomyopathies in which the patient exhibits severe hypoperfusion would benefit from the improvement in cardiac output, reduced afterload, reduced preload, and reduced capillary wedge pressure. Congenital heart disease with severe hemodynamic compromise that permits adequate anatomical positioning of IABP and without significant aortic regurgitation could also benefit from counterpulsation.

Valvular disease of any nature can cause or worsen acute heart failure. Ischemia can also contribute to ADHF caused by valvular disease. Because of the compromise on forward flow, patients with aortic stenosis benefit from measures that reduce afterload such as IABP. Augmentation of the diastolic filling gradient also helps improve stroke volume and cardiac output.[42] Mitral regurgitation and mitral stenosis derive much of the hemodynamic benefits afforded to aortic stenosis by use of IABP. However, moderate to severe aortic regurgitation is a counterindication for use of IABP as the amount of regurgitant volume can be increased and worsen the hemodynamic status of the patient.

Undoubtedly, it is the clinician's assessment of the patient's history, physical findings, and hemodynamic parameters that should ultimately determine the use of IABP. The use of a Swan–Ganz catheter will provide further hemodynamic information to help assess the patient's need for IABP implantation and, once implanted, assess the patient's response to therapy. The combination of clinical findings and hemodynamics can help further guide therapeutic choices.[48] Figure 27.1 offers a useful clinical paradigm in the acute heart failure patient. Patients with unstable, low-output heart failure (in a state of hypoperfusion, whether "wet" or "dry") comprise the group who would benefit from IABP support. The clinician should have a clear plan of the patient's management after stabilization with IABP, as this therapy alone is often not enough in the setting of cardiogenic shock. Exceptions to this may be the patient with an acute

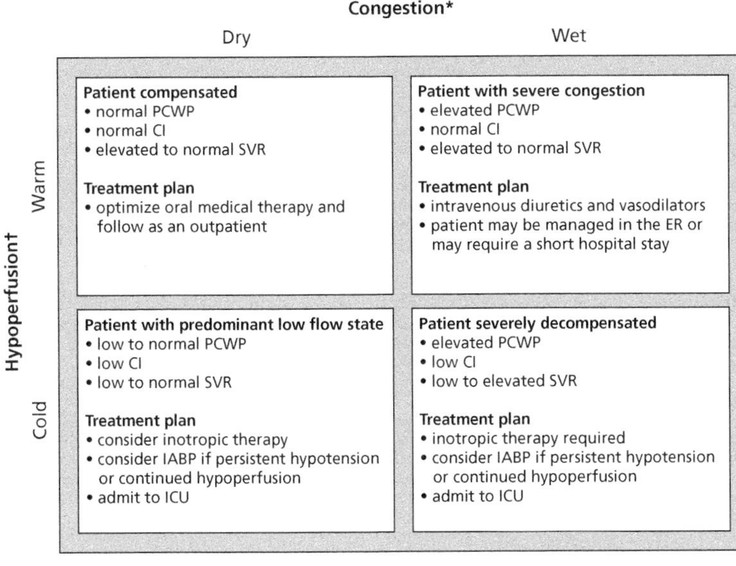

Congestion*
Dry
Wet
Hypoperfusion†
Warm
Cold
Patient compensated
• normal PCWP
• normal CI
• elevated to normal SVR
Treatment plan
• optimize oral medical therapy and follow as an outpatient
Patient with severe congestion
• elevated PCWP
• normal CI
• elevated to normal SVR
Treatment plan
• intravenous diuretics and vasodilators
• patient may be managed in the ER or may require a short hospital stay
Patient with predominant low flow state
• low to normal PCWP
• low CI
• low to normal SVR
Treatment plan
• consider inotropic therapy
• consider IABP if persistent hypotension or continued hypoperfusion
• admit to ICU
Patient severely decompensated
• elevated PCWP
• low CI
• low to elevated SVR
Treatment plan
• inotropic therapy required
• consider IABP if persistent hypotension or continued hypoperfusion
• admit to ICU
Adapted from Stevenson.48

Figure 27.1. *Clinical and hemodynamic characterization of the heart failure patient*

*Symptoms of congestion include shortness of breath, orthopnea, paroxysmal nocturnal dyspnea, morning cough, peripheral edema, rales, ascites, hepatic congestion, or jugular venous distention
†Symptoms of hypoperfusion include nausea, vomiting, early satiety, altered mental status, acidosis, worsening renal or hepatic function, reduced capillary refill, cold and clammy skin, hypotension, narrow pulse pressure
Abbreviations: CI = cardiac index; ER = emergency room; ICU = intensive care unit; IABP = intraaortic balloon pump; PCWP = pulmonary capillary wedge pressure; SVR = systemic vascular resistance.

reversible cause of heart failure, such as myocarditis,[43] and the patient with established heart failure with an acute decompensation.[3,4] These two groups of patients may also benefit from IABP as a short-term bridge to transplantation when available. Findings that would prompt IABP use in these patients would be persistent hypotension (mean arterial pressure [MAP] < 60 mm Hg), cardiac index < 1.5 L/min/m^2, signs of worsening hypoperfusion (altered mental status, worsening renal or hepatic function), despite maximal medical therapy including inotropic agents when appropriate.

If in spite of IABP support the patient remains unstable, surgical implantation of a ventricular assist device (VAD) should be considered if the patient is an adequate candidate for transplantation or VAD destination therapy. An experimental form of permanent IABP is also being explored as a long-term bridge to transplant or as palliative therapy for those patients who are not transplant candidates.[49] In general, there is no role for palliative use of IABP in end-stage patients when it is anticipated that weaning from IABP support may not be possible. Instead, other palliative measures and end-of-life issues should be discussed with patients and their families.

Contraindications

There are few absolute contraindications to the use of IABP (Table 27.5). Of the relative contraindications, peripheral vascular disease (PVD) of the lower extremities can be overcome by alternate modes of implantation via axillary or subclavian arteries.[50] However, access to these arterial sites requires surgery. The sheathless insertion technique

Table 27.5. *Contraindications for use of intraaortic balloon pump*

Absolute contraindications
Moderate to severe aortic regurgitation
Abdominal or thoracic aortic aneurysm
Aortic dissection
Uncontrolled bleeding diathesis
End-stage heart disease without further therapeutic alternatives
Relative contraindications
Severe aortic or femoral atherosclerosis
Severe symptoms of peripheral vascular disease

can also be used to reduce peripheral occlusion and limb ischemia caused by a vascular sheath.[51,52] IABP should be used cautiously in patients who may need mechanical circulatory support indefinitely and who are not candidates for further therapies, such as transplantation or VAD destination therapy.

Intraaortic Balloon Pump Insertion Technique

The most common setting for implantation is the cardiac catheterization laboratory, followed by the operating room and intensive care unit (ICU).[1] IABP can be implanted at the bedside with use of percutaneous technique and fluoroscopy. The most common access site is the right femoral artery approach. The correct position for the IABP is that the tip of the balloon is 1 cm below the origin of the subclavian, and the bottom should not occlude the origin of the renal arteries. The most common insertion technique is percutaneous access using a vascular sheath through which the IABP catheter is inserted.[1] There is also a sheathless approach in which the skin is pre-dilated and the IABP catheter is inserted over the guidewire and advanced to the correct aortic position. The sheathless approach and other arterial sites should be considered in patients with PVD. The size of the balloon is determined by patient size and manufacturer specifications. Once the IABP catheter is in place, a mark should be made with a permanent pen across both the balloon catheter and skin near the site of skin insertion to determine if there is balloon migration later on. The balloon catheter and, if used, the vascular sheath are then sutured into place. After successful implantation, anticoagulation with heparin is initiated at a loading dose of 60 U/kg to a maximum of 5000 U with a maintenance infusion of 12 U/kg/h to a maximum of 1000 U/h. One recent study reported comparable complications and less bleeding in patients on IABP without anticoagulation if IABP was used for ≤ 48 hours.[53]

The IABP timing is initially set at a 1:2 ratio—1 counterpulsation for every 2 heartbeats—to assess the proper timing cycle. Once timing parameters are judged to be adequate (see the "Hemodynamic Effects of Intraaortic Balloon Pumps" section of this chapter), IABP is set at a 1:1 ratio, at which every beat is assisted with counterpulsation.

Hemodynamic Effects of Intraaortic Balloon Pumps

During IABP counterpulsation, the balloon is inflated during diastole and deflated during systole to improve circulatory hemodynamics and reduce workload on the failing heart (Table 27.6). As a result, the effects of balloon counterpulsation are seen through the entire cardiac cycle (Figure 27.2).

During diastole, balloon inflation displaces into the coronary and peripheral circulation a volume of blood equal to the volume of the balloon. This is represented on the monitor as a peak in arterial waveform that is taller than the peak systolic pressure. This displaced blood improves systemic circulation and especially coronary circulation since

Table 27.6 *Hemodynamic effects of intraaortic balloon pump*

Increase	Decrease
Systemic blood flow	Pulmonary capillary wedge pressure
Coronary blood flow	Afterload
Stroke volume	Preload
Cardiac output	Cardiac wall stress
Left ventricular emptying	Cardiac oxygen consumption

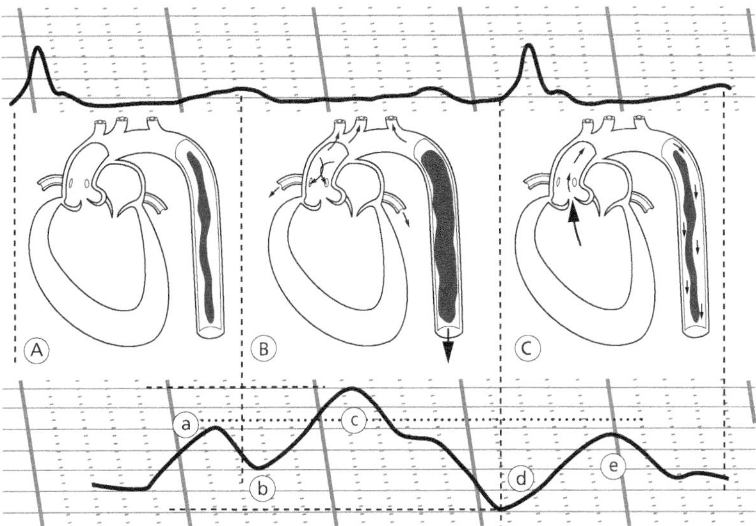

Figure 27.2. *Electrocardiogram (ECG) tracing with simultaneous depiction of intraaortic balloon pump (IABP) set at 2:1 ratio and arterial wave form. (A)* **Unassisted systole:** *the balloon is deflated during previous diastole and present systole and is seen as the* ***a*** *peak on pressure wave form. (B)* **Diastole:** *balloon inflated at peak of T-wave correlates with closure of aortic valve,* **b** *dip, which is unassisted end-diastolic pressure (EDP).There is improved coronary and systemic blood flow. The* **c** *peak is augmented diastolic pressure which is always higher than* ***a****. (C)* **Assisted systole:** *permits improved left ventricular unloading, improved stroke volume and reduces cardiac oxygen consumption. The* **d** *dip is balloon deflation at beginning of ECG R-wave and represents assisted EDP which is always less than* **b***. The* **e** *peak is assisted systolic pressure which should always be lower than* ***a****.*

80% of coronary arterial perfusion occurs during diastole. It is this mechanism of improved coronary perfusion that contributes to the reduction of infarct extension and reduction of ischemia.[19] Inflation of the balloon is timed with the peak of the T wave on electrocardiogram (ECG) monitor and 40 ms before the dicrotic notch on the arterial pressure tracing (Figure 27.3A).

Timing errors can be caused by either early or late balloon inflation. Early balloon inflation has dangerous hemodynamic consequences as it causes premature closure of the aortic valve, which results in increased aortic pressure, increased aortic regurgitation, increased afterload, increased preload, increased pulmonary capillary wedge pressure (PCWP), increased myocardial oxygen consumption, reduced stroke volume, and reduced cardiac output. Early balloon inflation can be seen in the arterial pressure tracing by a rapid peak diastolic upstroke that is followed by a clearly visible dicrotic notch (Figure 27.3B). Late inflation is not dangerous, but it does not permit the patient to receive the maximum benefit of counterpulsation, as there is less diastolic augmentation, which in turn reduces systemic and coronary perfusion. This is seen on the monitor as a long flat U-shaped dip preceding the diastolic augmentation upstroke, and the dicrotic notch is seen preceding the upstroke (Figure 27.3C). Diastolic augmentation must always be higher than the systolic pressure peak; the absence of this can indicate timing errors, hypovolemia, decreased vascular resistance, inadequate balloon size for patient's aorta, or hypertension.[9]

During systole, the balloon is deflated just before

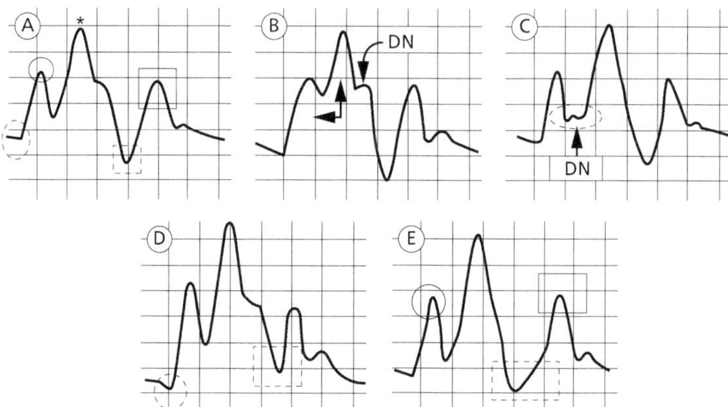

Figure 27.3. *Systemic pressure wave tracings of balloon inflation timing errors. (A)* **Normal IABP pressure tracing at 2:1 ratio:** *Diastolic augmentation (*). Unassisted systolic peak (○) is higher than assisted systolic peak (□). Unassisted end-diastolic pressure (dotted ○) is higher than the assisted end-diastolic pressure (dotted □). (B)* **Early inflation:** *There is a rapid diastolic upstroke (bidirectional arrow) and the dicrotic notch (DN) is visible. (C) Late inflation. Long, flat, U-shaped dip (dotted ○) preceding the diminished diastolic augmentation and the DN precedes the upstroke. (D)* **Late deflation:** *The assisted end-diastolic pressure (dotted □) is higher than the unassisted end-diastolic pressure (dotted ○). (E)* **Early deflation:** *Prolonged U-shaped dip after augmented diastolic upstroke (dotted □) with assisted systolic peak (□) equal to unassisted systolic peak (○).*

the aortic valve opens, causing a virtual vacuum equivalent to the volume of the balloon. This is timed to the beginning of the R wave on the ECG when the assisted systolic pressure is the lowest possible, resulting in a lower assisted end-diastolic pressure when compared to the patient's baseline. This has multiple effects. The first effect is a reduction of afterload which permits improved emptying of the left ventricle; therefore, reducing its oxygen consumption and wall stress. Second, there is increased stroke volume and cardiac output and decreased preload with a subsequent decrease in PCWP; thus, improved hemodynamics in the failing heart.

As in diastole, there can be two timing errors in systole, namely, early and late deflation. In contrast to late inflation in diastole, late deflation in systole is a dangerous timing error as it causes obstruction to LV emptying, thereby increasing afterload and reducing stroke volume and cardiac output. These effects cause increased oxygen consumption that can lead to further hemodynamic deterioration. This timing error can be seen on the monitor as an assisted end-diastolic pressure that is higher than the unassisted end-diastolic pressure on the arterial waveform (Figure 27.3D). In contrast, early deflation is not dangerous but causes reduced augmentation with less improvement of peripheral and coronary circulation. There can even be retrograde flow from higher-pressure peripheral systems into the aorta. This timing error is seen on the monitor as a flat prolonged U shape after the augmented diastolic upstroke with the resulting assisted systolic pressure being equal rather than less than the unassisted systolic pressure (Figure 27.3E).

In summary, early balloon inflation during diastole and late deflation during systole are dangerous timing errors that can cause further hemodynamic compromise. Late deflation during diastole and early inflation during systole are timing errors which prevent the patient from getting the most benefit out of IABP yet do not worsen the patient's hemodynamic state.

Complications

The major complications with IABP are major limb ischemia with possible loss of limb, arterial dissection, bleeding, balloon leak with helium embolization, balloon rupture, cerebrovascular accident (CVA) and sepsis.[1,4,10] Risk factors for complications have been age ≥ 75 years, PVD, body surface area of < 1.65 m^2, and female gender.[1,10] The rate of complications with IABP has been improving. The Benchmark Registry in 2003 reported a major complication rate of 2.7% and an in-hospital mortality of 0.05% in a population of 22 663 patients.[10] These complication rates are much lower than those seen in previous trials or previously reported in the literature and are most likely due to technological improvements, such as improved materials that reduce leaks and balloon ruptures, smaller diameter catheters, and the use of sheathless insertion, which reduces ischemia and bleeding. The rate of unsuccessful IABP insertion was 2.3% in the Benchmark registry.[10]

Patient Monitoring

Patients on IABP should always be in an ICU with personnel who are familiar with the IABP system and the management of critically ill patients. Patients must be in bed with a head elevation of no more than a 30° angle and limited movement of the limb where the IABP is inserted. If the balloon is inserted in one of the upper extremities, the patient is permitted to sit and even ambulate.[50] Daily chest radiography is performed to evaluate the position of the balloon tip, which should be 1 cm below the aortic origin of the subclavian artery or at the level of the carina. Pulses must be monitored at least once every 8-hour shift. Anticoagulation with heparin must be monitored with a target partial thromboplastin time (PTT) kept between 50 seconds and 70 seconds or 1.5 to 2 times baseline. Platelet count should be monitored as a certain degree of mild thrombocytopenia (80 000/mm^3 to 150 000/mm^3) is expected while on IABP. Otherwise additional causes for thrombocytopenia should be considered, such as heparin-induced thrombocytopenia or disseminated intravascular coagulation. Swan–Ganz measurements should also be performed at least once or twice per 8-hour shift to evaluate the patient's response to therapy. The IABP console must be followed for ECG, arterial pressure, and balloon pressure at least once or twice per 8-hour shift to evaluate timing errors or balloon malfunction. The data should be printed and placed in the patient's chart.

The intraaortic balloon catheter pressure curve should resemble the one shown in Figure 27.4A. The baseline of the balloon pressure curve will be incorrectly elevated if there is restriction or obstruction of gas flow through the lumen or overpressurization (Figure 27.4B). A helium leak or timing errors can cause a depression of the baseline (Figure 27.4B). The IABP system should detect helium leaks by sounding an alarm and automatically shutting off, to prevent helium embolization and possible subsequent ischemia or CVA. If helium embolization does occur, immediate hyperbaric oxygen therapy must be started.[54] Heart rate variations cause changes in plateau length which correlate with duration of diastole in the cardiac cycle (Figure 27.4C). A change in heart rate with no change in plateau length indicates a timing error. The arterial pressure waveform should be evaluated and the timing error corrected.

Discontinuation of Intraaortic Balloon Pump

Once the patient is deemed to be clinically and hemodynamically stable, the process of weaning IABP should be initiated. Weaning begins by reducing the frequency of beat-to-beat augmentation with a reasonable time period between each change. Most physicians discontinue therapy at ratios of 1:3 or 1:4. Before the IABP can be removed, heparin should be discontinued so that the patient's PTT is ≤ 50 seconds, or the activated clotting time is < 160 seconds. Prior to removing the IABP catheter, the balloon must be deflated via aspiration with a syringe from the inflation port. The balloon should be withdrawn towards the sheath, but not into it as this may tear the balloon and cause helium embolization. A backflow of blood is permitted to leak from the vascular site while mild upstream pressure is applied to the artery, as both the sheath and the balloon catheter are pulled simultaneously in one gentle yet swift

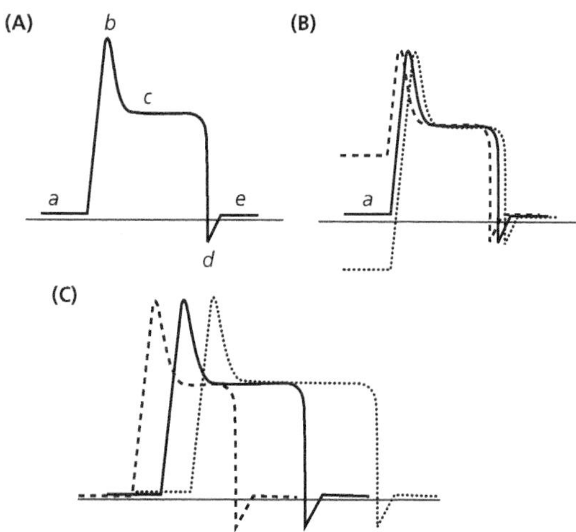

Figure 27.4. *Intraaortic balloon pump catheter pressure curves. (A)* **Normal balloon pressure waveform:** *a, Baseline pressure measured at deflation usually 2.5 to 10 mm Hg. b, Rapid balloon inflation. Overshoot reflects pressure generated by balloon lumen. c, Pressure plateau of inflation during diastole correlates with length of diastole. Height of plateau from baseline correlates directly with blood pressure. d, Rapid deflation and undershoot artifact. e, Return to baseline. (B)* **Restriction of gas flow**, *such as catheter kink, causes elevation of baseline pressure at deflation,* **a** *(dashed line). Gas leakage, such as balloon rupture, causes lowering of* **a** *(dotted line). (C)* **Changes in heart rate** *correlate directly with length of plateau. Slower heart rates (dotted line) have longer plateaus. Rapid heart rates (dashed line) have shortened plateaus. Heart rate variations without changes in plateau length indicate timing errors.*

motion. Manual pressure is applied by hand to the puncture site for 30 to 60 minutes, after which the patient is instructed to remain in bed for the next 24 hours with limited movement of the limb where the IABP was inserted.

Conclusion

Cardiogenic shock and other forms of ADHF respond to the mechanical hemodynamic support offered by IABP, after conventional medical therapy has failed. IABP is cost-effective, readily available, and simple to implant. IABP can provide temporary hemodynamic stability while further therapeutic measures, such as surgery or PCI, can be performed. With the mechanical counterpulsation from IABP, ADHF patients can benefit from afterload reduction, improved emptying of the left ventricle, reduced oxygen consumption and wall stress, increased stroke volume and cardiac output, and decreased preload with a consequent decrease in PCWP. The rate of complications is very low and the rate of successful implantation is high. In more than 30 years of use, the IABP has become a standard of care and has routinely demonstrated its clinical value as an adjunctive or single therapy in patients with the highest of risks. IABP is an essential tool that can help stabilize the most critically ill of heart failure patients and permit further lifesaving procedures.

References

1. Ferguson JJ 3rd, Cohen M, Freedman RJ Jr., *et al.* The current practice of intra-aortic balloon counterpulsation: results from the Benchmark Registry. J Am Coll Cardiol 2001; 38: 1456–1462.
2. Schmid C, Wilhelm M, Reimann A, *et al.* Use of an intraaortic balloon pump in patients with impaired left ventricular function. Scand Cardiovasc J 1999; 33: 194–198.
3. Francis G, Frazier O, Delgado R. Management of acute and decompensated heart failure: use of mechanical devices in treating heart failure. In: Hosenpud J, Greenberg B (eds) Congestive Heart Failure: Pathophysiology, Diagnosis, and Comprehensive Approach to Management. (Lippincott, Williams & Wilkins: Philadelphia, PA, 2000), 553–573.
4. Aroesty J. Intraaortic balloon counterpulsation and other circulatory assist devices. In: Baim DS, Grossman W (eds) Grossman's Cardiac Catheterization, Angiography, and Intervention, 6th edition (Lippincott, Williams & Wilkins: Philadelphia, PA, 2000).
5. Waksman R, Weiss AT, Gotsman MS, Hasin Y. Intraaortic balloon counterpulsation improves survival in cardiogenic shock complicating acute myocardial infarction. Eur Heart J 1993; 14: 71–74.

6. Kovack PJ, Rasak MA, Bates ER, Ohman EM, Stomel RJ. Thrombolysis plus aortic counterpulsation: improved survival in patients who present to community hospitals with cardiogenic shock. J Am Coll Cardiol 1997; 29: 1454–1458.
7. Sanborn TA, Sleeper LA, Bates ER, *et al.* Impact of thrombolysis, intra-aortic balloon pump counterpulsation, and their combination in cardiogenic shock complicating acute myocardial infarction: a report from the SHOCK Trial Registry. SHould we emergently revascularize Occluded Coronaries for cardiogenic shocK? J Am Coll Cardiol 2000; 36: 1123–1129.
8. Menon V, Webb JG, Hills LD, *et al.* Outcome and profile of ventricular septal rupture with cardiogenic shock after myocardial infarction: a report from the SHOCK Trial Registry. SHould we emergently revascularize Occluded Coronaries for cardiogenic shocK? J Am Coll Cardiol 2000; 36: 1110–1116.
9. Darovic G. Intraaortic balloon counterpulsation. In: Darovic G (ed) Hemodynamic Monitoring (W.B. Saunders Company: Philadelphia, PA, 2002), 347–349.
10. Stone GW, Ohman EM, Miller MF, *et al.* Contemporary utilization and outcomes of intra-aortic balloon counterpulsation in acute myocardial infarction: the Benchmark Registry. J Am Coll Cardiol 2003; 41: 1940–1945.
11. Dietl CA, Berkheimer MD, Woods EL, *et al.* Efficacy and cost-effectiveness of preoperative IABP in patients with ejection fraction of 0.25 or less. Ann Thorac Surg 1996; 62: 401–409.
12. Christenson JT, Simonet F, Schmuziger M. Economic impact of preoperative intraaortic balloon pump therapy in high-risk coronary patients. Ann Thorac Surg 2000; 70: 510–515.
13. Talley JD, Ohman EM, Mark DB, *et al.* Economic implications of the prophylactic use of intraaortic balloon counterpulsation in the setting of acute myocardial infarction. Am J Cardiol 1997; 79: 590–594.
14. Kantrowitz A. Experimental augmentation of coronary flow by retardation of the arterial pressure pulse. Surgery 1953; 34: 678–687.
15. Clauss RH, Birtwell WC, Albertal G, *et al.* Assisted circulation. I. The arterial counterpulsator. J Thorac Cardiovasc Surg 1961; 41: 447–458.
16. Moulopoulos SD, Topaz S, Kolff WJ. Diastolic balloon pumping (with carbon dioxide) in the aorta—a mechanical assistance to the failing circulation. Am Heart J 1962; 63: 669–675.
17. Kantrowitz A, Tjonneland S, Freed PS, *et al.* Initial clinical experience with intraaortic balloon pumping in cardiogenic shock. JAMA 1968; 203: 113–118.
18. Christenson JT, Simonet F, Badel P, Schmuziger M. The effect of preoperative intra-aortic balloon pump support in patients with coronary artery disease, poor left-ventricular function (LVEF < 40%), and hypertensive LV hypertrophy. Thorac Cardiovasc Surg 1997; 45: 60–64.
19. Stone GW, Marsalese D, Brodie BR, *et al.* A prospective, randomized evaluation of prophylactic intra-aortic balloon counterpulsation in high risk patients with acute myocardial infarction treated with primary angioplasty. Second Primary Angioplasty in Myocardial Infarction (PAMI-II) Trial Investigators. J Am Coll Cardiol 1997; 29: 1459–1467.
20. van't Hof AW, Liem AL, de Boer MJ, *et al.* randomized comparison of intra-aortic balloon pumping after primary coronary angioplasty in high risk patients with acute myocardial infarction. Eur Heart J 1999; 20: 659–665.
21. Torchiana DF, Hirsch G, Buckley MJ, *et al.* Intraaortic balloon pumping for cardiac support: trends in practice and outcome, 1968 to 1995. J Thorac Cardiovasc Surg 1997; 113: 758–764.
22. Lazar JM, Ziady GM, Dummer SJ, Thompson M, Ruffner RJ. Outcome and complications of prolonged intraaortic balloon counterpulsation in cardiac patients. Am J Cardiol 1992; 69: 955–958.
23. Hagemeijer F, Laird JD, Haalebos MM, Hugenholtz PG. Effectiveness of intraaortic balloon pumping without cardiac surgery for patients with severe heart failure secondary to a recent myocardial infarction. Am J Cardiol 1977; 40: 951–956.
24. Tobias MA, Challen PD, Franklin CB, Phillips G, Varley EM. Intra-aortic balloon counterpulsation. Clinical experience. Anaesthesia 1979; 34: 844–854.
25. Birovljev S, Radovancevic B, Burnett CM, *et al.* Heart transplantation after mechanical circulatory support: four years' experience. J Heart Lung Transplant 1992; 11: 240–245.
26. Masters RG, Hendry PJ, Davies RA, *et al.* Cardiac transplantation after mechanical circulatory support: a Canadian perspective. Ann Thorac Surg 1996; 61: 1734–1739.
27. Scanlon PJ, O'Connell J, Johnson SA, *et al.* Balloon counterpulsation following surgery for ischemic heart disease. Circulation 1976; 54: 90–93.
28. Macoviak J, Stephenson LW, Edmunds LH Jr., Harken A, MacVaugh H. The intraaortic balloon pump: an analysis of five years' experience. Ann Thorac Surg 1980; 29: 451–458.
29. Golding LA, Loop FD, Peter M, *et al.* Late survival following use of intraaaortic ballon pump in revascularization operations. Ann Thorac Surg 1980; 30: 48–51.

30. Downing TP, Miller DC, Stinson EB, *et al.* Therapeutic efficacy of intraaortic balloon pump counterpulsation. Analysis with concurrent "control" subjects. Circulation 1981; 64: II108–II113.
31. Kafrouni G. Intraaortic balloon counterpulsation. Am J Surg 1984; 147: 731–734.
32. McGeehin W, Sheikh F, Donahoo JS, Lechman MJ, MacVaugh H 3rd. Transthoracic intraaortic balloon pump support: experience in 39 patients. Ann Thorac Surg 1987; 44: 26–30.
33. Creswell LL, Rosenbloom M, Cox JL, *et al.* Intraaortic balloon counterpulsation: patterns of usage and outcome in cardiac surgery patients. Ann Thorac Surg 1992; 54: 11–20.
34. Mueller DK, Stout M, Blakeman BM. Morbidity and mortality of intra-aortic balloon pumps placed through the aortic arch. Chest 1998; 114: 85–88.
35. Arafa OE, Geiran OR, Svennevig JL. Transthoracic intra-aortic balloon pump in open heart operations: techniques and outcome. Scand Cardiovasc J 2001; 35: 40–44.
36. Hausmann H, Potapov EV, Koster A, *et al.* Predictors of survival 1 hour after implantation of intra-aortic balloon pump in cardiac surgery. J Card Surg 2001; 16: 72–77.
37. Castelli P, Condemi A, Munari M, *et al.* Intra-aortic balloon counterpulsation: outcome in cardiac surgical patients. J Cardiothorac Vasc Anesth 2001; 15: 700–703.
38. Meco M, Gramegna G, Yassini A, *et al.* Mortality and morbidity from intra-aortic balloon pumps. Risk analysis. J Cardiovasc Surg 2002; 43: 17–23.
39. Ryan TJ, Antman EM, Brooks NH, *et al.* 1999 update. ACC/AHA guidelines for the management of patients with acute myocardial infarction. A report of the American College of Cardiology/American Heart Association Task Force on Practice Guidelines (Committee on Management of Acute Myocardial Infarction). J Am Coll Cardiol 1999; 34: 890–911.
40. Van de Werf F, Ardissino D, Betriu A, *et al.*, Task Force on the Management of Acute Myocardial Infarction of the European Society of Cardiology. Management of acute myocardial infarction in patients presenting with ST-segment elevation. Eur Heart J 2003; 24: 28–66.
41. Braunwald E, Antman EM, Beasley JW, *et al.* ACC/AHA 2002 guideline update for the management of patients with unstable angina and non-ST-segment elevation myocardial infarction—summary article: a report of the American College of Cardiology/American Heart Association Task Force on Practice Guidelines (Committee on the Management of Patients with Unstable Angina). J Am Coll Cardiol 2002; 40: 1366–1374.
42. Folland ED, Kemper AJ, Khuri SF, Josa M, Parisi AF. Intraaortic balloon counterpulsation as a temporary support measure in decompensated critical aortic stenosis. J Am Coll Cardiol 1985; 5: 711–716.
43. Dembitsky WP, Moore CH, Holman WL, *et al.* Successful mechanical circulatory support for non-coronary shock. J Heart Lung Transplant 1992; 11: 129–135.
44. Killip T 3rd, Kimball JT. Treatment of myocardial infarction in a coronary care unit. A two year experience with 250 patients. Am J Cardiol 1967; 20: 457–464.
45. Craver JM, Murrah CP. Elective intraaortic balloon counterpulsation for high-risk off-pump coronary artery bypass operations. Ann Thorac Surg 2001; 71: 1220–1223.
46. Kim KB, Lim C, Ahn H, Yang JK. Intraaortic balloon pump therapy facilitates posterior vessel off-pump coronary artery bypass grafting in high-risk patients. Ann Thorac Surg 2001; 71: 1964–1968.
47. Roe M. Intraaortic balloon counterpulsation. In: Marso SP, Griffin BP, Topol EJ (eds) Manual of Cardiovascular Medicine, 2nd edition (Lippincott, Williams & Wilkins: Philadelphia, PA, 2000), 687–699.
48. Stevenson LW. Tailored therapy to hemodynamic goals for advanced heart failure. Eur J Heart Fail 1999; 1: 251–257.
49. Jeevanandam V, Jayakar D, Anderson AS, *et al.* Circulatory assistance with a permanent implantable IABP: initial human experience. Circulation 2002; 106: I183–I188.
50. H'Doubler PB Jr., H'Doubler WZ, Bien RC, Jansen DA. A novel technique for intraaortic balloon pump placement via the left axillary artery in patients awaiting cardiac transplantation. Cardiovasc Surg 2000; 8: 463–465.
51. Tatar H, Cicek S, Demirkilic U, *et al.* Vascular complications of intraaortic balloon pumping: unsheathed versus sheathed insertion. Ann Thorac Surg 1993; 55: 1518–1521.
52. Gol MK, Bayazit M, Emir M, Tasdemir O, Bayazit K. Vascular complications related to percutaneous insertion of intraaortic balloon pumps. Ann Thorac Surg 1994; 58: 1476–1480.
53. Jiang CY, Zhao LL, Wang JA, Mohammod B. Anticoagulation therapy in intra-aortic balloon counterpulsation: does IABP really need anticoagulation? J Zhejiang Univ Sci 2003; 4: 607–611.
54. Frederiksen JW, Smith J, Brown P, Zinetti C. Arterial helium embolism from ruptured intraaortic balloon. Ann Thorac Surg 1988; 46: 690–692.

CHAPTER 28

Ultrafiltration as a therapy for acute heart failure

Jonathan D Sackner-Bernstein, Maurizio Porcu, Rimbida Obeleniene

Introduction

Fluid overload is a common clinical marker of patients hospitalized with heart failure. "Wet" patients, who represent 70% of all patients admitted with decompensated heart failure,[1,2] should be treated with sodium and fluid restriction along with incremental doses of intravenous diuretics to normalize body fluids and cardiac preload,[3–5] which is generally accomplished within hours or days. However, volume overload in sicker patients may prove refractory to increasing doses of loop diuretics, even with the addition of adrenergic agonists, phosphodiesterase (PDE) inhibitors, nitrates (or nitroprusside), or nesiritide. While calcium sensitizers (levosimendan)[6] and vasopressin antagonists (tolvaptan[7,8] or conivaptan[9]) appear promising, even their ongoing clinical development programs are unlikely to eliminate the clinical scenario of refractory volume overload. Although their role is less clearly defined, mechanical approaches, specifically ultrafiltration, provide an additional therapeutic opportunity.

The Pathophysiology of Volume Overload

Overhydration is induced by several neurohormonal mechanisms, each mediated and/or triggered by reduced organ perfusion.[10] This reduces the inhibitory activity of the mechanoreceptors located in the arterial circulation (carotid sinus, aortic arch, renal afferent arterioles), releasing the brake from adrenergic outflow.[11] The resulting increase in sympathetic activity stimulates the activation of the renin-angiotensin-aldosterone system (RAAS) and leads to arginine vasopressin (AVP) release.[12] The level of activation of these different systems is directly related to the severity of heart failure[13] and these systems synergistically cause salt and fluid retention, in addition to their direct adverse effects on ventricular remodeling.

Vasopressin, also known as antidiuretic hormone (ADH), is an important mechanism in the control of body fluids. Recent studies focusing on this role of vasopressin have been stimulated as much by its pathophysiologic importance as by the development of vasopressin antagonists.[7–9] This peptide regulates free water reabsorption in the collecting duct of the nephron to maintain the stability of the circulating volume. In heart failure, an inappropriately high AVP level is related to both normal osmoregulatory mechanisms and non-osmotic mechanoreceptor-mediated mechanisms.[14] Vasopressin potently stimulates reabsorption of free water, which, when it exceeds the degree of salt retention, can lead to significant hyponatremia. ADH can also enhance both peripheral and coronary artery tone as well as aggravate neurohormonal activation.[15] The overall result is a significant increase in preload and afterload that further stimulates ventricular remodeling, thus amplifying neurohormonal activation.

The effects of these mechanisms can be aggravated by thirst, stimulated by these neurohormones,[14] and serve as a direct contributor to volume overload by leading to increased fluid intake. The synergism of these negative mechanisms can increase the body fluid by several liters in a short time, leading to clinical signs and symptoms of congestion. Dyspnea on exertion, orthopnea, nocturnal dyspnea, and cough are common symptoms of an abnormal elevation of left ventricular (LV) filling pressure and pulmonary congestion. In this context acute pulmonary edema may be a dramatic clinical event, presenting as the first manifestation of acute or subacute heart failure or following a progressive worsening of chronic heart failure.

Clinical Evaluation of "Wet" Patients

Whether due to a progressive chronic course or a new onset process, the presence and degree of fluid overload can be assessed with the clinical examination.[2] A simple estimation may be obtained with a serial determination of body weight, which can increase by several pounds within a few days. Wet patients generally are characterized by lower limb edema, lung crackles, and liver and abdominal congestion, largely governed by the effects of gravity. Yet, congestion does not necessarily present as dependent edema. Isolated thoracic or abdominal congestion may be the sole manifestation of fluid overload on clinical examination, even in the presence of very high water retention. Although imaging studies (such as chest x-ray, echocardiography, abdominal ultrasound or computed tomography [CT] scan) can localize and quantify excess fluids, the physical examination can be just as reliable. In this context, simple evaluations such as the jugular venous pressure (JVP), are very helpful bedside-detectable signs of excess preload and may represent reliable clinical prognostic indicators[16,17] able to drive therapeutic decisions. At times, patients may present with orthopnea as the dominant clinical symptom without any detectable pulmonary congestion on examination. This clinical symptom may respond to diuresis but the associated neurohormonal activation could represent subsequent risk.[18]

Standard Medical Management

Various critical pathways have been advocated for the heart failure patient hospitalized with acutely decompensated heart failure (ADHF),[3–5] each of which starts with the assessment of volume status as the key first step. Treatment strategies are largely guided by the cause of AHF, based on three different paths: (1) pulmonary congestion without total body volume excess; (2) volume overload with maintained end-organ perfusion; and (3) volume overload with hypotension or shock, reflecting impaired organ blood flow (Figure 28.1). The recommendations found in standard guidelines, review articles, and chapters on ADHF must be interpreted and applied differently from those for chronic heart failure. Fewer randomized clinical trials exist for ADHF and the published results tend to be less compelling than those investigating chronic heart failure. Although typically patients with ADHF are categorized into one of four groups based on volume status and organ perfusion,[2] organizing treatments based on the three pathways is merely another way to describe the same construct. The advantage is that many physicians consider patients volume overloaded with any signs of congestion and may react by administering diuretics. This raises the clinical scenario of patients with pulmonary congestion where aggressive diuresis could have adverse effects.

Prompt recognition of a patient with acute myocardial ischemia who presents with dyspnea and pulmonary congestion is crucial. While diuretics are useful, the key to treatment is reversing the underlying ischemia. Pulmonary congestion in this setting represents a shift of volume into the pulmonary system rather than total body volume excess. Extreme cases are familiar to invasive cardiologists. Heart failure manifesting as shock may require support devices including intraaortic balloon pumps (IABPs). Whether or not the patient presents with extremely decompensated heart failure, overly aggressive diuresis can lead to

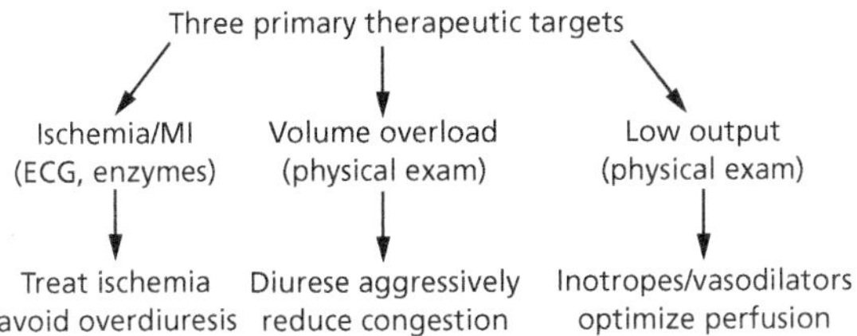

Figure 28.1. *Underlying pathophysiology determines therapeutic strategy*

Abbreviations: MI = myocardial infarction; ECG = electrocardiogram.

hypotension and impaired perfusion, which may worsen ischemia. A similar risk of overdiuresis exists for heart failure patients in whom the oliguric state results from an inappropriate high-dose and long-term diuretic regimen (the so-called "dry" low-output patients or possibly a patient who has been overdiuresed). This scenario can present independently of the cause of heart failure. In these patients, any effort to increase urine output by increasing diuretic doses will lead to rapid hemodynamic deterioration, without improving diuresis, while controlled fluid and sodium administration may improve renal function. Such a patient, however, does not typically present with organ congestion.

Perhaps the most common clinical situation is the patient who is admitted to the hospital for decompensated chronic heart failure or for ADHF, with clinical evidence of significant volume overload. Such patients are managed with sodium and fluid restriction and aggressive diuretic therapy, and in most cases, this is a sufficient first step towards long-term management with an angiotensin converting enzyme (ACE) inhibitor and beta-blocker, along with additional therapies as indicated, including an aldosterone antagonist, defibrillator, and biventricular pacemaker.

When treating excess volume, the first step is to rapidly find the effective dose of diuretics. Although most physicians use increments of 20 mg or 40 mg when dosing, based on familiarity with oral formulations, our experience is that too many choices of doses may slow down the dose-finding process. Even more problematic is that the selection of a diuretic dose may prove sub-therapeutic, leaving a patient with severe symptoms. Consider a hypothetical patient with severe volume overload. If 40 mg of furosemide is inadequate, the physician could choose to repeat the 40-mg dose or increase it to 60 mg or 80 mg. Is there any harm in selecting the higher dose? The major short-term problems with diuretics are excess volume depletion and electrolyte derangement.[19] In a severely volume overloaded patient, these are findings that occur after much of the volume overload has been successfully treated. They are not major risks early in treatment. Therefore, instead of repeating or slightly increasing the dose, it would be reasonable to double the dose (80 mg). Practically speaking, if a physician had the choice of 50 mg, 100 mg or 200 mg as unit doses of furosemide, the process of dose augmentation could prove more efficient, leading to prompt improvement of symptoms (Figure 28.2).

Due to the rapid effect of intravenous loop diuretics, assessment of the adequacy of dose can be determined within 2 to 3 hours. Many physicians may advocate that there should be a certain minimum urine output in order to consider the dose adequate. However, a simpler rule of thumb may prove as useful, and not depend upon whether there is adequate recording of such information. If the dose is appropriate, patients will notice that they are producing significantly more

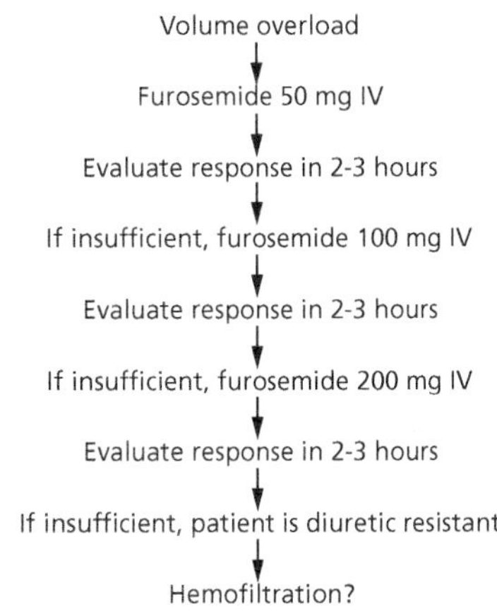

Figure 28.2. *Escalation of diuretic therapy leading to the consideration of hemofiltration (With permission from Sackner-Bernstein and Obeleniene.[49])*

urine than usual, and if they pay attention, they should notice that it is very dilute, appearing clear like water. If both criteria are met, the dose is adequate, and should be administered 2 or 3 times a day until the patient is free of congestion. Then the diuretic should be changed to an oral regimen. However, if after 2 to 3 hours, a patient is not responding appropriately, the dose should be doubled and administered immediately (not the next day). Then the patient should be reassessed in 2 to 3 hours. Continuous intravenous loop diuretic infusion preceded by a loading dose may be more effective in some patients than intermittent administration.[20] Oral and parenteral daily fluid and salt restrictions should also be kept in mind.[21]

A subset of patients remains refractory to increasing doses of diuretic therapy. Hyponatremia is a common cause of diuretic resistance, which can be due either to an excess of sodium dispersion with prolonged aggressive diuretic treatments (particularly when thiazides are used) or, more frequently, to sodium-overdilution in patients with fluid overload.[22,23] An additional effect of hyponatremia is resistance to further diuretic doses. Because loop diuretics produce hypotonic urine, continued diuresis could worsen hyponatremia, and if severe, be a reasonable basis for withholding diuretic therapy. In such a case, an alternative is needed beyond merely holding diuretics. Increasing doses of loop diuretics in chronically treated patients may lead to a reduction in efficacy, with a mechanism known as "the braking phenomenon."[24] Frequently, when a lack of effect of loop diuretics is due to hypochloremic metabolic alkalosis, this metabolic abnormality can be reversed by using acetazolamide,[25] and the loop diuretics may work more effectively. In the typical scenario, with rapid clinical evolution, common reasons for diuretic refractoriness should be investigated (Table 28.1).

Table 28.1. *Causes of refractoriness to diuretic therapy in heart failure patients*

Patient-related causes
- low compliance to drug prescriptions
- excessive sodium intake

Physician-related causes
- inappropriately low dosage
- inappropriate type of diuretic
- competitive inhibition by other drugs (aspirin, nonsteroidal antiinflammatory drugs)

Pharmacological causes
- reduced gastrointestinal absorption (enteral edema)
- reduced renal response (tubular necrosis or fibrosis)

Insufficient renal perfusion
- low cardiac output
- hypovolemia
- renal artery stenosis
- reduced filtration rate (angiotensin-converting enzyme inhibitors, angiotensin receptor blockers)

Defining Diuretic Refractoriness and Alternative Strategies

One problem with defining a treatment strategy in these patients is the lack of a consistent definition of diuretic resistance. Several alternative definitions could be used based on insufficient response to specific thresholds for pharmacotherapies or the lack of effectiveness of diuretics combined with adjunctive vasodilator or inotropic therapy. Alternatively, a definition could embrace the importance of metabolic derangements or azotemia as a result of diuretic therapies. Any such definition could be considered arbitrary, but for the purpose of this chapter, we define diuretic resistance as the state of having an insufficient clinical response to maximally-tolerated medical therapy. By some standards, a lack of response to 200 mg to 250 mg of furosemide, or an equivalent, could define a patient as diuretic resistant. Also a failing response to the addition of metolazone to high-dose loop diuretics, which generally improves diuresis, may be advocated as a resistance to the treatment. However, because such high doses are associated with increased risk,[18] patients without clinical resolution of volume overload in response to at least

80 mg of furosemide could be defined as diuretic refractory.

Diuretic resistance is more than merely a clinical inconvenience.[18,26] Patients requiring more intense therapeutic regimens generally seem sicker, and a recent report demonstrated that such patients are at increased risk of death, independent of the usual prognostic factors.[18] For that reason, even if no controlled clinical trials have defined the optimal treatment strategy for volume overloaded heart failure patients, diuretic refractory patients must be considered for pharmacologically more aggressive approaches, including the use of inotropes or vasodilators, or for mechanical LV assistance and urgent heart transplantation, when indicated.[27] However, despite the mandate for evidence-based medicine, the relative paucity of randomized clinical trials in ADHF means that decision making must depend upon less definitive data sources, as these will represent the best data available. Although the literature supports several strategies for volume management, the clinical focus to date has been primarily pharmacologic.

Although no trial has specifically evaluated the effect of inotropes on diuretic-resistant volume overloaded patients, OPTIME-CHF is the closest study to focus on this population in that it enrolled hospitalized patients with volume overload who were hemodynamically stable.[28] There was no reduction in length of stay when milrinone was added, suggesting that inotropes did not resolve volume overload significantly better than diuretics alone. The effects of long-term vasodilator therapies are mixed at best, with benefits with some[29] and increased risk of death with others,[30,31] despite the fact that vasodilator therapies are known to acutely lower cardiac filling pressures and reduce symptoms. Short-term use of nesiritide, a natriuretic peptide, appeared promising.[32] Although nesiritide has been shown to reduce symptoms within 3 hours, as compared with placebo, and lowers filling pressures faster than nitroglycerin, recent evidence suggests an 80% higher risk of death after its use.[33] Despite the expectation that a natriuretic peptide would promote natriuresis—a desirable effect in a volume-overloaded patient—nesiritide does not have natriuretic effects at the doses approved for use clinically.[34] In addition, nesiritide appears to be associated with worsening renal function,[35] a harbinger for increased risk.[36–38] Similarly, renal-dose dopamine appears to have physiological effects suggesting that it should improve diuresis, yet the only comprehensive assessment of the utility of renal dopamine excludes patients with heart failure,[39] due to the paucity of literature examining its effects in such patients. One study evaluated the effects on renal function in heart failure patients admitted with volume excess.[40] Although the addition of dopamine to diuretics was associated with marked improvement in renal function after 5 days, this assessment was made in patients who were not refractory to diuretics. Patients treated with diuretics had the same urine production as those patients in whom dopamine was added to their 1 mg b.i.d. of bumetanmide (equivalent to furosemide 40 mg b.i.d.). Further, dopamine can impair ventilatory responsiveness in heart failure patients via effects on the chemoreflex sensitivity.[41] Therefore, even though one study suggests its utility,[40] the relatively widespread use of renal dopamine should not be advocated until definitive data can support its safety and efficacy.

Combination therapy with these vasoactive intravenous medications can overcome resistance, in essence by improving renal blood flow. Options include high-dose nitroprusside or the combination of nitroprusside with a positive inotropic agent.[42–45] Investigational options include the development of vasopressin antagonists, potentially useful for their aquaretic effects, and positive inotropic agents including the calcium-sensitizing drug levosimendan.[6] Despite some of these approaches appearing advantageous over others, none of the available inotropic agents has been proven safe in patients with ADHF[28,46,47] even though they are able to improve patient status acutely,[42–45] and similar concerns exist for direct-acting vasodilators.[30,31,33]

Management of Refractory Patients with Dialytic Techniques

One reason that heart failure has received so much attention is the frequency and cost of hospitalizations. This includes a significant burden on system resources and costs focused on the management of these patients who are refractory to the use of loop diuretics alone. For the past three decades, the literature has described a treatment modality for volume overloaded heart failure patients that has not become part of the mainstream.[48–50] This approach rests on the principles of hemofiltration, using dialytic techniques, including hemodialysis, peritoneal dialysis, and extracorporeal ultrafiltration, either via an arterio-venous or veno-venous configuration (Table 28.2).

In hemodialysis and peritoneal dialysis, toxic substances are removed from the blood across semipermeable membranes. This is achieved by the presence of a solute separated from the blood by the membrane. This membrane allows molecules of sufficiently small size to traverse it, the amount removed from the blood being controlled by the concentration gradient across the membrane. Varying the constitution and concentration of the solute, therefore, determines the amount of water and toxic substances removed. For hemodialysis, the membrane is synthetic, while for peritoneal dialysis the peritoneum serves as a natural membrane. Because hemodialysis can be implemented immediately but peritoneal dialysis cannot, hemodialysis seems preferable. However, critically ill patients, and those with heart failure in particular, may not tolerate the metabolic changes, electrolyte shifts, and hemodynamic stress occurring during hemodialysis.[51]

In contrast to dialysis, ultrafiltration (or hemofiltration) is an extracorporeal technique by which an ultrafiltrate of plasma essentially consisting of water and minerals, particularly sodium and potassium, is produced by hydrostatic pressure exerted across a semipermeable membrane. Ultrafiltration, based on the principle of convective solute transport, differs from dialysis, wherein solutes diffuse across a semipermeable membrane into dialysate bath. Initial use of the technique used an arterial-to-venous connection configuration and, therefore, the rate of fluid removal was determined by the arterial pressure. This system worked well in patients with higher blood pressures, but was less useful when blood pressure was lower. An adaptation allowed connections from vein to vein, with the rate of fluid removal determined by a blood pump within the extracorporeal apparatus.[49] When used in this veno-venous configuration, ultrafiltration does not produce marked changes in blood pressure,[52,53] minimizing the risk of hemodynamic instability.

Veno-venous ultrafiltration appears to be an ideal approach for a heart failure patient with resistant volume overload. It avoids the risk of hemodynamic instability associated with hemodialysis, yet permits tight control of blood flow, and therefore fluid filtration rate. The principle is simple—blood is pumped from the patient, anticoagulated, and passed through a porous filter where fluid is removed according to the desired goal. The blood is then retuned to the patient without large fluctuations in electrolytes or acid-base balance. In fact, because the ultrafiltrate has a potassium concentration similar to that of plasma, there are no concerns about replacing potassium.[53]

In 1974, ultrafiltration was first reported as a modality for the treatment of volume overload, with several investigators reporting its utility for the treatment of patients with cardiac disease,[48,49,52–66] including those with contrast nephropathy after coronary intervention.[66] Heart failure patients with refractory volume overload are an ideal target for this therapy. It works independent of blood pressure, since it has a built-in pump for veno-venous flow, and does not produce marked swings in blood pressure or volume.[53,58,67] Ultrafiltration has been shown to be effective and well tolerated with up to 500 mL of ultrafiltrate removed per hour,[48,54,55,61–64] although initial rates are usually 100 mL/h to 200 mL/h. Initially, patients were instrumented and hemofiltration was continued until the right atrial pressure dropped by 50% or the hematocrit rose above 50.[54,61–65] Currently, hemofiltration can be implemented to treat patients to clinical goals, such as reduction in symptoms or congestion, and invasive assessment of right atrial pressure is not necessary.[53,67] Table 28.2 lists several of the studies using ultrafiltration in patients with heart failure, and in general, indicates that the technique is well tolerated even during large volume removal.

In most cases, the studies focused on the technical aspects of performing hemofiltration, while in several, the clinical impact was evaluated as well.

Table 28.2. *Experience with hemofiltration in patients with volume overload or heart failure*

Study, Year	No. of patients	Population	Therapy	Volume effects	Clinical effects
Silverstein, 1974[48]	5	Heart failure and end-stage renal failure	CAVH, 200–500 mL/h	3.6 L removed	Cramps, headaches, hypotension with rates of 400–500 mL/h filtered
Asaba, 1978[49]	9	Volume overload (3 with primarily heart failure)	CVVH, 200–300 mL/h	Average 5.5 L over 260 min	2/9 patients regained diuretic responsiveness after treatments; 3 HF patients responded as did the others
Rimondini, 1987[54]	11	Unresponsive to inotropes and diuretics, average of 289 mg furosemide in prior 24 h	CVVH, 500 mL/h until RAP reaches 2–3 mm Hg or hematocrit increases to 50	Over 4–6 h, removed 2450 mL	Diuretic responsiveness reported post treatments—urine output increased from 605/24 h to 1965/24 h, while diuretic decreased from 289 to 40 mg/24 h
DiLeo, 1988[55]	19	Refractory to up to 750 mg/day furosemide	CAVH, target 2–3 L/session over 2 h	1680–3500 mL/session, average weight loss 6.5 kg/session	
Inoue, 1988[56]	8	Oliguric	CAVH 1–14 days, average 5 days		Report that urine output increases after completing CAVH treatment course
Akiba, 1989[57]	17	Unresponsive to diuretics and vasodilators	Hemodialysis, peritoneal dialysis or filtration		The worse the fractional excretion of sodium, (more severe "prerenal" azotemia), the less likely to respond clinically
Canaud, 1991[58]	35	Unresponsive to diuretics and inotropes	CVVH	3.3 days, 19% decrease in body weight, 4.3 kg/day	Increased diuresis after treatment course
Biasioli, 1992[59]	8	"Refractory" or "intractable heart failure"	CVVH, with fluid exchange: Out: 10–40 mL/min In: 0–30 mL/min	Averages: Out:19 mL/min In: 8.7 mL/min Net:11.3 mL/min, 678 mL/h $\times$ 6+ h Total out: 4.5 L	

Table 28.2. *continued*

Study, Year	No. of patients	Population	Therapy	Volume effects	Clinical effects
Inoue, 1992[60]	15	Oliguric after 420 mg furosemide within prior 24 h	CAVH in 9, CVVH in 6		
Pepi, 1993[61]	24, randomized 1:1	Ambulatory, clinically silent but radiographically present pulmonary congestion	CVVH until RAP decreased by 50%, at 600 mL/h (single session)	Total net out: 1926 mL	Significantly increased VO_{2max} compared to control, better diastolic function by echocardiogram
Agostoni, 1993[62]	36, randomized 1:1	Ambulatory stable NYHA Class II-III heart failure patients	CVVH, 600 mL/h until RAP decreased 50%		Significantly improved VO_{2max} (sustained over 6 months)
Agostoni, 1994[63]	16, randomized 1:1	Ambulatory stable NYHA class II or III heart failure patients	CVVH, 600 ml/h until RAP decreased 50%		Significantly improved VO_{2max} (sustained over 3 months)
Marenzi, 1995[65]	26	No clinical congestion	CVVH until RAP decreased 50%	~ 2 L removed	Trends toward increased VO_{2max} at 3 months post treatment
Agostoni, 1995[64]	42, randomized 1:1	Ambulatory stable patients	CVVH, 600 mL/h until RAP decreased 50%	~1.8 L removed	Trends toward increased VO_{2max} at 3 months post treatment
Ramos, 1996[66]	30	Unresponsive to diuretics and inotropes	CVVH, up to 2 L/session	Average 2.4 sessions/patient, ranged from 1 to 5.5 L per session	Responders had more fluid removed (9.6 L vs. 3.2 L) yet had net fall in BUN/creatinine. Non-responders had worsened azotemia
Sacco, 1998[68]	31, non-randomized	Volume overloaded	CAPD (n = 20), Intermittent Dobutamine (n = 11) for 12 h/week to 12 h/day		Trend for worse survival in dobutamine patients (6 months, 55 vs. 36%, 12 months 35 vs. 18%)

Table 28.2. *continued*

Study, Year	No. of patients	Population	Therapy	Volume effects	Clinical effects
Marenzi, 2003[67]	33	Contrast induced oligoanuric renal failure after cardiac catheterization	CVVH + furosemide 500–1000 mg/24 h + dopamine at 2 mg/kg/min	0–400 ml/h, started 76 h post catheterization, continued for 4.7 days	No hypotension, 2 in-hospital deaths (9.1%) with 27% 1-year mortality (they argue this is better than other reports of outcomes without CVVH)
Jaski, 2003[53]	21	Volume overloaded	Peripheral access CVVH, up to 500 mL/h for up to 8 h	2611 mL over almost 7 h (6:43)	No change in heart rate, blood pressure, serum chemistry or hematology parameters.

Abbreviations: BUN = blood urea nitrogen; CAPD = continuous ambulatory peritoneal dialysis; CAVH = continuous arterio-venous hemofiltration; CVVH = continuous veno-venous hemofiltration; HF = heart failure; NYHA = New York Heart Association; RAP = right atrial pressure; VO_{2max} = maximal oxygen consumption.

In two out of three reports by Agostoni *et al.*,[62–64] ambulatory, apparently optimized patients were randomized to a single session of continuous veno-venous hemofiltration (CVVH) or additional intravenous bolus diuretic therapy. In each group, patients averaged nearly 2 liters net fluid removal. Over the following 3 to 6 months, maximum oxygen consumption (VO_{2max}) improved significantly in the hemofiltered group compared to the furosemide bolused group.[61–65] Another interesting clinical observation is the restoration of responsiveness to diuretics after treatment in these diuretic-resistant patients,[49,54,56–58] although the frequency and predictors remain undefined. In fact, the response can be quite dramatic, with one series reporting that the average urine output increased from 605 mL in the 24 hours prior to hemofiltration to 1965 mL in the 24 hours after completing treatment. This increase occurred despite marked reduction in the furosemide doses during those time periods, from 289 mg to 40 mg.[54] Although the cardiac effects of hemofiltration have not been studied specifically in patients with heart failure, the long-term safety relative to inotropic support were reported based upon a comparison of the experiences of two hospitals. In one hospital, patients (n = 11) were treated with intermittent dobutamine, while the other hospital (n = 20) used intermittent hemofiltration.[68] Despite the caveats warranted by such a comparison between two separate populations treated with unblinded therapy in a non-randomized trial, the better 1-year survival with hemofiltration suggested a potential effect worthy of investigation in a prospective trial.

The mechanisms for clinical improvement are incompletely defined. For example, while negative fluid balance will result in less pulmonary congestion, lung mechanics are not normalized as a result of acute ultrafiltration.[64,69] Despite reductions in cardiac filling pressures and total body volume, the improvement in spirometry is not paralleled by such an effect on diffusing capacity.[69] Further studies are required to delineate the mechanisms for improved functional status while verifying the data from the preliminary studies.

A recent advance is the development of an apparatus that permits CVVH to be performed without central venous access. Twenty-one patients were treated with this device, leading to United States Food and Drug Administration (FDA) approval for the treatment of severe volume overload.[53] This system uses catheters placed in the antecubital veins, one similar to a peripherally inserted central catheter (PICC) for withdrawal, and the other a short, large-bore intravenous catheter placed typically in the opposite arm. Sensors control the blood flow rates to prevent vein collapse, and can yield up to 500 mL/h of ultrafiltrate removal. Treatment was up to 8 hours in duration and fluid removal averaged 3725 mL. Patients felt better and experienced little change in serum electrolytes.[53]

Conclusion

Heart failure patients with volume overload refractory to diuretics have few options. Patients treated with high-dose diuretics are at increased risk of death,[18] as are those with persistent congestion[26,70] and those who develop worsening azotemia as therapy is intensified.[36–38] While the long-term effects of ultrafiltration for patients with heart failure have not been established, the literature supports the utility of ultrafiltration in ADHF with refractory volume overload.

In patients admitted for progressive, refractory heart failure and severe congestion unresponsive to appropriate pharmacological and dietary measures, as well as in less compromised patients, ultrafiltration generally demonstrates effectiveness in large fluid removal, while improving functional status[61–65] and diuretic responsiveness.[49,54,56–58] The available technical procedures seem to be safe and well tolerated even in patients with hemodynamic instability. Even if data are still inconclusive on the long-term benefits of this treatment, ultrafiltration should always be kept in mind for acute refractory congestive heart failure patients. Despite the available encouraging data, the use of this technique has not been widespread for three primary reasons. First, central access requirements have made intensive care unit (ICU) admission and logistical considerations a barrier. Second, the techniques have traditionally been viewed as dialytic/nephrologic ones, and cardiologists have been hesitant to embrace them as their own. Third, heart failure specialists as well as clinical cardiologists and primary care providers treating heart failure do not generally consider mechanical treatments as a primary option, in contrast to invasive cardiologists. With the development of peripheral access systems for CVVH, the logistical barriers are reduced markedly. New lower-cost devices are now available that can be managed in the ICU under the supervision of either nephrologists or cardiologists, and perhaps managed as safely and effectively as outpatient infusions of vasoactive agents in observation units. Although a randomized controlled trial would be ideal to demonstrate the clinical and pharmacoeconomic impact on heart failure, current data does support a more widespread use of ultrafiltration in volume overloaded diuretic refractory patients.

References

1. Kittleson M, Hurwitz S, Shah MR, *et al.* Development of circulatory-renal limitations to angiotensin-converting enzyme inhibitors identifies patients with severe heart failure and early mortality. J Am Coll Cardiol 2003; 41: 2029–2035.
2. Nohria A, Tsang SW, Fang JC, *et al.* Clinical assessment identifies hemodynamic profiles that predict outcomes in patients admitted with heart failure. J Am Coll Cardiol 2003; 41: 1797–1804.
3. Heart Failure Society of America (HFSA) practice guidelines. HFSA guidelines for management of patients with heart failure caused by left ventricular systolic dysfunction—pharmacological approaches. J Card Fail 1999; 5: 357–382.
4. Hunt SA, Baker DW, Chin MH, *et al.* ACC/AHA Guidelines for the Evaluation and Management of Chronic Heart Failure in the Adult: Executive Summary A Report of the American College of Cardiology/American Heart Association Task Force on Practice Guidelines (Committee to Revise the 1995 Guidelines for the Evaluation and Management of Heart Failure): Developed in Collaboration With the International Society for Heart and Lung Transplantation; Endorsed by the Heart Failure Society of America. Circulation 2001; 104: 2996–3007.
5. Remme WJ, Swedberg K., Task Force for the Diagnosis and Treatment of Chronic Heart Failure. European Society of Cardiology. Guidelines for the diagnosis and treatment of chronic heart failure. Eur Heart J 2001; 22: 1527–1560.
6. Follath F, Cleland JG, Just H, *et al.* Steering Committee and Investigators of the Levosimendan Infusion versus Dobutamine (LIDO) Study. Efficacy and safety of intravenous levosimendan compared with dobutamine in severe low output heart failure (the LIDO study): a randomised double-blind trial. Lancet 2002; 360: 196–202.
7. Gheorghiade M, Gattis WA, O'Connor CM, *et al.* Acute and Chronic Therapeutic Impact of a Vasopressin Antagonist in Congestive Heart Failure (ACTIV in CHF) Investigators. Effects of tolvaptan, a vasopressin antagonist, in patients hospitalized with worsening heart failure: a randomized controlled trial. JAMA 2004; 291: 1963–1971.
8. Gheorghiade M, Niazi I, Ouyang J, *et al.*, Tolvaptan Investigators. Vasopressin V2-receptor blockade with tolvaptan in patients with chronic heart failure: results from a double-blind, randomized trial. Circulation 2003; 107: 2690–2696.
9. Udelson JE, Smith WB, Hendrix GH, *et al.* Acute hemodynamic effects of conivaptan, a dual V(1A) and V(2) vasopressin receptor antagonist, in patients with advanced heart failure. Circulation 2001; 104: 2417–2423.
10. Schrier RW, Abraham WT. Hormones and hemodynamics in heart failure. N Engl J Med 1999; 341: 577–585.
11. Harris P. Congestive cardiac failure: central role of the arterial blood pressure. Br Heart J 1987; 58: 190–203.
12. Francis GS, Goldsmith SR, Levine TB, Olivari MT, Cohn JN. The neurohumoral axis in congestive heart failure. Ann Intern Med 1984; 101: 370–377.
13. Francis GS, Benedict C, Johnstone DE, *et al.* Comparison of neuroendocrine activation in patients with left ventricular dysfunction with and without congestive heart failure. A substudy of the Studies of Left Ventricular Dysfunction (SOLVD). Circulation 1990; 82: 1724–1729.
14. Antunes-Rodrigues J, de Castro M, Elias LL, Valenca MM, McCann SM. Neuroendocrine control of body fluid metabolism. Physiol Rev 2004; 84: 169–208.
15. Lilly LS, Dzau VJ, Williams GH, Rydstedt L, Hollenberg NK. Hyponatremia in congestive heart failure: implications for neurohumoral activation and responses to orthostasis. J Clin Endocrinol Metab 1984; 59: 924–930.
16. Drazner MH, Rame JE, Dries DL. Third heart sound and elevated jugular venous pressure as markers of the

subsequent development of heart failure in patients with asymptomatic left ventricular dysfunction. Am J Med 2003; 114: 431–437.
17. Drazner MH, Rame JE, Stevenson LW, Dries DL. Prognostic importance of elevated jugular venous pressure and a third heart sound in patients with heart failure. N Engl J Med 2001; 345: 574–581.
18. Neuberg GW, Miller AB, O'Connor CM, *et al.*, Prospective Randomized Amlodipine Survival Evaluation (PRAISE) Investigators. Diuretic resistance predicts mortality in patients with advanced heart failure. Am Heart J 2002; 144: 31–38.
19. Cody R, Pickworth KK. Approaches to diuretic therapy and electrolyte imbalance in congestive heart failure. Cardiol Clin 1994; 12: 37–50.
20. Lahav M, Regev A, Ra'anani P, Theodor E. Intermittent administration of furosemide vs continuous infusion preceded by loading dose for congestive heart failure. Chest 1992; 102: 725–731.
21. Kramer BK, Schweda F, Riegger GA. Diuretic treatment and diuretic resistance in heart failure. Am J Med 1999; 106: 90–96.
22. Riegger GA, Liebau G, Kochsiek K. Antidiuretic hormone in congestive heart failure. Am J Med 1982; 72: 49–52.
23. Friedman E, Shadel M, Halkin H, Farfel Z. Thiazide-induced hyponatremia. Reproducibility by single dose rechallenge and an analysis of pathogenesis. Ann Intern Med 1989; 110: 24–30.
24. Loon NR, Wilcox CS, Unwin RJ. Mechanism of impaired natriuretic response to furosemide during prolonged therapy. Kidney Int 1989; 36: 682–689.
25. Knauf H, Mutschler E. Sequential nephron blockade breaks resistance to diuretics in edematous states. J Cardiovasc Pharmacol 1997; 29: 367–372.
26. Lucas C, Johnson W, Hamilton MA, *et al.* Freedom from congestion predicts good survival despite previous class IV symptoms of heart failure. Am Heart J 2000; 140: 840–847.
27. Stevenson LW, Kormos RL, Bourge RC, *et al.* Mechanical cardiac support 2000: current applications and future trial design. June 15–16, 2000 Bethesda, Maryland. J Am Coll Cardiol 2001; 37: 340–370.
28. Cuffe MS, Califf RM, Adams KF Jr., *et al.* Outcomes of a Prospective Trial of Intravenous Milrinone for Exacerbations of Chronic Heart Failure (OPTIME-CHF) Investigators. Short-term intravenous milrinone for acute exacerbation of chronic heart failure: a randomized controlled trial. JAMA 2002; 287: 1541–1547.
29. Taylor AL, Ziesche S, Yancy, C *et al.* Combination of isosorbide dinitrate and hydralazine in blacks with heart failure. N Engl J Med 2004; 351: 2049–2057.
30. Califf RM, Adams KF, McKenna WJ, *et al.* A randomized controlled trial of epoprostenol therapy for severe congestive heart failure: The Flolan International Randomized Survival Trial (FIRST). Am Heart J 1997; 134: 44–54.
31. Moe GW, Rouleau JL, Charbonneau L, *et al.* Neurohormonal activation in severe heart failure: relations to patient death and the effect of treatment with flosequinan. Am Heart J 2000; 139: 587–595.
32. Publication Committee for the VMAC Investigators (Vasodilation in the Management of Acute CHF). Intravenous nesiritide vs. nitroglycerin for treatment of decompensated congestive heart failure: a randomized controlled trial. JAMA 2002; 287: 1531–1540.
33. Sackner-Bernstein JD, Kowalski M, Fox M, Aaronson K. Short-term risk of death after treatment with nesiritide for decompensated heart failure. A pooled analysis of randomized controlled trials. JAMA 2005; 293: 1900–1905.
34. Katz SD. Nesiritide (hBNP): a new class of therapeutic peptide for the treatment of decompensated congestive heart failure. Congest Heart Fail 2001; 7: 78–87.
35. Sackner-Bernstein JD, Skopicki HA, Aaronson KD. Risk of worsening renal function with nesiritide in patients with acutely decompensated heart failure. Circulation 2005. In press.
36. Krumholz HM, Chen YT, Vaccarino V, *et al.* Correlates and impact on outcomes of worsening renal function in patients > or =65 years of age with heart failure. Am J Cardiol 2000; 85: 1110–1113.
37. Smith GL, Vaccarino V, Kosiborod M, *et al.* Worsening renal function: what is a clinically meaningful change in creatinine during hospitalization with heart failure? J Card Fail 2003; 9: 13–25.
38. Forman DE, Butler J, Wang Y, *et al.* Incidence, predictors at admission, and impact of worsening renal function among patients hospitalized with heart failure. J Am Coll Cardiol 2004; 43: 61–67.
39. Marik PE. Low-dose dopamine: a systematic review. Intensive Care Med 2002; 28: 877–883.
40. Varriale P, Mossavi M. The benefit of low-dose dopamine during vigorous diuresis for congestive heart failure associated with renal insufficiency: does it protect renal function? Clin Cardiol 1997; 20: 627–630.
41. Van De Borne P, Somers VK. Dopamine and congestive heart failure: pharmacology, clinical use, and precautions. Congest Heart Fail 1999; 5: 216–221.
42. Monrad ES, Baim DS, Smith HS, Lanoue AS.

Milrinone, dobutamine, and nitroprusside: comparative effects on hemodynamics and myocardial energetics in patients with severe congestive heart failure. Circulation 1986; 73: III168–III174.

43. Kieback AG, Iven H, Stolzenburg K, Baumann G. Saterinone, dobutamine, and sodium nitroprusside: comparison of cardiovascular profile in patients with congestive heart failure. J Cardiovasc Pharmacol 1998; 32: 629–636.
44. Yamani MH, Haji SA, Starling RC, *et al.* Comparison of dobutamine-based and milrinone-based therapy for advanced decompensated congestive heart failure: hemodynamic efficacy, clinical outcome, and economic impact. Am Heart J 2001; 142: 998–1002.
45. Capomolla S, Febo O, Opasich C, *et al.* Chronic infusion of dobutamine and nitroprusside in patients with end-stage heart failure awaiting heart transplantation: safety and clinical outcome. Eur J Heart Fail 2001; 3: 601–610.
46. O'Connor CM, Gattis WA, Uretsky BF, *et al.* Continuous intravenous dobutamine is associated with an increased risk of death in patients with advanced heart failure: insights from the Flolan International Randomized Survival Trial (FIRST). Am Heart J 1999; 138: 78–86.
47. Silver MA, Horton DP, Ghali JK, Elkayam U. Effect of nesiritide versus dobutamine on short-term outcomes in the treatment of patients with acutely decompensated heart failure. J Am Coll Cardiol 2002; 39: 798–803.
48. Silverstein ME, Ford CA, Lysaght MJ, Henderson LW. Treatment of severe fluid overload by ultrafiltration. N Engl J Med 1974; 291: 747–751.
49. Asaba H, Bergstrom J, Furst P, Shaldon S, Wiklund S. Treatment of diuretic-resistant fluid retention with ultrafiltration. Acta Med Scand 1978; 204: 145–149.
50. Sackner-Bernstein JD, Obeleniene R. How should diuretic-refractory, volume-overloaded heart failure patients be managed? J Invasive Cardiol 2003; 15: 585–590.
51. Dormans TP, Huige RM, Gerlag PG. Chronic intermittent haemofiltration and haemodialysis in end stage chronic heart failure with oedema refractory to high dose frusemide. Heart 1996; 75: 349–351.
52. Marenzi G, Lauri G, Grazi M, *et al.* Circulatory response to fluid overload removal by extracorporeal ultrafiltration in refractory congestive heart failure. J Am Coll Cardiol 2001; 38: 963–968.
53. Jaski BE, Ha J, Denys BG, *et al.* Peripherally inserted veno-venous ultrafiltration for rapid treatment of volume overloaded patients. J Card Fail 2003; 9: 227–231.
54. Rimondini A, Cipolla C, Della Bella P, *et al.* Hemofiltration as short-term treatment for refractory congestive heart failure. Am J Med 1987; 83: 43–48.
55. DiLeo M, Paciti A, Bergerone S, *et al.* Ultrafiltration in the treatment of refractory congestive heart failure. Clin Cardiol 1988; 11: 449–452.
56. Inoue T, Morooka S, Hayashi T, *et al.* Effectiveness of continuous arteriovenous hemofiltration for patients with refractory heart failure. Jpn Heart J 1988; 29: 595–602.
57. Akiba T, Taniguchi K, Marumo F, Matsuda O. Clinical significance of renal hemodynamics in severe congestive heart failure: responsiveness to ultrafiltration therapies. Jpn Circ J 1989; 53: 191–196.
58. Canaud B, Cristol JP, Klouche K, *et al.* Slow continuous ultrafiltration: a means of unmasking myocardial functional reserve in end-stage cardiac disease. Contrib Nephrol 1991; 93: 79–85.
59. Biasoli S, Barbaresi F, Barbiero M, *et al.* Intermittent venovenous hemofiltration as a chronic treatment for refractory and intractable heart failure. ASAIO J 1992; 38: M658–663.
60. Inoue T, Sakai Y, Morooka S, *et al.* Hemofiltration as treatment for patients with refractory heart failure. Clin Cardiol 1992; 15: 514–518.
61. Pepi M, Marenzi GC, Agostoni PG, *et al.* Sustained cardiac diastolic changes elicited by ultrafiltration in patients with moderate congestive heart failure: pathophysiological correlates. Br Heart J 1993; 70: 135–140.
62. Agostoni PG, Marenzi GC, Pepi M, *et al.* Isolated ultrafiltration in moderate congestive heart failure. J Am Coll Cardiol 1993; 21: 424–431.
63. Agostoni P, Marenzi G, Lauri G, *et al.* Sustained improvement in functional capacity after removal of body fluid with isolated ultrafiltration in chronic cardiac insufficiency. Am J Med 1994; 96: 191–199.
64. Agostoni PG, Marenzi GC, Sganzerla P, *et al.* Lung-heart interaction as a substrate for the improvement in exercise capacity after body fluid depletion in moderate congestive heart failure. Am J Cardiol 1995; 76: 793–798.
65. Marenzi GC, Lauri G, Guazzi M, Perego GB, Agostoni PG. Ultrafiltration in moderate heart failure. Exercise oxygen uptake as a predictor of the clinical benefits. Chest 1995; 108: 94–98.
66. Ramos R, Salem B, DePawlikowsky MP, *et al.* Outcome predictors of ultrafiltration in patients with refractory congestive heart failure and renal failure. Angiology 1996; 47: 447–454.
67. Marenzi G, Bartorelli AL, Lauri G, *et al.* Continuous veno-venous hemofiltration for the treatment of

contrast-induced acute renal failure after percutaneous coronary interventions. Catheter Cardiovasc Interv 2003; 58: 59–64.

68. Sacco A, Agliata S, Schweiger K, *et al.* Peritoneal dialysis and chronic dobutamine, two experiences contrasted. Possible role and indications in refractory cardiac decompensation. Minerva Urol Nefrol 1998; 50: 91–95.

69. Agostoni PG, Guazzi M, Bussotti M, *et al.* Lack of improvement of lung diffusing capacity following fluid withdrawal by ultrafiltration in chronic heart failure. J Am Coll Cardiol 2000; 36: 1600–1604.

70. Shah MR, O'Connor CM. The congestion score: a simple tool for a complicated disease? Am Heart J 2000; 140: 824–826.

CHAPTER 29

Mechanical circulatory support for acute heart failure

Ashish S Shah, Carmelo A Milano

Introduction

Mechanical circulatory support (MCS) represents an important therapeutic modality for patients with acute decompensated cardiac failure (ADHF). As early as 1957, MCS in the form of pump oxygenators was used to support patients with acute myocardial infarction (AMI).[1] During this period, Clarence Dennis showed the effectiveness of left heart bypass in reducing myocardial oxygen demand experimentally, but clinical success remained elusive.[1,2] The first use of an implantable ventricular assist device (VAD) was in 1963. A VAD was used to save a patient following aortic valve replacement. The patient ultimately sustained an irreversible neurological injury and died, but even as early as 1963 the stage was set for a mechanical solution to the problem of acute heart failure (AHF).[3]

Patient Selection and Timing of Device Implantation

> I would like to emphasize one main point, namely the use of objective guides for the evaluation of assisted circulation. Unless such guides are employed both the indications for and the results from assisted circulation remain unclear.
>
> (Frank C Spencer, MD)[4]

A tremendous amount of time, effort, and financial resources are required to support patients with MCS. Furthermore, MCS represents a highly invasive treatment with significant surgical risk. Therefore, patient selection and the timing of device implantation remain challenging issues.

Patients with AHF who are considered for MCS must have objective evidence for ventricular failure—usually echocardiography can rapidly provide this information. Other treatable etiologies for ventricular failure such as acute coronary occlusion, acute valve dysfunction, or cardiac tamponade should be identified and corrected before MCS is considered. Circulatory failure should be defined with Swan–Ganz catheter measurements. Vasodilatory or septic shock must not be confused with cardiogenic shock. The hemodynamic picture is typically one of low cardiac index (CI < 2 L/m/m^2), elevated ventricular filling pressures (central venous pressure [CVP] or pulmonary capillary wedge pressure [PCWP] > 20 mm Hg), increased systemic vascular resistance, and reduced systemic blood pressure. Any patient considered for MCS should first receive a trial of noninvasive treatment usually consisting of intravenous inotropic support. These are general concepts that should guide the initial evaluation of AHF patients being considered for MCS. These hemodynamic criteria are certainly relevant, and defining noninvasive strategies is institution dependent. Furthermore, trends in hemodynamics and response to inotropes are more predictive than single time point assessment.

Careful assessment of end-organ dysfunction is critical in the evaluation of patients with AHF. Neurological function is the most important assessment. Devastating neurological injury is not uncommon, particularly in the setting of cardiac arrest, prolonged hypotension, or prolonged extracorporeal circulation during cardiac surgery. Patients who are unable to actively participate in their recovery, which includes walking and coughing, should not be offered MCS. On the other hand, it may be impossible to determine the neurological status with a patient *in extremis*. All sedation should be stopped, imaging of the brain performed, if possible, and evaluation by a neurologist may also be helpful. MCS is not warranted if significant anoxic brain injury has occurred.

Age is also an important consideration. Elderly patients (age > 65 years) may be excluded from device consideration for institutional reasons since cardiac transplantation may ultimately not be available for this group. Nevertheless, the elderly are an important group presenting commonly with AHF particularly after MI or cardiac surgery. Smedira and Blackstone reviewed data from the Cleveland Clinic Foundation (CCF) experience with MCS following cardiac surgery and found that age > 70 years was a risk factor for low cardiac output syndrome after heart surgery, but that younger age was associated with more aggressive use of extracorporeal membrane oxygenation (ECMO).[5] While age may preclude bridge to transplantation, it does not exclude the possibility of weaning the device or even destination therapy with a left ventricular assist device (LVAD). Furthermore, strong data demonstrating reduced outcomes with MCS in the elderly are lacking.

Psychosocial status of the patient is also a key issue. Patients in shock represent emotionally challenging situations for families. Nonetheless, good long-term results depend on strong social support and access to resources. Thus an assessment of the patient's ability to manage a device both physically and psychologically is important. It is however, difficult to deny MCS solely on the basis of the patient's psychosocial status.

Renal function is a significant predictor of outcome following LVAD placement. Farrar *et al.* showed that blood urea nitrogen (BUN) greater than 40 mg/dL was associated with increased mortality.[6] Furthermore, Williams and Oz reported that reduced urine output was predictive of poor outcome.[7] Renal impairment may, however, improve with device support. Therefore, renal impairment is not an absolute contraindication to MCS. Pagani *et al.* showed that even in patients requiring continuous veno-venous hemodialysis (CVVHD) preoperatively, long-term survival was possible following LVAD support.[8] In a series from the CCF, McCarthy *et al.* were unable to show that urine output was predictive of operative and long-term risk, but baseline serum creatinine was a risk factor.[9] A more recent report from CCF detailed the outcome of patients with preoperative creatinine > 3.0 mg/dL who had LVAD placement as a bridge to transplantation. In a cohort of 18 patients, 11 were successfully bridged to transplantation. None of these patients required permanent dialysis. Overall, the report stresses improved outcomes with continuous veno-venous hemofiltration (CVVH) versus conventional intermittent dialysis.[10] This conflicting literature reflects small patient cohorts and institutional practices. However, it does emphasize that advanced renal dysfunction (i.e. anuria, need for dialysis) is associated with poor outcomes but that some renal injury is reversible and should not be the sole contraindication to MCS. Although CVVHD has been a true improvement in acute dialysis, the ultimate goal is to initiate MCS prior to renal injury. Future work will have to identify better predictors of irreversible renal injury. Recent reports suggest that postoperative fenaldopam (a dopamine receptor agonist) may help promote renal recovery.

Hepatic function may be significantly compromised in patients with AHF. This dysfunction results from liver hypoperfusion or congestion, and can result in significant coagulopathy. Usually hepatic insufficiency is reversible with MCS. The presence of severe hepatic impairment however, may represent a relative contraindication for MCS. A prothrombin time (PT) > 16 s predicted an increase in post-operative bleeding requiring re-exploration.[11] A PT > 16 s was also identified by Williams and Oz as a predictor of early mortality post LVAD implantation.[7] Patients with elevated PT should be treated aggressively with preoperative vitamin K and fresh frozen plasma. Furthermore, elevated CVP and hepatic congestion may be predictors of right heart failure after LVAD placement and such patients may be better managed with biventricular support. Patients with underlying chronic liver disease, such as advanced cirrhosis are not candidates for MCS.

Patients with intrinsic lung disease are at increased risk for postoperative complications but this is difficult to assess preoperatively. Patients with primary lung disease may also have increased pulmonary vascular resistance that may contribute to right-sided circulatory failure after MCS. Thus, some determination of lung function should be performed preoperatively. In general, patients with severe primary lung disease or primary pulmonary hypertension are poor candidates for MCS.

AHF patients may have superimposed infection such as pneumonia, urinary tract infections, or catheter-related sepsis. These infections may complicate the management of a patient's heart failure, resulting in greater decompensation. These conditions should be identified and aggressively treated. Such infections should not preclude consideration for MCS since this may be the only mechanism to stabilize the patient. On the other hand, primary septic shock or active bacteremia represents a general contraindication to MCS.

Several groups have devised risk-scoring systems to stratify patients and provide a prospective tool to predict operative risk with MCS. A system devised by the group at Columbia Presbyterian Medical Center assigns a score to several factors (Table 29.1) and they report an operative mortality of 67% in patients with a preoperative score > 5.[7] Unfortunately, this risk-scoring system has not been proven in a prospective study. However, it does highlight the major variables associated with outcome. Most retrospective studies examine MCS implanted as a bridge to transplant with a minority of studies concentrating on MCS for AHF.[7,9] Nevertheless, these scoring systems emphasize that the presence of end-organ dysfunction at the time of LVAD implantation predicts poor outcome. A more aggressive strategy and earlier intervention with MCS will predictably yield better outcomes. Identifying the proper window of time in which conventional inotropes have failed but before end-organ damage takes place remains the goal. Achieving this goal requires a thorough and repeated clinical evaluation of the AHF patient. A number of signs may be helpful in predicting which patients are failing inotropic support and need urgent MCS. One of these signs is the development of confusion or delirium as a manifestation of early cerebral hypoperfusion. Dull abdominal pain or elevation of pancreatic enzymes may also be early signs of splanchnic hypoperfusion. Metabolic acidosis is an important finding that heralds systemic hypoperfusion. Sinus tachycardia and atrial or ventricular arrhythmias may be preterminal signs. Worsening hyponatremia may also indicate unresponsive heart failure. These physical signs may herald failure of inotropic therapy and warrant an urgent intervention with MCS. Failure to offer the patient MCS during such a window may lead to more severe end-organ dysfunction and preclude successful outcome even after adequate circulation is restored.

Table 29.1. *Columbia-Presbyterian left ventricular assist device scoring system*

Risk factor	Score
Mechanical ventilation	4
Postcardiotomy shock	2
Pre-left ventricular assist device	2
Prothrombin time > 16 s	1
Central venous pressure 16 mmHg	1

Traditionally, implantable LVADs were utilized for patients with chronic heart failure (CHF) who had been extensively evaluated and accepted for cardiac transplant. These patients usually have either ischemic or idiopathic dilated cardiomyopathy. Implantable LVADs are utilized when patients become decompensated and fail to stabilize with intravenous inotropic agents. These implantable systems enable complete physiologic recovery. Furthermore, the systems are wearable and enable hospital discharge and an active lifestyle. More recently, many forms of AHF have been treated with implantable LVADs. This strategy resulted from the observation that patients with acute presentations are often relatively young and ultimately suitable for transplantation. In these cases, however, LVAD implantation is often required before a complete transplant evaluation is possible. Williams *et al.* found no statistical difference in survival to transplant and post-transplant survival between patients implanted emergently as compared to non-emergently. Of the patients implanted, 19% died emergently of multisystem organ failure and 4 patients had device removal for irreversible neurological injury.[12] From 1994 to 2003 at Duke University Medical Center (DUMC), a total of 69 patients underwent implantation of a wearable LVAD. Of these 69 patients, 33 had chronic heart failure and complete transplant evaluation and listing prior to device implant. The other 36 presented acutely and could not undergo complete transplant evaluation. The etiologies for the acute group included post-MI shock, viral myocarditis, and postpartum as well as post-cardiotomy heart failure. Table 29.2 compares the outcomes for the two groups. Thirty-day post-LVAD survival, survival-to-transplant, and post-transplant survival were similar between the two groups. These observations emphasize that patients with AHF who cannot be fully evaluated should not be excluded from treatment with implantable LVADs as a bridge to transplant. Patients presenting with AHF ultimately did well with cardiac transplantation despite the lack of the complete transplant evaluation at the time of presentation and LVAD placement (Figure 29.1).

Device Selection

Once the decision has been made to initiate MCS, attention is turned to selecting the proper device. The current options are extensive and in the future may be even more complicated. There are several fundamental questions that need to be answered (Figure 29.2). First, is the patient a transplant candidate or a potential destination LVAD candidate? Second, how big is the patient? Third, what is the status of the right-sided circulation and will right-sided support be necessary? Finally, are there potential contraindications to anticoagulation?

Even in patients with AHF where there is a possibility of short-term support, all of these questions must be addressed. Several devices are designed for short-term use only, while others may be transitioned easily to longer-term devices. Thus, a review of currently available MCS devices will help shed light on the right device for the job.

Short-term devices

Intraaortic balloon counterpulsation

Since its introduction in the 1960s, intraaortic balloon pump (IABP) support has been the workhorse of devices. It was experimentally described in 1962 and then utilized clinically by Kantrowitz in 1968.[13] Approximately 100 000 IABPs are placed in patients in the United States annually. IABP sup-

Table 29.2. *Implantable left ventricular assist device and bridge to transplant for patients with acute vs. chronic heart failure*

	Acute heart failure (n = 36)	Chronic heart failure (n = 33)
Duration of LVAD support	59 ± 8 days	53 ± 7 days
30-day post-LVAD survival	89%	82%
Survival to transplantation	88%	76%
90-day post-transplant survival	97%	92%

Abbreviations: LVAD = left ventricular assist device.

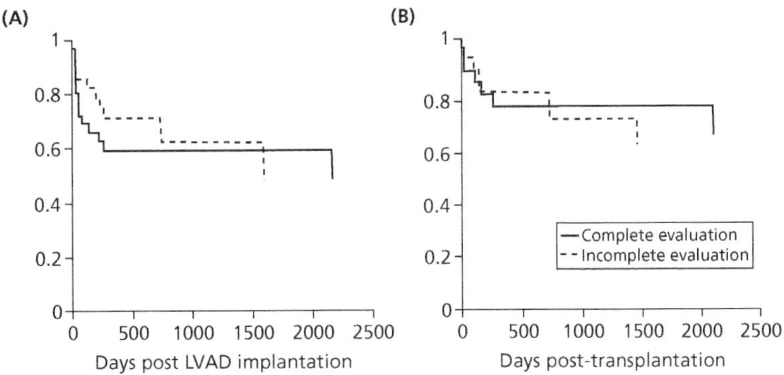

Figure 29.1. *A review of left ventricular assist device implantation at Duke University Medical Center from 1994 to 2003 for acute heart failure shows similar survival between patients with complete and incomplete preoperative transplant evaluations. (A) Actuarial survival from the time of LVAD implantations; (B) Actuarial survival from the time of transplantation in patients bridged with a device*

port should be first-line therapy for patients with medically refractory heart failure. IABP devices are safe and allow for rapid application via a percutaneous femoral arterial approach. Hemodynamically, IABP augments diastolic coronary perfusion and provides LV afterload reduction. Typically, used in patients with ischemic cardiomyopathy, we recommend its use in patients with nonischemic AHF and have had impressive results in some patients, eliminating the need for further device support. The

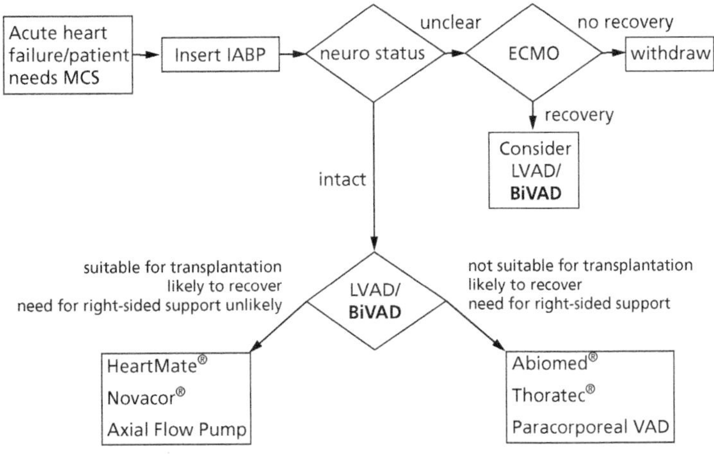

Figure 29.2. *Algorithm for ventricular assist device selection at Duke University Medical Center. In patients who are better candidates for cardiac transplantation, an implantable left ventricular assist device system enables long-term support and potential bridging. Patients who are poor candidates for transplant, or those patients for whom recovery is anticipated, are supported with paracorporeal left and/or right-sided devices. In general paracorporeal devices are less expensive but provide shorter duration of support*

Abbreviations: BiVAD = biventricular assist device; ECMO = extracorporeal membrane oxygenation; IABP = intraaortic balloon pump; LVAD = left ventricular assist device; MCS = mechanical circulatory support; neuro = neurological; VAD = ventricular assist device.

most important limitation of the IABP is that it provides indirect and incomplete circulatory support. The other potential complications include limb complications, thrombocytopenia, and patient immobilization. There are reports of transaxillary artery placement allowing patients to ambulate, but the most common approach still involves percutaneous femoral arterial introduction. IABP may allow for temporary hemodynamic stabilization, and preservation of end-organ function allowing for more elective LVAD placement.

Centrifugal pumps and extracorporeal membrane oxygenation

Pump oxygenators were used for patients with cardiogenic shock after MI as early as 1957. As cardiac surgery has progressed, conventional pump oxygenators have demonstrated a predicable track record. In patients with post-cardiotomy failure, they may be easily implemented to provide ventricular support. A centrifugal pump can be used, allowing transportation of the patient and conversion to an oxygenating circuit to provide ECMO. Access to the circulation may be via femoral or central cannulation. Pagani *et al.* have detailed the use of ECMO as a bridge to permanent VAD support and they make a compelling argument for its increased use. In acute patients in whom neurological or renal recovery is unclear, initial ECMO support represents a sensible option.[14] ECMO offers biventricular support as well as pulmonary replacement and it can be easily modified to provide continuous hemofiltration or dialysis. However, ECMO is associated with a number of potential complications. ECMO may activate inflammatory mediators which negatively impact renal and pulmonary function. ECMO requires significant systemic anticoagulation and bleeding complications may ensue. Additionally, thrombotic complications are frequent and cannulation-related problems such as limb ischemia may also be limiting.

ABIOMED BVS 5000®

The ABIOMED BVS 5000® biventricular support system is a pneumatically-driven assist device used for temporary circulatory support. The device gained United States Food and Drug Administration (FDA) approval in 1992 for use in patients with shock following cardiac surgery.[15] The BVS 5000® is composed of two compliant chambers housed in a rigid casing attached to a pneumatic driveline. Air driven into the rigid casing achieves pulsatile blood flow. The pump is filled by gravity and filling may be altered by changing the height of the pump relative to the patient. The heart can be cannulated in a number of ways depending on the type of support (biventricular or univentricular). The BVS 5000® does require significant systemic anticoagulation and is prone to thrombosis. Duration of support is usually 1 to 2 weeks and pump replacement may be required due to thrombus formation.

Today, the indications for BVS 5000® use have broadened and include short-term support for patients with shock complicating viral myocarditis, MI, intractable arrhythmia, and following cardiac transplantation. The BVS 5000® has a limit of 6 L/min output and patients are generally immobile. The device is relatively easy to use and troubleshoot and does not require additional personnel. Major limitations include a high thromboembolic rate and reduced patient mobility. Recently, our group reported successful use of the BVS 5000® in patients who had cardiac transplantation and AHF due to primary graft failure or severe rejection.[16] Success with the BVS 5000® in this group reflected the high likelihood of rapid ventricular recovery.

Recently, the ABIOMED AB 5000™ has been introduced for short-term support. This consists of a paracorporeal device which is also pneumatically driven. The AB 5000™ pump is compatible with the BVS 5000® cannulae. The AB 5000™ eliminates extensive blood tubing and provides assisted drainage. It is more mobile, less thrombogenic, and may provide safer long-term support (Figure 29.3). Generally, the ABIOMED systems are designed for support as a bridge to ventricular recovery.

Long-term devices

Thoratec® extracorporeal ventricular assist device

The Thoratec® extracorporeal VAD has been used since 1982 for post-cardiotomy support and as a bridge to transplant (Figure 29.4).[17] This device is composed of two cannulae and a pump that is

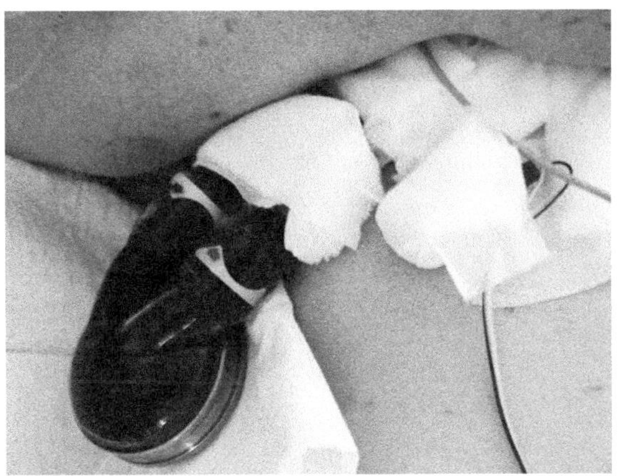

Figure 29.3. *A newer paracorporeal device, compatible with the ABIOMED BVS 5000®, the AB 5000™ circulatory support system eliminates extensive blood tubing and may be less prone to thromboembolic complications. See color plate section.*

placed in a paracorporeal position. The pump is pneumatically driven and utilizes two mechanical tilting disc valves. The drive console monitors pump output and operating pressures. Univentricular and biventricular support is possible and may be offered to smaller patients with a body surface area (BSA) as low as 0.75 m^2. Although it uses an external drive line, the console does allow the patient greater mobility. Recently, a smaller console has been developed and has led to FDA approval of the device for home discharge (Figure 29.5). The Thoratec® pump also requires long-term anticoagulation and patients with a contraindication to anticoagulation or bleeding diathesis may not be candidates for the device. As with the BVS 5000, there is some flexibility with respect to cannulation options. The inflow cannulae may be placed in the atria or ventricle, each with advantages and disadvantages. In general, ventricular cannulation enables better drainage and improved LVAD flows. In patients who are bridged to recovery, atrial cannulation enables easier LVAD explant.

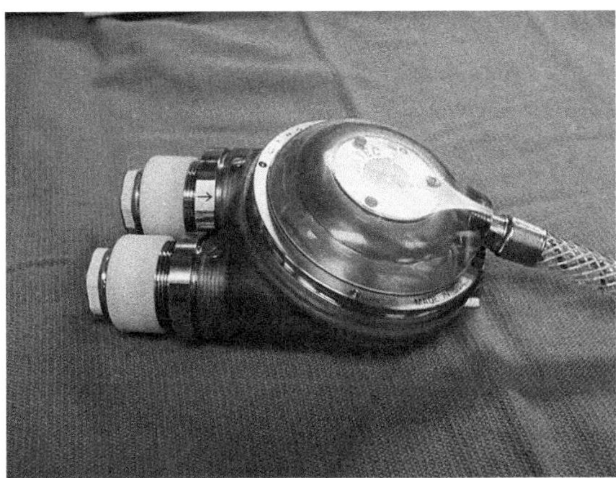

Figure 29.4. *The Thoratec® extracorporeal ventricular assist device (Reprinted with permission from Thoratec Corporation.) See color plate section.*

Novacor®

The WorldHeart Novacor® left ventricular assist system is an implantable, pulsatile electric pump. It was a product of research beginning in the 1970s

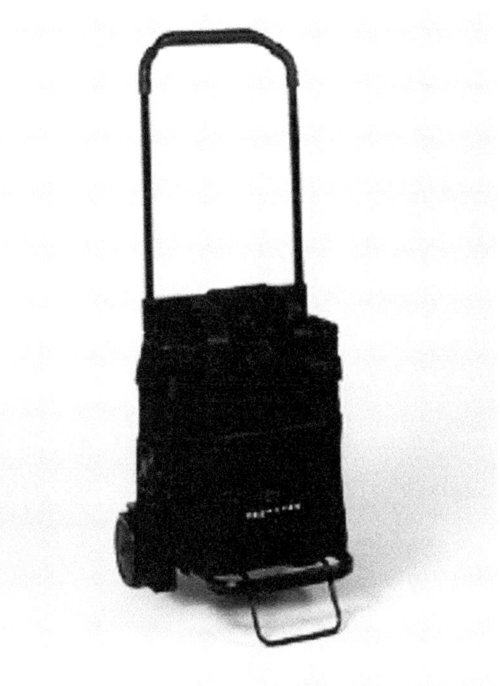

Figure 29.5. *A newer console allows patients greater mobility and the potential for home discharge (Reprinted with permission from Thoratec Corporation.) See color plate section.*

and culminating in its use as a bridge to transplantation in 1984 at Stanford. There have been several modifications to the device, and by 1993, it had evolved to its present design. It achieved FDA approval in 1998 as a bridge to transplant. It is an electrically-powered device that utilizes a pusher-plate design. An externalized drive line attaches to a small wearable battery allowing for complete patient mobility. Recently, modifications of the inflow conduit have been introduced to address problems with pannus ingrowth and subsequent embolization. Unlike extracorporeal devices, the pump is placed in a pre-peritoneal left subcostal pocket. The inflow graft is attached to the LV apex while the outflow graft is sewn to the ascending aorta. The device does require long-term systemic anticoagulation, generally with Coumadin. Patients may be discharged from the hospital with the Novacor® device and the longest period of support now exceeds 3 years.[18]

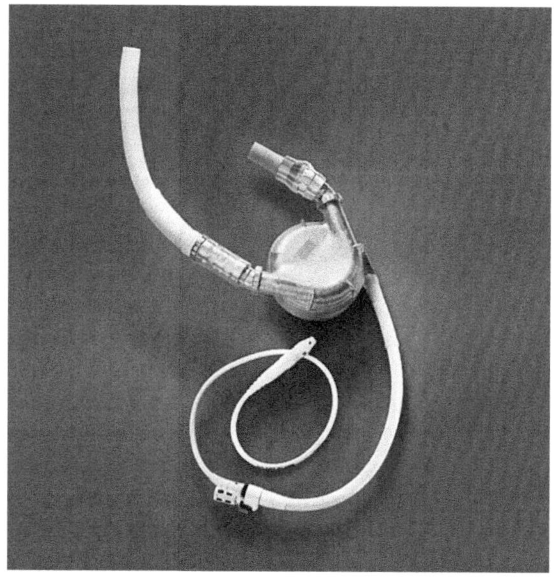

Figure 29.6. *The textured lining of the HeartMate® ventricular assist device generates a pseudointimal layer and contributes to decreased thromboembolic complications (Reprinted with permission from Thoratec Corporation.) See color plate section.*

HeartMate®

The Thoratec HeartMate® left ventricular assist system is another implantable, pulsatile electric pump, which began its clinical use in 1990 and was developed into a wearable model by 1995. The HeartMate® device has undergone extensive modification. In its original form, it was a pneumatically-driven, pusher-plate device. Later the VE model was developed and offered a vented electric-drive system with an external portable battery.[19] Most recently the XVE model offers modified inflow and outflow designs as well as software changes to reduce bearing wear and improve durability. The pump can generate up to 10 L/min and is implanted into a subcostal pre-peritoneal pocket. Unique to this design is a textured lining on the blood contact surfaces (Figure 29.6). Platelet and fibrin deposition on the textured surface results in the development of a pseudointimal layer. This layer appears to limit thromboembolism, and as a result, patients do not require systemic anticoagulation. As with the Novacor® device, patients may be supported for years. The device is limited to patients with a BSA greater than 1.5 m^2.[19]

The HeartMate® device is the most commonly-used long-term device on the market and was the subject of a large randomized trial looking at LVAD as destination therapy. The Randomized Evaluation of Mechanical Assistance for the Treatment of Congestive Heart Failure (REMATCH) trial randomized patients with end-stage chronic congestive heart failure (CHF) to optimal medical management or device support with the HeartMate® LVAD. Preliminary results showed a marked improvement in survival and quality of life at 2 years in the LVAD group.[20] The success and dependability of the HeartMate® LVAD has led to its FDA approval as destination therapy in patients with chronic heart failure. Hopefully, future studies will examine the utility of LVADs like the HeartMate® for destination therapy for AHF.

Axial flow pumps

While the current generation of implantable pumps produces pulsatile cardiac support, a newer variety of implantable devices generates continuous flow. These devices are smaller (3 inches), quieter and potentially more power efficient, relative to pusher-plate designs. The physiologic effects of non-pulsatile flow over long periods of time is unknown, although trials of the Jarvik 2000 and DeBakey® LVAD in Europe suggest adequate preservation of end-organ function after months of support.[21,22] The cardiac output is determined by rotational speed of the pump, thus lending itself to device weaning and recovery. The pumps are typically attached to the LV apex with an outflow graft to the ascending or descending aorta. The Jarvik 2000 has been implanted without bypass via a left thoracotomy.[23] These axial flow pumps represent the next generation of devices and may be attractive options for patients with AHF (Figure 29.7).

Device Use in Specific Forms of Acute Heart Failure

Acute myocardial infarction

MCS following AMI initially met with poor results. However, as experience with device support improved, several centers have reported encouraging outcomes. Approximately 10% of patients with AMI present with cardiogenic shock, yet this accounts for 50% of the mortality.[24] The conventional approach to patients in cardiogenic shock includes reperfusion therapy, inotropes, and IABP. Almost half of patients treated with this conventional approach will die. As detailed in the Should We Emergently Revascularize Occluded Coronaries for Cardiogenic Shock (SHOCK) trial, even very aggressive revascularization strategies in younger patients have resulted in 40% mortality.[24] LVAD support should be considered for the cohort which fails to show hemodynamic improvement. Device type selection depends on age and comorbidities. Older patients, or those with extensive comorbidities, are probably not candidates for long-term device support or transplantation. For these patients, short-term support with the ABIOMED BVS 5000® or AB 5000™ may sustain end-organ function and enable sufficient ventricular recovery to allow for device removal.

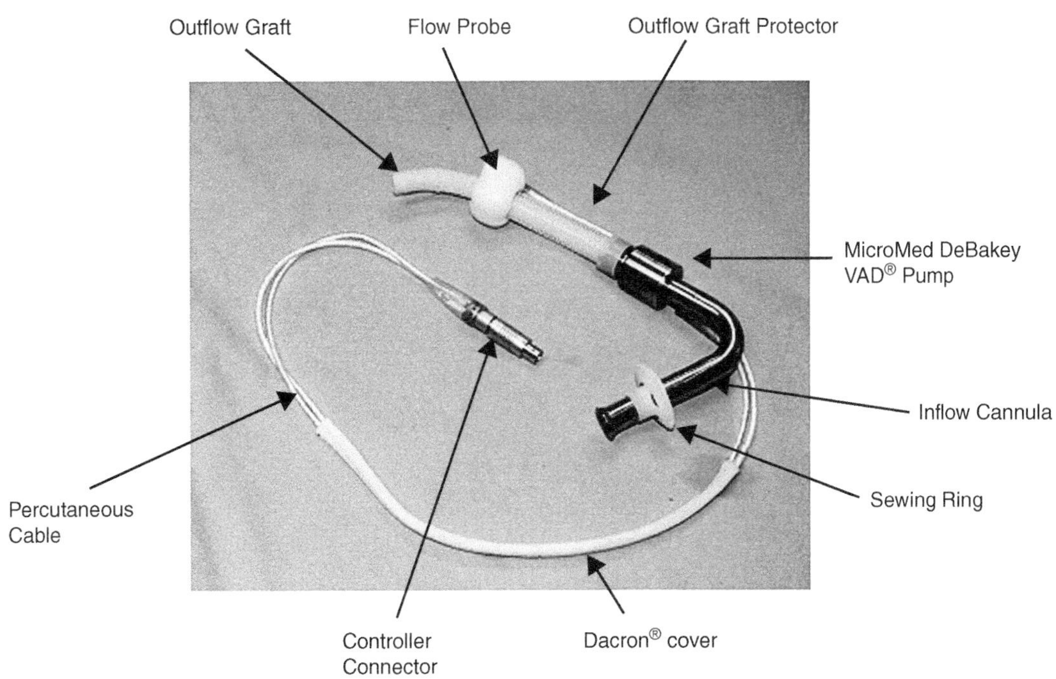

Figure 29.7. *The MicroMed DeBakey® ventricular assist device axial flow pump represents the next generation in devices. These blood pumps are smaller, quiet and more efficient then previous devices (Reprinted with permission from MicroMed Technology, Inc.) See color plate section.*

Younger patients or those without comorbidities should have implantable devices placed with the plan for a bridge to transplant. Several groups have described positive outcomes for AMI cardiogenic shock patients in whom implantable LVAD, bridge to transplant, strategies were employed.[25,26] Figure 29.8 details our algorithm at DUMC.

Post-cardiotomy failure

Shock following cardiac surgery is a rare phenomenon. Intraaortic balloon counterpulsation, which represents the most common form of device support, is used in up to 4% of cardiac operations and its use appears to be increasing.[27] More advanced support may be necessary in 0.5% of patients.[5] Patients should be supported with an IABP, inotropic support, and inhaled nitric oxide as indicated and if this is insufficient, advanced mechanical support may be initiated in the operating room. Importantly, careful inspection of the bypass grafts and prosthetic valve function should be done prior to MCS. Surgical correction of mechanical problems may obviate the need for MCS. Using ECMO, Media and colleagues at the Cleveland Clinic reported overall survival to discharge of 35%.[5] Infection was a common complication and limb complications occurred in nearly one-third of patients. ECMO has the advantage of providing support for failing lungs in patients with pulmonary insufficiency. Similarly, Samuels *et al.* reported a 31% hospital discharge rate in a series of 45 patients supported with the BVS 5000® following AHF. Over 50% of these patients had post cardiac surgery AHF.[15]

A more elaborate strategy had been devised by the Columbia Presbyterian University Medical Center group. Cardiac surgery programs in the area refer patients with post-cardiotomy shock to Columbia for evaluation of mechanical support. In 1999, the group reported their results from 1993 to 1998 and were able to show an impressive survival to discharge of 66%. Patients received temporary support initially after screening and about half went on to receive implantable support (HeartMate®). Mean duration of support using the implantable device was 76 days with 15 days in the intensive care unit (ICU). One-third of patients required inhaled nitric oxide and 22% required dialysis. Most of these patients failed to experience ventricular recovery and were bridged to cardiac transplant.[28]

Myocarditis

Myocarditis may be associated with significant hemodynamic instability and the need for inotropic therapy or MCS. Nonetheless ventricular recovery is common and long-term outcomes are good.[29] Thus patients with acute myocarditis, excluding giant cell myocarditis, should be supported aggressively with short-term devices. In these cases,

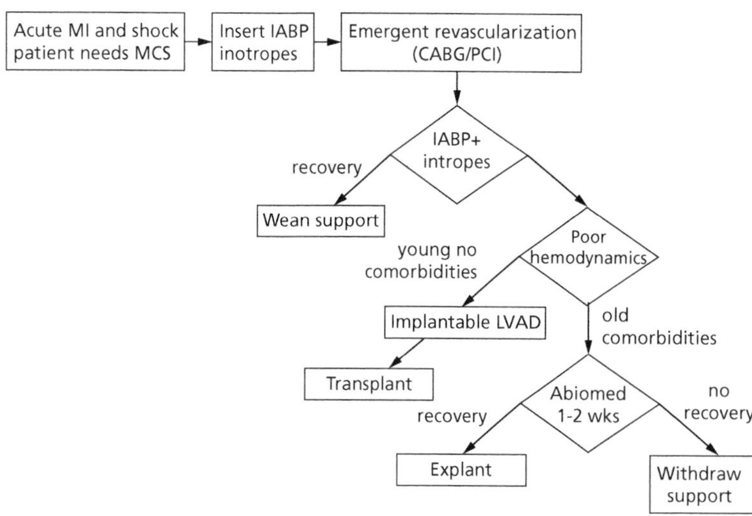

Figure 29.8. *Algorithm for management of patients with acute cardiogenic shock following myocardial infarction*

Abbreviations: CABG = coronary artery bypass grafting; IABP = intra aortic balloon pump; LVAD = left ventricular assist device; MCS = mechanical circulatory support; MI = myocardial infarction; PCI = percutaneous coronary intervention.

myocardial recovery is expected and short-term devices may be easier to explant. In a review by Acker, using short-term devices, less than 20% of patients went on to require transplantation. Special consideration should be given to patients with giant cell myocarditis. This histologically distinct entity carries a poor prognosis without transplantation, and may even recur in the transplanted organ.[30–32]

Post-transplant

AHF following cardiac transplantation may be due to primary graft failure secondary to preservation or reperfusion injury, or due to immunologic rejection. Most patients may be supported with inotropes or IABP. However, a small number of patients may require complete mechanical support. In a review of our experience at DUMC, after cardiac transplantation, 7 patients required MCS due to severe rejection (n = 4) or primary graft dysfunction (n = 3). Using the BVS 5000®, all patients experienced ventricular recovery and were weaned from the device; 5 out of 7 patients went on to long-term survival.[16]

Peripartum cardiomyopathy

Peripartum cardiomyopathy is an uncommon complication of pregnancy occurring in the third trimester or shortly after birth. It accounts for less than 10% of pregnancy related deaths and disproportionately affects African-American women.[33] MCS may be an option for advanced cases. There is no information on prognostic factors associated with ventricular recovery among patients with postpartum cardiomyopathy undergoing MCS. Our practice has been to use IABP support initially, followed by either a ABIOMED or Thoratec® device, if needed.

Weaning the Patient from the Device

When ventricular recovery occurs, VAD support can be weaned and the clinician may consider explanting the device. Proper evaluation of ventricular function requires that the VAD rate be substantially decreased and the native ventricle be allowed to fill. In general, increased systemic anticoagulation is warranted during this testing to avoid pump thrombosis. We recommend heparin to achieve an activated clotting time (ACT) > 300 s. For many of the devices, the pump is disconnected from its power source and manually activated to achieve a pump flow of 1 L/min to 2 L/min. During this period of reduced VAD support, blood pressure and heart rate are carefully monitored. Ventricular function is assessed with transesophageal echocardiography (TEE) and hemodynamics are measured with Swan–Ganz catheters. In addition, formal exercise testing may be accomplished in select patients with measurement of maximum oxygen consumption (VO_2max). General guidelines for weaning and pump explantation are provided in Table 29.3, but these decisions also depend on patient variables and the etiology of the patient's AHF.

Table 29.3. *Considerations for weaning the ventricular assist device*

A. Increase systemic anticoagulation (ACT ≥ 300)

B. Decrease VAD flow to enable adequate ventricular filling
   VAD flow < 2 L/min

C. Assess multiple hemodynamic and functional parameters
   1. Heart rate and blood pressure response
   2. Transesophageal echocardiogram
   3. Swan–Ganz measurements
   4. Exercise testing (VO_2max), if possible

D. Ideal conditions for VAD removal
   1. Acceptable heart rate and blood pressure (HR < 100 bpm, MAP > 70)
   2. Ejection fraction > 40%
   3. Cardiac index > 2.2 L/min/m^2
   4. Filling pressure < 15 mm Hg
   5. VO_2max > 15 cc/kg/min

Abbreviations: ACT = activated clotting time; bpm = beats per minute; MAP = mean arterial pressure; VAD = ventricular assist device.

Conclusion

MCS for AHF was first attempted in the 1950s. Substantial progress has been made since these early pioneering efforts. Several trends can be observed in our current practice. Each of the devices cited earlier in this chapter has undergone modifications in response to clinical experience. Improved devices and increased experience have resulted in more aggressive and earlier application of device therapy for patients with AHF. This represents an important step since end-organ dysfunction has been identified as a strong predictor of mortality post-LVAD placement. Identifying the proper window before significant end-organ damage has taken place remains critical. Greater confidence in device therapy will continue to encourage earlier application and better outcomes.

Another important trend is the utilization of long-term LVAD support for patients with AHF. This approach is developing because many etiologies of AHF are not readily reversible and ultimately require cardiac transplantation. The best example of this is AMI and cardiogenic shock. The physical loss of myocardium often precludes native LV recovery. Furthermore, even for types of AHF in which recovery has been described, this is often a delayed process requiring prolonged mechanical support (for weeks or even months). An example is viral myocarditis in which most patients experience ventricular recovery but many required prolonged support. The trend toward longer duration of LVAD support for AHF has led to the use of implantable or wearable systems for these patients. Such devices enable not only extubation and discharge from the ICU but may ultimately enable patients to return home. With extended support, some patients may experience LV recovery but many may require a bridge to cardiac transplantation. Finally, the recent FDA approval of the HeartMate® device for destination therapy in patients with chronic heart failure who do not qualify for transplantation raises hope that similar approval may be extended to patients with AHF. For example, a patient who presents with cardiogenic shock and acute MI may undergo urgent implantable LVAD procedure as a life-saving step. If it is determined later that the patient is not a suitable candidate for transplant, then they could continue with the device as a destination therapy.

Important frontiers still remain. The ideal device for AHF does not exist. While there are currently multiple options in terms of devices, the ideal device would combine the best features offered by the existing devices. Such a device would be easy to implant and it would subject the patient to minimal surgical risk. Perhaps such a device could be percutaneously installed like an IABP. The ideal device would be capable of complete ventricular unloading and complete circulatory support and would be applicable for both left and right ventricular support. Such a device would also feature a low thromboembolic rate like the HeartMate® device. It would be durable and portable; enabling ambulation and even discharge. Such features would be important for patients who do not experience ventricular recovery. In addition, the magnitude of device support would be variable, enabling partial support and partial ventricular loading. In addition, the device would explant easily. These later features would be important for patients who experience ventricular recovery and could be weaned from mechanical support. Obviously, such a device does not currently exist but many of these features are present in the different devices currently available. This provides hope for the development of such an "ideal device" for AHF.

While we stated earlier that most forms of AHF requiring MCS do not experience recovery, this reflects a very limited understanding of the recovery process. The fundamental molecular and cellular events required for functional recovery are poorly understood. This area represents another frontier but important efforts have been initiated. The concept of combining a period of LVAD support with adjunctive treatments for ventricular reverse remodeling has been introduced. Yacoub *et al.* have described the drug clenbuterol as a pharmacological treatment to potentiate ventricular reverse remodeling in chronic heart failure patients supported on LVADs.[34] Experimental genetic therapies have been described which appear to enhance ventricular function in acute failure models.[35] Such treatments could be potentially administered at the time of LVAD implantation. Finally, cellular therapies have already been tested clinically in the setting of heart failure and LVAD implantation.[36] Better understanding of the reverse remodeling process and application of some of these adjunctive treatments may result in an increased incidence of recovery, obviating the need for cardiac transplantation or prolonged LVAD support.

References

1. Stuckey JH, Newman MM, Dennis C, *et al.* The use of the heart-lung machine in selected cases of acute myocardial infarction. Surg Forum 1957; 8: 342–344.
2. Dennis C, Hall DP, Moreno JR, Senning A. Reduction of the oxygen utilization of the heart by left heart bypass. Circ Res 1962; 10: 298–305.
3. Liotta D, Hall CW, Henly WS, *et al.* Prolonged assisted circulation during and after cardiac or aortic surgery. Prolonged partial left ventricular bypass by means of intracorporeal circulation. Am J Cardiol 1963; 12: 399–405.
4. Spencer FC, Eiseman B, Trinkle JK, Rossi NP. Assisted circulation for cardiac failure following intracardiac surgery with cardiopulmonary bypass. J Thorac Cardiovasc Surg 1965; 49: 56–73.
5. Smedira NG, Blackstone EH. Postcardiotomy mechanical support: risk factors and outcomes. Ann Thorac Surg 2001; 71: S60–S66.
6. Farrar DJ. Preoperative predictors of survival in patients with Thoratec ventricular assist devices as a bridge to heart transplantation. Thoratec Ventricular Assist Device Principal Investigators. J Heart Lung Transplant 1994; 13: 93–100.
7. Williams MR, Oz MC. Indications and patient selection for mechanical ventricular assistance. Ann Thorac Surg 2001; 71: S86–S91.
8. Aaronson KD, Patel H, Pagani FD. Patient selection for left ventricular assist device therapy. Ann Thorac Surg 2001; 75: S29–S35.
9. McCarthy PM, Smedira NO, Vargo RL, *et al.* One hundred patients with the HeartMate left ventricular assist device: evolving concepts and technology. J Thorac Cardiovasc Surg 1998; 115: 904–912.
10. Khot UN, Mishra M, Yamani MH, *et al.* Severe renal dysfunction complicating cardiogenic shock is not a contraindication to mechanical support as a bridge to cardiac transplantation. J Am Coll Cardiol 2003; 41: 381–385.
11. Kaplon RJ, Gillinov AM, Media NG, *et al.* Vitamin K reduces bleeding in left ventricular assist device recipients. J Heart Lung Transplant 1999; 18: 346–350.
12. Williams M, Casher J, Joshi N. Insertion of a left ventricular assist device in patients without thorough transplant evaluation: a worthwhile risk? J Thorac Cardiovasc Surg 2003; 126: 436–441.
13. Kantrowitz A, Tjonneland S, Freed PS, *et al.* Initial clinical experience with intraaortic balloon pumping in cardiogenic shock. JAMA 1968; 203: 113–118.
14. Pagani FD, Lynch W, Swaniker F, *et al.* Extracorporeal life support to left ventricular assist device bridge to heart transplant: a strategy to optimize survival and resource utilization. Circulation 1999; 100: II206–II210.
15. Samuels LE, Holmes EC, Thomas MP, *et al.* Management of acute cardiac failure with mechanical assist: experience with the ABIOMED BVS 5000. Ann Thorac Surg 2001; 71: S67–S72.
16. Petrofski JA, Patel VS, Russell SD, Milano CA. BVS 5000 support after cardiac transplantation. J Thorac Cardiovasc Surg 2003; 126: 442–447.
17. Pennigton DG, Oaks TE, Lohmann DP. Extracorporeal support: the Thoratec device. In: Goldstein DJ, Oz MC (eds) Cardiac Assist Devices (Futura Publishing: New York, 2000), 251–262.
18. Ramasamy N, Vargo RL, Kormos RL, Portner PM. Intracorporeal support: Novacor left ventricular assist device system. In: Goldstein DJ, Oz MC (eds) Cardiac Assist Devices (Futura Publishing: New York, 2000), 323–339.
19. Goldstein DJ. Intracorporeal support: Thermo Cardiosystems ventricular assist. In: Goldstein DJ, Oz MC (eds) Cardiac Assist Devices (Futura Publishing: New York, 2000), 307–321.
20. Rose EA, Gelijns AC, Moskowitz AJ, *et al.*, Randomized Evaluation of Mechanical Assistance for the Treatment of Congestive Heart Failure (REMATCH) Study Group. Long-term mechanical left ventricular assistance for end-stage heart failure. N Engl J Med 2001; 345: 1435–1443.
21. Frazier OH, Myers TJ, Westaby S, Gregoric ID. Clinical experience with an implantable, intracardiac, continuous flow circulatory support device: physiologic implications and their relationship to patient selection. Ann Thorac Surg 2004; 77: 133–142.
22. Goldstein DJ. Worldwide experience with the MicroMed DeBakey Ventricular Assist Device as a bridge to transplantation. Circulation 2003; 108: II272–II277.
23. Westaby S, Frazier OH, Pigott DW, Saito S, Jarvik RK. Implant technique for the Jarvik 2000 Heart. Ann Thorac Surg 2002; 73: 1337–1340.

24. Hochman JS, Sleeper LA, Webb JG, *et al.* Early revascularization in acute myocardial infarction complicated by cardiogenic shock. SHOCK Investigators. Should we emergently revascularize occluded coronaries for cardiogenic shock? N Engl J Med 1999; 341: 625–634.
25. Chen JM, DeRose JJ, Slater JP, *et al.* Improved survival rates support left ventricular assist device implantation early after myocardial infarction. J Am Coll Cardiol 1999; 33: 1903–1908.
26. Park SJ, Nguyen DQ, Bank AJ, Ormaza S, Bolman RM 3rd. Left ventricular assist device bridge therapy for acute myocardial infarction. Ann Thorac Surg 2000; 69: 1146–1151.
27. Baskett RJ, O'Connor GT, Hirsch GM, *et al.*, Northern New England Cardiovascular Disease Study Group. A multicenter comparison of intraaortic balloon pump utilization in isolated coronary artery bypass graft surgery. Ann Thorac Surg 2003; 76: 1988–1992.
28. Helman DN, Morales DL, Edwards NM, *et al.* Left ventricular assist device bridge-to-transplant network improves survival after failed cardiotomy. Ann Thorac Surg 1999; 68: 1187–1194.
29. McCarthy RE 3rd, Boehmer JP, Hruban RH, *et al.* Long-term outcome of fulminant myocarditis as compared with acute (nonfulminant) myocarditis. N Engl J Med 2000; 342: 690–695.
30. Acker MA. Mechanical circulatory support for patients with acute-fulminant myocarditis. Ann Thorac Surg 2001; 71: S73–S76.
31. Davies JE, Kirklin JK, Pearce FB, Rayburn BK, Winokur TS, Holman WL. Mechanical circulatory support for myocarditis: how much recovery should occur before device removal? J Heart Lung Transplant 2002; 21: 1246–1249.
32. Davies RA, Veinot JP, Smith S, *et al.* Giant cell myocarditis: clinical presentation, bridge to transplantation with mechanical circulatory support, and long-term outcome. J Heart Lung Transplant 2002; 21: 674–679.
33. Whitehead SJ, Berg CJ, Chang J. Pregnancy-related mortality due to cardiomyopathy: United States, 1991–1997. Obstet Gynecol 2003; 102: 1326–1331.
34. Hon JK, Yacoub MH. Bridge to recovery with the use of left ventricular assist device and clenbuterol. Ann Thorac Surg 2003; 75: S36–S41.
35. Shah AS, White DC, Emani S, *et al.* In vivo ventricular gene delivery of a beta-adrenergic receptor kinase inhibitor to the failing heart reverses cardiac dysfunction. Circulation 2001; 103: 1311–1316.
36. Pagani FD, DerSimonian H, Zawadzka A, *et al.* Autologous skeletal myoblasts transplanted to ischemia-damaged myocardium in humans: histological analysis of cell survival and differentiation. J Am Coll Cardiol 2003; 41: 879–888.

Chapter 30

Left ventricular reconstruction for ischemic failing ventricle

Vincent Dor

During the past two decades, in spite of progress in the diagnosis and treatment of acute myocardial infarction (MI) (angiography-recommended, arterial recanalization by thrombolysis or percutaneous coronary intervention [PCI]) with a significant decrease in mortality, there exists an apparent paradox, as at the same time, the number of patients with ischemic congestive heart failure (CHF) has increased. In reality, this is logical as the survivors of MIs are more numerous but they are left with a scarred left ventricular (LV) wall.

More than 30 years ago, Gorlin[1] demonstrated that when 20% of the myocardium is necrosed, an irreversible evolution to progressive ventricular dilatation and failure occurs (now called remodeling). During the same time period, the same institution announced[2] that classical linear resection of LV aneurysm is not a technique for improving LV hemodynamic and function. In absence of documented ischemia, potentially controlled by coronary revascularization, cardiologists are considering that surgery is not indicated in the treatment of CHF with large asynergic scar.

Since the 1980s, modification of the surgical technique with circular rebuilding of the LV by a endoventricular patch[3] allows improvement in both morphology and hemodynamics of the scarred left ventricle. This LV reconstruction (LVR) is efficient even in very large asynergia with heart failure and in the end stage of this disease, when acute CHF occurs a few weeks or months after MI with inefficient medical therapy, and without the possibility for immediate heart transplantation.

Therefore, to be practical and efficient, it is essential to do the following: First, assess the LV wall after infarct with the same accuracy as arterial patency, in order to see and size the asynergic percentage of the LV circumference, which is the trigger of the remodeling initiation. Cardiovascular magnetic resonance (CMR) imaging appears to be the more reliable tool for this. Second, rebuild the scarred ventricle toward a more normal shape and curvature, in order to prevent, improve, or limit the remodeling consistent with White's description, "treatment of infarction should be aimed at the limitation of infarct size and prevention of ventricular dilatation."[4]

Left Ventricular Wall After Infarct

Infarcted areas

Even early reopening of the occluded coronary artery leaves some amount of infarcted necrotic LV wall. This was shown in the Mayo Clinic studies in 1991, where 18 out of 20 patients (90%) post recanalization had a scar affecting from 11% to 59% of the left ventricle.[5] In another series[6] in 1995, all 14 patients had necrotic LV wall scarring ranging from 6% to 8%. In our institution in 2002, only 2 of 26 early recanalized patients had no gadolinium late enhancement (GLE) fixing at CMR post-procedure control.

Type of lesion

The scar can be transmural or not. In the latter situation, there is often a subendocardial location of the necrosis. Bogaert mentioned[7] that recanalization of the occluded artery leads to this type of lesion with the obvious corollary of a decrease in the large bulging transmural scar. The healing of the infarcted areas is in three phases: the necrotic period, the fibrotic evolution, and finally calcification of the scar. The wall can be dyskinetic or akinetic and Gorlin mentioned "myocardial fibrosis, calcification within the scar, thickened overlaying pericardium, mural thrombosis, and endocardial thickening may rigidify the aneurysmal wall and prevent its extension. Thus, there is possibly a continuum between pure dyskinesis and pure akinesis as mechanical defects."[1]

Finally, transmural or subendocardial, dyskinetic, or akinetic, the scarred LV wall is asynergic with loss of contraction, and this loss of contraction depends on the size of the scar (Figure 30.1).

Localization

Even though disease in the right coronary artery (RCA) is the leading cause of infarction, the anteroapical septal region is the most common location for LV scar. This is probably due to the detrimental effect of occlusion of the left anterior descending (LAD) artery and its branches compared with the consequences of occlusion of the RCA or circumflex arteries with their balanced anatomy. The septum is not correctly analyzed by the right oblique projection of an angiogram. Echocardiography, and more precisely CMR with 4 projections (2 chambers, 4 chambers, left ventricular outflow tract (LVOT), and short axis), illustrates in the majority of cases, the involvement of the septum (Figure 30.2).

Prognosis of the post-infarct evolution

The prognosis of the post-infarct evolution depends on the extent of the asynergic wall.[1] This extension can be assessed by radionuclide outcome measurement essentially by technetium-99 m sestamibi single-photon emission computed tomography (SPECT).[8] Infarct size is calculated as the summed proportion of points < 60% of peak counts, expressed as a percentage of the left ventricle. By echocardiography or angiography with the centerline method,[9] the asynergic area is expressed as a percentage of LV circumference; and more easily/precisely, if there is no contraindication (e.g., implantable pacer or defibrillator), by CMR.[10–13] Analyzing the LV wall and the presence of this necrotic scar (white line traced by GLE) on 4 projections, the extension of the asynergic wall can be expressed as the ratio between the length of the necrotic scarred wall and the total length of the LV circumference (Figure 30.3). In Mayo Clinic reports with sestamibi measurement, the 6-month mortality was higher when infarct size was above 20%. In our center in 2002

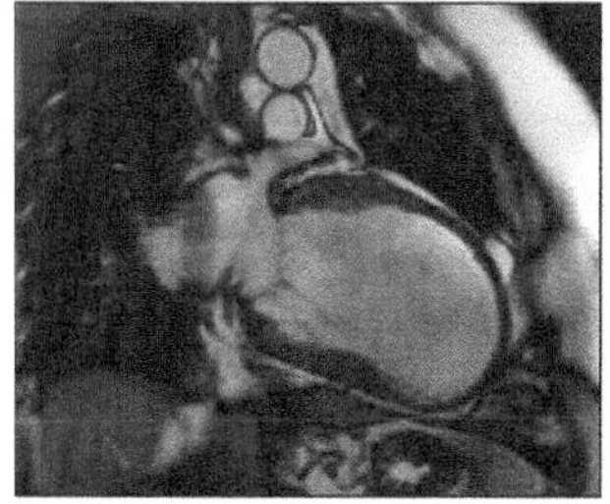

EDVI : 180 ml/m²
ESVI : 138 ml/m²
LVEF : 23 %

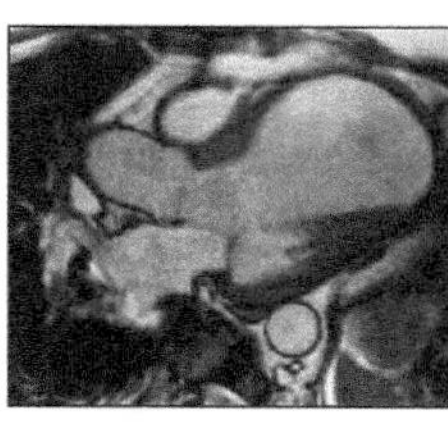

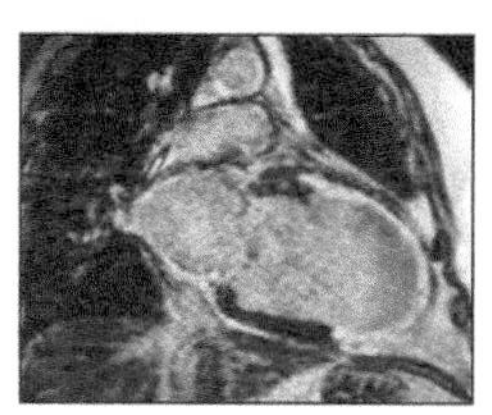

Gadolinium LH>50%

Figure 30.1. *Large asynergia (dyskinesis). Gadolinium late enhancement (GLE) shows that the scar is transmural in the apex and subendocardial on anterior wall. In spite of this layer of normal myocardium, the wall is totally dyskinetic*

Abbreviations: EDVI = end-diastolic volume index; ESVI = end-systolic volume index; LVEF = left ventricular ejection fraction.

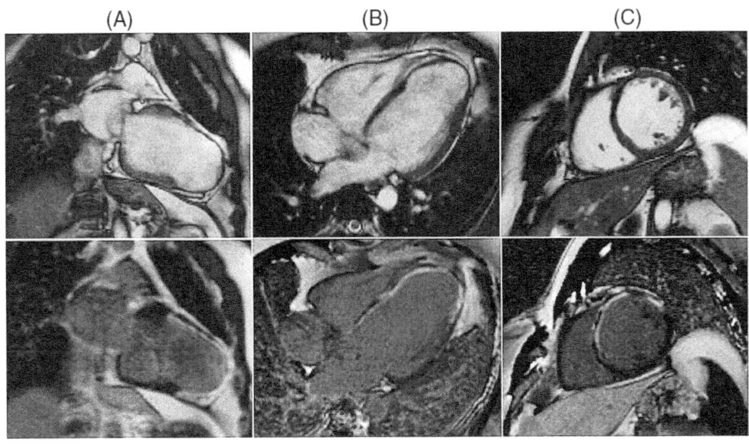

GLE

Figure 30.2. *Cardiac magnetic resonance (CMR) assessment of an anteroseptal apical aneurysm. (A) long-axis view; (B) 4 chambers; (C) short-axis view*

Abbreviations: GLE = Gadolinium Late Enhancement detected on the same 3 projections.

and 2003, among 55 patients proposed for LVR and with preoperative CMR, 41 (75%) had a GLE length ≥ 50% of LV circumference length.

The undamaged area—"remodeling"

The undamaged area is first normal, then hypertrophied to compensate for the lack of contractility of the necrotic wall, and finally dilated by physical mechanical forces. The dilatation increases the stroke volume and temporarily improves the cardiac index (Starling Law). However, the increased wall tension has a detrimental effect on myocardial contractility (Law of Laplace). This physical and mechanical explanation of the progressive dilatation of the heart, called LV remodeling, is based on a complex inflammatory and neurohormonal process[14,15] which in reality is due to the reaction (the fight) of the organism against the lack of contractility of a large scar when the remaining nonischemic area is not able to assume and maintain a normal cardiac output. This reaction might explain the progressive dilatation (remodeling), but is more a consequence than a cause of it. The real cause of remodeling is anatomical—the extension of the asynergic scarred area of the LV wall after infarct and all. The problem is to detect it early and to precisely assess its size. The aim for cardiology would be to precisely analyze the percentage of asynergic LV wall circumference, which can be considered as a critical trigger of the progressive remodeling. The end of this process is a dilatation of the non-infarcted area with a spherical shape and akinesia.

LV volume is a sensitive marker of post-infarction ventricular dysfunction, and LV end-systolic volume index (ESVI) is an important predictor of prognosis after MI.[16]

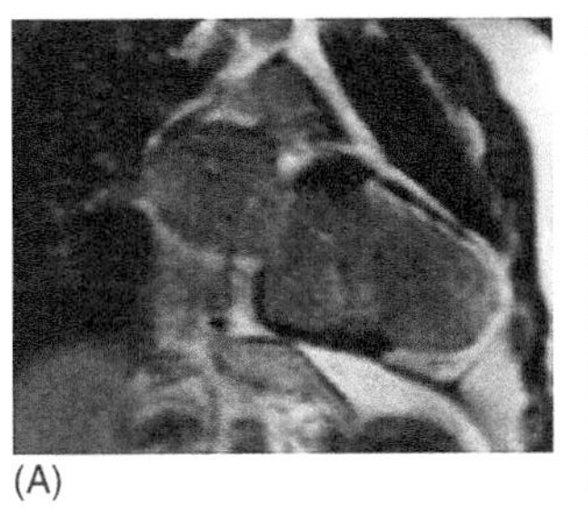

(A)

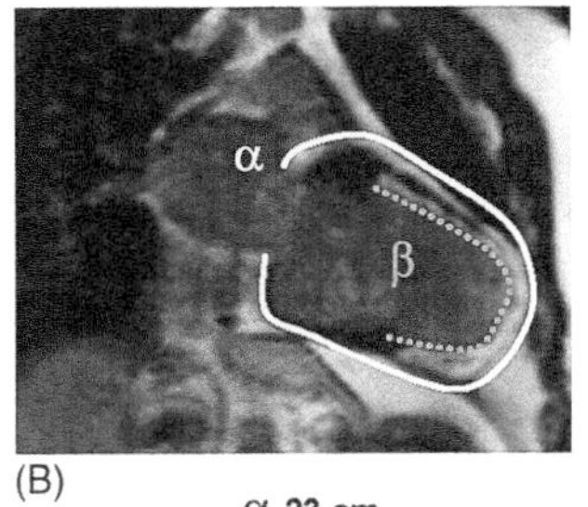

(B)

α **23 cm**
β **14.2 cm**
β**=61%** α

Figure 30.3. *Asynergic scar extension. (A) Gadolinium Late Enhancement of the same patient in long-axis view. (B) Assessment of the length of the asynergic wall (β = 14.2 cm) as compared with the total left ventricular circumference (α = 23 cm), proportion 61%.*

If 25/30 mL/m^2 for ESVI and 50/60 mL/m^2 for end diastolic volume (EDVI) are considered as normal values, doubling these indices can be considered as severe. In the recent Collaborative Organization for RheothRx Evaluation (CORE) study,[17] it was found that ejection fraction (EF) was superior to ESVI and infarct size (IS) in predicting 6-month mortality, but the investigators recognized that radionuclide assessment of EF and volume is less accurate than x-ray or magnetic resonance imaging (MRI) techniques.

Assessing precisely and regularly the evolving process of remodeling by repetitive measurement of LV volumes and performances, either by echocardiography or CMR, is mandatory after the initial period of healing of the infarcted area.

It can be characterized as large asynergia with (potential or already present) severe CHF and the need for reconstructive surgery in patients with: asynergia reaching 50% of LV circumference; ESVI > 50 to 60 mL/m^2; LVEF < 35%; cardiac index < 2 L/m^2; mitral regurgitation > 30% or mitral annulus > 40 mm in diameter; and patients, in a great majority of cases, with spontaneous ventricular tachycardia (VT).

Conservative Surgery for Ischemic Failing Ventricle

Heart transplantation has been and remains the ideal and more radical solution for ischemic failing ventricle at the end stage of the disease. However, progress in operative techniques, anesthesia, and post-operative care in the past 20 years allows us, in many cases, to try more conservative surgery with the hope of improvement above the volume expected of possible heart transplantation.

It has been mentioned previously that surgery of LV resection initiated in 1955[18] and 1958[19] has a poor reputation, as linear suture of the LV wall after resection of exteriorized scarred wall left a disorganized LV cavity without hemodynamic improvement, except for limited apical anterior dyskinetic lesions.

The aim of LVR by endoventricular circular patch plasty (EVCPP), described in 1985[3] and 1989,[20] was to rebuild a normal curvature of dilated LV wall by anchorage inside the ventricle, on contractile myocardium of a circular patch excluding non-resectable asynergic areas with maintenance of a "physiological" diastolic capacity. This concept of endoventricular patch, was also proposed again in 1989 by Cooley and called endoaneurysmorrhaphy.[21] In 1985, Jatene presented a large series of 1200 cases of treatment of LV aneurysm by external circular reorganization of the LV wall, which has the same effect on the curvature, but the scarred septum plicated is let inside the LV cavity, a patch is used only in 10% of cases, and revascularization due to external epicardial sutures done only in 20% of cases.[22]

Standard technique of endoventricular circular patch plasty

Transesophageal echocardiography (TEE) is used to assess the mitral valve. Surgery is conducted with a totally arrested heart (Figure 30.4). Coronary revascularization and mitral annuloplasty, if needed, are accomplished first, and then the LV wall is opened at the center of the depressed fibrous area. The clots are removed and the endocardial scar is dissected and resected if the scar is calcified or if there is spontaneous or inducible VT. In such circumstances, cryotherapy is applied also at the edge of the resection. The rebuilding of the LV cavity is initiated by continuous purse string suture of 2/0 monofilament set at the limit between fibrous and normal muscle (Figure 30.4B) and tied over a balloon inflated inside the LV cavity at the theoretical diastolic capacity of the patient (40 to 50 mL/m^2 body surface area) (Figure 30.4C). The endoventricular circular suture, in addition to restoring the curvature of myocardium to what it was before the infarct, also helps in the selection of the shape, size, and orientation of the patch. When the infarct scar is located in the anteroapical region, the septum and the apex are more involved than the lateral wall. The suture is placed far back and high in the septum, excluding also the totality of the apex and the posterior wall below the posterior papillary muscle root, but only a small portion of lateral wall above the anterolateral papillary muscle root, so that the orientation of this new neck (and of the

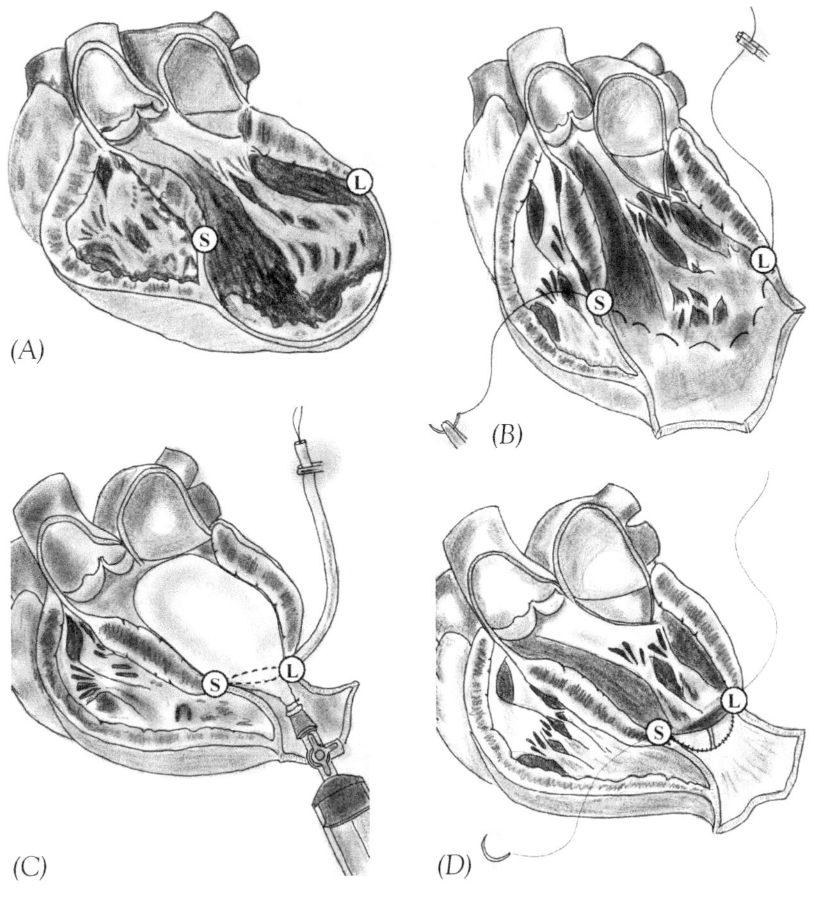

Figure 30.4. *Left ventricular reconstruction. (A) Anteroseptal apical aneurysm. The anteroseptal apical aneurysm with mural thrombi, the dilatation also affects the non-scarred myocardium on the septum (S) and lateral wall (L). (B) Endoventricular purse-string suture The continuous purse string suture at the limit between fibrous and normal myocardium. (C) Curvature restoration and balloon sizing. The suture is tied on a rubber balloon inflated with 50 mm per square meter of the body surface area (normal diastolic volume). The shortening of the SL length illustrates the reorganization of the curvature. (D) Endoventricular patch reconstruction. The Dacron patch anchored on the suture. The right ventricle apex overtakes the new left ventricular apex*

patch) is roughly aligned in the direction of the septum (Figure 30.4D). A patch of Dacron is fashioned to the size of this neck and fixed to the "clothesline" (the endoventricular circular suture) with the same suture. Exteriorized excluded fibrous areas are either resected or, more often, sutured above the patch.

Concomitant procedures

Coronary revascularization

Coronary revascularization of all significantly stenosed coronary arteries supplying the contractile area is mandatory. Revascularization of the infarcted area is almost always possible, even with a thrombosed LAD artery not filled by homologous or heterologous collaterals on the preoperative coronary angioplasty. With the introduction of early angioplasty 10 years ago, the problem is now whether or not to bypass the culprit artery that was successfully recanalized by PCI, leaving an asynergic wall on the corresponding territory which has to be excluded or rebuilt.

Mitral insufficiency

Mitral insufficiency is commonly associated with LV scar and the mitral valve must be assessed carefully before and during surgery by TEE. The valve is inspected using the atrium approach and eventually the ventricular approach. If necessary, a reconstructive procedure is performed, either posterior annuloplasty, Goretex neo cordae, Alfieri E-to-E suture, or mitral valve replacement if the posterior papillary muscle is totally diseased. When regurgitation is quantified as grade II or above 30 mL, and mitral annulus is sized above 35 mm, it seems that annuloplasty is advisable in all circumstances.

Ventricular arrhythmias

Spontaneous VT (13% of patients in our series) and inducible VT (25% in our series) are frequent and, in such circumstances, subtotal non-guided endocardectomy is conducted on all the endoventricular scar. Cryotherapy at the limit of this resection completes the surgical excision.

Particular cases of large failing ventricle

In the case of large dyskinesia or akinesia, VT is present in nearly 50% of cases. Mitral insufficiency has to be repaired in more than 30% of cases. The exclusion of all scarred areas leads to too small a LV cavity with a high risk of immediate or delayed diastolic noncompliance. The continuous suture is, therefore, placed above the limit of the sound muscle on the "transitional" fibrous area, and the use of a balloon inside the left ventricle, inflated at the "theoretical" end diastolic volume of the patient is mandatory before tightening of the suture. The patch is often larger (3 to 4 cm in diameter) than in the usual technique.

The excluded septum often cannot be sutured with lateral wall (destruction of revascularized LAD and restraint of right ventricle). The fibrous tissues are simply folded on the patch. In such cases, surgical glue is useful to reinforce the excluded septum and the patch is left uncovered.

Results

LVR by EVCPP is no longer an experimental technique as it has been applied for almost 20 years. The technique has been presented by many investigators in numerous publications. More and more surgical teams in Europe, North and South America, Australia, and Japan have adopted this technique (with variation in the details) as it produces better results than classical simple resection.[23–25] In the past decade, only a few presentations[26–28] based on the retrospective analysis of shorts series, without reliable data in term of LV volume, EF, localization and size of the lesion, have tried to give credit to the linear suture technique.

LV reconstruction enhances the beneficial, but partial, effects of coronary revascularization and of mitral valve repair (if necessary) by improving LV function, for the following reasons: the septal scar is excluded and the LV curvature is remodeled. This suppresses the increase in wall tension in remote myocardial areas and improves contraction of these areas. This is clearly shown by the analysis of pressure–volume curves. The morphology of pressure–length regional loops of regions remote from the scarred area are normalized after LVR, whereas they were totally disorganized before. This is true for both dyskinesia and akinesia.[29]

The patch sized at the theoretical diastolic volume of the patient avoids excessive reduction of volume and maintains a reasonable physiological cavity.

Based on the recent literature and our experience with more than 1100 LVR procedures, the results must be analyzed regarding the operative risk, hemodynamic data, and late evolution at 1 to 10 years.

Immediate results

This technique is feasible with an acceptable risk. In our global series, from April 1984 to December 2002, 77 out of 1050 patients who underwent surgery died during the first postoperative month (7.7%). But with increasing experience, improvement in the management of severely ill patients, and recognition of the importance of the residual diastolic volume by balloon sizing, operative risk in our recent series (1998 to 2002) was 4.8%. In the group of patients with severely depressed LV function (EF < 30%) with extensive akinesia, it was 7.7%. The operative risk published by other groups, with a series of 20 to 90 patients, varies from 0%,[23] to 4.6%,[24] 9.1%,[25] or 15% when emergency indications are included.[30]

Postoperative LV angiogram or CMR (Figure 30.5) shows a return to a normalization of the LV shape, particularly in relation to the septal exclusion. In the case of very large LV dilatation with acute CHF, the postoperative assessment (Figures

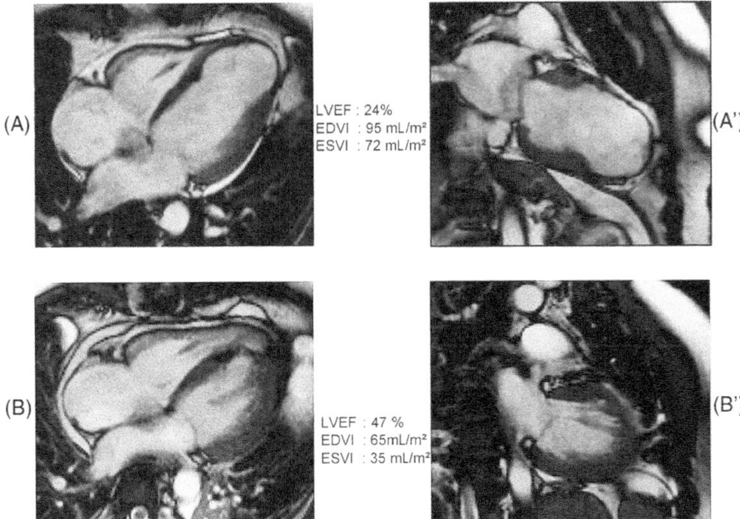

Figure 30.5. *Preoperative and postoperative view in the same patient as Figure 30.1. (A) Preoperative 4-chamber view, and (A') long-axis view in systole. (B) Postoperative (1 week) 4-chamber view, and (B') long-axis view with reorganization of the left ventricular curvature. Note the right ventricle overtaking the left ventricular apex*

Abbreviations: EDVI = end-diastolic volume index; ESVI = end-systolic volume index; LVEF = left ventricular ejection fraction.

30.6A and 30.6B) illustrates the effect of LVR on the decrease of asynergic areas, curvature, volume, and performance.

Both systolic and diastolic function are improved. The mean increase of LVEF is between 10% and 15%,[31] confirmed by Jakob (9%),[23] Grossi (12%),[24] and Salati (19%).[25] This improvement is noted for dyskinetic as well as akinetic lesions.[32] Diastolic function is also improved. Analysis by echocardiography showed peak filling rate which rose from 1.79/s EDV/s preoperatively to 3.07 EDV/s at 1 month and remained at 2.73 EDV/s after 1 year, when time-to-peak filling rate decreased from 190 ms to 110 ms and 90 ms, respectively. The tagging of the LV wall thickness is also a promising technique used with CMR to precisely check the diastolic function.

Ventricular arrhythmias, chiefly spontaneous or inducible VT are controlled by LVR associated with extended endocardectomy and completed by cryotherapy at immediate and late delayed control in 90% of cases.[33] Only 10% of these patients required implantation of an intraventricular defibrillator because they still had inducible ventricular arrhythmia after surgery.

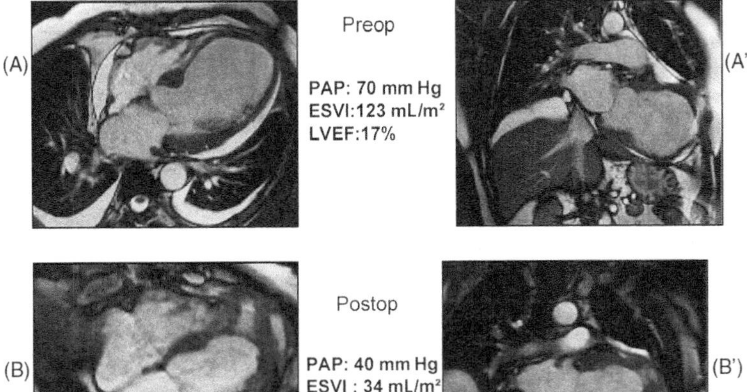

Figure 30.6. *Very large asynergia with acute congestive heart failure. (A) and (A') 4-chamber and long-axis views in systole. Note pericardial and bilateral pleural effusions. (B) and (B') 4-chamber and long-axis views in systole. Note the excluded necrotic chambers of the left ventricle*

Abbreviations: ESVI = end-systolic volume index; LVEF = left ventricular ejection fraction; PAP = pulmonary artery pressure.

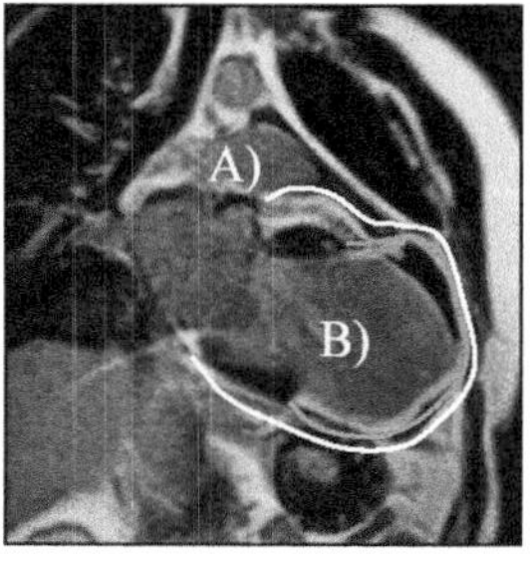

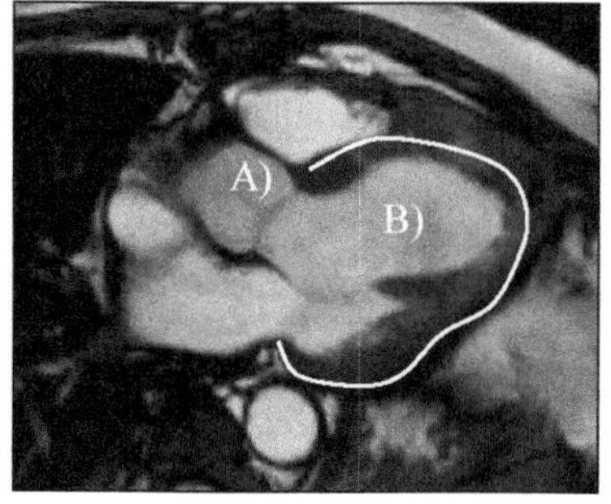

Figure 30.6 (contd). *Preoperative and postoperative Gadolinium Late Enhancement of the same patient. Note the reduction of asynergic area*

Secondary and late results

Secondary and late results are more often analyzed in global series,[34] where LVR can be indicated or complement coronary revascularization or for severe congestive heart failure.

In this latter situation, follow-up was conducted in some series: very poor EF with a mean LVEF of 17%, ESVI 125 mL/m^2, the hospital mortality was 20% and survival rate at 5 years of 70%;[30] patients with New York Heart Association (NYHA) class IV CHF, after a 12% hospital mortality, survival rate at 5 years was 60%[35]; and a cohort of 72 patients with very large ESVI above 120 mL/m^2 was followed from 1988 to 1998 with a 10-year life expectancy of 50%, similar to the survey after heart transplantation.[36]

The global 5-year life expectancy, including hospital mortality, was 85% in a cohort of 250 patients who underwent surgery at our center between 1998 and 2003, with the balloon-sizing technique, a group of 87 "hopeless patients" was selected according to the following indications: emergency procedure for mechanical complication of MI—24 cases; mandatory surgery within the first 8 weeks after MI for irreversible CHF—11 cases; extremely poor LV below 15%—7 cases; chronic CHF requiring in-hospital dobutamine intravenous therapy or intraaortic balloon pump—32 cases; and patients scheduled for heart transplantation or LVAD—13 cases.

Eight patients died during hospital stay (9%), and 9 patients died during the follow-up (11.5%). The survival curve at 5 years, hospital mortality included, was 75%.

In this category of indication, without any possible randomization to other techniques, like medical therapy or revascularization alone, some patients are surviving but with disappointing results (lack of hemodynamic improvement, persistent CHF) which is noticed in roughly 10% of cases or early during the months following surgery, or with delay of one or two years. If they are suitable candidates, these patients must undergo heart transplantation. Two patients in our group of 87 "hopeless cases" were transplanted 3 months and 6 months after surgery. But in a large majority of cases, the postoperative improvement is noted in values of LV performance and volume; stable, and often with progression of this improvement after 1 year (reversible remodeling).

Conclusion

In the case of patients with severe ischemic cardiomyopathy, who have failed full medical therapy and who are poor candidates for heart transplantation, conservative surgery has to be considered before palliative treatment, such as multi-chamber pacing, defibrillator, or temporary LV assist device. The results can be positive in roughly 80% of cases.

LVR in patients with a large ischemic failing ventricle at the late stage of remodeling, with NYHA class IV CHF, is possible with an acceptable risk (below 10%) and life expectancy at 2, 5 and 10 years, which is better than the natural evolution.

To regularly follow-the size of asynergia and LV volumes, weeks and months after infarct, even when coronary recanalization was successful (Thrombolysis in Myocardial Infarction [TIMI] III flow), MRI is the simplest, most reliable, and most easily reproducible non-invasive technique. In the same sense as the recommendation by Bigger,[37] it would be logical and fair, in the case of severe ischemic cardiomyopathy, with an EF < 30%, to await CMR assessment and analysis of the possibility for surgical repair before prophylactic defibrillator implantation as proposed in the Multicenter Automatic Defibrillator Implantation Trial (MADIT).[38]

In the same way that indications for surgery in valvular diseases have changed (surgery before permanent cardiac enlargement and failure, when regurgitation or gradient are severe), indications for LVR for ischemic wall motion abnormality must also change. In addition to classical indications for symptomatic LV aneurysms, there is a place for LVR in the treatment of large ischemic wall motion asynergy (when this asynergy reaches 40% to 50% of the circumference). This surgery may be more efficient in the weeks or months following MI than in the years following MI.

References

1. Klein MD, Herman MV, Gorlin R. A hemodynamic study of left ventricular aneurysm. Circulation 1967; 35: 614–630.
2. Cohen M, Packer M, Gorlin R. Indications for left ventricular aneurysmectomy. Circulation 1983; 67: 717–722.
3. Dor V, Kreitmann P, Jourdan J, *et al.* Interest of "physiological closure (circumferential plasty on contractile areas) of left ventricle after resection and endocardectomy for aneurysm of akinetic zone comparison with classical technique about a series of 209 left ventricular resections. J Cardiovasc Surg 1985; 26: 73 (Abstract).
4. White HD, Norris RM, Brown MA, *et al.* Left ventricular end-systolic volume as the major determinant of survival after recovery from myocardial infarction. Circulation 1987; 76: 44–51.
5. Christian TF, Behrenbeck T, Gersh BJ, Gibbons RJ. Relation of left ventricular volume and function over one year after acute myocardial infarction to infarct size determined by technetium–99 m sestamibi. Am J Cardiol 1991; 68: 21–26.
6. Chareonthaitawee P, Christian TF, Hirose K, Gibbons RJ, Rumberger JA. Relation of initial infarct size to extent of left ventricular remodeling in the year after acute myocardial infarction. J Am Coll Cardiol 1995; 25: 567–573.
7. Bogaert J, Maes A, Van de Werf F, *et al.* Functional recovery of subepicardial myocardial tissue in transmural myocardial infarction after successful reperfusion, an important contribution to the improvement of regional and global left ventricular function. Circulation 1999; 1: 36–43.
8. Miller TD, Christian TF, Hopfenspirger MR, *et al.* Infarct size after acute myocardial infarction measured by quantitative tomographic 99mTc sestamibi imaging predicts subsequent mortality. Circulation 1995; 92: 334–341.
9. Sheehan FH, Bolson EL, Dodge HT, *et al.* Advantages and applications of the centerline method for characterizing regional ventricular function. Circulation 1986; 74: 293–305.
10. Kim RJ, Wu E, Rafael A, *et al.* The use of contrast-enhanced magnetic resonance imaging to identify reversible myocardial dysfunction. N Engl J Med 2000: 343: 1445–1453.
11. Klein C, Nekolla SG, Bengel FM, *et al.* Assessment of myocardial viability with contrast-enhanced magnetic resonance imaging: comparison with positron emission tomography. Circulation 2002; 105: 162–167.
12. Mahrholdt H, Wagner A, Judd RM, Sechtem U. Assessment of myocardial viability by cardiovascular magnetic resonance imaging. Eur Heart J 2002; 23: 602–619.
13. Bello D, Shah DJ, Farah GM, *et al.* Gadolinium cardiovascular magnetic resonance predicts reversible myocardial dysfunction and remodeling in patients with heart failure undergoing beta-blocker therapy. Circulation 2003; 108: 1945–1953.
14. McAlpine HM, Morton JJ, Leckie B, *et al.* Neuroendocrine activation after acute myocardial infarction. Br Heart J 1988; 60: 117–124.
15. Packer M. The neurohormonal hypothesis: a theory to explain the mechanism of disease progression in heart failure. J Am Coll Cardiol 1992; 20: 248–254.

16. Yamaguchi A, Ino T, Adachi H, *et al.* Left ventricular volume predicts postoperative course in patients with ischemic cardiomyopathy. Ann Thorac Surg 1998; 65: 434–438.
17. Burns RJ, Gibbons RJ, Yi Q, *et al.*, CORE Study Investigators. The relationships of left ventricular ejection fraction, end-systolic volume index and infarct size to six-month mortality after hospital discharge following myocardial infarction treated by thrombolysis. J Am Coll Cardiol 2002; 39: 30–36.
18. Likoff W, Bailey CP. Ventriculoplasty: excision of myocardial aneurysm; report of a successful case. JAMA 1955; 158: 915–920.
19. Cooley DA, Collins HA, Morris GC Jr., Chapman DW. Ventricular aneurysm after myocardial infarction: surgical excision with use of temporary cardiopulmonary bypass. JAMA 1958; 167: 557–560.
20. Dor V, Saab M, Coste P, Komaszewska M, Montiglio F. Left ventricular aneurysm: a new surgical approach. Thorac Cardiovasc Surg 1989; 37: 11–19.
21. Cooley D. Ventricular endoaneurysmorrhaphy: a simplified repair for extensive postinfarction aneurysm. J Card Surg 1989; 4: 200–205.
22. Jatene AD. Left ventricular aneurysmectomy resection or reconstruction. J Thorac Cardiovasc Surg 1985; 89: 321–331.
23. Jakob H, Zölch B, Schuster S, *et al.* Endoventricular patch plasty improves results of LV aneurysmectomy. Eur J Cardiothorac Surg 1993; 7: 428–436.
24. Salati M, Di Biasi P, Pajè A, Santoli C. Left ventricular geometry after endoventriculoplasty. Eur J Cardiothorasc Surg 1993; 7: 574–579.
25. Grossi EA, Chinitz LA, Galloway AC, *et al.* Endoventricular remodeling of left ventricular aneurysm: functional, clinical, and electrophysiological results. Circulation 1995; 92: II98–II100.
26. Eleftriades JA, Solomon LW, Salazar AM, *et al.* Linear left ventricular aneurysmectomy: modern imaging studies reveal improved morphology and function. Ann Thorac Surg 1993; 56: 242–252.
27. Kesler KA, Fiore AC, Naunheim KS, *et al.* Anterior wall left ventricular aneurysm repair: a comparison of linear versus circular closure. J Thorac Cardiovasc Surg 1992; 103: 841–848.
28. Tavakoli R, Bettex A, Weber A, *et al.* Repair of post infarction dyskinetic LV aneurysm with either linear or patch technique. Eur J Cardiothorasc Surg 2002; 22: 129–134.
29. Di Donato M, Sabatier M, Montiglio F, *et al.* Outcome of left ventricular aneurysmectomy with patch repair in patients with severely depressed pump function. Am J Cardiol 1995; 76: 557–561.
30. Dor V, Sabatier M, Di Donato M, *et al.* Late hemodynamic results after left ventricular patch repair associated with coronary grafting in patients with postinfarction akinetic or dyskinetic aneurysm of the left ventricle. J Thorac Cardiovasc Surg 1995; 110: 1291–1301.
31. Dor V, Sabatier M, Di Donato M, *et al.* Efficacy of endoventricular patch plasty in large postinfarction akinetic scar and severe left ventricular dysfunction: comparison with a series of large dyskinetic scars. J Thorac Cardiovasc Surg 1998; 116: 50–59.
32. Dor V, Sabatier M, Montiglio F, *et al.* Results of nonguided subtotal endocardiectomy associated with left ventricular reconstruction in patients with ischemic ventricular arrhythmias. J Thorac Cardiovasc Surg 1994; 107: 1301–1308.
33. Di Donato M, Sabatier M, Toso A, *et al.* Regional myocardial performance of non-ischaemic zones remote from anterior wall left ventricular aneurysm. Effects of aneurysmectomy. Eur Heart J 1995; 16: 1285–1292.
34. Di Donato M, Toso A, Maioli M, *et al.*, RESTORE Group. Intermediate survival and predictors of death after surgical ventricular restoration. Semin Thorac Cardiovasc Surg 2001; 13: 468–475.
35. Lundblad R, Abdelnoor M, Svennevig J. Repair of left ventricular aneurysm: surgical risk and long-term survival. Ann Thorac Surg 2003; 76: 719–725.
36. Hertz M, Mohacsi P, Taylor D, *et al.* The registry of the International Society for Heart and Lung Transplantation: introduction to the Twentieth Annual Reports—2003. J Heart Lung Transplant 2003; 22: 610–615.
37. Bigger JT. Expanding indications for implantable cardiac defibrillators. N Engl J Med 2002; 346: 931–933.
38. Moss AJ, Zareba W, Hall WJ, *et al.*, Multicenter Automatic Defibrillator Implantation Trial II Investigators. Prophylactic implantation of a defibrillator in patients with myocardial infarction and reduced ejection fraction. N Engl J Med 2002; 346: 877–883.

Chapter 31

The Acorn Cardiac Support Device as a therapy for heart failure

Hani N Sabbah, Elaine J Tanhehco, Victor G Sharov, Robert Brewer, Norman A Silverman

Introduction

Heart failure is a disorder characterized by progressive left ventricular (LV) dysfunction, dilation, and increased LV chamber size, invariably accompanied by increased LV wall stress and myocardial stretch.[1,2] Increased LV wall stress leads to increased myocardial oxygen consumption and myocardial stretch can activate stretch-response proteins that may play an important role in the development of maladaptive cardiomyocyte hypertrophy.[3] Progressive chamber sphericity is a determinant of functional mitral regurgitation,[4] a condition which, depending on its severity, can have a major impact on reducing LV stroke output which is already impaired in heart failure. Among clinical indicators of progressive LV remodeling, LV dilation and increased LV sphericity are sensitive indicators of poor long-term outcome.[5,6] For these reasons, preventing or reversing remodeling has emerged as important target in the treatment of dilated cardiomyopathies.[7] Treatment with angiotensin-converting enzyme (ACE) inhibitors, beta-adrenergic receptor blockers, and more recently aldosterone antagonists has improved survival in patients with heart failure partly as a result of attenuating, and in some cases reversing, LV remodeling.

In recent years, several surgical approaches have been implemented with the objective of improving LV function through amelioration of progressive LV remodeling. These include surgical reduction of LV size, the so-called Batista procedure,[8] dynamic cardiomyoplasty[9] and mitral valve repair to limit or eliminate functional mitral regurgitation.[10] While the Batista procedure and dynamic cardiomyoplasty have for all practical purposes been abandoned, the lessons learned from these procedures gave rise to a new generation of devices aimed at preventing progressive LV dilation and restoring LV shape by passive mechanical containment of the failing LV. One such device is the Acorn Cardiac Support Device (CSD) or the CorCap™. The CSD consists of a flexible polyester mesh that is designed to fit snugly around the left ventricle. The fabric is high-strength, yet allows for bi-directional compliance. It is available in six sizes and can be adjusted to custom fit each heart. The device conforms to the ventricle and supports its reshaping to an ellipsoid. This chapter will focus on experimental and clinical studies examining the effects of the Acorn CSD in heart failure and the possible mechanisms underlying its ability to attenuate the progression of the disease.

Experimental Evidence Supporting Cardiac Support Device Therapy

Two animal models of heart failure have been primarily used to determine the efficacy of the Acorn CSD experimentally—the canine model of intracoronary microembolization-induced heart failure, and the ovine model of heart failure induced by ventricular pacing.[11–13] These are the models that will be referred to in the remainder of this section. Although both models elicit heart failure through different mechanisms, the Acorn CSD diminishes the decline in cardiac function associated with the heart failure state in both models.

Hemodynamic improvement following cardiac support device therapy

In dogs with heart failure, 3 months of therapy with the CSD prevented the progressive increases in LV end-diastolic and end-systolic volumes that were seen in the control dogs with untreated heart failure (Figure 31.1).[14–16] This observation confirmed that the CSD prevented ongoing LV enlargement. Over the course of 3 months, the CSD decreased both LV end-diastolic and end-systolic volumes in this model.[14–16] In contrast, sheep outfitted with the CSD did not experience any change in LV long axis area and short axis dimensions.[13] While unexpected, treatment with the CSD significantly improved LV ejection fraction (EF) in dogs and sheep (Figure 31.1).[13–16] In fact, the improvement seen in the ovine heart failure model persisted through ongoing pacing.[13] Therapy with the CSD also significantly reduced LV end-diastolic circumferential wall stress (Figure 31.1).[14–16] This observation in and of itself could partly explain the improvement in LV function, possibly through a reduction in myocardial oxygen consumption. The significant fall in circulating plasma norepinephrine that was observed in dogs following CSD therapy[16] (Figure 31.1) which signals a lesser need for compensatory sympathetic support, lends further support to the finding that an overall improvement of the heart failure state has indeed taken place. Incidentally, this improvement has been shown to occur in the absence of any hemodynamic or Doppler echocardiographic evidence of constrictive or restrictive physiology.[14,17]

In addition, in an ovine model of acute myocardial infarction, treatment with the CSD reduced the area of akinesis and increased minimum wall thickness.[18] This suggests that the CSD may be beneficial in situations other than dilated cardiomyopathy.

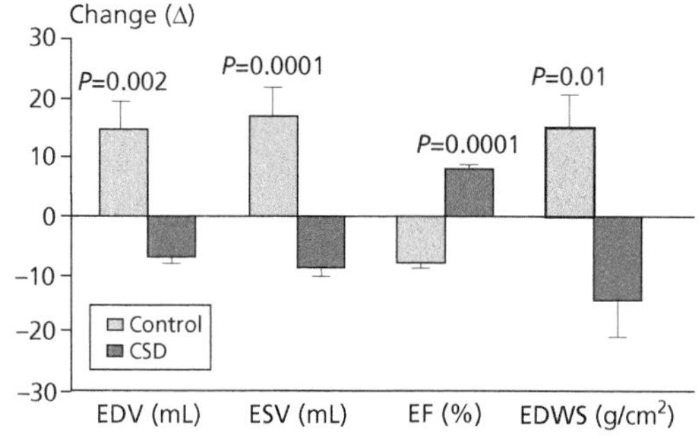

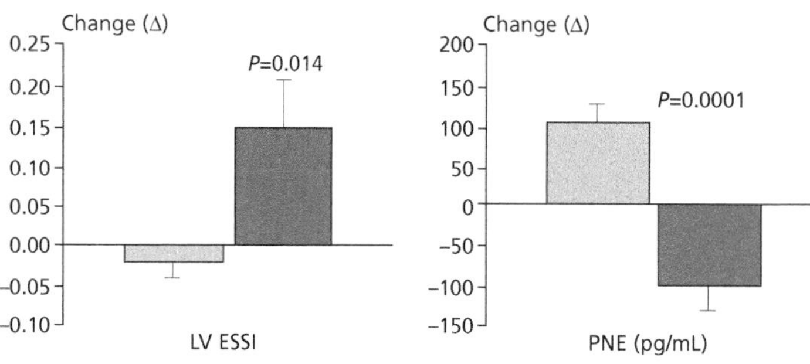

Figure 31.1. *Comparison of the change (Δ) from pre-treatment to post-treatment (3-month interval) in angiographic and neurohumoral measurement between dogs with untreated heart failure (Control, gray bars) and dogs with heart failure treated with the cardiac support device (CSD; black bars) (treatment effect). Top panel: left ventricular (LV) end-diastolic volume (EDV), end-systolic volume (ESV), ejection fraction (EF), and end-diastolic circumferential wall stress (EDWS). Bottom panel left: LV end-systolic sphericity index (ESSI). Bottom panel right: Circulating plasma norepinephrine concentration (PNE)*

Impact of cardiac support device therapy on functional mitral regurgitation

Long-term therapy with the CSD has also been shown to improve functional mitral regurgitation in sheep and nearly eliminate this problem in dogs with heart failure.[13,14] This observation is consistent with the finding that therapy with the CSD also restores, albeit in part, the normal physiological ellipsoidal shape of the left ventricle. It was previously shown that therapy with the CSD in dogs with heart failure significantly increases the LV end-systolic sphericity index (Figure 31.1).[14,16] An increase in this index implies a change in the shape of the left ventricle away from a sphere and more closely approximating an ellipsoid. A reduction in the sphericity index, or as the index approaches unity, has been shown to be directly associated with the development of functional mitral regurgitation.[4] The design of the CSD is such that it partly mandates the normalization of LV shape. For the same applied load, the CSD is more compliant in the longitudinal direction (LV apex to base) than it is in the circumferential direction, thus possessing the ability to restore the failing, more spherical, ventricle to one that is more ellipsoidal.[14,16]

Myocardial structural changes elicited by cardiac support device application

Post-mortem examination of CSD-treated dogs after 3 months of implantation showed the device fibers to be encapsulated in a translucent thin layer of mature connective tissue that was approximately 0.3 to 0.5 mm in thickness.[14,16] There was a clear demarcation, evident both at light microscopy as well as on scanning electron microscopy, between the CSD and the epicardial myocardium without encroachment of the connective tissue into the epicardial myocardium (Figure 31.2). Long-term implantation of the CSD in dogs with heart failure

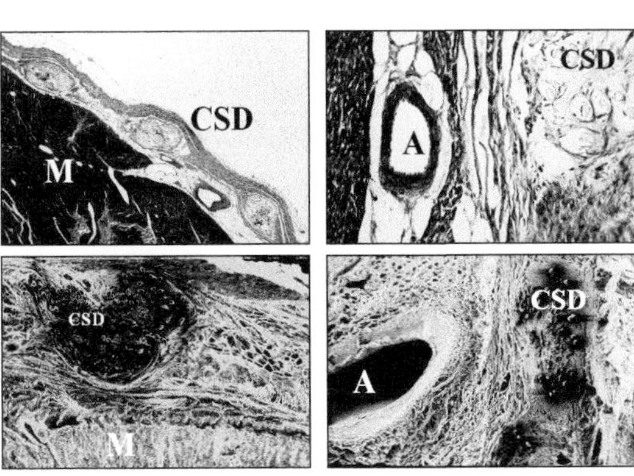

Figure 31.2. *Top left: Trichrome stained section of left ventricular myocardium from a dog treated for 3 months with the cardiac support device (CSD). The CSD is encapsulated by thin layers of mature connective tissue (blue-green). There is a clear demarcation between the CSD and the myocardium (M, dark red) with no evidence of invasion of the myocardium by connective tissue. Top right: An epicardial artery (A) coursing between the CSD and the epicardial myocardium is normal in appearance. Bottom panels: Scanning electron micrograph from a dog with heart failure treated for 3 months with the CSD. The micrograph depicts a single CSD fiber consisting of multiple filaments, the adjacent connective tissue, underlying epicardial myocardium and an epicardial artery (A) coursing between the CSD and the epicardial myocardium. See color plate section.*

was also shown to have no effect on the integrity of the lumen of either epicardial coronary arteries or epicardial coronary veins[16] (Figure 31.2). The patency of the epicardial coronary arteries was confirmed by coronary arteriography as well as by histology. Histology also confirmed complete patency of epicardial coronary veins underlying the CSD (Figure 31.2).

At the cellular level, passive containment of the failing LV with the CSD resulted in observations that are consistent with reverse LV cellular remodeling. Contraction and relaxation of cardiomyocytes isolated from LV myocardium of normal dogs, LV myocardium of control dogs with untreated heart failure, and from LV myocardium of dogs with heart failure treated for 3 months with the CSD was evaluated in-vitro using an edge detection algorithm and contraction evoked by electrical field stimulation.[15] Concordant with the observation of improved LVEF with CSD therapy, percent shortening, rate of change of shortening, and rate of change of relaxation all increased significantly in cardiomyocytes of CSD-treated dogs compared to untreated controls.[15] These observations clearly suggest that long-term therapy with the CSD improves the intrinsic contractile function of cardiomyocytes.

Measurements made using cardiomyocytes isolated from LV myocardium of normal dogs, dogs with untreated heart failure, and dogs with heart failure treated with CSD, showed that treatment with the CSD leads to normalization of cardiomyocyte size as evidenced by normalization of cardiomyocyte cross-sectional area, cardiomyocyte length, and cardiomyocyte width (Table 31.1). The attenuation of myocardial hypertrophy in the setting of heart failure appears to favor improvement of intrinsic cardiomyocyte contractile function and may contribute to the improvement in global LV function seen with chronic CSD therapy.

Histomorphometric studies from these dogs also suggest that chronic CSD therapy induces reverse remodeling at the cellular level.[14] Therapy with the CSD significantly reduced the accumulation of collagen in the cardiac interstitium,[14] a phenomenon termed "reactive interstitial fibrosis." Interstitial fibrosis can lead to LV diastolic dysfunction and ultimately to systolic dysfunction.[19] Treatment with the CSD was also associated with increased myocardial capillary density and reduced oxygen diffusion distance,[14] which are certain to alleviate cardiomyocyte hypoxia that is often attributed to reduced function of the failing heart.[19]

Table 31.1. *Histomorphometric measurements of cardiac tissue from normal dogs, control dogs with untreated heart failure and dogs with heart failure treated with the CSD (n=6)*

	Normal	Heart failure controls*	Heart failure CSD-treated†
MCSA (μm^2)	610 ± 15	820 ± 4	647 ± 4
C-Length (μm)	103 ± 2	169 ± 2	116 ± 2
C-Width (μm)	28 ± 0.4	32 ± 0.1	28 ± 0.4
VFIF (%)	3.5 ± 0.7	12.2 ± 0.9	10.2 ± 1.5
CD (Cap/fiber)	1.00 ± 0.05	0.95 ± 0.01	1.14 ± 0.13
ODD (μm)	11.8 ± 0.3	13.5 ± 0.6	11.8 ± 0.6

*P < 0.05 vs. normals
†P < 0.05 vs. heart failure controls
Abbreviations: Cap = capillary; CD = capillary density; CSD = cardiac support device; C-Length = cardiomyocyte length; C-Width = cardiomyocyte width; MCSA = cardiomyocyte cross-sectional area; ODD = oxygen diffusion distance; VFIF = volume fraction of interstitial fibrosis.

Effects of cardiac support device therapy at the cellular and molecular levels

Effect of cardiac support device therapy on cardiomyocyte apoptosis

Cardiomyocyte loss via apoptosis in the failing left ventricle can contribute to the progression of LV dysfunction characteristic of the heart failure state.[20,21] Treatment with the CSD in dogs with heart failure was shown to reduce cardiomyocyte apoptosis as evidenced by a significant reduction in terminal deoxynucleotidyl transferase-mediated dUTP-biotin end labeling (TUNEL) positive cardiomyocytes in LV myocardium compared to dogs with untreated heart failure.[22] Treatment with the CSD also decreased the expression of apoptosis inducing factor (AIF) as well as Bax, both of which are pro-apoptotic proteins while increasing the expression of Bcl-2 and Bcl-XL, both of which are anti-apoptotic proteins.[22,23]

Modulation of stretch response protein by cardiac support device therapy

Myocardial stretch in heart failure can activate stretch response proteins such as p21ras, c-fos, and p38 α/β mitogen activated protein kinase (MAPK).[24–26] The latter may play an important role in the development of maladaptive cardiomyocyte hypertrophy. p21ras, c-fos, and p38 α/β MAPK were shown to be upregulated in dogs with coronary microembolization-induced heart failure.[15] Long-term treatment with the CSD was shown to downregulate these proteins returning their expression to near normal levels.[15] The observed decrease in these stretch-response proteins is consistent with the observations of reduced LV wall stress and reduced cardiomyocyte hypertrophy following long-term treatment with the CSD.

Effects of chronic cardiac support device therapy on sarcoplasmic reticulum calcium cycling

Abnormal calcium cycling within the sarcoplasmic reticulum (SR) is a maladaptation that occurs during heart failure and plays a key role in the systolic and diastolic dysfunction that characterizes this disease syndrome. In the failing canine left ventricle, SERCA2a activity and expression are reduced as is the affinity of SERCA2a for calcium. In addition, expression of phosphorylated phospholamban at serine 16 and threonine 17 is also decreased in failing LV myocardium.[15,27,28] In dogs with heart failure treated with the CSD, SERCA2a expression (V_{max}) and total phospholamban were unchanged compared to untreated heart failure dogs.[15] The affinity of SERCA2a for calcium ($k_{0.5}$), however, increased significantly in the LV myocardium of dogs with heart failure after CSD therapy compared to dogs with untreated heart failure.[15] Dogs with treated heart failure also exhibited significantly increased expression of phosphorylated phospholamban.[15] Increased affinity of SERCA2a for calcium in dogs with heart failure treated with the CSD most likely resulted from increased expression of phosphorylated phospholamban. Increased affinity of SERCA2a for calcium can lead to improved calcium cycling within the SR, particularly at low cytosolic calcium concentrations.[15]

Effects of chronic cardiac support device therapy on expression of myosin heavy chain isoforms

Cardiomyocytes express both the α- and β-myosin heavy chain (MHC) isoforms. Compared to β-MHC, cardiac α-MHC is associated with faster velocity of shortening.[29] Studies obtained from explanted failed human hearts showed a reduction in the ratio of α-MHC to β-MHC[29]—a condition that favors diminished cardiomyocyte contractility. A similar reduction was also reported in dogs with coronary microembolization-induced heart failure.[15] Chronic therapy with the CSD in dogs with heart failure was associated with restoration of cardiac α-MHC/β-MHC ratios that were close to normal levels,[15] suggesting that therapy with the CSD can reverse this molecular maladaptation.

Clinical evidence supporting cardiac support device therapy

Randomized and non-randomized clinical trials with the Acorn CSD remain ongoing worldwide. Initial safety studies were completed without reports of adverse device-related events.[30] These included patients who were outfitted with the CSD alone and those who required additional cardiac surgery. The device does not cause cardiac constriction or reduce coronary flow capacity.[30] Initial results indicate that the CorCap reduces ventricular enlargement and mitral regurgitation, and increases EF in patients with dilated cardiomyopathy (Table 31.2) (Figure 31.3).[30–34] Favorable changes in LV function, end-diastolic dimension, and New York Heart Association (NYHA) class emerge as early as 3 months after implantation, and continue to improve at subsequent follow-up visits, up to 24 months.[30,32] The effects of the Acorn CSD on human cardiomyocyte structure and biochemistry remain to be explored.

The placement of the device is relatively simple, does not require cardiac cross clamping and can be accomplished in less than an hour, reducing the possibility of surgical complications.[30] In addition, the CSD does not prevent the execution of additional cardiac operations, such as coronary artery bypass grafting and mitral valve repair, if necessary. Thus, the Acorn CSD lends itself as a practical and potentially efficacious therapy to halt the progression of heart failure.

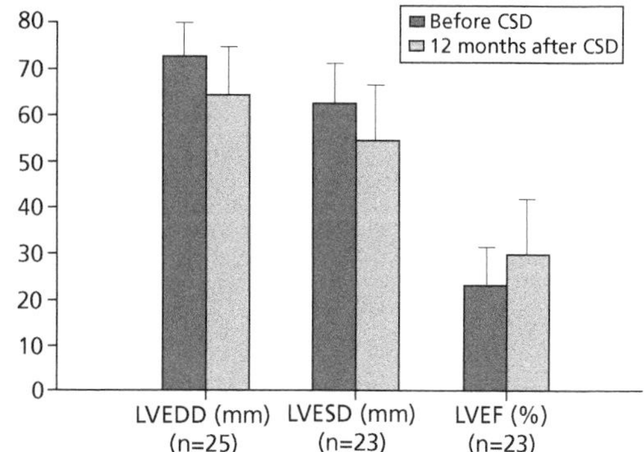

Figure 31.3. *Changes in left ventricular dimensions and ejection fraction after implantation of the CSD device in patients with dilated cardiomyopathy (Adapted from Oz,* et al.[30])

Abbreviations: LVEDD = left ventricular end-diastolic dimension; LVESD = left ventricular end-systolic dimension; LVEF = left ventricular ejection fraction.

Conclusion

The improvement in LV function seen with chronic CSD therapy may be explained by observed alterations of several factors at the global, cellular, and molecular levels (Figure 31.4). Reducing LV wall stress alone can lead to functional improvement as a consequence of reduced myocardial oxygen consumption and possibly through alleviation of LV subclinical subendocardial ischemia. In addition, chronic CSD therapy could have improved LV function by limiting interstitial fibrosis and reversing potential hypoxia of viable cardiomyocytes. This can lead to augmented intrinsic cardiomyocyte function and limit ongoing cell death through apoptosis (Figure 31.4). Another possible explanation that can contribute

Table 31.2. *Cardiac support device patients at 12 months of follow-up (n=12)*

	Before implantation	12 months after implantation
LVEDD (mm)	72.7 ± 5.5	64.4 ± 5.4
LVESD (mm)	64.4 ± 5.4	56.9 ± 5.7
LVEF (%)	22.7 ± 5.7	28.6 ± 8.2
MR (0-4+)	1.1 ± 0.5	0.5 ± 0.8
NYHA Class	2.5 ± 0.5	1.8 ± 0.7

Adapted from Oz *et al.*[30] Mean ± SD.
Abbreviations: LVEDD = left ventricular end-diastolic dimension; LVEF = left ventricular ejection fraction; LVESD = left ventricular end-systolic dimension; MR = mitral regurgitation; NYHA = New York Heart Association.

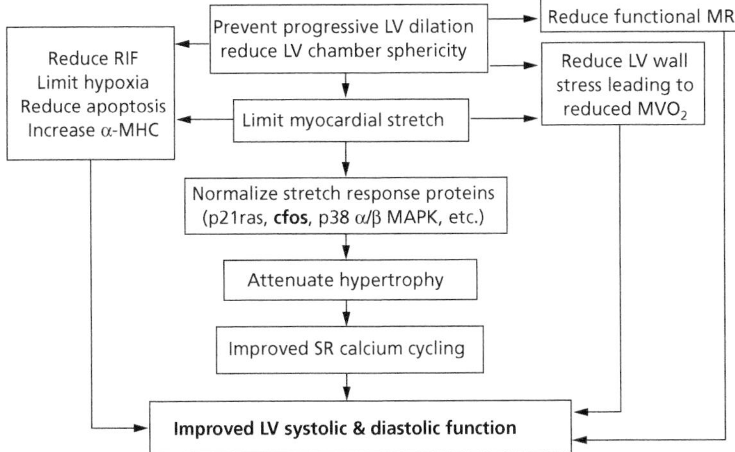

Figure 31.4. *Diagram illustrating possible mechanisms through which prevention of progressive left ventricular (LV) remodeling and attenuation of LV sphericity and LV myocardial stretch with the CSD can lead to long-term improvement in LV systolic and diastolic function*

Abbreviations: RIF = reactive interstitial fibrosis; MHC = myosin heavy chain; MR = mitral regurgitation; MVO_2 = myocardial oxygen consumption; MAPK = mitogen activated protein kinase; SR = sarcoplasmic reticulum.

to functional improvement is the fact that CSD therapy appears to normalize stretch response proteins. This can lead to attenuation of maladaptive cardiomyocyte hypertrophy. Finally, improvement in LV function with CSD therapy could have resulted, in part, from normalization in the ratio of cardiac α-MHC to β-MHC, a condition that favors faster velocity of shortening. All these factors could contribute to the improvement in LV function; however, it is unlikely that any single factor dominates. It is remarkable that preventing progressive LV dilation and stretch by passive mechanical containment of the failing LV can in itself lead to reversal of many of the maladaptive structural, cellular, biochemical, and molecular changes that culminate in intractable end-stage heart failure.

Acknowledgment

This chapter was supported, in part, by research grants from Acorn Cardiovascular, Inc., and by a grant from the National Heart, Lung, and Blood Institute (HL49090-09).

References

1. Sabbah HN, Goldstein S. Ventricular remodelling: consequences and therapy. Eur Heart J 1993; 14 (Suppl C): 24–29.
2. Cohn JN, Ferrari R, Sharpe N. Cardiac remodeling—concepts and clinical implications: a consensus paper from an international forum on cardiac remodeling. J Am Coll Cardiol 2000; 35: 569–582.
3. Sadoshima J, Jahn L, Takahashi T, Kulik TJ, Izumo S. Molecular characterization of the stretch-induced adaptation of cultured cardiac cells. An in vitro model of load-induced cardiac hypertrophy. J Biol Chem 1992; 267: 10 551–10 560.
4. Kono T, Sabbah HN, Rosman H, *et al.* Left ventricular shape is the primary determinant of functional mitral regurgitation in heart failure. J Am Coll Cardiol 1992; 20: 1594–1598.
5. White HD, Norris RM, Brown MA, *et al.* Left ventricular end-systolic volume as the major determinant of survival after recovery from myocardial infarction. Circulation 1987; 76: 44–51.
6. Douglas PS, Morrow R, Ioli A, Reicheck N. Left ventricular shape; afterload and survival in idiopathic dilated cardiomyopathy. J Am Coll Cardiol 1989; 13: 311–315.
7. Margulies KB. Blocking stretch-induced myocardial remodeling. Circ Res 2003; 93: 1020–1022.
8. Batista RJ, Santos JL, Takeshita N, *et al.* Partial left ventriculectomy to improve left ventricular function in end-stage heart disease. J Card Surg 1996; 11: 96–97.
9. Kass DA, Baughman KL, Pak PH, *et al.* Reverse remodeling from cardiomyoplasty in human heart failure: External constraint versus active assist. Circulation 1995; 91: 2314–2318.
10. Bolling SF, Pagani FD, Deeb GM, Back DS. Intermediate-term outcome of mitral reconstruction in cardiomyopathy. J Thorac Cardiovasc Surg 1998; 115: 381–386.

11. Sabbah HN, Stein PD, Kono T, *et al.* A canine model of chronic heart failure produced by multiple sequential coronary microembolizations. Am J Physiol 1991; 260: H1379–H1384.
12. Power JM, Raman J, Dornom A, *et al.* Passive ventricular constraint amends the course of heart failure: a study in an ovine model of dilated cardiomyopathy. Cardiovasc Res 1999; 44: 549–555.
13. Raman JS, Byrne MJ, Power JM, Alferness CA. Ventricular constraint in severe heart failure halts decline in cardiovascular function associated with experimental dilated cardiomyopathy. Ann Thorac Surg 2003; 76: 141–147.
14. Chaudhry PA, Mishima T, Sharov VG, *et al.* Passive epicardial containment prevents ventricular remodeling in heart failure. Ann Thorac Surg 2000; 70: 1275–1280.
15. Sabbah HN, Sharov VG, Gupta RC, *et al.* Reversal of chronic molecular and cellular abnormalities due to heart failure by passive mechanical ventricular containment. Circ Res 2003; 93: 1095–1101.
16. Sabbah HN. The cardiac support device and the myosplint: treating heart failure by targeting left ventricular size and shape. Ann Thorac Surg 2003; 75: S13–S19.
17. Saavedra WF, Paolocci N, Mishima T, *et al.* Reverse remodeling and enhanced adrenergic reserve from passive external support in experimental dilated heart failure. J Am Coll Cardiol 2002; 39: 2069–2076.
18. Pilla JJ, Blom AS, Brockman DJ, *et al.* Ventricular constraint using the Acorn cardiac support device reduces myocardial akinetic area in an ovine model of acute infarction. Circulation 2002; 106 (Suppl 1): I207–211.
19. Sabbah HN, Sharov VG, Lesch M, Goldstein S. Progression of heart failure: a role for interstitial fibrosis. Mol Cell Biochem 1995; 147: 29–34.
20. Sabbah HN. Apoptotic cell death in heart failure. Cardiovasc Res 2000; 45: 704–712.
21. Sabbah HN, Sharov VG, Goldstein S. Cell death, tissue hypoxia and progression of heart failure. Heart Fail Rev 2000; 5: 131–138.
22. Gupta RC, Sharov VG, Mishra S, Todor A, Sabbah HN. Chronic therapy with the Acorn Cardiac Support Device (CSD) attenuates cardiomyocyte apoptosis in dogs with heart failure. J Am Coll Cardiol 2001; 37: 478A (Abstract).
23. Todor A, Sharov VG, Fanous NH, *et al.* Chronic therapy with the Acorn Cardiac Support Device (CSD) is associated with downregulation of apoptosis-inducing factor and upregulation of the anti-apoptotic protein Bcl-XL. Eur J Heart Fail 2002; 1: 83 (Abstract).
24. Sadoshima J, Izumo S. Mechanical stretch rapidly activates multiple signal transduction pathways in cardiac myocytes: potential involvement of an autocrine/paracrine mechanism. EMBO J 1993; 12: 1681–1692.
25. Sadoshima J, Izumo S. Signal transduction pathways of angiotensin-II induced c-fos gene expression in cardiac myocytes in vitro, roles of phospholipid-derived second messengers. Circ Res 1993; 73: 424–438.
26. Sadoshima J, Qiu Z, Morgan JP, Izumo S. Angiotensin II and other hypertrophic stimuli mediated by G protein-coupled receptors activate tyrosine kinase, mitogen-activated protein kinase, and 90-kD S6 kinase in cardiac myocytes: the critical role of Ca^{2+}-dependent signaling. Circ Res 1995; 76: 1–15.
27. Gupta RC, Shimoyama H, Tanimura M, *et al.* SR Ca^{2+}-ATPase activity and expression in ventricular myocardium of dogs with heart failure. Am J Physiol 1997; 273: H12–H18.
28. Gupta RC, Mishra S, Mishima T, Goldstein S, Sabbah HN. Reduced sarcoplasmic reticulum Ca^{2+}-uptake and expression of phospholamban in left ventricular myocardium of dogs with heart failure. J Mol Cell Cardiol 1999; 31: 1381–1389.
29. Miyata S, Minobe W, Bristow MR, Leinwald LA. Myosin heavy chain isoform expression in the failing and nonfailing human heart. Circ Res 2000; 86: 386–390.
30. Oz MC, Konertz WF, Kleber FX, *et al.* Global surgical experience with the Acorn cardiac support device. J Thorac Cardiovasc Surg 2003; 126: 983–991.
31. Oz MC. Passive ventricular constraint for the treatment of congestive heart failure. Ann Thorac Surg 2001; 71: S185–S187.
32. Konertz WF, Shapland JE, Hotz H, *et al.* Passive containment and reverse remodeling by a novel textile cardiac support device. Circulation 2001; 104 (Suppl 1): I270–I275.
33. Lembcke A, Wiese TH, Dushe S, *et al.* Effects of passive cardiac containment on left ventricular structure and function: verification by volume flow measurements. J Heart Lung Transplant 2004; 23: 11–19.
34. Raman JS, Power JM, Buxton BF, Alferness C, Hare D. Ventricular containment as an adjunctive procedure in ischemic cardiomyopathy: early results. Ann Thorac Surg 2001; 70: 1124–1126.

CHAPTER 32

The role of continuous positive airway pressure in the management of decompensated heart failure complicated by acute pulmonary edema

Michael D Faulx, Mark E Dunlap

Introduction

Decompensated heart failure is a highly prevalent condition associated with significant morbidity and mortality, especially when heart failure is complicated by acute cardiogenic pulmonary edema (ACPE).[1] Although many patients presenting with decompensated heart failure complicated by ACPE respond to the time-honored regimen of intravenous furosemide, nitroglycerine, morphine, and oxygen, a number of these patients, especially those with significant hypoxia, will progress to respiratory failure requiring endotracheal intubation and mechanical ventilation. Unfortunately, much of the morbidity associated with severe ACPE arises from the mechanical ventilation used to treat it, with barotrauma and ventilator-acquired pneumonia being of particular concern.[2,3] Not surprisingly, interest in the use of noninvasive ventilation (NIV) in the management of ACPE has grown recently. This chapter provides an overview of current research and uses of NIV in the treatment of ACPE.

Overview of Noninvasive Ventilation

NIV provides positive airway pressure to the patient by means of a tight-fitting face or nasal mask connected most commonly to a flow-triggered, pressure-cycled ventilator system.[4] NIV has been used successfully to treat chronic ventilatory disorders such as obstructive sleep apnea, as well as acute respiratory failure due to acute exacerbations of chronic obstructive pulmonary disease (COPD) and acute hypoxemia of diverse etiology.[5,6] Although NIV can be provided to patients with acute respiratory failure in a variety of ways, the two most commonly described modalities are continuous positive airway pressure (CPAP) and bilevel positive airway pressure (BLPAP), often inappropriately referred to by the proprietary term BiPAP® (Respironics, Inc., Murrysville, PA, USA).[7] With CPAP, the amount of pressure delivered to the airways remains constant throughout the entire respiratory cycle, whereas with BLPAP the amount of applied pressure is greater during inspiration than during expiration. Both modalities have theoretical advantages in treating diffuse pulmonic processes such as cardiogenic pulmonary edema. NIV improves alveolar ventilation while reducing the work of breathing in patients with respiratory failure.[8] BLPAP also appears to facilitate gas exchange in patients with respiratory failure complicated by hypercapnia.[9]

Both CPAP and BLPAP are used to treat patients with heart failure complicated by ACPE. Although both modalities appear to produce favorable hemodynamic and clinical effects, a few small studies suggest that CPAP may be the safer modality in subjects with ACPE. One study randomized 27 patients presenting to an emergency department with acute respiratory distress, of which 10 (37%) had cardiogenic pulmonary edema, to receive conventional medical therapy plus BLPAP or conventional therapy alone.[10] There was no difference between the two groups with respect to the need for endotracheal intubation. In post-hoc subgroup, analysis mortality was increased in patients with cardiogenic pulmonary edema receiving BLPAP.[7,10] Another randomized study compared BLPAP and CPAP in 27 patients with acute pulmonary edema.[11] Although BLPAP resulted in more immediate improvement in heart rate, blood pressure, and hypercapnia than CPAP, the study was terminated early due to an increased rate of myocardial infarction (MI) among patients treated with BLPAP (71%, versus 31% for CPAP and 38% for historic controls). Finally, Sharon *et al.* randomized 40 patients with severe pulmonary edema to receive treatment with intravenous isosorbide dinitrate (ISDN) plus BLPAP or ISDN alone.[12] BLPAP therapy was associated with significantly higher rates of endotracheal intubation, and the combined endpoints of death, mechanical ventilation, and MI, prompting early termination of the study. Therefore, although some data exist supporting the safe use of BLPAP in ACPE,[13] until its safety has been better established in larger randomized trials, BLPAP should not be used to treat decompensated heart failure with acute pulmonary edema. Accordingly, the remainder of this chapter will focus on the use of CPAP in ACPE.

Physiologic Effects of Continuous Positive Airway Pressure

CPAP is a fundamentally simple intervention; it increases intrathoracic pressure. The hemodynamic consequences of this pressure increase, however, vary substantially with differences in left ventricular (LV) systolic function and left ventricular LV loading (both preload and afterload) conditions. In animal and human subjects without heart failure the introduction of positive intrathoracic pressure has been shown to *reduce* cardiac output, stroke volume, and systolic blood pressure, largely via a reduction in venous return to the heart with subsequent underfilling of the left ventricle.[14,15] However, the failing myocardium has been shown to be far more sensitive to changes in afterload than preload,[16] and in the setting of LV failure complicated by pulmonary edema, CPAP is felt to promote a number of favorable changes in respiratory and cardiovascular mechanics (Table 32.1).

Effects on respiratory mechanics

In the setting of heart failure with pulmonary edema, CPAP has been shown to result in a number of positive changes in respiratory function. First, CPAP improves arterial oxygenation in patients with pulmonary edema.[17] Improved oxygenation with CPAP may be due to several mechanisms, including displacement of

Table 32.1. *Potential beneficial effects of continuous positive airway pressure in the management of acute decompensated heart failure*

Organ system	Mechanism of benefit	Observed clinical response
Cardiovascular	Reduced afterload Reduced preload*	Improved stroke volume
Pulmonary	Increased airway compliance Increased alveolar recruitment Reduced pulmonary shunt	Improved oxygenation Reduced work of breathing
Neurohormonal	Reduced cardiac adrenergic activity Reduced endothelin-1 expression	Reduced heart rate and blood pressure

*In patients with low pulmonary capillary wedge pressure, continuous positive airway pressure (CPAP) may cause a decrease in stroke volume.

intra-alveolar fluid with recruitment of alveoli, increased functional residual capacity and decreased right-to-left intrapulmonary shunting of blood.[15,17–19] Lin *et al.* randomized 100 patients admitted to an intensive care unit (ICU) with ACPE to conventional medical therapy plus either oxygen alone or oxygen therapy plus CPAP.[17] Intrapulmonary shunt, calculated from arterial, mixed venous, and end-pulmonary capillary blood oxygen saturation measurements, was significantly reduced in patients receiving CPAP after 3 hours, with a concurrent rise in arterial oxygen saturation. This trend was not observed among patients treated with oxygen alone.

A second positive effect of CPAP on respiratory function may be reduction in the work of breathing secondary to improved lung compliance. Increased work of breathing raises the oxygen cost of breathing, which may increase oxygen consumption while reducing delivery.[16] In patients with acute respiratory failure being weaned from mechanical ventilation, CPAP treatment has been shown to increase both dynamic and effective lung compliance while reducing total and nonelastic pulmonary energy requirements.[18] CPAP treatment in patients with decompensated heart failure and pulmonary edema results in a reduction in respiratory rate and subjective respiratory effort, with simultaneous improvement in oxygenation and hypercapnia.[17,20] This, coupled with a significant reduction in intrapulmonary shunt, provides indirect evidence of decreased work of breathing. However, CPAP has also been shown to reduce the work of breathing more directly. Lenique *et al.* studied 9 patients with decompensated, New York Heart Association (NYHA) class IV heart failure complicated by pulmonary edema.[16] The work of breathing, computed using esophageal pressure and tidal volume measurements and from transpulmonary pressure measurements, was significantly reduced by CPAP at 10 cm H_2O with no demonstrable change in cardiac index or stroke volume. Upon withdrawal of CPAP therapy, the work of breathing returned to baseline levels. Third, CPAP may supply some of the pressure required for lung inflation during inspiration, which may assist the respiratory muscles and improve fatigue.[21] Lastly, CPAP may reduce airway resistance.[16]

Effects on cardiovascular mechanics

While studies concerning the effects of CPAP on respiratory mechanics in patients with cardiogenic pulmonary edema appear fairly consistent, studies exploring the influence of CPAP on cardiovascular performance and hemodynamics have produced more varied results.

CPAP appears to reduce afterload by increasing intrathoracic pressure, thus decreasing the force required to eject blood against systemic arterial pressure. In patients who underwent coronary artery bypass surgery but who were without signs of heart failure, increased (20 cm H_2O) intrathoracic pressure by Valsalva maneuver reduced cardiac output, stroke volume, LV end-diastolic filling and LV transmural pressure, a determinant of LV afterload.[22] More recently, Naughton *et al.* treated 15 patients with chronic heart failure and 9 healthy controls with graduated CPAP (0 to 10 cm H_2O) for 75 minutes while estimating LV transmural pressure from arterial and mid-esophageal transducer measurements.[23] Cardiac index was also measured with Doppler echocardiography. CPAP treatment in patients with heart failure resulted in a significant decrease in LV transmural pressure with no significant change in cardiac index. In contrast, healthy control subjects experienced no change in LV transmural pressure but cardiac index decreased significantly.

Studies measuring hemodynamic changes associated with CPAP therapy in patients with heart failure and acute pulmonary edema have shown variable results, with studies demonstrating that cardiac output and stroke volume may increase, decrease, or remain unchanged in response to CPAP.[16,20,24,25] Much of this difference may be related to the effects that CPAP has on preload in patients with ACPE. As mentioned above, CPAP impedes venous return to the heart by increasing the pressure gradient between the venous circulation and the right side of the heart. In both animals and humans, CPAP has been shown to result in underfilling of the left ventricle, with reduced preload and a subsequent reduction in stroke volume and cardiac output.[14,22] However, the failing left ventricle appears to be less sensitive to changes in venous return than to changes in afterload.[16,26] Thus, while CPAP reduces both preload *and* afterload, in patients with impaired LV function, the contribution of afterload reduction to improved cardiac function overrides any negative effect of decreased preload, provided that filling pressures are adequate. For example, one study of patients presenting with ACPE revealed that patients treated with CPAP who had baseline wedge pressures < 12 mm Hg experienced a reduction in cardiac output and stroke volume, while similar patients with wedge pressures > 12 mm Hg actually increased their cardiac outputs on CPAP.[25] Similar dichotomous findings were seen in another study in which pulmonary capillary wedge pressure was not directly measured, though the authors acknowledged that differences in cardiac output with CPAP could be due to differences in preload.[23] Since the failing left ventricle requires increased end-diastolic pressure to maintain cardiac output (in accordance with the Frank–Starling mechanism), the reduction in venous return seen with CPAP therapy appears to benefit patients with high filling pressures, but it may further reduce cardiac output in those with low filling pressures.

Effects on neurohormonal regulation

Neurohormonal activation plays a major role in the pathophysiology of heart failure. In particular, the adrenergic nervous system has a significant negative influence on the failing left ventricle, and this pathway represents a key target for pharmacotherapy.[27,28] Both indirect and direct evidence suggests that CPAP reduces sympathetic input to the myocardium during ACPE. Several studies involving patients with ACPE have shown significant decreases in heart rate, an indirect correlate of cardiac sympathetic tone, in response to CPAP versus conventional oxygen therapy. However, this has not been a universal observation.[20,29,30] Additionally, despite a favorable clinical response to CPAP in patients presenting with ACPE, one study observed no detectable change in serum epinephrine or norepinephrine concentration compared to patients treated with oxygen alone.[30] However, CPAP may influence sympathetic tone in decompensated heart failure in a more cardiac-specific fashion. Kaye *et al.* recently evaluated the effect of short-term CPAP therapy (10 minutes) on systemic and cardiac sympathetic activity in patients with NYHA class III heart failure using a norepinephrine spillover technique.[31] Patients treated with CPAP demonstrated a significant decrease in cardiac norepinephrine spillover rate, while the systemic spillover rate remained unchanged. This observation led the investigators to believe that CPAP therapy inhibits cardiac sympathetic nervous activity. Additionally, another study showed that levels of endothelin-1 (ET-1) were significantly lowered in patients presenting with acute MI complicated by ACPE who were treated with conventional therapy plus CPAP versus oxygen therapy. ET-1 is a potent endothelium-derived vasoconstrictor that is felt to play a major role in endothelial dysfunction.[29] Finally, one study observed that serum levels of B-type natruretic peptide (BNP) did not differ between patients treated with CPAP or oxygen therapy for acute pulmonary edema, although elevated BNP was associated with an increased likelihood of death or MI regardless of treatment group.[30]

Clinical Utility of Continuous Positive Airway Pressure in Decompensated Heart Failure

Since the mid-1980s several investigators have approached the question of whether CPAP therapy, in conjunction with conventional medical therapy (diuretics, opiates, nitrates, and oxygen), could reduce or eliminate the need for endotracheal intubation and mechanical ventilation, or possibly reduce mortality in patients presenting with decompensated heart failure complicated by pulmonary edema. Although most published materials appear as case reports or retrospective surveys, a growing number of small, randomized controlled trials have provided some insight into the usefulness of CPAP to treat heart failure.

CPAP appears to reduce the need for endotracheal intubation in patients with decompensated heart failure. In the early 1990s, three small, randomized studies of patients presenting with acute pulmonary edema (160 total patients) each demonstrated a significant reduction in the need for endotracheal intubation with CPAP and conventional therapy versus oxygen and conventional therapy.[17,20,32] Data from these trials were pooled in a subsequent meta-analysis, which showed that CPAP therapy was associated with a 26% reduction in risk for intubation (95% confidence interval [CI], 14–38%), or 1 intubation avoided for every 4 patients treated with CPAP (number needed to treat [NNT] 4, 95% CI, 3–8).[33] More recent randomized studies continue to illustrate this trend.[29,30]

CPAP is associated with a strong trend toward reduced mortality in patients presenting with decompensated heart failure. Although several studies of CPAP in the setting of ACPE have included mortality as an endpoint, individually these studies were too small to detect meaningful differences in mortality between patients treated with CPAP versus those treated with conventional therapy.[17,20,32] When survival data were pooled in a recent review, a trend toward decreased mortality was observed for patients treated with CPAP.[33] In this review, CPAP therapy was associated with a 7% reduction in the risk for death, although the 95% CI was broad enough that one cannot exclude a potential small (3%) increase in mortality. However, subsequent studies, though small, have continued to demonstrate reduced mortality in patients treated with CPAP. For example, Takeda *et al.* studied 22 patients presenting with acute MI complicated by pulmonary edema.[29] Patients randomized to receive conventional therapy plus CPAP had a significantly reduced mortality rate compared to those assigned to receive conventional therapy plus oxygen (9% vs. 64%, respectively, $P = 0.02$). Similarly, Kelly *et al.* noted a trend toward reduced mortality among 58 consecutive patients randomized to receive standard therapy plus CPAP versus standard therapy plus oxygen in patients with acute pulmonary edema.[30] The investigators comment that when data from a previous study were combined with the data from their study, the results suggested a survival benefit with CPAP.[34]

Finally, CPAP in the treatment of cardiogenic pulmonary edema does not appear to be associated with significant adverse effects. Although facial discomfort and aspiration are potential risks with CPAP therapy, overall tolerability of the procedure was high in the aforementioned trials, and no major adverse events were attributed to CPAP therapy.[17,20,30,32] As mentioned previously, although a number of case reports suggest that BLPAP is effective and safe for the treatment of pulmonary edema, a number of recent randomized studies of patients with acute pulmonary edema have suggested an increased risk for MI and death with this modality.[10,12]

Technical Considerations

At the present time, no published guidelines exist regarding the use of CPAP for the treatment of decompensated heart failure complicated by pulmonary edema. However, recently published trials evaluating the use of CPAP in heart failure, in addition to a recent review article provide enough information to address a number of technical concerns.[7,17,20,30,32]

Patient selection

There are several clinical factors that may be used to determine which patients with pulmonary edema may benefit the most from CPAP therapy. First, the "ideal" candidate for CPAP in the setting of ACPE should be hemodynamically stable. Studies of CPAP in acute heart failure generally excluded patients with evidence for cardiogenic shock, so the efficacy of CPAP in these patients has not been established. The patient should be at risk for, but not require, endotracheal intubation. Second, based on available data, patients with severe pulmonary edema tend to derive more benefit from CPAP therapy than those with mild or moderate pulmonary edema.[7] To make this criterion more objective, one investigator has suggested that a respiratory rate ≥ 30/min, oxygen saturation < 90% on at least 4 L/min of supplemental oxygen, and mild hypercapnia may be considered indications for CPAP therapy.[7] Third, the patient should be cooperative. Individuals with impaired mentation or inability to protect their airways are not good candidates for CPAP therapy, and CPAP use in these patients may delay needed endotracheal intubation.[7] Finally, CPAP appears to be beneficial in patients with pulmonary edema complicating acute MI.[29] In contrast, patients with a cardiogenic shock, mental obtundation or an obvious need for endotracheal intubation are poor candidates for CPAP therapy (Table 32.2).

Administration of continuous positive airway pressure

Given the risk for aspiration and the general acuity of illness in patients with acute pulmonary edema, CPAP should be administered in a monitored setting by personnel who are specifically experienced with CPAP, such as a dedicated respiratory therapist. One drawback to CPAP therapy is that its administration places significant time demands on healthcare providers, especially in the first few hours of therapy when pressure uptitration generally occurs.[4] Most studies have shown benefit with CPAP within an hour to several hours after presentation with pulmonary edema, and therapy is usually initiated in the emergency department or upon arrival to the intensive care unit.[11,17,24,29] However, one retrospective review has suggested that CPAP may benefit patients with acute pulmonary edema in the pre-hospital (mobile ICU) setting.[35]

Although CPAP may be administered via face mask or nasal mask, some data suggest that using a face mask, especially in the initial hours of therapy, may be a better option.[36,37] In patients with COPD complicated by hypercapneic respiratory failure, the nasal mask has been associated with significant mouth leak in a large number of patients, especially edentulous patients.[36] The nasal passages themselves may increase resistance to flow.[37] CPAP is generally started using 5 cm H_2O pressure, with most studies demonstrating beneficial effects at levels between 7.5 cm H_2O and 12.5 cm H_2O.[33] CPAP is generally titrated upward as tolerated, and using increments of 2 cm H_2O pressure has been recommended until the desired effect is reached.[7] One investigator has suggested targeting CPAP therapy to achieve a respiratory rate < 25/min with arterial oxygen saturation $> 90\%$ in the setting of hemodynamic stability.[7] Although no guidelines exist regarding the duration of CPAP therapy in the setting of acute pulmonary edema, response to CPAP was evaluated over a period of hours (6 to 48 hours), with improvement often seen within the first hour.[17,20,32] Once the desired response has been achieved, it is recommended that CPAP be gradually weaned off in a manner similar to its initial uptitration.[7]

Conclusion

Decompensated heart failure complicated by acute pulmonary edema is a common problem associated

Table 32.2. *Relative indications and contraindications for use of continuous positive airway pressure in acute decompensated heart failure*

Indications	Contraindications
Severe cardiogenic pulmonary edema	Indication for endotracheal intubation
■ oxygen saturation < 90%*	■ severe respiratory acidosis (pH < 7.2)
■ respiratory rate > 25/min*	■ severe respiratory distress
■ mild respiratory acidosis (pH ≥ 7.3)	Cardiogenic shock
■ mild to moderate respiratory distress	Depressed mental status
Stable hemodynamics	High aspiration risk
Cooperative patient	Facial trauma or deformity
	Inability to tolerate mask

*Despite conventional therapy with supplemental oxygen, diuretics, and nitrates.

with considerable morbidity and mortality. CPAP has been shown to improve respiratory mechanics in heart failure patients with ACPE, with resultant improvements in arterial oxygenation and the work of breathing. CPAP has also been shown to reduce preload and afterload in patients with heart failure, and there is some evidence that cardiac output and stroke volume improve with CPAP. In cooperative patients, presenting with severe pulmonary edema, who appear to be at risk for endotracheal intubation but who are without evidence of cardiogenic shock, CPAP therapy has been shown to significantly reduce heart rate, respiratory rate, subjective breathlessness, and the need for endotracheal intubation. Furthermore, a strong trend toward reduced in-hospital mortality has been shown for these patients. CPAP also appears to be safe and generally well tolerated in heart failure patients with acute pulmonary edema. Presently, enough data exist to support the use of CPAP as an adjunct to conventional therapy in patients with decompensated heart failure complicated by severe pulmonary edema. A large, multicenter randomized controlled trial of CPAP is certainly indicated to establish whether CPAP improves survival in patients with cardiogenic pulmonary edema.

References

1. Felker GM, Adams KF Jr., Konstam MA, *et al.* The problem of decompensated heart failure: nomenclature, classification, and risk stratification. Am Heart J 2003; 145: S18–S25.
2. Craven DE, Steger KA. Epidemiology of nosocomial pneumonia. New perspectives on an old disease. Chest 1995; 108: 1S–16S.
3. Schnapp LM, Chin DP, Szaflarski N, Matthay MA. Frequency and importance of barotrauma in 100 patients with acute lung injury. Crit Care Med 1995; 23: 272–278.
4. International Consensus Conferences in Intensive Care Medicine: noninvasive positive pressure ventilation in acute respiratory failure. Organized jointly by the American Thoracic Society, the European Respiratory Society, the European Society of Intensive Care Medicine, and the Société de Réanimation de Langue Française, and approved by ATS Board of Directors, December 2000. Am J Respir Crit Care Med 2001; 163: 283–291.
5. Antonelli M, Conti G, Moro ML, *et al.* Predictors of failure of noninvasive positive pressure ventilation in patients with acute hypoxemic respiratory failure: a multicenter study. Intensive Care Med 2001; 27: 1718–1728.
6. Brochard L, Mancebo J, Wysocki M, *et al.* Noninvasive ventilation for acute exacerbations of chronic obstructive pulmonary disease. N Engl J Med 1995; 333: 817–822.
7. Panacek EA, Kirk JD. Role of noninvasive ventilation in the management of acutely decompensated heart failure. Rev Cardiovasc Med 2002; 3: S35–S40.
8. Mehta S, Hill NS. Noninvasive ventilation. Am J Respir Crit Care Med 2001; 163: 540–577.
9. Diaz O, Iglesia R, Ferrer M, *et al.* Effects of noninvasive ventilation on pulmonary gas exchange and hemodynamics during acute hypercapnic exacerbations of chronic obstructive pulmonary disease. Am J Respir Crit Care Med 1997; 156: 1840–1845.
10. Wood KA, Lewis L, Von Harz B, Kollef MH. The use of noninvasive positive pressure ventilation in the emergency department: results of a randomized clinical trial. Chest 1998; 113: 1339–1346.
11. Mehta S, Jay GD, Woolard RH, *et al.* Randomized, prospective trial of bilevel versus continuous positive airway pressure in acute pulmonary edema. Crit Care Med 1997; 25: 620–628.
12. Sharon A, Shpirer I, Kaluski E, *et al.* High-dose intravenous isosorbide-dinitrate is safer and better than Bi-PAP ventilation combined with conventional treatment for severe pulmonary edema. J Am Coll Cardiol 2000; 36: 832–837.
13. Masip J, Betbese AJ, Paez J, *et al.* Non-invasive pressure support ventilation versus conventional oxygen therapy in acute cardiogenic pulmonary oedema: a randomised trial. Lancet 2000; 356: 2126–2132.
14. Fewell JE, Abendschein DR, Carlson CJ, Murray JF, Rapaport E. Continuous positive-pressure ventilation decreases right and left ventricular end-diastolic volumes in the dog. Circ Res 1980; 46: 125–132.
15. Sturgeon CL, Douglas ME, Downs JB, *et al.* PEEP and CPAP: cardiopulmonary effects during spontaneous ventilation. Anesth Analg 1977; 56: 633–641.
16. Lenique F, Habis M, Lofaso F, *et al.* Ventilatory and hemodynamic effects of continuous positive airway pressure in left heart failure. Am J Respir Crit Care Med 1997; 155: 500–505.
17. Lin M, Yang YF, Chiang HT, *et al.* Reappraisal of continuous positive airway pressure therapy in acute cardiogenic pulmonary edema. Short-term results and long-term follow-up. Chest 1995; 107: 1379–1386.

18. Katz JA, Marks JD. Inspiratory work with and without continuous positive airway pressure in patients with acute respiratory failure. Anesthesiology 1985; 63: 598–607.
19. Rizk NW, Murray JF. PEEP and pulmonary edema. Am J Med 1982; 72: 381–383.
20. Rasanen J, Heikkila J, Downs J, *et al.* Continuous positive airway pressure by facemask in acute cardiogenic pulmonary edema. Am J Cardiol 1985; 55: 296–300.
21. Martin JG, Shore S, Engel LA. Effect of continuous positive airway pressure on respiratory mechanics and pattern of breathing in induced asthma. Am Rev Respir Dis 1982; 126: 812–817.
22. Buda AJ, Pinsky MR, Ingels NB Jr., Daughters GT 2nd, Stinson EB, Alderman EL. Effect of intrathoracic pressure on left ventricular performance. N Engl J Med 1979; 301: 453–459.
23. Naughton MT, Rahman MA, Hara K, Floras JS, Bradley TD. Effect of continuous positive airway pressure on intrathoracic and left ventricular transmural pressures in patients with congestive heart failure. Circulation 1995; 91: 1725–1731.
24. Baratz DM, Westbrook PR, Shah PK, Mohsenifar Z. Effect of nasal continuous positive airway pressure on cardiac output and oxygen delivery in patients with congestive heart failure. Chest 1992; 102: 1397–1401.
25. Bradley TD, Holloway RM, McLaughlin PR, *et al.* Cardiac output response to continuous positive airway pressure in congestive heart failure. Am Rev Respir Dis 1992; 145: 377–382.
26. Guyton AC, Jones CE, Coleman TG. Circulatory Physiology I: Cardiac Output and Its Regulation (W. B. Saunders: Philadelphia, PA, 1973), 258–296.
27. Packer M, Bristow MR, Cohn JN, *et al.* The effect of carvedilol on morbidity and mortality in patients with chronic heart failure. U.S. Carvedilol Heart Failure Study Group. N Engl J Med 1996; 334: 1349–1355.
28. Effect of metoprolol CR/XL in chronic heart failure: Metoprolol CR/XL Randomized Intervention Trial in Congestive Heart Failure (MERIT-HF). Lancet 1999; 353: 2001–2007.
29. Takeda S, Nejima J, Takano T, *et al.* Effect of nasal continuous positive airway pressure on pulmonary edema complicating acute myocardial infarction. Jpn Circ J 1998; 62: 553–558.
30. Kelly CA, Newby DE, McDonagh TA, *et al.* Randomised controlled trial of continuous positive airway pressure and standard oxygen therapy in acute pulmonary oedema; effects on plasma brain natriuretic peptide concentrations. Eur Heart J 2002; 23: 1379–1386.
31. Kaye DM, Mansfield D, Aggarwal A, Naughton MT, Esler MD. Acute effects of continuous positive airway pressure on cardiac sympathetic tone in congestive heart failure. Circulation 2001; 103: 2336–2338.
32. Bersten AD, Holt AW, Vedig AE, Skowronski GA, Baggoley CJ. Treatment of severe cardiogenic pulmonary edema with continuous positive airway pressure delivered by face mask. N Engl J Med 1991; 325: 1825–1830.
33. Pang D, Keenan SP, Cook DJ, Sibbald WJ. The effect of positive pressure airway support on mortality and the need for intubation in cardiogenic pulmonary edema: a systematic review. Chest 1998; 114: 1185–1192.
34. Kelly C, Newby DE, Boon NA, Douglas NJ. Support ventilation versus conventional oxygen. Lancet 2001; 357: 1126.
35. Kallio T, Kuisma M, Alaspaa A, Rosenberg PH. The use of prehospital continuous positive airway pressure treatment in presumed acute severe pulmonary edema. Prehosp Emerg Care 2003; 7: 209–213.
36. Soo Hoo GW, Santiago S, Williams AJ. Nasal mechanical ventilation for hypercapnic respiratory failure in chronic obstructive pulmonary disease: determinants of success and failure. Crit Care Med 1994; 22: 1253–1261.
37. Hess D. Noninvasive positive pressure ventilation: predictors of success and failure for adult acute care applications. Respir Care 1997; 42: 424–431 (Abstract).

CHAPTER 33

Exercise training in advanced heart failure: a need for more data

Ileana L Piña, David J Whellan, Christopher M O'Connor

Introduction

Despite significant advances in the medical treatment of heart failure, those patients who suffer from the advanced form of the syndrome remain among the most symptomatic of patients with chronic disease. Prone to the "revolving door" dilemma of frequent hospital admissions, these patients go through periods of decompensation during which symptoms limit activity and deconditioning worsens. It may be difficult to distinguish the symptoms of fatigue and dyspnea due to deconditioning from the heart failure syndrome itself. Coupled with frequent hospitalizations, which utilize intermittently aggressive therapy, is the fear that exercise training or simple physical conditioning might worsen the progression of the disease.

Because the symptoms of deconditioning can be confused with the symptoms of heart failure, this patient population might derive significant benefits from better conditioning. As in populations with less severe disease, resting ventricular function (i.e., ejection fraction [EF]) bears no correlation to exercise capacity whether measured by duration or by cardiopulmonary testing.[1]

Although data are scant regarding exercise training in patients with advanced heart failure, this chapter attempts to differentiate and clarify the areas where information is available as opposed to those areas where there is only speculation. This section combines New York Heart Association (NYHA) class III and IV heart failure since these functional classes are fluid and patients move from one to the other; both represent the more advanced chronic disease process.

Bed Rest

Due to periods of bed rest, the advanced heart failure patient will be more deconditioned and debilitated than the NYHA class II patient who remains out of the hospital. Bed rest is deleterious to normal subjects and it is certainly deleterious to patients with chronic diseases such as heart failure. Table 33.1 depicts the changes incurred by bed rest. After 10 days of continuous bed rest in normal subjects, peak oxygen uptake (VO_2) decreases by 8.4% in men and 6.8% in women and total exercise tolerance decreases by 8.1% in men and 7.3% in women.[2] Peak heart rate increases in both men and women. In addition, there is a direct correlation between the drop in peak VO_2 and the number of days of bed rest.[3]

Not only is there a loss of functional capacity, but changes in muscle and bone also occur, particularly in the lower extremities. These changes can occur after 4 to 6 weeks of bed rest, accompanied by a loss of contractile strength by as much as 40%.[4]

Inactivity also increases maximal heart rate with a decrease in vagal tone, increased sympathetic

Table 33.1. *Deleterious effects of bed rest*

Loss of functional capacity (peak VO_2)
Loss of muscle mass
Loss of contractile strength
Loss of bone
Decreased mitochodrial oxidative enzymes
Muscle atrophy with loss of fiber size
Decreased vagal tone
Increased beta receptor sensitivity
Increased heart rate at rest and with activity

catecholamine secretion, and enhanced beta-receptor sensitivity to circulating catecholamines. Although heart rate is elevated, the peak VO_2 falls due to a lower stroke volume and decrease in cardiac output.[5]

The arteriovenous oxygen (AV O_2) difference is not altered by bed rest. However, there are reductions in baseline and exercise blood flow to working skeletal muscles with a loss of capillarization. These mechanisms will ultimately affect peak VO_2. Fiber type may not change but fiber area does, resulting in muscle atrophy. The volume density of mitochondria is reduced by as much as 28% with a concomitant decrease in oxidative enzymes.[6] Advanced heart failure patients who enter a period of bed rest with pre-existing subnormal muscle and bone mass, particularly if they are elderly, are likely to incur risk of injury upon re-ambulation whether in the hospital or at home. For elderly patients, other comorbidities augment the risk of injury.

General Role of Exercise Training in Heart Failure

Benefits of exercise training

The potential benefits of exercise training in heart failure patients include increases in exercise capacity, plasma catecholamines, ventilatory response, endothelial function, survival, and quality of life.

Exercise Capacity

The benefits of exercise training in patients with heart failure include an improvement in exercise duration as measured by time on the treadmill or bicycle, and more importantly in functional capacity as measured by peak VO_2.[2,3,7–14] Training programs have varied and include supervised or home-based training; treadmill or bicycle; durations of 8 weeks to 3 months; and levels of intensity ranging from low to moderate. Improvements in peak VO_2 have ranged from a low of 12% to a high of 31%. Most of the improvement occurs by week 3 but can still be noted at 6 months, if compliance with the training program continues.[4,6] Indices of submaximal exercise, as measured by the 6-minute walk or ventilatory threshold, can also improve.[7] Changes in peak VO_2 have been reported to be greater in patients with non-ischemic than ischemic cardiomyopathy.[12] These studies have included a variety of patients with NYHA class II–III heart failure primarily. Medical therapy has varied over the years with early trials devoid of significant beta-blocker therapy.

Catecholamines

Since increased plasma catecholamines are associated with poor prognosis in patients with heart failure, investigators have sought to measure changes in catecholamines in response to exercise training. The results of these studies, however, have been variable. Kiilavuori *et al.* found a 19% drop in resting epinephrine after a 3-month training program.[15] In contrast, Keteyian *et al.* found no changes in resting norepinephrine after 24 weeks of training.[16] Hambrecht *et al.* found a significant drop in resting epinephrine levels with a trend toward decreased norepinephrine levels at rest but also during submaximal exercise.[17] Enhanced vagal control with a shift away from sympathetic activity has been documented in a small but well-designed cross-over trial of 8 weeks of home training.[8] Other investigators have found that local muscle training could improve not only aerobic activity but also lower catecholamine levels.[18] The variability in these findings are probably due to the duration and severity of disease, intensity and duration of exercise training, and presence of sympathetic activity modulating drugs (e.g., angiotensin-converting enzyme [ACE] inhibitors or especially beta-adrenergic blockers). Some of these findings may be different in a population that would be studied today due to the increasing use of beta-blockers in clinical practice, especially after the findings of the Carvedilol Prospective Randomized Cumulative Survival (COPERNICUS) trial.[19]

Ventilatory response

Symptoms in patients with heart failure are related to an excessive increase in blood lactate during low exercise levels, with reduction in VO_2 at peak exercise, and disproportionate increases in ventilation at submaximal and peak work loads. Several investigators have shown that the relationship of ventilatory equivalent (VE) to carbon dioxide output (VCO_2) is abnormal and related to prognosis as well. The increased ventilatory requirement assessed by the hyperventilatory response to exercise and increase in pulmonary dead space leads to rapid and shallow breathing during exercise. Since skeletal muscles become deconditioned all over, deconditioning in the respiratory muscles should occur as well.

Mancini *et al.* have studied the effect of respiratory muscle training in patients with chronic heart failure.[20] In a group of 14 patients with an average EF of 22%, maximal sustainable ventilatory capacity increased from 48.6 L/min to 76.9 L/min, which was accompanied by an increase in inspiratory and expiratory respiratory muscle strength. There was also a concomitant increase in peak exercise VO_2 from 11.4 mL/min/kg to 13.3 mL/min/kg. Loss of ventilatory muscles accompanied overall muscle atrophy with bed rest and deconditioning.

Endothelial function

One of the possible mechanisms of functional capacity increase in heart failure patients could be attributed to endothelial functional improvement. In an exercise training trial, Hambrecht *et al.* enrolled 40 patients with severe heart failure and a mean EF of 19%. Subjects were randomized to one of three treatment groups: one group received L-arginine daily and underwent resistance training with daily handgrip exercises; the second group underwent resistance training alone; and the third group was an inactive control group. The mean internal radial artery diameter increased in response to endothelium-dependent and independent stimuli in both the training-only group and in the training + L-arginine group. When compared to the control group, these increases were significant ($P < 0.001$).[21]

This same group of investigators has now demonstrated improvement in endothelium-dependent vasodilation in epicardial vessels as well as in resistance vessels in patients with known coronary artery disease (CAD). After 4 weeks of training, the exercise group had a 29% increase in coronary artery flow reserve as compared to the non-exercise control group.[22] Therefore, there is mounting evidence of improvement in endothelial function in the peripheral vessels as well as in the coronary tree. Whether these endothelial changes will lead to survival benefits is yet to be proven.

Survival

Although multiple factors can improve with exercise training, they are nonetheless, surrogates. In the past, multiple pharmacologic agents have demonstrated increases in exercise function, but then failed to improve mortality (e.g., flosequinan, pimobendan, milrinone). In addition, an exercise regimen of short duration may fail to show any improvement in survival beyond 6 months or 1 year. Belardinelli *et al.* studied the effects of a longer-term (14-month) exercise program of moderate intensity in 99 patients with stable chronic heart failure (NYHA class I–IV).[23] Of the 99 patients, 85% had heart failure with an ischemic etiology. At 2 months, the percentage of myocardial perfusion defects with improved thallium activity and reversible defects were significantly higher in the patients who underwent training than in the patients in the control group. An improved thallium uptake was noted in 75% of the trained subjects and only 2% of the untrained subjects, and this level was maintained at 14 months. Of interest, cardiac events, including cardiac deaths and non-fatal events, were more frequent in the control group (37 vs. 17 events, $P = 0.006$). In addition, the rate of hospital readmission for heart failure was significantly lower in the trained subjects than in the control subjects ($P = 0.02$).

Cardiac mortality was also significantly lower in the trained subjects than in the untrained subjects ($P = 0.01$).

Small trials, although tantalizing, should not be taken as proof of survival benefits. Prospective data are needed. Currently, a National Institutes of Health (NIH) supported trial, Heart Failure: A Controlled Trial Investigating Outcomes of Exercise Training (HF-ACTION) is enrolling patients and randomizing them to either a control group or an exercise training group. The primary endpoint of this trial is a composite of all-cause mortality and all-cause hospitalization. The targeted enrollment is 3000 patients with NYHA class II–IV heart failure over age 18, regardless of etiology. If the trial successfully enrolls a sufficient number of patients with NYHA class III or IV, the impact of exercise training on outcome in heart failure patients will be better understood.

Quality of life

Studies that address quality of life in heart failure patients who are participating in an exercise program have had inconsistent results. Tools that focus on symptoms, such as dyspnea and fatigue, as well as psychosocial status, such as emotional function and mastery or perceived control over symptoms, are more likely to show a good outcome.

The commonly used Minnesota Living With Heart Failure Questionnaire (MLWHFQ)[24] assesses disease-specific health-related quality of life by including the patient's perceptions of the effects of heart failure and its treatment on his or her daily life. However, two randomized prospective exercise training studies and one observational study failed to show significant improvement in quality of life when utilizing this questionnaire.[6,16] Other randomized, controlled studies of heart failure patients have ranged in sample size from 25 to 99 and consisted predominantly of men aged 30 to 76 years undergoing 3 to 12 months of exercise training. Several different tools were used.[23,25–28] All of these studies showed improvement in exercise capacity as well as improvement in most measures of quality of life for patients randomized to exercise training.

In summary, there is limited research on quality of life improvement in patients with heart failure who are participating in exercise training and little data on those with advanced disease. However, most of the existing data support an improvement in quality of life with exercise training in this population. Future trials should include health status instruments which are specifically designed to test the group of heart failure patients that is continuing to grow—the elderly. The HF-ACTION trial will evaluate the use of the Kansas City Cardiomyopathy Questionnaire (KCCQ) in both the training and control groups. The KCCQ correlates well with functional indices such as the 6-minute walk.[29]

Exercise Trials in Advanced Heart Failure

The majority of randomized controlled trials have excluded patients with more advanced disease. Others have classified the patient cohorts as "moderate to severe" but have not divided the groups into NYHA classes. Most have excluded any unstable patients. Others have considered severity based on left ventricular ejection fraction (LVEF) and have not provided a clear definition of functional class, while others have considered NYHA class III as moderate to severe. This lack of consistency in defining advanced heart failure makes interpretation of study results even more difficult for patients with advanced heart failure. The small number of patients enrolled in each study makes an analysis of mortality impractical. Annual mortality, however, could help characterize the level of sickness. Furthermore, medical therapy has continued to evolve and patients in some of these trials were not on beta-blocker therapy. Due to the severity of symptoms, concerns about safety, and potential risks are expected. Table 33.2 illustrates the number or inclusion of the advanced chronic heart failure patients described as NYHA class III and IV and the results of functional capacity changes in a selection of randomized controlled trials of exercise training in heart failure.[7–9,15,16,18,20,23,30] All of these trials report no significant complications secondary to the exercise training.

A few studies, however, are worth discussing

Table 33.2. *Controlled trials of exercise training in heart failure with improvements in peak VO_2*

Author (year)	No. of patients	NYHA class III/IV	Exercise program	% VO_2 increase outcome vs. controls
Jette (1991)[30]	18	8 EF < 30%	4 wk program, Monday-Friday, AM: Jog at 70-80% max HR, 5 min, 3×/wk; 30 min calisthenics; cycle 15 min 70-80% max HR. PM: Walk 30-60 min	22 in group with EF < 30%
Coats (1992)[8]	17	All moderate to severe	Cycle 20 min 3×/wk at 60-80% max HR, 8 wk	18
Belardinelli (1995)[34]	55	17/0	Cycle 40 min 3×/wk at 60% VO_2max; 8 wk	12; cardiac event with larger LV
Hambrecht (1995)[7]	22	10/0	0 min 6×/day at 70% VO_2max; 13 wk	31; no differences between NYHA class; improvement in NYHA class
Keteyian (1996)[16]	40	13/0	RPE 12-14. 60% exercise capacity 33 min 3×/wk × 24 wk	16.3; no mention of differences between II and III
Radaelli (1996)[18]	6	All moderate to severe	Cycle 20 min × 5 days/wk × 5 wk	15
Tyni-Lenne (1997)[9]	16	7/0	Knee extensor for 8 wk	14; all women; no mention of differences between II and III
Belardinelli (1999)[23]	99	34/19	Cycle at 60% peak VO_2, 8 wk, 3×/wk; maintenance, 12 mo, 2×/wk.	18 at 2 mo 23 at 14 mo; more events in control with larger LV
Sturm (1999)[35]	26	12/0	50% capacity × 12 wk, then 100 min step aerobics/wk + cycle 50 min/wk	23.3; EF = 17%; no mention of differences between II and III

Abbreviations: b/w = between; EF = ejection fraction; HR = heart rate (bpm); LV = left ventricle; mo = months; NYHA = New York Heart Association; RPE= rate of perceived exertion; VO_2 = oxygen uptake; wk = week(s).

individually. Fonarow *et al.* selected a group of patients that had been referred for cardiac transplantation candidacy.[22] All patients, therefore, were considered NYHA class III (44%) or IV (56%). In a "package" of medication adjustment, extensive education, and close follow-up, no formal exercise program was included. Patients were, nonetheless instructed to walk or use a stationary bicycle 4 times per week to a target of 30 to 45 minutes duration. All patients underwent a baseline cardiopulmonary test to determine their baseline functional capacity. Mean baseline peak VO_2

was 11.0 cc/min/kg, placing the population at a limited functional capacity level. Functional class improved significantly after 6 months, with 49% of patients classified as NYHA class I or II. Peak VO_2 improved to 15.2 cc/min/kg. As expected, rehospitalizations also decreased significantly.

Erbs *et al.* have performed seminal trials that have furthered our understanding of the benefits of exercise in heart failure.[31] The Leipzig Heart Failure Training Trial used the same entry criteria as the COPERNICUS carvedilol trial—chronic advanced heart failure patients—and enrolled 73 patients who were randomized to either training or control.[19] Nine out of 37 patients in the exercise group and 10 out of 36 patients in the control group had symptoms of advanced heart failure. Six months of training improved most patients by one NYHA class with a 49% increase in VO_2 and ventilatory threshold and a 32% increase in peak VO_2. In addition, the authors noted a small but significant reduction in LV end-diastolic diameter of 7%.

Most exercise training programs have used a low to moderate intensity prescription. Sturm *et al.* examined the level of intensity recommended in training.[20] This group of investigators recruited a group of 26 heart failure patients (12 were NYHA class III) whose VO_2 was less than 50% predicted and whose EF was < 25% (mean 19% and 17% respectively) and randomized them either to control or a combined moderate intensity program of cycling with step aerobics. Work capacity, peak VO_2 and exercise time increased in the exercise group. The value of this study is the use of a moderate intensity program in patients with chronic heart failure which the authors describe as severe. Only one patient required an increase in diuretics and no complications were encountered.

Recommendations

Given the deleterious effects of bed rest and deconditioning, added to the severity of symptoms due to the advanced heart failure syndrome, a commonsense approach to improving conditioning in this population is essential. Table 33.3 lists possible benefits of exercise training in advanced heart failure. Given the paucity of data, there are no set rules or guidelines for the sicker patients.[25] However, a preliminary exercise test is recommended to determine the hemodynamic response to activity and symptoms induced with exercise, to exclude ischemia or arrhythmias, and to better define an exercise prescription. In heart failure patients, a cardiopulmonary exercise test is ideal since it also provides prognostic information.[32]

Table 33.3. *Potential benefits of exercise training in patients with advanced heart failure.*

Improved functional capacity
Improved onset of ventilatory threshold
Improved exercise duration
Increase in muscle tone
Improved stability
Improved transfer from bed to chair and vice versa
Improved ventilatory capacity
Better quality of life
Improved function for activities of daily living
More independence and self-care

Telemetry monitoring is reasonable early on during the exercise program. Although there have been few arrhythmias in the trials noted previously, none of these trials have included a very sick population which may be more prone to arrhythmias. Certainly, supervised training should be recommended in the early sessions of a program to be continued at home. The transition to home-based training is critical since stopping training will result in deconditioning again. A home-based training program must be tailored to fit the lifestyle and living situation of the individual patient. Recommended activities may include hobbies, such as gardening or bowling. Walking is always recommended since it does not require any expensive equipment and can be performed in multiple locations, such as parks or shopping malls. Extremes of temperature and humidity should be avoided. Times of day when the patient feels less fatigued may be more suitable for an enjoyable experience. For example, many patients feel that early in the morning, after a good night's rest, may be their most energetic period. With proper instruction, small weights or elastic bands may be added to strengthen upper body muscles which are so critical in performing the activities of daily living (ADLs).

Intensity

The intensity may be the most difficult aspect to prescribe given the probable debilitated state of the advanced heart failure patient. Exercise testing is very useful in this regard for documenting heart rate and blood pressure response as well as workload. With cardiopulmonary exercise testing (CPX), a value below the ventilatory threshold is reasonable. If CPX testing is not available, the Borg scale can be invaluable for assessing total body work and assigning a value between 13–15, which indicates moderate intensity as described by the patient.[33] Alternatively, and importantly in the era of beta-blockade, a percent of the heart rate reserve (peak heart rate–resting heart rate) can also be applied. Most commonly a 60% to 70% of heart rate reserve will allow a reasonable amount of activity. The patient would need education about pulse measurements. Other forms of intensity can include activity to the point of symptoms.

The most debilitated patients may need periods of rest between exercise intervals. Intensity can be gradually increased as the program ensues.

Duration

Most exercise sessions should last for 20 to 30 minutes; the lighter the intensity, the longer the duration. The goal is to make these minutes continuous. However, some patients may need 5-minute training intervals interspersed with 5 minutes of rest. The goal should be to achieve continuous exercise activity. In advanced heart failure patients, this may take several sessions to achieve. Warm-up and cool-down periods are essential. The warm-up may consist of stretching, calisthenics, or walking at a slower pace. Likewise, the cool-down period is important for gradually diminishing the heart rate and avoiding sudden blood pressure drops. Cool-down can be achieved with slower walking or cycling.

Frequency

A supervised exercise training program should occur 3 times per week. On the other days, the patient should be instructed to walk for at least 20 to 30 minutes at their own pace. If the patient only exercises 2 times per week, then the total time for training needs to be extended. In this patient population, marked by frequent readmissions, the program may need to restart after each hospitalization, since the patient may lose the training effect when admitted and placed on bed rest.

Conclusion

In summary, the advanced heart failure patient may be among the most deconditioned of all patients with chronic diseases, due to frequent admissions characterized by periods of bed rest and loss of function. Bed rest can be deleterious. Although not directly the subject of any given large trial, exercise conditioning seems to benefit patients with heart failure, albeit best tested in the mild to moderate population. However, the risks have been low and patients with chronic advanced heart failure should not be deprived of some form of exercise conditioning, if for no other reason than to improve their performance of ADLs and quality of life. We will not know whether or not outcomes, such as mortality and hospitalizations, are decreased with exercise training until the conclusion of the HF-ACTION trial. We eagerly await the results.

References

1. Franciosa JA, Park M, Levine TB. Lack of correlation between exercise capacity and indexes of resting left ventricular performance in heart failure. Am J Cardiol 1981; 47: 33–39.
2. Convertino VA, Goldwater DJ, Sandler H. Bedrest-induced peak VO_2 reduction associated with age, gender, and aerobic capacity. Aviat Space Environ Med 1986; 57: 17–22.
3. Hung J, Goldwater D, Convertino VA, *et al.* Mechanisms for decreased exercise capacity after bed rest in normal middle-aged men. Am J Cardiol 1983; 51: 344–348.

4. Bloomfield SA. Changes in musculoskeletal structure and function with prolonged bed rest. Med Sci Sports Exerc 1997; 29: 197–206.
5. Convertino VA. Cardiovascular consequences of bed rest: effect on maximal oxygen uptake. Med Sci Sports Exerc 1997; 29: 191–196.
6. Ferretti G. The effect of prolonged bed rest on maximal instantaneous muscle power and its determinants. Int J Sports Med 1997; 18: S287–S289.
7. Hambrecht R, Niebauer J, Fiehn E, *et al.* Physical training in patients with stable chronic heart failure: effects on cardiorespiratory fitness and ultrastructural abnormalities of leg muscles. J Am Coll Cardiol 1995; 25: 1239–1249.
8. Coats AJ, Adamopoulos S, Radaelli A, *et al.* Controlled trial of physical training in chronic heart failure. Exercise performance, hemodynamics, ventilation, and autonomic function. Circulation 1992; 85: 2119–2131.
9. Tyni-Lenne R, Gordon A, Jansson E, Bermann G, Sylven C. Skeletal muscle endurance training improves peripheral oxidative capacity, exercise tolerance, and health-related quality of life in women with chronic congestive heart failure secondary to either ischemic cardiomyopathy or idiopathic dilated cardiomyopathy. Am J Cardiol 1997; 80: 1025–1029.
10. Short KR, Sedlock DA. Excess postexercise oxygen consumption and recovery rate in trained and untrained subjects. J Appl Physiol 1997; 83: 153–159.
11. Picozzi NM, Clark AL, Lindsay KA, McCann GP, Hillis WS. Responses to constant work exercise in patients with chronic heart failure. Heart 1999; 82: 482–485.
12. Riley M, Stanford CF, Nicholls DP. Ventilatory and heart rate responses after exercise in chronic cardiac failure. Clin Sci (Lond) 1994; 87: 231–238.
13. Riley M, Porszasz J, Stanford CF, Nicholls DP. Gas exchange responses to constant work rate exercise in chronic cardiac failure. Br Heart J 1994; 72: 150–155.
14. Francis GS, Goldsmith SR, Levine TB, Olivari MT, Cohn JN. The neurohumoral axis in congestive heart failure. Ann Intern Med 1984; 101: 370–377.
15. Kiilavuori K, Naveri H, Leinonen H, *et al.* The effect of physical training on hormonal status and exertional hormonal response in patients with chronic congestive heart failure. Eur Heart J 1999; 20: 456–464.
16. Keteyian SJ, Levine AB, Brawner CA, *et al.* Exercise training in patients with heart failure. A randomized, controlled trial. Ann Intern Med 1996; 124: 1051–1057.
17. Hambrecht R, Gielen S, Linke A, *et al.* Effects of exercise training on left ventricular function and peripheral resistance in patients with chronic heart failure. JAMA 2000; 283: 3095–3101.
18. Radaelli A, Coats AJ, Leuzzi S, *et al.* Physical training enhances sympathetic and parasympathetic control of heart rate and peripheral vessels in chronic heart failure. Clin Sci (Lond) 1996; 91: 92–94.
19. Packer M, Fowler MB, Roecker EB, *et al.*, Carvedilol Prospective Randomized Cumulative Survival (COPERNICUS) Study Group. Effect of carvedilol on the morbidity of patients with severe chronic heart failure: results of the carvedilol prospective randomized cumulative survival (COPERNICUS) study. Circulation 2002; 106: 2194–2199.
20. Mancini DM, Henson D, LaManca J, *et al.* Benefit of selective respiratory muscle training on exercise capacity in patients with chronic congestive heart failure. Circulation 1995; 91: 320–329.
21. Hambrecht R, Hilbrich L, Erbs S, *et al.* Correction of endothelial dysfunction in chronic heart failure: additional effects of exercise training and oral L-arginine supplementation. J Am Coll Cardiol 2000; 35: 706–713.
22. Fonarow GC, Stevenson LW, Walden JA, *et al.* Impact of a comprehensive heart failure management program on hospital readmission and functional status of patients with advanced heart failure. J Am Coll Cardiol 1997; 30: 725–732.
23. Belardinelli R, Georgiou D, Cianci G, Purcaro A. Randomized, controlled trial of long-term moderate exercise training in chronic heart failure: effects on functional capacity, quality of life, and clinical outcome. Circulation 1999; 99: 1173–1182.
24. Rector TS, Cohn JN. Assessment of patient outcome with the Minnesota Living with Heart Failure questionnaire: reliability and validity during a randomized, double-blind, placebo-controlled trial of pimobendan. Pimobendan Multicenter Research Group. Am Heart J 1992; 124: 1017–1025.
25. Pina IL, Apstein CS, Balady GJ, *et al.*, American Heart Association Committee on exercise, rehabilitation, and prevention. Exercise and heart failure: A statement from the American Heart Association Committee on exercise, rehabilitation, and prevention. Circulation 2003; 107: 1210–1225.
26. Thompson PD, Buchner D, Pina IL, *et al.*, American Heart Association Council on Clinical Cardiology Subcommittee on Exercise, Rehabilitation, and Prevention; American Heart Association Council on Nutrition, Physical Activity, and Metabolism Subcommittee on Physical Activity. Exercise and physical activity in the prevention and treatment of atherosclerotic cardiovascular disease: a statement

from the Council on Clinical Cardiology (Subcommittee on Exercise, Rehabilitation, and Prevention) and the Council on Nutrition, Physical Activity, and Metabolism (Subcommittee on Physical Activity). Circulation 2003; 107: 3109–3016.

27. Pina IL. Physical activity needs to be a lifelong commitment. J Cardiopulm Rehabil 2003; 23: 107–108.
28. Whellan DJ, O'Connor CM, Pinã I. Training trials in heart failure: time to exercise restraint? Am Heart J 2004; 147: 190–192.
29. Cohn JN, Tognoni G, Valsartan Heart Failure Trial Investigators. A randomized trial of the angiotensin-receptor blocker valsartan in chronic heart failure. N Engl J Med 2001; 345: 1667–1675.
30. Jette M, Heller R, Landry F, Blumchen G. Randomized 4-week exercise program in patients with impaired left ventricular function. Circulation 1991; 84: 1561–1567.
31. Erbs S, Linke A, Gielen S, *et al.* Exercise training in patients with severe chronic heart failure: impact on left ventricular performance and cardiac size; a retrospective analysis of the Leipzig Heart Failure Training Trial. Eur J Cardiovasc Prev Rehabil 2003; 10: 336–344.
32. Chua TP, Ponikowski P, Harrington D, *et al.* Clinical correlates and prognostic significance of the ventilatory response to exercise in chronic heart failure. J Am Coll Cardiol 1997; 29: 1585–1590.
33. Borg GA. Psychophysical bases of perceived exertion. Med Sci Sports Exerc 1982; 14: 377–381.
34. Belardinelli R, Georgiou D, Cianci G, *et al.* Exercise training improves left ventricular diastolic filling in patients with dilated cardiomyopathy. Clinical and prognostic implications. Circulation 1995; 91: 2775–2784.
35. Sturm B, Quittan M, Wiesinger GF, *et al.* Moderate-intensity exercise training with elements of step aerobics in patients with severe chronic heart failure. Arch Phys Med Rehabil 1999; 80: 746–750.

CHAPTER 34

Calcium sensitizers in acute heart failure

John G F Cleland, Krishna M Lalukota, Anne-Marie Seymour

Introduction

Acute heart failure is heterogeneous in its pathophysiology, etiology, and presentation. Classic pathophysiological features are an increase in systemic vascular resistance (SVR) and pulmonary capillary pressure, which may be accompanied by a fall in cardiac output. The etiology of acute heart failure is complex and can result from systolic and diastolic ventricular dysfunction or valve disease. There are, in addition, many precipitating factors including myocardial ischemia, arrhythmias (especially atrial fibrillation), hypertension, infection, anemia, adverse effects from taking inappropriate therapy, not taking appropriate therapy, or excess dietary salt. Presentations include acute cardiogenic pulmonary edema or shock, with or without a preceding history of chronic heart failure, and subacute decompensation, often characterized by salt and water retention, leading to progressive fatigue, exertional breathlessness, orthopnea and edema. Many patients present with a mixture of the above.

There are few adequately designed trials with any group of agents directed at the treatment of acute heart failure. Treatment is based largely on theoretical principles. Acute pulmonary edema is managed by either reducing the pulmonary capillary wedge pressure (PCWP) rapidly by altering hemodynamics or more slowly using diuretics, or by increasing alveolar pressure using continuous positive airways pressure (CPAP) devices. Cardiogenic shock is managed by trying to reduce the load on the failing heart while maintaining or increasing organ perfusion pressure and flow. Medical therapy has shown limited success in the management of shock. Treatment targeted at removing the underlying problem (e.g., myocardial ischemia [MI], ruptured ventricular septum) or mechanical interventions (e.g., intraaortic balloon pump [IABP]) should be considered. Patients with pre-existing chronic heart failure due to left ventricular systolic dysfunction (LVSD) are more likely to present with severe breathless raised pulmonary capillary pressures, low-normal blood pressure and a low cardiac output. In contrast, patients with preserved LV systolic function are more likely to present with marked increases in SVR, raised pulmonary capillary pressures, raised blood pressure, and a relatively normal cardiac output. Until the gaps in knowledge are plugged, treatment options should be tailored to the known or likely pathophysiology on an individual patient basis.

An important feature of heart failure is a reduction in ventricular contractility. Abnormalities in myocardial intracellular calcium handling are thought to be major factors underlying this dysfunction. Specifically, altered expression and function of key proteins involved in excitation–contraction coupling and relaxation have been observed in patients with heart failure. These include a decrease in expression of the ryanodine receptor (RyR2), the calcium release channel of the sarcoplasmic reticulum (SR) and inappropriate phosphorylation, in response to chronic beta-adrenergic stimulation. In consequence, hyperphosphorylation of RyR2 can lead to abnormal calcium release from the SR, a subsequent depletion of calcium stores, and ultimately decreased myocardial contractility and impaired systolic function.

In the relaxation phase, there is strong evidence from both clinical and experimental studies for a reduction in expression and function of the key calcium uptake protein, sarcoplasmic reticulum calcium ion adenosine triphosphatase (Ca^{2+} ATPase [SERCA2a]), in cardiac hypertrophy and heart failure, which correlates with impaired contractility. Reduction in this calcium pump results in a decreased rate of calcium removal from the cytosol, thus prolonging the relaxation phase. In addition, altered expression and regulation of the SERCA regulatory protein, phospholamban, have been shown to modify both SERCA activity and SR Ca^{2+} loading, with decreased phosphorylation inhibiting SERCA activity and prolonging relaxation. This can lead to a rise in intracellular diastolic calcium concentrations. It is controversial whether there is a loss of sensitivity of the actin-myosin-troponin-tropomyosin complex to calcium when other factors have been controlled for, including inadequate calcium ion re-uptake or changes in calcium ionization due to changes in intracellular hydrogen ion concentration (pH). The force–frequency relationship describes the increase in contractility observed in the normal myocardium as the frequency of contraction increases. This is depressed or lost in heart failure, providing some clinical evidence to support the theory of calcium desensitization in the failing heart.

Theoretically, calcium sensitizers should increase myocardial contractility without increasing myocardial energy consumption, which could be highly beneficial in the failing heart. Unfortunately, as they might act in both diastole and systole they could also impair myocardial relaxation, which would be undesirable. Agents with ancillary properties that either increase the re-uptake of calcium into the SR, thus reducing calcium ion concentration during diastole, or act only in systole might have more desirable effects.

Currently, no agent that acts as a specific calcium sensitizer without any other potentially important mode of action has been tested in patients. A variety of agents may sensitize the actin-myosin complex to calcium but this has not been their primary mode of action. There is little evidence that these agents are useful, or even safe, for the management of patients with heart failure. So far, only one agent, levosimendan, that appears to mediate a positive inotropic effect primarily through calcium sensitization, has been tested in patients. It is also a vasodilator and, therefore, the benefits of the drug may not be mediated entirely, or indeed predominantly, through calcium sensitization.

Levosimendan: Mechanisms of Action

Levosimendan has multiple mechanisms of action (Table 34.1). From animal and in-vitro experiments, it appears to exert its inotropic effect mainly by keeping troponin C stabilized for longer in the conformation that triggers and maintains contraction in the presence of calcium ions. Sensitization is calcium-concentration dependent,[1–5] so that the contractile apparatus is sensitized in systole but not in diastole, leading to an inotropic effect without impairing diastolic relaxation.[5–7] Agents which act through adrenergic pathways may cause a rise in cytosolic calcium concentration, which might provoke cardiac myocyte dysfunction, arrhythmias, and cell death. Unlike these agents, levosimendan may not cause this rise in cytosolic calcium concentration. With agents that exert part of their action through calcium sensitization (e.g., pimobendan, which is also a phosphodiesterase [PDE] inhibitor), the affinity of troponin C for calcium is increased in both systole and diastole, so although contractility is enhanced, diastolic function may be impaired.[8] Levosimendan may also increase calcium-dependent inotropic effects by enhancing the release and re-uptake of calcium into the SR.[9] Levosimendan exerts positive

Table 34.1. *Mechanisms of action of levosimendan*

Calcium-concentration-dependent enhancement of binding of calcium to tropomyosin
Stabilizing troponin C in "contraction" phase
Increased myocardial contractility
No increase in cytosolic calcium concentration or calcium sensitivity during diastole
No impairment of relaxation
Possible increase in sarcoplasmic reticulum calcium re-uptake
Potential improvement in diastolic function
Activation of adenosine triphosphate (ATP)-sensitive potassium channels in vascular smooth muscle
Coronary, peripheral, and pulmonary arterial vasodilatation
Potent metabolite with similar profile of action and an 80-hour half-life

inotropic and lusitropic effects when infused directly into the coronary circulation at concentrations that do not have peripheral vascular effects, suggesting that the hemodynamic effects of levosimendan are mediated, at least in part, directly on the myocardium.[10,11] OR-1986 is an active, potent, acetylated metabolite of levosimendan with a long half-life. OR-1986 is also a calcium sensitizer, which may be responsible for most of levosimendan's longer-term effects.[12] It is not yet clear whether the actions of OR-1896 are calcium-concentration-dependent or whether it interacts with potassium channels in the same way as its parent compound.

Levosimendan causes arteriolar and venous dilatation due to its ability to open ATP-sensitive potassium channels on vascular smooth muscle.[13–15] Levosimendan is also a selective PDE III inhibitor in vitro although this effect probably only occurs at concentrations above the therapeutic dose range.[16] Levosimendan is very specific for PDE III rather than PDE IV and therefore may not increase intracellular calcium or cyclic adenosine monophosphate (cAMP).

Improved contractile performance and vasodilatation may lead to a reduction in the preload and afterload of the failing heart. Improved cardiac efficiency means that improved performance does not increase oxygen consumption and may even reduce it.[17–19] Combined with coronary vasodilatation,[11,20] this may have anti-ischemic effects. Right ventricular function and efficiency may also improve.[19]

The increase in cardiac output is distributed to the heart, liver and kidneys, whilst that to resting skeletal muscle is maintained but not increased.[19–21] Anecdotal reports that an increase in renal blood flow may result in a diuresis are yet to be confirmed objectively, although a reduction in weight was noted in one study during a 7-day infusion.[12] Venous capacitance may also increase, as expected given the ability of levosimendan to cause venous dilatation. Preliminary data suggest that pulmonary vascular resistance may also fall.[19]

No tolerance to the effects of levosimendan has been observed, despite infusions lasting up to 7 days.[22] Additionally, no rebound decline in hemodynamic variables has been observed after withdrawal of levosimendan.

In healthy subjects, levosimendan does not appear to increase heart rate directly.[23] However, in patients with heart failure, an increase in heart rate has been observed with infusions lasting for several hours.[24,25] This effect is less marked in patients with severe heart failure. Increases in heart rate may reflect a reflex response to excessive lowering of filling pressures in patients without markedly elevated baseline values and may be mediated partly through sympathetic activation,[25] although beta-blockers do not prevent the increase in heart rate.[26–28] It is also possible that OR-1896 has a more marked chronotropic effect than the parent compound, as heart rate changes may be more closely related to the metabolite and remain elevated for some days after stopping the infusion, by which time levosimendan has disappeared from the circulation.[26] Levosimendan shortens sinus node recovery time, which may be responsible for a direct chronotropic effect of the drug.[29] Levosimendan shortens atrial (20 to 30 ms), atrioventricular nodal (40 to 60 ms), and ventricular (5 to 10 ms) effective refractory periods and ventricular monophasic action potential by 5 to 20 ms in patients with normal cardiac function.[29,30] These properties indicate that levosimendan might accelerate atrioventricular conduction which might increase the ventricular rate in patients with atrial fibrillation, suggesting that special care may be required to control ventricular rate in this population. Shortening of the ventricular refractory period could improve ventricular dyssynchrony.[31,32] Levosimendan has little or no direct effect on the QT interval, although QTc (QT corrected for the increase in heart rate using Bazett's formula) is increased by up to 50 ms.[12,22,29] This may reflect the inadequacy of Bazett's formula.[22] There is no evidence of a pro-arrhythmic effect either clinically or on ambulatory electrocardiogram (ECG) monitoring.[29,30]

Reductions in myocardial ischemia and infarct size have been demonstrated in animal experiments.[33] In an experimental canine model of ventricular stunning, levosimendan improved contractile function and synchrony.[11] In humans, levosimendan improved the function of stunned myocardium in patients with acute myocardial infarction (AMI) undergoing angioplasty.[34] In studies of heart failure, infusion of levosimendan did not cause elevations in troponin-T, a sensitive marker of myocardial damage.[25]

Levosimendan reduces plasma concentrations of endothelin-1 (ET-1) in patients with severe heart failure but does not increase plasma norepinephrine.[35] However, in patients with mild heart failure, levosimendan may increase plasma concentrations of norepinephrine.[25] Levosimendan reduces plasma concentration of brain (B-type) natriuretic peptide (BNP),[25] an effect that persists for several days after cessation of the infusion, implying a sustained reduction in cardiac filling pressures or improved renal clearance. These data suggest that levosimendan may exert beneficial neuroendocrine effects in patients with severe heart failure but that reflex activation of the sympathetic nervous system may occur in patients who do not have markedly elevated filling pressures. Heart rate variability and autonomic function appear unaffected, at least during a short-term (6-hour) infusion.[36]

Pharmacokinetics and Metabolism

Levosimendan was developed as an intravenous agent. Despite high oral bioavailability (85%), levosimendan's complex pharmacokinetics have delayed development of an oral preparation.[12,37–39]

Levosimendan is rapidly distributed. Steady state is achieved within 4 hours of a constant dose infusion. A loading dose can be used to obtain a more rapid effect. There is a linear relationship between the dose administered and plasma concentrations achieved. About 97% of levosimendan is bound to plasma proteins, particularly albumin. Elimination is mainly by conjugation and excretion in urine and feces with an elimination half-life of about 1 hour.

About 5% of levosimendan is acetylated to form the active metabolite, OR-1896. This metabolite is formed from an intermediate metabolite OR-1855, which may also have some activity. OR-1855 is formed mainly by the action of intestinal bacteria on levosimendan excreted presumably by the biliary route. Reabsorbed OR-1855 is then acetylated to OR-1896. Formation of OR-1896 is slow, with peak metabolite concentrations occurring 1 to 2 days after cessation of a 24-hour infusion of levosimendan.[22,27] About 40% of OR-1896 is bound to plasma proteins. The elimination half-lives of OR-1896 and OR-1855 are both about 80 hours.[12] Accordingly, the pharmacological effects of the OR-1896 metabolite may persist for about 1 week.[22,27]

Potential Interactions with Drugs and Disease

Acetylator status does not influence the pharmacokinetics of levosimendan but rapid acetylators appear to form more of the active metabolite OR-1896. This does not appear to influence the short-term pharmacodynamic response to levosimendan, but it may further prolong the duration of effect.

Cytochrome P-450 enzymes do not appear to play a role in the metabolism of levosimendan or its active metabolite as indicated by a lack of interaction with itraconazole,[40] warfarin,[41] and felodipine.[42]

The severity of heart failure and the presence of renal dysfunction have little effect on the pharmacokinetics of levosimendan,[43,44] but these factors may have an effect on the pharmacokinetics of OR-1896. Liver cirrhosis prolongs the elimination half-life of levosimendan slightly, but the effects on production or metabolism of OR-1896 are unknown. Although definitive data are lacking, the potential for agents that suppress the gastrointestinal flora to interfere with the production of this metabolite exist.

The positive inotropic and chronotropic effects of levosimendan were not affected by carvedilol,[28] a beta-blocker, or felodipine,[42] a calcium antagonist. No significant interaction has been observed with captopril,[45] an angiotensin-converting enzyme (ACE) inhibitor, or oral isosorbide mononitrate.[46] However, in each case the hypotensive effects of each agent was additive and with nitrates this led to some postural hypotension.

Clinical Studies

A number of randomized controlled trials primarily investigating the hemodynamic effects of levosimendan as compared to placebo or dobutamine have been reported. Clinical outcome data have also been reported from 4 medium-sized trials including more than 1000 patients overall, although at least one of these trials, Levosimendan Infusion versus Dobutamine in Severe Low Output Heart Failure (LIDO), focused primarily on patients with worsening chronic heart failure rather than acutely symptomatic patients.

Hemodynamic studies

Three substantial randomized placebo or active-comparator controlled hemodynamic studies with infusions lasting 6 to 48 hours have been reported (Table 34.2 and Table 34.3).[24,25,47] One further study compared 2 doses of levosimendan infused for up to 7 days.[22] Another study used only a 5-minute infusion and is reported only briefly.[48] These studies demonstrate that, at recommended doses, levosimendan reduces PCWP by 4 to 6 mm Hg and increases cardiac output by 0.4 to 0.8 L/min. The increase in cardiac output reflects both an increase in stroke volume and heart rate. SVR falls significantly and systolic blood pressure tends to decline. Pulmonary artery pressures and vascular resistance decline although the transpulmonary gradient is not markedly affected.

Dose-ranging study

A double-blind, dose-ranging study including 151 patients with mainly stable New York Heart Association (NYHA) class II to IV heart failure and comparing 5 different doses of levosimendan to a placebo, open-label dobutamine, and an ethanol "vehicle" group infused over 24 hours, was conducted (Table 34.2 and Table 34.3, Figure 34.1).[24] The dose of levosimendan ranged from 0.05 μg/kg/min to 0.6 μg/kg/min and each dose was preceded by a 10-minute loading infusion, which was also dose ranged. Dose-dependent effects of levosimendan on cardiac output and PCWP were noted with significant hemodynamic effects even at the lowest dose. All doses of levosimendan exerted a greater reduction in PCWP as compared to placebo or dobutamine. Levosimendan and dobutamine exerted similar effects on stroke volume but higher doses of levosimendan had a greater effect on cardiac output due to greater increases in heart rate. SVR fell equally with levosimendan and dobutamine at recommended doses, although further vasodilatation occurred with higher doses of levosimendan. A fall in mean systemic arterial pressure of 5 to 10 mm Hg was noted with higher doses of levosimendan. Pulmonary vascular resistance (PVR) declined with higher doses of levosimendan although the transpulmonary gradient was not reduced.

Dose-escalation study

A double-blind, dose-escalation study randomized 146 patients with NYHA class III-IV heart failure

Table 34.2. *Entry criteria and baseline characteristics of patients in substantial trials of levosimendan for heart failure**

	Dose-ranging study[35] (n = 151)	**Dose escalation study[34] (n = 146)**	**LIDO study[56] (n = 203)**	**RUSSLAN study[49] (n = 504)**	**REVIVE-I[57] (n = 100)**	**CASINO[58] (n = 299)**	**REVIVE-II (target n = 700)**	**SURVIVE (target n = 1300+)**
Levosimendan compared with	Placebo and dobutamine	Placebo	Dobutamine	Placebo	Placebo	Placebo and dobutamine	Placebo	Dobutamine
NYHA class	III (98%) IV (2%)	III (66%) IV (34%)	III/IV	IV	IV	IV	IV	IV
LVEF	< 40% (26%)	≤ 30% (21%)	< 35%	NReq	< 35%	≤ 35%	< 35%	< 35%
Hospital admission for worsening heart failure	NReq	Yes	Yes	Yes (AMI)	Yes	Yes	Yes	Yes
Diuretics (% used)	NReq (74%)	Required (NR)	NReq (76%)	NReq (75%)	Required		Required	NReq
ACE inhibitors	NReq (61%)	Required (NR)	NReq (90%)	NReq (47%)				NReq
Beta-blockers	NReq (28%)	NReq (NR)	NReq (38%)	NReq (39%)				NReq
PCWP (mm Hg)	NReq (16)	> 15	> 15	Not measured				NReq (> 18†)
Cardiac output (L/min) or Cardiac Index (L/min/m²)	NReq (4.8)	CI < 2.5	CI < 2.5	Not measured				NReq (CI < 2.2†)
Age (years)	62	58	59	67	59	71	TBR	TBR
Gender (% female)	9	18	12	49	23	29	TBR	TBR
Etiology (% CAD)	100	60	48	100	47	54 prior MI	TBR	TBR
Rapid AF excluded	Yes	Yes	Yes	Yes		TBR		Yes

Table 34.2. *continued*

	Dose-ranging study[35] (n = 151)	Dose escalation study[34] (n = 146)	LIDO study[56] (n = 203)	RUSSLAN study[49] (n = 504)	REVIVE-I[57] (n = 100)	CASINO[58] (n = 299)	REVIVE-II (target n = 700)	SURVIVE (target n = 1300+)
Serious arrhythmias excluded	Yes	Yes	Yes	Yes		TBR		Torsades de pointe
Systolic blood pressure excluded (mm Hg)	< 100	< 85	< 85	< 90		TBR		< 80
Severe angina excluded	Yes	Yes	Yes	No		TBR		No
Valve stenosis or LVOT excluded	Yes	Yes	Yes	Yes		TBR		Yes
Serum creatinine excluded (µmol/L)	> 150	> 200	> 450	> 250		TBR		> 450

*Hemodynamic effects at 0.1 ug/kg/min.
†When measured.
Abbreviations: ACE = angiotensin-converting enzyme; AF = atrial fibrillation; AMI = acute myocardial infarction; CI = cardiac index; LVOT = left ventricular outflow tract obstruction; LVEF = left ventricular ejection fraction; NYHA = New York Heart Association; NR = not reported; NReq = not required as entry criterion;
PCWP = pulmonary capillary wedge pressure; TBR = to be reported.

Table 34.3. *Hemodynamic effects of levosimendan at 0.1 μg/kg/min*

	Dose-ranging study (~24 hours)[@]			Dose-escalation study (1 hour)			LIDO study (24 hours)				
	Baseline	Placebo	Levosimendan	Baseline	Placebo	Levosimendan	Baseline	Dobutamine		Levosimendan	
								1 h	24 h	1 h	24 h
HR	72	+7	+7	81	−1	+1	82	NR	+4	NR	+6
sSAP	NA			NA			115	NR	NR	NR	NR
MSAP	86	+1	−3	84	0	−1	NR	NR	NR	NR	NR
PCWP	14	+1	−5[†]	27	−1	−3*	25	−3	−3	−5	−7[†]
CO or CI[#]	4.8	−0.3	+0.4[†]	1.8[#]	0	+0.3**	3.7	+1.3	+0.8	+1.2	+1.1*
SV	67	−7	−2	46	+1	+7*	48	+11	+8	+12	+10
SVR	NR	NR	Reduced[†]	1700	0	−220*		−6.5	−4.6	−6.2	−5.8
PVR	NR	NR	Reduced[†]	Na	+20	−15	NR	NR	NR	NR	NR
TPG	16	−1	0	11	+1m	+1	NR	NR	NR	NR	NR
ANP (ng/L)	150	−5	−36	NR	RN	NR	NR	NR	NR	NR	NR
NE (nmol/L)	2.3	0	+0.6	NR	NR	NR	NR	NR	NR	NR	NR

[@]Little difference was noted in hemodynamics at 1–hour and 24–hour measurements. * $P < 0.05$; ** $P < 0.01$; [†] $P < 0.001$

Abbreviations: ANP = atrial natriuretic peptide; CI = cardiac index; CO = cardiac output; HR = heart rate; MSAP = mean systemic arterial pressure; NA = not available; NE = norepinephrine; NR = not reported; PCWP = pulmonary capillary wedge pressure; PVR = pulmonary vascular resistance; sSAP = systolic systemic arterial pressure; SV = stroke volume; SVR = systemic vascular resistance; TPG = transpulmonary gradient.

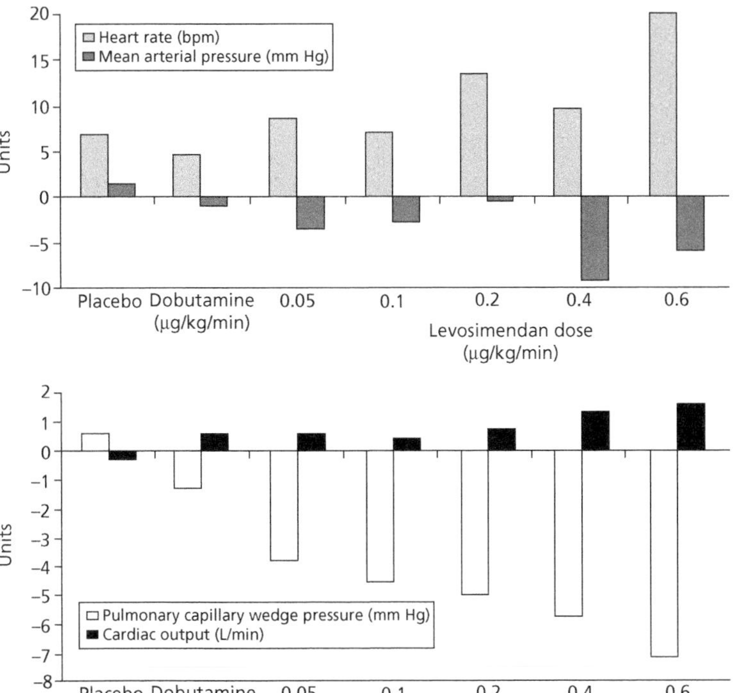

Figure 34.1. *Dose-ranging study of the hemodynamic effects of levosimendan as compared to placebo and dobutamine*

hospitalized for treatment of worsening heart failure guided by invasive hemodynamic monitoring to levosimendan or placebo (Table 34.2 and Table 34.3).[25] Levosimendan was initiated as a 6 μg/kg bolus followed by an infusion at 0.1 μg/kg/min for 1 hour followed by hourly increments of 0.1 μg/kg/min up to a maximum of 0.4 μg/kg/min (each preceded by a further bolus of 6 μg/kg) or matching placebo for 6 hours. Of the patients, 70% were titrated to the maximum dose of levosimendan. Reduction in PCWP to ≤ 10 mm Hg was the commonest reason for not attaining the top dose, followed by an increase in heart rate above baseline of ≥ 15 bpm. Patients randomized to levosimendan then received open-label drug for the remainder of the 24 hours. Subsequently, patients were randomized to continue levosimendan for a further 24 hours or to have it withdrawn. Further hemodynamic measurements were made at 48 hours.

Levosimendan increased stroke volume by about 12 mL (baseline 46 mL) and cardiac index by 0.7 L/min/m^2 (baseline 1.8 L/min/m^2) with significant effects even at the lowest dose. Heart rate increased by an average of 6 bpm at higher doses, although this could also reflect the effect of more prolonged infusion. SVR and PVR declined while mean systemic arterial pressure dropped by 4 mm Hg. Transpulmonary gradient was not affected. For those who remained on the infusion, hemodynamic effects persisted or increased over the subsequent 48 hours. However, amongst patients in whom levosimendan had been withdrawn after 24 hours of infusion, the hemodynamic effects at 48 hours were as great as in patients who had continued to receive the drug. The sustained effect after cessation of infusion appeared to be related to the active metabolite, concentrations of which continued to rise for at least 24 hours after stopping the infusion.[26]

The Levosimendan Infusion versus Dobutamine in Severe Low Output Heart Failure study

The Levosimendan Infusion versus Dobutamine in Severe Low Output Heart Failure (LIDO) study, a double-blind study comparing infusion over 24 hours of levosimendan (24 μg/kg over 10 minutes followed by 0.1 μg/kg/min) with dobutamine (initially 5 μg/kg/min), was conducted on 203 patients mainly with an exacerbation of severe chronic heart failure; few patients with acute heart failure were included (Table 34.2 and Table 34.3, Figure 34.2).[47] Infusion rates were doubled after 2 hours in 69 patients randomized to levosimendan and 40 patients randomized to dobutamine whose cardiac output had not risen by more than 30%. Further hemodynamic measurements were made at 30 hours. At the doses used, levosimendan increased cardiac output and reduced PCWP to a greater extent than dobutamine. Levosimendan reduced systolic blood pressure more and tended to cause more vasodilatation. The effects of dobutamine were markedly attenuated by beta-blockers but the effects of levosimendan tended to be enhanced. Six hours after stopping the infusion, the hemodynamic effects of dobutamine had disappeared but those of levosimendan persisted.

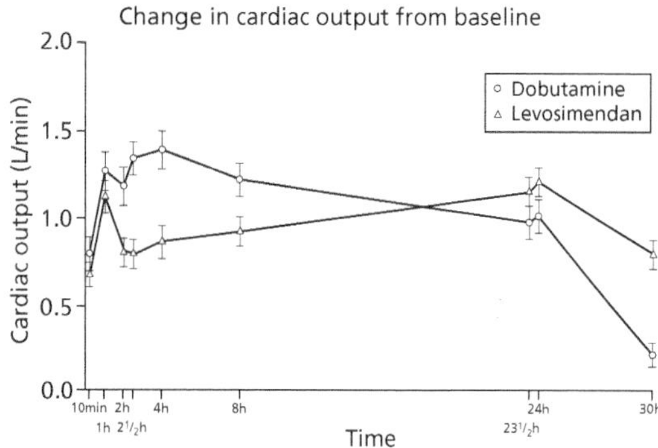

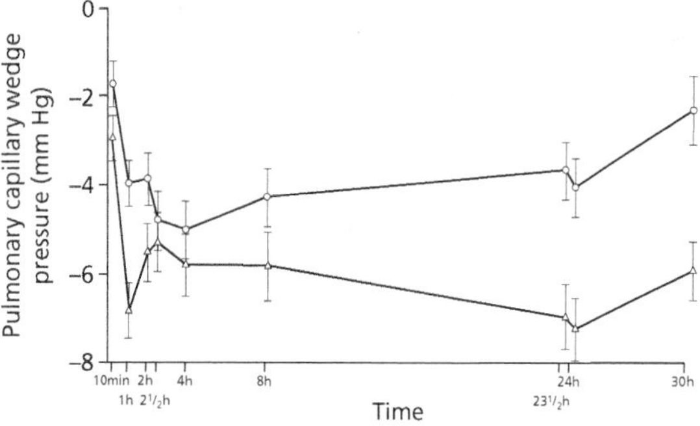

Figure 34.2. *Time of course of the hemodynamic effects of levosimendan and dobutamine in the Levosimendan Infusion versus Dobutamine in Severe Low Output Heart Failure (LIDO) study. Levosimendan was given as 24 μg/kg/min for 10 min then 0.1 μg/kg/min and could be titrated to 0.2 μg/kg/min if inadequate hemodynamic response after 2 hours. Dobutamine was given as 5 μg/kg/min initially and titrated to 10 μg/kg/min if inadequate hemodynamic response after 2 hours*

†Primary endpoint.

‡Secondary endpoint.

Seven-day study

Twenty-four patients with NYHA class III or IV heart failure were randomized to an infusion of 0.05 μg/kg/min or 0.1 μg/kg/min for 7 days, during which time heart rate, blood pressure, and ECG were monitored.[22] Heart rate rose progressively over 7 days, with a maximum increase of 18 bpm and 26 bpm with the lower and higher dose of levosimendan respectively. Heart rate was still increased by about 10 bpm, 14 days after cessation of the infusion. Blood pressure fell by 6 mm Hg and 11 mm Hg during infusions, with lower and higher doses respectively, but returned to baseline within 3 days of stopping therapy. PR and QTc intervals declined by 10 to 20 ms and 40 to 50 ms respectively, although absolute QT interval did not change. Hemoglobin declined by about 1 g/dL during infusion. With the higher dose of levosimendan, weight dropped by 1.9 kg, suggesting that a diuresis may have occurred. Steady state for the formation of the active metabolite was not reached by 7 days. Metabolite concentrations peaked about 24 hours after stopping the infusion. Plasma concentrations declined slowly thereafter and were detectable and probably still at therapeutic concentrations 2 weeks after cessation of infusion.

Bolus study

The Bolus study randomized 24 patients to 5-minute bolus infusions of levosimendan ranging from 0.25 mg to 4 mg.[48] The study showed increases in heart rate and cardiac output with reductions in filling pressure, peaking at about 10 minutes. Effects were observed with the lowest dose and were broadly dose related. Higher doses of levosimendan did not increase stroke volume, perhaps reflecting a excessive fall in filling pressures.

Effects on symptoms

Symptoms were assessed in the dose-escalation[25] and LIDO[47] studies and in a large safety study called Randomized Study on Safety and Effectiveness of Levosimendan in Patients with Left Ventricular Failure After an Acute Myocardial Infarct (RUSSLAN).[49] Symptoms were also assessed in a pilot study called Randomized Multicenter Evaluation of Intravenous Levosimendan Efficacy vs. Placebo in the Short-term Treatment of Acute Heart Failure (REVIVE)-I[57] (Table 34.2).

Effects on symptoms in the dose-escalation study

In the dose escalation study, both patients and doctors judged that the patient's symptoms were more often improved on levosimendan compared to placebo at the end of the 6-hour double-blind phase. Similar trends were observed for fatigue.

Effects on symptoms in the LIDO study

In the LIDO study, non-significant trends for a greater improvement in breathlessness and fatigue were noted among patients receiving levosimendan compared to dobutamine. However, many of these patients were not markedly symptomatic at rest. It is possible that patients with more severe symptoms would have shown clearer benefit. Also, the judgement of both patient and physician may have been influenced by their knowledge of changes in hemodynamic measurements in these studies and any apparent change in symptoms should be interpreted with caution.

Effects on symptoms in the RUSSLAN study

The RUSSLAN study (Table 34.2) enrolled 504 patients with radiological pulmonary congestion or edema, the vast majority of whom were reported to be breathless and have rales (suggesting clinically acute pulmonary edema), within 5 days of an MI. Patients were randomized to either placebo or 1 of 4 different 6-hour dosing regimens of levosimendan (initial 10-min bolus of 6 µg/kg, 12 µg/kg, or 24 µg/kg followed by infusion of 0.2 µg/kg/min or a bolus of 24 µg/kg followed by infusion of 0.4 µg/kg/min) in addition to usual background therapy with the exception of other intravenous inotropic agents. The primary objective of the study was to examine the safety of levosimendan in this high-risk population, targeting particularly the risk of hypotension and ischemia. Levosimendan was found not to exacerbate these conditions except possibly at the highest dose (Figure 34.3) Hemodynamic monitoring was discouraged. Overall, there was no impact of levosimendan on symptoms. In each group, 48% of patients reported an improvement. However, an outcome of death or worsening heart failure was less likely with levosimendan compared with placebo at 6 hours (5.9% vs. 2.0%; $P = 0.033$) and at 24 hours (8.8% vs. 4.0%; $P = 0.044$). Also, if a worst outcome analysis was done, including death, worsening heart failure, or need for rescue therapy over the first 6 hours, then patients treated with levosimendan experienced less worsening (17.0% vs. 10.8%; $P = 0.042$). Using patient self-assessment, probably the most relevant method for assessment, levosimendan was again associated with fewer reports of worsening symptoms (16.7% vs. 11.0%; $P = 0.056$). Worsening fatigue was also reported less often by patients taking levosimendan (16.7% vs. 10.08%; $P = 0.045$).

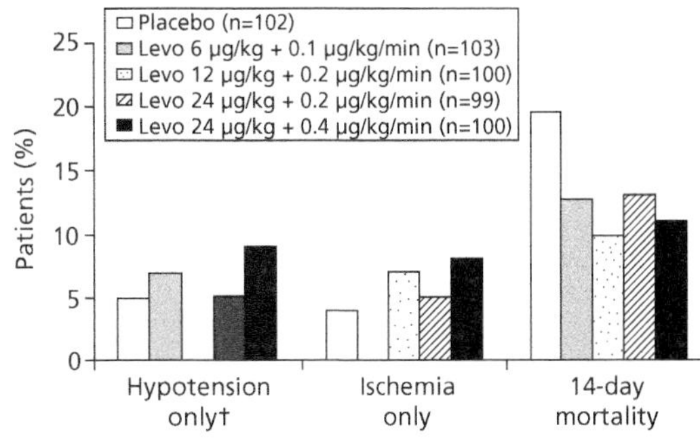

Figure 34.3. *Relationship between dose of levosimendan, side effects, and mortality in patients with post-infarction heart failure (Randomized Study on Safety and Effectiveness of Levosimendan in Patients with Left Ventricular Failure After an Acute Myocardial Infarct [RUSSLAN] study). Note lack of increase in mortality despite use of high doses of levosimendan*

Effects on symptoms in the REVIVE-1 study

The REVIVE-I pilot study enrolled 100 patients with worsening heart failure leading to breathlessness at rest despite administration of an intravenous bolus of diuretic. Patients were randomized to either placebo or levosimendan (12 μg/kg bolus followed by 0.1 μg/kg/min for 1 hour and then 0.2 μg/kg/min for 23 hours). The principal aim of this pilot study was to test the definition of a proposed primary outcome measure for a larger study, REVIVE-II, which was clinical status at 24 hours and 5 days after randomization. Patients were asked to record on a 7-point scale whether they were markedly, moderately, or mildly improved; worse; or unchanged. Patients who had deteriorated at either time point or had not improved by 24 hours were considered to have met the definition of worsening but only if they required "rescue" therapy. Intravenous diuretics were considered rescue therapy only after 3 days. Clinical deterioration also included deteriorating invasively-assessed hemodynamics, worsening renal function, or death. Patients had to be moderately or markedly better to be considered improved. Outcomes were also adjudicated separately according to the protocol-defined outcome by an expert panel.

By intention to treat and using the predefined criteria, 47% of patients improved on levosimendan and 20% deteriorated, whilst 31% improved on placebo and 27% met the definition of worsening. The trend toward greater improvement with levosimendan was not significant, but the study was not adequately powered for this outcome. However, if change in status at 6 hours or the use of intravenous rescue diuretics at any time was included, and if hemodynamic data were ignored, then 33% of patients were reported to have improved with levosimendan and 24% worsened, compared to 14% improved and 37% worsened on placebo ($P = 0.029$). Levosimendan was associated with an increase in adverse events such as headache and dizziness and a trend toward more hypotension, mostly asymptomatic. There were few deaths reported by 5 days. The investigator concluded that patients were a better judge of treatment effect than their physicians, which may come as a surprise to some. This definition is now the primary outcome measure for REVIVE-II.

Effects on morbidity and mortality

The effect of levosimendan on morbidity and mortality was a pre-specified secondary outcome in the LIDO[47] and RUSSLAN[49] studies and the primary outcome measure in the Calcium Sensitizer or Inotrope or None in Low Output Heart Failure (CASINO) trial (Figure 34.4 and Figure 34.5).

Effects on morbidity and mortality in the LIDO study

In the LIDO study, 3 deaths occurred during infusion of dobutamine but none on levosimendan. At the pre-specified 31-day time point, there was a significantly lower mortality with levosimendan compared to dobutamine and a reduction in the composite of death or worsening heart failure reported as an adverse event. Regulatory authorities requested that 6-month mortality should also be reported. Retrospective acquisition of these data

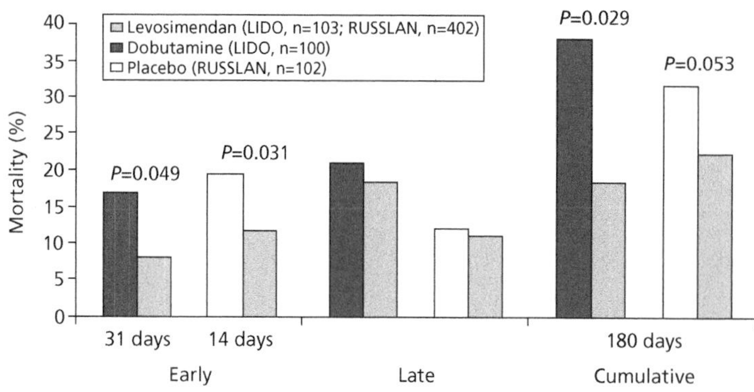

Figure 34.4. *Early (prospectively declared endpoint) and late (retrospectively requested by regulators) mortality in the RUSSLAN (compared to placebo) and LIDO (compared to dobutamine) studies. Note that early mortality on levosimendan was lower in both studies without any evidence of 'catch-up' before 6 months*

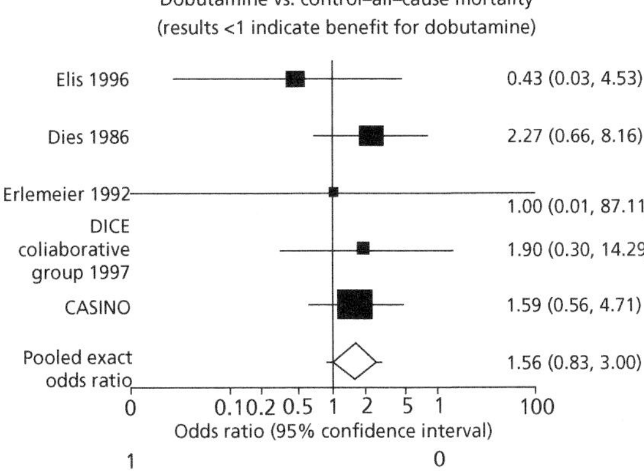

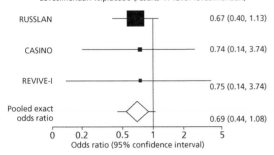

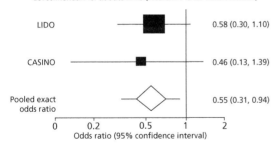

Figure 34.5. *Meta-analysis of published or presented randomized controlled studies of levosimendan or dobutamine compared to inactive control, placebo, or each other. These data suggest a powerful trend toward increased mortality with dobutamine and a powerful trend toward reduced mortality with levosimendan. However, only the difference between dobutamine and levosimendan is significant*

suggested that the early mortality benefit was sustained out to 6 months; no "catch-up" increase in mortality was observed. By 180 days, 27 patients (26%) who were randomized to a single 24-hour infusion of levosimendan had died versus 38 patients (38%) who received dobutamine (hazard ratio [HR], 0.57; 95% CI, 0.34–0.95; $P = 0.029$). A reduction in the composite outcome of death or hospitalization with heart failure and an increase in the number of days alive and out of the hospital over 180 days was also observed.

The results of the LIDO study have led to much speculation, especially since it is the largest randomized trial of dobutamine for heart failure ever conducted.[50] The difference between levosimendan and dobutamine may have arisen by chance. Alternatively, dobutamine may have had an adverse effect on survival as has been observed previously in repetitive dosing studies.[50] Acute exposure to powerful adrenergic stimulants may not only provoke arrhythmias but also accelerate programmed cell death of cardiac myocytes, thus worsening both short-term and long-term outcome. A third possibility is that levosimendan might exert a sustained beneficial effect on hemodynamics, with possible secondary neuroendocrine benefits without the hazards of arrhythmogenesis, cellular calcium overload and induction of cell death. This combination of effects may lead to an improvement in medium- and long-term survival.

Effects on morbidity and mortality in the RUSSLAN study

In the RUSSLAN study, the composite outcome of death or worsening heart failure at 24 hours was reduced from 8.8% to 4.0% ($P = 0.04$). Early reduction in mortality may have been related primarily to a reduction in myocardial rupture (3.9% vs. 0.25%; $P = 0.027$). All-cause mortality at 14 days was reduced from 19.6% to 11.7% ($P = 0.03$). At 180 days, mortality on levosimendan was 22.6% (91 of 402) compared to 31.4% (32 of 102) on placebo (HR, 0.67; 95% CI, 0.45–1.00; $P = 0.05$). Importantly, the reduction in mortality appeared similar regardless of the dose of levosimendan used in this study.

Effects on morbidity and mortality in the REVIVE-I study

A preliminary report from the REVIVE-I study indicated only 5 deaths on placebo and 4 deaths on levosimendan at 90 days.

Effects on morbidity and mortality in the CASINO study

The CASINO trial was an investigator-initiated study designed to compare the safety and efficacy of levosimendan, dobutamine, and placebo in patients with decompensated heart failure, with mortality as the primary endpoint.

Hospitalized patients with NYHA class IV heart failure and LVEF ≤ 35% were randomized to treatment with levosimendan, dobutamine, or placebo, infused intravenously over 24 hours. The study was originally designed to recruit 600 patients. However, the study was stopped prematurely after 299 patients had been enrolled, due to lower mortality on levosimendan compared to dobutamine. Although recruitment was stopped, follow-up continued. As further data became available, it appeared that survival was also significantly better on levosimendan compared to placebo. However, it should be noted that these data might not be complete and the number of deaths was not large; 28 deaths at 31 days (14 after dobutamine, 8 after placebo, and 6 after levosimendan) and after 6-month follow-up, 88 deaths (42 after dobutamine, 28 after placebo, and 18 after levosimendan) reported so far.

Safety concerns

Levosimendan increases ventricular rate and steps should be taken to control any pre-existing tachycardia prior to or concomitant with the introduction of levosimendan.

Levosimendan may cause hypotension due to vasodilatation. This may be aggravated by an inadequate rise in cardiac output in patients who do not have sufficiently elevated ventricular filling pressures initially or when a marked reduction in filling pressure occurs with levosimendan. Levosimendan should generally not be used in patients with a systolic blood pressure < 85 mm Hg or patients with clinical shock, at least until further research has been conducted. If use of levosimendan is contemplated in such patients, hemodynamic monitoring is mandatory to ensure that filling pressures are initially high and do not fall excessively.

Levosimendan reduces hematocrit, possibly reflecting an increase in circulating blood volume due to redistribution of fluid into the vascular compartment secondary to venous and arterial vasodilatation. Levosimendan may cause serum potassium to fall, possibly reflecting activation of the sympathetic nervous system, which drives potassium from the extracellular to intracellular compartment.

Levosimendan generally does not appear to precipitate or exacerbate myocardial ischemia or stunning and may actually improve it. However, excessive reduction in arterial pressure should be avoided as it may reduce coronary perfusion pressure to critical levels, provoking ischemia.

Clinical utility of levosimendan

Overall, these data provide compelling evidence that levosimendan is the safest intravenous inotropic agent for the management of worsening heart failure. This partly reflects the paucity of data from well-designed trials that support the use of other agents. Further randomized controlled trials are required to show conclusively that levosimendan should become part of the routine management of patients with acute or severe worsening of heart failure to improve symptoms or prognosis. However, when an inotropic agent is considered necessary, then in the absence of contraindications such as hypotension (systolic blood pressure < 85 mm Hg), levosimendan could be considered the agent of choice. Lack of data with dobutamine is not a reasonable basis for the continued use of this agent. Although well-conducted, placebo-controlled randomized trials exist with milrinone, a popular alternative to dobutamine, these trials have usually failed to show benefit.[51,52] Lack of benefit is also not a reasonable basis for giving a treatment.

There is also more evidence for the safety and efficacy of levosimendan in randomized controlled trials of patients with acute or severe heart failure than with any other vasodilator agent including sodium nitroprusside, organic nitrates, or nesiritide. Nesiritide, a synthetic BNP, acts as a short-acting vasodilator and natriuretic, and is probably the next best studied intravenous agent for heart failure. This agent has shown evidence of benefit on hemodynamics (a reduction in filling pressures), probably improves symptoms (although the data are probably less robust than with levosimendan) but has not shown reduced morbidity or mortality in randomized trials so far.[53,54]

Currently, the obvious target groups for levosimendan are patients with an exacerbation of chronic heart failure secondary to LVSD who are not obviously fluid overloaded or who do not respond readily to increased doses of diuretics as well as patients with acute pulmonary edema, perhaps especially in the aftermath of an MI. Patients receiving beta-blockers may gain a special advantage. Patients with rapid atrial fibrillation or a marked sinus tachycardia should have treatment for ventricular rate control first or concomitantly with levosimendan. Until further data are available, patients with a systolic blood pressure < 85 mm Hg and those with shock should not be treated with levosimendan except in the context of a clinical trial. Levosimendan could be effective in patients with diastolic heart failure but data are still lacking.

The limited post-operative experience with the use of levosimendan for patients with ventricular dysfunction after coronary bypass surgery is encouraging.[20,55]

It is not clear for how long levosimendan may be given. Few patients have received levosimendan for > 24 hours.[22] Longer infusions will lead to greater production of the active metabolite and a prolonged effect after cessation of the infusion. Conversely, short infusions may be associated with a rapid loss of effect upon ceasing infusion. Few patients have had a repeat dose of levosimendan and there are no data to indicate how frequently it may be given. The hemodynamic effects of a 24-hour infusion will probably last about 1 week, but the effect on morbidity and mortality may last longer. Shorter infusions may need to be given more frequently. However, levosimendan could prove to be the ideal agent for pulsed inotropic therapy.

Health economics

A health economic appraisal of the use of levosimendan rather than dobutamine for the management of severe heart failure suggested that, although levosimendan was more expensive to purchase, the cost per life-year saved over 3 years was only 4000 euros which is rather similar to the cost per life-year saved of ACE inhibitors and beta-blockers for heart failure.[56]

Ongoing Studies

At least two further large, double-blind, multicenter randomized controlled trials have been initiated to further assess the effects of levosimendan on morbidity and mortality in patients with very severe heart failure. The REVIVE-II trial, being conducted in the United States, is comparing levosimendan and placebo, while, in Europe, the SURVIVE trial is comparing levosimendan and dobutamine. The protocols of these studies have not yet been published. One key study being planned is a repetitive dosing trial. If this study proves positive, pulsed intravenous therapy will finally come of age for the management of severe chronic heart failure. This could revolutionize the way that heart failure is managed.

Conclusions

Levosimendan is a promising new inodilator agent for the management of severe heart failure. Its pharmacokinetic profile is complex. If further studies confirm that, uniquely among inotropic agents, it reduces mortality, it is likely to become the intravenous inotropic, and possibly vasodilator, agent of first choice in acute or severe heart failure.

Many clinicians do not currently use inotropic agents for the management of acute or severe heart failure. Instead, they focus on the manipulation of diuretic, neuroendocrine, and conventional vasodilator therapies. Levosimendan could be the first agent that convinces this group of clinicians that there is a role for inotropic agents in the management of heart failure.

References

1. Haikala H, Kaivola J, Nissinen E, *et al.* Cardiac troponin C as a target protein for a novel calcium sensitizing drug, levosimendan. J Mol Cell Cardiol 1995; 27: 1859–1866.

2. Pollesello P, Ovaska M, Kaivola J, *et al.* Binding of a new Ca^{2+} sensitizer, levosimendan, to recombinant human cardiac troponin C. A molecular modelling, fluorescence probe, and proton nuclear magnetic resonance study. J Biol Chem 1994; 269: 28584–28590.
3. Sorsa T, Heikkinen S, Abbott MB, *et al.* Binding of levosimendan, a calcium sensitizer, to cardiac troponin C. J Biol Chem 2001; 276: 9337–9343.
4. Haikala H, Levijoki J, Linden IB. Troponin C-mediated calcium sensitization by levosimendan accelerates the proportional development of isometric tension. J Mol Cell Cardiol 1995; 27: 2155–2165.
5. Haikala H, Nissinen E, Etemadzadeh E, Levijoki J, Linden IB. Troponin C-mediated calicum sensitization induced by levosimendan does not impair relaxation. J Cardiovasc Pharmacol 1995; 25: 794–801.
6. Hasenfuss G, Pieske B, Castell M, *et al.* Influence of the novel inotropic agent levosimendan on isometric tension and calcium cycling in failing human myocardium. Circulation 1998; 98: 2141–2147.
7. Pagel PS, Harkin CP, Hettrick DA, Warltier DC. Levosimendan (OR-1259), a myofilament calcium sensitizer, enhances myocardial contractility but does not alter isovolumic relaxation in conscious and anesthetized dogs. Anesthesiology 1994; 81: 974–987.
8. Haikala H, Linden IB. Mechanisms of action of calcium-sensitizing drugs. J Cardiovasc Pharmacol 1995; 26: S10–S19.
9. Edes I, Kiss E, Kitada Y, *et al.* Effects of levosimendan, a cardiotonic agent targeted to troponin C, on cardiac function and on phosphorylation and Ca^{2+} senstivity of cardiac myofibrils and sarcoplasmic reticulum in guinea pig heart. Circ Res 1995; 77: 107–113.
10. Givertz MM, Conrad CH, Andreou C. Direct myocardial effects of levosimendan, a novel calcium sensitizing agent, in humans with left ventricular dysfunction. Circulation 1998; 17: I-579 (Abstract).
11. Jamali IN, Kersten JR, Pagel PS, Hettrick DA, Warltier DC. Intracoronary levosimendan enhances contractile function of stunned myocardium. Anesth Analg 1997; 85: 23–29.
12. Louis AA, Manousos IR, Coletta AP, Clark AL, Cleland JGF. Clinical trials update: The Heart Protection Study, IONA, CARISA, ENRICHD, ACUTE, ALIVE, MADIT II and REMATCH. Eur J Heart Fail 2002; 4: 111–116.
13. Bowman P, Haikala H, Paul RJ. Levosimendan, a calcium sensitizer in cardiac muscle, induces relaxation in coronary smooth muscle through calcium desensitization. J Pharmacol Exp Ther 1999; 288: 316–325.
14. Kaheinen P, Pollesello P, Levijoki J, Haikala H. Levosimendan increases diastolic coronary flow in isolated guinea-pig heart by opening ATP-sensitive potassium channels. J Cardiovasc Pharmacol 2001; 37: 367–374.
15. Pataricza J, Hohn J, Petri A, Balogh A, Papp JG. Comparison of the vasorelaxing effect of cromakalim and the new inodilator, levosimendan, in human isolated portal vein. J Pharm Pharmacol 2000; 52: 213–217.
16. Haikala H, Kaheinen P, Levijoki J, Linden IB. The role of cAMP- and cGMP-dependent protein kinases in the cardiac actions of the new calcium sensitizer, levosimendan. Cardiovasc Res 1997; 34: 536–546.
17. Todaka K, Wang J, Yi GH, *et al.* Effects of levosimendan on myocardial contractility and oxygen consumption. J Pharmacol Exp Ther 1996; 279: 120–127.
18. Ukkonen H, Saraste M, Akkila J, *et al.* Myocardial efficiency during calcium sensitization with levosimendan: a noninvasive study with positron emission tomography and echocardiography in healthy volunteers. Clin Pharmacol Ther 1997; 61: 596–607.
19. Ukkonen H, Saraste M, Akkila J, *et al.* Myocardial efficiency during levosimendan infusion in congestive heart failure. Clin Pharmacol Ther 2000; 68: 522–531.
20. Lilleberg J, Nieminen MS, Akkila J, *et al.* Effects of a new calcium sensitizer, levosimendan, on haemodynamics, coronary blood flow and myocardial substrate utilization early after coronary artery bypass grafting. Eur Heart J 1998; 19: 660–668.
21. Pagel PS, Hettrick DA, Warltier DC. Influence of levosimendan, pimobendan, and milrinone on the regional distribution of cardiac output in anaesthetized dogs. Br J Pharmacol 1996; 119: 609–615.
22. Kivikko M, Antila S, Eha J, Lehtonen L, Pentikainen PJ. Pharmacodynamics and safety of a new calcium sensitizer, levosimendan, and its metabolites during an extended infusion in patients with severe heart failure. J Clin Pharmacol 2002; 42: 43–51.
23. Lilleberg J, Sundberg S, Hayha M, Akkila J, Nieminen MS. Haemodynamic dose-efficacy of levosimendan in healthy volunteers. Eur J Clin Pharmacol 1994; 47: 267–274.
24. Slawsky MT, Colucci WS, Gottlieb SS, *et al.* Acute hemodynamic and clinical effects of levosimendan in patients with severe heart failure. Circulation 2000; 102: 2222–2227.
25. Nieminen M, Akkila J, Hasenfuss G, *et al.* Hemodynamic and neurohumoral effects of continuous infusion of levosimendan in patients with congestive heart failure. J Am Coll Cardiol 2000; 36: 1903–1912.
26. Kivikko M, Lehtonen L, Colucci WS. Sustained hemodynamic effects of intravenous levosimendan. Circulation 2003; 107: 81–86.

27. Kivikko M, Antila S, Eha J, Lehtonen L, Pentikainen PJ. Pharmacokinetics of levosimendan and its metabolites during and after a 24-hour continuous infusion in patients with severe heart failure. Int J Clin Pharmacol Ther 2002; 40: 465–471.
28. Lehtonen L, Sundberg S. The contractility enhancing effect of the calcium sensitiser levosimendan is not attenuated by carvedilol in healthy subjects. Eur J Clin Pharmacol 2002; 58: 449–452.
29. Toivonen L, Viitasalo M, Sundberg S, Akkila J, Lehtonen L. Electrophysiologic effects of a calcium sensitizer inotrope levosimendan administered intravenously in patients with normal cardiac function. J Cardiovasc Pharmacol 2000; 35: 664–669.
30. Singh BN, Lilleberg J, Sandell E-P, *et al.* Effects of levosimendan on cardiac arrhythmia: electrophysiologic and ambulatory electrocardiographic findings in phase II and phase III clinical studies in cardiac failure. Am J Cardiol 1999; 83 (Suppl 12B): I16–I20.
31. Cleland JG, Thackray S, Goodge L, Kaye G, Cooklin M. Outcome studies with device therapy in patients with heart failure. J Cardiovasc Electrophysiol 2002; 13: S73–S91.
32. Cleland JG, Daubert JC, Erdmann E, *et al.*, CARE-HF Study Steering Committee and Investigators. The CARE-HF study (Cardiac Resynchronization in Heart Failure study): rationale, design, and endpoints. Eur J Heart Fail 2001; 3: 481–489.
33. Kersten JR, Montgomery MW, Pagel PS, Warltier DC. Levosimendan, a new positive inotropic drug, decreases myocardial infarct size via activation of K(ATP) channels. Anesth Analg 2000; 90: 5–11.
34. Sonntag S, Opitz C, Wellnhofer E, *et al.* Effects of the calcium sensitizer levosimendan on stunned myocardium after percutaneous transluminal coronary angioplasty. Eur Heart J 2000; 21: 40 (Abstract).
35. Nicklas JM, Monsur JC, Bleske BE. Effects of intravenous levosimendan on plasma neurohormone levels in patients with heart failure: relation to hemodynamic response. Am J Cardiol 1999; 83 (Suppl 12B): I12–I15.
36. Binkley PF, Nunziata E, Hatton PS, Leier CV. The positive inotropic agent levosimendan mediates increased cardiac output without progression of sympathovagal imbalance in patients with heart failure. Circulation 2000; 102: II720 (Abstract).
37. Sandell EP, Hayha M, Antila S, *et al.* Pharmacokinetics of levosimendan in healthy volunteers and patients with congestive heart failure. J Cardiovasc Pharmacol 1995; 26: S57–S62.
38. Sundberg S, Antila S, Scheinin H, *et al.* Integrated pharmacokinetics and pharmacodynamics of the novel calcium sensitizer levosimendan as assessed by systolic time intervals. Int J Clin Pharmacol Ther 1998; 36: 629–635.
39. Antila S, Huuskonen H, Nevalainen T, *et al.* Site dependent bioavailability and metabolism of levosimendan in dogs. Eur J Pharm Sci 1999; 9: 85–91.
40. Antila S, Honkanen T, Lehtonen L, Neuvonen PJ. The CYP3A4 inhibitor itraconazole does not affect the pharmacokinetics of a new calcium-sensitizing drug levosimendan. Int J Clin Pharmacol Ther 1998; 36: 446–449.
41. Antila S, Jarvinen A, Honkanen T, Lehtonen L. Pharmacokinetic and pharmacodynamic interactions between the novel calcium sensitiser levosimendan and warfarin. Eur J Clin Pharmacol 2000; 56: 705–710.
42. Lehtonen L, Antila S, Eha J, *et al.* No pharmacodynamic interactions between a new calcium sensitizing agent levosimendan and a calcium antagonist drug felodipine. Eur J Clin Pharmacol 1997; 52: A136 (Abstract).
43. Pentikainen PJ, Antila S, Kivikko M, *et al.* Pharmacokinetics of levosimendan in patients with severe congestive heart failure. J Card Fail 1999; 5: 48 (Abstract).
44. Sandell E-P, Antila S, Koistinen H, Pentikainen PJ. The effects of renal failure on the pharmacokinetics of levosimendan. Therapie 1995; Abstracts of EACPT (Suppl) (Abstract).
45. Antila S, Eha J, Heinpalu M, *et al.* Haemodynamic interactions of a new calcium sensitizing drug levosimendan and captopril. Eur J Clin Pharmacol 1996; 49: 451–458.
46. Sundberg S, Lehtonen L. Haemodynamic interactions between the novel calcium sensitiser levosimendan and isosorbide-5-mononitrate in healthy subjects. Eur J Clin Pharmacol 2000; 55: 793–799.
47. Follath F, Cleland JG, Just H, *et al.*, Steering Committee and Investigators of the Levosimendan Infusion versus Dobutamine (LIDO) study. Efficacy and safety of intravenous levosimendan compared with dobutamine in severe low-output heart failure (the LIDO study): a randomised double-blind trial. Lancet 2002; 360: 196–202.
48. Lilleberg J, Sundberg S, Nieminen M. Dose-range study of a new calcium sensitizer, levosimendan, in patients with left ventricular dysfunction. J Cardiovasc Pharmacol 1995; 26: S63–S69.
49. Moiseyev VS, Poder P, Andrejevs N, *et al.*, RUSSLAN Study Investigators. Safety and efficacy of a novel calcium sensitiser, levosimendan, in patients with left ventricular failure due to an acute myocardial infarc-

tion. A randomized, placebo-controlled, double-blind study (RUSSLAN). Eur Heart J 2002; 23: 1422–1432.

50. Thackray S, Eastaugh J, Freemantle N, Cleland JG. The effectiveness and relative effectiveness of intravenous inotropic drugs acting through the adrenergic pathways in patients with heart failure—a meta-regression analysis. Eur J Heart Fail 2002; 4: 515–529.
51. Thackray S, Coletta A, Jones P, *et al.* Clinical trials update: Highlights of the Scientific Sessions of Heart Failure 2001, a meeting of the Working Group on Heart Failure of the European Society of Cardiology. CONTAK-CD, CHRISTMAS, OPTIME-CHF. Eur J Heart Fail 2001; 3: 491–494.
52. Publication Committee for the VMAC Investigators (Vasodilation in the Management of Acute CHF). Intravenous nesiritide vs nitroglycerin for treatment of decompensated congestive heart failure: a randomized controlled trial. JAMA 2002; 287: 1531–1540.
53. Colucci WS, Elkayam U, Horton DP, *et al.*, Nesiritide Study Group. Intravenous nesiritide, a natriuretic peptide, in the treatment of decompensated congestive heart failure. N Engl J Med 2000; 343: 246–253.
54. Cuffe MS, Califf RM, Adams KF, *et al.*, Outcomes of a Prospective Trial of Intravenous Milrinone for Exacerbations of Chronic Heart Failure (OPTIME-CHF) Investigators. Short-term intravenous milrinone for acute exacerbation of congestive heart failure: a randomized controlled trial. JAMA 2002; 287: 1541–1547.
55. Cleland JGF. Beta-blockers for heart failure. In: Amiel S (ed.) Horizons in Medicine (Royal College of Physicians: London, 2002), 13–38.
56. Cleland JG, Takala A, Apajasalo M, Zethraeus N, Kobelt G. Intravenous levosimendan treatment is cost-effective compared with dobutamine in severe low-output heart failure: an analysis based on the international LIDO trial. Eur J Heart Fail 2003; 5: 101–108.
57. Packer M, Colucci WS, Fisher L, *et al.* Development of a comprehensive new endpoint for the evaluation of new treatments for acute decompensated heart failure: results with levosimendan in the REVIVE-1 study. J Card Fail 2003; 9: S61 (Abstract).
58. Zairis MN, Apostolatos C, Anastassiadis P, *et al.* Comparison of the effect of levosimendan, or dobutamine or placebo in chronic low output decompensated heart failure. CAlcium Sensitizer or Inotrope or NOne in low output heart failure (CASINO) study. Eur J Heart Fail 2004; 3: S66.

CHAPTER 35

Vasopressin antagonists

Cesare Orlandi, Wendy Gattis Stough, Christopher M O'Connor, Kirkwood F Adams, Jr, Mihai Gheorghiade

Introduction

The role and importance of neuroendocrine imbalances in the pathophysiology of chronic heart failure have become evident in the past decade. Modulation of excessive angiotensin II and beta-adrenergic stimulation has produced impressive benefits in the clinical outcomes of chronic heart failure patients. However, despite decreased mortality and morbidity rates associated with the use of angiotensin-converting enzyme (ACE) inhibitors, beta-blockers, and anti-aldosterone drugs, the risk of these events remains high in this patient population. It is still not clear whether blockade of other neurohormones could provide additional improvements.

Data from the Studies of Left Ventricular Dysfunction (SOLVD) neuroendocrine study have shown that arginine vasopressin (AVP) levels are also elevated in chronic heart failure patients even when they are asymptomatic and even prior to demonstrable elevations of plasma renin activity.[1] However, assessment of the potential benefit associated with AVP receptor blockade in chronic heart failure has been hampered until recently by the lack of orally-active, effective, and well-tolerated non-peptide agents. Newly developed compounds targeting the V_1 (vascular) and V_2 (renal) vasopressin receptors are currently being studied in chronic heart failure patients. These agents may represent the next generation of neuroendocrine modulators to show a beneficial impact in this syndrome.

Arginine Vasopressin

Vasopressin, also known as arginine vasopressin (AVP) or antidiuretic hormone (ADH), is a neuropeptide produced in the supraoptic and paraventricular nuclei of the hypothalamus. AVP is transported from the hypothalamus to the pituitary gland and released into the bloodstream. Secretion of this hormone from hypothalamic neurons is regulated by baroreceptors and osmoreceptors and is affected by such factors as malignancies, cardiopulmonary disease, central nervous system (CNS) disorders, endocrinopathies, and some pharmacologic agents. A decrease in blood pressure, as well as an increase in plasma osmolality, leads to marked increases in AVP blood levels.

Two AVP receptors have been isolated: the V_1 and V_2 receptors. The V_1 receptor is localized in the vasculature, uterus, and brain, while the V_2 receptor is primarily localized in the collecting duct of the renal nephron where it mediates changes in water permeability.

AVP causes vasoconstriction via cyclic adenosine monophosphate (cAMP)-independent vascular V_{1a} receptors and promotes water reabsorption in the kidneys via cAMP-dependent

V_2 receptors, thus having an antidiuretic effect.[2] Absence of vasopressin, or its blockade by antagonists, leads to the excretion of large volumes of dilute urine and to an increase in plasma sodium concentration if water intake is unchanged.

As mentioned previously, increased AVP levels have been demonstrated in patients with heart failure since the early 1980s.[1,3] These changes are similar to those observed for plasma levels of renin and norepinephrine, with values that become higher as the severity of the disease increases. The neurohormone may contribute to the genesis and maintenance of congestive heart failure (CHF) through a number of mechanisms mediated by activation of the V_{1a} and V_2 receptors. The activation of the V_{1a} vascular receptor produces vasoconstriction resulting in increased peripheral vascular resistance and afterload. Activation of the V_2 renal tubular receptor produces water retention with consequent increased intracellular and extracellular volumes and fluid overload. Vasopressin has also been shown to stimulate cell growth and to contribute to the genesis of cardiac hypertrophy. Protein synthesis, as well as the protein/deoxyribonucleic acid (DNA) ratio, is increased in cultured neonatal myocytes,[4] and enhanced DNA synthesis has also been observed in fibroblasts.

Many of the potentially negative effects of AVP in heart failure are similar to those described for angiotensin II, and include vasoconstriction, cardiac hypertrophy, vascular smooth muscle cell remodeling and growth, CNS effects, and fluid retention. Whether or not blockade of the vasopressin receptors will have a positive impact on clinical outcomes remains to be determined.

In a multivariate analysis from the Survival and Ventricular Enlargement (SAVE) study, Rouleau *et al.*[5] demonstrated that circulating vasopressin concentrations correlated independently with the occurrence of severe CHF, recurrent myocardial infarction (MI), and combined mortality, heart failure and recurrent MI. These data are enticing, but large well-controlled outcome studies with AVP receptor blockers are necessary to fully establish their potential role.

Arginine Vasopressin and Serum Sodium in Congestive Heart Failure

Several reports have highlighted the common association between CHF and sodium and water retention.[6–10] Increased AVP release is one of the postulated mechanisms for this imbalance.[11] In heart failure, the decreases in "effective" blood volume and arterial filling would be sensed by the aortic and carotid sinus baroreceptors resulting in stimulation of AVP release.[12–14] The importance of this mechanism is stressed in experimental models of heart failure, where abnormal dilution is also observed. Indeed, correction of the observed water excretory defect by a vasopressin receptor antagonist has been reported in rats with chronic heart failure induced by inferior vena cava constriction.[15]

Also, of particular interest is the role played by AVP in the genesis and maintenance of hyponatremia in heart failure. Studies have demonstrated that patients with heart failure and hyponatremia have inappropriately elevated AVP levels, indicating that in this condition the normal osmotic control of vasopressin release is dysfunctional.[16,17] In these circumstances, non-osmotic regulatory pathways of vasopressin release, via aortic and carotid baroreceptors among other pathways, likely predominate. These inappropriately elevated AVP levels contribute to the development and maintenance of the hyponatremic and volume overloaded state due to ongoing stimulation of V_2 renal receptors mediating water retention. The problem becomes more evident in patients with worsening chronic heart failure. In these patients, the concomitant presence of fluid overload and hyponatremia represents a particular challenge. Current treatment strategies for patients with decompensated heart failure and hyponatremia consist of additional loop diuretics to remove excess fluid and free-water restriction to correct the sodium imbalance. This approach is often inadequate. The effect of fluid restriction is limited and, additionally, diuretic therapy produces further stimulation of AVP secretion, and may result in maintenance or worsening of hyponatremia.[18] Indeed, loop diuretics produce reductions in plasma osmolality due to the excretion of isosmolar urine. The resulting elevated vasopressin levels will provide a continuing stimulus to renal water retention, maintaining or even worsening the state of hyponatremia, even with a restriction of water intake.

Thus, more than just improving a marker of the clinical state (i.e., correction of hyponatremia), treatment of this syndrome with a V_2 receptor antagonist has the potential to directly address an important component of the pathophysiologic state which is driving the clinical signs of both hyponatremia and volume overload.

Vasopressin Receptor Antagonists in Acute Heart Failure

Patients hospitalized for heart failure commonly have a history of progressive fluid retention/congestion (often manifested by an increase in body weight) leading to worsening symptoms requiring hospitalization. The overwhelming majority of these patients are normotensive and have signs and symptoms of pulmonary and/or systemic congestion. Congestion in these patients has been associated with high mortality rates.[19,20]

Current management of pulmonary and systemic congestion resulting in heart failure hospitalization often does not result in substantial decreases in body weight, nor in an improvement in signs and symptoms.[19,20]

Six-month post-discharge readmission and mortality rates are as high as 50% and 25%, respectively.[19,20] This unacceptably high event rate occurs in spite of the fact that most patients are normotensive, without renal failure, and appear to respond well to therapy. Non-potassium-sparing diuretics are the mainstay of pharmacological therapy for congestion. Their use is often associated with hypotension, electrolyte abnormalities, and worsening renal function. The ideal drug to treat congestive symptoms should significantly increase fluid loss and lower filling pressures without negatively affecting blood pressure, heart rate, electrolytes, renal function, neurohormones, or clinical outcomes. Non-potassium-sparing loop diuretics do not have these characteristics. Based on mechanism of action and preliminary proof-of-concept studies,[21–23] vasopressin V_2 receptor antagonists may be ideally suited.

Vasopressin Receptor Antagonists in Development

Several orally-active, non-peptide AVP antagonists are currently in clinical development and include selective V_2 receptor blockers and mixed V_{1a}/V_2 receptor blockers. Limited published data are available on three compounds: the V_2 blockers VPA-985 (lixivaptan) and OPC-41061 (tolvaptan), and the mixed V_{1a}/V_2 receptor blocker YM-087 (conivaptan). Clinical data have shown the ability of all three agents to mobilize fluid and increase serum sodium levels in heart failure patients.

In chronic heart failure patients with signs of mild fluid overload and on stable standard therapy including diuretics, chronic oral administration of tolvaptan showed an increase in urine volume accompanied by an acute, statistically significant reduction in body weight that was maintained for 25 days.[21] In the same study, a differential effect on serum sodium was observed in patients with normonatremia and hyponatremia at baseline. In normonatremic patients, an acute and non-sustained elevation in sodium levels was observed at day 1. However, patients with hyponatremia demonstrated statistically significant and sustained increases in serum sodium often leading to normalization.

Acute intravenous administration of the V_{1a}/V_2 receptor blocker, conivaptan, has been shown to produce hemodynamic effects.[22] However, the observed reduction in pulmonary capillary wedge pressure (PCWP) did not appear to be related to V_{1a} receptor-mediated vasodilation, but to the V_2 receptor-mediated reduction in blood volume. Indeed, large and dose-dependent increases in urine volume have been reported, but no changes in systemic vascular resistance.

The effects of these agents on renal physiology and hemodynamics also highlight the striking differences between V_2 receptor blockers and loop diuretics. Unlike furosemide, tolvaptan has been shown to increase renal blood flow and glomerular filtration rate, as well as decrease renal vascular resistance.[24]

The expected effects of tolvaptan on fluid balance led to the Acute and Chronic Therapeutic Impact of a Vasopressin Antagonist in Congestive

Heart Failure (ACTIV in CHF) study, a trial conducted to evaluate the short-term (in-hospital) and intermediate-term (outpatient, after hospital discharge) effects of the compound in patients hospitalized for worsening heart failure.[23] Compared with placebo, tolvaptan resulted in significant improvements in body weight at 24 hours (one of the primary endpoints of the study), at hospital discharge, and at 60 days not associated with changes in heart rate or blood pressure, nor hyponatremia (Figure 35.1).[23] A rapid and sustained improvement in serum sodium was observed (Figure 35.2). Tolvaptan treatment did not significantly affect the other primary endpoint of worsening heart failure, defined as death, rehospitalization, or unscheduled visits for heart failure. In retrospect, there was a trend toward lower total mortality in the combined tolvaptan groups compared with placebo, particularly in patients with hyponatremia, renal dysfunction, or severe congestion at baseline (Figure 35.3).

Conclusion

In acute heart failure, non-potassium-sparing diuretics remain the only available pharmacological tool to treat fluid overload. However, they have

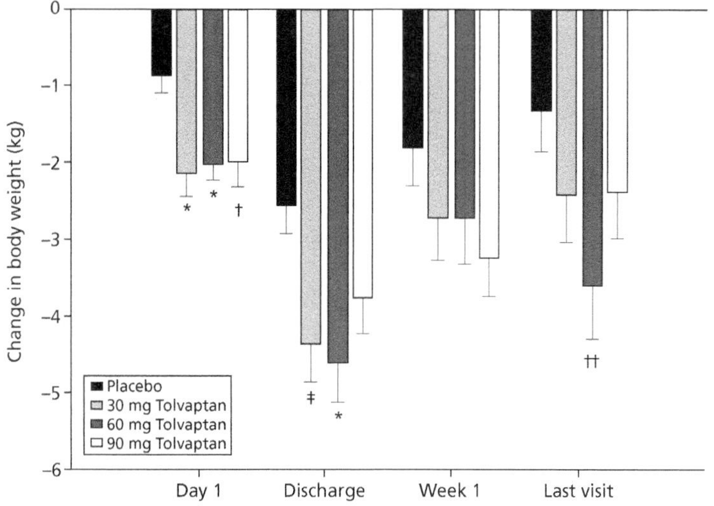

Figure 35.1. *Median changes in body weight over time (From Gheorghiade* et al.[23]*)*
$^{*}P = 0.002$;
$^{\dagger}P = 0.009$;
$^{\ddagger}P = 0.006$;
$^{\dagger\dagger}P = 0.008$.

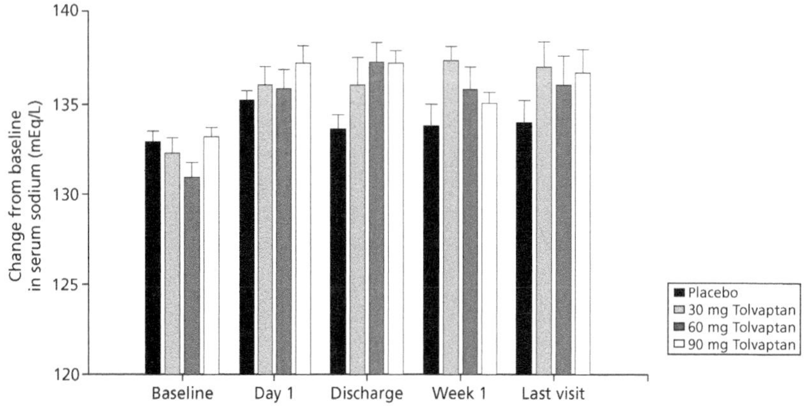

Change from baseline in serum sodium (mEq/L)
140
135
130
125
120
Baseline
Day 1
Discharge
Week 1
Last visit
Placebo
30 mg Tolvaptan
60 mg Tolvaptan
90 mg Tolvaptan

Figure 35.2. *Change in serum sodium from baseline (From Gheorghiade* et al.[23]*)*

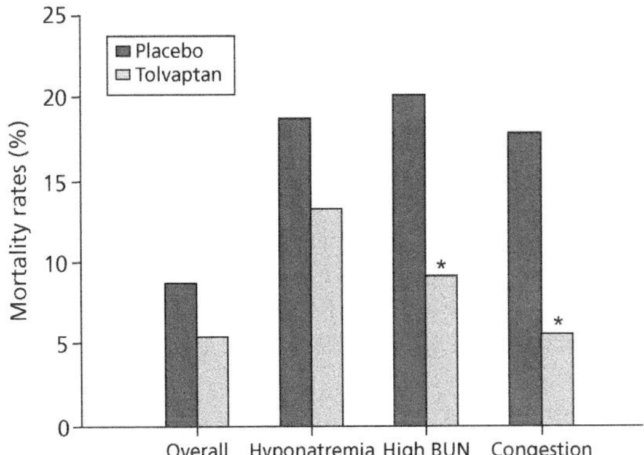

Figure 35.3. *Mortality rates of placebo versus tolvaptan in higher-risk subgroups (From Gheorghiade* et al.[23])

*$P < 0.05$.

Hyponatremia = serum sodium < 136 mEq/L

High BUN = BUN > 29 mg/dL

Congestion = dyspnea + peripheral edema + rales

Abbreviations: BUN = blood urea nitrogen.

substantial limitations. Their ability to effectively reduce systemic congestion and decrease edema may be limited, since they are known to decrease plasma osmolarity and renal blood flow, resulting in prerenal azotemia even in patients who continue to be fluid overloaded. Hospitalized patients with worsening heart failure and congestion often have hyponatremia, elevated blood urea nitrogen (BUN), and low systolic blood pressure, which are major predictors of poor prognosis. Those abnormalities can be further worsened by non-potassium-sparing diuretic use. In this setting, vasopressin V_2 receptor antagonists appear to be particularly promising. Definitive studies are still needed. However, at least one large outcome study is currently underway (Efficacy of Vasopressin Antagonism in Heart Failure: Outcome Study with Tolvaptan [EVEREST]) which should help clarify their potential in patients hospitalized with worsening heart failure in both the acute and post-discharge setting.

References

1. Francis GS, Benedict C, Johnstone DE, *et al.* Comparison of neuroendocrine activation in patients with left ventricular dysfunction with and without congestive heart failure. A substudy of the Studies of Left Ventricular Dysfunction (SOLVD). Circulation 1990; 82: 1724–1729.
2. Michell RH, Kirk CJ, Billah MM. Hormonal stimulation of phosphatidylinositol breakdown with particular reference to the hepatic effects of vasopressin. Biochem Soc Trans 1979; 7: 861–865.
3. Goldsmith SR, Francis GS, Cowley AW Jr., *et al.* Increased plasma arginine vasopressin levels in patients with congestive heart failure. J Am Coll Cardiol 1983; 1: 1385–1390.
4. Nakamura Y, Haneda T, Osaki J, *et al.* Hypertrophic growth of cultured neonatal rat heart cells mediated by vasopressin V(1A) receptor. Eur J Pharmacol 2000; 391: 39–48.
5. Rouleau JL, Packer M, Moye L, *et al.* Prognostic value of neurohumoral activation in patients with an acute myocardial infarction: effect of captopril. J Am Coll Cardiol 1994; 24: 583–591.
6. Dzau VJ, Colucci WS, Williams GH, *et al.* Sustained effectiveness of converting-enzyme inhibition in patients with severe congestive heart failure. N Engl J Med 1980; 302: 1373–1379.
7. Nitter-Hauge S, Brodwall EK, Rootwelt K. Renal function studies in hyponatremic cardiac patients with edema (dilution syndrome). Am Heart J 1974; 87: 33–40.
8. Paller MS, Schrier RW. Pathogenesis of sodium and water retention in edematous disorders. Am J Kidney Dis 1982; 2: 241–254.
9. Dzau VJ, Packer M, Lilly LS, *et al.* Prostaglandins in severe congestive heart failure. Relation to activation of the renin—angiotensin system and hyponatremia. N Engl J Med 1984; 310: 347–352.
10. Bichet DG, Schrier RW. Water metabolism in edematous disorders. Semin Nephrol 1984; 4: 325.
11. Anderson RJ, Cadnapaphornchai P, Harbottle JA, *et al.* Mechanism of effect of thoracic inferior vena cava constriction on renal water excretion. J Clin Invest 1974; 54: 1473–1479.
12. Schrier RW. Pathogenesis of sodium and water retention in high-output and low-output cardiac failure, nephrotic syndrome, cirrhosis, and pregnancy (1). N Engl J Med 1988; 319: 1065–1072.
13. Schrier RW. Pathogenesis of sodium and water retention in high-output and low-output cardiac failure, nephrotic syndrome, cirrhosis, and pregnancy (2). N Engl J Med 1988; 319: 1127–1134.
14. Schrier RW, Humphreys MH, Ufferman RC. Role of cardiac output and the autonomic nervous system in the antinatriuretic response to acute constriction of the thoracic superior vena cava. Circ Res 1971; 29: 490–498.

15. Ishikawa S, Saito T, Okada K, *et al.* Effect of vasopressin antagonist on water excretion in inferior vena cava constriction. Kidney Int 1986; 30: 49–55.
16. Riegger GA, Liebau G, Kochsiek K. Antidiuretic hormone in congestive heart failure. Am J Med 1982; 72: 49–52.
17. Szatalowicz VL, Arnold PE, Chaimovitz C, *et al.* Radioimmunoassay of plasma arginine vasopressin in hyponatremic patients with congestive heart failure. N Engl J Med 1981; 305: 263–266.
18. Ikram H, Chan W, Espiner EA, *et al.* Haemodynamic and hormone responses to acute and chronic frusemide therapy in congestive heart failure. Clin Sci (Lond) 1980; 59: 443–449.
19. Fonarow GC. The Acute Decompensated Heart Failure National Registry (ADHERE™): opportunities to improve care of patients hospitalized with acute decompensated heart failure. Rev Cardiovasc Med 2003; 4: S21–S30.
20. Lucas C, Johnson W, Hamilton MA, *et al.* Freedom from congestion predicts good survival despite previous class IV symptoms of heart failure. Am Heart J 2000; 140: 840–847.
21. Gheorghiade M, Niazi I, Ouyang J, Czerwiec F. Chronic effects of vasopressin receptor blockade with tolvaptan in heart failure: a randomized, double-blind trial. Circulation 2000; 102: II592 (Abstract).
22. Udelson JE, Smith WB, Hendrix GH, *et al.* Acute hemodynamic effects of conivaptan, a dual V(1A) and V(2) vasopressin receptor antagonist, in patients with advanced heart failure. Circulation 2001; 104: 2417–2423.
23. Gheorghiade M, Gattis WA, O'Connor CM, *et al.* Effects of tolvaptan, a vasopressin antagonist, in patients hospitalized with worsening heart failure: a randomized controlled trial. JAMA 2004; 291: 1963–1971.
24. Burnett JC, Smith WB, Ouyang J, *et al.* Tolvaptan (OPC-41061), a V2 vasopressin receptor antagonist protects against the decline in renal function observed with loop diuretic therapy. J Card Fail 2003; 9: 36 (Abstract).

Chapter 36

Endothelin receptor antagonists in the treatment of acute heart failure

John R Teerlink, Christopher M O'Connor

Introduction

Advances in therapeutics and treatment strategies have had a dramatic impact on morbidity and mortality in the chronic heart failure population. Until recently, however, patients admitted with acute decompensated heart failure (ADHF) have been largely ignored. In the United States, heart failure is the primary hospital discharge diagnosis in 1 million patients per year, and it is listed as a contributing diagnosis in 2 million more patients, accounting for $14 billion in hospital costs annually.[1] The therapeutic approach to these patients has remained essentially unchanged for decades, with diuretics, vasodilators and positive inotropic agents being used as the standard of care, despite the relative absence of clinical trial evidence. Recent surveys have demonstrated that with these therapies, patients admitted for heart failure have a 45% chance of readmission[2] and a 20% to 40% risk of death in the following 6 months. These figures have encouraged the medical community to reevaluate the current approach to the acute heart failure (AHF) syndrome and to search for new therapies to treat these patients, with a goal of favorably influencing clinical outcomes. As a result of this reassessment, ADHF has been recognized as a vascular disorder and consequently the need to develop therapies that can provide vascular protection has also been recognized. Endothelin receptor antagonists (ERAs) hold the promise of providing a novel approach to the treatment of ADHF by addressing the underlying pathophysiologic abnormalities in this syndrome. This chapter discusses the new paradigm of AHF as a vascular disorder, the role of endothelin in AHF with specific reference to its effects as a vascular toxin, and the experimental and clinical evidence of the utility of ERAs in the treatment of AHF.

A New Paradigm: Acute Heart Failure as a Vascular Disorder

AHF is a term of questionable value in describing the pathophysiology of the patients who present to hospitals afflicted with this syndrome. First, the development of the symptoms comprising the syndrome is not typically acute, but rather it usually results from a gradual increase in peripheral or pulmonary edema and the vascular responses to this fluid accumulation. In Randomized Evaluation of Strategies for Left Ventricular Dysfunction (RESOLVD),[3] 143 out of 768 heart failure patients with an ejection fraction (EF) of less than 40% required hospitalization during the 43 weeks of the study. The most frequent precipitant was noncompliance with salt restriction, occurring in 27% of these patients, while 10% had inappropriate reductions in congestive heart failure (CHF) therapy. In cases where there is an acute presentation, another type of vascular abnormality is often to blame, such as an acute coronary syndrome (ACS).

Second, the heart often does not appear to be the central organ in the pathophysiology of the syndrome. In approximately half of the patients, there is preserved left ventricular (LV) systolic function. While an underlying abnormality of LV diastolic or systolic dysfunction may instigate the syndrome, most of the symptoms, signs and even therapies are directed to the vasculature. Pathologic vasoconstriction can be viewed as the central abnormality in AHF (Figure 36.1). Peripheral venoconstriction redistributes blood centrally, increasing pulmonary venous congestion and edema, resulting in the symptoms of dyspnea and fatigue. Peripheral arterial vasoconstriction results in increased afterload on the heart, elevation of LV filling pressures, and increased post-capillary pulmonary venous pressures, which results in worsening of pulmonary edema and dyspnea. This increased afterload results in elevation of ventricular wall stress and increased myocardial ischemia and cardiac arrhythmias. In addition, systemic vasoconstriction contributes to poor organ perfusion, such as the kidney, brain, and gut, contributing to renal failure and symptoms of fatigue, confusion, anorexia, and abdominal discomfort. Elevations in peripheral venous pressures and pathologic "leakiness" of the vessels result in the peripheral edema that often represents the most obvious sign of AHF.

Third, therapies that are effective in the treatment of AHF are not necessarily directed at the heart, but rather influence the vasculature. Diuretics, such as furosemide, are the most commonly used therapies for these patients. The main effect of these agents is to reduce central venous pressures through diuresis and possibly via direct vasodilating properties,[4] not via any direct effect on the heart. The other commonly used agents, nitroglycerin, nitroprusside and, more recently, nesiritide, are all vasodilators—achieving symptom relief through their actions on the vasculature. None of these agents have significant direct myocardial effects. Positive inotropes are used in a minority of AHF patients, about 8% of the patients in the Acute Decompensated Heart Failure (ADHERE™) registry.[5] However, even the positive inotropes in common use, such as dobutamine and milrinone, have significant vasodilating effects. Thus, the main therapeutic target of current therapies has been the vasculature using non-specific vasodilation.

This new paradigm of AHF as a vascular syndrome has important implications for the clinical

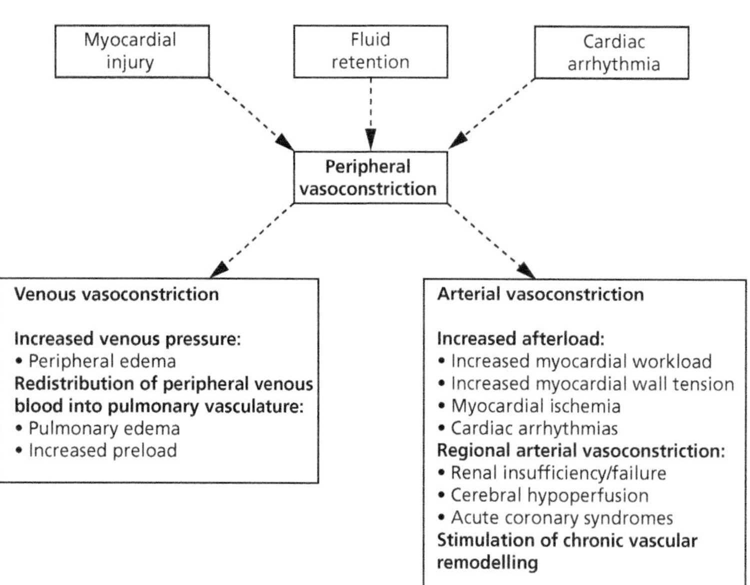

Figure 36.1. *A central role for the vasculature in the pathogenesis of acute decompensated heart failure*

development of new AHF therapies. For acute symptom resolution, the new therapy must be an effective vasodilator, relieving the elevated venous pressures that lead to congestion and dyspnea, and reducing the abnormally high afterload that results in organ hypoperfusion and increased cardiac wall stress with the attendant increases in ischemia and arrhythmias. Yet, the new therapy must also target the underlying mediators of these vascular abnormalities to prevent acute and chronic damage. The neurohormonal hypothesis has been well established in chronic heart failure, where agents antagonizing the deleterious effects of neurohormones, such as angiotensin and adrenergic hormones, have improved clinical outcomes. AHF is accompanied by stimulation of these same neurohormones, as well as other toxic agents, such as endothelin. New therapies for AHF need to improve clinical outcomes and a vasodilating agent that can antagonize vascular and end-organ damage has the potential to have both short-term and long-term benefits for patients. Over 15 years of basic science and clinical research suggest that the ERAs have this potential.

Preclinical Studies

Preclinical studies: endothelin as a vascular toxin

Endothelin-1 (ET-1)[6] is a 21 amino acid peptide, homologous to the extraordinarily potent vascular toxins, known as sarafotoxins, isolated from the venom of *Atractaspis engadensis* or the Israeli burrowing asp. ET-1 is the most important and prevalent member of the endothelin family of gene products, which includes three isopeptides encoded from separate genes known as ET-1, ET-2 and ET-3. Although the brain and kidney also produce significant amounts of this peptide, ET-1 is synthesized predominantly by cardiovascular tissues in response to cardiovascular stressors, including vascular damage, other neurohormones (angiotensin II, epinephrine or norepinephrine), cytokines (interleukin-1 [IL-1] or tumor growth factor-beta [TGF-β]), and other stimuli (acidosis, thrombin, hypoxia, and shear stress). ET-1 signals via two main types of receptors, known as ET_A and ET_B on the basis of their relative affinities for the endothelin isopeptides (Table 36.1). ET receptors are members of the family of 7-transmembrane spanning G-protein coupled receptors.

Endothelin is present in abnormally high concentrations in both acute and chronic heart failure. Plasma ET-1 levels were first shown to be increased in patients with AHF due to cardiogenic shock,[7] but subsequent studies have found increases in acute and chronic heart failure, pulmonary hypertension, systemic hypertension, and all forms of ACS, as well as many other conditions. Margulies and colleagues[8] provided the first evidence of elevated endothelin concentrations in an experimental setting using the rapid ventricular pacing canine heart failure model and these findings were subsequently confirmed in the rat coronary artery

Table 36.1. *Characteristics of endothelin receptors*

	Relative affinities	Cardiovascular distribution	Selected effects of receptor stimulation
ET_A	ET-1=ET-2>>ET-3	Vascular smooth muscle cells	Vasoconstriction, hyperplasia
		Heart (myocytes > fibroblasts)	"Pathologic" hypertrophy and fibrosis
		Vascular fibroblasts	Fibrosis
ET_B	ET-1=ET-2=ET-3	Vascular endothelium	Vasorelaxation, ET clearance
		Heart (fibroblast > myocytes)	Fibrosis, ? Apoptosis, hypertrophy
		Vascular fibroblasts	Fibrosis
		Vascular smooth muscle cell	Vasoconstriction

Abbreviations: ET = endothelin.

ligation heart failure model.[9] In patients with chronic heart failure (CHF), endothelin concentrations were found to be markedly elevated in a number of studies[10–12] and correlated with the extent of pulmonary hypertension,[10] severity of symptoms and ventricular dysfunction,[13] and predictive of mortality.[14] In patients with ADHF, elevated plasma endothelin levels have been shown to be very strong predictors of severe ventricular arrhythmias[15] and even long-term survival.[16] Thus, the endothelin system appears to be up-regulated in the setting of AHF and predictive of adverse outcomes. More importantly, there is substantial evidence demonstrating that these alterations have important effects on the vasculature, as well as the myocardium.

The most apparent effect of endothelin is potent arterial and venous vasoconstriction,[17] a lethal mechanism of sarafotoxin, the deadly snake venom to which endothelin is related. The potent vasoconstricting effects of ET-1 are mediated predominantly by the vascular smooth muscle cell ET_A receptors, as well as the vascular smooth muscle cell ET_B receptors.[18,19] The increased afterload caused by ET-1 is significant and at least additive to that caused by other neurohormones, such as angiotensin,[9,20] presenting a major specific target for afterload reduction therapy in the ADHF patient. However, many non-specific vasodilators, such as nitroglycerin and nesiritide, already exist. It is the more specific actions of endothelin that make it such a dangerous toxin for patients with AHF. Endothelin can induce marked regional vasoconstriction, which seems to be more specific for the renal, cerebral, and coronary vascular beds,[21] and plays an important role in end-organ damage.

Peripheral edema and pulmonary edema are prominent symptoms in AHF, and endothelin exacerbates edema not only through changes in capillary hemodynamics, but also by promoting increased vascular permeability. Unlike other vasoconstrictors, endothelin causes an increase in capillary pressure and a decreased pre-capillary/post-capillary resistance ratio resulting in net transcapillary fluid filtration with increased interstitial edema.[22,23] In addition to these hemodynamic effects, a part of this increased vascular permeability is thought to be due to local recruitment of inflammatory factors. In study by Filep *et al.*,[24] administration of endothelin to guinea pigs resulted in a 2-fold to 4-fold increase in pulmonary albumin extravasation, which appeared to be both ET_A and ET_B receptor-dependent. Thus, endothelin's unique vascular effects contribute to increased peripheral and pulmonary edema.

ET-1 also acts as a potent mitogen on the vasculature and is important to the pathogenesis of arterial remodeling. Endothelin initiates hypertrophic remodeling of capacitance[25] and resistance arteries in multiple disease models,[26] resulting in hypertension and end-organ damage. This mitogenic effect is mediated by both ET_A[27] and ET_B receptors,[28] although their relative contributions remain unclear. The vascular remodeling and resulting end-organ damage, such as kidney injury,[29] can occur in the absence of elevated blood pressure,[30,31] and requires only a brief exposure to endothelin to produce sustained pathologic remodeling.[32] In addition, endothelin induces remodeling of the vascular extracellular matrix[33,34] and promotes fibroblast hyperplasia.[35] Thus, in the absence of antagonism, the transient marked elevations in ET-1 during AHF could instigate deleterious long-term vascular remodeling.

Endothelin exerts other effects on the vasculature by stimulating inflammation and promoting atherosclerosis. Endothelin causes greater vasoconstriction in atherosclerotic than normal coronary vessels,[36] indicative of the role that it has in contributing to endothelial dysfunction. It also facilitates the progression of atherosclerosis,[37] through increasing the cellular content of the plaque (vascular smooth muscle hypertrophy,[38] and inhibition of apoptosis of vascular smooth muscle cells[39] and fibroblasts[40,41]), stimulating neutrophil adhesion,[42] and increasing local inflammatory cytokines[43] and adhesion molecules.[44,45] Endothelin concentrations are elevated and predictive of mortality in patients with acute myocardial infarction (AMI),[46,47] and seem to play an important role in myocardial ischemia and ACS. Thus, endothelin has many effects on the vasculature that are relevant to the pathophysiology and clinical outcomes of patients with AHF, but there are additional effects beyond the vasculature to consider as well.

Preclinical studies: other effects of endothelin

The central role of endothelin in ventricular remodeling is supported by a number of studies.[48] Endothelin concentrations correlate with measures of ventricular remodeling in both the rat coronary artery ligation model of heat failure[49] and in patients.[50] In the myocardium, ET-1 directly stimulates "pathologic" hypertrophy with early gene expression and mediates apoptosis in pathologic conditions. Endothelin directly promotes vascular and myocardial fibrosis by stimulating fibroblast proliferation[51] and the synthesis of the extracellular matrix components fibronectin, collagen and laminin. ET-1 has also been shown to play a role in inflammation by increasing vascular permeability, inducing the release of cytokines, stimulating lipoxygenase activity, and increasing production of monocyte chemoattractant protein-1 and several adhesion molecules. Most of these effects appear to be mediated, to some extent, by both the ET_A and ET_B receptors and are clearly related to the process of ventricular remodeling.

Endothelin also has a role in the pathogenesis of heart failure via interactions with other neurohormones. Endothelin stimulates the secretion of neurohormones known to be important in AHF, such as norepinephrine, angiotensin II, vasopressin[52] and aldosterone.[53] Conversely, vasopressin,[54] angiotensin II and norepinephrine also stimulate endothelin production. In addition, endothelin potentiates[55] and mediates[56] the effects of these neurohormones. Other studies have demonstrated a central role of endothelin in the pressor and renal effects of angiotensin II[57] and in both angiotensin II and aldosterone-induced LV fibrosis.[58] Thus, endogenous ET-1 mediates the effects of many neurohormones known to be involved in heart failure.

The effects of endothelin on myocardial contractility are complicated, since its primary hemodynamic effect is as a vasodilator. In some studies of normal hearts, ET-1 acts as a mild positive inotrope, increasing contractility in reconstructed rat cardiac tissue,[59] as well as isolated guinea pig[60] or human[61] atrial muscle strips and the in vivo mouse heart.[62] However, ET-1 had no beneficial effect on contractility of in vivo pig[63] hearts. ET-1 has been shown to increase contractility in hamsters[64] and rats[65] with heart failure, while in other studies of CHF, antagonism of ET-1 in rats,[66–68] mice,[62] and dogs[69] actually improved LV function. In a study in humans,[70] intracoronary infusion of the ET_A receptor antagonist, BQ-123, increased contractility in heart failure patients while it decreased contractility in patients with normal EFs. These studies suggest that ET-1 supports myocardial contractility in healthy subjects, but acts as a myocardial depressant in heart failure patients. The importance of these findings is unclear for patients with AHF, but it suggests that endothelin-receptor antagonism would have minimal effect on patients with preserved LV function and, if anything, would improve contractility in patients with decreased function.

Endothelin has proarrhythmic effects[71] on both ventricular[72] and atrial[73] tissue. Many underlying mechanisms for this effect have been suggested, including prolongation or dispersion of the action potential, QT prolongation, and instigation of early after-depolarizations. Arrhythmias are a frequent and important complication of AHF, and in a recent study of 83 patients hospitalized for AHF, there was a very significant positive relationship between plasma endothelin concentrations and multiple measures of ventricular ectopy, including total premature ventricular complexes, frequency of ventricular pairs and number of ventricular tachycardia episodes.[15]

Endothelin is also known to have profound adverse effects on renal function. In the rat kidney, ET-1 increases renal vascular resistance and reduces renal blood flow and glomerular filtration rate via afferent and efferent arteriolar vasoconstriction.[74] In healthy human subjects, ET-1 infusion resulted in similar findings with decreased renal blood flow, glomerular filtration rate, and urinary sodium excretion, and marked increases in sodium retention and renal vasoconstriction.[75,76] In rat models, increases in urinary ET-1 excretion correlated with the development of proteinuria, renal insufficiency, and glomerular sclerosis.[77,78] ET-1 overexpression in transgenic mice produced interstitial renal fibrosis, glomerulosclerosis, and renal vascular hypertrophy.[29] In addition, multiple studies have demonstrated increased ET-1 urinary excretion and abnormal renal function in patients with heart failure.[79] There is growing evidence for a significant interaction between renal failure and heart failure,[80] and renal function is among the most important prognostic variables in patients with heart failure.[81] Furthermore, there is evidence that therapeutic interventions that favorably influence renal function might be beneficial.[82]

Preclinical studies of endothelin antagonism: vascular protection and beyond

Preclinical studies have clearly established endothelin as an important potential target for therapeutic intervention. With the development of ERAs, researchers were able to evaluate this new strategy in in vivo preclinical studies. A number of ERAs have been developed and they may be broadly categorized as ET_A-selective and dual (ET_A and ET_B) receptor antagonists. ERAs have been demonstrated to reduce systemic[9] and pulmonary[83] vasoconstriction, as well as decreasing LV filling pressures[84] in rats with heart failure. Administration of an ERA has also been shown to decrease vascular permeability[22,85] and pulmonary edema,[84] while decreasing inflammation and release of adhesion molecules.[86,87] ERAs have also been shown to be protective against vascular-induced end-organ damage, such as progressive renal dysfunction[88] and cerebral injury[89,90] in a number of animal models. ERAs have had beneficial effects on renal function in a variety of models of intrinsic renal disease and in experimental models of heart failure,[91–94] as well as in healthy human volunteers.[95] Thus, there is ample preclinical evidence that ERAs can provide vascular protection in multiple pathophysiologic disorders. In addition, there have been many studies performed in heart failure models.

The ET_A-selective peptide antagonist BQ-123 was the first agent to be widely available to investigate the role of endothelin in heart failure. Early studies suggested that administration of either BQ-123[96] or FR 139317,[97] another ET_A-selective agent, at the time of MI resulted in significant reduction in myocardial infarct size. In a landmark study by Sakai and colleagues,[68] BQ-123 treatment of rats with chronic MI due to coronary artery ligation resulted in a significant reduction in left ventricular hypertrophy (LVH) and chamber enlargement, as well as increased survival. Other studies in the Pfeffer rat coronary artery ligation heart failure model with different ET_A-selective ERAs have found conflicting results. In a study by Mulder and colleagues,[98] after 10 weeks of LU 135252 treatment, the treated rats had reduced LV enlargement and collagen density, but no difference in hypertrophy. However, LU 135252 administered chronically from 24 hours after coronary ligation increased LV filling pressures, lung congestion, ventricular dilation, and scar thinning 4 weeks later.[99] Treatment with EMD 94246 in rats with large MIs resulted in worsening of LV dilation.[100] In a more recent study,[101] sitaxsentan treatment resulted in a favorable leftward shift in the passive diastolic pressure–volume curve compared to untreated heart failure in rats, almost normalizing ventricular volumes, and markedly decreased matrix metalloproteinase (MMP) activation. Experimental studies using the rapid ventricular pacing heart failure model also showed some conflicting results with ET_A-selective agents. Spinale and co-investigators[102] demonstrated that PD 156707 treatment of rabbits attenuated progressive LV enlargement and improved myocyte function, but treatment with LU 135252 had no significant effect on canine rapid ventricular-pacing-induced ventricular enlargement.[103]

The other group of endothelin antagonists is the dual ET_A/ET_B receptor antagonists. Bosentan[104] is an oral non-peptide, dual ERA, currently approved for the treatment of pulmonary arterial hypertension. Administration of bosentan to rats with CHF resulted in significant reductions in blood pressure and this blood pressure reduction was at least additive, and possibly potentiating, to that caused by administration of maximal doses of the angiotensin-converting enzyme (ACE) inhibitor cilazapril.[9] Chronic administration of bosentan in the Pfeffer rat heart failure model significantly reduced adverse ventricular remodeling, including decreasing LV filling pressures, volumes, and fibrosis, while increasing cardiac output and decreasing circulating catecholamines.[67] Bosentan given chronically from 3 hours[66] or 24 hours[105] after coronary artery ligation also improved long-term LV ventricular remodeling and hemodynamics. Most importantly, bosentan has been demonstrated to increase survival in rats with chronic heart failure.[67] Bosentan also prevented adverse ventricular remodeling in Dahl salt-sensitive rat[106] and the rapid ventricular pacing models of heart failure in dogs.[107]

Tezosentan is structurally related to bosentan and is also a dual (ET_A/ET_B) ERA, designed specifically for intravenous use in hospitalized patients.[108] Acute administration of tezosentan to rats with heart failure effectively reduced systemic and LV filling pressures with no effect on contractility (dP/dt), and these effects were additive to acute enalapril treatment.[109] In addition, acute tezosentan administration decreased renal vascular resistance and increased renal plasma flow, glomerular filtration rate, urine flow rate, and sodium excretion in rats with heart failure.[93] In rats with MI,[84] two doses of tezosentan at 1 hour and 24 hours after coronary artery ligation resulted in attenuation of the increase in left ventricular end-diastolic pressure (LVEDP) and marked decrease in pulmonary edema at 48 hours after ligation. Consistent with the hypothesis that short-term therapy for AHF can provide long-term benefit, rats receiving these two doses of tezosentan during the first 24 hours had significantly reduced LVH and improved survival 5 months later. These preclinical studies provided strong support for using the vascular protective therapies of ERAs in patients with AHF.

Clinical Studies

Clinical studies of acute effects of endothelin antagonism in chronic heart failure

The recognition of endothelin as an important target in the pathogenesis of AHF and the beneficial effects of ERAs in experimental models encouraged the rapid investigation of these agents in patients. However, these drugs were initially tested in patients with more stable, chronic heart failure. As noted above, ERAs have been shown to reduce vasoconstriction, and in general, systemically-administered agents have decreased systemic vascular resistance (SVR) and pulmonary vascular resistance (PVR), pulmonary arterial pressures (PAPs), and pulmonary capillary wedge pressure (PCWP), while increasing cardiac output. However, there are relatively few published studies with these agents and some differences among ERAs have emerged (Tables 36.2 and 36.3).[110]

Bosentan was the first ERA to be tested in heart failure patients. In a study[111] of 24 patients with stable symptomatic chronic heart failure, left ventricular ejection fraction (LVEF) $\leq 30\%$, PCWP ≥ 15 mm Hg, and a cardiac index ≤ 2.5 L/min/m^2, bosentan infusion resulted in significant reductions in mean arterial pressure (MAP), mean pulmonary artery pressure (MPAP), right atrial pressure (RAP), and PCWP, as well as SVR and PVR (Table 36.2). Cardiac index increased significantly, but there was no change in heart rate. Plasma endothelin concentrations increased with bosentan infusion, presumably due to receptor displacement or decreased clearance by the ET_B receptors. The beneficial effects, not only on systemic and pulmonary vascular beds, but also on LV filling pressures and cardiac output, confirmed the promise of these agents for AHF. A subsequent study[112] administered 1 gram b.i.d. of oral bosentan (24 patients) or placebo (12 patients) to heart failure patients with similar hemodynamic effects as noted for the previous study, with no change in heart rate (Table 36.2). Thus, bosentan, given orally or intravenously, produced favorable acute hemodynamic responses in patients with stable chronic heart failure.

As noted previously, tezosentan is also a dual-receptor ERA, designed as an intravenous formulation for acute use.[108] Initial pharmacokinetic and pharmacodynamic studies in healthy patients suggested that doses from 5 to 100 mg/h would be appropriate for further study,[113] and that there were no clinically relevant adverse effects or need for dose adjustments with this tezosentan dose range in patients with markedly reduced renal function.[114] In 38 patients with chronic stable heart failure (Table 36.2),[115] reduced EF and cardiac index, and mildly-elevated PCWP, tezosentan was administered in an ascending dose protocol (5 mg, 20 mg, 50 mg, and 100 mg over 1 hour each). Invasive hemodynamic measurements demonstrated significant increases in cardiac

Table 36.2. *Acute hemodynamic effects of dual endothelin receptor antagonists (ET_A/ET_B) in heart failure patients from selected studies*

% Change from baseline	Study				
	Bosentan (IV)[111‡]	Bosentan (PO)[112§]	Tezosentan (IV)[115‖]	Tezosentan (IV)[116¶]	Tezosentan (IV)[117**]
Heart rate	0	−1	+3	+2	+1
Mean arterial pressure	−8[†]	−14[†]	−7	−10*	N/A
Right atrial pressure	−18[†]	−20*	−11	N/A	−15[†]
Mean pulmonary artery pressure	−14[†]	−13*	−10	−18*	N/A
Pulmonary capillary wedge pressure	−9*	−14*	−10	−13*	−17[†]
Cardiac index	+14*	+15[†]	+27[†]	+50[†]	+19*
Systemic vascular resistance	−16[†]	−24[†]	−25[†]	−34[†]	N/A
Pulmonary vascular resistance	−33*	−20*	−39[†]	−51[†]	N/A

Adapted, with permission, from Seed *et al.*[110]
*$P < 0.05$ versus baseline within study.
[†]$P < 0.01$ versus baseline within study, otherwise P = not significant.
[‡]100-mg dose, then 200-mg dose 60 minutes later, 2-hour measurement.
[§]1-gram dose, 3-hour measurement.
[‖]5 to 100-mg/h ascending dose, 4-hour measurement, placebo-corrected.
[¶]5 to 100-mg/h parallel dose, 100-mg/h dose, 6-hour measurement, placebo-corrected.
**20-mg/h and 50-mg/h groups combined, 48-hour hemodynamic measurement by Doppler echocardiography.
Abbreviations: ET = endothelin; N/A = data not available.

index, and decreases in PVR and SVR, with strong trends toward decreases in PCWP, RAP, PAP, and MAP. Dose-dependent increases in plasma endothelin and epinephrine were noted, but there was no evidence of rebound or significant adverse events. Another study of 61 patients with New York Heart Association (NYHA) class III or IV heart failure, LVEF < 35%, PCWP > 18 mm Hg, and cardiac index < 2.5 L/min/m^2 evaluated the hemodynamic effects of 6-hour infusions of tezosentan in a placebo-controlled, parallel group design with doses of 5, 20, 50, and 100 mg/h (Table 36.2).[116] Tezosentan caused up to a 50% dose-dependent increase in cardiac index, as well as significant decreases in PCWP. Plasma endothelin levels were quite markedly increased in the 50 to 100 mg/h groups, although only mildly elevated with the 5 mg/h dose and there were no significant adverse events. Another study of 14 patients[117] assessed the safety of a 48-hour infusion of 20 mg/h and 50 mg/h tezosentan compared to dobutamine (Table 36.2) and it demonstrated no episodes of hypotension requiring discontinuation, although headache was quite common. There was no evidence of tachyphylaxis during, or rebound after, the infusion. Despite the significant increases in cardiac index and decreases in PCWP, SVR and PVR, there were no significant increases in heart rate in any of these trials. These studies demonstrated that tezosentan was effective in improving hemodynamics, but larger studies would need to be performed to evaluate clinical efficacy.

The ERAs that are selective for the ET_A receptor were the first to be developed, and BQ-123 was the prototypical agent of this class. BQ-123 was infused in 10 patients with stable CHF,[118] resulting in significant decreases in MAP, PAP, and SVR, with increased cardiac index. There was a trend toward decreased PVR, as well, and no comment is made in the publication of effects on right atrial or

Table 36.3. *Acute hemodynamic effects of ET_A-selective endothelin receptor antagonists in heart failure patients from selected studies*

% Change from baseline	Study					
	BQ-123[118‡]	Darusentan (LU135252)[119§]	Darusentan (LU135252)[120‖]	Sitaxsentan (TBC11251)[121¶]	BMS 193884[123**]	ABT-627[132††]
Heart rate	+1	0	NS	−1	N/A	N/A
Mean arterial pressure	−8†	−10†	NS	−7	N/A	N/A
Right atrial pressure	−14	−19†	NS	−15*	N/A	N/A
Mean pulmonary artery pressure	−14†	−20†	NS	−12*	N/A	N/A
Pulmonary capillary wedge pressure	−18	−25†	NS	−7	−33*	−33*
Cardiac index	+5*	+22†	+13%	+11	+28*	+28*
Systemic vascular resistance	−12†	−27†	NS	−3	−26*	−26*
Pulmonary vascular resistance	−14	−26†	NS	−20*	N/A	N/A

Adapted, with permission, from Seed *et al.*[110]
*$P < 0.05$ versus baseline within study.
†$P < 0.01$ versus baseline within study, otherwise P = not significant.
‡100/200 nmol/min dose, 60–minute measurement.
§300-mg dose, 2-hour measurement.
‖300-mg dose, 2-hour measurement.
¶6-mg/kg dose, 2-hour measurement.
**100-mg dose, 4-hour measurement.
††7 to 30-mg dose, time of measurement not given.
Abbreviations: N/A = data not available; NS = no statistically significant difference compared to placebo.

ventricular filling pressures (Table 36.3). Although this study was uncontrolled, the marked hemodynamic effects of BQ-123 were supportive of a beneficial response in these patients. Darusentan (LU135252) is an orally available highly-selective ET_A receptor antagonist that has been investigated in a number of studies (Table 36.3). In a study by Spieker *et al.*,[119] 95 NYHA class II–III heart failure patients with an LVEF $\leq 35\%$ and PCWP ≥ 14 mm Hg, or cardiac index ≤ 2.8 L/min/m^2 were randomized to 1 of 5 oral doses of darusentan (1 mg, 10 mg, 30 mg, 100 mg, or 300 mg). The 30-mg to 300-mg doses of darusentan produced significant reductions in all pertinent hemodynamic measures and increased cardiac index with minimal adverse effects. Plasma endothelin concentrations also increased in a dose-dependent fashion, supporting a mechanism of receptor displacement. In the Heart Failure ET_A Blockade Trial,[120] 157 NYHA class III patients with LVEF $\leq 35\%$, PCWP ≥ 12 mm Hg, and cardiac index ≤ 2.6 L/min/m^2 were randomized to either placebo or 1 of 3 doses of darusentan (30 mg, 100 mg, or 300 mg p.o. q.d.). These patients all took their regular medications on the morning of the study, and although definite trends were evident, there were no significant changes in any of the hemodynamics measured at 4 hours after oral administration of darusentan. Sitaxsentan (TBC 11251) is also a non-peptide, highly-selective ET_A receptor antagonist that appeared to have preferential effects on the pulmonary vasculature in preclinical studies. In a multicenter, double-blind, placebo-controlled study of 48 NYHA III–IV heart failure patients with LVEF $\leq 35\%$, PCWP ≥ 15 mm Hg, and cardiac index ≤ 2.5 L/min/m^2, 3 doses of a 15-minute sitaxsentan infusion (1.5 mg/kg, 3.0 mg/kg, and 6.0 mg/kg) were compared to placebo.[121] The infusion of sitaxsentan resulted in significant decreases in RAP and mean PAP, as well as in PVR, but no significant effects on heart rate, MAP, PCWP, SVR or cardiac index (Table 36.3). A smaller study confirmed the acute pulmonary vasodilating effects of sitaxsentan in 8 heart failure patients, while there was no effect in 4 controls with normal LV systolic function.[122] Two other ET_A-selective antagonists (BMS-193884 and ABT-627) have been used in studies reported only as abstracts to date (Table 36.3).

These studies, and others,[123] on ERAs in patients with stable chronic heart failure have demonstrated favorable acute hemodynamic effects. However, few of these studies were placebo-controlled and few investigated the full-dose response of these agents or the time course of their effects. In addition, most drug development programs proceeded under the assumption that beneficial hemodynamic effects would translate into clinical benefit, an assumption that has proven wrong with other drug classes (i.e., phosphodiesterase [PDE] inhibitors). Nonetheless, the findings from these acute studies encouraged some development programs to proceed to Phase III clinical trials.

Clinical trials of endothelin antagonists in acute heart failure

The hemodynamic effects of tezosentan have been investigated in a number of trials, enrolling over 100 patients with advanced chronic heart failure using doses ranging from 5 to 100 mg/h as infusions for up to 48 hours.[115–117,124] These studies confirmed the predicted beneficial hemodynamic effects of tezosentan, which acutely reduced PAPs, LV filling pressures, and afterload, while increasing cardiac index with no change in heart rate. These studies were the basis for the design of the Randomized Intravenous TeZosentan (RITZ) trials.[125] This program was designed to have two pivotal trials, with RITZ-1 assessing symptom improvement without confounding from invasive hemodynamic monitoring and RITZ-2 investigating the effect of tezosentan on invasive hemodynamics. Two other trials evaluated the safety of tezosentan in 2 specific high-risk groups: AHF in patients with ACS (RITZ-4) and AHF associated with fulminant pulmonary edema (RITZ-5).

The RITZ-2 trial[126] randomized 184 patients hospitalized for ADHF (NYHA class III/IV, CI < 2.5 L/min/m^2, PCWP > 15 mm Hg) to 24-hour infusions of placebo or tezosentan (increased from 25 mg/h to either 50 mg/h or 100 mg/h). Both doses of tezosentan decreased PCWP by about 4 mm Hg (placebo-corrected; $P < 0.0001$) and increased cardiac index by about 0.4 L/min/m^2 (placebo-corrected; $P < 0.0001$), and there was a significant improvement in dyspnea at 24 hours

($P = 0.048$). There was also a strong trend toward improving the time to worsening of heart failure or death at 30 days in the tezosentan-treated patients ($P = 0.06$). The most frequent side effects were related to vasodilation and included hypotension and headache, all of which were much more frequent in the high-dose group. Interestingly, most of the hemodynamic benefit in this trial was achieved by the initial 25 mg/h dose within the first hour of treatment, suggesting that lower doses could have fewer side effects and potentially equivalent hemodynamic effects.

The RITZ-1 trial randomized 669 patients with ADHF to at least 24 hours of tezosentan (50 mg/h intravenous) or placebo on top of standard therapy.[127,128] Due to concerns in previous trials with the potential confounding effects of invasive hemodynamic monitoring on symptom assessment, patients with pulmonary artery (PA) catheter monitoring were excluded. The primary endpoint, the change in dyspnea between baseline and at 24 hours, was not statistically different between the two treatment groups. In addition, there was no difference in the main secondary endpoint of time to worsening of heart failure or death. However, adverse events related to excessive vasodilation, such as hypotension, nausea, headache, dizziness, and renal impairment were significantly more frequent in tezosentan-treated patients. These results were surprising in view of the findings from RITZ-2, and are probably explained by the RITZ-1 patient population being less acutely ill than the RITZ-2 patient groups (therefore less likely to show benefit), the absence of invasive monitoring, and the dose of tezosentan still being too high.

The RITZ-4 study investigated the effects of tezosentan in patients with ADHF and ACS,[129] randomizing 193 patients to placebo or tezosentan (50 mg/h). The composite primary endpoint (death, worsening of heart failure, recurrent ischemia, and recurrent or new MI within 72 hours) was not significantly different between the two groups, an anticipated result given the marginal power of the study. Although symptomatic hypotension was greater in the patients treated with tezosentan, there was no evidence for pro-ischemic effects. Other adverse events related to vasodilation, such as headache, dizziness, nausea, and renal failure or impairment, were more common in the tezosentan treated patients. This study reassured the investigators that tezosentan was relatively safe in patients with ACS, and reinforced the impression from the other trials that the dose used in these trials was probably too high.

RITZ-5[130] studied the effect of tezosentan on changes in oxygen saturation in patients with AHF and fulminant pulmonary edema. This study randomized 84 patients to either placebo or tezosentan, and tezosentan could be up-titrated from 50 to 100 mg/h at the investigator's discretion. The primary endpoint was the change in oxygen saturation as measured by pulse oximetry from baseline to 60 minutes after study drug administration. There was no difference between the placebo and tezosentan-treated groups with regard to the primary endpoint, but in a post-hoc analysis, patients receiving tezosentan at 50 mg/h had better outcomes, as assessed by time to death, cardiac failure, pulmonary edema, or cardiogenic shock, than those on placebo. Patients in the group receiving tezosentan at 100 mg/h had a high incidence of hypotensive episodes and worse outcomes. Once again, RITZ-5 suggested that the tezosentan dose was too high, yet despite significant hypotension, there was no evidence of pro-ischemic or pro-arrhythmic effects.

The evidence from the RITZ studies revealed a number of important lessons for clinical development programs for new AHF therapies. First, tezosentan clearly produces favorable hemodynamic effects in patients with AHF. Second, demonstrating improved clinical outcomes can be very difficult in this patient population. Third, despite significant hypotension and related adverse effects, tezosentan was relatively safe and well tolerated. Fourth, the dose of tezosentan used in the RITZ program did not have a favorable risk-to-benefit profile, given the excess symptomatic hypotension and related renal failure observed in the studies. To address this issue, a recent dose-ranging study demonstrated that tezosentan doses of 1 to 5 mg/h (compared to 50 and 100 mg/h in the RITZ studies) improved cardiac index and PCWP with no hypotension or renal insufficiency or failure in patients with AHF.[131] This low-dose, dose-ranging study strongly suggested that a lower dose of tezosentan would have a better risk-to-benefit profile.

The potential for providing improvement in clinical outcomes by administering a vascular-protective agent such as tezosentan has led to the initiation of a large, international, multicenter, randomized, placebo-controlled investigation of low-dose tezosentan—Value of Endothelin Receptor Inhibition with Tezosentan in Acute heart failure Study (VERITAS). The goal of VERITAS is to demonstrate the efficacy and safety of endothelin-receptor antagonism in ADHF. The VERITAS program consists of two identical, double-blind, randomized, placebo-controlled trials. The two trials (VERITAS-1 and VERITAS-2) will enroll approximately 1760 patients, within 24 hours of hospital admission, with dyspnea at rest due to heart failure and a respiratory rate of over 24 breaths per minute in need of intravenous therapy. In addition, the patient must also demonstrate objective signs of pulmonary congestion or heart failure. Patients will be randomized to 24 to 72 hours of tezosentan (5 mg/h intravenous for 30 min followed by 1 mg/h) or placebo and stratified based on the presence or absence of a Swan–Ganz catheter. The primary endpoints are: (1) incidence of death or worsening heart failure at 7 days in the combined trials; and (2) area under the curve of the change in dyspnea assessment (measured using a visual analog scale) from baseline over the first 24 hours of treatment in each trial. Secondary endpoints include hemodynamic data, time-to-event analysis for death or worsening heart failure, hospitalizations, and mortality, as well as other safety endpoints. This trial will definitively address the question of whether ERAs will fulfill their promise as therapeutic agents for patients with AHF.

References

1. American Heart Association. Heart Disease and Stroke Statistics—2004 Update. (American Heart Association: Dallas, TX, 2003).
2. Krumholz HM, Parent EM, Tu N, *et al.* Readmission after hospitalization for congestive heart failure among Medicare beneficiaries. Arch Intern Med 1997; 157: 99–104.
3. Tsuyuki RT, McKelvie RS, Arnold JM, *et al.* Acute precipitants of congestive heart failure exacerbations. Arch Intern Med 2001; 161: 2337–2342.
4. Dikshit K, Vyden JK, Forrester JS, *et al.* Renal and extrarenal hemodynamic effects of furosemide in congestive heart failure after acute myocardial infarction. N Engl J Med 1973; 288: 1087–1090.
5. Scios, Inc. ADHERE™ Acute Decompensated Heart Failure National Registry. Second Quarter 2003 National Benchmark Report. Available at: http://www.adhereregistry.com/national_bmr/q2_03_national_adhere_bmr.pdf. Accessed November 30, 2004.
6. Yanagisawa M, Kurihara H, Kimura S, *et al.* A novel potent vasoconstrictor peptide produced by vascular endothelial cells. Nature 1988; 332: 411–415.
7. Cernacek P, Stewart DJ. Immunoreactive endothelin in human plasma: marked elevations in patients in cardiogenic shock. Biochem Biophys Res Commun 1989; 161: 562–567.
8. Margulies KB, Hildebrand FL Jr., Lerman A, Perrella MA, Burnett JC Jr. Increased endothelin in experimental heart failure. Circulation 1990; 82: 2226–2230.
9. Teerlink JR, Löffler BM, Hess P, *et al.* Role of endothelin in the maintenance of blood pressure in conscious rats with chronic heart failure. Acute effects of the endothelin receptor antagonist Ro 47–0203 (bosentan). Circulation 1994; 90: 2510–2518.
10. Cody RJ, Haas GJ, Binkley PF, Capers Q, Kelley R. Plasma endothelin correlates with the extent of pulmonary hypertension in patients with chronic congestive heart failure. Circulation 1992; 85: 504–509.
11. McMurray JJ, Ray SG, Abdullah I, Dargie HJ, Morton JJ. Plasma endothelin in chronic heart failure. Circulation 1992; 85: 1374–1379.
12. Lerman A, Kubo SH, Tschumperlin LK, Burnett JC Jr. Plasma endothelin concentrations in humans with end-stage heart failure and after heart transplantation. J Am Coll Cardiol 1992; 20: 849–853.
13. Wei CM, Lerman A, Rodeheffer RJ, *et al.* Endothelin in human congestive heart failure. Circulation 1994; 89: 1580–1586.
14. Pacher R, Stanek B, Hülsmann M, *et al.* Prognostic impact of big endothelin-1 plasma concentrations compared with invasive hemodynamic evaluation in severe heart failure. J Am Coll Cardiol 1996; 27: 633–641.
15. Aronson D, Burger AJ. Neurohumoral activation and ventricular arrhythmias in patients with decompensated congestive heart failure: role of endothelin. Pacing Clin Electrophysiol 2003; 26: 703–710.

16. Aronson D, Burger AJ. Neurohormonal prediction of mortality following admission for decompensated heart failure. Am J Cardiol 2003; 91: 245–248.
17. McNeill JR. Role of endothelin in regulation of resistance, fluid-exchange, and capacitance functions of the systemic circulation. Can J Physiol Pharmacol 2003; 81: 522–532.
18. Gray GA, Löffler BM, Clozel M. Characterization of endothelin receptors mediating contraction of rabbit saphenous vein. Am J Physiol 1994; 266: H959–H966.
19. Teerlink JR, Breu V, Sprecher U, Clozel M, Clozel JP. Potent vasoconstriction mediated by endothelin ETB receptors in canine coronary arteries. Circ Res 1994; 74: 105–114.
20. Dohi Y, Hahn AW, Boulanger CM, Buhler FR, Luscher TF. Endothelin stimulated by angiotensin II augments contractility of spontaneously hypertensive rat resistance arteries. Hypertension 1992; 19: 131–137.
21. Clozel M, Clozel JP. Effects of endothelin on regional blood flows in squirrel monkeys. J Pharmacol Exp Ther 1989; 250: 1125–1131.
22. Ekelund U, Albert U, Edvinsson L, Mellander S. In-vivo effects of endothelin-1 and ETA receptor blockade on arterial, venous and capillary functions in skeletal muscle. Acta Physiol Scand 1993; 148: 273–283.
23. Ekelund U, Adner M, Edvinsson L, Mellander S. Effects of selective ETB-receptor stimulation on arterial, venous and capillary functions in cat skeletal muscle. Br J Pharmacol 1994; 112: 887–894.
24. Filep JG, Fournier A, Foldes-Filep E. Acute proinflammatory actions of endothelin-1 in the guinea-pig lung: involvement of ETA and ETB receptors. Br J Pharmacol 1995; 115: 227–236.
25. Yang Z, Krasnici N, Luscher TF. Endothelin-1 potentiates human smooth muscle cell growth to PDGF: effects of ETA and ETB receptor blockade. Circulation 1999; 100: 5–8.
26. Schiffrin EL. Endothelin: potential role in hypertension and vascular hypertrophy. Hypertension 1995; 25: 1135–1143.
27. Kanse SM, Wijelath E, Kanthou C, Newman P, Kakkar VV. The proliferative responsiveness of human vascular smooth muscle cells to endothelin correlates with endothelin receptor density. Lab Invest 1995; 72: 376–382.
28. Davie N, Haleen SJ, Upton PD, *et al.* ET(A) and ET(B) receptors modulate the proliferation of human pulmonary artery smooth muscle cells. Am J Respir Crit Care Med 2002; 165: 398–405.
29. Hocher B, Thone-Reineke C, Rohmeiss P, *et al.* Endothelin-1 transgenic mice develop glomerulosclerosis, interstitial fibrosis, and renal cysts but not hypertension. J Clin Invest 1997; 99: 1380–1389.
30. Moreau P, Dao HH. Endothelin receptor antagonists: novel agents for the treatment of hypertension? Expert Opin Investig Drugs 1999; 8: 1807–1821.
31. Schiffrin EL. Role of endothelin-1 in hypertension and vascular disease. Am J Hypertens 2001; 14: 83S–89S.
32. Dao HH, Martens FM, Lariviere R, *et al.* Transient involvement of endothelin in hypertrophic remodeling of small arteries. J Hypertens 2001; 19: 1801–1812.
33. Hocher B, Schwarz A, Fagan KA, *et al.* Pulmonary fibrosis and chronic lung inflammation in ET-1 transgenic mice. Am J Respir Cell Mol Biol 2000; 23: 19–26.
34. Shi-Wen X, Denton CP, Dashwood MR, *et al.* Fibroblast matrix gene expression and connective tissue remodeling: role of endothelin-1. J Invest Dermatol 2001; 116: 417–425.
35. Cambrey AD, Harrison NK, Dawes KE, *et al.* Increased levels of endothelin–1 in bronchoalveolar lavage fluid from patients with systemic sclerosis contribute to fibroblast mitogenic activity in vitro. Am J Respir Cell Mol Biol 1994; 11: 439–445.
36. Kinlay S, Behrendt D, Wainstein M, *et al.* Role of endothelin-1 in the active constriction of human atherosclerotic coronary arteries. Circulation 2001; 104: 1114–1118.
37. Luscher TF, Barton M. Endothelins and endothelin receptor antagonists: therapeutic considerations for a novel class of cardiovascular drugs. Circulation 2000; 102: 2434–2440.
38. Filippatos GS, Gangopadhyay N, Lalude O, *et al.* Regulation of apoptosis by vasoactive peptides. Am J Physiol Lung Cell Mol Physiol 2001; 281: L749–L761.
39. Wu-Wong JR, Chiou WJ, Dickinson R, Opgenorth TJ. Endothelin attenuates apoptosis in human smooth muscle cells. Biochem J 1997; 328: 733–737.
40. Shichiri M, Kato H, Marumo F, Hirata Y. Endothelin-1 as an autocrine/paracrine apoptosis survival factor for endothelial cells. Hypertension 1997; 30: 1198–1203.
41. Shichiri M, Sedivy JM, Marumo F, Hirata Y. Endothelin-1 is a potent survival factor for c-Myc-dependent apoptosis. Mol Endocrinol 1998; 12: 172–180.
42. Helset E, Lindal S, Olsen R, Myklebust R, Jorgensen L. Endothelin-1 causes sequential trapping of

platelets and neutrophils in pulmonary microcirculation in rats. Am J Physiol 1996; 271: L538–L546.
43. Browatzki M, Schmidt J, Kubler W, Kranzhofer R. Endothelin-1 induces interleukin-6 release via activation of the transcription factor NF-kappaB in human vascular smooth muscle cells. Basic Res Cardiol 2000; 95: 98–105.
44. Sanz MJ, Johnston B, Issekutz A, Kubes P. Endothelin-1 causes P-selectin-dependent leukocyte rolling and adhesion within rat mesenteric microvessels. Am J Physiol 1999; 277: H1823–H1830.
45. Parissis JT, Venetsanou KF, Mentzikof DG, *et al.* Plasma levels of soluble cellular adhesion molecules in patients with arterial hypertension. Correlations with plasma endothelin-1. Eur J Intern Med 2001; 12: 350–356.
46. Omland T, Lie RT, Aakvaag A, Aarsland T, Dickstein K. Plasma endothelin determination as a prognostic indicator of 1-year mortality after acute myocardial infarction. Circulation 1994; 89: 1573–1579.
47. Ray SG, McMurray JJ, Morton JJ, Dargie HJ. Circulating endothelin in acute ischaemic syndromes. Br Heart J 1992; 67: 383–386.
48. Teerlink JR. Reversal of left ventricular remodeling: role of the endothelin pathway. J Card Fail 2002; 8: S494–S499.
49. Loennechen JP, Støylen A, Beisvag V, Wisløff U, Ellingsen O. Regional expression of endothelin-1, ANP, IGF-1, and LV wall stress in the infarcted rat heart. Am J Physiol Heart Circ Physiol 2001; 280: H2902–H2910.
50. Tsutamoto T, Wada A, Maeda K, *et al.* Transcardiac extraction of circulating endothelin-1 across the failing heart. Am J Cardiol 2000; 86: 524–528.
51. Piacentini L, Gray M, Honbo NY, *et al.* Endothelin-1 stimulates cardiac fibroblast proliferation through activation of protein kinase C. J Mol Cell Cardiol 2000; 32: 565–576.
52. Yamamoto T, Kimura T, Ota K, *et al.* Central effects of endothelin-1 on vasopressin release, blood pressure, and renal solute excretion. Am J Physiol 1992; 262: E856–E862.
53. Belloni AS, Rossi GP, Andreis PG, *et al.* Endothelin adrenocortical secretagogue effect is mediated by the B receptor in rats. Hypertension 1996; 27: 1153–1159.
54. Imai T, Hirata Y, Emori T, *et al.* Induction of endothelin-1 gene by angiotensin and vasopressin in endothelial cells. Hypertension 1992; 19: 753–757.
55. Yoshida K, Yasujima M, Kohzuki M, *et al.* Endothelin-1 augments pressor response to angiotensin II infusion in rats. Hypertension 1992; 20: 292–297.
56. Kaddoura S, Firth JD, Boheler KR, Sugden PH, Poole-Wilson PA. Endothelin-1 is involved in norepinephrine-induced ventricular hypertrophy in vivo. Acute effects of bosentan, an orally active, mixed endothelin ETA and ETB receptor antagonist. Circulation 1996; 93: 2068–2079.
57. Riggleman A, Harvey J, Baylis C. Endothelin mediates some of the renal actions of acutely administered angiotensin II. Hypertension 2001; 38: 105–109.
58. Ramires FJA, Sun Y, Mady C, Ramires JAF, Weber KT. Effect of endothelin on myocardial fibrosis in response to chronic administration of angiotensin II or aldosterone. Circulation 1999; 100: I-474 (Abstract).
59. Zolk O, Munzel F, Eschenhagen T. Effects of chronic endothelin-1 stimulation on cardiac myocyte contractile function. Am J Physiol Heart Circ Physiol 2004; 286: H1248–H1257.
60. Ishikawa T, Yanagisawa M, Kimura S, Goto K, Masaki T. Positive inotropic action of novel vasoconstrictor peptide endothelin on guinea pig atria. Am J Physiol 1988; 255: H970–H973.
61. Zerkowski HR, Broede A, Kunde K, *et al.* Comparison of the positive inotropic effects of serotonin, histamine, angiotensin II, endothelin and isoprenaline in the isolated human right atrium. Naunyn Schmiedebergs Arch Pharmacol 1993; 347: 347–352.
62. Pandey AS, Stewart DJ, Cernacek P, Dawood F, Wen WH, Liu P. Chronic endothelin-1 blockade preserves myocardial contractility in dilated cardiomyopathy. J Cardiovasc Pharmacol 1998; 31: S306–S308.
63. Ricou FJ, Murata K, Oh BH, Kambayashi M, Peterson KL. Evaluation of inotropic effect of endothelin-1 in vivo. J Cardiovasc Pharmacol 1992; 20: 671–677.
64. Fontaine ER, Viau S, Jasmin G, Dumont L. Effects of phosphoramidon, BQ 788, and BQ 123 on coronary and cardiac dysfunctions of the failing hamster heart. J Cardiovasc Pharmacol 1998; 32: 12–20.
65. Sakai S, Miyauchi T, Sakurai T, *et al.* Endogenous endothelin-1 participates in the maintenance of cardiac function in rats with congestive heart failure. Marked increase in endothelin-1 production in the failing heart. Circulation 1996; 93: 1214–1222.
66. Fraccarollo D, Hu K, Galuppo P, Gaudron P, Ertl G. Chronic endothelin receptor blockade attenuates progressive ventricular dilation and improves cardiac function in rats with myocardial infarction: possible

involvement of myocardial endothelin system in ventricular remodeling. Circulation 1997; 96: 3963–3973.
67. Mulder P, Richard V, Derumeaux G, *et al.* Role of endogenous endothelin in chronic heart failure: effect of long-term treatment with an endothelin antagonist on survival, hemodynamics, and cardiac remodeling. Circulation 1997; 96: 1976–1982.
68. Sakai S, Miyauchi T, Kobayashi M, *et al.* Inhibition of myocardial endothelin pathway improves long-term survival in heart failure. Nature 1996; 384: 353–355.
69. Onishi K, Ohno M, Little WC, Cheng CP. Endogenous endothelin-1 depresses left ventricular systolic and diastolic performance in congestive heart failure. J Pharmacol Exp Ther 1999; 288: 1214–1222.
70. MacCarthy PA, Grocott-Mason R, Prendergast BD, Shah AM. Contrasting inotropic effects of endogenous endothelin in the normal and failing human heart: studies with an intracoronary ET(A) receptor antagonist. Circulation 2000; 101: 142–147.
71. Duru F, Barton M, Lüscher TF, Candinas R. Endothelin and cardiac arrhythmias: do endothelin antagonists have a therapeutic potential as antiarrhythmic drugs? Cardiovasc Res 2001; 49: 272–280.
72. Yorikane R, Shiga H, Miyake S, Koike H. Evidence for direct arrhythmogenic action of endothelin. Biochem Biophys Res Commun 1990; 173: 457–462.
73. Burrell KM, Molenaar P, Dawson PJ, Kaumann AJ. Contractile and arrhythmic effects of endothelin receptor agonists in human heart in vitro: blockade with SB 209670. J Pharmacol Exp Ther 2000; 292: 449–459.
74. Katoh T, Chang H, Uchida S, Okuda T, Kurokawa K. Direct effects of endothelin in the rat kidney. Am J Physiol 1990; 258: F397–F402.
75. Rabelink TJ, Kaasjager KA, Boer P, *et al.* Effects of endothelin-1 on renal function in humans: implications for physiology and pathophysiology. Kidney Int 1994; 46: 376–381.
76. Sorensen SS, Madsen JK, Pedersen EB. Systemic and renal effect of intravenous infusion of endothelin-1 in healthy human volunteers. Am J Physiol 1994; 266: F411–F418.
77. Orisio S, Benigni A, Bruzzi I, *et al.* Renal endothelin gene expression is increased in remnant kidney and correlates with disease progression. Kidney Int 1993; 43: 354–358.
78. Lariviere R, D'Amours M, Lebel M, *et al.* Increased immunoreactive endothelin-1 levels in blood vessels and glomeruli of rats with reduced renal mass. Kidney Blood Press Res 1997; 20: 372–380.
79. Modesti PA, Cecioni I, Costoli A, *et al.* Renal endothelin in heart failure and its relation to sodium excretion. Am Heart J 2000; 140: 617–622.
80. Silverberg D, Wexler D, Blum M, Schwartz D, Iaina A. The association between congestive heart failure and chronic renal disease. Curr Opin Nephrol Hypertens 2004; 13: 163–170.
81. Dries DL, Exner DV, Domanski MJ, Greenberg B, Stevenson LW. The prognostic implications of renal insufficiency in asymptomatic and symptomatic patients with left ventricular systolic dysfunction. J Am Coll Cardiol 2000; 35: 681–689.
82. Gottlieb SS, Abraham W, Butler J, *et al.* The prognostic importance of different definitions of worsening renal function in congestive heart failure. J Card Fail 2002; 8: 136–141.
83. Hess P, Clozel M, Clozel JP. Telemetry monitoring of pulmonary arterial pressure in freely moving rats. J Appl Physiol 1996; 81: 1027–1032.
84. Clozel M, Qiu C, Qiu CS, Hess P, Clozel JP. Short-term endothelin receptor blockade with tezosentan has both immediate and long-term beneficial effects in rats with myocardial infarction. J Am Coll Cardiol 2002; 39: 142–147.
85. Filep JG. Endogenous endothelin modulates blood pressure, plasma volume, and albumin escape after systemic nitric oxide blockade. Hypertension 1997; 30: 22–28.
86. Finsnes F, Skjonsberg OH, Tonnessen T, *et al.* Endothelin production and effects of endothelin antagonism during experimental airway inflammation. Am J Respir Crit Care Med 1997; 155: 1404–1412.
87. Verma S, Li SH, Badiwala MV, *et al.* Endothelin antagonism and interleukin-6 inhibition attenuate the proatherogenic effects of C-reactive protein. Circulation 2002; 105: 1890–1896.
88. Lariviere R, Lebel M. Endothelin-1 in chronic renal failure and hypertension. Can J Physiol Pharmacol 2003; 81: 607–621.
89. Hino A, Weir BK, Macdonald RL, *et al.* Prospective, randomized, double-blind trial of BQ-123 and bosentan for prevention of vasospasm following subarachnoid hemorrhage in monkeys. J Neurosurg 1995; 83: 503–509.
90. Kwan AL, Lin CL, Chang CZ, *et al.* Oral administration of an inhibitor of endothelin-converting enzyme attenuates cerebral vasospasm following experimental subarachnoid haemorrhage in rabbits. Clin Sci (Lond) 2002; 103: 414S–417S.
91. Ohnishi M, Wada A, Tsutamoto T, *et al.* Chronic effects of a novel, orally active endothelin receptor

antagonist, T-0201, in dogs with congestive heart failure. J Cardiovasc Pharmacol 1998; 31: S236–S238.
92. Bauersachs J, Braun C, Fraccarollo D, *et al.* Improvement of renal dysfunction in rats with chronic heart failure after myocardial infarction by treatment with the endothelin A receptor antagonist, LU 135252. J Hypertens 2000; 18: 1507–1514.
93. Qiu C, Ding SS, Hess P, Clozel JP, Clozel M. Endothelin mediates the altered renal hemodynamics associated with experimental congestive heart failure. J Cardiovasc Pharmacol 2001; 38: 317–324.
94. Ding SS, Qiu C, Hess P, *et al.* Chronic endothelin receptor blockade prevents renal vasoconstriction and sodium retention in rats with chronic heart failure. Cardiovasc Res 2002; 53: 963–970.
95. Fleisch M, Sutsch G, Yan XW, *et al.* Systemic, pulmonary, and renal hemodynamic effects of endothelin ET(A/B)-receptor blockade in patients with maintained left ventricular function. J Cardiovasc Pharmacol 2000; 36: 302–309.
96. Grover GJ, Dzwonczyk S, Parham CS. The endothelin-1 receptor antagonist BQ-123 reduces infarct size in a canine model of coronary occlusion and reperfusion. Cardiovasc Res 1993; 27: 1613–1618.
97. Burke SE, Nelson RA. Endothelin-receptor antagonist FR 139317 reduces infarct size in a rabbit model when given before, but not after, coronary artery occlusion. J Cardiovasc Pharmacol 1997; 29: 87–92.
98. Mulder P, Richard V, Bouchart F, *et al.* Selective ETA receptor blockade prevents left ventricular remodeling and deterioration of cardiac function in experimental heart failure. Cardiovasc Res 1998; 39: 600–608.
99. Nguyen QT, Cernacek P, Calderoni A, *et al.* Endothelin A receptor blockade causes adverse left ventricular remodeling but improves pulmonary artery pressure after infarction in the rat. Circulation 1998; 98: 2323–2330.
100. Hu K, Gaudron P, Schmidt TJ, Hoffmann KD, Ertl G. Aggravation of left ventricular remodeling by a novel specific endothelin ET(A) antagonist EMD94246 in rats with experimental myocardial infarction. J Cardiovasc Pharmacol 1998; 32: 505–508.
101. Podesser BK, Siwik DA, Eberli FR, *et al.* ET(A)-receptor blockade prevents matrix metalloproteinase activation late postmyocardial infarction in the rat. Am J Physiol Heart Circ Physiol 2001; 280: H984–H991.
102. Spinale FG, Walker JD, Mukherjee R, *et al.* Concomitant endothelin receptor subtype-A blockade during the progression of pacing-induced congestive heart failure in rabbits. Beneficial effects on left ventricular and myocyte function. Circulation 1997; 95: 1918–1929.
103. Moe GW, Albernaz A, Naik GO, Kirchengast M, Stewart DJ. Beneficial effects of long-term selective endothelin type A receptor blockade in canine experimental heart failure. Cardiovasc Res 1998; 39: 571–579.
104. Clozel M, Breu V, Gray GA, *et al.* Pharmacological characterization of bosentan, a new potent orally active nonpeptide endothelin receptor antagonist. J Pharmacol Exp Ther 1994; 270: 228–235.
105. Oie E, Bjonerheim R, Grogaard HK, *et al.* ET-receptor antagonism, myocardial gene expression, and ventricular remodeling during CHF in rats. Am J Physiol Heart Circ Physiol 1998; 275: H868–H877.
106. Iwanaga Y, Kihara Y, Inagaki K, *et al.* Differential effects of angiotensin II versus endothelin-1 inhibitions in hypertrophic left ventricular myocardium during transition to heart failure. Circulation 2001; 104: 606–612.
107. Mishima T, Tanimura M, Suzuki G, *et al.* Effects of long-term therapy with bosentan on the progression of left ventricular dysfunction and remodeling in dogs with heart failure. J Am Coll Cardiol 2000; 35: 222–229.
108. Clozel M, Ramuz H, Clozel JP, *et al.* Pharmacology of tezosentan, new endothelin receptor antagonist designed for parenteral use. J Pharmacol Exp Ther 1999; 290: 840–846.
109. Qiu CB, Qiu CS, Hess P, Clozel JP, Clozel M. Additional effects of endothelin receptor blockade and angiotensin converting enzyme inhibition in rats with chronic heart failure. Acta Pharmacol Sin 2001; 22: 541–548.
110. Seed A, Love MP, McMurray JJ. Clinical experience with endothelin receptor antagonists in chronic heart failure. Heart Fail Rev 2001; 6: 317–323.
111. Kiowski W, Sutsch G, Hunziker P, *et al.* Evidence for endothelin-1-mediated vasoconstriction in severe chronic heart failure. Lancet 1995; 346: 732–736.
112. Sütsch G, Kiowski W, Yan XW, *et al.* Short-term oral endothelin-receptor antagonist therapy in conventionally treated patients with symptomatic severe chronic heart failure. Circulation 1998; 98: 2262–2268.
113. Dingemanse J, Clozel M, van Giersbergen PL. Pharmacokinetics and pharmacodynamics of tezosentan, an intravenous dual endothelin receptor antagonist, following chronic infusion in healthy subjects. Br J Clin Pharmacol 2002; 53: 355–362.

114. van Giersbergen PL, Dingemanse J. Effect of severe renal impairment on the pharmacokinetics and tolerability of the parenteral endothelin antagonist tezosentan. Int J Clin Pharmacol Ther 2003; 41: 261–266.
115. Schalcher C, Cotter G, Reisin L, *et al.* The dual endothelin receptor antagonist tezosentan acutely improves hemodynamic parameters in patients with advanced heart failure. Am Heart J 2001; 142: 340–349.
116. Torre-Amione G, Young JB, Durand J, *et al.* Hemodynamic effects of tezosentan, an intravenous dual endothelin receptor antagonist, in patients with class III to IV congestive heart failure. Circulation 2001; 103: 973–980.
117. Torre-Amione G, Durand JB, Nagueh S, *et al.* A pilot safety trial of prolonged (48 h) infusion of the dual endothelin-receptor antagonist tezosentan in patients with advanced heart failure. Chest 2001; 120: 460–466.
118. Cowburn PJ, Cleland JG, McArthur JD, *et al.* Short-term haemodynamic effects of BQ-123, a selective endothelin ET(A)-receptor antagonist, in chronic heart failure. Lancet 1998; 352: 201–202.
119. Spieker LE, Mitrovic V, Noll G, *et al.* Acute hemodynamic and neurohumoral effects of selective ET(A) receptor blockade in patients with congestive heart failure. ET 003 Investigators. J Am Coll Cardiol 2000; 35: 1745–1752.
120. Lüscher TF, Enseleit F, Pacher R, *et al.* Hemodynamic and neurohumoral effects of selective endothelin A (ET(A)) receptor blockade in chronic heart failure: the Heart Failure ET(A) Receptor Blockade Trial (HEAT). Circulation 2002; 106: 2666–2672.
121. Givertz MM, Colucci WS, LeJemtel TH, *et al.* Acute endothelin A receptor blockade causes selective pulmonary vasodilation in patients with chronic heart failure. Circulation 2000; 101: 2922–2927.
122. Ooi H, Colucci WS, Givertz MM. Endothelin mediates increased pulmonary vascular tone in patients with heart failure: demonstration by direct intrapulmonary infusion of sitaxsentan. Circulation 2002; 106: 1618–1621.
123. Smith W, Iteld B, LeJemtel T, *et al.* Improved hemodynamics with the ETA selective receptor antagonist BMS-193884 in patients with heart failure. J Am Coll Cardiol 2000 35: 241 (Abstract).
124. Cotter G, Kiowski W, Kaluski E, *et al.* Tezosentan (an intravenous endothelin receptor A/B antagonist) reduces peripheral resistance and increases cardiac power therefore preventing a steep decrease in blood pressure in patients with congestive heart failure. Eur J Heart Fail 2001; 3: 457–461.
125. Teerlink JR, Torre-Amione G. A new strategy for a clinical development program in acute decompensated heart failure: The Randomized Intravenous TeZosentan (RTIZ) trials. J Cardiac Fail 2000; 6: 48 (Abstract).
126. Torre-Amione G, Young JB, Colucci WS, *et al.* Hemodynamic and clinical effects of tezosentan, an intravenous dual endothelin receptor antagonist, in patients hospitalized for acute decompensated heart failure. J Am Coll Cardiol 2003; 42: 140–147.
127. Teerlink JR, Massie BM, Cleland JGF, Tzivoni D, for the RITZ-1 Investigators. A double-blind, parallel-group, multicenter, placebo-controlled study to investigate the efficacy and safety of tezosentan in reducing symptoms in patients with acute decompensated heart failure. Circulation 2001; 104: II-526 (Abstract).
128. Coletta AP, Cleland JG. Clinical trials update: highlights of the scientific sessions of the XXIII Congress of the European Society of Cardiology—WARIS II, ESCAMI, PAFAC, RITZ-1 and TIME. Eur J Heart Fail 2001; 3: 747–750.
129. O'Connor CM, Gattis WA, Adams KF Jr., *et al.* Tezosentan in patients with acute heart failure and acute coronary syndromes: results of the Randomized Intravenous TeZosentan Study (RITZ-4). J Am Coll Cardiol 2003; 41: 1452–1457.
130. Kaluski E, Kobrin I, Zimlichman R, *et al.* RITZ-5: randomized intravenous TeZosentan (an endothelin-A/B antagonist) for the treatment of pulmonary edema: a prospective, multicenter, double-blind, placebo-controlled study. J Am Coll Cardiol 2003; 41: 204–210.
131. Coletta AP, Clark AL, Seymour AM, Cleland JG. Clinical trials update from the European Society of Cardiology Heart Failure meeting: COMET, COMPANION, Tezosentan and SHAPE. Eur J Heart Fail 2003; 5: 545–548.
132. Chen HH, Salz LM, McKinley LJ, *et al.* Safety and efficacy of an orally active selective endothelin-A receptor antagonist in moderate-severe human chronic heart failure. J Cardiac Fail 1999; 5: 172 (Abstract).

Part V

Issues in the Management of Acute Heart Failure

CHAPTER 37

Advanced nursing aspects of acute heart failure

Laura H Gaulden, Jana Glotzer

Introduction

The management of patients with acute decompensated heart failure (ADHF) can be a challenging process, and evidence is lacking from clinical trials to guide therapy. The care of these patients, therefore, depends on the sound clinical judgment of the care team. In the past, the care of these complicated patients lay solely in the medical domain with physician management. With the advent of multidisciplinary team management of heart failure patients, promoted by both the American Heart Association and the Agency for Healthcare Reform, the advanced practice nurse (APN) has become an important component in the care of heart failure patients.[1,2]

Advanced Practice Nursing

An advanced practice nurse (APN), as defined by the American Nurses Association (ANA), is a registered nurse (RN) who has "a masters or doctoral education concentrating in a specific area of advanced nursing practice, had supervised practice during graduate education, and has ongoing clinical experiences."[3] APNs are expected to "provide comprehensive health assessments and demonstrate a high level of autonomy and expert skill in the diagnosis and treatment of the complex human responses of individuals, families, or communities to actual or potential health problems."[3] The ANA recognizes four types of APNs: (1) nurse practitioners (NPs); (2) clinical nurse specialists (CNSs); (3) certified registered nurse anesthetists; and (4) certified nurse midwives. For the purposes of this discussion, we will use APNs to mean NPs and CNSs.

APNs bring added value to the clinical care of the heart failure patient because they are able to incorporate the art of nursing into the medical model. Respecting the patient's values and acting as patient advocate are core principles of nursing care. APNs practice in a collaborative, multidisciplinary fashion with physicians and other health care providers to provide a high quality of care. APNs are trained to care for patients across the continuum of illness and are, therefore, uniquely qualified to treat patients in inpatient, as well as outpatient, settings.[4] With their holistic approach to care, APNs are trained not only to manage the medical aspects of the disease itself, but also to treat the person as a whole and include family and caregivers in the plan of care. APNs often practice in both outpatient and inpatient settings and can assist patients in navigating the complexities of the medical arena. Patients with decompensated heart failure may receive their care in either setting. Knowledge of their baseline functional status and social support are key elements to providing optimal care in the decompensated state.

Inpatient Care

A number of investigators have explored the role of the APN in the inpatient setting. Dahle *et al.* developed an inpatient service that was managed by an NP.[5] Patients with uncomplicated heart failure were admitted to the NP service, while patients with hypotension, symptomatic arrhythmias, hypoxia, or cardiac ischemia were admitted to the house officer team. Although there was no difference in the 30-day readmission rate between the services, total hospital cost of care was lower and length of stay trended toward shorter stays on the NP service. Knaus *et al.* reported high levels of patient and physician satisfaction with quality of care in a study of a collaborative rounding service utilizing acute care NPs.[6] In another study by Constantini *et al.*, a consult service composed of an NP and a faculty cardiologist was shown to significantly increase adherence to guideline-based care, decrease length of stay, and lower cost of care.[7] By participating in the inpatient management of advanced heart failure patients, APNs are able to better anticipate their outpatient needs and enhance continuity of care.

Congestive heart failure (CHF) is the most common indication for admission among older adults.[8] It has been estimated that anywhere from 20% to 50% of patients with CHF are readmitted within 60 days to 6 months of discharge.[9] A number of investigators have explored the factors leading to the high readmission rate among heart failure patients. Precipitating or contributing causes that are largely preventable include noncompliance with medications and diet, poor social support, inadequate discharge planning, inadequate medical treatment, and limited understanding of the disease and the symptoms of worsening failure.[8,10,11] Iatrogenic causes including adverse drug reactions, nosocomial infections, procedural complications, and overhydration have also been implicated.[12] Comorbid conditions including anemia, arrhythmias, infections, and coronary ischemia also contribute to the high readmission rate. Prognosis for patients who are readmitted is poor.[12] In a large multicenter observational study, Krumholz *et al.* were able to identify predictors of readmission, including male gender, presence of comorbidities, at least one admission within 6 months of the index admission, and length of stay for the index hospitalization of more than 7 days. Although heart failure was the most common cause for readmission, accounting for 18% of all hospitalizations, a number of comorbid conditions including infection and coronary ischemia lead to the rest of the unplanned admissions.[9] Assessment for and prevention of these contributing factors should, therefore, be included in the plan of care. Health care providers should tailor patient and family education to address the risk factors identified for each individual patient.

A multidisciplinary approach to patient care using APNs has the potential to reduce these hospitalizations, as APNs practice a holistic model of care, providing care to the whole person rather than just targeting the disease process. APNs are uniquely qualified to assist patients in managing the risk factors and comorbidities that often contribute to exacerbation of their disease. Ongoing assessment of the patient in the chronic stable state is critically important. These factors should also be evaluated in the inpatient setting as treatment of exacerbating factors is important in stabilization of the disease. In addition to reinforcing patient education performed in the outpatient setting, an evaluation should be performed to determine whether gaps in the patient's knowledge might have contributed to the episode of decompensation.

When patients are admitted to the hospital with CHF exacerbation, it is vital that the APN not only begin the process of managing the acute episode, but also start the discharge planning process. The study by Nayor *et al.*, which included a comprehensive discharge planning protocol involving coordination of services during the hospitalization and for 2 weeks after discharge by nurse specialists, resulted in an increase in time between initial discharge and readmission, a decrease in total length of stay during rehospitalization, and decreased cost of care for readmission.[13] A multicenter Veterans Administration (VA) study of unplanned readmissions within 2 weeks of discharge found a link between the quality of the inpatient care and risk for readmission.[14] A list of criteria indicating readiness for discharge was developed, and non-adherence to these criteria was associated with early readmission. The criteria for heart failure readiness for discharge included stable weight, stable medical regimen (no significant change for at least 24 hours), documentation of patient and family understanding of medications and dietary restrictions, significant symptomatic improvement, and documentation of scheduled hospital follow-up.[14] By completing a comprehensive assessment of the patient at the time of admission, detecting potential discharge concerns, communicating effectively with team members, providing education to the patient and family, and ensuring cost-effective and streamlined care, the APN plays a valuable role in improving quality of care and preventing hospital readmissions.[4,15]

Multidisciplinary Outpatient Care

With the current limitations of pharmacologic therapy, it is clear that additional strategies are needed to augment the care of these complex patients. Strategies to optimize medical management, reduce cost, and improve quality of life have been evaluated in multiple studies. The most successful strategies have used APNs in collaborative practice interventions, with reduction in readmissions for heart failure of up to 56%.[16,17] These programs are typically multidisciplinary, nurse driven, and place a heavy emphasis on patient education. Outpatient management of these complex patients by APNs has been shown to positively impact a number of factors important to both quality of patient care and the cost of providing that care. These benefits include reduction in length of stay, decreased readmission rate, decreased cost of hospitalization, and increased patient satisfaction with the quality of care. Despite a number of attempts at exploring the components of the different variations of disease management, to date no evidence has been found that clearly defines a combination of components or duration of intervention that ensures success. Interestingly, a study of increased access to primary care and nurse intervention resulted in an improvement in patient satisfaction, but also resulted in an increase in readmission rate.[18] These results would suggest that in order to significantly impact length of stay, readmissions, and cost of care, disease management programs should ideally be staffed with physicians and APNs with expertise in heart failure management.

Multidisciplinary management can take many forms, depending on the needs of the community and the resources available to the institution or practice implementing the program. Ansari *et al.* evaluated three interventions designed to increase the use of beta-blockers. Strategies included educating providers, computerized reminders for patients and providers, and nurse initiation and titration of beta-blocker. The number of patients who were initiated on beta-blockers and achieved target dose was highest in the nurse intervention arm.[19]

Home-based nurse interventions with telephone follow-up have successfully reduced readmission rates and cost of care.[20–22] Home visits can uncover barriers to compliance that are difficult to assess in the inpatient setting and facilitate assessment of early warning signs of decompensation. Key components of these interventions included educating patients about heart failure, optimizing their medical regimen, and monitoring symptom progression through close follow-up. However, the number and frequency of visits necessary to derive the most benefit are still not clear.

Telephone interventions have been successful in enhancing compliance with lifestyle modifications, improving quality of life, and decreasing hospitalization and outpatient visits.[23] A pilot study of a computerized home monitoring system resulted in a decrease in cost of care and total days hospitalized for the intervention arm. This system including monitoring of daily weights, blood pressure, and symptoms that would trigger a telephone call to the patient by a nurse in combination with weekly educational mailings and telephone calls from a nurse.[24]

Rich *et al.* reported a decrease in readmissions by 56% and decreased cost of care for inpatients with heart failure in a prospective randomized trial of a complex nurse-directed multidisciplinary intervention consisting of comprehensive education on diet and medications, early discharge planning, social service consultation, and intensive post-discharge follow-up.[16] A multicenter, multidisciplinary intervention involving a telephone nurse coordinator, CHF nurse, heart failure cardiologist, and primary care physician (PCP) resulted in improvement in symptom management, increased adherence to evidence-based medicine, and a trend towards reduction in the primary endpoint of mortality plus hospitalization.[25]

Education and Counseling

Ultimately, the best management strategy is prevention of ADHF. Optimal medical management and use of state of the art technologies clearly have a role. However, without the active participation of patients and their caregivers, medical management will ultimately fail. By providing the knowledge needed to manage their disease, nurses can empower patients to improve their quality of life, reduce their likelihood of rehospitalization, and prolong their lives. Patient education should happen throughout the course of the disease—from the relative asymptomatic stage to advanced heart failure—in the outpatient setting as well as in the hospital.[26]

Symptoms and symptom management

Common symptoms of heart failure include dyspnea, fatigue, lower extremity edema, orthopnea, paroxysmal nocturnal dyspnea, and dizziness. Patients need to understand how to differentiate between their symptoms of chronic stable heart failure and changes in their symptoms that may indicate worsening heart failure. Patients should be provided with contact numbers for the appropriate health care providers to call and report their symptoms. If they are prompted to call before their symptoms progress to decompensation, patients can potentially avoid hospitalization. For patients with comorbidities that have symptom profiles similar to heart failure, such as chronic obstructive pulmonary disease (COPD), additional counseling to help differentiate between the symptoms of heart failure and other illnesses can be helpful. The importance of daily weight monitoring should be stressed, and contact numbers for the appropriate health care provider to call in the event of weight gain or loss of more than 2 pounds in 1 day or 5 pounds in 1 week should be provided.

Lifestyle modification

Patients and their families should be counseled about lifestyle modifications that are essential to ensuring the stability of their disease process. Patients should adhere to a 2-gram sodium-restricted diet. Because this dietary restriction is difficult to comply with, patients can benefit from detailed instructions on how to read nutritional labels and make decisions when dining out. All patients should be instructed to avoid adding salt to their food when cooking or at the table. They should be cautioned that the overuse of salt substitutes can result in hyperkalemia. Abstinence from alcohol should also be encouraged, especially in those patients with an alcohol-induced cardiomyopathy. Fluid restrictions of 2 liters or less may be beneficial in patients requiring high doses of diuretics, patients requiring frequent adjustments in their diuretic regimen, or patients who remain symptomatic despite optimization of their medical therapy. The importance of balancing activity and rest should be stressed and patients should be encouraged to remain as active as possible, unless contraindicated by active ischemia or a recent myocardial infarction (MI).[26]

Social issues

Patients with heart failure are often elderly and may be on fixed incomes. Optimal medical therapy for their heart failure can require taking up to 5 different medications: angiotensin-converting enzyme (ACE) or angiotensin-receptor blocker (ARB), beta-blocker, diuretic, digoxin, or spironolactone. When we include medications for comorbidities, such as diabetes, hypertension, and hyperlipidemia, these patients can end up taking more than 10 medications each month. An assessment of the patient's ability to pay for these medications is a key element to improving compliance. If financial issues are a concern, patients should be directed to programs that can assist them in paying for their medications. Patients and their families should be educated about the medications in their heart failure regimen. Understanding the reason for taking these medications and knowing about the side effects that they might experience can improve compliance. If side effects are creating barriers to medication compliance, a reassessment of the drug of choice, timing, or dosage might help reduce or eliminate these barriers.

End-of-life care

Throughout the course of treatment, patients should be provided with information regarding the pathophysiology and prognosis of heart failure in terms they can understand. Information about long-term care options should also be available. Additionally, patients should be encouraged to discuss end-of-life issues with their families while they are in a chronic stable state. This might reduce the likelihood that decisions regarding resuscitation and aggressiveness of care will have to be made by family members in a crisis state. All patients should be encouraged to fill out an advanced directive and health care power of attorney. Although this topic can be awkward and uncomfortable for patients and their loved ones, the psychosocial consequences of an unexpected decline in functional ability or death can be devastating. Patient preferences about how much they want to know about their condition and prognosis and their desire, or lack thereof, for active participation in treatment planning should be included in their plan of care.

Conclusion

Heart failure is a devastating disease which is associated with significant morbidity and mortality. Despite advances in pharmacologic and technologic interventions, the effects that these treatments have on overall patient prognosis remain modest. Adjunctive strategies are necessary to prevent and treat this complex disease. APNs promote a collaborative multidisciplinary approach to care that has been shown to increase adherence to guideline-based therapies and decrease length of stay, readmissions, and cost of care, as well as improve quality of life. Although no specific strategy or model of multidisciplinary care has been shown to consistently affect these outcomes, promoting patient empowerment through education, increasing access to care, and providing holistic care are essential components to any successful intervention. Because APNs view health on a continuum of wholeness for their patients, they are ideally suited to coordinate a collaborative model of care.

References

1. Konstam M, Dracup K, Baker D, *et al.* Clinical Practice Guideline Number 11: Heart Failure: Evaluation and Care of Patients with Left-Ventricular Systolic Dysfunction. (Agency for Health Care Policy and Research, U.S. Depart of Health and Human Services: Rockville, MD, 1994). AHCPR publication 94–0612.
2. Grady KL, Dracup K, Kennedy G, *et al.* Team management of patients with heart failure: A statement for healthcare professionals from The Cardiovascular Nursing Council of the American Heart Association. Circulation 2000; 102: 2443–2456.
3. American Nurses Association. Scope and Standards of Advanced Practice Registered Nursing (American Nurses Association: Washington, DC, 1996).
4. Figueira M. ACNPs' role in heart failure management. Nurse Pract 2003; 28: 57–58.
5. Dahle KL, Smith JS, Ingersoll GL, Wilson JR. Impact of a nurse practitioner on the cost of managing inpatients with heart failure. Am J Cardiol 1998; 82: 686–688.
6. Knaus VL, Felten S, Burton SM, Fobes P, Davis K. The use of nurse practitioners in the acute care setting. J Nurs Adm 1997; 27: 20–27.
7. Costantini O, Huck K, Carlson MD, *et al.* Impact of a guideline-based disease management team on outcomes of hospitalized patients with congestive heart failure. Arch Intern Med 2001; 161: 177–182.
8. Michalsen A, Konig G, Thimme W. Preventable causative factors leading to hospital admission with decompensated heart failure. Heart 1998; 80: 437–441.
9. Krumholz HM, Parent EM, Tu N, *et al.* Readmission after hospitalization for congestive heart failure among Medicare beneficiaries. Arch Intern Med 1997; 157: 99–104.
10. Chin MH, Goldman L. Factors contributing to the hospitalization of patients with congestive heart failure. Am J Public Health 1997; 87: 643–648.
11. Balk AH. The "heart failure nurse" to help us close the gap between what we can and what we do achieve. Eur Heart J 1999; 20: 632–633.

12. Rich MW, Shah AS, Vinson JM, Freedland KE, Kuru T, Sperry JC. Iatrogenic congestive heart failure in older adults: clinical course and prognosis. J Am Geriatr Soc 1996; 44: 638–643.
13. Naylor M, Brooten D, Jones R, *et al.* Comprehensive discharge planning for the hospitalized elderly: a randomized clinical trial. Ann Intern Med 1994; 120: 999–1006.
14. Ashton CM, Kuykendall DH, Johnson ML, Wray NP, Wu L. The association between the quality of inpatient care and early readmission. Ann Intern Med 1995; 122: 415–421.
15. Urban N. Managed care challenges and opportunities for cardiovascular advanced practice nurses. AACN Clin Issues 1997; 8: 78–89.
16. Rich MW, Beckham V, Wittenberg C, *et al.* A multidisciplinary intervention to prevent the readmission of elderly patients with congestive heart failure. N Engl J Med 1995; 333: 1190–1195.
17. Cintron G, Bigas C, Linares E, Aranda JM, Hernandez E. Nurse practitioner role in a chronic congestive heart failure clinic: in-hospital time, costs, and patient satisfaction. Heart Lung 1983; 12: 237–240.
18. Weinberger M, Oddone EZ, Henderson WG. Does increased access to primary care reduce hospital readmissions? Veterans Affairs Cooperative Study Group on Primary Care and Hospital Readmission. N Engl J Med 1996; 334: 1441–1447.
19. Ansari M, Shlipak MG, Heidenreich PA, *et al.* Improving guideline adherence: a randomized trial evaluating strategies to increase beta blocker use in heart failure. Circulation 2003; 107: 2799–2804.
20. Krumholz HM, Amatruda J, Smith GL, *et al.* Randomized trial of an education and support intervention to prevent readmission of patients with heart failure. J Am Coll Cardiol 2002; 39: 83–89.
21. Blue L, Lang E, McMurray JJ, *et al.* Randomised controlled trial of specialist nurse intervention in heart failure. Heart 2001; 323: 715–718.
22. Stewart S, Marley JE, Horowitz JD. Effects of a multidisciplinary, home-based intervention on planned readmissions and survival among patients with chronic congestive heart failure: a randomised controlled study. Lancet 1999; 354: 1077–1083.
23. West JA, Miller NH, Parker KM, *et al.* A comprehensive management system for heart failure improves clinical outcomes and reduces medical resource utilization. Am J Card 1997; 79: 58–63.
24. Heidenreich PA, Ruggerio CM, Massie BM. Effect of a home monitoring system on hospitalization and resource use for patients with heart failure. Am Heart J 1999; 138: 633–640.
25. Kasper EK, Gerstenblith G, Hefter G, *et al.* A randomized trial of the efficacy of multidisciplinary care in heart failure outpatients at high risk of hospital readmission. J Am Coll Cardiol 2002; 39: 471–480.
26. Dracup K, Baker DW, Dunbar SB, *et al.* Management of heart failure II. Counseling, education, and lifestyle modifications. JAMA 1994; 272: 1442–1446.

CHAPTER 38

The role of the pharmacist in caring for patients with acute heart failure

Wendy Gattis Stough, J Herbert Patterson

Introduction

In patients with acute heart failure (AHF), managing pharmacotherapy is a complex process. Focus should be placed on ensuring that evidence-based therapies are prescribed, and are prescribed appropriately. Many medication errors and adverse effects occur because of a failure to recognize pharmacodynamic and pharmacokinetic alterations which are present in patients with advanced heart failure.

Pharmacists are uniquely qualified to focus on the appropriate use of drugs in challenging clinical scenarios. These individuals can be extremely helpful in selecting and monitoring drug regimens, as well as providing focused patient education.

This chapter reviews the role of the pharmacist in the care of patients with AHF. In addition, it provides an overview of pharmacokinetic alterations that occur in AHF.

Pharmacists as Care Providers in Heart Failure

A multidisciplinary approach to managing heart failure has been proven to reduce rehospitalization.[1] While most studies evaluated a nurse-directed multidisciplinary intervention, a few studies have also evaluated the advantages of adding a pharmacist to the heart failure team. These studies have been conducted in the chronic outpatient setting. No data are available in the acute setting for review. However, the contributions of pharmacists are similar in both settings, and perhaps even more pronounced in the acute setting. In the absence of acute data, we shall review the literature supporting pharmacists in the outpatient setting.

The Pharmacist Assessment Recommendation and Monitoring (PHARM) study was the first randomized trial to evaluate the effect of including a clinical pharmacist on the heart failure team.[2] The study randomized 192 patients to either pharmacist intervention or usual care. For the patients randomized to the intervention arm, a pharmacist reviewed their medical regimen and current symptoms, recommended changes in pharmacotherapy to the attending cardiologist, provided patient education, and contacted the patient by telephone to identify new symptoms and side effects, and reinforce education principles. Patients in the usual care arm received standard follow-up, but they did not receive a pharmacist's involvement in their care. The primary endpoint of the study was all-cause mortality and hospitalization or emergency department visit for heart failure. Secondary endpoints included an evaluation of angiotensin-converting enzyme (ACE) inhibitor use and dose prescribed.

Patients randomized to the intervention group had a lower rate of death or hospitalizations for heart failure as compared to the usual care group (odds ratio [OR], 0.22; 95% confidence interval [CI], 0.07–0.65; $P = 0.005$). This effect was primarily due to a decrease in rehospitalization. Additionally, patients in the intervention group were closer to the target ACE-inhibitor dose as compared to the usual care group ($P < 0.001$).[2]

In a similar study, conducted by Rainville *et al.*,[3] all patients hospitalized for heart failure from July 1996 to July 1997 were evaluated for inclusion. Patients were randomly assigned to either a control group or an intervention group. Patients in the control group received routine care and discharge procedures and a nurse reviewed their diet and medications. The intervention group received the same care; however, for these patients, the pharmacist also reviewed their medication regimen, recommended changes to their physicians, and provided patient education. The primary endpoint of this study was death or hospital readmission for heart failure within 1 year following discharge. With only 38 patients, the study was small. However, the investigators did observe a readmission rate of 58.8% in the control group as compared to 23.5% in the intervention group ($P < 0.05$). The endpoint of death or readmission was 82.3% in the control group and 29.4% in the intervention group ($P < 0.01$).

Other studies have evaluated the impact of pharmacists on medication appropriateness,[3] diuretic compliance,[4] and patient education.[5] These studies have consistently found that the addition of a pharmacist to the heart failure team was effective at improving outcomes, medication use, and patient knowledge of their condition.

Specific Aspects of Pharmacist Interventions

There are several areas where the pharmacist's expertise can be particularly useful in the management of patients with heart failure:

- *Drug selection.* The pharmacologic properties of drugs differ, even among drugs within the same class. Pharmacists can participate in selecting the right drug for the patient. For example, by avoiding or dose adjusting a drug that is renally excreted in a patient with renal failure or selecting a beta-1-selective beta-blocker in a patient with pulmonary disease, side effects can be minimized and drug tolerability improved.
- *Dose initiation and titration.* Pharmacists can ensure that drugs are dosed appropriately by accounting for patient-specific characteristics, comorbid conditions, concomitant medications, and patient response to therapy.
- *Pharmacokinetic drug interactions.* The potential for drug interactions is high in heart failure patients because of the number of drugs that they are prescribed. Interactions may also occur with non-cardiac drugs that the heart failure patient is taking. The pharmacist can recognize these potential drug interactions and offer suggestions to avoid or minimize them. Heart failure patients are commonly treated with digoxin, amiodarone, and warfarin, all of which have a high potential for drug interactions. Including a team member with the ability to recognize such interactions can protect against medication errors related to drug interactions.
- *Pharmacokinetic alterations.* The pharmacokinetics of drugs can be altered in heart failure patients due to changes in absorption, distribution, metabolism, and excretion. Because they understand the potential for these changes, pharmacists can aid in selecting appropriate drugs and doses for patients.
- *Pharmacodynamic interactions.* Heart failure patients are treated with multiple drugs that have similar pharmacodynamic effects. ACE-inhibitors, beta-blockers, and diuretics all lower blood pressure. ACE-inhibitors and aldosterone antagonists can cause hyperkalemia and these patients may also be on potassium supplementation or no-salt substitutes which can increase their potassium levels. Diuretics can increase the renin-angiotensin-aldosterone system making patients more sensitive to the blood pressure lowering effects of ACE-inhibitors and beta-blockers. Pharmacists can develop strategies for the timing of drug administration or make other recommendations to minimize the risk for pharmacodynamic interactions.
- *Comorbidities.* Patients with heart failure may have many comorbidities, including diabetes,

ischemic heart disease, pulmonary disease, arthritis, or other conditions, which increase the difficulty in managing their heart failure. The pharmacist can be helpful in selecting drugs such as beta-blockers in the patients with diabetes mellitus or pulmonary disease. In patients with arthritis, the pharmacist can offer alternatives to nonsteroidal antiinflammatory drugs (NSAIDs). The pharmacist can monitor fluid retention and weight gain in the diabetic patient treated with thiazolinediones. In addition, the pharmacist can help manage adverse effects and develop a care plan to minimize the adverse effects of drugs to ultimately improve tolerability and patient adherence.

- *Patient education.* Patient education is a key component of successful heart failure management. Patients need to know more than that their ACE-inhibitor or beta-blocker is "a heart pill." Educating patients on the purpose of their medications, how to take their medications appropriately, and how to identify drug-related side effects is extremely important to successful patient management.
- *Patient assistance.* Most heart failure patients are over the age of 65, and many do not have prescription coverage. Thus, identifying cost-effective regimens and applying for pharmaceutical company sponsored patient assistance programs is a valuable contribution that the clinical pharmacist can make to the heart failure patient.
- *Process implementation.* In health care systems, implementing processes and pathways is a successful approach that ensures that patients receive evidence-based therapies. Pharmacists can aid in writing drug protocols, standard orders, and participating in quality improvement teams to ensure that the best care is given in managing heart failure patients.

Mechanisms by which Acute Heart Failure Affects Pharmacokinetics

Absorption

The absorption of medications in patients with advanced heart failure can be altered by several mechanisms. These alterations typically result in a lower systemic bioavailability. As heart failure progresses, cardiac output is reduced, leading to organ hypoperfusion. Blood flow is redirected to vital organs such as the brain and kidneys. Some organ systems, such as the gastrointestinal tract, may remain hypoperfused and drug absorption may be reduced as a result. Reduced gastrointestinal motility and delayed gastric emptying may also contribute to reduced absorption, which may be responsible for gastrointestinal discomfort symptoms reported by many patients with advanced heart failure. Intestinal edema is also a factor in the lower absorption and bioavailability of drugs, and it may particularly impact lipophilic compounds.

The efficacy of oral loop diuretics often declines in patients with advanced or decompensated heart failure. Clinicians often observe worsening heart failure symptoms despite increasing diuretic doses. Reduced absorption results in lower systemic bioavailability of loop diuretics, and this process may be partially responsible for the inadequate diuretic response that commonly occurs in this population.

Advanced heart failure may also affect the absorption of topically administered drugs. Because peripheral perfusion may be compromised in patients with low cardiac output, oral administration may be favored in these patients. For example, oral isosorbide dinitrate or isosorbide mononitrate may be preferable to nitroglycerin patches.

The effect of advanced heart failure on drug absorption is likely most important for drugs which have low bioavailability even in normal patients. Data are not widely available that evaluate drug absorption in advanced heart failure patients, but decreased absorption should be considered as a potential cause of inadequate response to drug therapy in patients with advanced or decompensated heart failure.

Distribution

The volume of distribution (V_d) for drugs can be altered in patients with advanced heart failure. The V_d can be increased or decreased. Most commonly, V_d is reduced in both central and peripheral compartments, which may be due to reduced cardiac output. Theoretically, the V_d may be increased for hydrophilic drugs in patients with volume overload and preserved cardiac output because these drugs may be widely distributed in the periphery. Conversely, V_d may be reduced for lipophilic drugs in these patients. Data evaluating changes in V_d in advanced heart failure patients is not widely available for the drugs commonly used to treat these patients.

Protein binding can affect V_d for highly protein-bound drugs. As heart failure progresses, patients may become cachectic. The decreased albumin may affect drugs that are highly protein bound, and result in a higher free fraction of active drug. The clinical significance of this has not been well described in the literature. Drugs with a narrow therapeutic index that are highly protein bound, such as phenytoin, should be closely monitored in patients with advanced heart failure.

Metabolism

Drugs that are highly protein bound may be affected by the AHF state. Hepatic metabolism may decrease due to volume overload and hepatic congestion. It may also be reduced in the low cardiac output state due to decreased perfusion. In these scenarios, decreased metabolism, higher levels of free drug, and long half-lives may be observed. Patients treated with drugs such as warfarin, beta-blockers, amiodarone, and phenytoin, among others should receive close monitoring during episodes of AHF. Patients receiving warfarin for anticoagulation may experience significant elevations in international normalized ratio (INR) during episodes of AHF. The exact reactions to pharmacokinetic alterations are extremely difficult to predict, and close monitoring is warranted.

Excretion

Patients with AHF may also experience changes in the excretion of drugs, particularly those excreted renally. In the low-output state, renal perfusion may be decreased, resulting in a decline in renal function. In addition, high doses of diuretics given to decompensated heart failure patients may also worsen renal function. Thus, serum creatinine should be closely monitored, and doses of drugs that are excreted renally should be adjusted. This focused monitoring approach may be particularly important with drugs such as digoxin, aldosterone antagonists, aminoglycosides, and other renally eliminated drugs that heart failure patients may be receiving.

Recommendations for Drug Monitoring in the Acute Heart Failure Patient

An accurate drug history should be obtained as soon as possible after a patient is admitted for AHF. The history may provide insight into factors that precipitated the admission. Additionally, it will ensure that all components of the patient's therapy are addressed during the admission.

The clinical importance of potential pharmacokinetic alterations should be assessed for each drug. In addition, the clinical need for each drug should be evaluated. Patients may be on drugs which are unnecessary or which worsen their heart failure state.

Obtaining drug levels may be indicated for drugs with narrow therapeutic windows in which a pharmacokinetic alteration is expected. For example, obtaining digoxin levels would be appropriate in a patient with new or worsening renal insufficiency, particularly in elderly patients. Drug doses should be adjusted as indicated to account for significant alterations in absorption, distribution, metabolism, and excretion, as well as the presence of other interacting drugs.

Therapies should also be readjusted once the AHF symptoms, such as congestion, have been treated. Often, patients are discharged on higher doses of diuretics than needed on a chronic basis because they were receiving higher doses during the admission to overcome gut edema. Similarly, if doses of other drugs were decreased (such as warfarin) because of hepatic congestion or decreased metabolism, they may need to be increased to the preadmission dose. For therapies such as warfarin, the INR should be monitored and the dose adjusted as indicated.[6]

Conclusion

Specific considerations must be given to drug therapy in the AHF setting. To date, these considerations have not been well described in the literature, and data are generally unavailable to guide decision-making. Thus, having a health care provider knowledgeable in pharmacology can be extremely helpful in managing these patients successfully. Pharmacists can play a key role as a member of the heart failure management team. Their unique expertise regarding drug therapy can impact multiple components of heart failure management.

References

1. Rich MW, Beckham V, Wittenberg C, Leven CL, Freedland KE, Carney RM. A multidisciplinary intervention to prevent the readmission of elderly patients with congestive heart failure. N Engl J Med 1995; 333: 1190–1195.
2. Gattis WA, Hasselblad V, Whellan DJ, O'Connor CM. Reduction in heart failure events by the addition of a clinical pharmacist to the heart failure management team: results of the Pharmacist in Heart Failure Assessment Recommendation and Monitoring (PHARM) Study. Arch Intern Med 1999; 159: 1939–1945.
3. Rainville EC. Impact of pharmacist interventions on hospital readmissions for heart failure. Am J Heath Syst Pharm 1999; 56: 1339–1342.
4. Bucci C, Jackevicius C, McFarlane K, Liu P. Pharmacist's contribution in a heart function clinic: patient perception and medication appropriateness. Can J Cardiol 2003; 19: 391–396.
5. Bouvy ML, Heerdink ER, Urquhart J, *et al.* Effect of a pharmacist-led intervention on diuretic compliance in heart failure patients: a randomized controlled study. J Cardiac Fail 2003; 9: 404–411.
6. Fradette M, Bungard TJ, Simpson SH, Tsuyuki RT. Development of educational materials for congestive heart failure patients. Am J Health Syst Pharm 2004; 61: 386–389.

CHAPTER 39

Economics and quality of life in the advanced heart failure patient

David J Whellan, Jonathan E E Yager, Joëlle Y Friedman, Kevin A Schulman

Introduction

It was estimated in 1990 that congestive heart failure affected 4 million people in the United States, with 400 000 new cases being diagnosed each year.[1] Disease prevalence is expected to grow to over 10 million by 2007.[2] In 1994, heart failure was the highest-volume Medicare diagnosis related group and represented 4.8% of total Medicare Part A expenditures ($5.45 billion),[3,4] greater than expenditures for all types of cancer ($2.24 billion) and for myocardial infarction (MI) ($3.18 billion).[4] Medicare beneficiaries with heart failure had 2 668 440 hospitalizations in 1995, of which 619 080 were for the primary diagnosis of heart failure. Analysis by our group found that total Medicare expenditures in 1995 for patients with heart failure totaled $22.8 billion (unpublished data, 2002).

The ability to reduce the economic burden of caring for patients with heart failure may be limited. Decreases in total hospital costs may be difficult to achieve—even with therapies that reduce mean length of stay for heart failure admissions (6.46 days in 1995)—because 75% of the costs associated with a heart failure admission are incurred in the first 2 days.[5] Moreover, although readmission rates are high (36% to 57% at 90 days) and present a promising target for cost containment, any reduction in inpatient resource use may shift the costs of care to the outpatient setting, where patient expenses can exceed $4000 per patient per year.[5–7]

In this chapter, we present a review of the literature on the economic and quality-of-life impact of drugs and devices in patients with heart failure.

Drug Therapies

A limited number of drugs have proven beneficial to patients with left ventricular (LV) dysfunction in large, randomized, controlled trials. Those medications include angiotensin-converting enzyme (ACE) inhibitors, digoxin, beta-blockers, diuretics, spironolactone, and angiotensin II receptor blockers (ARBs).

Angiotensin-converting enzyme inhibitors

A number of studies, including the Studies of Left Ventricular Dysfunction (SOLVD) treatment and prevention trials, the Veterans Administration Cooperative Vasodilator Heart Failure Trial (V-HeFT II), and the Cooperative North Scandinavian Enalapril Survival Study (CONSENSUS), have shown that ACE inhibitors decrease mortality, reduce hospitalizations, and improve quality of life in patients with systolic dysfunction.[8–11] However, none of these studies included an economic substudy as part of the original trial design. The only economic data come from models based on resource use data collected from the randomized trials.

The first study to examine resource use was the SOLVD treatment trial,[8] a multicenter, randomized, double-blind, placebo-controlled trial conducted in the United States, Belgium, and Canada. The study randomized 2569 patients with symptomatic heart failure with an ejection fraction (EF) of ≤ 35% to receive either enalapril or placebo. Over a mean follow-up of 41.4 months, enalapril reduced mortality by 16% ($P = 0.0036$). Total hospitalizations were 971 in the placebo group vs. 683 in the enalapril group ($P < 0.001$). CONSENSUS, which enrolled a cohort of patients with New York Heart Association (NYHA) class IV heart failure, found an even greater reduction in mortality for patients taking enalapril vs. placebo (26% vs. 44%; $P = 0.002$).[11] No data on hospitalizations were reported. In both CONSENSUS and the SOLVD treatment trial, the majority of patients were taking digitalis (93% in CONSENSUS and 67% in SOLVD) and diuretics (98% in CONSENSUS and 86% in SOLVD). In V-HeFT II, enalapril significantly improved mortality compared to hydralazine-isosorbide dinitrate (HID) (18% vs. 25%; $P = 0.016$) at 2 years of follow-up in 804 men receiving digoxin and a diuretic.[10] Compared to HID, enalapril did not reduce total hospitalizations.

The Assessment of Treatment with Lisinopril and Survival (ATLAS) trial provided evidence that higher doses of ACE inhibitors (33.2 ± 5.4 mg vs. 4.5 ± 1.1 mg) in a cohort of primarily NYHA class II and III patients decreased total hospitalizations by 13% ($P = 0.021$).[12] There was no significant change in mortality (42.5% for high-dose therapy vs. 44.9% for low-dose therapy; $P = 0.128$). It is worth noting that 22.1% of patients in the low-dose group were initiated on open-label ACE inhibition. The investigators did not report background use of digoxin, diuretic, or beta-blocker.

ACE inhibitors have also proven beneficial for asymptomatic heart failure patients. In the SOLVD prevention trial, enalapril significantly reduced the number of hospitalizations for heart failure (184 vs. 273; risk reduction, 36%; $P < 0.001$) and the time to development of heart failure symptoms (22.3 months vs. 8.3 months; $P < 0.001$). However, enalapril did not significantly reduce mortality (313 for enalapril vs. 334 for control; $P = 0.30$) or total hospitalizations (2645 for enalapril vs. 2839 for control; $P = 0.12$).[13] In this study, very few patients were on digoxin (12.5%) or diuretics (16.6%), which is expected given the heart failure population enrolled.

Economics of angiotensin-converting enzyme inhibitors

Most economic evaluations of ACE-inhibitor use have relied on clinical outcome data from the SOLVD treatment trial to create models to predict the costs and benefits of ACE-inhibitor therapy. Glick *et al.* used outcomes and clinical resource use data from SOLVD and cost data derived from Medicare reimbursement rates.[14] The number of hospitalizations for participants was categorized into 9 primary causes of admission. Hospital costs for admissions were estimated by multiplying the diagnosis related group (DRG) weight for each of the 9 hospitalization categories with the mean Medicare reimbursement rate for that DRG, excluding adjustments for capital expenditures, free care, and medical education. In this analysis, enalapril saved $717 over the follow-up period of SOLVD. When the analysis was continued over a patient's lifetime using decision-analysis techniques, enalapril was found to be cost-additive, producing a cost-utility ratio of $115 per quality-adjusted life-year. In a follow-up substudy of hypertensive patients with LV dysfunction, the investigators found an even greater impact of enalapril, with a $1656 reduction per patient over the follow-up period and a $1456 reduction per patient over the projected lifetime.[15]

Using data from SOLVD and V-HeFT II, Paul *et al.* developed a model that estimated the incremental cost of enalapril at $2569 for 3 months of additional life as compared to standard therapy,[16] yielding a cost-effectiveness ratio of $9700 per life-year gained. The authors performed a similar analysis for HID and found a cost-effectiveness ratio of $5600 per life-year gained ($119 incremental cost for 8 additional days of life). In this analysis, the estimated cost of each hospitalization for heart failure was $6750. The annual cost was $959 for enalapril and $437 for HID. If the cost of enalapril became less than 1.6 times that of HID, enalapril became more cost-effective than HID. This analysis did not take into account the total hospitalization rate for patients treated with enalapril in SOLVD, in which 1285 patients treated with enalapril experienced 683 hospitalizations (53%).[8] Paul *et al.* estimated a probability of admission of only 39%. In addition, the cost per hospitalization was derived from heart failure admissions at a single hospital. The investigators did perform sensitivity analyses of the duration of treatment benefit, efficacy, heart failure mortality, cost of vasodilators, cost of hospitalization, and discounting.

The cost-effectiveness analysis of the ATLAS trial provided evidence that high-dose ACE-inhibitor use resulted in greater cost savings compared to low-dose ACE-inhibitor use.[17] Data on resource use and ACE-inhibitor dose were collected prospectively in the clinical trial. Given the absence of any difference in the incidence of adverse events (reported only for side effects of ACE inhibitors), the investigators did not include concomitant medication use (not reported in the ATLAS trial) or degree of symptomatic relief (also not reported in the original study).[12] Estimated costs for resource use came from 1997 to 1998 unit costs for hospitals in the United Kingdom. Days in the hospital for ATLAS patients were valued using the mean cost per inpatient day. The number of day-cases and their mean costs were included in the model. Hospitalizations and the mean cost per day were allocated to a specific specialty. The estimated cost of medications was based on British National Formulary prices. Both study drug use and open-label ACE-inhibitor use were valued. The cost-effectiveness analysis used the mean life expectancy in the 2 arms of the study. Using the UK Department of Health recommendations, costs were discounted at 6% and effects were discounted at 2%. All costs were reported in pounds sterling (£).

Patients in the high-dose group spent a mean of 18.5 days in the hospital (as compared to 22.5 days for the low-dose group) and had 0.38 day-cases per patient (as compared to 0.44 day-cases for the low-dose group). The mean cost per patient for the high-dose group was £397 lower than for the low-dose group (95% confidence interval [CI], –£1263 to –£436). The higher cost of the drug was offset by the reduction in hospitalizations. Since high-dose lisinopril was more effective in both increasing life-years per patient (mean difference [high-dose–low-dose], 0.085 years; 95% CI, −0.0074 to 0.1706) and decreasing costs, high-dose ACE inhibitor was considered the dominant treatment.

For symptomatic patients with heart failure, ACE inhibitors are a cost-saving therapy at best and an economically attractive, cost-additive therapy at worst. In addition to the two studies above, economic analyses using the SOLVD data and modeling to non-US markets concluded that enalapril would reduce costs over the lifetime of a patient outside of the United States.[13,18,19] There are strong economic and clinical arguments for ACE-inhibitor use in symptomatic heart failure patients.[20–22]

Quality of life with angiotensin-converting enzyme inhibitors

ACE inhibitors improve quality of life for patients with heart failure, but the magnitude of the documented effect is modest. This modest effect could be explained by the lack of sensitive measures available to examine quality of life, high mortality rates in some studies which preclude quality-of-life analysis, or the fact that ACE inhibitors may not, in fact, offer substantial improvements in quality of life.

In the SOLVD treatment trial (symptomatic patients with EF ≤ 35%), enalapril yielded greater quality-of-life improvements than placebo. Specifically, quality of life improved with respect to ability to perform activities of daily living, social functioning, general life satisfaction, general health perception, and dyspnea. These domains improved at 6 weeks after initiation of therapy. When measured again at 1 year, however, only the social functioning and dyspnea domains remained different between the two groups. Also at 1 year, patients receiving enalapril had higher productivity measures than patients receiving placebo. At 2 years, however, none of the differences remained significant, and there were no detectable differences in quality of life. It is noteworthy that quality of life was measured in SOLVD with a battery of self-report instruments that included questions from the Short Form-36 (SF-36), a common generic quality-of-life instrument, and that 40% of the quality-of-life responses were missing at 2 years, whether due to death or to failure of surviving patients to return the questionnaires.

Although the SOLVD treatment trial found some short-term quality-of-life benefit for enalapril, the SOLVD prevention trial found only that social functioning was better in the enalapril arm, and only at 6 weeks. Given the asymptomatic nature of the patients enrolled in the prevention trial, however, it is not surprising that no major advances were seen in quality of life, because neither group felt limited by their heart failure.

The CONSENSUS trial examined quality of life with enalapril using the Quality of Life in Severe Heart Failure Questionnaire. In this case, the study found no differences between the treated and placebo groups. Patients in the trial had NYHA class IV heart failure, and the high mortality rate prevented the investigators from obtaining sufficient data to achieve statistical significance.[23]

In the V-HeFT II trial, investigators used the Minnesota Living with Heart Failure (MLWHF) questionnaire, a 21-question instrument with a 5-point Likert scale for responses. Possible scores ranged from 0 (best quality of life) to 105 (worst quality of life). As patients improve, scores fall. Using this measure, no difference was seen in quality of life between the enalapril group and patients treated with hydralazine and nitrates.

Beta-blockers

Beta-blocker therapy for heart failure is now recognized as the next line of therapy after ACE inhibitors. Prior to the 1990s, these drugs were considered to be contraindicated in heart failure due to short-term effects noted in small studies.[24] Starting in the late 1970s and 1980s, small studies of long-term beta-blocker therapy demonstrated improved hemodynamics, LV function, functional capacity, and symptoms in patients with LV dysfunction.[25–30]

In the 1990s, a number of trials found that beta-blockers improved clinical outcomes, including hospitalization and mortality for patients with LV dysfunction and mild to moderate symptoms. The Metoprolol in Dilated Cardiomyopathy (MDC) trial randomized 383 patients with idiopathic heart failure, primarily NYHA class II and III symptoms, and EF of < 40% to metoprolol or placebo.[31] Approximately 80% of participants were taking an ACE inhibitor and digitalis, and 75% were on a diuretic. There was a nonsignificant decrease of 34% in the primary endpoint of death or transplantation in patients taking metoprolol (95% CI, −6 to 62; $P = 0.058$). Readmissions per patient decreased significantly from 0.47 to 0.28 in the metoprolol group ($P < 0.04$).

The Cardiac Insufficiency Bisoprolol Study (CIBIS) continued the evaluation of beta-selective adrenergic receptor antagonists in patients with LV dysfunction.[32] This study randomized 641 patients (95% NYHA class III) with any etiology to either bisoprolol or placebo. Although there was no significant difference in survival between patients treated with bisoprolol or placebo, subgroup analysis revealed a significant decrease in mortality in patients without a history of MI taking bisoprolol (12% vs. 22.5%; $P = 0.01$). There was a significant decrease in heart failure decompensation requiring hospitalization in the bisoprolol group (61 vs. 90; $P < 0.01$).

MDC and CIBIS were followed by two larger randomized trials, CIBIS II and the Metoprolol CR/XL Randomized Intervention Trial in Congestive Heart Failure (MERIT-HF).[33–35] Both studies confirmed the initial findings of the smaller studies regarding hospitalization and found significant improvement in mortality. CIBIS II included 2647 patients with NYHA class III and IV (83% class III) heart failure and an EF of < 35%. After a mean follow-up of 1.3 years, the study was stopped early for significant reduction in mortality (11.8% vs. 17.3%; $P < 0.0001$).[33] All-cause hospitalizations also decreased significantly (440 vs. 513; hazard ratio [HR], 0.80; $P = 0.0006$), due entirely to a decrease in hospitalizations for worsening heart failure (159 vs. 232; HR, 0.64; $P = 0.0001$).

MERIT-HF investigators enrolled 3991 patients with chronic LV dysfunction (EF of < 40%) and NYHA class II to IV (96% classes II and III).[34] As with CIBIS II, the steering committee for MERIT-HF stopped the study early, after a mean follow-up time of only 1 year, due to a 34% reduction in mortality (relative risk [RR], 0.66; $P < 0.0001$). Metoprolol reduced all-cause hospitalizations (1021 vs. 1149; $P = 0.005$). As with CIBIS II, the reduction in hospitalizations was due primarily to a reduction in the number of patients hospitalized for worsening heart failure (−35%; $P < 0.001$).[36] Approximately 90% of patients were taking an ACE inhibitor and diuretic in MERIT-HF, and more than 95% of patients in CIBIS II were taking an ACE inhibitor and diuretic. Only 50% of patients in CIBIS II and 63% of patients in MERIT-HF were taking digitalis.

Carvedilol, a nonselective beta-blocker, has also been proven effective in patients with LV dysfunction. In the US Carvedilol Study, patients were randomized to four separate protocols with mortality as a secondary endpoint.[36] The study was stopped early by the data and safety monitoring board due to a significant decrease in mortality. After a median follow-up of 6 months, carvedilol reduced the risk of death by 65% in a pooled analysis of the 4 studies (3.2% vs. 7.8% for placebo; $P < 0.001$). Due to the unequal randomization of patients into each arm of the 4 protocols, it is difficult to use the absolute number of hospitalizations as an indicator of carvedilol's impact. Carvedilol significantly reduced the risk of a patient being hospitalized at least once by 27% (14.1% vs. 19.6%; $P = 0.036$). In a follow-up study by Fowler *et al.*, carvedilol reduced hospitalizations per patient for all causes from 0.40 ± 0.78 to 0.30 ± 0.78 ($P = 0.003$).[37] The majority of this change came from a reduction in heart failure hospitalizations per patient, which decreased from 0.15 ± 0.54 to 0.07 ± 0.34 ($P = 0.028$). Carvedilol was associated with a shorter length of stay for cardiovascular admissions (7.4 days vs. 10.8 days for placebo; $P = 0.298$) and heart failure admissions (6.8 days vs. 10.8 days; $P = 0.025$). The reduction in length of stay was also associated with a decrease in the mean number of days per patient spent in an intensive/coronary care unit, which was significantly reduced for cardiovascular admissions (0.33 days vs. 1.46 days; $P = 0.011$) and for heart failure admissions (0.07 days vs. 0.68 days; $P < 0.001$).

Carvedilol benefits appear to extend to patients with LV dysfunction and severe heart failure symptoms (NYHA class IV).[38] The Carvedilol Prospective Randomized Cumulative Survival (COPERNICUS) Study enrolled 2289 patients and included follow-up for a mean duration of 10.4 months. The data and safety monitoring board stopped the study early due to a significant beneficial effect of carvedilol on survival. Mortality was reduced by 35% (95% CI, 19–48%; $P = 0.00014$ [adjusted]). Hospitalizations were not reported separately, but there was a 24% lower risk of death or first hospitalization for patients treated with carvedilol ($P < 0.001$).

Somewhat complicating the story of beta-blockers is the Beta-Blocker Evaluation of Survival Trial (BEST).[39] A total of 2078 patients with LV dysfunction (EF ≤ 35%) and NYHA class III or IV symptoms (92% class III) were randomly assigned treatment with bucindolol or placebo. Bucindolol is a nonselective beta-blocker without intrinsic sympathomimetic activity in the human heart. The data and safety monitoring board stopped the trial after a mean follow-up of 2 years due to the results of other studies of beta-blockers in heart failure patients and to address concerns about the equipoise of the trial. Bucindolol treatment was found to have a nonsignificant trend for improved survival, with 30% mortality vs. 33% mortality in the placebo group (HR, 0.90; 95% CI, 0.78–1.02; $P = 0.13$). The lack of a significant outcome when other studies of beta-blockers had significant outcomes over shorter periods of follow-up was felt to be due to differences in cohorts and pharmacological differences between agents. Similar to the other studies, bucindolol reduced all-cause hospitalizations (829 vs. 875; $P = 0.08$) primarily by reducing admissions for heart failure (476 vs. 569; $P < 0.001$). However, bucindolol appears to have increased the number of hospitalizations for non-heart failure causes.

Economics of beta-blockers

At present, very little economic data other than hospitalizations have been reported regarding beta-blocker therapy. Fowler *et al.*[37] modeled costs using the results of the US Carvedilol Trials Program. Although all occurrences of any hospitalization were collected prospectively, detailed data—

including diagnoses, selected cardiac procedures, and intensive/coronary care unit time—were collected only for admissions deemed cardiovascular in nature. Unit cost data were assigned to each cardiovascular hospitalization based on total hospitalization costs from 153 hospitals in the United States. Given the reductions in admissions, length of stay, and intensive care unit time for hospitalizations due to cardiovascular disease and heart failure, the investigators found a corresponding reduction in mean cost per patient for cardiovascular inpatient resource use ($1912 vs. $4463; $P = 0.016$) and for heart failure-related inpatient resource use ($452 vs. $2338; $P = 0.022$). The cost reductions were due to a reduction in admissions (55% and 63% for cardiovascular and heart failure hospitalizations, respectively) and in cost per admission (45% and 37%). Carvedilol decreased the cost per hospitalization due to any cardiovascular cause ($9318 vs. $16 426; $P = 0.097$) and due to heart failure ($5632 vs. $15 258; $P = 0.002$). This analysis did not consider the effect of carvedilol on all-cause hospitalization or outpatient costs, including the cost of carvedilol, and did not consider the long-term effect on cost.

Delea *et al.*[40] evaluated the long-term economic impact of carvedilol by using a Markov model to project life expectancy and lifetime medical care costs, with the US Carvedilol Heart Failure Trials Program serving as a baseline for treated patients. Two scenarios were used: "limited benefit," in which benefits persisted for 6 months (i.e., the duration of follow-up in the trial) and ended abruptly; and "extended benefit," in which the benefits persisted for 6 months and then declined gradually over time, vanishing by the end of 3 years. Long-term outcomes for patients on conventional therapy alone were estimated using the SOLVD Treatment Trial results. Outpatient costs, including medication costs and clinic visits, were estimated based on wholesale drug prices and reported clinic costs. Inpatient costs for hospitalizations secondary to heart failure were estimated from all hospitalizations with the primary diagnosis of heart failure found in a national database. Non-heart failure medical care costs were estimated using annual per capita personal health care expenditures from 1980 data and were assumed to be equivalent for patients treated with and without carvedilol. Heart failure-related costs were estimated to be 40% of the total costs in the conventionally treated patients. Based on the above assumptions, the incremental cost per life-year saved for carvedilol was $29 477 and $12 799 under limited and extended benefit assumptions, respectively.

Quality of life with beta-blockers

Data supporting quality-of-life improvements with beta-blockers are less compelling than data supporting the mortality benefit. Quality-of-life studies of beta-blockers in patients with heart failure are heterogeneous. Some have used exercise tolerance or distance walked in 6 minutes as an endpoint; others have used instruments such as the MLWHF questionnaire. Some studies have examined beta-blocker use in patients with mild to moderate heart failure, and others have examined their use in patients with more severe disease.

The US Carvedilol Heart Failure Study Group[41] examined MLWHF scores in patients receiving carvedilol who had EF < 35%. Eighty-five percent of patients had NYHA class II symptoms, and 15% had class III symptoms. At 12 months of follow-up, MLWHF scores for patients receiving placebo improved by 2.4 points, whereas scores for patients receiving carvedilol improved 4.9 points. This difference was not statistically significant. When a global clinical score was used, however, more carvedilol patients improved than did placebo patients. Physicians believed that 69% of the patients treated with carvedilol had improved, as compared with 47% of the patients receiving placebo ($P = 0.001$). Whereas 60% of the patients receiving placebo rated themselves as "improved," 75% of the patients receiving carvedilol thought that they were better ($P = 0.013$).

The PRECISE study[42] examined MLWHF scores in patients treated with carvedilol and placebo and found no difference between the two groups, both in overall scores and in the emotional and physical components. The MOCHA study[43] also found no difference in MLWHF scores for patients treated with carvedilol compared to placebo. When measured at 6 months, scores improved by 7.3 points for the placebo group, whereas patients receiving 6.25 mg b.i.d. carvedilol improved their scores by 7.9 points, patients receiving 12.5 mg b.i.d. improved by 7.3 points, and patients receiving 25 mg b.i.d. improved by 5.5 points. These differences were not statistically significant. As with the PRECISE study, there was also no difference in MLWHF scores when the physical and emotional components were examined separately.

Just as studies with carvedilol have not demonstrated improved quality of life with the MLWHF scale, nor have they shown improvements with metoprolol. Patients with NYHA class II to IV heart failure were studied by the RESOLVD investigators,[44] who found that controlled-release metoprolol did not significantly affect MLWHF scores at 24 weeks. The MERIT-HF investigators[45] performed a quality-of-life substudy of 741 patients (out of 3991 patients studied) and found that MLWHF scores, which were available for 670 patients, were not significantly different between the metoprolol and placebo groups. At the same time, however, more metoprolol patients in the MERIT-HF trial reported improvement in the McMaster Overall Treatment Evaluation score (50% compared with 40%; $P = 0.009$). Similarly, more patients receiving metoprolol were found to improve at least one NYHA class, and fewer were found to deteriorate, than were those receiving placebo (28.6% compared with 25.8% for improvement, and 6.0% vs. 7.5% for deterioration; $P = 0.003$).

Bucindolol was also studied in patients with NYHA class II and III heart failure, and MLWHF results were obtained at baseline and at 12 weeks.[46] The drug was administered at three doses (12.5 mg per day, 50 mg per day, or 200 mg per day), and a placebo group was included. Physical scores improved by 3.2 ± 1.4 in the placebo group, and emotional scores improved by 1.2 ± 0.8, for a total improvement of $4.5 + 2.0$ points. Results for the groups taking bucindolol were not significantly different from those of the placebo group. Combining the three doses of bucindolol studied, treated patients improved by 5.0 ± 1.1 overall, with a 1.2 ± 0.5 point improvement in the emotional score and a 3.7 ± 0.8 point improvement in the physical score.

In addition to data regarding the MLWHF questionnaire, beta-blockers have been studied with regard to their effect on exercise tolerance. Some studies have found no difference between baseline values and values at the conclusion of the trial, while others have shown absolute increases. None have shown statistical benefit over placebo. In the Australia–New Zealand study,[47] patients with class I to III heart failure were randomized to carvedilol or placebo. At 6 months, there was no difference in the distance walked in 6 minutes between the two groups. Similarly, the MOCHA study cited earlier found no difference in either the 6-minute walk distance or the distance walked on a 9-minute self-powered treadmill for carvedilol or placebo groups, and this was the same result found by the PRECISE investigators. The RESOLVD Pilot study found no difference at 24 weeks for 6-minute walk differences for patients randomized to either placebo or metoprolol, and the bucindolol study mentioned above found no difference between patients on placebo or those taking active drug.

As opposed to the above studies that found no difference in exercise tolerance, however, Metra *et al.*[48] found that patients randomized to both metoprolol and carvedilol improved their absolute 6-minute walk distance at 12 months. The metoprolol patients increased an average of 63 meters, and the carvedilol patients 50 meters, although statistically there was no difference between the two groups. Both groups did show statistically significant and clinically relevant absolute improvement.

Finally, NYHA class has been used as a quality-of-life endpoint in trials of beta-blockers, and the findings with this more subjective endpoint do seem to favor beta-blockers. The CIBIS investigators[49] noted that 21% of bisoprolol patients improved by at least one NYHA class as compared with only 15% of the placebo patients ($P < 0.03$). The MERIT-HF trial showed that 28.6% of metoprolol patients improved, whereas 65.4% were unchanged and 6.0% deteriorated, as compared with 25.8% of placebo patients who improved, with 66.7% remaining the same and 7.5% deteriorating ($P = 0.003$). Similarly, Colucci *et al.*[41] found that 12% of carvedilol patients improved by at least one

NYHA class and only 4% worsened as compared with 9% of placebo patients who improved while 15% worsened ($P = 0.003$).

On the other hand, the Australia–New Zealand study cited above showed a trend toward less improvement with carvedilol. At 6 months, 23% of the carvedilol patients improved by one NYHA class, compared with 28% of the placebo patients ($P = 0.05$). At 12 months the difference was not statistically significant (26% improvement for the carvedilol group and 28% for the placebo group).

Overall, the quality-of-life data for beta-blockers is not overwhelmingly positive. While some studies show benefit in NYHA functional status, most do not demonstrate harder endpoint significance, such as MLWHF scores or exercise tolerance. Regardless, patients treated with beta-blockers as well as those treated with placebo tend to improve their quality of life overall, and this speaks to the need to enroll more patients in clinical trials. Whatever the placebo effect may be in these trials, patients are feeling better, and that in and of itself is a good endpoint.

Digoxin

Digoxin has been a therapeutic option in the care of heart failure patients for over 200 years. A number of studies in the 1980s showed a beneficial effect of digoxin on symptoms and exercise tolerance in patients with LV systolic dysfunction and normal sinus rhythm.[50–52] In 1993, the Randomized Assessment of Digoxin and Inhibitors of Angiotensin-Converting Enzyme (RADIANCE) trial and the Prospective Randomized Study of Ventricular Failure and Efficacy of Digoxin (PROVED) examined the effect of withdrawing digoxin from patients with LV systolic dysfunction.[53–55] In both studies, the withdrawal of digoxin caused a worsening of symptoms, exercise tolerance, and quality of life in patients with mild to moderate heart failure symptoms. The Digitalis Investigation Group (DIG) study evaluated the benefit of initiating digoxin in 6800 patients with LV systolic dysfunction.[56] Most patients had NYHA class II or III symptoms (84%) and were taking a diuretic (82%) and an ACE inhibitor (94%). Although digoxin had no effect on mortality (34.8% vs. 35.1%; risk ratio with digoxin, 0.99; $P = 0.80$), digoxin treatment resulted in a significant decrease in hospitalizations per patient (1.87 vs. 1.99; $P = 0.01$) over the mean follow-up period of 37 months. As in other heart failure studies, the most significant decrease in hospitalization was for heart failure hospitalizations (910 vs. 1180; RR, 0.72; $P < 0.001$). In fact, digoxin caused an increase in noncardiac and nonvascular hospitalizations (1126 vs. 1079; RR, 1.06; 95% CI, 0.98 to 1.15).

Using data from the RADIANCE and PROVED trials, Ward *et al.*[57] modeled the impact of withdrawing or continuing digoxin in patients with heart failure (NYHA class II or III), normal sinus rhythm, and LVEF ≤ 35%. The investigators assumed that digoxin had no effect on mortality and only decreased the incidence of heart failure exacerbations requiring medical intervention. For the economic analysis, they included the cost of digoxin, monitoring digoxin concentration every 3 months, and treatment of episodes of digoxin toxicity. The investigators assumed the prevalence of heart failure at the time of their analysis to be 2.5 million patients, of whom 50% would be in normal sinus rhythm and have NYHA class II or III symptoms. Based on internal analysis of a single managed care organization, they estimated that only 46% of patients would be taking ACE inhibitors. Cost estimates for digoxin therapy, digoxin concentration monitoring, a clinic visit, emergency department visit, and admission for digoxin toxicity came from Henry Ford Hospital. The investigators used the Medicare reimbursement rate (claims paid) for heart failure admissions to estimate that each heart failure admission would cost $3844. They assumed no difference in length of stay per heart failure hospitalization resulting from digoxin therapy. The investigators extended the follow-up of the 2 clinical trials from 12 weeks to 1 year by assuming that digoxin would be 75% as effective in reducing the risk of treatment failures during the 13-week to 52-week period. The 12-week RR for treatment failures adjusted for follow-up duration was 0.50 in PROVED and 0.23 in RADIANCE.

It is important to note that there were only 20 hospital admissions for worsening heart failure in both studies for both cohorts and only 4 emergency department visits. Using these assumptions, the investigators extrapolated the results of the 2 studies to 1.25 million Americans with heart failure who would meet the criteria for digoxin use. They estimated that the net savings resulting from continuing digoxin to be $406 million per year, including $247 million for patients with ACE-inhibitor therapy and $159 million for those without. Not surprisingly, sensitivity analysis showed that the largest source of uncertainty in the results came from the epidemiologic assumptions about the prevalence of heart failure in the United States, the proportion of patients with heart failure meeting criteria for digoxin use, and the baseline incidence of hospital admissions for patients meeting the criteria. The most important sensitivity analysis was the one assuming digoxin had no effect during weeks 13 to 52. Even in this situation, $21 million dollars would be saved. In the Monte Carlo approach for sensitivity analysis, more than 99% of the 10 000 model iterations yielded a net savings with continuation of digoxin therapy.

Diuretics

Diuretics are a mainstay of heart failure treatment and are recommended by all of the guidelines for the management and treatment of heart failure.[58–60] Diuretics are used to control symptoms. Given the likely outcome of patients with volume overload not being treated with a diuretic, an argument could easily be made regarding survival. However, there is limited information regarding diuretics and outcomes. This may be due in part to the ethical dilemma of performing a placebo-controlled trial of this therapy. It may also be due to the effectiveness of furosemide—which is inexpensive—as a diuretic. In addition, there is indirect evidence that increasing diuretic dosing may increase mortality.[61]

There have been comparisons between furosemide and torsemide, a newer loop diuretic with a potentially better pharmacokinetic profile (improved absorption profile, longer elimination half-life, more rapid onset, and longer duration of action).[62–64] Initial pharmacoeconomic assessments comparing the two diuretics found significant cost reduction when torsemide was used, but these studies were retrospective and had significant limitations.[65,66] The PharmacoEconomic Assessment of Torsemide and Furosemide in Congestive Heart Failure (PEACH) was a prospective, open-label, randomized comparison of torsemide and furosemide.[67] Patients with NYHA class II or III symptoms and with a hospital, emergency department, or clinic visit for heart failure-related treatment in the previous 12 months (n = 240) participated in the study. LVEF was not an inclusion or exclusion criterion and was not reported in the results. In addition, the cohort had a higher prevalence of diabetes (39%) and a lower prevalence of coronary artery disease (42% with previous MI, 30% with previous coronary artery bypass) than in other randomized controlled trials enrolling heart failure patients.

Over 6 months, the investigators found no significant difference in quality of life, number of clinic visits, telephone calls, hospitalizations, or length of stay for heart failure-related or all-cause hospitalizations. Although torsemide was approximately 300% more expensive over 6 months ($121 vs. $42), there was no significant difference in overall costs between the cohorts. (This study may not have been powered to detect an $80 cost difference between treatment arms.)

Spironolactone

Spironolactone improves clinical outcomes, including resource use.[68] Although spironolactone has a mild natriuretic effect, initial evidence suggested that at low doses it has no apparent diuretic effect. Spironolactone may also block aldosterone-mediated myocardial and vascular fibrosis, baroreceptor dysfunction, and inhibition of norepinephrine uptake by the myocardium. The Randomized Aldactone Evaluation Study (RALES) enrolled patients with LV dysfunction (mean EF of 25%) and NYHA class III or IV symptoms (99%). The average dose was 26 mg. All patients were taking a loop diuretic, 95% were on an ACE inhibitor, and 72% were taking digitalis. Only 10% of patients were taking a beta-blocker, which reflects the treatment guidelines at the time of enrollment (1995 to 1996). Spironolactone reduced the risk of death by 30% (35% vs. 46%; RR, 0.70; 95% CI, 0.60–0.82; $P < 0.001$). The annual death rate of approximately 20% reflects the more severe profile of patients participating in the study. In addition, a 30% reduction in hospitalizations for cardiovascular causes among patients in the spironolactone cohort was reported (515 vs. 753; RR, 0.70; 95% CI, 0.59–0.82; $P < 0.001$). The decrease in all-cause hospitalizations was due entirely to a decrease in heart failure-related hospitalizations. In the evaluation of cost-effectiveness of spironolactone in the RALES trial, Glick *et al.*[69] reported that spironolactone therapy was associated with an increase of 0.13 quality-adjusted life-years and a net savings of $1500.

Angiotensin II receptor blockers

ARBs were initially considered a potential alternative to ACE inhibitors. By not increasing bradykinin levels, ARBs avoided some of the side effects seen with ACE inhibitors. Losartan was the first ARB evaluated in a cohort of heart failure patients. The Evaluation of Losartan in the Elderly (ELITE) was a randomized controlled trial comparing losartan to captopril in patients over the age of 65 years (mean age, 74 years).[70] The majority of the 722 randomized patients were taking diuretics (74%) and digitalis (56%). Ischemia was the underlying etiology of cardiomyopathy in 68% of the patients in the study. Although there was no significant difference in the primary outcome of worsening renal function (10.5% in each group) or the secondary outcome of death or heart failure admission (9.4% vs. 13.2%; risk reduction, 32%; 95% CI, −4 to 55; $P = 0.075$), there was a 46% reduction in risk of death for patients in the losartan group (4.8% vs. 8.7%; 95% CI, 5–69; $P = 0.035$). All-cause hospitalizations decreased significantly from 29.7% to 22.2% (26% risk reduction; 95% CI, 4–43; $P = 0.014$). In contrast to other heart failure clinical trials, there was no difference in heart failure-related hospitalizations between treatment arms (5.7% in both arms).

ELITE II compared losartan with captopril using mortality as the primary outcome.[71] Using similar inclusion criteria (patients over the age of 60 years were enrolled), 3152 patients were randomized to either captopril or losartan. The investigators stratified patients based on beta-blocker use. The median follow-up period was 1.5 years. In contrast to ELITE, there was a trend toward a higher mortality rate in patients taking losartan (17.7% vs. 15.9%; HR 1.13; 95% CI, 0.95–1.35; $P = 0.16$). When patients were taking a beta-blocker, there was a significant improvement in survival for patients receiving captopril compared to patients taking losartan (HR, 1.77). For patients not receiving a beta-blocker, there was no difference between the 2 therapies (HR, 1.05). In addition, all-cause and heart failure-related hospital admissions did not decrease (all-cause hospitalizations, 41.8% for losartan vs. 40.5% for captopril; heart failure-related hospitalizations, 17.1% for losartan vs. 18.6% for captopril; P-value not significant). Although the investigators acknowledged that ELITE II was designed as a superiority trial and not as an equivalence trial between the two therapies, they suggested that ARBs might be considered as an alternative therapy to ACE inhibitors. They also stated that the results of ELITE II should not be extrapolated to other ARBs or to other cohorts, such as post-MI patients.

The Valsartan Heart Failure Trial (Val-HeFT) provided further information regarding ARBs.[72] Investigators from more than 302 centers in 16 countries randomized 5010 patients to receive valsartan or placebo. The majority of patients had symptoms categorized as NYHA class II (61.7%) or III (36.2%) at baseline and were taking ACE inhibitors (93%). Only 35% of patients were taking a beta-blocker. After 2 years of follow-up, there was no difference in mortality, one of the primary outcomes (19.7% for valsartan vs. 19.4% for placebo; RR, 1.02; 95% CI, 0.90–1.15; $P = 0.8$).[73] However, patients treated with valsartan had a significant reduction in the second primary endpoint of all-cause mortality and morbidity (28.8% vs. 32.1% for placebo; RR, 0.87; 95% CI, 0.79–0.96; $P < 0.009$). Treatment was associated with a 24% reduction in heart failure hospitalizations as a first event (13.8% vs. 18.2% for placebo; $P < 0.001$). As with other clinical trials, the reduction in heart failure hospitalizations contributed the most to the reduction in the combined endpoint. Since hospitalizations for other causes were not significantly different, the rate of all-cause hospitalizations was not significantly reduced. It is interesting to note that, unlike other clinical trials enrolling heart failure patients, hospitalizations represented a minority of the combined endpoint. Quality of life was significantly better for patients in the valsartan cohort as compared to patients taking placebo, in terms of improvement in NYHA classification (23.1% vs. 20.7%; $P < 0.001$), worsening NYHA classification (10.1% vs. 12.8%; $P < 0.001$), and MLWHF score (no change vs. −1.9; $P = 0.005$).

The effect of valsartan did depend on the type of background therapy. There was a significant interaction between the use of valsartan and the use or nonuse of ACE inhibitors and the use of beta-blockers ($P = 0.009$).[73] If patients were on neither drug (n = 226) or on either an ACE inhibitor (n = 3034) or beta-blocker alone (n = 140), valsartan improved the combined endpoint of mortality or morbidity. If a patient was receiving both an ACE inhibitor and beta-blocker as baseline therapy (n = 1610), valsartan had a significant adverse effect on mortality ($P = 0.009$) and was associated with a trend toward an increase in the combined endpoint ($P = 0.10$).

Devices

In the past few years, implantable cardiac devices have become more common in managing the heart failure patient. Specifically, biventricular pacemakers (known also as cardiac resynchronization therapy), implantable cardioverter-defibrillators (ICDs), and LV assist devices (LVADs) are being used in patients with heart failure because of their effect on mortality and quality of life.

Implantable cardioverter-defibrillators

The clinical trial history of ICDs has been one of expanding use, from very high-risk heart failure patients to broader indications. The Antiarrhythmic Versus Implantable Defibrillators (AVID) study was a secondary prevention study of patients with reduced LV function and a history of near-fatal ventricular fibrillation or sustained ventricular tachycardia.[74] The investigators estimated that the control group would have a 40% mortality rate over an average follow-up of 2.6 years. The study was terminated early by the data and safety monitoring committee when the benefit of the ICD crossed the statistical boundary for early termination. Patients assigned to the ICD arm had significant improvement in overall survival compared to patients treated with antiarrhythmic drugs at 1 year (89.3% vs. 82.3%), 2 years (81.6% vs. 74.7%), and 3 years (75.4% vs. 64.1%). There was a slight increase in rehospitalization for patients treated with ICD compared to patients treated with antiarrhythmic therapy (60% vs. 56%; $P = 0.04$).

The Multicenter Automatic Defibrillator Trial (MADIT) enrolled a cohort of patients with LVEF ≤ 35%, prior MI, asymptomatic nonsustained ventricular tachycardia, and inducible ventricular tachyarrhythmia at electrophysiology testing that was not suppressed by procainamide.[75] Based on previous studies, the investigators estimated that 2-year mortality for patients randomized to conventional therapy alone was 30%. As in the AVID study, MADIT was terminated early after an average follow-up of 27 months due to a 54% reduction in the risk of death for patients receiving ICD compared to patients receiving conventional therapy (HR, 0.46; 95% CI, 0.26–0.82; $P = 0.009$).

The Multicenter Automatic Defibrillator Implantation II (MADIT II) Trial broadened the potential candidate pool for ICD therapy by enrolling patients with LVEF ≤ 30% and prior MI in the absence of electrophysiologic testing to induce arrhythmias.[76] As with the previous ICD trials in heart failure patients, MADIT II was terminated by the data and safety monitoring committee. For the randomized cohort, ICD reduced the risk of death by 31% (HR, 0.69; 95% CI, 0.51–0.93; $P = 0.016$). The investigators estimated a 2-year mortality rate of 19% for patients in the conventional treatment arm; actual mortality was 19.8% over 20 months. Thus, at the time the trial was stopped, 1232 patients were randomized, a significant increase over the 196 patients required to see a significant difference in MADIT.

Although the findings were not published, the Sudden Cardiac Death in Heart Failure Trial (SCD-HeFT) was presented at the American

College of Cardiology 2004 Scientific Meeting. This study had the broadest inclusion criteria of all the studies, enrolling patients with LVEF of ≤ 35% in the absence of a history of MI or inducible arrhythmias during an electrophysiology test.

According to the clinical trial evidence, there is little doubt that ICDs improve survival for appropriate patients, but it is less clear if the improvement in survival yields a reasonable cost-effectiveness ratio for this expensive therapy. A significant driver of the cost-effectiveness ratio is the type of patient population selected to receive the therapy. Clinical trials of ICDs have moved from high-risk cohorts to lower-risk cohorts, weakening the potential cost-effectiveness of ICDs. In a study of secondary prevention (patients who have already experienced lethal arrhythmias), the AVID investigators calculated a cost-effectiveness ratio of \$66 677 per life-year saved (95% CI, \$30 761 to \$154 768) using hospital bills (supplemented by detailed health care cost data from a subgroup of patients).[77] Using billing information from patients participating in MADIT, Mushlin *et al.*[78] calculated an incremental cost-effectiveness ratio of \$27 000 per life-year saved. The importance of risk stratification has been shown using a Markov model.[79] Investigators found that the cost-effectiveness of ICD vs. amiodarone was influenced strongly by the total annual cardiac mortality rate and by the proportion of deaths that were sudden, with cost-effectiveness being unfavorable at both low and high total cardiac mortality rates. The study found the most favorable cost-effectiveness ratios for ICD were in patients at high risk of sudden cardiac death and low rates of non-sudden cardiac death. Cost-effectiveness analyses for SCD-HeFT and MADIT II have not yet been published.

Quality of life has also been a concern for patients with ICDs. By definition, patients receiving ICDs have experienced major cardiac events, and often the ICD has been implanted because of aborted sudden cardiac death. Overall, studies of quality of life in patients receiving ICDs have found wide variability in the level of clinically significant psychological distress. Between 24% and 33% of patients with ICDs have depressive symptoms, and between 24% and 87% have symptoms of anxiety, with 13% to 38% experiencing a clinically significant anxiety disorder.[80] Much of this distress might be attributable to the underlying condition of the patient; one study found no difference in quality-of-life scores between patients with ICDS and patients in the general population with coronary artery disease.[81] In general, the patient population with heart failure or coronary artery disease has lower quality-of-life scores than age-matched controls in the general population. However, some investigators have studied whether the ICD itself is related to lower quality of life.

The Coronary Artery Bypass Graft (CABG) Patch trial randomized 262 patients undergoing CABG to receive an ICD and 228 patients to usual care. Review of the quality-of-life data from this trial revealed no difference in quality of life for patients with and without ICDs who did not receive shocks, but that those who did receive shocks had worse quality-of-life scores.[82] The authors suggested that ICD shocks may reinforce a patient's sense of illness, although patients who received shocks may have been sicker to begin with.

The AVID Trial also followed quality of life in patients randomized to ICD or amiodarone as secondary prevention and found that there were no differences in overall quality of life between the two groups.[83] There was, however, an independent association between lower quality-of-life scores and having received a shock, as well as having received more frequent shocks compared with less frequent shocks. Also, as the authors pointed out, frequent ICD shocks are associated with increased risk of death, again implying a sicker population overall.

The Canadian Implantable Defibrillator Study, on the other hand, found improved quality of life at 12 months for patients with ICDs compared to patients on amiodarone.[84] Improvements were seen in the overall mental health index and in the psychological distress and psychological well-being components of the measure. For patients with ICDs, those who did not receive shocks had no difference in quality-of-life scores compared to patients who received 1 to 4 shocks. Patients who received ≥ 5 shocks, however, scored lower on the measures than those who had received 1 to 4 shocks.

Overall, it seems that quality of life for patients with ICDs is lower than that of the general population, which is not surprising given their disease state. Patients with ICDs appear to have quality of life that is not worse, and is better in some cases, than patients receiving amiodarone. Most studies have found that the more shocks a patient receives, the lower the quality of life. As ICD therapy improves—with fewer inappropriate shocks and nonshock therapies such as antitachycardic pacing—quality of life may also improve.

Biventricular pacemakers

Biventricular pacemakers work by providing cardiac resynchronization therapy, a simultaneous contraction of the left and right ventricles during systole. In heart failure, roughly 30% of patients have intraventricular conduction delays. Often the septum and the lateral wall receive electrical impulses at different times, leading to inefficient contraction and worsening mitral regurgitation (MR). By threading a pacing lead into the coronary sinus, electrophysiologists can pace the left ventricle simultaneously with the right, leading to a more efficient contraction pattern, improved MR, and consequently better exercise tolerance and quality of life.

The MUSTIC trial[85] was one of the first to use quality-of-life endpoints to show the benefit of biventricular pacemakers. Sixty-seven patients with NYHA class III heart failure received the devices. All had a QRS duration of ≥ 150 ms. In the study design, each patient acted as his or her own control, with a 12-week period of active biventricular pacing and a 12-week period of no pacing. The patient was blinded to the order of the active and inactive periods. Patients had a 23% improvement in distance walked in 6 minutes (399 ± 100 vs. 326 ± 134 meters in active vs. inactive pacing modes, with a baseline of 320 ± 97 meters). While patients were actively paced, their MLWHF scores improved by 32%. At the end of the study, patients were asked which time period they preferred (while still blinded to the order of their active or inactive pacing), and 85% preferred the active pacing mode. Peak oxygen uptake increased by 8% during active pacing (baseline of 13.7 mL/kg/min, paced mode 16.2 mL/kg/min, inactive mode 15 mL/kg/min). Hospitalizations decreased by 66% during modes of active pacing.

In the following year, the MIRACLE trial was published.[86] This was a larger trial with a sicker patient population and had similarly positive results. The trial enrolled 453 patients with NYHA class III/IV heart failure, EF of ≤ 35%, QRS duration of ≥ 130 ms, and clinically stable heart failure over a 6-month period. All patients had biventricular pacemakers implanted and were randomized to active pacing or an inactive mode. Those randomized to active pacing had a 39-meter improvement in their 6-minute walk test, compared with a 10-meter improvement in the inactive pacing group. The MLWHF score improved by 18 points in the paced group compared with 9 points in the control group. The treatment group also had a better peak oxygen uptake and a longer total exercise time. Treated patients had a better overall clinical composite score and fewer hospitalizations.

More recently, the COMPANION trial[87] compared optimal medical therapy with biventricular pacing and biventricular ICDs. Both groups showed a reduction in time to hospitalization or death, which was the primary endpoint of the study. The 12-month rate of the primary endpoint was 68% in the optimal medical therapy group, compared to 56% in the biventricular pacing group (HR, 0.81; $P = 0.014$) and 56% in the biventricular ICD group (HR, 0.80; $P = 0.010$), The ICD group also had a statistically significant reduction in all-cause mortality, with 12-month mortality of 19% in the placebo group, 15% in the biventricular pacing group (HR, 0.76; $P = 0.059$), and 12 % in the biventricular ICD group (HR, 0.64; $P = 0.003$). Patients with devices had a statistically significant improvement in their 6-minute walk distance, at both 3 months and 6 months, compared with the placebo group. At 3 months, placebo patients improved by 9 meters, compared with 33 meters for the biventricular pacing group and 44 meters for the biventricular ICD group, and this carried forward to 6 months, with improvements of 1 meter, 40 meters, and 46 meters for each of the groups, respectively. At 3 months, 24% percent of the placebo patients improved by at least one NYHA symptom class, compared with 58% of the biventricular pacing patients and 55% of the biventricular

ICD patients. These differences remained equally significant at 6 months. MLWHF scores improved by 9 points in the placebo group at 3 months and by 24 points in the device groups. These differences remained significant at 6 months.

Because of the relatively recent development of cardiac resynchronization therapy for heart failure, there is limited information about the cost-effectiveness of these strategies. All of the analyses have relied on modeling clinical trial outcomes using a number of assumptions. An analysis by Nichol *et al.*[88] used the probabilities of death, hospitalization, and adverse events from 9 randomized controlled trials of cardiac resynchronization therapy in a Markov model to estimate cost-effectiveness. They found that cardiac resynchronization therapy added 0.28 quality-adjusted life-years (QALYs) for patients with NYHA class III symptoms for an additional median cost of $30 000, and a cost-effectiveness ratio of $107 800 per QALY. The results were sensitive to risk of death, likelihood of complications from therapy, and degree of improvement in quality of life from cardiac resynchronization therapy. It is important to note that the analysis was performed from a health care system perspective rather than a societal perspective.

Left ventricular assist devices

LVADs are now being considered as "destination therapy" for some patients who are otherwise ineligible for cardiac transplantation. The Randomized Evaluation of Mechanical Assistance for the Treatment of Congestive Heart Failure (REMATCH)[89] studied 129 such patients, randomizing them to optimal medical therapy (n = 61) or destination LVAD (n = 68). The primary endpoint was mortality, and 52% of the LVAD patients were alive at 12 months, compared with only 25% of the medically treated group. At 2 years, however, most patients in both groups were dead.

LVADs also seemed to show a quality-of-life benefit. Baseline MLWHF scores were 75, indicating poor quality of life. At 1 year, scores improved to 41 for the LVAD group and 58 for the medically treated group, but given the small numbers tested at 1 year, this was not statistically significant. SF-36 scores also improved more for the LVAD patients (46 vs. 21 for the physical function component [$P = 0.01$] and 64 vs. 17 for the emotional component [$P = 0.03$]) at 1 year. While medically treated patients remained with NYHA class IV symptoms, those receiving LVADs improved to NYHA class II symptoms. Almost all of the patients treated medically died of progressive pump failure, while those with LVADs died of device-related complications such as sepsis, stroke, or device failure. As the technology improves for these devices, outcomes are likely to improve even more for the advanced heart failure patient.

Comment

A number of pharmaceutical and device therapies have been tested and found to be beneficial in patients with chronic left systolic dysfunction over the past 15 years. ACE inhibitors, beta-blockers, digoxin, diuretics, and ARBs (in patients intolerant of ACE inhibition) are now considered evidence-based therapy for patients with LV dysfunction who can tolerate those medicines (only ACE inhibitor and beta-blocker for asymptomatic patients[50]). These medications improve survival and quality of life and decrease hospitalization. In addition, findings from studies of ICDs and chronic resynchronization therapy have made these strategies standard options for appropriate heart failure patients.

Unfortunately, most of the clinical trials evaluating pharmaceutical therapies for patients with LV dysfunction did not include a prospective economic analysis, thus requiring investigators to model the potential economic impact of specific therapies. Although most of these models were created using the trial results, a number of assumptions had to be incorporated into such analyses. As pointed out in this chapter, some of the assumptions, including omissions of important variables, may limit the usefulness of some analyses.

The extrapolation of clinical trial results to the general heart failure population can lead to over-estimating benefits, owing to differences between community practice patterns and clinical trial protocols. In clinical trials, investigators and their staff follow protocols that dictate background therapies and the initiation and titration of the study medication. It is difficult for practicing physicians to replicate this type of interaction. Patients participating in clinical trials are highly selected and may not be representative of the majority of heart failure patients in the United States. On average, most patients with heart failure are older than patients participating in clinical trials. Almost 75% of the nearly 5 million patients with heart failure in the United States are older than 65.[64,65] It is not surprising, therefore, that studies have documented the underutilization of ACE inhibitors by primary care physicians and cardiologists.[66–70]

As therapies have improved, trials have shifted their endpoints from mortality to both hospitalization and mortality, with reductions in heart failure hospitalizations frequently the most significant results. An exception to this rule is found in studies of ICD therapy, which have used mortality as the primary endpoint, in part because of the potential for worsening quality of life and increased hospitalizations.[74,90] Changes in primary outcome from a single mortality endpoint to a combined endpoint may be due in part to the limited ability of additional therapies to have a further impact on mortality, and the need to identify outcomes with higher event rates so as to detect smaller effects. There is remarkable consistency in how triple to quadruple therapy affects heart failure hospitalizations across therapeutic classes. Unfortunately, diverse combinations of therapies make comparisons of quadruple therapy problematic and make it difficult to prioritize fourth agents.

New therapeutic strategies targeting the neurohormonal imbalance found in heart failure patients may be reaching a threshold at which significant improvements in outcomes are not achievable. The results of Val-HeFT showed that the addition of valsartan to background therapy of ACE inhibitor and beta-blocker not only provided no additional benefit, but was in fact deleterious. Endothelin receptor antagonists are not proving to be effective in improving outcomes. Results from recent studies of bosentan (the ENABLE trial) and tezosentan (RITZ-1 and RITZ-4) have shown that these agents do not improve outcomes in heart failure patients. As it becomes more difficult to show improved outcomes, including reductions in hospitalizations, it will also become more difficult to show that new therapies are cost-effective.

Conclusion

Recommended pharmaceutical therapies for patients with LV dysfunction appear to be economically attractive. Proven therapies for heart failure are economically dominant because they decrease heart failure hospitalizations; however, a change in heart failure hospitalization is not the same as a reduction in total hospitalizations. Thus, a decrease in heart failure hospitalization may not translate into cost savings. Economic evaluation should remain an essential component of the overall evaluation of heart failure therapies. The quality of this literature is improving, but better data in the clinical trial setting and in clinical practice are needed, especially as the ability to show significant changes in clinical outcomes decreases and regulatory approval relies increasingly on such outcomes as cost-effectiveness.

References

1. Massie BM, Packer M. Congestive heart failure: current controversies and future prospects. Am J Cardiol 1990; 6: 429–430.
2. Rich MW. Epidemiology, pathophysiology, and etiology of congestive heart failure in older adults. J Am Geriatr Soc 1997; 45: 968–974.
3. Medicare Provider Analysis and Review. 100% MEDPAR Inpatient Hospital Fiscal Year 1994 (Health Care Financing Administration: Baltimore, MD, 1995).
4. O'Connell JB, Bristow MR. Economic impact of heart failure in the United States: time for a different approach. J Heart Lung Transplant 1994; 13: S107–S112.
5. O'Connell JB. The economic burden of heart failure. Clin Cardiol 2000; 23: III6–III10.
6. Vinson JM, Rich MW, Sperry JC, Shah AS, McNamara T. Early readmission of elderly patients with congestive heart failure. J Am Geriatr Soc 1990; 38: 1290–1295.
7. Gooding J, Jette AM. Hospital readmissions among the elderly. J Am Geriatr Soc 1985; 33: 595–601.

8. The SOLVD Investigators. Effect of enalapril on survival in patients with reduced left ventricular ejection fractions and congestive heart failure. N Engl J Med 1991; 325: 293–302.
9. The SOLVD Investigators. Effect of enalapril on mortality and the development of heart failure in asymptomatic patients with reduced left ventricular ejection fractions. N Engl J Med 1992; 327: 685–691.
10. Cohn JN, Johnson G, Ziesche S, *et al.* A comparison of enalapril with hydralazine-isosorbide dinitrate in the treatment of chronic congestive heart failure. N Engl J Med 1991; 325: 303–310.
11. The CONSENSUS Trial Study Group. Effects of enalapril on mortality in severe congestive heart failure, results of the Cooperative North Scandinavian Enalapril Survival Study (CONSENSUS). N Engl J Med 1987; 316: 1429–1435.
12. Packer M, Poole-Wilson PA, Armstrong PW, *et al.* Comparative effects of low and high doses of the angiotensin-converting enzyme inhibitor, lisinopril, on morbidity and mortality in chronic heart failure. ATLAS Study Group. Circulation 1999; 100: 2312–2318.
13. Scott WG, Scott HM. Heart failure, a decision analytic analysis of New Zealand data using the published results of the SOLVD Treatment Trial. Studies of Left Ventricular Dysfunction. Pharmacoeconomics 1996; 9: 156–167.
14. Glick HA, Cook JR, Kinosian B, *et al.* Costs and effects of enalapril therapy in patients with symptomatic heart failure: an economic analysis of the Studies of Left Ventricular Dysfunction (SOLVD) Treatment Trial. J Card Fail 1995; 1: 371–380.
15. Cook JR, Glick HA, Gerth W, Kinosian B, Kostis JB. The cost and cardioprotective effects of enalapril in hypertensive patients with left ventricular dysfunction. Am J Hypertens 1998; 11: 1433–1441.
16. Paul SD, Kuntz KM, Eagle KA, Weinstein MC. Costs and effectiveness of angiotensin converting enzyme inhibition in patients with congestive heart failure. Arch Intern Med 1994; 154: 1143–1149.
17. Sculpher MJ, Poole L, Cleland J, *et al.* Low doses vs. high doses of the angiotensin converting-enzyme inhibitor lisinopril in chronic heart failure: a cost-effectiveness analysis based on the Assessment of Treatment with Lisinopril and Survival (ATLAS) study. The ATLAS Study Group. Eur J Heart Fail 2000; 2: 447–454.
18. van Hout BA, Wielink G, Bonsel GJ, Rutten FF. Effects of ACE inhibitors on heart failure in The Netherlands: a pharmacoeconomic model. Pharmacoeconomics 1993; 3: 387–397.
19. Butler JR, Fletcher PJ. A cost-effectiveness analysis of enalapril maleate in the management of congestive heart failure in Australia. Aust N Z J Med 1996; 26: 89–95.
20. Cleland JG, Walker A. Is medical treatment for angina the most cost-effective option? Eur Heart J 1997; 18: B35–B42.
21. McMurray J, Davie A. The pharmacoeconomics of ACE inhibitors in chronic heart failure. Pharmacoeconomics 1996; 9: 188–197.
22. Jonsson B, Johannesson M, Kjekshus J, *et al.* Cost-effectiveness of cholesterol lowering, results from the Scandinavian Simvastatin Survival Study (4S). Eur Heart J 1996; 17: 1001–1007.
23. Wiklund I, Swedberg K. Some methodological problems in analyzing quality of life data in severe congestive heart failure. J Clin Res Pharmacoepidemiol 1991; 5: 265–273.
24. Epstein SE, Braunwald E. Beta-adrenergic receptor blocking drugs, mechanisms of action and clinical applications. N Engl J Med 1966; 275: 1106–1112.
25. Waagstein F, Hjalmarson A, Varnauskas E, Wallentin I. Effect of chronic beta-adrenergic receptor blockade in congestive cardiomyopathy. Br Heart J 1975; 37: 1022–1036.
26. Swedberg K, Hjalmarson A, Waagstein F, Wallentin I. Prolongation of survival in congestive cardiomyopathy by beta-receptor blockade. Lancet 1979; 1: 1374–1376.
27. Lowes BD, Tsvetkova T, Eichhorn EJ, Gilbert EM, Bristow MR. Milrinone versus dobutamine in heart failure subjects treated chronically with carvedilol. Int J Cardiol 2001; 81: 141–149.
28. Eichhorn EJ, Heesch CM, Barnett JH, *et al.* Effect of metoprolol on myocardial function and energetics in patients with nonischemic dilated cardiomyopathy: a randomized, double-blind, placebo-controlled study. J Am Coll Cardiol 1994; 24: 1310–1320.
29. Woodley SL, Gilbert EM, Anderson JL, *et al.* Beta-blockade with bucindolol in heart failure caused by ischemic versus idiopathic dilated cardiomyopathy. Circulation 1991; 84: 2426–2441.
30. Metra M, Nardi M, Giubbini R, Dei CL. Effects of short- and long-term carvedilol administration on rest and exercise hemodynamic variables, exercise capacity and clinical conditions in patients with idiopathic dilated cardiomyopathy. J Am Coll Cardiol 1994; 24: 1678–1687.
31. Waagstein F, Bristow MR, Swedberg K, *et al.* Beneficial effects of metoprolol in idiopathic dilated cardiomyopathy, Metoprolol in Dilated Cardiomyopathy (MDC) Trial Study Group. Lancet 1993; 342: 1441–1446.

32. CIBIS Investigators and Committees. A randomized trial of beta-blockade in heart failure. The Cardiac Insufficiency Bisoprolol Study (CIBIS). Circulation 1994; 90: 1765–1773.
33. The Cardiac Insufficiency Bisoprolol Study II (CIBIS-II): a randomised trial. Lancet 1999; 353: 9–13.
34. Effect of metoprolol CR/XL in chronic heart failure: Metoprolol CR/XL Randomised Intervention Trial in Congestive Heart Failure (MERIT-HF). Lancet 1999; 353: 2001–2007.
35. Hjalmarson A, Goldstein S, Fagerberg B, *et al.* Effects of controlled-release metoprolol on total mortality, hospitalizations, and well-being in patients with heart failure: the Metoprolol CR/XL Randomized Intervention Trial in congestive heart failure (MERIT-HF), MERIT-HF Study Group. JAMA 2000; 283: 1295–1302.
36. Packer M, Bristow MR, Cohn JN, *et al.* The effect of carvedilol on morbidity and mortality in patients with chronic heart failure. U.S. Carvedilol Heart Failure Study Group. N Engl J Med 1996; 334: 1349–1355.
37. Fowler MB, Vera-Llonch M, Oster G, *et al.* Influence of carvedilol on hospitalizations in heart failure: incidence, resource utilization and costs. U.S. Carvedilol Heart Failure Study Group. J Am Coll Cardiol 2001; 37: 1692–1699.
38. Packer M, Coats AJ, Fowler MB, *et al.* Effect of carvedilol on survival in severe chronic heart failure. N Engl J Med 2001; 344: 1651–1658.
39. Beta Blocker Evaluation of Survival Trial Investigators. A trial of the beta-blocker bucindolol in patients with advanced chronic heart failure. N Engl J Med 2001; 344: 1659–1667.
40. Delea TE, Vera-Llonch M, Richner RE, Fowler MB, Oster G. Cost effectiveness of carvedilol for heart failure. Am J Cardiol 1999; 83: 890–896.
41. Colucci WS, Packer M, Bristow MR, *et al.* Carvedilol inhibits clinical progression in patients with mild symptoms of heart failure. U.S. Carvedilol Heart Failure Study Group. Circulation 1996; 94: 2800–2806.
42. Packer M, Colucci WS, Sackner-Bernstein JD. Double-blind, placebo-controlled study of the effects of carvedilol in patients with moderate to severe heart failure. The PRECISE Trial, Prospective Randomized Evaluation of Carvedilol on Symptoms and Exercise. Circulation 1996; 94: 2793–2799.
43. Bristow MR, Gilbert EM, Abraham WT. Carvedilol produces dose-related improvements in left ventricular function and survival in subjects with chronic heart failure. MOCHA Investigators. Circulation 1996; 94: 2807–2816.
44. Effects of metoprolol CR in patients with ischemic and dilated cardiomyopathy: the randomized evaluation of strategies for left ventricular dysfunction pilot study. Circulation 2000; 101: 378–384.
45. Hjalmarson A, Goldstein S, Fagerberg B, *et al.* Effects of controlled-release metoprolol on total mortality, hospitalizations, and well-being in patients with heart failure: the Metoprolol CR/XL Randomized Intervention Trial in congestive heart failure (MERIT-HF), MERIT-HF Study Group. JAMA 2000; 283: 1295–1302.
46. Bristow MR, O'Connell JB, Gilbert EM, *et al.* Dose-response of chronic beta-blocker treatment in heart failure from either idiopathic dilated or ischemic cardiomyopathy, Bucindolol Investigators. Circulation 1994; 89: 1632–1642.
47. Australia/New Zealand Heart Failure Research Collaborative Group. Randomised, placebo-controlled trial of carvedilol in patients with congestive heart failure due to ischaemic heart disease. Lancet 1997; 349: 375–380.
48. Metra M, Giubbini R, Nodari S, *et al.* Differential effects of beta-blockers in patients with heart failure: A prospective, randomized, double-blind comparison of the long-term effects of metoprolol versus carvedilol. Circulation 2000; 102: 546–551.
49. CIBIS Investigators and Committees. A randomized trial of beta-blockade in heart failure. The Cardiac Insufficiency Bisoprolol Study (CIBIS). Circulation 1994; 90: 1765–1773.
50. Lee DC, Johnson RA, Bingham JB, *et al.* Heart failure in outpatients: a randomized trial of digoxin versus placebo. N Engl J Med 1982; 306: 699–705.
51. Guyatt GH, Sullivan MJ, Fallen EL, *et al.* A controlled trial of digoxin in congestive heart failure. Am J Cardiol 1988; 61: 371–375.
52. The Captopril-Digoxin Multicenter Research Group. Comparative effects of therapy with captopril and digoxin in patients with mild to moderate heart failure. JAMA 1988; 259: 539–544.
53. Packer M, Gheorghiade M, Young JB, *et al.* Withdrawal of digoxin from patients with chronic heart failure treated with angiotensin-converting-enzyme inhibitors. RADIANCE Study. N Engl J Med 1993; 329: 1–7.
54. Uretsky BF, Young JB, Shahidi FE, *et al.* Randomized study assessing the effect of digoxin withdrawal in patients with mild to moderate chronic congestive heart failure: results of the PROVED trial. PROVED Investigative Group. J Am Coll Cardiol 1993; 22: 955–962.
55. Adams KF Jr., Gheorghiade M, Uretsky BF, *et al.*

Patients with mild heart failure worsen during withdrawal from digoxin therapy. J Am Coll Cardiol 1997; 30: 42–48.
56. The Digitalis Investigation Group. The effect of digoxin on mortality and morbidity in patients with heart failure. N Engl J Med 1997; 336: 525–533.
57. Ward RE, Gheorghiade M, Young JB, Uretsky B. Economic outcomes of withdrawal of digoxin therapy in adult patients with stable congestive heart failure. J Am Coll Cardiol 1995; 26: 93–101.
58. Agency for Health Care Policy and Research. Heart Failure: Evaluation and Care of Patients With Left-Ventricular Systolic Dysfunction. Clinical Practice Guideline (11) (US Dept of Health and Human Services, Agency for Health Care Policy and Research: Rockville, MD, 1994), AHCPR Publication Number 94–0612.
59. Consensus recommendations for the management of chronic heart failure: on behalf of the membership of the advisory council to improve outcomes nationwide in heart failure. Am J Cardiol 1999; 83: 1A–38A.
60. Hunt SA, Baker DW, Chin MH, *et al.* ACC/AHA Guidelines for the Evaluation and Management of Chronic Heart Failure in the Adult: Executive Summary: A Report of the American College of Cardiology/American Heart Association Task Force on Practice Guidelines (Committee to Revise the 1995 Guidelines for the Evaluation and Management of Heart Failure): Developed in Collaboration with the International Society for Heart and Lung Transplantation; Endorsed by the Heart Failure Society of America. Circulation 2001; 104: 2996–3007.
61. Neuberg GW, Miller AB, O'Connor CM, *et al.* Diuretic resistance predicts mortality in patients with advanced heart failure. Am Heart J 2002; 144: 31–38.
62. Scheen AJ, Vancrombreucq JC, Delarge J, Luyckx AS. Diuretic activity of torasemide and furosemide in chronic heart failure: a comparative double blind cross-over study. Eur J Clin Pharmacol 1986; 31: 35–42.
63. Broekhuysen J, Deger F, Douchamps J, Ducarne H, Herchuelz A. Torasemide, a new potent diuretic, double-blind comparison with furosemide. Eur J Clin Pharmacol 1986; 31: 29–34.
64. Dodion L, Ambroes Y, Lameire N. A comparison of the pharmacokinetics and diuretic effects of two loop diuretics, torasemide and furosemide, in normal volunteers. Eur J Clin Pharmacol 1986; 31: 21–27.
65. Heaton AH, Bryant J, Berman BN, Trotter JP. Pharmacoeconomic comparison of loop diuretics in the treatment of congestive heart failure. Med Interface 1996; 9: 101–107.
66. Spannheimer A, Goertz A, Dreckmann-Behrendt B. Comparison of therapies with torasemide or furosemide in patients with congestive heart failure from a pharmacoeconomic viewpoint. Int J Clin Pract 1998; 52: 467–471.
67. Noe LL, Vreeland MG, Pezzella SM, Trotter JP. A pharmacoeconomic assessment of torsemide and furosemide in the treatment of patients with congestive heart failure. Clin Ther 1999; 21: 854–866.
68. Pitt B, Zannad F, Remme WJ, *et al.* The effect of spironolactone on morbidity and mortality in patients with severe heart failure, Randomized Aldactone Evaluation Study Investigators. N Engl J Med 1999; 341: 709–717.
69. Glick HA, Orzol SM, Tooley JF, Remme WJ, Sasayama S, Pitt B. Economic evaluation of the randomized aldactone evaluation study (RALES): treatment of patients with severe heart failure. Cardiovasc Drugs Ther 2002; 16: 53–59.
70. Pitt B, Segal R, Martinez FA, *et al.* Randomised trial of losartan versus captopril in patients over 65 with heart failure (Evaluation of Losartan in the Elderly Study, ELITE). Lancet 1997; 349: 747–752.
71. Pitt B, Poole-Wilson PA, Segal R, *et al.* Effect of losartan compared with captopril on mortality in patients with symptomatic heart failure: randomised trial—the Losartan Heart Failure Survival Study ELITE II. Lancet 2000; 355: 1582–1587.
72. Cohn JN, Tognoni G, Glazer R, Spormann D. Baseline demographics of the Valsartan Heart Failure Trial. Val-HeFT Investigators. Eur J Heart Fail 2000; 2: 439–446.
73. Konstam MA. Comment—Val-HeFT and angiotensin-receptor blockers in perspective: a tale of the blind man and the elephant. J Card Fail 2002; 8: 56–58.
74. The Antiarrhythmics versus Implantable Defibrillators (AVID) Investigators. A comparison of antiarrhythmic-drug therapy with implantable defibrillators in patients resuscitated from near-fatal ventricular arrhythmias. N Engl J Med 1997; 337: 1576–1584.
75. Moss AJ, Hall WJ, Cannom DS, *et al.* Improved survival with an implanted defibrillator in patients with coronary disease at high risk for ventricular arrhythmia. Multicenter Automatic Defibrillator Implantation Trial Investigators. N Engl J Med 1996; 335: 1933–1940.
76. Moss AJ, Zareba W, Hall WJ, *et al.* Prophylactic implantation of a defibrillator in patients with myocardial infarction and reduced ejection fraction. N Engl J Med 2002; 346: 877–883.
77. Larsen G, Hallstrom A, McAnulty J, *et al.* Cost-effectiveness of the implantable cardioverter-

defibrillator versus antiarrhythmic drugs in survivors of serious ventricular tachyarrhythmias: results of the Antiarrhythmics Versus Implantable Defibrillators (AVID) economic analysis substudy. Circulation 2002; 105: 2049–1057.

78. Mushlin AI, Hall WJ, Zwanziger J, *et al.* The cost-effectiveness of automatic implantable cardiac defibrillators: results from MADIT. Multicenter Automatic Defibrillator Implantation Trial. Circulation 1998; 97: 2129–2135.
79. Owens DK, Sanders GD, Heidenreich PA, McDonald KM, Hlatky MA. Effect of risk stratification on cost-effectiveness of the implantable cardioverter defibrillator. Am Heart J 2002; 144: 440–448.
80. Sears SF Jr., Todaro JF, Lewis TS, Sotile W, Conti JB. Examining the psychosocial impact of implantable cardioverter defibrillators: a literature review. Clin Cardiol 1999; 22: 481–489.
81. Herrmann C, von zur Muhen F, Schaumann A, *et al.* Standardized assessment of psychological well-being and quality-of-life in patients with implanted defibrillators. Pacing Clin Electrophysiol 1997; 20: 95–103.
82. Namerow PB, Firth BR, Heywood GM, Windle JR, Parides MK. Quality-of-life six months after CABG surgery in patients randomized to ICD versus no ICD therapy: findings from the CABG Patch Trial. Pacing Clin Electrophysiol 1999; 22: 1305–1313.
83. Schron EB, Exner DV, Yao Q, *et al.* Quality of life in the antiarrhythmics versus implantable defibrillators trial: impact of therapy and influence of adverse symptoms and defibrillator shocks. Circulation 2002; 105: 589–594.
84. Irvine J, Dorian P, Baker B, *et al.* Quality of life in the Canadian Implantable Defibrillator Study (CIDS). Am Heart J 2002; 144: 282–289.
85. Cazeau S, Leclercq C, Lavergne T, *et al.* Effects of multisite biventricular pacing in patients with heart failure and intraventricular conduction delay. N Engl J Med 2001; 344: 873–880.
86. Abraham WT, Fisher WG, Smith AL, *et al.* Cardiac resynchronization in chronic heart failure. N Engl J Med 2002; 346: 1845–1853.
87. Bristow MR, Saxon LA, Boehmer J, *et al.* Cardiac-resynchronization therapy with or without an implantable defibrillator in advanced chronic heart failure. N Engl J Med 2004; 350: 2140–2150.
88. Nichol G, Kaul P, Huszti E, Bridges JF. Cost-effectiveness of cardiac resynchronization therapy in patients with symptomatic heart failure. Ann Intern Med 2004; 141: 343–351.
89. Rose EA, Gelijns AC, Moskowitz AJ, *et al.* Long-term mechanical left ventricular assistance for end-stage heart failure. N Engl J Med 2001; 345: 1435–1443.
90. Wilkoff BL, Cook JR, Epstein AE, *et al.* Dual-chamber pacing or ventricular backup pacing in patients with an implantable defibrillator: the Dual Chamber and VVI Implantable Defibrillator (DAVID) Trial. JAMA 2002; 288: 3115–3123.

CHAPTER 40

Disease management in the advanced heart failure patient

David J Whellan

Introduction

The growing epidemic of heart failure has been well described in the heart failure literature.[1,2] This fact has led the federal government and private industry to spend millions of dollars on identifying new therapies that improve mortality and morbidity for heart failure patients.[3] Unfortunately, as highlighted in a recent report from the Institute of Medicine, these life-saving therapies remain significantly underused in clinical practice.[4] The gap between what we know and what we do in heart failure management has been described as a "quality chasm."[4]

Heart failure disease management has been proposed as a care strategy that bridges the "quality chasm" for heart failure patients. Since the publication of the landmark study by Rich *et al.*, a number of studies have shown the benefit of providing additional interactions with health care providers for heart failure patients (including discharge planning, clinic visits, telephone calls, and home visits).[5] The consistent theme in disease management interventions is an attempt to shift patient care responsibilities, particularly patient education and monitoring, to non-physicians. The message from these studies is that intensifying interaction with a multidisciplinary team significantly decreases hospitalizations (relative risk [RR], 0.77; 95% confidence interval [CI], 0.68–0.86).[6]

The primary focus of this review chapter is randomized controlled study design. A number of studies have used non-randomized study designs, including pre-enrollment versus post-enrollment comparisons and retrospective chart review.[7–17] Since significant limitations exist in this type of analysis, including regression to the mean, these studies will only be referenced to highlight significant points throughout the discussion. Not surprisingly, all these studies found significant improvement in clinical outcomes for participating patients.

It is critical to recognize that disease management has a variety of definitions and designs throughout the literature and in practice.[18] Interventions can be as simple as patient education or vital-sign monitoring, or as complex as multidisciplinary approaches to care that include a pharmacist, nutritionist, nurse practitioner (NP), and physician. Some interventions incorporate protocols to provide specific guidelines for care; others only provide information or identify at-risk patients, allowing care decisions to fluctuate based on the individual choices of caregivers. Due to the variety of interventions evaluated, classification schemes have been developed in an attempt to categorize heart failure disease management.[19] Using location as the discriminating characteristic, Grady *et al.* identified the following settings for disease management: inpatient, specialty heart failure care, specialty heart failure care outside the clinic setting (home visits, telephone calls, or telemonitoring), and primary care clinic.

This review will attempt to categorize studies based on the classification system proposed by Grady *et al.* (Table 40.1). It is critical to recognize that most disease management interventions involve patient care in multiple locations; assignment of an intervention to a particular category of disease management intervention was based on what appeared to be the primary intervention. Since all of the interventions involve physician extenders, an attempt was made to identify the type of physician supervising the intervention, cardiologist versus primary care physician (PCP). For the interventions involving home visits and telephone follow-up, we considered the supervising physician to be a PCP unless the study specified that a cardiologist was involved.

Inpatient Disease Management Strategies

The majority of disease management interventions described in this review included some form of inpatient intervention. Given that a heart failure hospitalization is a crude means to identify a heart failure cohort at risk for future events and an inpatient stay is an excellent opportunity to interact with a "captive" audience, providing a disease management intervention during a hospitalization makes intuitive sense.[20] Depending on the study, the intensified inpatient care was considered part of the intervention or provided as standard of care.[5,10,21–23]

One randomized controlled trial has evaluated an inpatient heart failure intervention with no post-discharge care plan.[24] The study by Constantini *et al.* evaluated an intervention that included inpatient guidelines for the use of angiotensin-converting enzyme (ACE) inhibitors, echocardiogram, daily weights, and a consultative service provided by a nurse care manager and cardiologist. The consults included patient education, treatment recommendations, and discharge planning. The intervention significantly improved ACE inhibitor use at discharge, percentage with daily weights, and percentage with documented left ventricular ejection fraction (LVEF). Although the intervention achieved a significant decrease in length of stay and

Table 40.1. *Classification scheme for heart failure disease management interventions*

Location	Cardiology supervision		Primary care supervision
Inpatient	Constantini (2001)[24] IMPACT (2003)[25]		
Clinic based	**Post-discharge** Cline (1998)[69] Doughty (2002)[70] Kasper (2002)[71] McDonald (2002)[21] Capomolla (2002)[72]	**Chronic outpatient** Gattis (1999)[73] Ansari (2003)[31]	**Post-discharge** Oddone (1996, 1999)[74,75] Ekman (1998)[30]
Home visit	Rich (1995)[76] Blue (2001)[22]		Stewart (1998, 1999)[57,58] Stewart (1999)[77] Harrison (2001)[78] Hughes (2000)[79] Jaarsma (1999)[80]
Telephone follow-up	Krumholz (2002)[81] Laramee (2003)[34]		Naylor (1994)[82] Naylor (1999)[83] Riegel (2002)[84]

cost per case, there was a non-significant increase in 30-day readmissions for patients receiving the intervention, lending support to the recommendation by McDonald *et al.*[21]

A second randomized controlled trial, the IMPACT-HF study, assessing an inpatient care strategy, evaluated the benefit of initiating beta-blocker therapy during heart failure hospitalization.[25] Intervention patients had low-dose carvedilol, a beta-blocker shown to improve survival and decrease hospitalization in heart failure patients, initiated prior to discharge.[26–28] Patients in this arm of the study were more likely to be taking a beta-blocker at 60 days post discharge (91.2% vs. 73.4%; $P < 0.0001$) with no significant increase in readmissions.

Based on these studies, investigators have proposed extending the inpatient stay to include 2 days of stabilization to achieve improved outcomes.[29] Although the value of extending patient stays may make intuitive sense, the impact on outcomes of longer or more intensive inpatient care is difficult to assess due to the continuation of most interventions in the outpatient setting. In addition, in the current reimbursement environment, it is unattractive for hospitals and health care systems in the United States to promote longer hospital stays, both in terms of additional costs for the initial hospitalization and the lost revenue for reducing future hospitalizations.

Clinic Visits

Due to the commonality with ongoing clinical services, disease management interventions based in the clinic setting represent the most feasible type of intervention for a provider or health care system to implement. Two non-randomized controlled studies were extensions of ongoing cardiac transplant programs.[11,12] Reimbursement for physician extender services is available depending on state and third party regulations; thus providing some mechanism to cover part of the cost.

Clinic-based disease management studies can be categorized based on the type of heart failure patient enrolled (post-discharge or chronic outpatient) and the type of physician supervising the intervention. Nine randomized controlled trials evaluated clinic-based disease management interventions (Table 40.2). All of these studies involved the supervision of a physician extender (NP, nurse, or PharmD) by a cardiologist or PCP. The intensity of the interventions ranged from a single visit to multiple visits over a 12-month period. As described in the introduction, the clinic-based interventions included components of the other types of disease management interventions; all of the interventions included telephone follow-up ranging from 1 to 10 calls per patient. Most studies only described the number of clinic visits, telephone calls, or use of home visits dictated by the study protocol, and did not document the actual number of visits; making the true assessment of intensity and cost of providing the program difficult to ascertain.

The success of the programs varied considerably between the different studies. Patients in the intervention arm had significant increases in their ACE inhibitor or beta-blocker use or dose in 4 out of the 9 randomized controlled trials of clinic-based interventions; medication use was not reported in 2 of the studies.[21,30] Quality of life (QOL), which was measured with a variety of instruments and methods, improved in 3 of the 7 studies reporting QOL endpoints.[31] All-cause hospitalization improved in 3 studies, with the primary mechanism being a decrease in heart failure hospitalizations. Care within clinic-based interventions supervised by PCPs was associated with an increase in all-cause hospitalizations. An improvement in medication use did not appear to correlate with an improvement in QOL or readmissions.

The two interventions enrolling patients in the outpatient setting (as opposed to enrollment at the time of discharge) specifically focused on medication use, and not surprisingly, identified improvement in the primary outcome of improved use of heart failure medications.[31,32] Possibly due to the lower risk of hospitalization, only one of the studies found a significant reduction in heart failure hospitalizations (odds ratio [OR] 0.22; 95% CI, 0.07–0.65; $P = 0.005$).[33] Despite a fairly intensive interaction with an NP, no change in readmissions was noted in the study by Ansari *et al.* in the nurse facilitator, provider/patient notification or control arms (9% vs. 14% vs. 10%; $P = 0.66$).[31]

Table 40.2. *Randomized controlled trials using clinic follow-up*

Author (year)	Country	Follow-up (months)	Number of patients randomized	Mean age (years)	Readmissions/LOS (days) (intervention vs. control)
Clinic follow-up, cardiologist supervision					
Cline (1998)[85]	Sweden	12	190	75.6	AC per pt: 0.7 ± 1.1 vs. 1.1 ± 1.8 AC LOS: 4.2 vs. 8.2
Doughty (2002)[70]	New Zealand	2	197	73	AC: 120 vs. 154; CHF: 36 vs. 65 LOS AC: 8.9 vs. 7.6; CHF: 9.9 vs. 8.6
Kasper (2002)[71]	United States, Maryland	6	200	63.5	AC: 77 vs. 96; CHF: 43 vs. 59 LOS: 6.3 vs. 4.8
McDonald (2002)[21]	Ireland	3	98	71	CHF: 1 vs. 11† Index LOS: 13.7 vs. 14.6
Capomolla (2002)[72]	Italy	12	234	56	AC: 13 vs. 78, $P < 0.00001$
Clinic follow-up, PCP supervision					
Oddone (1996, 1999)[75,86]	United States, VA centers	6	504	65	AC: 56 vs. 44†; CHF: 29 vs. 30 LOS: 9.1 vs. 7.3*
Ekman (1998)[30]	Sweden	6	158	80	AC: 61 vs. 57; LOS: 15 vs. 11 AC day/pt: 6.9 vs. 9.5
Stable HF patient clinic follow-up, cardiologist supervision					
Gattis (1999)[87]	United States, North Carolina	6	181	67	HF: 1 vs. 11†
Ansari (2003)[31]	United States, California	6	169	70	CHF: 12% vs. 10% AC: 44% vs. 49%

*$P \leq 0.05$
†$P \leq 0.01$
Abbreviations: AC = all-cause; CHF = congestive heart failure; HF = heart failure; LOS = length of stay; PCP = primary care physician; pt = patient; VA = Veterans Affairs.

Home Visits

Recognizing that the best possible location to evaluate a heart failure patient is in the home, 7 randomized controlled trials evaluated the use of home visits in the care of heart failure patients (Table 40.3). Similar to the clinic-based heart failure disease management approaches, this concept utilizes an existing paradigm of current medical practice (home nursing) that has an existing reimbursement structure, making the adoption of this intervention more feasible for individual provider groups or health care organizations.

Similar to the clinic-based interventions, the home-visit-based interventions varied significantly in terms of structure and intensity. Although all of the interventions appear to involve a specialist's input in terms of design, the type of physician that the home nurse contacted for issues was a cardiologist in only two of the studies. In the other five studies, the PCP was contacted, which could either be a general internist or cardiologist. The number of home visits dictated by the protocol varied from 1 visit to as many as required. Most of the interventions also had telephone calls as part of the protocol. As expected, clinic visits were part of the

Table 40.3. *Randomized controlled trials using home visit follow-up*

Author (year)	Country	Follow-up (months)	Number of patients randomized	Mean age (years)	Readmissions/LOS (days) (intervention vs. control)
Rich (1995)[88]	United States, Missouri	3	282	79	AC: 53 vs. 94*; CHF: 24 vs. 54* ALOS: 10.5 vs. 9.2
Stewart (1998, 1999)[57,58]	Australia	0.25	97	75	AC unplanned: 36 vs. 63* / 64 vs. 125* ER visit: 48 vs. 87* / 2.5 vs. 4.5†
Stewart (1999)[89]	Australia	0.25–0.5	200	75	AC: 68 vs. 118*; HF: 34 vs. 58 ALOS: 6.8 vs. 9.9
Jaarsma (1999)[80]	Netherlands	0.375	186	73	AC: 37 vs. 50; CV: 29 vs. 39 AC day/pt: 9 vs. 9, *P* = NS
Hughes (2000)[79]	United States, VA centers	12 (average 6)	1966	70	AC: 3.6 vs. 2.0
Harrison (2001)[78]	Canada	0.5	192	76	AC % pt: 23% vs. 31%, *P* = NS ER % pt: 29% vs. 46%, *P* = 0.03
Blue (2001)[22]	Scotland	12	165	75	AC: 86 vs. 114*; CHF 19 vs. 45‡ Days/pt AC: 10 vs. 17; CHF: 3.4 vs. 7.6†

$^{*}P \leq 0.05$
$^{\dagger}P \leq 0.01$
$^{\ddagger}P \leq 0.001$
Abbreviations: AC = all-cause; ALOS = average length of stay; CHF = congestive heart failure; CV = cardiovascular; ER = emergency room; LOS = length of stay; NS = not significant; pt = patient; VA = Veterans Affairs.

intervention but most studies left the decision regarding the need for a clinic visit up to the discretion of the home nurse and supervising physician. Unfortunately, none of the studies provided information on the number of home visits, telephone calls, or clinic visits required during the study.

Unlike the clinic-based approach, home visits consistently decreased all-cause and heart failure-related hospitalizations (Table 40.3). In one intervention by Stewart *et al.*, a significant increase in survival was identified (RR, 0.72; 95% CI, 0.54–0.97; $P \leq 0.05$). For the studies reporting QOL outcomes, patients had significant improvement in heart failure-specific QOL scores but no significant change in general QOL scores (SF-36-Medical Outcome Study Short Form). Unfortunately, none of the studies reported medication changes.

Telephone Follow-Up

The limitation of clinic-based and home-visit-based programs as disease management interventions is the inability to easily expand these services to a large population of heart failure patients and to provide a consistent process of care to those patients. Telephone follow-up with a centralized call-in center addresses these issues, but with a few limitations (Table 40.4). The patient–physician relationship can be undermined or circumvented with telephone follow-up interventions. One study found that the lack of personal familiarization between the nurses who called the patients and the physicians involved in the direct care of the patients decreased the benefit of telephone follow-up intervention.[34] The investigators suggested that it was the ability of case managers to communicate easily with providers and the providers' trust in

Table 40.4. *Randomized controlled trials using telephone follow-up**

Author (year)	Country	Follow-up (months)	Number of patients randomized	Mean age (years)	Readmissions/LOS (days) (intervention vs. control)
Riegel (2002)[90]	United States, California	6	358	72	AC/pt: 0.62 vs. 0.87; HF/pt: 0.21 vs. 0.41† Day/pt AC: 3.5 vs. 4.8; HF: 1.1 vs. 2.1†
Krumholz (2002)[91]	United States, Connecticut	12	88	74	AC: 49 vs. 80; HF: 22 vs. 42 Day/pt AC: 10 vs. 15; HF: 4.1 vs. 7.6
Laramee (2003)[34]	United States, Vermont	3	287	70.7	AC: 70 vs. 61

*Data from the Naylor studies were not included due to lack of reporting specific to heart failure.[83,92]
†$P \leq 0.05$
Abbreviations: AC = all-cause; HF = heart failure; pt = patient.

familiar case managers that created a benefit when telephone follow-up was performed by local NPs, which would decrease the capability of such an intervention to expand to multiple centers.

Three published randomized controlled trials of heart failure disease management using primarily telephone follow-up have been published.[34–36] Although each of these studies were performed at only 1 or 2 sites, their designs are similar, which is consistent with the concept of expansion to multiple centers. Patients were called within 7 days of discharge and then weekly for some defined interval, with an increase in time between telephone calls taking place the longer the patients remained at home. The calls certainly identified issues requiring clinic visits but the number of visits was not reported by the studies. The study by Krumholz *et al.* mandated 2 clinic visits post-discharge.[37]

In the published studies, the impact of telephone follow-up on outcomes for heart failure patients remains unanswered. A significant decrease in all-cause and heart failure-related hospitalizations was found in two of the studies (n = 446, with a study follow-up of 6 and 12 months). In the study by Laramee *et al.* (n = 287, 3 months of follow-up time), there was a trend for worse outcomes.[34] None of the studies provide outcomes for QOL; and only the study by Laramee *et al.* provided results for medication use (ACE inhibitor use was 84% vs. 80%, intervention vs. control, P = not significant).

The Randomized Trial of Telephone Intervention in Chronic Heart Failure (DIAL) is the first large randomized controlled trial of telephone follow-up. The study randomized 1518 patients at 51 centers in Argentina.[38] Patients were required to be stable, in ambulatory care, and on optimal medical therapy for at least 2 months prior to enrollment. Patients with either normal LV function or decreased LV function (defined as an LVEF of less than 40%) were included in the study. Randomization was stratified by attending cardiologist; only cardiologists participated in the study.

The intervention involved a centralized calling center staffed by nurses trained in the management of heart failure patients. Nurses contacted intervention patients within 7 days of randomization. The calling center made all telephone calls; patients could not initiate telephone calls to the calling center. The protocol for the study set a minimum calling frequency of 1 call every 14 days for the first 4 calls. This could be modified at the discretion of the nursing staff. The calling center nurses used a questionnaire to track 5 goals of the treatment: (1) diet compliance; (2) drug compliance;

(3) monitoring of symptoms and early notification of provider; (4) control of volume symptoms (daily weight and edema); and (5) daily physical activity. In addition, the nurses reviewed a patient education manual which was provided to only the intervention patients. Answers to questions were collected using software and analyzed by the system to identify at-risk patients. Nurses contacted a patient's cardiologist as needed during the intervention.

The DIAL trial was completed in August 2002 and was presented at the American Heart Association Scientific Meetings in the fall of 2002. Over a 2-year follow-up period, the investigators found a significant reduction in the primary endpoint of all-cause mortality and heart failure admission (20% RR reduction, 26.3% vs. 31%; intervention vs. usual care, $P = 0.026$). There was no significant difference in all-cause mortality (15.3% vs. 16.1%, $P = 0.69$). The benefit seen in the primary endpoint was primarily due to a significant reduction in heart failure admissions (16.8% vs. 22.3%, $P = 0.005$). Unfortunately, the results of this study have yet to be published and no further information is available on secondary outcomes, including cardiovascular and all-cause hospitalizations, QOL, or cost.

Automated Telemonitoring

A number of companies have developed telemonitoring systems to collect patient biometrics (weight, blood pressure, blood oxygen saturation, and heart rate and rhythm) and, in some cases, answers to questions. These devices then send the collected data to a server where they can be reviewed by a provider. One study evaluated a system that included a video system that allowed providers and patients to see each other during visits.[39] A second study had patients input physiologic parameters using a computerized voice answering system.[40] A number of non-randomized studies have evaluated a number of different systems.[39–43] As expected, these non-controlled trials found a significant decrease in hospitalizations and cost, with improvements in patient QOL, understanding of disease state, and satisfaction with health care.

Eight-month data from the first large-scale randomized, prospective clinical trial, Trans-European Network Homecare Monitoring Study (TEN-HMS), was recently presented at the 2003 Heart Failure Society of America Scientific Sessions.[44] This study compared three treatment arms: usual care and telephone support with home telemonitoring (twice-daily home measurements of blood pressure, ECG device, and weight), usual care and telephone support alone (monthly calls by a nurse), and usual care. Physicians accessed the patient information via the internet. During the course of the trial, 428 heart failure patients with New York Heart Association (NYHA) class II to IV symptoms were randomized.

There was consistent improvement in the primary outcome (number of days lost to hospitalization or death) as the intensity of care increased from usual care to telephone contact to home telemonitoring (19.5% vs. 15.9% vs. 13.0%, respectively), with the only significant difference being between usual care and telemonitoring. When looking at the individual components of the primary outcomes, the benefit of home telemonitoring is less clear. The home telemonitoring significantly decreased the number of days lost due to death, which may be due to greater adherence to heart failure medical therapies (ACE inhibitors, beta-blockers, and spironolactone). However, the percentage of patient days lost due to hospitalization was less in the usual care group (4.1%) versus the telephone support alone group (6.3%) and the telephone support plus home monitoring group (4.9%). Based on the other randomized controlled trials of heart failure disease management in which a significant benefit was seen for hospitalizations, not for mortality, this outcome is difficult to explain. One would have expected twice-daily monitoring to detect episodes of decompensation earlier and avoid hospitalization.

Although the intent is to decrease provider burden, it remains unclear whether these systems achieve this goal or create more work in terms of following up on abnormal readings. In 1 study, 57 alerts were created for 27 patients; 22 of the alerts were for the wrong buttons being pushed.[43] Physicians were called for the 57 alerts and modified the clinical plan (medication change, unscheduled clinic visit, or hospitalization) for 21 cases.

Only 57% of the physicians found the information regarding patient status useful for the management of patients. A similar finding was detected by Heindenreich *et al.*[40] In this study, there were 294 physician notifications, of which only 13% resulted in a medication change within 3 days and only 10% resulted in an admission within 2 weeks. For every physician notification, 6 other computer-detected abnormalities required a nurse to contact the patient to determine that vital sign or symptom data were not accurately entered. The initial presentation of the TEN-HMS trial did not provide any insight regarding provider time and false alarms.[44]

Who Should Be In Charge? Cardiologists or Primary Care Providers

This is a critical question since the majority of heart failure patients in the United States are cared for by PCPs.[45–47] Given the expected increase in heart failure patients over the next 30 years and the current shortage of cardiologists, it is unlikely that a greater percentage of heart failure patients will be cared for by cardiologists.[48,49] It is for this reason that the results of studies like the DIAL trial must be viewed cautiously, since all the physicians being called by the call-in center were cardiologists. The application of this intervention in the United States using the current study design would miss a number of heart failure patients. If this intervention were expanded to include heart failure patients cared for by PCPs, the benefit seen in the original study might not be seen.

From the group of studies included in this review, it remains unclear which type of physician, cardiologist or PCP, should supervise heart failure disease management interventions. The outcomes for the post-discharge interventions depended on the type of provider providing supervision. Supervision by a cardiologist consistently provided a decrease in all-cause and heart failure hospitalizations. This was not the case when PCPs provided the supervision. Recognizing that only 2 studies included PCP supervision in a clinic setting, there are potential explanations for this finding in the literature.

Differences in the quality of care provided by specialists versus generalists have been identified. A number of studies have identified a significant difference in heart failure guideline adherence between cardiologists and non-cardiologists, including the use of heart failure medications and diagnostic testing.[45,50–52] One possible explanation is the greater experience that cardiologists have in a clinical practice with a higher percentage of heart failure patients. Although the majority of heart failure patients are cared for by PCPs, the experience of the PCPs is diluted by the other conditions that they see during their daily clinical activity.[46] This lack of experience has been identified as a significant predictor for outcomes in the treatment of patients experiencing myocardial infarctions (MIs) or unstable angina and for peri-procedural outcomes for patients undergoing angioplasty.[53] In addition, internists may lack some of the infrastructure cardiologists have to take care of heart failure patients, such as intravenous administration of diuretics in the clinic setting.

Despite the identified differences between cardiologists and non-cardiologists regarding heart failure patient care, the differences in outcomes have been reported primarily for survival—not hospitalization.[50] Recent studies using administrative databases have found survival benefit for heart failure patients treated by cardiologists.[45,46,50–52,54,55] The impact of cardiology care on readmission is less clear. A number of studies have found a significant decrease in readmissions for heart failure patients seen by a cardiologist.[46,50,56] However, in a study by Jong *et al.* using a Canadian administrative database, the benefit for the composite endpoint of death and readmission for heart failure was not statistically significant at 1 year for the cardiologists compared with general internists (54.7% vs. 55.4%, $P = 0.39$), although there were significant differences between cardiologists and family practitioners (54.7% vs. 58.1%, $P = 0.001$).[45]

Another possible reason for the lack of benefit by the PCP-supervised interventions is the lower intensity of follow-up in the studies using clinic follow-up with PCP supervision. All of the clinic-based interventions using a cardiologist included at least 2 visits, with some being extremely intensive. Both clinic-based interventions with PCP supervision only required 1 patient visit. Unfortunately, the correlation of intensity to outcome does not appear to hold up when evaluating disease management interventions using home visits. The studies by Stewart *et al.* found significant benefit in hospitalization rates and mortality by having only 1 home visit after being discharged from the hospital.[57–59]

Making any final conclusion regarding the supervision by PCPs should be withheld since only two studies were used in this category of heart failure disease management. Many of the studies with home visits or telephone follow-up had PCPs (along with cardiologists) as the main contact physician for the physician extenders performing the intervention. One potential difference regarding the non-clinic interventions versus the clinic interventions is that the initial training received by the physician extenders for the non-clinic based intervention included working with cardiologists.[22,34,60,61]

Who Should Be Enrolled in Heart Failure Disease Management Programs?

It is clear from the current randomized controlled trials of heart failure disease management that a wide variety of patients benefit from participating in disease management interventions. Due to the entry criteria of a heart failure hospitalization, many of the patients had a normal LVEF. In addition, the increased average age of 70.6 years in the randomized controlled trials of heart failure disease management reflects the true epidemiology of heart failure. Consistent with this increased age is the higher percentage of women participating in these trials (40.2%).

It is important to recognize that patients participating in the randomized controlled trials of disease management are not like the patients randomized in recent therapeutic clinical trials.[62] As was true in the National Heart Failure Project database used by Masoudi *et al.*, the mean age, percentage of female patients (excluding studies performed within the Veterans Administration Health System) and percentage of minority patients (for studies performed in the United States and Australia) are all greater than those found in clinical trials. Since a number of disease management studies enrolled heart failure patients with preserved LV function, the mean EF is higher in this group of patients. ACE inhibitor and beta-blocker use, when reported, are significantly less than expected when compared to percentages in recent clinical trials. This is possibly due to the difference in patient characteristics versus pharmacological randomized controlled trials enrolling heart failure patients.[63]

Economic Impact of Disease Management

Although heart failure disease management improves the quality of care and decreases hospitalization for heart failure patients (the primary driver of cost for heart failure care) in a number of studies, the impact on cost is less certain.[1,64] Although many of the randomized controlled trials of heart failure disease management provided personnel costs, few included cost estimates for patient medications (increased utilization of medications), patient time, additional clinic visits potentially generated by the intervention, patient materials, and personnel training. One study of telephone follow-up estimated that training involved 95 hours of personnel time.[65] At $26.51 per hour, training cost $2518 per case manager. In addition, the increased surveillance of patients by interventions identifies a number of issues that may have gone undetected and subsequently increase physician time. One economic model of heart failure disease management based in the United Kingdom, which attempted to account for the cost of the intervention, changes in pharmacotherapy, and increases in clinic visits, estimated that £49 000 per year could be generated for each heart failure nurse hired to provide a heart failure disease management intervention.[66]

Although many providers and health care systems would like to offer disease management services to heart failure patients, current reimbursement can create a disincentive to provide disease management interventions.[67] The lack of reimbursement has been identified as a significant reason for the limited the use of disease management by providers.[68] Gaining the ability to reimburse for disease management services will be difficult based on the current randomized controlled trials. The diversity of interventions will not allow payers to easily define which services they will cover and at what intensity. The differences between patients enrolled in disease management interventions and clinical trials make it difficult to identify appropriate clinical benchmarks to declare an intervention successful. The Centers of Medicare and Medicaid Services (CMS) have decided to use historical benchmarks of expenditures in the CMS Heart Failure Disease Management Demonstration Projects as a mechanism to reimburse for services. Unfortunately, the study design of demonstration projects shifts the financial risk of providing care from CMS to the organizations delivering the disease management services.

Conclusion

Underlying all the different approaches to heart failure disease management is the general concept that providing increased access to health care providers for an at-risk group of heart failure patients will improve outcomes. In the majority of studies, this rings true; heart failure disease management improves clinical outcomes. The real questions are: can this concept be implemented beyond a single center; and how much will it cost patients, their providers, health care systems, and payers? Certainly, recent studies in Argentina and Europe suggest that large-scale disease management interventions can be implemented, at least within a research study design. If the initial randomized controlled trial results can be replicated in community practice, certainly patients and third-party payers will benefit from a reduction in hospitalizations. Less clear is the impact on providers and health care systems that lose significant revenues, from decreased hospitalizations, by providing services without reimbursement. There is a clear need to prove the concept of heart failure disease management in a large-scale clinical trial based in the United States in which patients are randomized to usual care and various disease management interventions.

Acknowledgment

Reprinted with permission from *Cardiology in Review*.[93]

References

1. American Heart Association. Heart Disease and Stroke Statistics—2002 Update. (American Heart Association: Dallas, TX, 2001).
2. Haldeman GA, Croft JB, Giles WH, *et al.* Hospitalization of patients with heart failure: National Hospital Discharge Survey, 1985 to 1995. Am Heart J 1999; 137: 352–360.
3. Hunt SA, Baker DW, Chin MH, *et al.* ACC/AHA guidelines for the evaluation and management of chronic heart failure in the adult: executive summary. A report of the American College of Cardiology/American Heart Association Task Force on Practice Guidelines (Committee to revise the 1995 Guidelines for the Evaluation and Management of Heart Failure). J Am Coll Cardiol 2001; 38: 2101–2113.
4. Committee on Quality Health Care in America, Institute of Medicine. Crossing the Quality Chasm: A New Health System for the 21st Century (National Academy Press: Washington, DC, 2001).
5. Rich MW, Beckham V, Wittenberg C, *et al.* A multidisciplinary intervention to prevent the readmission of elderly patients with congestive heart failure. N Engl J Med 1995; 333: 1190–1195.
6. McAlister FA, Lawson FM, Teo KK, *et al.* A systematic review of randomized trials of disease management programs in heart failure. Am J Med 2001; 110: 378–384.
7. Cintron G, Bigas C, Linares E, *et al.* Nurse practitioner role in a chronic congestive heart failure clinic: in-hospital time, costs, and patient satisfaction. Heart & Lung 1983; 12: 237–240.
8. Kornowski R, Zeeli D, Averbuch M, *et al.* Intensive home-care surveillance prevents hospitalization and improves morbidity rates among elderly patients with severe congestive heart failure. Am Heart J 1995; 129: 762–766.
9. Lasater M. The effect of a nurse-managed CHF clinic on patient readmission and length of stay. Home Healthc Nurse 1996; 14: 351–356.
10. West JA, Miller NH, Parker KM, *et al.* A comprehensive management system for heart failure improves clinical outcomes and reduces medical resource utilization. Am J Cardiol 1997; 79: 58–63.

11. Fonarow GC, Stevenson LW, Walden JA, *et al.* Impact of a comprehensive heart failure management program on hospital readmission and functional status of patients with advanced heart failure. J Am Coll Cardiol 1997; 30: 725–732.
12. Hanumanthu S, Butler J, Chomsky D, *et al.* Effect of a heart failure program on hospitalization frequency and exercise tolerance. Circulation 1997; 96: 2842–2848.
13. Smith L, Fabbri S, Pai R, *et al.* Symptomatic improvement and reduced hospitalization for patients attending a cardiomyopathy clinic. Clin Cardiol 1997; 20: 949–954.
14. Shah NB, Der E, Ruggerio C, *et al.* Prevention of hospitalizations for heart failure with an interactive home monitoring program. Am Heart J 1998; 135: 373–378.
15. Dennis L, Blue C, Stahl S, *et al.* The relationship between hospital readmissions of medicare beneficiaries with chronic illnesses and home care nursing interventions. Home Healthc Nurse 1996; 14: 303–309.
16. Martens K, Mellor S. A study of the relationship between home care services and hospital readmission of patients with congestive heart failure. Home Healthc Nurse 1997; 15: 123–129.
17. Whellan DJ, Gaulden L, Gattis WA, *et al.* The benefit of implementing a heart failure disease management program. Arch Intern Med 2001; 161: 2223–2228.
18. Whellan DJ, Cohen EJ, Matchar DB, *et al.* Disease management in healthcare organizations: results of in-depth interviews with disease management decision makers. Am J Manag Care 2002; 8: 633–641.
19. Grady KL, Dracup K, Kennedy G, *et al.* Team management of patients with heart failure: A statement for healthcare professionals from The Cardiovascular Nursing Council of the American Heart Association. Circulation 2000; 102: 2443–2456.
20. Krumholz HM, Parent EM, Tu N, *et al.* Readmission after hospitalization for congestive heart failure among Medicare beneficiaries. Arch Intern Med 1997; 157: 99–104.
21. McDonald K, Ledwidge M, Cahill J, *et al.* Heart failure management: multidisciplinary care has intrinsic benefit above the optimization of medical care. J Card Fail 2002; 8: 142–148.
22. Blue L, Lang E, McMurray JJ, *et al.* Randomised controlled trial of specialist nurse intervention in heart failure. BMJ 2001; 323: 715–718.
23. Naylor M, Brooten D, Jones R, *et al.* Comprehensive discharge planning for the hospitalized elderly: a randomized clinical trial. Ann Intern Med 1994; 120: 999–1006.
24. Costantini O, Huck K, Carlson MD, *et al.* Impact of a guideline-based disease management team on outcomes of hospitalized patients with congestive heart failure. Arch Intern Med 2001; 161: 177–182.
25. Gattis WA, O'Connor CM, Gallup DS, *et al.* Predischarge initiation of carvedilol in patients hospitalized for decompensated heart failure: results of the IMPACT-HF (Initiation Management Pre-discharge: process for Assessment of Carvedilol Therapy in Heart Failure) trial. J Am Coll Cardiol 2004. In press.
26. Colucci WS, Packer M, Bristow MR, *et al.* Carvedilol inhibits clinical progression in patients with mild symptoms of heart failure. U.S. Carvedilol Heart Failure Study Group. Circulation 1996; 94: 2800–2806.
27. Krum H, Roecker EB, Mohacsi P, *et al.* Effects of initiating carvedilol in patients with severe chronic heart failure: results from the COPERNICUS Study. JAMA 2003; 289: 712–718.
28. Poole-Wilson PA, Swedberg K, Clelandsa JG, *et al.* Comparison of carvedilol and metoprolol on clinical outcomes in patients with chronic heart failure in the Carvedilol Or Metoprolol European Trial (COMET): randomised controlled trial. Lancet 2003; 362: 7–13.
29. McDonald K, Ledwidge M. Heart failure management programs: can we afford to ignore the inpatient phase of care? J Card Fail 2003; 9: 258–262.
30. Ekman I, Andersson B, Ehnfors M, *et al.* Feasibility of a nurse-monitored, outpatient-care programme for elderly patients with moderate-to-severe, chronic heart failure. Eur Heart J 1998; 19: 1254–1260.
31. Ansari M, Shlipak MG, Heidenreich PA, *et al.* Improving guideline adherence: a randomized trial evaluating strategies to increase beta-blocker use in heart failure. Circulation 2003; 107: 2799–2804.
32. Gattis WA, Hasselblad V, Whellan DJ, *et al.* Reduction in heart failure events by the addition of a clinical pharmacist to the heart failure management team: results of the Pharmacist in Heart Failure Assessment Recommendation and Monitoring (PHARM) Study. Arch Intern Med 1999; 159: 1939–1945.
33. Gattis WA, Hasselblad V, Whellan DJ, *et al.* Reduction in heart failure events by the addition of a clinical pharmacist to the heart failure management team: results of the Pharmacist in Heart Failure Assessment Recommendation and Monitoring (PHARM) Study. Arch Intern Med 1999; 159: 1939–1945.
34. Laramee AS, Levinsky SK, Sargent J, *et al.* Case management in a heterogeneous congestive heart failure population: a randomized controlled trial. Arch Intern Med 2003; 163: 809–817.

35. Riegel B, Carlson B, Kopp Z, *et al.* Effect of a standardized nurse case-management telephone intervention on resource use in patients with chronic heart failure. Arch Intern Med 2002; 162: 705–712.
36. Krumholz HM, Amatruda J, Smith GL, *et al.* Randomized trial of an education and support intervention to prevent readmission of patients with heart failure. J Am Coll Cardiol 2002; 39: 83–89.
37. Krumholz HM, Amatruda J, Smith GL, *et al.* Randomized trial of an education and support intervention to prevent readmission of patients with heart failure. J Am Coll Cardiol 2002; 39: 83–89.
38. Grancelli H, Varini S, Ferrante D, *et al.* Randomized Trial of Telephone Intervention in Chronic Heart Failure (DIAL): study design and preliminary observations. J Card Fail 2003; 9: 172–179.
39. Johnston B, Wheeler L, Deuser J, *et al.* Outcomes of the Kaiser Permanente Tele-Home Health Research Project. Arch Fam Med 2000; 9: 40–45.
40. Heidenreich PA, Ruggerio CM, Massie BM. Effect of a home monitoring system on hospitalization and resource use for patients with heart failure. Am Heart J 1999; 138: 633–640.
41. Baer CA, DiSalvo TG, Cail MI, *et al.* Electronic home monitoring of congestive heart failure patients: design and feasibility. Congest Heart Fail 1999; 5: 105–113.
42. Mehra MR, Uber PA, Chomsky DB, *et al.* Emergence of electronic home monitoring in chronic heart failure: rationale, feasibility, and early results with the HomMed Sentry-Observer system. Congest Heart Fail 2000; 6: 137–139.
43. Nanevicz T, Piette J, Zipkin D, *et al.* The feasibility of a telecommunications service in support of outpatient congestive heart failure care in a diverse patient population. Congest Heart Fail 2000; 6: 140–145.
44. Cleland, JG. TEN-HMS: Telemonitoring cost-effective in light of reductions in days lost to hospitalizations and death. Heart Wire. Available at: http://www.heartwire.org. Accessed March 17, 2004.
45. Jong P, Gong Y, Liu PP, *et al.* Care and outcomes of patients newly hospitalized for heart failure in the community treated by cardiologists compared with other specialists. Circulation 2003; 108: 184–191.
46. Indridason OS, Coffman CJ, Oddone EZ. Is specialty care associated with improved survival of patients with congestive heart failure? Am Heart J 2003; 145: 300–309.
47. Cleland JG, Cohen-Solal A, Aguilar JC, *et al.* Management of heart failure in primary care (the IMPROVEMENT of Heart Failure Programme): an international survey. Lancet 2002; 360: 1631–1639.
48. Rich MW. Epidemiology, pathophysiology, and etiology of congestive heart failure in older adults. J Am Geriatr Soc 1997; 45: 968–974.
49. Fye WB. Cardiology workforce: there's already a shortage, and it's getting worse! J Am Coll Cardiol 2002; 39: 2077–2079.
50. Reis SE, Holubkov R, Edmundowicz D, *et al.* Treatment of patients admitted to the hospital with congestive heart failure: specialty-related disparities in practice patterns and outcomes. J Am Coll Cardiol 1997; 30: 733–738.
51. Chin MH, Wang JC, Zhang JX, *et al.* Utilization and dosing of angiotensin-converting enzyme inhibitors for heart failure. Effect of physician specialty and patient characteristics. J Gen Intern Med 1997; 12: 563–566.
52. Stafford RS, Saglam D, Blumenthal D. National patterns of angiotensin-converting enzyme inhibitor use in congestive heart failure. Arch Intern Med 1997; 157: 2460–2464.
53. Jollis JG, Peterson ED, Nelson CL, *et al.* Relationship between physician and hospital coronary angioplasty volume and outcome in elderly patients. Circulation 1997; 95: 2485–2491.
54. Jollis JG, Peterson ED, Nelson CL, *et al.* Relationship between physician and hospital coronary angioplasty volume and outcome in elderly patients. Circulation 1997; 95: 2485–2491.
55. Auerbach AD, Hamel MB, Davis RB, *et al.* Resource use and survival of patients hospitalized with congestive heart failure: differences in care by specialty of the attending physician. SUPPORT Investigators. Study to Understand Prognoses and Preferences for Outcomes and Risks of Treatments. Ann Intern Med 2000; 132: 191–200.
56. Philbin EF, Jenkins PL. Differences between patients with heart failure treated by cardiologists, internists, family physicians, and other physicians: analysis of a large, statewide database. Am Heart J 2000; 139: 491–496.
57. Stewart S, Pearson S, Horowitz JD. Effects of a home-based intervention among patients with congestive heart failure discharged from acute hospital care. Arch Intern Med 1998; 158: 1067–1072.
58. Stewart S, Vandenbroek AJ, Pearson S, *et al.* Prolonged beneficial effects of a home-based intervention on unplanned readmissions and mortality among patients with congestive heart failure. Arch Intern Med 1999; 159: 257–261.
59. Stewart S, Marley JE, Horowitz JD. Effects of a multidisciplinary, home-based intervention on unplanned readmissions and survival among patients with chronic congestive heart failure: a randomised controlled study. Lancet 1999; 354: 1077–1083.

60. Rich MW, Beckham V, Wittenberg C, *et al.* A multidisciplinary intervention to prevent the readmission of elderly patients with congestive heart failure. N Engl J Med 1995; 333: 1190–1195.
61. Krumholz HM, Amatruda J, Smith GL, *et al.* Randomized trial of an education and support intervention to prevent readmission of patients with heart failure. J Am Coll Cardiol 2002; 39: 83–89.
62. Masoudi FA, Havranek EP, Wolfe P, *et al.* Most hospitalized older persons do not meet the enrollment criteria for clinical trials in heart failure. Am Heart J 2003; 146: 250–257.
63. Abraham WT, Fisher WG, Smith AL, *et al.* Cardiac resynchronization in chronic heart failure. N Engl J Med 2002; 346: 1845–1853.
64. O'Connell JB. The economic burden of heart failure. Clin Cardiol 2000; 23: III6–III10.
65. Riegel B, Carlson B, Kopp Z, *et al.* Effect of a standardized nurse case-management telephone intervention on resource use in patients with chronic heart failure. Arch Intern Med 2002; 162: 705–712.
66. Stewart S, Horowitz JD. Specialist nurse management programmes: economic benefits in the management of heart failure. Pharmacoeconomics 2003; 21: 225–240.
67. Havranek EP, Krumholz HM, Dudley RA, *et al.* Aligning quality and payment for heart failure care: defining the challenges. J Card Fail 2003; 9: 251–254.
68. Casalino L, Gillies RR, Shortell SM, *et al.* External incentives, information technology, and organized processes to improve health care quality for patients with chronic diseases. JAMA 2003; 289: 434–441.
69. Cline CM, Israelsson BY, Willenheimer RB, *et al.* Cost effective management programme for heart failure reduces hospitalisation. Heart 1998; 80: 442–446.
70. Doughty RN, Wright SP, Pearl A, *et al.* Randomized, controlled trial of integrated heart failure management: The Auckland Heart Failure Management Study. Eur Heart J 2002; 23: 139–146.
71. Kasper EK, Gerstenblith G, Hefter G, *et al.* A randomized trial of the efficacy of multidisciplinary care in heart failure outpatients at high risk of hospital readmission. J Am Coll Cardiol 2002; 39: 471–480.
72. Capomolla S, Febo O, Ceresa M, *et al.* Cost/utility ratio in chronic heart failure: comparison between heart failure management program delivered by day-hospital and usual care. J Am Coll Cardiol 2002; 40: 1259–1266.
73. Gattis WA, Hasselblad V, Whellan DJ, *et al.* Reduction in heart failure events by the addition of a clinical pharmacist to the heart failure management team: results of the Pharmacist in Heart Failure Assessment Recommendation and Monitoring (PHARM) Study. Arch Intern Med 1999; 159: 1939–1945.
74. Weinberger M, Oddone EZ, Henderson WG. Does increased access to primary care reduce hospital readmissions? Veterans Affairs Cooperative Study Group on Primary Care and Hospital Readmission. N Engl J Med 1996; 334: 1441–1447.
75. Oddone EZ, Weinberger M, Giobbie-Hurder A, *et al.* Enhanced access to primary care for patients with congestive heart failure. Veterans Affairs Cooperative Study Group on Primary Care and Hospital Readmission. Eff Clin Pract 1999; 2: 201–209.
76. Rich MW, Beckham V, Wittenberg C, *et al.* A multidisciplinary intervention to prevent the readmission of elderly patients with congestive heart failure. N Engl J Med 1995; 333: 1190–1195.
77. Stewart S, Marley JE, Horowitz JD. Effects of a multidisciplinary, home-based intervention on unplanned readmissions and survival among patients with chronic congestive heart failure: a randomised controlled study. Lancet 1999; 354: 1077–1083.
78. Harrison MB, Browne GB, Roberts J, *et al.* Quality of life of individuals with heart failure: a randomized trial of the effectiveness of two models of hospital-to-home transition. Med Care 2002; 40: 271–282.
79. Hughes SL, Weaver FM, Giobbie-Hurder A, *et al.* Effectiveness of team-managed home-based primary care: a randomized multicenter trial. JAMA 2000; 284: 2877–2885.
80. Jaarsma T, Halfens R, Huijer Abu-Saad H, *et al.* Effects of education and support on self-care and resource utilization in patients with heart failure. Eur Heart J 1999; 20: 673–682.
81. Krumholz HM, Amatruda J, Smith GL, *et al.* Randomized trial of an education and support intervention to prevent readmission of patients with heart failure. J Am Coll Cardiol 2002; 39: 83–89.
82. Naylor M, Brooten D, Jones R, *et al.* Comprehensive discharge planning for the hospitalized elderly. A randomized clinical trial. Ann Intern Med 1994; 120: 999–1006.
83. Naylor MD, Brooten D, Campbell R, *et al.* Comprehensive discharge planning and home follow-up of hospitalized elders: a randomized clinical trial. JAMA 1999; 281: 613–620.
84. Riegel B, Carlson B, Kopp Z, *et al.* Effect of a standardized nurse case-management telephone intervention on resource use in patients with chronic heart failure. Arch Intern Med 2002; 162: 705–712.
85. Cline CM, Israelsson BY, Willenheimer RB, *et al.* Cost effective management programme for heart failure reduces hospitalisation. Heart 1998; 80: 442–446.

86. Weinberger M, Oddone EZ, Henderson WG. Does increased access to primary care reduce hospital readmissions? Veterans Affairs Cooperative Study Group on Primary Care and Hospital Readmission. N Engl J Med 1996; 334: 1441–1447.
87. Gattis WA, Hasselblad V, Whellan DJ, *et al.* Reduction in heart failure events by the addition of a clinical pharmacist to the heart failure management team: results of the Pharmacist in Heart Failure Assessment Recommendation and Monitoring (PHARM) Study. Arch Intern Med 1999; 159: 1939–1945.
88. Rich MW, Beckham V, Wittenberg C, *et al.* A multidisciplinary intervention to prevent the readmission of elderly patients with congestive heart failure. N Engl J Med 1995; 333: 1190–1195.
89. Stewart S, Marley JE, Horowitz JD. Effects of a multidisciplinary, home-based intervention on unplanned readmissions and survival among patients with chronic congestive heart failure: a randomised controlled study. Lancet 1999; 354: 1077–1083.
90. Riegel B, Carlson B, Kopp Z, *et al.* Effect of a standardized nurse case-management telephone intervention on resource use in patients with chronic heart failure. Arch Intern Med 2002; 162: 705–712.
91. Krumholz HM, Amatruda J, Smith GL, *et al.* Randomized trial of an education and support intervention to prevent readmission of patients with heart failure. J Am Coll Cardiol 2002; 39: 83–89.
92. Naylor M, Brooten D, Jones R, *et al.* Comprehensive discharge planning for the hospitalized elderly. A randomized clinical trial. Ann Intern Med 1994; 120: 999–1006.
93. Whellan DJ. Heart failure disease management: implementation and outcomes. Cardiol Rev 2005; 13: 1–9.

CHAPTER 41

End-of-life care in the acute heart failure patient

Cheryl H Zambroski, Lynn P Roser, Debra K Moser

Introduction

Despite recent data suggesting that heart failure is more malignant than many common types of cancer,[1] the most ignored aspect of heart failure management is end-of-life care. Over 250 000 people in the United States die prematurely each year as a result of heart failure.[2] Across all classes of heart failure, approximately 20% of individuals die within 1 year of diagnosis.[1] The yearly incidence of death is higher in patients with the most advanced heart failure and may near 50% in that subgroup. Patients experiencing an episode of acute decompensated heart failure (ADHF) are at increased risk for death during and in the aftermath of such an episode. Nonetheless, patients with heart failure and their families rarely receive assistance from their physicians and nurses regarding end-of-life issues. The purpose of this chapter is to provide clinicians with the background and information needed to help them address end-of-life care in their patients with heart failure.

What is End-of-life Care for Patients with Heart Failure?

A major problem impeding clinicians' ability to provide appropriate end-of-life care is a lack of understanding about what is meant by end-of-life care. For many clinicians, end-of-life care means giving up hope and abandoning usual care. However, end-of-life care refers to care that is delivered in order to provide symptom relief, comfort, and support for patients and their families as they cope with managing an illness when optimal treatments have failed to halt progression of the illness or relieve symptoms. End-of-life care is recommended when the likelihood is thought to be high that death is imminent within the coming weeks to months. For patients with heart failure, optimal care, particularly drug therapy, is not necessarily discontinued. The major component of appropriate end-of-life care is palliative care.

Palliative care refers to holistic care processes in which the primary goal is improving the quality of life of patients facing a life-threatening illness, and their families, through the relief of suffering and provision of comfort.[3] It is an interdisciplinary approach aimed at the treatment of pain and other physical, psychosocial, and spiritual symptoms or problems, as well as support for the patient and family at the end of life. The goals of palliative care are to improve quality of life, promote psychological and spiritual well-being, improve symptom management, and support family members. The World Health Organization indicates that palliative care is appropriate early in the course of an illness in conjunction with therapies that may be intended to prolong a patient's life. Palliative care is viewed as total care of a person's mind, body, and spirit, wherein all physical, social, emotional, and spiritual needs are addressed.

The concept of palliative care has continued to evolve and the practice of palliative care has been extended to provide comfort and increased quality of life in terminal disease, as well as in non-terminal disease.[4,5] Palliative care should be used to control symptoms and provide psychological support of both patients and families in conjunction with life-prolonging and curative efforts, and should not be limited to cancer patients.[6] Reasonable efforts should be made to prolong life until death is imminent, and then those efforts may also continue at the same time that palliative care is provided. Above all, while palliative care openly acknowledges death, it should not be characterized by less care or withdrawal of care in the face of death.[4,7] Palliative care experts advocate for the use of both curative and palliative therapies in conditions such as heart failure, and they suggest the use of palliative care earlier in the course of chronic illnesses that are likely to result in premature death.[8,9]

Placing End-of-life Care in the Context of Optimal Heart Failure Management

With optimal medical management, quality of life and survival may be increased for many patients with heart failure. Patients can remain symptomatic with poor functional status and may be labeled, inappropriately, as end-stage when evidence-based and guideline-driven pharmacologic and non-pharmacologic therapies are not delivered. Any decision to institute end-of-life care should only be made after consideration of a number of factors, including assurance that therapy has been optimized appropriately (Table 41.1). Despite evidence that heart failure disease management improves patient outcomes substantially compared to usual care, most patients do not receive care using these superior models of care and thus do not have access to optimal management strategies.[10] It is critical for clinicians to realize that institution of end-of-life care does not necessitate discontinuation of heart failure therapies. Symptom management strategies include the use of appropriate heart failure medications and thus these medications should be continued to maintain the patient's quality of life.

Candidates for End-of-life Care

Patients with acute heart failure (AHF) are considered potential candidates for end-of-life care when they have advanced heart failure with persistent, refractory symptoms at rest and remain classified as New York Heart Association (NYHA) functional class III or IV despite optimal medical therapy (Table 41.1). Such patients usually have a history of frequent (three or more per year) hospitalizations for ADHF, rate their quality of life as

Table 41.1. *Issues to be addressed prior to instituting end-of-life care for patients with heart failure*

Patient referred to clinician with expertise in the management of heart failure
Optimal pharmacological and nonpharmacologic therapy attempted for sufficient time to see benefit
Reversible causes of heart failure and heart failure exacerbation identified and treated
Psychological problems, such as depression, treated
Social support enhanced
Reasons for persistent non-adherence determined and addressed, if possible
Adequate patient and family or caregiver education and counseling delivered
Patient and family wishes identified and respected

With permission[17]

poor, are unable to accomplish activities of daily living, or require intermittent or continuous intravenous support to maintain an acceptable quality of life.

Why End-of-life Care Needs Greater Attention from Clinicians: Symptom Burden

There is limited research available in the area of end-of-life care and the needs of patients with heart failure. What is known is that for most patients heart failure is a progressive condition that results in premature death. The course of heart failure is often marked by periods of decompensation with acute exacerbations of symptoms, and poor quality of life.[11] While researchers have made marked advances in management, in the end stages of heart failure, patients often suffer from poor quality of life and a constellation of distressing symptoms including dyspnea, pain, fatigue, anxiety, and depression.[12,13] Families report that patients with heart failure are either "extremely ill" or "very ill" during their last days of life.[14] Yet, specific care directed at relieving physical and psychological symptoms and their associated distress in patients with advanced, refractory heart failure has received little attention from researchers, is ill-defined, and rarely implemented systematically.

Symptom burden at the end of life

A major goal of end-of-life care is relief of unnecessary suffering by decreasing the physical and emotional symptoms associated with a life-threatening illness. In fact, relief of symptoms is the foundational cornerstone on which appropriate end-of-life care models are built. Inadequate symptom relief is distressing to patients, and adversely affects quality of life, as well as the ability of patients to complete life closure tasks at the end of their life.[15] Despite knowledge of the importance of symptom relief among patients with advanced heart failure, little data exist that adequately describe symptom prevalence and severity among patients dying from this condition.

Symptom burden is the accumulation of physical and emotional sensations perceived by patients as causing undue distress. Most of the research related to symptom burden among patients dying from cardiac disease or advanced heart failure come from two large-scale, multicenter studies completed in the early to mid-1990s—the Regional Study of Care for the Dying (RSCD)[16] and the Study to Understand Prognoses and Preferences for Outcomes and Risks of Treatment (SUPPORT).[12]

McCarthy *et al.* reviewed data from the RSCD, a regional population-based survey that consisted of interviews with family members of 600 people who died of heart disease.[16] The focus of these interviews was the last year of the patient's life. The most commonly reported symptoms during the 12 months prior to death were pain (78%), dyspnea (61%), low mood (59%), sleeplessness (45%), and anxiety (30%). Additional symptoms included loss of appetite (43%), constipation (37%), nausea and vomiting (32%), urinary incontinence (29%), and confusion (40%). The family rated pain, dyspnea, low mood, anxiety, urinary incontinence, and confusion as being the most distressing to patients in the last year of their life. Over half of the patients died in the hospital. Additionally, pain and symptom management in the hospital was considered to be poor overall, with little or no relief in as many as 24% to 36% of the patients.

Data from the SUPPORT study was used to describe the last 6 months of life for patients admitted for AHF and considered to be end-stage.[12] The heart failure cohort in SUPPORT consisted of 539 patients who died within 12 months of entry into the study. Data were collected by interviews with patients and their identified surrogates on numerous variables, including symptoms and quality of life, during various points in time up to 6 months prior to death. Although patient interviews were the preferred source of information, all data about the patient's last 3 days of life were obtained after death using interviews with identified surrogates. The three most commonly-reported symptoms were dyspnea, pain, and confusion. Although the minority of patients experienced severe pain or dyspnea during the last 6 months of life, the percentage of patients experiencing increasing rates of severe dyspnea and pain increased significantly as death approached. In the last 3 days of life, 63% of all heart failure patients experienced severe dyspnea. In the last week of life, 70% of patients rated their quality of life as poor to fair. Additionally, increases in emotional symptoms such as anxiety and depression were reported during the last 3 days prior to death.

A subsequent retrospective study demonstrated similar findings.[7] Analysis of medical records of 80 patients diagnosed with heart failure revealed that the most common symptoms experienced in the last 6 months of life were breathlessness (88%), followed by pain (75%), and fatigue (69%). Patients also suffered from anxiety, sleeplessness, nausea, edema, and constipation. In fact, on average, each patient reported 6.7 symptoms. At least 25% of the patients who reported pain did not receive any treatment for it, regardless of origin, and over 67.5% of the patients died in the hospital. The investigators concluded that end-stage heart failure patients experience similar symptoms to end-stage cancer patients. However, unlike cancer patients who have access to palliative care services, heart failure patients are frequently excluded from these services and must seek emergency care to receive treatment when the symptoms become severe.

Symptoms during the last seven days of life

Because there have been no studies to date concentrating on the last week of life for patients dying of heart failure, we conducted a study of all patients who died from heart failure and who were enrolled in a regional hospice service over an 18-month period.[17] Although less than 5% of all heart failure patients are referred for hospice care, we chose to study this group of patients because they provide one of the few opportunities for systematically examining the end of life in heart failure. The purposes of this study were to: (1) describe the characteristics of patients with heart failure who died while receiving hospice care; (2) identify symptoms most commonly reported by patients with heart failure in hospice during the last 7 days of life; and (3) identify interventions used by hospice nurses to manage the symptoms of patients with heart failure who died while receiving hospice care.

A total of 90 records of patients were included in the study (Table 41.2). These heart failure patients were referred for hospice care and received it (as is usual for hospice patients) in a variety of environments. Upon referral, patients received hospice care in their own homes (42%), long-term care facilities (31%), or inpatient hospice units (21%). Patients in these 3 groups did not differ in age, gender, marital status, ethnicity, ejection fraction (EF), comorbidities, heart failure etiology, admission medications, or heart failure symptoms experienced. They did differ in primary caregiver and functional status. Patients without a primary caregiver more commonly received hospice care in a long-term care facility than those with a close relation as a primary caregiver ($P = 0.001$). Functional status for patients referred to the inpatient hospice care unit (mean Palliative Performance Scale [PPS] $= 21 \pm 8$) was worse than that of patients receiving hospice care either at home (mean PPS $= 35 \pm 9$) or in long-term care (mean PPS $= 34 \pm 11$, $P = 0.001$) (see Table 41.2 for an explanation of PPS ratings).

Patients received hospice care (from admission to death) for an average of 37 ± 56 days. This number was skewed by the 25% of patients who received hospice care for longer than 2 months, although only 3 individuals received hospice care for longer than 6 months. The median time receiving hospice care was 10 days (25th percentile = 3 days; 75th percentile = 58 days).

With regard to symptom status, the mean functional status score by PPS on admission was 32 ± 11, indicating that patients had markedly decreased functional status characterized by remaining mostly in bed to being totally bedbound. The highest individual PPS score on referral to hospice care was 50, while the lowest was 10 (indicating a moribund state). Functional status score declined substantially from admission (32 ± 11) to day of death (22 ± 12, $P = 0.001$).

Upon admission for hospice care, 75% of patients reported no pain while 3% reported chest pain and 20% reported other pain (no documentation was available for this symptom in the remaining 2%). The primary symptoms documented during the last week of life included shortness of breath (60%), edema (43%), incontinence of bowel or bladder (37%), and confusion at least

Table 41.2. *Characteristics of with heart failure dying while receiving hospice care*

Characteristic	Number of patients (%) (n = 90)
Age, yr (mean ± SD)	81 ± 8 (range 54-96)
Female	54 (60)
Race	
Caucasian	74 (84)
African American	11 (12)
Other	1 (4)
Marital status	
Widowed	51 (57)
Married	30 (33)
Single/divorced/separated	9 (10)
Living with another person	
Yes	46 (51)
No	25 (28)
Long-term care	19 (21)
Primary caregiver	
Spouse	25 (28)
Other	22 (24)
Daughter	17 (19)
None	17 (19)
Son	8 (9)
Friend	1 (1)
Heart failure etiology	
Ischemic	42 (55)
Unspecified	24 (31)
Hypertension	8 (10)
Valvular	2 (3)
Idiopathic	1 (1)
Ejection fraction, % (mean ± SD)	25 ± 13 (range 10-65)
Charlson Comorbidity Index (mean ± SD)	10 ± 2 (range 4-14)
PPS* (mean ± SD)	32 ± 11 (range, 10-50)
Medications prescribed for heart failure on admission to hospice	
Diuretics	61 (68)
Nitrates	44 (49)
Digoxin	29 (32)
ACE inhibitors	22 (24)
Beta-blockers	18 (20)
Warfarin	18 (20)
Hydralazine	10 (11)

*Higher PPS ratings = greater functional status; theoretical range 0-100, 0 = dead, 100 = fully functional.
Abbreviations: ACE = angiotensin-converting enzyme; PPS = Palliative Performance Scale; SD = standard deviation.

some of the time (48%). Of note, 9% of patients were reported to be "actively dying" on admission for hospice care. The average length of stay for those patients was 1 day with a maximum of 2 days. Hospice nurses used the term "actively dying" to indicate symptoms such as decreased level of consciousness, labored and irregular breath sounds, pulmonary congestion with rattle, cool skin with mottled hands and feet, and little or no urinary output. Additional symptoms associated with actively dying included terminal restlessness, tachycardia with weak thready peripheral pulses, and a PPS score of 10 to 20.

Our findings about symptoms were similar to those found in SUPPORT in that 60% of patients experienced at least some degree of shortness of breath in the last week of life. Unlike the SUPPORT study, where pain was reported by a majority of patients, we found pain reported in only 23% of patients. Although it is difficult to determine the exact cause of this discrepancy, it is possible that the patient's lack of pain was related to their overall moribund condition at the time of admission compared to patients in SUPPORT, or the use of morphine in managing symptoms at the end of life.

Although pharmacologic management in this study included mainstay drugs for heart failure, few patients were prescribed these drugs at a level near that recommended by current heart failure care guidelines. Perhaps clinicians chose traditional hospice protocols for symptom management rather than using mainstay heart failure medications. Nevertheless, mainstay heart failure medications may enhance traditional hospice medications in symptom management and should not be overlooked when caring for patients with heart failure at the end of life.

To summarize, patients with heart failure experience many distressing physical and psychological symptoms as they near the end of life. These symptoms often are not well managed with the end result that patients may be suffering needlessly. A further consequence of failure to adequately address, and even ignore, end-of-life issues in heart failure include feelings of isolation for both patients and families at a time when support is most needed.[9]

Reasons for Lack of Adequate End-of-life Care in Heart Failure

Lack of adequate end-of-life care for patients with heart failure can be attributed to a wide variety of factors, including lack of communication between physicians and their patients regarding preferences about resuscitation,[18] and high preferences of patients with heart failure for resuscitation when compared to patients with cancer.[19] Additional reasons may be a lack of understanding (by providers and patients) of what end-of-life care entails. Further, providers often question their own ability to address the difficult questions surrounding end of life with patients and their families.[20]

The inability to accurately predict death in patients with heart failure may be the major reason for inadequate end-of-life care. While patients with heart failure have a high mortality, they typically experience a relatively unpredictable course of illness characterized by acute exacerbations of symptoms rather than by the progressive decline typical of conditions such as cancer.[21] Results from SUPPORT indicated that for many with heart failure, a 6-month survival rate was predicted at 54% even within 3 days of death.[12] This factor highlights the complexity of predicting the likelihood of death. Lynn and Forlini[22] agreed that for a variety of chronic illnesses (including end-stage heart failure), there is often no distinct terminal phase associated with the period just before death.

Trajectory of Illness

Patients at the end stage of a disease or chronic illness typically follow one of several trajectories.[21] The first trajectory is the more predictable course, where patients such as those suffering from a terminal malignancy are able to maintain their activities of daily living until late in the course of their illness. This trajectory is characterized usually by weight loss and decreased ability to function in the last 2 months, with death occurring soon after. In contrast to this well defined trajectory, patients with heart failure follow a different, unpredictable trajectory. Patients are usually ill for months to years with occasional acute exacerbations. Each exacerbation has the potential to cause death. However, heart failure patients usually survive numerous episodes and the timing of death is, for the most part, uncertain and difficult to predict.[23,24]

The high rate of sudden death among heart failure patients complicates the ability of health care providers to determine the course of illness. Heart failure patients experience sudden death at 6 to 9 times the rate of the general population.[2] Estimates vary as to the exact incidence of sudden death among patients with heart failure. Narang *et al.*[25] described a sudden death incidence of 31% to 35% from a total of 27 studies where a total of 3909 deaths were recorded. However, Kannel *et al.* analyzed data from the Framingham Heart Study in which a cohort of 5209 men and women were followed over 30 years.[26] These investigators concluded that 40% to 50% of heart failure deaths were sudden in nature occurring in the context of relatively compensated heart failure.

Predicting death

Determining the appropriate timing for initiating end-of-life care in heart failure is a dilemma, as currently used prognostic indicators have not proven to be consistently reliable. NYHA functional classification has been used traditionally as a guideline to classify severity of disease,[27] and patients in NYHA class III or IV are considered to be in the advanced stages of heart failure with a corresponding increased risk of death. The probability of mortality for NYHA class IV patients has been estimated as 20% to 50% per year, a wide range over a long period, which is not particularly helpful for clinicians trying to make decisions with individual patients. Moreover, patients commonly move among classes and these statistics do not speak to the immediate risk faced by patients in AHF. The lack of sensitivity and precision of this measure makes it unreliable for predicting mortality in individual patients.

To further confound the difficulty of predicting death, recent clinical trials have suggested that mortality rates associated with heart failure are improving. The most frequently cited annual mortality rates of 35% to 50 % are based on 2 major studies, the Framingham Study[28] and the Rochester study,[29] both published before angiotensin-converting enzyme (ACE) inhibitors were routinely prescribed. The Cooperative North Scandinavian Enalapril Survival Study,[30] in which only NYHA class IV heart failure patients were enrolled, demonstrated a crude mortality rate of 26% at 6 months for those patients receiving an ACE inhibitor. The Randomized Aldactone Evaluation Study[31] demonstrated that the addition of spironolactone improved survival in patients with severe heart failure, as did the Cardiac Insufficiency Bisoprolol Study (CIBIS) II.[32] Recently, the Carvedilol Prospective Randomized Cumulative Survival (COPERNICUS) study[33] demonstrated that the addition of carvedilol produced a 35% decrease in the risk of death in advanced heart failure patients with NYHA class III or IV. However, benefits and reported decreases in mortality in these studies could be misleading, as the studies were conducted for relatively short periods of time. Additionally, with the exception of the Cooperative North Scandinavian Enalapril Survival Study (CONSENSUS), the majority of the clinical studies have traditionally excluded heart failure patients with preserved left ventricular systolic function. Exclusion of patients with preserved systolic function from major clinical trials contributes to the inability of health care providers to accurately predict end of life.[34]

Even if use of optimal drug therapy has produced an improvement in survival, the net effect is more patients with advanced heart failure living longer in a state of functional decline. While cancer patients typically experience a rapid functional decline in the last 2 months of life, over 40% of patients dying from noncancerous causes such as heart failure experience significant functional impairments for at least 1 year prior to death.[35] They do not exhibit the same classic, rapid functional decline seen in cancer patients that has frequently served as a cue to physicians and family that the end of life is near. Lack of a rapid functional decline in patients with heart failure and the inability of practitioners to recognize end of life may account for the fact that only 3% of this population has been referred for palliative care before death.[12]

Data compiled from two studies that included patients hospitalized with exacerbations of heart failure provide specific information about mortality in AHF. Investigators analyzed data from the SUPPORT and the Acute Physiology and Chronic Health Evaluation III (APACHE III) study to evaluate various estimates of prognoses from physicians and from two multivariate survival models in the final days prior to death of numerous severely ill patients.[36] In SUPPORT, 9105 patients with 1 out of 9 serious diagnoses, including heart failure, were enrolled. The APACHE III database allowed estimation of survival from the physiology data of 16 622 intensive care patients. The likelihood of survival for patients with heart failure was predicted as a better than 50% chance to live an additional 2 months, even on the day before death. The prognosis was essentially the same throughout the week before death, as were prognosis estimates from physicians and using APACHE III scores. Although patients had severe baseline disability, they usually died from causes such as dysrhythmias and appeared to be no more ill on the day of death as on any other day. Thus, patients with heart failure often died within a few days of having a reasonably optimistic prognosis that allowed for some hope of recovery and survival.

Although the uncertain illness trajectory and high risk of sudden death have made prognostication of the end of life difficult in patients with heart failure, there have been limited efforts at developing other objective criteria to identify these patients.[37] Eichhorn reported that in a review of 96 studies, several variables appear to be strong predictors of mortality.[38] These variables include cardiac norepinephrine spillover, elevated plasma norepinephrine level, elevated B-type natriuretic peptide (BNP) level, left ventricular ejection fraction (LVEF) less than 35%, decreased peak oxygen consumption (VO_2max), advanced age, history of sudden death, and the lack of use of therapies such as ACE inhibitors, beta-blockers, spironolactone, and automatic internal cardiac defibrillators. Other prognostic markers such as circulating concentrations of cytokines, endothelins, atrial natriuretic peptides (ANPs), serum sodium, as well as heart rate variability, ability to perform a 6-minute walk, and other hemodynamic studies traditionally used to predict outcomes were noted to be moderate or weak predictors of mortality.

The Epidemiologie de l'Insuffisance Cardiaque Avancee en Lorraine (EPICAL) database was used to evaluate numerous variables believed to be prognostic markers.[39] These researchers identified 401 patients with severe heart failure, defined as NYHA class III or IV due to ischemic or dilated cardiomyopathy and developed a prognostic survival rating and algorithm with a multivariate analysis. They identified four prognostic markers in ischemic cardiomyopathy (serum sodium level, creatinine level, resting heart rate, and prior decompensation) and 6 prognostic markers in dilated cardiomyopathy (serum sodium level, creatinine level, resting heart rate, serious comorbidity, level of dependence, and advanced age). Patients who had 3 out of 4 markers in ischemic cardiomyopathy or 4 out of 6 markers in dilated cardiomyopathy were found to have a less than 25% chance of surviving 1 year. Although this model may provide some insight into prognostication, it lacks validation in prospective studies, and does not provide specific guidance for clinicians regarding AHF patients. Complexity of predicting death should not, however, be the rationale for inadequate end-of-life care.

Addressing End-of-life Care

Communication

In one of the few studies of a palliative care intervention, Rabow *et al.* describe the benefits of what they found to be a powerful intervention—simple communication.[9] These investigators included patients with advanced heart failure in their study and observed that anxiety, depression, loneliness, and isolation were common among patients who were at the "beginning of the end of life."[9] These patients did not feel as if they were being heard by their physicians and most valued the opportunity to be listened to as they told their stories and attempted to work through issues related to end of life, including establishing a meaning to their lives. Clinicians can take advantage of the opportunity to improve end-of-life care by taking the time to actively listen to patients, thereby promoting more effective communication.[3] Physicians often feel that patients do not want to discuss end-of-life issues. However, even though they found them difficult, the majority of patients desired these conversations.[9] Moreover, most patients believe that it is up to the physician to broach the subject.[9]

Timing

As previously discussed, determining the appropriate timing of discussions about end-of-life care is complicated by our inability to predict death in patients with heart failure. Although it is most difficult to predict those patients who will die suddenly from a fatal dysrhythmia in the context of relatively compensated heart failure, there are difficulties in predicting death even in those who will die from progressive heart failure. Nonetheless, death from progressive heart failure is commonly preceded by refractory symptoms and clinical deterioration, despite optimal heart failure therapy. These patients and their families are clearly ideal candidates for discussions about end-of-life care.

Relegating discussions about end-of-life issues to only patients who are severely clinically compromised limits the usefulness of such discussions by eliminating a large number of patients who do not follow such a clinical trajectory. In addition, by the time a patient's condition deteriorates to the point where clinicians may be more comfortable broaching the subject of end-of-life care, the patient's cognitive status may have deteriorated. Moreover, a time of crisis is not the optimal time to begin a discussion about end-of-life issues. For these reasons, it is recommended that clinicians discuss the prognosis of heart failure in the context of advances in treatment and the improvement in outlook with optimal treatment with all heart failure patients when they are in a relatively compensated state and can actively participate in the discussion.[3] An appropriate way to begin such discussions is to inquire about advance directives.

Advance directives are health care decisions by patients that are made known formally to healthcare providers and significant others. Using advance directives, patients make known their wishes about desired treatment in case they become incapacitated and incapable of expressing their wishes about care. All individuals are advised to make known their wishes about their future care and thus advance directives are not only for patients with terminal illnesses. Most patients with heart failure can benefit from discussion of their wishes regarding medical therapy in the event that their condition deteriorates substantially. It is part of reasonable decision-making for all individuals, regardless of their health status, to make their wishes known in the event that they become incapacitated.

For patients with AHF, the time during hospitalization after stabilization or during a follow-up visit after hospital discharge may represent an ideal time to broach the topic of advance directives. Many patients respond to such discussions with questions about their prognosis and naturally pave the way for a more wide-ranging discussion about end-of-life issues if appropriate. Discussion of prognosis and the possible impact of heart failure on quality of life, if heart failure progresses, is an appropriate discussion as part of the management of heart failure.

Symptom management

Despite the general belief that palliative care can help in the relief of symptom burden, very few studies are available documenting the effectiveness of symptom management for heart failure patients using any systematic approach, including the provision of palliative care. Hermann and Looney attempted to describe the efficacy of interventions used to treat symptoms of hospice patients in the last week of life.[40] The majority of the 100 patients in this study had a cancer diagnosis, while 5% had a cardiovascular diagnosis. Although there were a variety of symptoms reported in this population, the three most common symptoms were pain, dyspnea, and lethargy. Most of the interventions for pain were pharmacological, while dyspnea was treated with oxygen and an anxiolytic. However, conclusions could not be made about the effectiveness of treatment due to a lack of documentation in the medical records.

We encountered similar problems in our study of 90 heart failure patients receiving hospice care.[17] Symptoms of shortness of breath, edema, incontinence of bowel and bladder, and confusion were noted, but no other symptoms were consistently recorded. A number of different therapies were used by nurses while providing care. The most common therapies included supplemental oxygen administration (92%), skin care (62%), family reassurance or education (50% to 82%), and patient education (51%). Education typically involved information about hospice services, possible symptoms the patient might experience and how to best manage them, when to call the hospice nurse, when to call the doctor, and bereavement services.

Medications that were commonly prescribed to relieve the patient's physical and psychological symptoms included antianxiety medications (79%), morphine (74%) or other narcotics (42%), antidepressants (26%), haloperidol (24%), scopolamine (21%), and Thorazine (7%). Specific heart failure medications were prescribed as follows: diuretics (68%), nitrates (49%), digoxin (32%), ACE inhibitors (24%), and beta-blockers (20%). Calcium channel blockers were prescribed for 16% of patients.

Thus, heart failure patients received many of the traditional hospice medications. However, for a majority of the patients, specific heart failure medications that could relieve symptoms and help maintain quality of life were not prescribed. Unfortunately, there was little documentation regarding the effectiveness of any of the approaches used. Other studies concerning the efficacy of palliative care in reducing symptom burden are almost non-existent. This is a vital area for future research.

Despite the lack of a strong evidence base for managing symptoms at the end of life in patients with heart failure, evidence from other conditions and from centers with substantial experience in the management of advanced heart failure provides guidance. Although cancer patients usually experience more pain than heart failure patients,[16] other symptoms such as dyspnea, fatigue, nausea, emotional distress, and constipation are common to both. Palliative care interventions commonly employed to relieve these symptoms include analgesics, narcotics, antiemetics, anxiolytics, antidepressants, laxatives, and stool softeners, as well as the administration of oxygen.[27,40] Heart failure patients may benefit from the use of these agents in addition to maximizing traditional heart failure pharmacotherapy.

Specifically, dyspnea is one of the most distressing symptoms of heart failure. Oral or intravenous morphine (both short-acting and long-acting types) has been shown to help relieve dyspnea through a variety of mechanisms including reduction in preload, reduced responsiveness of the dominant respiratory control center, and decreased anxiety. Sedation may be helpful for refractory dyspnea and short-term mechanical ventilation can be considered for pulmonary edema.[3,37] Gastrointestinal problems such as nausea or vomiting, constipation, and fecal incontinence can be managed with medication and diet modifications, although anorexia may make the latter impractical. Urinary incontinence may be managed by changing the timing of diuretic doses, or by using a urinary catheter or external device.[3,37] Commonly, anxiety, depression, and sleeplessness overwhelm patients near the end of life, and such symptoms should not be accepted as "natural." Treating these symptoms can free patients to interact meaningfully with loved ones and engage in activities or contemplation important at this stage.[3,37] Antidepressants, anxiolytics, and hypnotics should be considered to manage these symptoms. Additionally, complementary therapies, such as relaxation, biofeedback, and stress reduction strategies have been shown to decrease anxiety and depression and increase quality of life in patients with advanced heart failure.[41–45]

Resuscitation

Because sudden death from a malignant dysrhythmia is common in patients with heart failure, it is helpful to discuss this possibility with patients and their families particularly during treatment for an acute exacerbation. Most sudden deaths occur while the patient is at home or with a family member. A common, unmet need of family members of high-risk cardiac patients is learning to respond appropriately in an emergency.[46] Cardiac patients want their families to know what to do in an emergency.[46,47] While discussing advance directives, clinicians can discuss resuscitation options with patients and their families. Clinicians can assist patients in this aspect of decision-making by providing information about resuscitation and the various options available to patients. It should also be clear to patients that they can change their minds as their condition changes. In fact, patient preferences regarding resuscitation commonly do change.[18] These decisions need to be made clear to all of the patient's caregivers.

When patients and families decide in favor of resuscitation, family members should be advised about obtaining cardiopulmonary resuscitation (CPR) training, in case the need arises. Many clinicians have expressed concerns over the ability of families of high-risk cardiac patients to learn CPR. They also worry that CPR training will burden families with excessive responsibility or feelings of guilt if resuscitation attempts are unsuccessful. To the contrary, we have demonstrated in studies of families of patients at risk for sudden death that the majority of family members can learn CPR, are not unduly burdened by responsibility or guilt, and use CPR appropriately when the occasion arises.[48–50] When their family members learn CPR, some patients may exhibit negative psychological responses.[51] These negative responses are attenuated when CPR training is combined with a simple, one-time social support intervention provided by the CPR instructor in which families are given the opportunity to discuss their fears about the possibility of having to perform CPR on their loved one.[51]

When patients decide against resuscitation, their families need to be told what steps to take if death occurs. The common response for most families is to call the emergency medical services number. However, they may not realize that in doing so they may set into motion undesired resuscitation activities. Clinicians should advise family members to call them or another health care provider who is aware of the patient's desire for no resuscitation efforts. Written confirmation of patient wishes regarding resuscitation increase the likelihood that these wishes will be honored.[9]

As more patients with heart failure have cardioverter defibrillators implanted, it is important to consider what actions to take when these patients approach the end of life. These devices can be inactivated for those end-stage patients who do not desire resuscitation. This option should be discussed with patients.

Honoring patient preferences at end of life

In order to provide high quality care for heart failure patients who are considered end stage, it is essential not only to elicit information on preferences regarding treatment, but to honor those wishes as well. Patients need to be given the opportunity to make well-informed decisions about what type of care they want, where they want it, and how aggressive they want it to be. At the end of life, patients must make decisions about treatment, resuscitation, and site of care. This is because family members and healthcare providers may not be able to accurately determine what treatments a patient may want or be willing to endure.

For example, when recovery was unlikely, patients with advanced heart failure preferred to receive treatment in a hospital rather than at home or in a hospice setting.[3,52] Frequently, patients are concerned with caregiver burden and felt better terminal care would be available in the hospital to relieve symptoms.[52] However, heart failure patients also tended to prefer treatment at the site where more aggressive treatment was available and chance of survival was greatest. Few patients with end-stage heart failure preferred treatment in a hospice setting.

Despite a progressive decline in quality of life, patients with advanced heart failure commonly report a desire for maximal medical treatment until death.[18] It is not unusual for patients with heart failure to receive more life-sustaining treatments than patients with other conditions.[14,53] The SUPPORT study demonstrated that most severely ill patients, including those with heart failure, wanted to be given every chance to live,[12,19] unless they were in severe pain or their condition was hopeless.[12,19] Although most patients reported poor quality of life in the SUPPORT study at the end of life, for some patients, despite increasing severity of illness, quality of life did not decline as death approached. Some believed that they enjoyed a good quality of life up until death. Another group of investigators found that 94% of patients with heart failure were willing to receive treatments that were considered burdensome, as long as there was a high probability of restoring current health.[54,55] However, this proportion decreased to 29.7% if the treatment had a high probability of functional or cognitive impairment, even if the treatment burden was low.

Because healthcare providers and families may not accurately determine a patient's wishes, it is imperative that clinicians discuss end-of-life issues with patients so that their wishes become known and can be acted upon. One discussion, however, will not suffice, as a patient's wishes regarding their care may change over time. As part of the SUPPORT study, Krumholz *et al.* described resuscitation preferences among 936 patients hospitalized with heart failure, as well as the perceptions of patient preferences by their physicians.[18] A total of 69% of patients expressed a desire for resuscitation in the event of a cardiac arrest, 23% reported that they did not want to be resuscitated, and 8% were unsure. Those that did not want to be resuscitated were older, had a worse perception of their prognosis, poorer functional status, and higher income. Quality of life was not a significant predictor of resuscitation preference. However, after 2 months, 19% of the patients in the study had changed their minds. Approximately 14% of the patients who had initially wanted to be resuscitated had decided against it, and of those who had initially opposed resuscitation, 40% expressed a desire for it. The physician's perception of the patient's preference was inaccurate in 24% of the cases.

Despite a desire to prolong life, when acknowledging death, most people express a desire for a "good death." In a study of the meaning of a good life, patients thought 6 components constituted a good death: pain and symptom management, clear decision-making, preparation for death, completion, contributing to others, and affirmation of the whole person.[56] Adequate pain and symptom management was the primary component of a good death.

Referral to hospice care

The American College of Cardiology and the American Heart Association recommended hospice care as appropriate to decrease suffering in patients with end-stage heart failure.[57] Yet, only about 10% of patients with end-stage heart failure enroll in formal hospice programs. Patients with cancer are routinely referred for hospice care and comprise the majority of hospice patients nationally. On the other hand, those with end-stage heart failure may be suffering unnecessarily at the end of life without the benefit of hospice care services. Although heart failure patients often do not express a desire for hospice care,[52] this may stem, in part, from misconceptions about such care.

For select patients, referral for hospice services may be an appropriate method of providing palliation when symptoms are refractory and quality of life is poor and associated with functional decline.[58] A Medicare benefit exists to pay for hospice services for end-stage heart failure patients. This benefit was developed so that individuals could choose to move from curative care to supportive care and still receive Medicare funding. Initially, the hospice benefit included 3 benefit periods with a maximum of 210 days of coverage. It was soon discovered that the difficulty in making an accurate prognosis for the terminally ill warranted reconsideration. In 1990, the limit was extended to add an additional period of unlimited usage. To be eligible for the hospice benefit, the patient's physician and the hospice medical director must believe that the patient has a life expectancy of 6 months or less, and the patient must consent to receive hospice in lieu of special treatments for their terminal illness. This agreement does not preclude other treatments for illnesses or injuries not related to their terminal illness, nor does it necessitate abandonment of appropriate heart failure medical therapy. In addition, patients may withdraw from the hospice program and reenroll at a later date with no penalty.[58]

The Medicare hospice benefit includes coverage for services such as prescription medications for pain relief and symptom management, homemaker and home health aid assistance, and bereavement counseling for the patient and their family. Physician management, nursing care, medical supplies, and medical appliances as well as a wide variety of other professional support services necessary to provide quality end-of-life care are also covered. Although a number of these services are individually available to patients and their family, hospices offer holistic and coordinated services, particularly addressing issues important at the end of life, beyond maintaining persons with advanced illnesses.

The Medicare Hospice Benefit remains one of Medicare's smallest programs accounting for about 1% of all program expenditures.[58] In our recent study of patients with end-stage heart failure referred for hospice services, only 3% of patients used more than 6 months of hospice services while the median length of stay in hospice for patients with end-stage heart failure was 10 days, clearly indicating an underutilization of services.[17] A total of 37% of patients were referred for hospice care 1 week or less prior to death and 9% of the patients with heart failure were admitted in a moribund state. Shorter hospice stays limited the opportunity for providers to reduce the suffering of patients and their families.[59]

Although some believe that heart failure patients will overuse hospice resources, patterns of use by patients with end-stage heart failure were similar to those of patients with other diagnoses such as breast and prostate cancer.[58] Cost savings are evident when patients are appropriately referred for hospice care services. During the 6 months prior to hospice enrollment, Medicare expenditures for patients with heart failure were greater than all other medical diagnoses, including lung cancer, colon cancer, and even Alzheimer's disease.[58] When compared with other patients enrolled in hospice, based on medical diagnoses, those with heart failure use lower payments per case and per day than the mean cost of care.

As hospice care has evolved, it is important to understand that "hospice" is not necessarily a "place." It is a method of care delivery in which palliative care is emphasized. Hospice care can be, and often is, delivered in patients' homes.[17] Hospice care can be delivered in extended care facilities, hospitals, and inpatient hospice units. The holistic approach of the hospice to the care of the dying patient and their family should contribute to the realization of a "good death" despite the medical diagnosis of the patient. The Institute of Medicine considered a good death to be one "free from avoidable distress and suffering for patients, families, and caregivers; in general accord with patients' and families' wishes; and reasonably consistent with clinical, cultural, and ethical standards."[60] For some patients, hospice may be the care model that most effectively achieves that goal.

While research efforts have been made to describe symptoms and quality of life for those with advanced heart failure, research efforts to better understand the impact of hospice care on patients with end-stage heart failure have lagged behind. In one of the few studies of hospice care for patients with heart failure, Lynn *et al.* found that in a small sample of hospice patients with heart disease, there was a decrease in inpatient hospital days and emergency room visits using cardiac protocols for symptom management.[61] They found that emergencies related to pain and shortness of breath could be managed more effectively at home while the patient was receiving hospice care, rather than admitting the patient to an acute care setting.

Conclusion

Additional research is needed to address changes in the healthcare environment to provide optimal curative and palliative care for patients with serious and complex illnesses, including end-stage heart failure, that cannot be placed in the traditional 6-month prognostic categories.[58] Advanced heart failure is associated with significant physical and emotional symptoms, decreased quality of life, poor functional status, and recurrent hospitalizations. During acute exacerbations, clinicians can take the opportunity to improve the quality of the care they deliver and improve the patient's quality of life by addressing end-of-life issues. The approach taken with each patient differs depending on the individual patient's condition and preferences. However, at a minimum, clinicians should engage each patient with heart failure in a discussion about the patient's prognosis and advance directives. Such discussions do require a fine balancing act as the clinician strives to maintain hope, yet provide patients with a realistic view of their condition. The benefits of such discussions far outweigh the difficulties. As clinicians begin to undertake these discussions and open communication with their patients, they pave the way for more difficult discussions that are needed to enhance decision-making as patients with heart failure near the end of life.

References

1. Stewart S. Prognosis of patients with heart failure compared with common types of cancer. Heart Fail Monit 2003; 3: 87–94.
2. American Heart Association. Heart Disease and Stroke Statistics—2004 Update (American Heart Association: Dallas, TX, 2004).
3. Funk M, Hudson K. Caring for the patient with end-stage heart failure: palliative care. In: Stewart S, Moser DK, Thompson DR (eds) Caring for the Heart Failure Patient: A Textbook for the Health Care Professional (Martin Dunitz: London, 2004), 189–195.
4. Billings JA. What is palliative care? J Palliat Med 1998; 1: 73–81.
5. Formiga F, Espel E, Chivite D, Pujol R. Dying from heart failure in hospital: palliative decision making analysis. Heart 2002; 88: 187.
6. Carney MT, Meier DE. Palliative care and end-of-life issues. Anesthesiol Clin North America 2000; 18: 183–209.
7. Nordgren L, Sorensen S. Symptoms experienced in the last six months of life in patients with end-stage heart failure. Eur J Cardiovasc Nurs 2003; 2: 213–217.
8. Lynn J. Caring at the end of our lives. N Engl J Med 1996; 335: 201–202.
9. Rabow MW, Petersen J, Schance K, Dibble SL, McPhee SJ. The comprehensive care team: a description of a controlled trial of care at the beginning of the end of life. J Palliat Med 2003; 6: 489–499.
10. Moser DK, Mann DL. Improving outcomes in heart failure: It's not unusual beyond usual care. Circulation 2002; 105: 2810–2812.
11. Juenger J, Schellberg D, Kraemer S, *et al.* Health related quality of life in patients with congestive heart failure: comparison with other chronic diseases and relation to functional variables. Heart 2002; 87: 235–241.
12. Levenson JW, McCarthy EP, Lynn J, Davis RB, Phillips RS. The last six months of life for patients with congestive heart failure. J Am Geriatr Soc 2000; 48: S101–S109.
13. Freeborne N, Lynn J, Desbiens NA. Insights about dying from the SUPPORT project. The Study to Understand Prognoses and Preferences for Outcomes and Risks of Treatments. J Am Geriatr Soc 2000; 48: S199–S205.
14. Lynn J, Teno JM, Phillips RS, *et al.* Perceptions by family members of the dying experience of older and seriously ill patients. SUPPORT Investigators. Study to Understand Prognoses and Preferences for Outcomes and Risks of Treatments. Ann Intern Med 1997; 126: 97–106.
15. Paolini CA, Family Medicine, Division of Geriatrics. Symptoms management at the end of life. J Am Osteopath Assoc 2001; 101: 609–615.
16. McCarthy M, Lay M, Addington-Hall J. Dying from heart disease. J R Coll Physicians Lond 1996; 30: 325–328.
17. Zambroski CH, Moser DK, Roser L, Heo S, Chung ML. Patients with heart failure who die in hospice. Am Heart J 2005; 149: 558–664,
18. Krumholz HM, Phillips RS, Hamel MB, *et al.* Resuscitation preferences among patients with severe congestive heart failure: results from the SUPPORT project. Study to Understand Prognoses and Preferences for Outcomes and Risks of Treatments. Circulation 1998; 98: 648–655.
19. Califf RM, Vidaillet H, Goldman L. Advanced congestive heart failure: What do patients want? Am Heart J 1998; 135: S320–S326.
20. Dracup K, Bryan-Brown CW. Asking difficult questions. Am J Crit Care 1998; 7: 399–401.
21. Lynn J. Perspectives on care at the close of life. Serving patients who may die soon and their families: the role of hospice and other services. JAMA 2001; 285: 925–932.
22. Lynn J, Forlini JH. "Serious and complex illness" in quality improvement and policy reform for end-of-life care. J Gen Intern Med 2001; 16: 315–319.
23. Jaarsma T, Leventhal M. End-of-life issues in cardiac patients and their families. Eur J Cardiovasc Nurs 2002; 1: 223–225.
24. Gibbs JS, McCoy AS, Gibbs LM, Rogers AE, Addington-Hall JM. Living with and dying from heart failure: the role of palliative care. Heart 2002; 88: ii36–39.
25. Narang R, Cleland JG, Erhardt L, *et al.* Mode of death in chronic heart failure. A request and proposition for more accurate classification. Eur Heart J 1996; 17: 1390–1403.
26. Kannel WB, Plehn JF, Cupples LA. Cardiac failure and sudden death in the Framingham Study. Am Heart J 1988; 115: 869–875.
27. Noyes D. Heart failure. In: Smith SA (ed.) Hospice and Palliative Nurses Association Monograph: Treatment of End-Stage Non-Cancer Diagnoses (Hospice and Palliative Nurses Association: Pittsburgh, PA, 2001), 31–35.
28. Ho KK, Pinsky JL, Kannel WB, Levy D. The epidemiology of heart failure: the Framingham Study. J Am Coll Cardiol 1993; 22: 6A–13A.

29. Rodeheffer RJ, Jacobsen SJ, Gersh BJ, *et al.* The incidence and prevalence of congestive heart failure in Rochester, Minnesota. Mayo Clin Proc 1993; 68: 1143–1150.
30. The CONSENSUS Trial Study Group. Effects of enalapril on mortality in severe congestive heart failure. Results of the Cooperative North Scandinavian Enalapril Survival Study (CONSENSUS). N Engl J Med 1987; 316: 1429–1435.
31. Pitt B, Zannad F, Remme WJ, *et al.* The effect of spironolactone on morbidity and mortality in patients with severe heart failure. Randomized Aldactone Evaluation Study Investigators. N Engl J Med 1999; 341: 709–717.
32. The Cardiac Insufficiency Bisoprolol Study II (CIBIS-II): a randomised trial. Lancet 1999; 353: 9–13.
33. Packer M, Coats AJ, Fowler MB, *et al.* Effect of carvedilol on survival in severe chronic heart failure. N Engl J Med 2001; 344: 1651–1658.
34. Rich MW. Epidemiology, pathophysiology, and etiology of congestive heart failure in older adults. J Am Geriatr Soc 1997; 45: 968–974.
35. Teno JM, Weitzen S, Fennell ML, Mor V. Dying trajectory in the last year of life: does cancer trajectory fit other diseases? J Palliat Med 2001; 4: 457–464.
36. Lynn J, Harrell F Jr., Cohn F, Wagner D, Connors AF Jr. Prognoses of seriously ill hospitalized patients on the days before death: implications for patient care and public policy. New Horiz 1997; 5: 56–61.
37. Ward C. The need for palliative care in the management of heart failure. Heart 2002; 87: 294–298.
38. Eichhorn EJ. Prognosis determination in heart failure. Am J Med 2001; 110: 14S–36S.
39. Alla F, Briancon S, Juilliere Y, *et al.* Differential clinical prognostic classifications in dilated and ischemic advanced heart failure: the EPICAL study. Am Heart J 2000; 139: 895–904.
40. Hermann C, Looney S. The effectiveness of symptom management in hospice patients during the last seven days of life. J Hospice Palliat Nurs 2001; 3: 88–95.
41. Moser DK, Dracup K, Woo MA, Stevenson LW. Voluntary control of vascular tone by using skin-temperature biofeedback-relaxation in patients with advanced heart failure. Altern Ther Health Med 1997; 3: 51–59.
42. Moser DK, Kim A, Baisden-O'Brien J. Impact of a nonpharmacologic cognitive intervention on clinical and psychosocial outcomes in patients with advanced heart failure. Circulation 1999; 100: I-99 (Abstract).
43. Moser DK, Lennie TA, Doering LV. Nonpharmacologic management of heart failure. In: Stewart S, Moser DK, Thompson D (eds) Caring for the Heart Failure Patient: A Textbook for the Healthcare Professional (Martin Dunitz: London, 2004).
44. Moser DK, Nelson SD. Impact of biofeedback-relaxation training on hemodynamics, neuroendocrine function and rehospitalizations in advanced heart failure. Am J Crit Care 1999; 8: 202 (Abstract).
45. Kostis JB, Rosen RC, Cosgrove NM, Shindler DM, Wilson AC. Nonpharmacologic therapy improves functional and emotional status in congestive heart failure. Chest 1994; 106: 996–1001.
46. Moser DK, Dracup KA, Marsden C. Needs of recovering cardiac patients and their spouses: compared views. Int J Nurs Stud 1993; 30: 105–114.
47. Hagenhoff BD, Feutz C, Conn VS, Sagehorn KK, Moranville-Hunziker M. Patient education needs as reported by congestive heart failure patients and their nurses. J Adv Nurs 1994; 19: 685–690.
48. Moser DK, Dracup K. Impact of cardiopulmonary resuscitation training on perceived control in spouses of recovering cardiac patients. Res Nurs Health 2000; 23: 270–278.
49. Moser DK, Dracup K, Guzy PM, Taylor SE, Breu C. Cardiopulmonary resuscitation skills retention in family members of cardiac patients. Am J Emerg Med 1990; 8: 498–503.
50. Dracup K, Moser DK, Guzy PM, Taylor SE, Marsden C. Is cardiopulmonary resuscitation training deleterious for family members of cardiac patients? Am J Public Health 1994; 84: 116–118.
51. Dracup K, Moser DK, Taylor SE, Guzy PM. The psychological consequences of cardiopulmonary resuscitation training for family members of patients at risk for sudden death. Am J Public Health 1997; 87: 1434–1439.
52. Fried TR, van Doorn C, O'Leary JR, Tinetti ME, Drickamer MA. Older persons' preferences for site of terminal care. Ann Intern Med 1999; 131: 109–112.
53. Tanvetyanon T, Leighton JC. Life-sustaining treatments in patients who died of chronic congestive heart failure compared with metastatic cancer. Crit Care Med 2003; 31: 60–64.
54. Fried TR, Bradley EH, Towle VR, Allore H. Understanding the treatment preferences of seriously ill patients. N Engl J Med 2002; 346: 1061–1066.
55. Fried TR, Bradley EH. What matters to seriously ill older persons making end-of-life treatment decisions? A qualitative study. J Palliat Med 2003; 6: 237–244.
56. Steinhauser KE, Clipp EC, McNeilly M, Christakis NA, McIntyre LM, Tulsky JA. In search of a good death: observations of patients, families, and providers. Ann Intern Med 2000; 132: 825–832.

57. Hunt SA, Baker DW, Chin MH, *et al.*, American College of Cardiology/American Heart Association. ACC/AHA guidelines for the evaluation and management of chronic heart failure in the adult: executive summary. A report of the American College of Cardiology/American Heart Association Task Force on Practice Guidelines (Committee to revise the 1995 Guidelines for the Evaluation and Management of Heart Failure). J Am Coll Cardiol 2001; 38: 2101–2113.
58. Zambroski CH. Hospice as an alternative model of care for older patients with end-stage heart failure. J Cardiovasc Nurs 2004; 19: 76–83; quiz 84–85.
59. Teno JM, Field MJ, Byock I. Preface: The road taken and to be traveled in improving end-of-life care. J Pain Symptom Manage 2001; 22: 713–716.
60. Field MJ, Cassell CK (eds). Committee on Care at the End of Life, Division of Health Care Services, Institute of Medicine. Approaching Death: Improving Care at the End of Life (National Academy of Sciences: Washington, DC, 1997).
61. Lynn J, Schuster JL, Kabcenell A. Offering end-of-life services to patients with advanced heart failure. In: Improving Care for the End of Life: A Sourcebook for Health Care Managers and Clinicians. Lynn J *et al.* (eds). Oxford University Press Inc. New York, 2000, 256–257.

Index

B

D

E

F

K

L

M

N

O

T

U

V

W

X

Y

T - #0977 - 101024 - C628 - 246/189/34 [36] - CB - 9781841843742 - Gloss Lamination